Jarvis's

Health Assessment

Fourth edition

Australia and New Zealand edition

Jarvis's Health Assessment

Fourth edition

ɿAROLYN JARVIS
PhD, APRN, CNP
ɿrofessor of Nursing Emerita
Illinois Wesleyan University
Bloomington, Illinois
and
Family Nurse Practitioner
Bloomington, Illinois

ANN ECKHARDT
PhD, RN
Chair and Associate Professor,
Department of Graduate Nursing
College of Nursing and Health Innovation
University of Texas at Arlington
Arlington, Texas

Australian Adapting Editors

ɦELEN FORBES
N, BAppSc (AdvNurs) (La Trobe
ersity), MEdSt (Monash University),
PhD (University of Sydney)
Nurse Consultant (Education)
ɔrmerly Associate Professor and
ciate Head of School (Teaching &
Learning)
School of Nursing & Midwifery,
Deakin University, Melbourne,
Victoria, Australia

ELIZABETH WATT
RN, DipN (College of Nursing Australia),
BAppSc (AdvNurs) (Lincoln Institute
of Health Sciences), MNS (La Trobe
University), Cert Prom Cont, FACN
Nurse Consultant (Education),
Senior Research Fellow,
National Ageing Research Institute,
Melbourne, Victoria, Australia

Original illustrations by Pat Thomas, CMI, FAMI
East Troy, Wisconsin

Assessment photographs by Kevin Strandberg
fessor of Art, Illinois Wesleyan University, Bloomington, Illinois

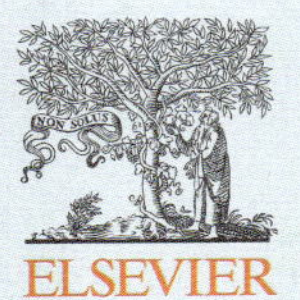

Australia and New Zealand edition

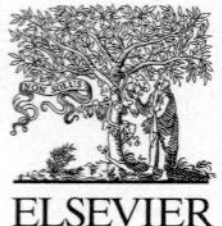

Elsevier Australia, ACN 001 002 357
(a division of Reed International Books Australia Pty Ltd)
Tower 1, 475 Victoria Avenue, Chatswood, NSW 2067

ISBN: 978-0-323-80984-9

This adaptation of Physical Examination and Health Assessment, ninth edition, by Carolyn Jarvis and Ann Eckhardt, was undertaken by Elsevier Australia and is published by arrangement with Elsevier Inc.

ISBN: 978-0-7295-4465-8

National Library of Australia Cataloguing-in-Publication Data

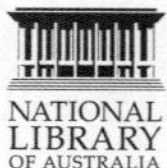

A catalogue record for this book is available from the National Library of Australia

Senior Content Strategist: Melinda McEvoy
Content Project Manager: Shruti Raj
Edited by Matt Davies
Proofread by Tim Learner
Cover by Georgette Hall
Internal design: Non-standard
Index by Innodata Indexing
Typeset by GW Tech
Printed in Chennai by Multivista Global Pvt. Ltd.

Last digit is the print number: 9 8 7 6 5 4 3 2 1

Contents

Text Features

Colour-coded structure

All health assessment chapters (Chapters 11–30) provide a clearly identified colour-coded structure to define the seven major sections of health assessment

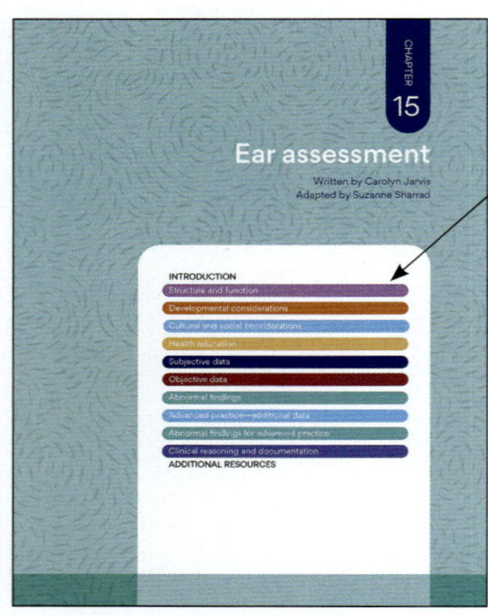
CHAPTER 15

Ear assessment

Written by Carolyn Jarvis
Adapted by Suzanne Sharrad

INTRODUCTION
Structure and function
Developmental considerations
Cultural and social considerations
Health education
Subjective data
Objective data
Abnormal findings
Advanced practice—additional data
Abnormal findings for advanced practice
Clinical reasoning and documentation
ADDITIONAL RESOURCES

Easy navigation tabs

Highlight the section within each chapter

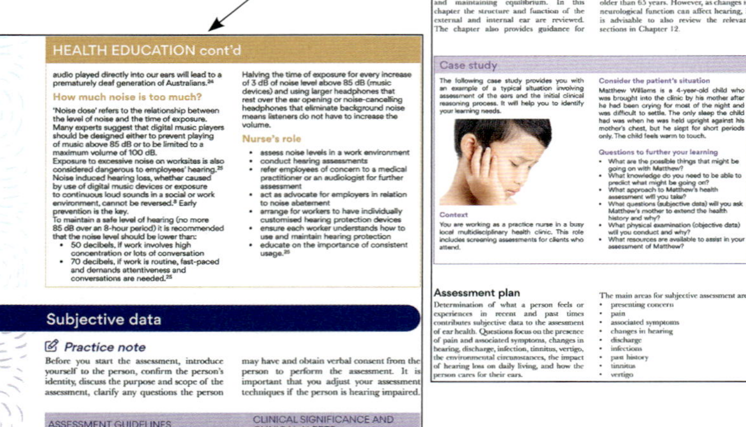
HEALTH EDUCATION cont'd

audio played directly into our ears will lead to a prematurely deaf generation of Australians.[24]

How much noise is too much?

'Noise dose' refers to the relationship between the level of noise and the time of exposure. Many experts suggest that digital music players should be designed either to prevent playing of music above 85 dB or to be limited to a maximum volume of 100 dB.

Exposure to excessive noise on worksites is also considered dangerous to employees' hearing.[25] Noise induced hearing loss, whether caused by use of digital music devices or exposure to continuous loud sounds in a social or work environment, cannot be reversed.[8] Early prevention is the key.

To maintain a safe level of hearing (no more 85 dB over an 8-hour period) it is recommended that the noise level should be lower than:

- 50 decibels, if work involves high concentration or lots of conversation
- 70 decibels, if work is routine, fast-paced and demands attentiveness and conversations are needed.[25]

Halving the time of exposure for every increase of 3 dB of noise level above 85 dB (music devices) and using larger headphones that rest over the ear opening or noise-cancelling headphones that eliminate background noise means listeners do not have to increase the volume.

Nurse's role

- assess noise levels in a work environment
- conduct hearing assessments
- refer employees of concern to a medical practitioner or an audiologist for further assessment
- act as advocate for employers in relation to noise abatement
- arrange for workers to have individually customised hearing protection devices
- ensure each worker understands how to use and maintain hearing protection
- educate on the importance of consistent usage.[25]

Subjective data

Practice note

Before you start the assessment, introduce yourself to the person, confirm the person's identity, discuss the purpose and scope of the assessment, clarify any questions the person may have and obtain verbal consent from the person to perform the assessment. It is important that you adjust your assessment techniques if the person is hearing impaired.

ASSESSMENT GUIDELINES	CLINICAL SIGNIFICANCE AND CLINICAL ALERTS
Presenting concern	
• *Do you have any problems concerning your hearing or your ears?* It is important to ascertain the person's perception of their presenting health concern. If the person does perceive a problem, ask: *How does this impact on your quality of life?*	During history taking, the following clues from normal conversation indicate possible hearing loss: • the person lip reading or watching your face and lips closely rather than your eyes • the person frowning or straining forwards to hear you

INTRODUCTION

The ear is the sensory organ for hearing and maintaining equilibrium. In this chapter the structure and function of the external and internal ear are reviewed. The chapter also provides guidance for conducting a comprehensive ear assessment for adults, infants and children and adults older than 65 years. However, as changes in neurological function can affect hearing, it is advisable to also review the relevant sections in Chapter 12.

Case study

The following case study provides you with an example of a typical situation involving assessment of the ears and the initial clinical reasoning process. It will help you to identify your learning needs.

Context

You are working as a practice nurse in a busy local multidisciplinary health clinic. This role includes screening assessments for clients who attend.

Consider the patient's situation

Matthew Williams is a 4-year-old child who was brought into the clinic by his mother after he had been crying for most of the night and was difficult to settle. The only sleep the child had was when he was held upright against his mother's chest, but he slept for short periods only. The child feels warm to touch.

Questions to further your learning

- What are the possible things that might be going on with Matthew?
- What knowledge do you need to be able to predict what might be going on?
- What approach to Matthew's health assessment will you take?
- What questions (subjective data) will you ask Matthew's mother to extend the health history and why?
- What physical examination (objective data) will you conduct and why?
- What resources are available to assist in your assessment of Matthew?

Assessment plan

Determination of what a person feels or experiences in recent and past times contributes subjective data to the assessment of ear health. Questions focus on the presence of pain and associated symptoms, changes in hearing, discharge, infection, tinnitus, vertigo, the environmental circumstances, the impact of hearing loss on daily living, and how the person cares for their ears.

The main areas for subjective assessment are:

- presenting concern
- pain
- associated symptoms
- changes in hearing
- discharge
- infections
- past history
- tinnitus
- vertigo

Case Studies

Most chapters use a case study early in the chapter to prompt the reader to adopt an inquiry based approach to their learning.

Case study

The following case study gives an example of a typical situation involving pain assessment and the initial clinical reasoning process. It will help you to identify your learning needs.

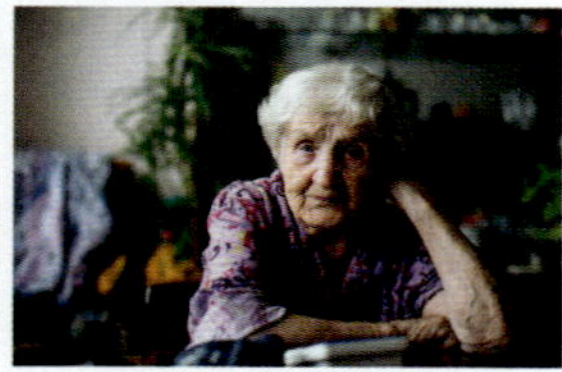

Context

You are nursing student on your third-year final clinical placement. Your clinical supervisor asks you to perform a pain assessment on Mrs Alberici.

Consider the patient's situation

Mrs Maria Alberici is an 85-year-old Italian-Australian female with a 20-year history of osteoarthritis.

Subjective

Mrs Alberici reports increased pain and stiffness in her hips and knees for the past year. However, she isn't experiencing any radiation of pain, tingling or numbness in the lower extremities.

Questions to further your learning

- What are the possible things that might be going on with Mrs Alberici?
- What knowledge do you need to be able to predict what might be going on?
- What approach to pain assessment will you take?
- What questions (subjective data) will you ask Mrs Alberici to extend the health history and why?
- What physical examination (objective data) will you conduct and why?
- What resources are available to assist in your assessment of Mrs Alberici?

Clear headings

User-friendly design makes the text easy to use

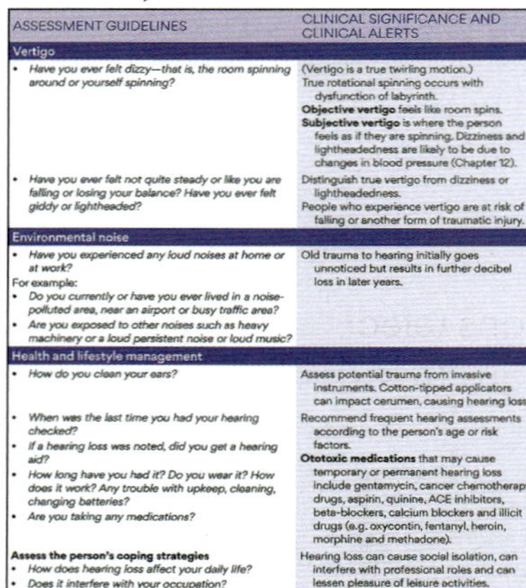

ASSESSMENT GUIDELINES	CLINICAL SIGNIFICANCE AND CLINICAL ALERTS
Vertigo	
• *Have you ever felt dizzy—that is, the room spinning around or yourself spinning?*	(Vertigo is a true twirling motion.) True rotational spinning occurs with dysfunction of labyrinth. **Objective vertigo** feels like room spins. **Subjective vertigo** is where the person feels as if they are spinning. Dizziness and lightheadedness are likely to be due to changes in blood pressure (Chapter 12).
• *Have you ever felt not quite steady or like you are falling or losing your balance? Have you ever felt giddy or lightheaded?*	Distinguish true vertigo from dizziness or lightheadedness. People who experience vertigo are at risk of falling or another form of traumatic injury.
Environmental noise	
• *Have you experienced any loud noises at home or at work?* For example: • *Do you currently or have you ever lived in a noise-polluted area, near an airport or busy traffic area?* • *Are you exposed to other noises such as heavy machinery or a loud persistent noise or loud music?*	Old trauma to hearing initially goes unnoticed but results in further decibel loss in later years.
Health and lifestyle management	
• *How do you clean your ears?*	Assess potential trauma from invasive instruments. Cotton-tipped applicators can impact cerumen, causing hearing loss.
• *When was the last time you had your hearing checked?* • *If a hearing loss was noted, did you get a hearing aid?* • *How long have you had it? Do you wear it? How does it work? Any trouble with upkeep, cleaning, changing batteries?* • *Are you taking any medications?*	Recommend frequent hearing assessments according to the person's age or risk factors. **Ototoxic medications** that may cause temporary or permanent hearing loss include gentamycin, cancer chemotherapy drugs, aspirin, quinine, ACE inhibitors, beta-blockers, calcium blockers and illicit drugs (e.g. oxycontin, fentanyl, heroin, morphine and methadone).
Assess the person's coping strategies • *How does hearing loss affect your daily life?* • *Does it interfere with your occupation?* • *Does it cause you to feel embarrassed or frustrated?* • *How do your family and friends react?*	Hearing loss can cause social isolation, can interfere with professional roles and can lessen pleasure of leisure activities.

Highly illustrated

Full colour illustrations show detailed anatomy and physiology, and demonstrate physical examination techniques and abnormal findings

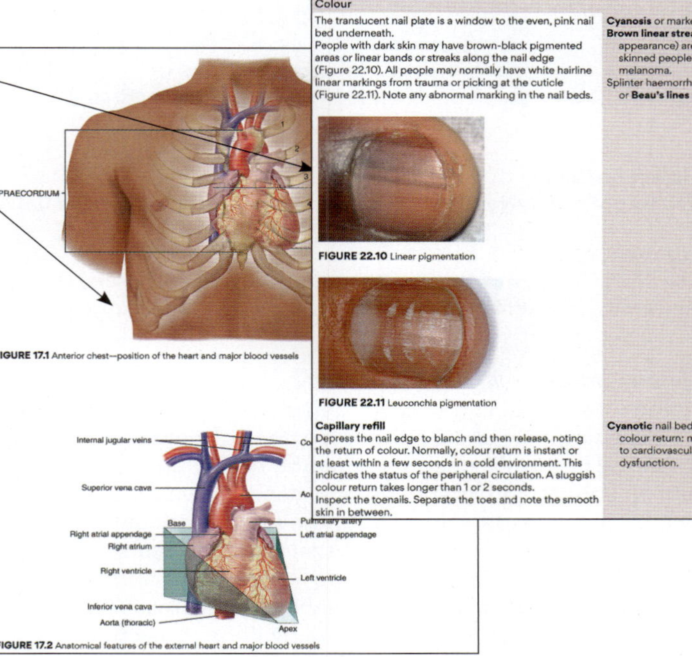

FIGURE 17.1 Anterior chest—position of the heart and major blood vessels

FIGURE 17.2 Anatomical features of the external heart and major blood vessels

PROCEDURES AND NORMAL FINDINGS	ABNORMAL FINDINGS AND CLINICAL ALERTS
The nail is firmly adherent to the nail bed, and the nail base is firm to palpation.	A spongy nail base accompanies clubbing.
Colour	
The translucent nail plate is a window to the even, pink nail bed underneath. People with dark skin may have brown-black pigmented areas or linear bands or streaks along the nail edge (Figure 22.10). All people may normally have white hairline linear markings from trauma or picking at the cuticle (Figure 22.11). Note any abnormal marking in the nail beds.	**Cyanosis** or marked pallor. **Brown linear streaks** (especially sudden appearance) are abnormal in light-skinned people and may indicate melanoma. Splinter haemorrhages, transverse ridges or **Beau's lines** (Table 22.11).
FIGURE 22.10 Linear pigmentation	
FIGURE 22.11 Leuconchia pigmentation	
Capillary refill Depress the nail edge to blanch and then release, noting the return of colour. Normally, colour return is instant or at least within a few seconds in a cold environment. This indicates the status of the peripheral circulation. A sluggish colour return takes longer than 1 or 2 seconds. Inspect the toenails. Separate the toes and note the smooth skin in between.	**Cyanotic** nail beds or sluggish colour return: may be related to cardiovascular or respiratory dysfunction.

Cultural and social considerations

Highlights specific cultural and social considerations relevant to the Australian and New Zealand context

Cultural and social considerations

As foods and eating customs are culturally distinct, each person has a unique cultural heritage that may affect nutritional status. Australia and Aotearoa New Zealand have had a continual influx of immigrants since the time of European settlement. Up until the second half of the 20th century, migrants to Australia and Aotearoa New Zealand were overwhelmingly from the British Isles. They throughout the latter half of the 20th century with European, Asian, Middle Eastern and African cuisines commonly found in restaurants and homes, particularly in Australia. Since about 2005, the increased immigration of peoples from Islamic backgrounds, from the African continent, has seen a growing cultural awareness of religious food practices such as halal diets (Table 21.1).

Developmental considerations

Highlight the needs of specific age groups

Developmental considerations

Infants and children

The inner ear starts to develop early in the fifth week of gestation. In early development, the ear is posteriorly rotated and lowset; it ascends later to its normal placement around eye level. A child may be born with impaired hearing. Post-lingual hearing loss develops **after** the acquisition of speech and language and usually **after** the age of 6 years.

An infant's Eustachian tube is relatively shorter and wider and its position is more

Clinical reasoning and documentation

Continues the clinical case study from early in the chapter, and illustrates the initial parts of the clinical reasoning process and documentation of health assessment.

Clinical reasoning and documentation

The following case studies give examples of typical situations involving ear assessment and the clinical reasoning process including problem/issue identification. Consult a fundamentals of nursing or medical-surgical nursing text for information about goal setting, nursing interventions and evaluation.

Case study 1 (continued)—Middle ear infection

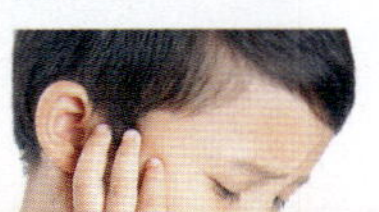

immunisations and has no significant previous medical history. His mother reports that Matthew has recently had a mild cold.

Matthew and his parents live in a small two-bedroom house approximately 40 km north of the central business district. He shares a bedroom with his older sister who is aged 6 years. Matthew's father works at the local council undertaking park and garden maintenance, and Matthew's mother works as a receptionist in a community centre. While the parents are working, the children are cared for by their maternal grandmother. The grandmother also cares for two other grandchildren every day. Both parents and Matthew's grandmother smoke up to 10 cigarettes each per day.

Yesterday, Matthew's grandmother put him to bed for his afternoon sleep. He did not sleep ... tugging ... nk only ... at solid ... the end ... erature

Health education

Provides health education information for key health concerns

Health Assessment Videos

The enhanced eBook features the following videos:

Abdominal Assessment

Respiratory Assessment

Cardiac Assessment

Neurological Assessment

Vital Signs (electronic)

Vital Signs (manual)

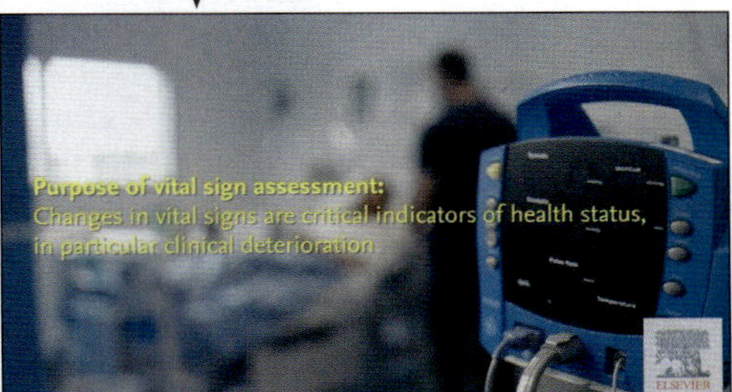

HEALTH EDUCATION

Stroke prevention

Stroke is a leading cause of long-term disability and death. A stroke occurs when the blood flow is interrupted to a part of the brain. The most common type is an ischaemic stroke, occurring when a blood clot blocks a blood vessel in the brain. Less common is a haemorrhagic stroke, which occurs when a blood vessel in the brain ruptures and causes bleeding.

Symptoms

The symptoms and after-effects of a stroke depend on which area of the brain is affected and to what extent. This can make a stroke difficult to diagnose. However, early recognition of symptoms and prompt treatment are essential.

The **most common** symptoms of stroke include sudden:

- weakness or numbness in the face, arms or legs, especially when it is on one side of the body
- confusion, trouble speaking or understanding speech
- changes in vision, such as blurry vision or

public in recognising the signs and symptoms of stroke quickly and calling for an ambulance.

The acronym is FAST:

- **F**ace—Check the person's face—has their mouth drooped?
- **A**rm—Can they lift both arms?
- **S**peech—Is their speech slurred? Do they understand you?
- **T**ime is critical—If you see any of these signs call the emergency number (Triple Zero [000] in Australia; 111 in Aotearoa New Zealand).

Stroke can strike anyone without warning. People need to be aware of their stroke risk and take steps to change the risk factors they can control.

Modifiable risk factors for stroke include:

- history of cardiovascular disease including hypertension, atrial fibrillation, dyslipidaemia and asymptomatic carotid stenosis
- cigarette smoking
- type 1 and type 2 diabetes
- sickle cell disease
- postmenopausal hormone therapy

About the Australian adapting editors

Helen Forbes
RN, BAppSc (AdvNurs) (La Trobe University), MEdSt (Monash University), PhD (University of Sydney)

Elizabeth Watt
RN, DipN (College of Nursing Australia), BAppSc (AdvNurs) (Lincoln Institute of Health Sciences), MNS (La Trobe University), CertPromCont, FACN

Helen Forbes
Helen has a background in general adult acute care nursing as well as a focus on care of patients following head and neck surgery. She has extensive higher education experience and has held various teaching and leadership roles at the undergraduate and postgraduate levels over the past 35 years. Previously she was Associate Professor and Associate Head of School (Teaching & Learning) at the School of Nursing & Midwifery, Deakin University, Melbourne. Helen's teaching interests include clinical education, health assessment and adult acute care nursing. She has taught health assessment at undergraduate and postgraduate level for many years locally and internationally. She has vast experience in curriculum design and development in nursing education. Helen is now a Nurse Education Consultant and accreditation reviewer with the Australian Nursing and Midwifery Accreditation Council and the Tertiary Education Quality and Standards Agency.

Elizabeth Watt
Liz has a background in adult acute care nursing and has practised in both hospital and community-based midwifery. She has more than 30 years' experience in higher education, teaching in undergraduate and postgraduate nursing programs. She has significant experience in curriculum design and development. Liz's current clinical and research interests include supporting carers of older people who have dementia and incontinence and improving urinary catheter care for older people living in residential aged care. She has taught health assessment at the undergraduate and postgraduate levels for many years. Liz is currently working as a Senior Research Fellow at the National Ageing Research Institute in Melbourne and is a Nurse Education Consultant. Liz is also a board member of the Continence Nurses Society of Australia.

About the US author

Carolyn Jarvis received her PhD from the University of Illinois at Chicago, with a research interest in the physiologic effect of alcohol on the cardiovascular system; her MSN from Loyola University (Chicago); and her BSN cum laude from the University of Iowa. She is Professor Emerita, School of Nursing at Illinois Wesleyan University, where she taught Health Assessment, Pathophysiology and Pharmacology. She earned Emerita status in 2020. Her current research interest concerns accuracy of pulse count methods, and she includes Honors students in this research.

In 2016, Illinois Wesleyan University honoured Dr. Jarvis for her contributions to the ever-changing field of nursing with the dedication of the Jarvis Center for Nursing Excellence. The Jarvis Center for Nursing Excellence equips students with laboratory and simulation learning so that they may pursue their nursing career with the same commitment as Dr. Jarvis.

Dr. Jarvis is the Student Senate Professor of the Year (2017) and was honoured to give remarks at commencement. She is a recipient of the University of Missouri's Superior Teaching

Award; has taught physical assessment to thousands of baccalaureate students, graduate students, and nursing professionals; has held 150 continuing education seminars; and is the author of numerous articles, textbook contributions, and this textbook and its ancillaries.

Dr. Jarvis's advanced practice roles included cardiovascular clinical specialist in various critical care settings, certified family nurse practitioner in primary care, as well as communicating in Spanish to provide health care in rural Guatemala and at the Community Health Care Clinic in Bloomington. Dr. Jarvis was instrumental in developing a synchronous teaching program for Illinois Wesleyan University students both in Barcelona, Spain, and at the home campus.

Ann Eckhardt received her PhD from the University of Illinois at Chicago with a research interest in cardiovascular disease symptomatology and her BSN magna cum laude from Illinois Wesleyan University. Dr. Eckhardt was an Endowed Associate Professor at Illinois Wesleyan University, where she taught for 10 years with a primary responsibility for health assessment, leadership and management, and senior seminars. She also served as the internship coordinator for the School of Nursing.

In 2021, Dr. Eckhardt accepted a position at University of Texas at Arlington as the Associate Chair of Clinical Education in the Department of Graduate Nursing. She is also an adjunct faculty member at Tokyo Medical Dental University in Tokyo, Japan. Her current research focuses on cardiovascular disease symptomatology, emergency department nurses' triage decision making, and conception of chest pain in the lay public.

In 2016, Dr. Eckhardt was named a 40 under 40 Emerging Nurse Leader by the American Nurses Association Illinois. She is an active member of the Honor Society of Phi Kappa Phi and Sigma Theta Tau International Nursing Honor Society and served as chapter presidents of both organisations. She has received numerous grants to support her scholarly pursuits and has published book chapters, peer-reviewed manuscripts, and editorials. Dr. Eckhardt mentors graduate students and includes students in her research whenever possible.

Dr. Eckhardt spent 15 years in clinical practice. Her first clinical position was in a cardiovascular intensive care unit where she cross-trained to the surgical ICU, pediatric ICU and neonatal ICU. She spent the last decade of her in-hospital career as a house officer.

Australian and New Zealand contributors

Helen Forbes
RN, BAppSc (AdvNurs) (La Trobe University), MEdSt (Monash University), PhD (University of Sydney)
Nurse Consultant (Education)
Formerly Associate Professor and Associate Head of School (Teaching & Learning)
School of Nursing & Midwifery,
Deakin University, Melbourne,
Victoria, Australia

Elizabeth Watt
RN, DipN (College of Nursing Australia), BAppSc (AdvNurs) (Lincoln Institute of Health Sciences), MNS (La Trobe University), CertPromCont, FACN
Nurse Consultant (Education)
Senior Research Fellow,
National Ageing Research Institute, Melbourne,
Victoria, Australia

Leonie Cox
RN (Baillie Henderson School of Psychiatric Nursing), PhD (Social Anthropology, University of Sydney), GCHEd (Queensland University of Technology)
Adjunct Associate Professor, School of Nursing,
Queensland University of Technology,
Kelvin Grove, Brisbane,
Queensland, Australia

Chris Taua
PhD, MN, PGCerMH, CertAdTch, DipN, CertDD, FNZCMHN
Director/Senior Consultant
Pumahara Consultants
North Canterbury, New Zealand

Catina Adams
BA(Hons), GDipEd, RN, RM, MClinNur, PhD, MACN, FHEA, CF
Course Coordinator – Child, Family and Community Nursing
Discipline Lead (Postgraduate Nursing)
School of Nursing and Midwifery,
La Trobe University, Bundoora,
Victoria, Australia

Elizabeth Pascoe
PhD, MSc(Nursing), BSc(Hons), DipEd
Casual Academic
Ethics, Integrity and Biosafety
La Trobe University, Bundoora,
Victoria, Australia

Rebecca Corbett
RPN, MANP
Psychiatric Nurse Consultant
Mental Health, Drugs and Alcohol Education Team
Barwon Health
Victoria, Australia

Josh Allen
RN, BN, BN(Hons), GDipNurPrac(CritCare), GCHEd, PhD
Senior Lecturer in Nursing
Department of Nursing
Faculty of Medicine Dentistry and Health Sciences
The University of Melbourne
Victoria, Australia

Amanda Wylie
RN, BN, MN, GCNur(ClinEd), GC(OphthalNurs)

Sue Sharrad
PhD, BEd, CCRN, GDipIC, MN
Senior Lecturer in Nursing
Clinical and Health Sciences Academic Unit
Rosemary Bryant AO Research Centre
University of South Australia, Adelaide,
South Australia, Australia

Niki Lillibridge
CCRN, BN, BN(Hons), MN, GCertHEd
Lecturer in Nursing
School of Nursing and Midwifery
La Trobe University,
Victoria, Australia

Amy N B Johnston
PhD, MEd, GCert(AdEd), BSc(Hons), BN
Conjoint Senior Research Fellow
Department of Emergency Medicine – Princess Alexandra Hospital and School of Nursing, Midwifery and Social Work
University of Queensland, Woolloongabba,
Queensland, Australia

Kate Schimmelbusch
RN, BN, PGCert(AcSurg/Ortho)
Nursing Education Department
Austin Health
Victoria, Australia

Trish Burton
DipAppSc, BSc, BAppSc, MEd, PhD, FACN
Senior Lecturer, Nursing, College of Healthcare Sciences
James Cook University, Cairns,
Queensland, Australia

David M Lee
DrPH, MPH, GDip(CCRN, Emerg/Trauma), BAppSc, DipAppSc(Nursing), FCNA
Nurse Practitioner (Primary Health)/Epidemiologist
Melbourne
Victoria, Australia

Nicki Hartney
RN, RM, MProfEdTrng (Deakin)
Senior Lecturer, School of Nursing and Midwifery
Deakin University, Geelong,
Victoria, Australia

Contributors to US edition

CHAPTER CONTRIBUTORS

Lydia Bertschi
DNP, APRN, ACNP-BC
Dr. Bertschi is the co-contributor for Chapter 19 (Thorax and Lungs), Chapter 20 (Heart and Neck Vessels), Chapter 21 (Peripheral Vascular System), and Chapter 22 (Abdomen). Dr. Bertschi is an Assistant Professor at Illinois Wesleyan University School of Nursing and a nurse practitioner in the intensive care unit at UnityPoint Health—Methodist.

Sarah Jarvis
DNP, APRN
Dr. Jarvis is the co-contributor for Chapter 14 (Head, Face, and Neck). Dr. Jarvis is a Certified Nurse Practitioner in Ann Arbor, Michigan.

ASSESSMENT PHOTOGRAPHERS

Chandi Kesler
BSN, RN
Chandi is a former Intensive Care Unit nurse and is an award-winning professional photographer. Chandi specialises in newborn and family photography in and around Central Illinois.

INSTRUCTOR AND STUDENT ANCILLARIES NGN CASE STUDIES

Kim Webb
MN, RN
Retired ADN Chair
Adjunct Faculty
Pioneer Technology Center
Ponca City, Oklahoma

KEY POINTS

Joanna Cain
RN, BSN
President & Founder
Global Academic Consultants, LLC
Boulder, Colorado

POWERPOINT PRESENTATIONS AND REVIEW QUESTIONS

Daryle Wane
PhD, APRN, FNP-BC
BSN Program Director
Professor of Nursing BSN Faculty
Department of Nursing and Health Programs
Pasco-Hernando State College
New Port Richey, Florida

TEACH FOR NURSES

Christian Richeson
MA, JD
Richeson Translations
Toledo, Ohio

TEST BANK

Heidi Monroe
PhD, RN, CAPA, CNE
Associate Professor of Nursing
NCLEX-RN Coordinator
Bellin College
Green Bay, Wisconsin

Preface

Health assessment is central to nursing practice. By practising and developing the knowledge and skills of health assessment you will develop confidence and competence in understanding and responding to each person's health situation. You need to listen to the cues from the person; these will guide and direct your questioning and physical examination. Whether you are an undergraduate nursing student, a newly qualified registered nurse or an experienced nurse seeking to advance your scope of practice, this text holds the content and resources you need to develop and refine your health assessment skills.

As a learner you should use this text in conjunction with the skills videos for self-directed learning. Also, you need to actively participate in formal on-campus skills development sessions and clinical placements. You need to be continuously reflecting on your learning and on the feedback provided by your learning facilitators and clinicians to refine your health assessment skills and knowledge. The fourth edition of this text is contextualised to suit the Australian and Aotearoa New Zealand healthcare environments. We hope this text will become an invaluable part of your professional library, and we look forward to ongoing feedback from you, our readers.

NEW TO THE FOURTH AUSTRALIAN AND NEW ZEALAND EDITION

The fourth ANZ edition of *Jarvis's Health Assessment* (note new title) has been fully revised and updated for the Australian and Aotearoa New Zealand contexts. It has been structured to enhance learning for undergraduate and postgraduate students, nurse practitioner candidates and clinicians.

This text differs from other health assessment texts by adopting a unique person-centred, enquiry-focused approach. In addition:

- Learners are provided with opportunities to adapt their assessment skills and to form clinical judgements by identifying the person's actual or potential health problems.
- The content has been restructured to support learning by using case studies and probing questions.
- There has been significant revision of the chapters on screening for family violence (Chapter 5) and screening for substance misuse (Chapter 6).
- The chapter on communication skills has also been significantly revised, with a new title and content on person-centred communication in health assessment.
- Approaches to gender diversity and inclusion have also been further developed.

APPROACH TO LEARNING HEALTH ASSESSMENT

This text, written by leading academics and clinicians, is the ideal learner guide to conducting health assessments in a range of healthcare settings. The learner will be guided to seamlessly apply their biomedical and nursing knowledge with clinical assessment and communication skills. Chapters have a logical structure covering key knowledge, frameworks and techniques, as well as specific areas of human structure and function, and finally, application of health assessment knowledge and skills in the clinical setting.

This text identifies the foundational knowledge and clinical skills every nurse needs to assess clients in a range of healthcare settings. Chapters 11–29 are divided into two main sections: entry-level health assessment expected of a newly graduated nurse; and an advanced knowledge and skills section for nurses wishing to advance their scope of practice.

This text applies an enquiry approach to learning, with a person-centred focus using case studies. Case studies in Chapters 2, 5–9 and 11–30 provide a clinical context to assist the learner to develop a deep understanding of the ways in which health assessment skills must be adapted relative to each person's needs. This approach is supported by probing questions aimed at guiding investigation of the impact of an altered health state on each person's day-to-day function.

KEY FEATURES

- Fully updated for the Australian and Aotearoa New Zealand contexts, reflecting current practice and guidelines
- Ideal for nursing students and those studying for advanced practice roles
- Clear separation of knowledge and skills—easy for teachers and students to identify content relevant to their level of learning
- An enquiry approach to learning with a person-centred focus
- Health education, inclusive practice and lifespan considerations embedded throughout
- Includes case studies to illustrate the initial parts of the clinical reasoning process and documentation of health assessment findings
- Easy to navigate—clearly structured and colour-coded
- Extensive use of learning and teaching resources, with illustrations to clarify important anatomical and physiological concepts to help learners grasp key concepts
- Accompanying resources include QR codes, Australian-produced videos showcasing physical examination skills, PowerPoints and a summative MCQ question bank

INSTRUCTOR RESOURCES ON EVOLVE

- Instructor teaching and learning guide
- PowerPoint presentations
- Skills videos
- Image collection
- Test bank
- New semester planner—embedding Elsevier solutions into your course
- New mapping guide—cross-references Elsevier foundation content

STUDENT AND INSTRUCTOR RESOURCES ON EVOLVE

- Australian-produced skills videos include vital signs measurement (manual and electronic), respiratory assessment, cardiac assessment, abdominal assessment and neurological assessment
- Access to Elsevier resources on Evolve including an eBook version of the text

ACKNOWLEDGEMENTS

We would like to acknowledge the people who made the fourth Australian and New Zealand edition of this text possible:

- Melinda McEvoy (Senior Content Strategist) for her support and leadership in developing this edition.

- Matt Davies (Editor) for his professional editorial skills.
- Shruti Raj (Content Project Manager) for her efforts in transforming the manuscript into a textbook.
- Deakin University, School of Nursing and Midwifery, who generously made simulation centre space available for the video shoot.

We would also like to thank our families for supporting us in developing this text over the past two and a half years. We thank our families and friends for their support, encouragement and for the endless cups of tea.

We would like to dedicate this edition to the nursing students and registered nurses who will use this text to develop their clinical skills. We encourage you to continually strive to develop and refine your health assessment skills. Your efforts will contribute to improving the person's experience and the overall quality and safety of nursing care.

To nursing curriculum designers, we encourage you to prioritise health assessment knowledge and skill development by ensuring a strong focus, particularly in undergraduate curricula. To the nursing lecturers, we thank you for your continuing motivation and encouragement of student learning in this critical area of nursing practice.

The publisher and editors would also like to thank each of the chapter authors and reviewers who ensured the relevance, accuracy and strong clinical application of the content. In this new edition we would also like to acknowledge past contributors and reviewers who provided a strong foundation on which we could build.

Helen Forbes
Elizabeth Watt

Contents

UNIT 1

Approaches and contexts of health assessment in nursing

CHAPTER 1

The context and frameworks of health assessment

Adapted by Helen Forbes and Elizabeth Watt

INTRODUCTION

Knowledge, skill and a professional approach are essential for nurses to be able to provide health care for a person. Knowledge or skill on their own is not enough, however. Nurses must be able to anticipate the problems or health issues that the person may have and guide them to either known medical diagnoses or situations where a medical diagnosis has not yet been established. Nurses also have an important role in identifying changes over time to a person's health state. Knowledge of health and underpinning health sciences are fundamental to identifying health issues.

Nurses have a range of health assessment frameworks to choose from depending on the situation. Using the most appropriate health assessment framework ensures all the relevant information is identified. Nurses focus on exploring the symptoms the person is reporting, the impact of symptoms on day-to-day functioning and any possible risks that the person may have in relation to their symptoms and altered function. Once all the person's problems are identified (symptoms, risk and altered function), nurses then identify health outcomes and prioritise and plan care. In this chapter, you will be introduced to health assessment, the concept of health, models of health, the concept of nursing, quality and safety in health care, lifespan and social and cultural considerations, approaches to health assessment in different situations and frameworks for health assessment.

Resources available

You will find additional resources and the reference list at the end of this chapter. There is a series of videos that accompany this text that show specific, focused assessments. We have developed and produced these videos to assist you in your skill development and to show how you can approach these areas of health assessment that learners often find difficult. The videos include vital sign measurement (manual and electronic), an aspect of neurological assessment (routine neurological screening), cardiac, respiratory and abdominal assessment. You will find a QR code in each relevant chapter that will enable you to easily access the relevant video on your device through Elsevier ClinicalKey.

What is health assessment?

Assessment is the collection of data about a person's health state. Throughout this text, you will be studying the techniques of collecting and analysing **subjective data** (i.e. what the person *says* about themselves during history taking) and **objective data** (i.e. what you as the health professional *observe* by inspecting, percussing, palpating and auscultating during the physical examination). Together with the patient's record and laboratory studies, these elements form the **database** of assessing the person's health.

Nurses make a clinical judgement or diagnosis about the person's health state. This diagnosis is based on the data nurses collect by asking the person questions (subjective data), conducting a physical examination and taking any relevant measurements (objective data). The problems (diagnoses) identified may be related to the person's symptoms (subjective data) or alterations in function and/or risks for further health issues. So, the purpose of a health assessment is to make a clinical judgement or diagnosis by identifying

TABLE 1.1 Nursing registration requirements relevant to health assessment

Nursing and Midwifery Board of Australia, Registered Nurse Standards for Practice[3]	Competencies for Registered Nurses, New Zealand Nursing Council[4]
Standard 4: Comprehensively conducts assessments.	***Competency 2.2: Undertakes a comprehensive and accurate nursing assessment of health consumers in a variety of settings.***
RNs accurately conduct comprehensive and systematic assessments. They analyse information and data and communicate outcomes as the basis for practice. The RN: • 4.1 conducts assessments that are holistic as well as culturally appropriate • 4.2 uses a range of assessment techniques to systematically collect relevant and accurate information and data to inform practice • 4.3 works in partnership to determine factors that affect, or potentially affect, the health and wellbeing of people and populations to determine priorities for action and/or for referral, and • 4.4 assesses the resources available to inform planning.	• Indicator: Undertakes assessment in an organised and systematic way. • Indicator: Uses suitable assessment tools and methods to assist the collection of data. • Indicator: Applies relevant research to underpin nursing assessment.

RN = registered nurse

the person's actual or potential health problems. Knowledge and skill in health assessment is a requirement of the Nursing and Midwifery Board of Australia[1] and the Nursing Council of New Zealand for Registered Nurse registration.[2] See Table 1.1.

Because all healthcare treatments and decisions are based on the data gathered during assessment, it is paramount that the assessment be factual and complete, providing the foundation for clinical decision making. Chapter 2 provides more detail about the process of clinical decision making that requires critical thinking and reasoning in health assessment.

What is health?

Assessment is the collection of data about a person's health state. Therefore, nurses need to have a clear idea of the concept of health because this determines which assessment data should be collected when assessing people for alterations in their health. In general, the list of data that must be collected has lengthened as our conception of health has broadened. The World Health Organization (WHO) defines health as 'a state of complete physical, mental, and social wellbeing and not merely the absence of disease or infirmity'.[5] While this is a broad definition, it is important to recognise that health is an emerging state and is not merely the absence of disease. In order to achieve an adequate quality of life in later years, actively promoting good health is vital throughout life. Further descriptions of health from a cultural perspective can be found in Chapter 4.

The situations in which people are born, grow, live and play have an important role in determining health. WHO states: 'The social determinants of health are the conditions in which people are born, grow, live, work and age. These circumstances are shaped by the distribution of money, power and resources at global, national and local levels. The social determinants of health are mostly responsible for health inequities—the unfair and avoidable differences in health status seen within and between countries.'[6]

Therefore, conducting a health assessment on a person requires acknowledgment of both the social and the environmental context in which they live. For example, consider the discharge needs of a homeless young male patient after a motorcycle accident. How could his wound care and nutritional needs be managed in the community if he has no fixed address?

Models of health

The **social model of health** acknowledges the effect of social, economic, cultural and political factors and conditions on a person's state of health and wellbeing. Using the model aims to improve health outcomes, prevent and reduce illness and address the inequalities and disadvantage that exist within the community. Community health care, as a part of primary health care, is informed by the values and principles supported in the Alma-Ata Declaration on Primary Health Care[7] and the Ottawa Charter for Health Promotion.[8]

The social model of health recognises:

- the social, economic and environmental determinants of health and illness
- the importance of health promotion and disease prevention
- the importance of community participation in decision making
- the importance of working with sectors outside the health sector
- that equity is an important outcome of health service intervention.

The **biomedical model** (the Western tradition) views health as the absence of disease. Health and disease are seen as opposites—extremes on a linear continuum. Disease is caused by specific agents or pathogens. So, the biomedical focus is on diagnosing and treating those pathogens and curing disease. Assessment factors are a list of biophysical symptoms and signs. The person is certified as healthy when these symptoms and signs have been eliminated. When disease does exist, medical diagnosis is worded to identify and explain the cause of disease.

Accurately diagnosing and treating illness is an important part of health care, but the medical model has limiting boundaries. While biomedical thinking and its approach to patient care is still the dominant model, the **biopsychosocial model of health care** is thought to have the potential to improve clinical outcomes for people with chronic diseases and functional illnesses. The biopsychosocial model of health care recognises the interrelationships between biological, psychological, sociocultural and spiritual factors on a person's health. However, remuneration schemes, clinical guidelines and clinical performance indicators are biomedically orientated, providing limited incentive for medical practitioners to adopt the biopsychosocial model in their practice.[9]

The public's concept of health has expanded since the 1950s. Now we view health in a wider context. We have an increasing interest in lifestyle, personal habits, exercise and nutrition and the social and natural environment. **Wellness** is a dynamic process, a move towards optimal functioning. Different levels of wellness exist, with optimal health described as 'high-level wellness'. Wellness is a direction of progress. Health professionals serve to maximise the person's potential and to assist the person to grow towards high-level wellness.

Considering the whole person is the essence of **holistic health**. Holistic health views the mind, body and spirit as interdependent and functioning as a whole within the environment.[10] Health depends on all these factors working together. The basis of disease is multifaceted, originating both from within the person and from the external environment. Treating disease therefore requires the services of numerous providers.

A natural progression to **health promotion** and disease prevention rounds out our concept of health. The leading causes of death among Australians aged 65 years and older are related to ischaemic heart disease, dementia, Alzheimer's disease, stroke, lung cancer and chronic obstructive pulmonary disease.[11] The causes of death for New Zealanders are similar.[12] Many of these chronic conditions can be modified by changes to lifestyle. Health promotion focuses on public policy change, counselling and support to motivate people to improve their health. Policy changes in recent times have focused on reducing smoking and alcohol and drug use, encouraging activity and exercise, healthy eating, safety in the home and on the road and safe sexual practices. Health promotion is a much broader concept than disease prevention. Health promotion was defined in the Ottawa Charter for Health Promotion and includes building public health policy, creating supportive environments for healthy living, strengthening community action, developing personal knowledge and skills and reorienting the healthcare system.[8,13] Chapter 4 extends this discussion of varying cultural conceptualisations of health.

What is nursing?

The International Council of Nurses states that nursing includes 'autonomous and collaborative care of individuals of all ages, families, groups and communities, sick or well and in all settings. Nursing includes the promotion of health, prevention of illness, and the care of ill, disabled and dying people. Advocacy, promotion of a safe environment, research, participation in shaping health policy and in-patient and health systems management, and education are also key nursing roles'.[14] This implies that the nursing approach to health care is holistic in nature and therefore health assessment should reflect that philosophy with its focus on the whole person and their context.

There is a range of clinical contexts in which you may work as a nurse. These include community health settings, mental health care, acute and critical care contexts, remote and rural settings, rehabilitation or residential aged care. The nature of the context will usually determine the type and focus of health assessment required. In the community, you may focus on assessing a person, a family or a community and be interested in gathering information about wellness as opposed to illness. In an acute setting, whether it is in a critical care or more general ward area, your focus will differ depending on the health status of the person. Patient problems may vary across the treatment trajectory, which means you will need to time and focus your health assessment accordingly.

In providing care, nurses and midwives are ethically responsible and accountable to the person who receives that care.[15] From an ethical point of view, it is expected that nurses and midwives will respect, promote, protect and uphold the rights of people either receiving care or providing health care. The nursing and midwifery codes of ethics outline minimum national standards of conduct that members of the professions are expected to uphold. These codes inform the community of the standards of professional conduct it can expect nurses and midwives to uphold and provide the consumer, regulatory, employing and professional bodies with a basis for evaluating their professional conduct. The Nursing and Midwifery Board of Australia[16] and Nursing Council of New Zealand[17] codes of professional conduct provide guidelines about expected behaviour of nurses and midwives. Nurses and midwives are expected to conduct their practice using exemplary standards of behaviour. In summary, it is expected that each professional will be safe and competent and practise in keeping with the standards of nursing and the broader health system. Nurses must conduct their practice according to laws relevant to nursing. Nurses and midwives are also legally responsible for their practice and answerable to the relevant professional registering body: the Nursing and Midwifery Board of Australia or the Nursing Council of New Zealand. All nurses and midwives in Australia and Aotearoa New Zealand must meet the professional standards in a range of domains, one of which relates to the conduct of comprehensive and systematic nursing health assessment.[3,4] Nurse practitioners also have legal requirements to meet in their specialist area related to advanced health assessment.[18,19]

Quality and safety in health care

Once a person accesses the healthcare system for treatment of illness, a number of factors pose a potential risk for harm. Examples include increasing age, comorbidity and the increasing use of complex technology, the use of numerous and complex interventions during an episode of illness, movement between community and hospital health sectors giving rise to possible duplication of, or gaps in care and/or communication breakdown. The Australian Charter of Healthcare Rights[20] and the New Zealand Code of Rights[21] describe the rights of patients and other people using the Australian or Aotearoa New Zealand health systems. One of the principles of these Charters is the recognition that every person has the right to the highest standard of care. While the solutions to decreasing risk to the person are complex, improving the use, availability and communication of health information is critical to providing high-quality and safe care.[22,23] Quality and safe care of people requires that nurses use assessment as part of their practice to determine care needs. Assessment is conducted in collaboration with the person and the multidisciplinary healthcare team to achieve positive goals and health outcomes for the recipient of care. See Chapter 2 for the processes involved in clinical decision making. There will be many opportunities throughout this text to practise clinical reasoning and clinical decision making.

Developmental considerations

Life span considerations

It is important to consider health assessment from a life cycle approach, no matter what clinical context you are working in. First, you must be familiar with the usual and expected developmental tasks for each age group (Chapter 3). This alerts you to which physical, psychosocial, cognitive and behavioural tasks are important for each person. For example, if you are assessing a 6-year-old child with asthma, your approach will need to take into account the developmental tasks for that child's age group, which include mastering skills that will be needed later as an adult, building self-esteem and a positive self-concept, adopting moral standards and taking a place in a peer group. This knowledge will guide how you collect subjective and objective data. The data from the physical examination is more accurate when you consider age-specific information about anatomy, method of examination, normal findings and abnormal findings. For example, an average normal respiratory rate for a 6-year-old child is 21 to 26 breaths per minute.

Cultural and social considerations

The population of Australia is in excess of 25 million; Aotearoa New Zealand is approximately 5 million. Both Aotearoa New Zealand and Australia are countries that are ethnically and culturally diverse. Cultural and social considerations are critical to health assessment: there is an introduction to these concepts in Chapter 4, and the concepts are emphasised throughout the text as they relate to specific chapters.

Assessment approaches for different situations

The approach you take to health assessment will depend on the context of care and the reason for the assessment. In many situations, assessment is guided by a pre-printed form—for example, an admission assessment and risk identification form. However, this should not restrict you from seeking additional information relevant to the person's situation and needs.

Comprehensive health assessment

A comprehensive health assessment is performed at a person's first entry in an outpatient setting or initial admission to a hospital. It includes a complete health history (Chapter 8) and relevant physical examination. It describes the current and past health state and forms a baseline against which all future changes can be measured. It yields the first cues to actual and potential health problems.

In community health or domiciliary care settings, nurses are usually the first health professional to see the person and has primary responsibility for monitoring the person's health care. In community settings, the comprehensive health assessment could also be conducted on a well person with the purpose of focusing on health maintenance and health promotion. In acute care settings, the comprehensive health assessment is performed on admission to the hospital. Often, the person has completed a standard pre-printed health history form before admission. Part of the admission assessment would then focus on clarifying and validating the information with the person and extending the health history where needed. In an admission assessment, you will go on to collect information on the person's perception/impact of illness, functional ability and impact on activities of daily living, health maintenance activities, coping patterns and health goals. An important outcome of a comprehensive assessment is to identify potential risk factors that may impact on the person's hospitalisation or discharge. (See Chapter 8 for taking a health history.)

Often a comprehensive assessment is also performed when a person moves from one area of a hospital to another—for example, from intensive care to a ward, or from a ward to a rehabilitation facility. This serves as a summary of the person's health state at that time and gives the next group of clinicians a new baseline on which future assessment and care decisions can be made.

Focused (episodic) assessment

Focused assessment is for a limited or short-term problem. Here, you complete a focused assessment, which is smaller in scope than the comprehensive health assessment. It concerns mainly one problem, one cue or one body system. The cue could be something that the person has told you ('*I feel very nauseated*' or '*I feel like I need to go to the toilet all the time*') or can be a sign that you observe—the person appears to be in pain, or the urine output is less per hour than expected. Focused assessment is used in all settings—hospital, primary care or long-term care. For example, 2 days after surgery, a hospitalised person suddenly has a congested cough, shortness of breath and fatigue. The history and physical examination focuses primarily on the respiratory and cardiovascular systems.

Ongoing assessment

In ongoing assessment the status of any identified problems should be evaluated at regular and appropriate intervals. For example, in the acute care setting, this would mean assessing a person after a surgical procedure, or frequent neurological observations (neuro obs) for a person who has an actual or potential for change in conscious state. In a primary care setting the assessment may be related to, for example, ongoing monitoring of an asthma or diabetes plan. In this situation, your assessment focuses on determining if any change in health state has occurred, whether an intervention is effective and how the person is managing their health. This type of assessment is used in all settings to follow up short-term or chronic health problems.

Primary survey

Primary survey is conducted in emergency and non-emergency situations. In an emergency situation, the assessment must be rapid and focused and is often conducted alongside life-saving measures to identify and manage impending or actual life threats for the person. A systematic approach using ABCDE is used (Table 1.2).

PRIMARY SURVEY IN A NON-EMERGENCY CLINICAL SETTING

When you take over the care of a person at the beginning of a shift it is important to do a primary survey that includes airway, breathing, circulation, level of consciousness and environment.

TABLE 1.2 Summary of primary survey (A, B, C, D, E)

A = airway	Ask the person their name and listen carefully for air movement. If they speak then the airway is considered to be open.
B = breathing	Is the person breathing without effort? Observe rate, depth and symmetry of breathing and use of accessory muscles.
C = circulation	Palpate the radial or carotid pulse for rate, strength and rhythm. Also check capillary refill time, skin colour and survey for obvious bleeding.
D = disability	Assess level of conscious state.
E =exposure and environment	Exposure of the body may need to be done sequentially, uncovering one body area at a time to maintain patient dignity and temperature control. The environment should be checked to ensure the person is not in danger of further trauma.

The following example focuses on hospitalised people and their immediate environment. Assessment may include:

- airway, breathing, circulation, level of consciousness
- location of emergency equipment and readiness to function
- check IV fluids, medications and/or gastric feeding that is in progress (syringe drivers, other pumps and drains) to make sure the correct solution is being infused at the prescribed rate (check against the medical orders)
- IV site is clean, covered and not inflamed or swollen
- oxygen is being delivered at the right rate and flow
- oxygen and suction equipment is available at the bedside and functioning correctly
- drains or drainage equipment are functioning correctly, noting the amount of drainage at the time of the assessment
- appearance and location of surgical and other wounds
- urinary catheter is draining correctly with no kinks in the tubing, the drainage bag is below the level of bladder and not touching the floor, and that the system is intact; note the amount and colour of urine in the drainage bag at the time of the assessment.

PRIMARY SURVEY IN A HOME SETTING

When working in a home environment the primary survey often includes elements listed in the acute care setting above, but the home environment is also surveyed for actual or potential risks to the person or yourself:

- access to the home
- state of the home—cleanliness, tidiness, presence of rubbish, etc.
- safety—presence of animals, trip hazards, electrical hazards, weapons
- availability of running water for handwashing, availability of a clean area to put equipment for procedures.

Table 1.3 summarises the main points for each of the assessment approaches.

TABLE 1.3 Summary of assessment approaches

Comprehensive Assessment	Focused Assessment	Ongoing Assessment	Primary Survey
• Performed at a person's first entry to the health setting • Includes complete health history and physical examination • Yields first clues to actual and potential health problems and risks during hospitalisation • May include use of a pre-printed form • Forms a baseline for future assessments • Usually performed by the first health professional to see the person on admission	• Used for limited or short-term problems • Concerns one health problem, one cue or one body system • Used in all settings • History and physical examination focuses on the relevant body system • Informs impact on function and risks to the person	• Assessment is performed at regular intervals, e.g. 2-hourly neuro obs • Related to a specific health problem, e.g. acute/chronic • Determines change in health state or effectiveness of an intervention • Used in all settings	• Conducted in emergency and non-emergency situations • In emergency situations ABCDE is used—see Table 1.1 • In non-emergency situations, i.e. start of a shift, ABC, level of consciousness and environment survey

Frameworks for assessment

There are several frameworks to guide health assessment. These frameworks guide the sequence of data collection and, to some extent, the type of data that is collected. The **head-to-toe** and **body systems** approaches tend to be medically rather than nursing focused and are commonly used in acute care settings. The **functional health approach** is used in acute, subacute, rehabilitation and community nursing settings. This approach is more focused on the whole person and aims to explore the impact of health issues on the person and their daily activities and to identify potential health risks. However, a body systems approach is evident in the functional approach and should not be seen as a separate framework. The content in this textbook has been arranged as a combination of functional and body systems approaches.

Regardless of the approach you choose, you need to include important aspects of the person's health status that are relevant to nursing practice, such as interpersonal relationships and resources, values and beliefs, coping and stress management, and sleep and rest (see Chapter 8 for details). These aspects of health assessment are often overlooked in the head-to-toe and body systems approaches and can lead to fragmented care and poor discharge planning.

Functional approach

The functional approach to health assessment is based on the functional health patterns as described by Marjorie Gordon.[24] This approach to assessment is designed to facilitate a comprehensive and person-focused assessment where the person's health status and health management practices are taken into account, leading to a holistic perspective.[25,26] See Table 1.4.

TABLE 1.4 Areas for assessment: functional approach

Areas for Assessment	Relevant Chapter(s)
Health perception and health management pattern (how the person perceives and manages their health)	11–29
Nutritional metabolic pattern	22
Elimination pattern (excretion patterns/problems)	13, 21, 23–25
Activity exercise pattern (capacity to do daily activities without any problem, self-care activities including cardiac, respiratory and musculoskeletal assessment)	10, 13, 16, 17, 19, 20
Sleep, rest–sleeping patterns	5, 6, 11–13, 16–22, 24, 25, 29
Cognitive–perceptual pattern (assessment of neurological function and pain)	10, 12, 13
Self-perception/self-concept pattern	3, 5, 6, 11
Roles/relationships pattern	3–6, 11
Sexuality/reproductive pattern	3–6, 11, 24, 26–28
Coping–stress tolerance pattern	5, 6, 11
Value–beliefs pattern	5, 6, 11–29

SUBJECTIVE DATA—THE HEALTH HISTORY

Collect the history, complete or limited, as relevant to the person's specific health concerns. Always start with asking the person and/or their carer about their presenting concern or the reason for their hospitalisation (if relevant) and their usual health management practices. Each area being assessed includes the impact of the health issues on the whole person, such as interpersonal relationships and resources, values and beliefs, coping and stress management, and sleep and rest (see Chapter 8 for details).

OBJECTIVE DATA—PHYSICAL EXAMINATION, MEASUREMENT AND SPECIMEN SCREENING

- While obtaining the history and throughout the assessment, note the person's general appearance.
- To further assess change in function or risk for change you will draw on information from relevant chapters identified in Table 1.4.
- In addition to the areas for assessment outlined in Table 1.4, you may also need to consider screening for family violence (Chapter 5) and/or substance misuse (Chapter 6).

Body systems approach

Using a body systems approach to health assessment aligns with the biomedical model where individual body systems (cardiac, respiratory, endocrine, renal, gastrointestinal, neurological) are assessed independently of each other. Inspection, palpation, percussion and auscultation techniques are used aimed at identifying abnormality.

SUBJECTIVE DATA—THE HEALTH HISTORY

Collect the history, complete or limited, as relevant to the person's specific health concerns. Always start with asking the person and/or their carer about their presenting concern or the reason for their hospitalisation (if relevant). This includes a psychosocial assessment such as their perception of their health status, interpersonal relationships and resources, values and beliefs, coping and stress management and sleep and rest.

OBJECTIVE DATA—PHYSICAL EXAMINATION

- While obtaining the history and throughout the assessment, note the person's general appearance.
- To further assess change in function or risk for change you will draw on information from relevant chapters identified in Table 1.5.

TABLE 1.5 Areas for assessment: body systems approach

Areas for Assessment	Relevant Chapter(s)
General survey, vital signs	10
Neurological	12–15
Mental health	5, 6, 11
Cardiovascular system	16, 17
Respiratory system	18, 19
Gastrointestinal system	21, 23, 25
Endocrine system	21
Renal/bladder	23, 24
Skin, hair, nails	22
Musculoskeletal	20
Reproductive system	26–29
Ears	15
Eyes	14

- In addition to the areas for assessment outlined in Table 1.5, you may also need to consider screening for family violence (Chapter 5) and/or substance misuse (Chapter 6).

Head-to-toe approach

Taking a head-to-toe approach to assessment generally means assessing body parts starting at the head and finishing at the toes, using a sequence of inspection, palpation, percussion and auscultation aimed at identifying abnormality.[27]

SUBJECTIVE DATA—THE HEALTH HISTORY

- Collect the history, complete or limited, as relevant to the person's specific health concerns. Always start with asking the person and/or their carer about their presenting concern or the reason for their hospitalisation (if relevant).

OBJECTIVE DATA—PHYSICAL EXAMINATION

- While obtaining the history and throughout the assessment, note the person's general appearance.
- To further assess change in function or risk for change you will draw on information from relevant chapters identified in Table 1.6.
- There is a risk with taking only a head-to-toe approach to assessment that conclusions drawn tend to be medically focused rather nursing-focused. You will need to keep this in mind as you approach your assessment.
- In addition to the areas for assessment outlined in Table 1.6, you may also need to consider screening for family violence (Chapter 5) and/or substance misuse (Chapter 6).

TABLE 1.6 Areas for assessment: head-to-toe assessment

Areas for Assessment	Relevant Chapter(s)
General appearance	10
Measurement of height and weight	10, 21
Vital signs	10
Nutritional assessment (including skin, hair and nails)	21, 22
Head (including eyes, ears, mouth and throat)	12, 14, 15, 18, 21
Upper extremities (musculoskeletal, peripheral, vascular)	16, 20
Neurological assessment	12
Mental health	11
Chest posterior and lateral (inspection, palpation and auscultation of breath sounds)	17, 19
Chest anterior (inspection, palpation and auscultation of breath sounds)	17, 19
Breasts	28
Heart (inspection, palpation and auscultation of apical rate and rhythm)	17
Abdomen (including bowel function)	23, 25
Anus, rectum, prostate	23–25, 27
Genito-urinary (external genitalia, urinary function)	24, 26, 27
Lower extremities (musculoskeletal, peripheral vascular)	16, 20

ADDITIONAL RESOURCES

You can further develop your knowledge and skills relevant to health assessment, related pathophysiology, common health issues and nursing interventions by:

- reading chapters of a fundamentals of nursing or medical-surgical nursing textbook
- answering chapter multiple choice questions online. Log onto ClinicalKey Student and search for the text 'Health Assessment, 4th edition'. Choose the section titled 'Teaching material'. In this section you will find question and answer documents for each chapter.
- visiting websites

  Australian Commission on Quality and Safety in Health Care: https://www.safetyandquality.gov.au

  New Zealand Health Quality and Safety Commission: https://www.hqsc.govt.nz

ADDITIONAL RESOURCES cont'd

International Council of Nurses. The ICN code of ethics for nurses. 2021. Available at: https://www.icn.ch/node/1401

Nursing and Midwifery Board of Australia. www.nursingmidwiferyboard.gov.au

Nursing and Midwifery Board of Australia. Code of conduct for nurses: https://www.nursingmidwiferyboard.gov.au/codes-guidelines-statements/professional-standards.aspx.

Nursing and Midwifery Board of Australia. Code of conduct for midwives: https://www.nursingmidwiferyboard.gov.au/Codes-Guidelines-Statements/Professional-standards.aspx

Nursing Council of New Zealand. www.nursingcouncil.org.nz

Midwifery Council of New Zealand. https://midwiferycouncil.health.nz/Public

Nursing Council of New Zealand. Code of conduct for nurses. 2012. Available at: https://www.nursingcouncil.org.nz/Public/Nursing/Standards_and_guidelines/NCNZ/nursing-section/Standards_and_guidelines_for_nurses.aspx?hkey=9fc06ae7-a853-4d10-b5fe-992cd44ba3de

REFERENCES

1. Nursing and Midwifery Board of Australia. Registered nurse standards for practice. 2016. Available at: https://www.nursingmidwiferyboard.gov.au/codes-guidelines-statements/professional-standards.aspx
2. Nursing Council of New Zealand. Competencies for Registered Nurses. 2016. Available at: https://www.nursingcouncil.org.nz/Public/Nursing/Standards_and_guidelines/NCNZ/nursing-section/Standards_and_guidelines_for_nurses.aspx?hkey=9fc06ae7-a853-4d10-b5fe-992cd44ba3de
3. Nursing and Midwifery Board of Australia. Registered nurse standards for practice. 2016. Available at https://www.nursingmidwiferyboard.gov.au/Codes-Guidelines-Statements/Professional-standards/registered-nurse-standards-for-practice.aspx
4. Nursing Council of New Zealand. Competencies for Registered Nurses. 2016. Available at: https://www.nursingcouncil.org.nz/Public/Nursing/Standards_and_guidelines/NCNZ/nursing-section/Standards_and_guidelines_for_nurses.aspx?hkey=9fc06ae7-a853-4d10-b5fe-992cd44ba3de
5. World Health Organization (WHO). Constitution of the World Health Organization: principles 2019. 2019. Available at: https://www.who.int/about/mission/en/
6. World Health Organization (WHO). Social determinants of health. 2023. Available at: https://www.who.int/health-topics/social-determinants-of-health#tab=tab_1
7. World Health Organization (WHO). Declaration of Alma-Ata. 1978. Available at: https://cdn.who.int/media/docs/default-source/documents/almaata-declaration-en.pdf?sfvrsn=7b3c2167_2
8. World Health Organization (WHO). The 1st International Conference on Health Promotion, Ottawa, 1986. 2023. Available at: https://www.who.int/teams/health-promotion/enhanced-wellbeing/first-global-conference
9. Kusnanto H, Agustian D, Hilmanto D. Biopsychosocial model of illnesses in primary care: A hermeneutic literature review. Journal of Family Medicine and Primary Care. 2018 May;7(3):497.
10. Frisch NC, Rabinowitsch D. What's in a definition? Holistic nursing, integrative health care, and integrative nursing: report of an integrated literature review. Journal of Holistic Nursing. 2019 Sep;37(3):260–272.

11. Australian Institute of Health and Welfare. Deaths in Australia [Internet]. Canberra: Australian Institute of Health and Welfare, 2023 [cited 2023 Nov. 9]. Available from: https://www.aihw.gov.au/reports/life-expectancy-deaths/deaths-in-australia
12. Ministry of Health, New Zealand. 2023. Health and Independence Report 2022. Wellington: Ministry of Health. Available at: https://www.health.govt.nz/publication/health-and-independence-report-2022
13. Talbot L, Verrinder G. Promoting health: the primary health care approach. 6th ed. Sydney: Elsevier; 2018.
14. International Council of Nurses. Nursing definitions 2002. Available at: https://www.icn.ch/resources/nursing-definitions
15. International Council of Nurses. The ICN code of ethics for nurses. Geneva: ICN; Revised 2021. Available at: https://www.icn.ch/sites/default/files/2023-06/ICN_Code-of-Ethics_EN_Web.pdf
16. Nursing and Midwifery Board of Australia. Code of conduct for nurses. 2018. Available at: https://www.nursingmidwiferyboard.gov.au/Codes-Guidelines-Statements/Professional-standards.aspx
17. Nursing Council of New Zealand. Tikanga Whanonga. Code of Conduct. 2012 Available at: https://www.nursingcouncil.org.nz/Public/Nursing/Code_of_Conduct/NCNZ/nursing-section/Code_of_Conduct.aspx#:~:text=The%20Code%20is%20framed%20around,cannot%20fulfil%20their%20role%20effectively
18. Nursing and Midwifery Board of Australia. Nurse Practitioner standards for practice. 2021 Availableat:https://www.nursingmidwiferyboard.gov.au/Codes-Guidelines-Statements/Professional-standards/nurse-practitioner-standards-of-practice.aspx
19. Nursing Council of New Zealand: Competencies for the mātanga tapuhi nurse practitioner scope of practice. 2017. Available at: https://www.nursingcouncil.org.nz/public/nursing/scopes_of_practice/nurse_practitioner/ncnz/nursing-section/nurse_practitioner.aspx
20. Australian Commission on Safety and Quality in Health Care. Australian Charter of Healthcare Rights. 2nd ed. 2019. Available at: https://www.safetyandquality.gov.au/sites/default/files/2019-06/Charter%20of%20Healthcare%20Rights%20A4%20poster%20ACCESSIBLE%20pdf.pdf
21. New Zealand Health and Disability Commissioner. Code of health & disability services: Consumers' rights. 1996. Available at: https://www.hdc.org.nz/your-rights/about-the-code/code-of-health-and-disability-services-consumers-rights/
22. Australian Commission on Quality and Safety in Health Care. 2023. Available at: https://www.safetyandquality.gov.au/
23. New Zealand Health Quality and Safety Commission. 2020. Available at: https://www.hqsc.govt.nz/news/?programme=43
24. Gordon M (1994). Nursing diagnosis: Process and application (3rd ed). Mosby.
25. Butcher RD, Jones DA. An integrative review of comprehensive nursing assessment tools developed based on Gordon's Eleven Functional Health Patterns. International Journal of Nursing Knowledge. 2021;32:294–307.
26. Karaca T. Functional health patterns model: a case study (2016). Case Studies Journal. 5(7), July 2016. Available at: https://ssrn.com/abstract=3415861
27. Haugh KH. Head-to-toe: organizing your baseline patient physical assessment. Nursing. 2015 Dec 1;45(12):58–61.

CHAPTER 2

Clinical decision making

Written by Carolyn Jarvis and Ann Eckhardt
Adapted by Helen Forbes

INTRODUCTION

Registered nurses provide evidence-based nursing care for people of varying ages who are experiencing physical or mental illness in a range of clinical contexts. Nursing care is aimed at promoting and maintaining health and preventing illness; that is, it focuses on health outcomes.[1] Nurses work collaboratively with healthcare team members to help the person/family/community meet their health outcomes.[2] Regardless of the role or context of care, nurses are responsible and accountable for making clinical decisions as part of their role in caring for people.[3,4] Nurses need to understand the roles of the different health professionals who will be involved in the care of the person (e.g. nurse, physician, surgeon and other medical specialists, physiotherapist, occupational therapist, speech therapist, diabetes educator, stomal therapist, dietitian, pharmacist, social worker) to achieve collaborative health outcomes.

Nurses must conduct their role within their scope of practice as defined by the Nursing and Midwifery Board of Australia,[5] the Nursing Council of New Zealand,[6] the health Acts in Australia[7] and Aotearoa New Zealand[8] and relevant hospital policies, all of which are aimed at keeping patients safe. There are several indicators of quality and safe care of which the incidence of medication error, infection, falls, pressure injuries, malnutrition and unrelieved pain are specifically relevant to nursing people in hospitals.[9] The National Safety and Quality Health Care Standards describe the standard of care consumers can expect from their health service organisations.[10] The aim of these standards is to minimise the likelihood of hospital-acquired complications such as infections, medication errors, pressure injuries, falls and clinical deterioration from occurring. These standards also encompass the need for clear and effective clinical governance, comprehensive care and effective clinical communication between all members of the healthcare team. The aims of the Health Quality and Safety Commission of New Zealand also focus on patient safety, describing their healthcare standards and indicators of safe care similarly.[11]

Critical thinking and clinical decision making

Whether you are a nursing student or a new graduate, you need to be clear about the *purpose* of health assessment in your clinical context. This will direct what information you collect, the time frame and frequency of assessment and what you do with the information. For example, when in an acute care context, you need to be clear about the person's reasons for admission and known medical diagnoses, the medical plan, the person's trajectory and the role of the multidisciplinary healthcare team. (See Chapter 1 for the different approaches to assessment.)

As outlined in Chapter 1, assessment is the ongoing collection of information about a person's health state. However, collecting information is not enough. You must also consider whether the person's health situation is stable or rapidly changing because a nurse's decisions affect the person's health outcomes. Nurses use clinical judgement to make decisions to help keep the person safe and to improve their situation.[1] Clinical decision-making skills help nurses to decide which information should be collected using a range of sources that includes the person and their medical and nursing history, which may also include laboratory test results and information provided by family.[12] The assessment information needs to be organised, compared and evaluated and critical thinking and reasoning used to make inferences or predictions about the meaning of the information.[13] Analysis of health assessment information and drawing conclusions to identify health issues or problems is based on the scientific method used by most health professionals.[13] See Figure 2.1 for an outline of the components of the clinical reasoning cycle. Table 2.1 describes in further detail the steps of the clinical reasoning cycle and has examples of each step.

More assessment may follow the initial assessment to identify the person's health problems, areas of risk and/or needs. Following problem/nursing diagnosis and needs identification, nurses judge the quality of evidence available to inform the selection of the most appropriate interventions.[14] Nurses also consider the context, level of evidence, availability of resources, preference of the person and level of expertise of the nurse when deciding which interventions are suitable for the person's problem(s). Finally, the effectiveness of nursing interventions is evaluated in terms of achievement or non-achievement of health outcomes.[13]

Clinical decision making is therefore a dynamic process that starts on the first encounter with the person and continues as the nurse plans and implements care and evaluates the person's responses to interventions.

Table 2.1 describes the steps of the clinical reasoning cycle in more detail.

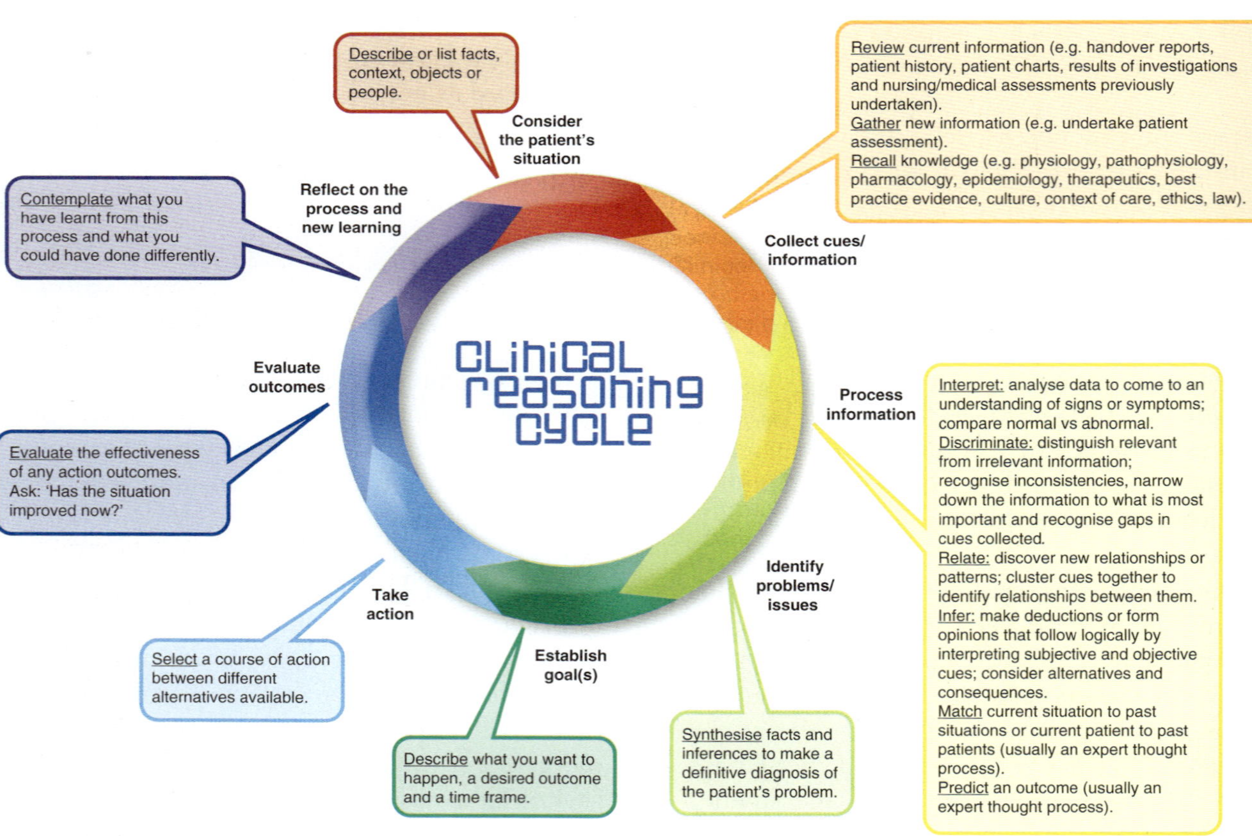

FIGURE 2.1 Clinical reasoning cycle

TABLE 2.1 Steps of the clinical reasoning cycle

Step	Description
1. To gain an understanding of the person's experience you will **identify available cues** (data) from a range of sources. This is the first step in clinical reasoning.	A ***cue*** is a piece of information provided by the person either in response to your questions (subjective) or determined by your physical assessment (objective). Cues will include a sign (objective, e.g. rash or cough) or symptom (subjective, e.g. headache or nausea) or a piece of laboratory data. ***Additional data*** may be collected from other sources (history, family, laboratory tests, hand over) in relation to a person's response to an actual or potential health alteration.
2. An important part of data **analysis** is to: • **discriminate** between relevant and irrelevant data. • identify **normal and abnormal data** • identify **relationships** between the data.	***Identify relevant and irrelevant data*** For example, for a person having a knee replacement, a history of appendicectomy is unlikely to be relevant during this episode of care. ***Identify normal data or abnormal data*** For example, normal data: afebrile, urine output is equal to input abnormal data: pain, tachycardia, tachypnoea, etc. ***Cluster or group related data***—this helps you see relationships between the data. For example, look for similar data such as that related to breathing, activity or urinary function. ***Identify patterns in the data***—this helps to fill in the whole picture and helps you identify missing pieces of information.
3. Draw conclusions **by making inferences/predictions/ hypotheses*** about the data by interpreting, validating and testing. (*Note that different nursing textbooks have a preference for one or the other of these terms.)	***Interpret*** the data by formulating inferences, predictions or forming hypotheses. An ***inference, prediction or hypothesis*** is a tentative explanation for a cue or a set of cues that can be used as a basis for further investigation, e.g. the person hasn't opened their bowels for 4 days. This triggers you to think about possible constipation. ***Draw on your clinical knowledge*** and question what you think might be going on. You know that when a person hasn't been moving about, taking opioid pain medications or not eating a normal diet they are at risk of constipation. ***Validate*** or check the accuracy and reliability of your inferences/hypotheses/predictions by gathering more information to *test* the tentative inferences/prediction/ hypotheses. Continuing the above example, you would ask more questions about normal bowel patterns, dietary intake, exercise, activity and medications and perform an abdominal assessment to confirm constipation.

Continued

TABLE 2.1 Steps of the clinical reasoning cycle cont'd

Step	Description
4. A **nursing diagnosis** is a statement of an actual or potential patient problem/health issue that registered nurses are licensed to treat as part of their scope of practice. The statement is identified by analysing the data/cues.	Assessment is aimed at ***diagnosing actual and potential (risk) health problems***. ***Actual problems/diagnoses:*** existing problems that are amenable to independent nursing interventions, e.g. constipation related to immobility and opioid medication. ***Potential health problems/diagnoses:*** problems that an individual does not currently have but is particularly vulnerable to developing, e.g. risk of a pressure injury related to immobility.
5. **Goals** of care are determined.	***Goals*** should be person-centred, achievable and measurable and have a suitable timeframe, e.g. the person will have a bowel movement within 24 hours. The person will resume a normal bowel movement (Bristol 3–4) within 3 days.
6. **Interventions** selected that are person-centred and evidence-based.	***Nursing interventions*** are selected to meet each of the identified problems and goals. Following the previous example, if constipation was confirmed on assessment, the interventions would focus on addressing the specific factors that have caused the problem, e.g. increasing fluid intake, mobility and dietary fibre.
7. **Outcomes** of interventions are evaluated.	***Evaluation*** is ongoing and is aimed at achieving the person's goals, e.g. has the person had a bowel movement within 24 hours that is soft and easily evacuated?

Case study

This case study further exemplifies the clinical reasoning and clinical decision-making cycle as described in Table 2.1 and Figure 2.1. The case study will also help you identify your learning needs.

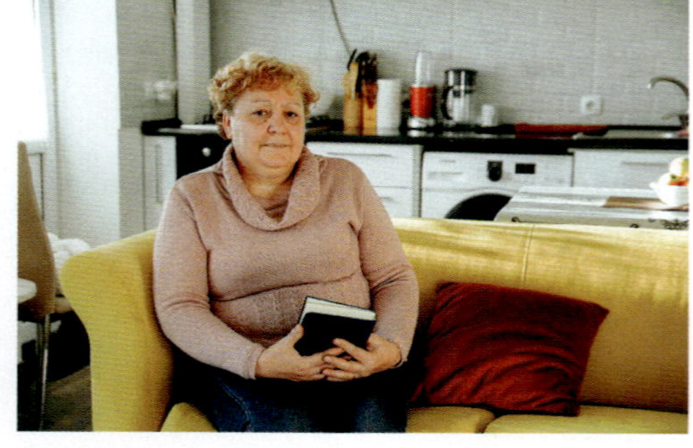

Context

You are the nurse who conducts the preoperative assessment in the preadmission clinic for Mrs Williams 1 week before surgery. Mrs Williams is accompanied by her daughter.

Consider the patient's situation

From your reading of Mrs Williams' health history, you discover the following information:

One month ago, Mrs Williams was referred to the hospital by her local GP for investigation of rectal discomfort and a positive faecal occult blood test (identified by the National Bowel Screening Program). A colonoscopy revealed the presence of a tumour in the rectum, which was biopsied. Visually, the

Continued

Case study cont'd

surgeon determined that it was likely to be adenocarcinoma. Histology confirmed the diagnosis. Subsequently, Mrs Williams was booked for a laparoscopic low anterior bowel resection and formation of a loop ileostomy for adenocarcinoma of the rectum to be performed next week.

Questions to further your learning

- What are the possible issues that might be going on with Mrs Williams?
- What knowledge do you need to be able to predict what might be going on?
- What approach to Mrs Williams' health assessment will you undertake?
- What questions (subjective data) will you ask Mrs Williams to extend the health history and why?
- What physical assessment (objective data) will you conduct and why?
- What resources are available to you to help in your assessment of Mrs Williams?

Assessment plan

The aim of the assessment is to:

- identify any significant issues that could impact on the person during and after surgery
- provide Mrs Williams with information about the surgical procedure and what to expect postoperatively
- begin the discharge plan.

To help you to identify issues that may have an impact on Mrs Williams, in the preop and postop stages, consider what the impact of impending surgery, the cancer diagnosis, the ileostomy and type 2 diabetes may have on her future functional status. Answers to these questions will be helpful in planning for Mrs Williams' discharge.

For example, will there be a change in:

- how Mrs Williams perceives her health and wellbeing and how she will manage her health in the future?
- the way Mrs Williams consumes food and fluid in the short term (preop and postop) and in the long term when she is home after discharge?
- her diabetes control after surgery?
- how Mrs Williams manages her bowel elimination?
- how Mrs Williams engages in her everyday activities immediately postop and once she is discharged? Will there be any changes in her breathing, circulation or mobility in the immediate postop period or once she is discharged?
- how Mrs Williams describes her level of physical comfort in the immediate postop period?
- Mrs Williams' sleep patterns in the short term (postop) and once she is back at home after discharge?
- the way Mrs Williams sees herself, particularly in the light of her cancer diagnosis and changes to her bowel elimination?
- the way Mrs Williams undertakes her role as a part-time sales assistant and carer of grandchildren?
- the impact that surgery may have on her sexual function?
- Mrs Williams' ability to cope? Will she experience periods of stress?
- Mrs Williams' values and beliefs?

The nurse in the preadmission clinic would *not* be able to fully evaluate Mrs Williams' nutritional status and management of her type 2 diabetes or begin the education process about stoma care. The plan would be to refer to specialist nurses or other clinicians for more comprehensive assessment and care planning.

Your assessment of Mrs Williams is detailed in Table 2.2. From this assessment you can see that Mrs Williams has several actual and potential health problems, but at the time of the assessment she is not in any acute discomfort.

TABLE 2.2 Assessment and clinical reasoning process example: Mrs Williams	
COLLECT SUBJECTIVE AND OBJECTIVE DATA FROM A RANGE OF SOURCES	
Cluster or group-related data—identify patterns in the data	**Subjective Data:** • Works part-time as a sales assistant. • Says: 'I don't know how I am ever going to manage the bag'. • Has never had abdominal surgery or a general anaesthetic. • Has had a gastroscopy and colonoscopy recently. • Is experiencing rectal discomfort. • Stopped smoking 1 month ago (smoked approximately 10 per day for 30 years). • Takes pantoprazole daily for gastro-oesophageal reflux disorder (GORD); no other regular medication. • Sensitive to codeine—causes nausea and vomiting. • Manages type 2 diabetes with diet. • Struggles to choose the right foods and to lose weight. • Has some knowledge of dietary requirements but doesn't really understand the effects of type 2 diabetes. • Rarely takes blood glucose measurement because she is 'too busy'. • Can climb stairs and had a negative stress echocardiogram 1 year ago. • Does not do any regular exercise. • Divorced, lives with her daughter, son-in-law and their three primary school–age children. • Provides some after-school care for her grandchildren. • Other daughter lives nearby, with whom she has a good relationship. **Objective Data:** • Age 66 years **Past medical history:** • Peptic ulcer disease—*Helicobacter pylori*—identified 3 years ago. Treated—no current symptoms • GORD—on 40 mg pantoprazole daily • Transient ischaemic attack three years ago • Type 2 diabetes—diet controlled • Two normal pregnancies and births **General inspection:** Obese middle-aged woman Current weight: 87 kg; height 164 cm; BMI 32 • Temp: 37.3 • HR rate: 120, regular • BP: 120/75 • RR: 24 per min • Random blood glucose level 7.9 mmol • ECG, full blood examination and chest x-ray no abnormalities detected.

TABLE 2.2 Assessment and clinical reasoning process example: Mrs Williams cont'd

	Learning Activity: • From the information provided in her health history, is there further objective data that could be included here that would add to your understanding of Mrs Williams' situation? • The subjective data has been grouped. Where will you insert the objective data into the groupings above?
Interpret the data by formulating inferences, predictions or forming hypotheses	**Key issues:** History of smoking, nutrition/exercise imbalance, expressed fear and anxiety about having surgery and ileostomy bag, inadequate diabetes management. **Strengths:** Exercise tolerance is adequate for her daily activities. Family support. **Recall of knowledge:** Your knowledge about the following will help you to make inferences/hypotheses/predictions from the available data: These may include: • impact of obesity and type 2 diabetes on health in general and potential risks in the perioperative period ***(risk for elevated blood glucose levels)*** • risk of chest infection in smokers following abdominal surgical procedures and general anaesthesia ***(risk for infection)***. You also know that: • It is normal for a person to feel anxious about forthcoming surgery, having a cancer diagnosis and the need to manage an ileostomy bag and stoma ***(anxiety)***. • Managing an ileostomy bag brings with it an impact on self-concept, body image and a need to refocus many activities of daily living ***(risk for altered self-image, knowledge deficit)***. • Adequate preparation of the person for surgery, pain management and other aspects of postoperative care are important ***(knowledge deficit)***.

***Validate* or check the accuracy and reliability of your inferences/ hypotheses/predictions by gathering more information to *test* the tentative inferences/ hypotheses/predictions.**	• You will then validate your inferences/hypotheses/predictions by collecting more information. Consider:
	  • Is her increased heart rate due to the stress of admission and prospective surgery?
	  • Is it related to obesity?
	• You will need to get more information about Mrs Williams' diet and her activity and exercise patterns. What other questions will you ask and what objective data will you collect?
	• Mrs Williams' daughter may be able to clarify some information, if necessary. Physical examination data can be compared with findings from other health professionals and data from diagnostic tests if needed.

Continued

TABLE 2.2 Assessment and clinical reasoning process example: Mrs Williams cont'd

NURSING DIAGNOSES/PATIENT PROBLEMS	
Actual potential (risk) health problems	**Actual Nursing Diagnoses/Patient Problems:** • Fear and anxiety related to upcoming surgery, new cancer diagnosis and ileostomy • Knowledge deficit: management of type 2 diabetes • Alteration in nutritional status: more than body requirements • Knowledge deficit: management of ileostomy • Knowledge deficit: surgical procedure and usual postoperative care **Potential (risk) Nursing Diagnoses/Patient Problems:** • Risk for unstable postoperative blood glucose levels related to stress response • Risk for chest infection related to surgery and recent smoking history • Risk for postoperative pain related to surgical incision
GOAL STATEMENTS	
Goals statements are person-centred, achievable, measurable and have a suitable timeframe.	**Mrs Williams will:** • be knowledgeable about the surgical procedure, anaesthesia, typical postoperative care and recovery including pain management using a patient-controlled pump, tubes, intravenous access, urinary catheter, etc., before surgery • always have postoperative pain less than 4/10. • always have postoperative blood glucose levels between 3.0 and 7.7 mmol/L • not develop a chest infection in the postoperative phase as demonstrated by effective deep breathing and coughing techniques, effective pain control and early postop mobility • be knowledgeable and confident with managing an ileostomy bag within 5 days after surgery • be knowledgeable about managing type 2 diabetes, including dietary requirements and activity and exercise requirements within 5 days after surgery.

Collaborative patient problems

The clinical reasoning process detailed above is one that nurses use to identify actual and potential patient problems and then plan and evaluate care. Collaborative problems are those in which the approach to treatment involves multiple disciplines. For example, Mrs Williams has several medical diagnoses (type 2 diabetes, bowel cancer and GORD). It is the medical practitioner's responsibility to diagnose and prescribe the treatments for these conditions. The nurse, the medical practitioner and other allied health team members work together in managing the patient's care during hospitalisation and after discharge. However, nurses also focus on managing specific nursing-related patient problems as described in Table 2.2.

Clinical reasoning and documentation

Throughout the text, examples are provided for documenting health assessment data. As you develop more knowledge and skills, you will become more efficient and accurate in your documentation. Always record the data from the patient interview (subjective data), the medical history and physical examination (objective data) as you conduct the assessment, but in such a way that does not get in the way of your communication with the person. The documentation of your findings should be systematic, comprehensive and detailed. This includes charting *relevant* normal or abnormal findings. The selected assessment framework as described in Chapter 1 will guide your documentation.

Electronic health records

The use of technology at the bedside extends far beyond the standard equipment. An increasing number of hospitals and clinics use a basic or comprehensive electronic health record system. The electronic health record replaces the paper health record, placing all relevant patient information in an easily accessible electronic system. The functions typically include clinical notes, medication charts, fluid balance and observation charts, consultation and referral requests, laboratory and diagnostic imaging requests and results and discharge summaries from all health professionals.

Electronic health records allow all providers, regardless of geographic location, to access the health information, place orders and receive timely patient status updates. No longer does a provider have to be on the clinical unit to retrieve test results, vital signs or the most recent nurse's or doctor's note. Well-designed electronic health records can notify providers of potential medication interactions, dosage adjustments for use in relevant situations and other required testing (e.g. laboratory tests). Nurses can benefit from using electronic health records in medication administration using barcode scanners, which identify both the person and the medication. Checklists built into electronic health records can help clinicians identify healthcare-associated infections or patients at risk for these infections. Although no system is perfect, well-designed electronic health records can increase patient safety when successfully integrated into the workflow of a clinic or hospital. As electronic health records use becomes the standard of care, more research is needed to determine the specific factors that contribute to patient safety and increased quality of care.

In Australia, My Health Record is aimed at providing personal health information available to nominated health professionals such as GPs, specialists and pharmacists.[15] A similar strategy is available in Aotearoa New Zealand.[16] The information includes:

- a shared health summary (overview of health)
- reports of tests and scans
- current medications
- discharge plan
- referral letters as relevant.

The general Australian and Aotearoa New Zealand public can opt in or opt out of this arrangement. The digital health record is a separate platform from the electronic health records of health services.

Developing your clinical reasoning skills

All healthcare treatments and decisions are based on the information you gather during assessment, and it is therefore important that your assessment be factual and complete. The way in which nurses make clinical decisions depends on the context in which they work, their level of knowledge and the extent of their experience.[14] *Novice* nurses usually have extensive knowledge but need to develop the ability to apply that knowledge; they may have little experience with specified populations and use rules to guide practice.[17] It takes time, perhaps 2 to 3 years in similar clinical situations, to achieve *proficiency*, where the nurse sees actions in the context of goals or daily plans for the people they care for. With more time and experience, a *proficient* nurse understands a person's situation as a whole rather than as a list of tasks. This nurse sees long-term goals for the person and how today's nursing actions apply to the point the nurse wants the person to be in, say, 6 weeks. Finally, it seems that *expert* nurses jump over the steps and arrive at a clinical decision or judgement in one leap. The expert has well-developed observational skills and trusts their physical assessment skills, even if this conflicts with technologically driven data. *Expert* nurses have an intuitive grasp of clinical situations and can quickly identify accurate solutions.[18]

The way to move from novice to expert practitioner is by using critical thinking. We all start as novices who need the familiarity of clear-cut rules to guide actions. Critical thinking is how we learn to assess and modify, if indicated, before acting. Critical thinking is required for sound clinical reasoning and clinical judgement. During your career, you will need to sort through vast amounts of data to make sound judgements to manage care of the person. This data will be dynamic and unpredictable. There will not be any one protocol you can memorise that will apply to every situation. This is true particularly with expert nurses in critical care or emergency situations in which a person's health status changes rapidly and accurate decisions are paramount. The stakes are high, and nursing autonomy is strong. In these cases, expert nurses focus on the person's responses and prevent complications through anticipation and vigilant monitoring.[19]

To be an effective critical thinker, the following attributes are needed (adapted from Levett-Jones[13]):

- **holistic and contextual perspective**: the whole person is considered, as well as their entire situation including background, relationships and environment
- **creativity**: capable of generating, discovering or restructuring ideas and being able to imagine other options
- **inquisitiveness**: carefully questions and investigates a range of possibilities
- **perseverance**: dedicated to trying to understand the person's situation
- **intuition**: recognises patterns based on past experiences
- **flexibility**: ability to adapt thinking and behaviours
- **academic integrity**: uses processes that are honest and truthful, even if the results are contrary to one's beliefs and assumptions
- **reflexivity**: thoughtfully reviews assumptions, thinking and approaches to ensure understanding
- **confidence**: belief in one's abilities
- **open-mindedness**: open and sensitive to other views.

RESOURCES AVAILABLE

To ensure the effectiveness and appropriateness of clinical decisions, there are several clinical tools, clinical guidelines, hospital/agency policies and protocols and best practice resources available to support your clinical decision making in future healthcare settings. Throughout this text, reference is made to a range of assessment tools to guide the type of questions you should ask and which aspects of physical examination should be undertaken. There are several videos provided to help you to develop some of the more difficult assessment skills. Most chapters include clinical case studies to assist you to practise gathering health assessment data, and to organise and use your critical thinking and reasoning skills to make inferences or predictions about the meaning of the information. You will find additional resources and a reference list at the end of this and all other chapters.

- visiting websites

  Australian Commission on Safety and Quality in Health Care: https://www.safetyandquality.gov.au/

REFERENCES

1. Manetti W (2019). Sound clinical judgment in nursing: a concept analysis. Nursing Forum, 54(1), 102–110. https://doi.org/10.1111/nuf.12303
2. Twohig PL (2018). The second ‘great transformation’: Renegotiating nursing practice in Ontario, 1945–70. Canadian Historical Review, 99(2), 169–195.
3. Nursing and Midwifery Board of Australia. Registered nurse standards for practice. 2016. Available at: https://www.nursingmidwiferyboard.gov.au/codes-guidelines-statements/professional-standards/registered-nurse-standards-for-practice.aspx
4. Nursing Council of New Zealand. Competencies for registered nurses. 2016. Available at: https://www.nursingcouncil.org.nz/Public/Nursing/Standards_and_guidelines/NCNZ/nursing-section/Standards_and_guidelines_for_nurses.aspx
5. Nursing and Midwifery Board of Australia. Scope of practice and capabilities of nurses and midwives. 2016. Available at: https://www.nursingmidwiferyboard.gov.au/Codes-Guidelines-Statements/FAQ/Fact-sheet-scope-of-practice-and-capabilities-of-nurses-and-midwives.aspx
6. Nursing Council of New Zealand. Scopes of practice 2016. Available at: https://www.nursingcouncil.org.nz/Public/Nursing/Scopes_of_practice/NCNZ/nursing-section/Scopes_of_practice.aspx
7. Australian Health Practitioners Registration Authority. Legislation. 2023. Available at: https://www.ahpra.gov.au/about-ahpra/what-we-do/legislation.aspx
8. The Ministry of Health New Zealand. The Health Practitioners Competence Assurance Act 2003. Available at: https://www.health.govt.nz/our-work/regulation-health-and-disability-system/health-practitioners-competence-assurance-act/about-health-practitioners-competence-assurance-act#:,:text=The%20Health%20Practitioners%20Competence%20Assurance%20Act%202003%20(the%20Act)%20is,long%20competence%20of%20health%20practitioners
9. Australian Commission on Safety and Quality in Health Care. The state of patient safety and quality in Australian hospitals 2019. Sydney. Available at: https://www.safetyandquality.gov.au/publications-and-resources/resource-library/state-patient-safety-and-quality-australian-hospitals-2019

10. Australian Commission on Safety and Quality in Health Care. National Safety and Quality Health Service Standards. 2nd ed. Sydney: ACSQHC; 2017.
    Available at: www.safetyandquality.gov.au/sites/default/files/migrated/National-Safety-and-Quality-Health-Service-Standards-second-edition.pdf
11. The Health Quality and Safety Commission, New Zealand. Quality and Safety Markers. 2023. Available at: https://www.hqsc.govt.nz/our-data/quality-and-safety-markers/
12. Wright J, Scardaville D (2021). A nursing residency program: a window into clinical judgement and clinical decision making. Nurse Education in Practice, 50, 102931. https://doi.org/10.1016/j.nepr.2020.102931
13. Levett-Jones T, editor. Clinical reasoning: learning to think like a nurse. 3rd ed. Frenchs Forest, NSW: Pearson Australia; 2022.
14. Connor J, Flenady T, Massey D, Dwyer T (2023). Clinical judgement in nursing: an evolutionary concept analysis. Journal of Clinical Nursing, 32, 3328–3340. https://doi.org/10.1111/jocn.16469
15. Australian Government, Australian Digital Health Agency. My Health Record. 2019. Available at: https://www.digitalhealth.gov.au/initiatives-and-programs/my-health-record
16. Health New Zealand. My Health Account. 2023. Available at: https://www.tewhatuora.govt.nz/our-health-system/digital-health/my-health-account/
17. Benner P, Tanner CA, Chesla CA. Expertise in nursing practice: caring, clinical judgment and ethics. 2nd ed. New York, NY: Springer; 2009.
18. Benner P, Tanner CA, Chesla CA. Becoming an expert nurse. American Journal of Nursing. 1997;97(6).
19. Hoffman KA, Aitken LM, Duffield C. A comparison of novice and expert nurses' cue collection during clinical decision-making: Verbal protocol analysis. International Journal of Nursing Studies. 2009;46(10):1335–1344.

CHAPTER 3

Developmental tasks across the life span

Written by Carolyn Jarvis

Adapted by Helen Forbes and Elizabeth Watt

INTRODUCTION

As you have learnt in the previous chapters, subjective and objective data is collected by interview and physical examination. The data is then used to promote health-related strengths and to identify and manage health concerns (Chapter 1). To have a better understanding of the person it is also necessary to consider the developmental stage relevant to that person.

Case study

The following case study offers an example of a typical situation involving the health assessment of an adolescent and the initial clinical reasoning process. It will help you identify your learning needs.

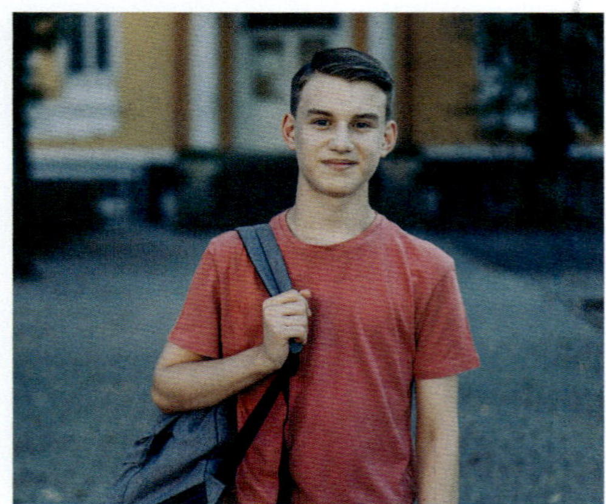

Context

You are working in a general practice clinic as a practice nurse. Part of your role includes monitoring health and providing advice to all people attending the clinic who are living with diabetes. The GP has asked you to follow up with Lachlan's care.

Consider the person's situation

Lachlan is a 15-year-old who was diagnosed with type 1 diabetes at the age of 5 years. Your initial interview reveals several concerns: Lachlan has been experiencing worsening glycaemic control, with frequent episodes of hyperglycaemia. His parents also say he has become increasingly withdrawn and moody over the past few months. Lachlan's parents explain that he has recently been diagnosed with mild depression by the family's GP.

Questions to further your learning

- What are the possible things that might be going on with Lachlan?
- What knowledge do you need to be able to plan a focused health assessment?
- What questions (subjective data) will you ask Lachlan to extend the health history and why?
- What physical examination (objective data) will you conduct and why?
- What resources are available to you to help you assess Lachlan?
- How might your approach to the health assessment change if Lachlan was an adult with diabetes?

Some things to consider

Managing Lachlan's diabetes will be influenced by his current mental state because there is a significant relationship between symptoms of depression, sleep difficulties and poor self-management of diabetes.[1] At the same time, Lachlan's chronic health condition may impact on his ability to achieve developmental tasks that are typical for adolescents. For example, Lachlan may have trouble developing a sense of independence if he relies on his parents for health care, or he may have difficulty forming close relationships with peers if he is constantly missing school due to illness. Lachlan may feel that his condition and its treatment makes him 'different' from his peers during a stage of development where fitting in and being 'normal' is prized.[2] Working with Lachlan and his parents to address the physical, developmental and psychosocial aspects of his condition is crucial.

Assessment plan

Growth can be conceptualised as an increase in the size and complexity of the physical being, while development extends beyond maturation of physical systems and includes changes to social, emotional and cognitive functioning. The following sections will explore growth and development to provide a picture of the person across the life span. Physical, psychosocial, cognitive and behavioural development will be examined at each developmental stage. These stages are:

1. Infancy (birth to 1 year)
2. Early childhood—toddler (1 to 3 years)
3. Early childhood—preschooler (3 to 5 or 6 years)
4. Middle childhood—school-aged child (6 to 10 or 11 years)
5. Preadolescence (10 to 12 or 13 years)
6. Adolescence (12 or 13 to 19 years)
7. Early adulthood (20 to 40 years)
8. Middle adulthood (40 to 64 years)
9. Late adulthood (65+ years).

Resources available

You will find additional resources and the reference list at the end of this chapter.

Infancy (birth to 1 year)

The first year of life represents the most dramatic and rapid period of growth and development. The infant changes from a totally dependent being into a person who interacts with the environment and forms close relationships with other people (Figure 3.1).

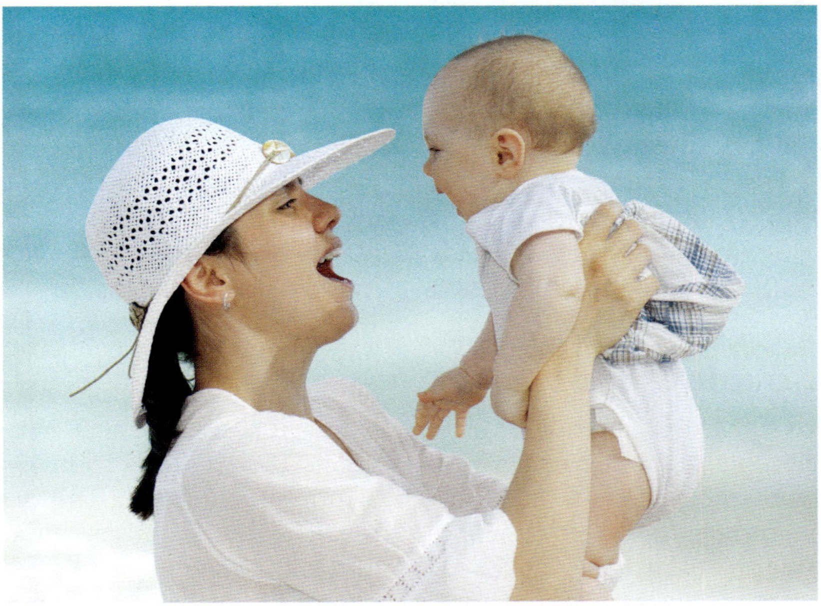

FIGURE 3.1 Infant forming relationships with other people

Physical development

Weight, length and head circumference reflect physical growth and are sensitive indicators of an infant's general health. The average healthy term infant weighs 3.4 kg, with 95% of full-term infants ranging from

2.5 to 4.6 kg.[3] In the first few days of life, most infants lose weight while excess extracellular fluid is lost and feeding is established,[4] but this weight is typically regained by day 10 of life. Growth spurts result in doubling of birth weight by 4 to 6 months and tripling of birth weight by 1 year. Length increases by 50% by 1 year.

Head circumference also increases rapidly across the first year, signifying an increase in brain size. At birth, the average head circumference is 35 cm, with about 95% of infants within the range of 32.6 to 37.2 cm.[3] Nutrition in this period is particularly critical because brain development during infancy is in part regulated by the availability of both macro and key micronutrients.[5]

Of all the organ systems, the central nervous system undergoes the most dramatic changes during infancy. Protective reflexes such as cough, sneeze and gag are present at birth and persist throughout life. However, maturation of the brain allows primitive reflexes, such as grasping, to be suppressed by the developing cerebral cortex. In a healthy infant, the appearance and extinction of primitive reflexes follows a predictable sequence (Chapter 12). Vision also develops rapidly across the first years of life; infants have poor visual acuity at birth (about 20/400) because their maculae are immature.[6,7] By 3 months of age, a typically developing infant can fix on an object and follow its movement, and visual acuity improves rapidly across the first year of life.

Cognitive development

Jean Piaget (1896–1980) described the stages of cognitive development in a growing child. Each stage represents new ways of thinking and behaving. According to Piaget's theory of cognitive development, each stage is a foundation for the next. Piaget believed that a child's thinking develops progressively from simple reflex behaviour into complex, logical and abstract thought where the child becomes capable of attending to information, developing concepts, applying reason and remembering past experiences.[8]

This development from simple to complex behaviours can be seen in a 6-month-old who has discovered his hands. Over time, the instinct to place all new objects into the mouth turns into a more detailed inspection, with the object being dropped, picked up and passed hand-to-hand before being mouthed. This more complex play indicates that the infant is testing their conceptual models (or **schema**) for new objects in their environment.

The first stage of cognitive development is described as the **sensorimotor** stage.[8,9] Very young infants interact with their world purely through reflex actions, but they quickly learn to repeat accidental behaviours that bring about positive sensory stimulation, such as accidentally sucking a thumb and repeating the activity for pleasure. Soon these behaviours extend beyond the self to include the external environment, and by the end of the first year infants can not only manipulate objects in their environment but also interact with others and plan activities to attain specific goals.[10]

A particularly important cognitive milestone in infants is developing **object permanence**. This is an understanding that objects out of sight continue to exist. At about 7 or 8 months of age, infants will start to look for objects that are hidden while they watch. For example, a child of this age will drop their spoon over the edge of the highchair and then look over the edge to see where it went but will give up their search unless the spoon is spotted immediately. By 9 months, the infant will continue searching for a hidden object, indicating that they understand the object still exists, even though it cannot be seen. At the same time, infants learn that they are an individual separate from others and to the objects in their environment.[10]

While Piaget's theory provides a useful framework for understanding the development of thought, more recent research indicates that Piaget may have underestimated the cognitive capacity of infants. For example, even young infants appear surprised and look longer at unexpected events, such as the unanticipated disappearance or appearance of an object, indicating they have already developed some understanding of the rules that govern their physical world.[7]

Psychosocial development

Erik Erikson (1902–1994) was concerned with the growth of the **ego**, the conscious, organised, rational part of the personality. He conceptualised a series of eight ego qualities that emerge due to 'crises' during critical periods of development.[11] The first psychosocial crisis the infant experiences is **trust versus mistrust**. The infant is completely dependent on the outside world to meet basic needs including food, warmth and comfort. When these basic needs are consistently met by a responsive caregiver, the infant learns that the world is a safe and reliable place. Conversely, if the primary caregivers are poorly attuned to the needs of the infant, or if care is unreliable, the infant learns to mistrust themselves and others. Perhaps most importantly, it is the quality of the parent–child relationship that enables the infant to develop a sense of trust, and ultimately to view the world as a benign and welcoming place.[11]

Another developmental theory that emphasises the relationship between caregiver and child is **attachment theory**. John Bowlby (1907–1990) described attachment behaviour as any behaviour that helps the person maintain proximity to a preferred person—usually the primary caregiver. These behaviours can be seen both in infants who visually 'check-in' with their mother while playing across the room to confirm she is still present, and in children who cling when the parent tries to leave the room. When proximity is threatened, the infant begins to experience **separation anxiety**. Separation anxiety (or separation distress) initially appears with protest, which may include crying, screaming, following or clinging to maintain or regain contact with the caregiver.[11,12] When this is unsuccessful, the child experiences despair, appearing withdrawn and depressed. If the caregiver fails to return, the child eventually becomes emotionally detached from the caregiver, sometimes forming superficial relationships with others as a survival strategy. Separation anxiety typically appears at around 6 months of age and peaks at around 8 or 9 months of age. Caregivers who consistently respond to the child's needs and show affection help the child develop a secure attachment.[13,14]

Motor development

Motor function across the first year of life transitions from reflexive responses to the environment, to purposeful, functional movements. **Gross motor skills** include gaining control of the head and trunk, learning to sit, to crawl, to stand and eventually to walk. The pattern of developing these skills is predictable, following the pattern of myelination of the spinal and peripheral nerves; development occurs from the centre of the body to the extremities (proximodistal development), and from the head to the toes (cephalocaudal development).[10]

Infants are born with rudimentary head control, enabling them to turn their head to the side when lying prone to avoid suffocation. However, at birth, this head control is underdeveloped, resulting in significant head lag when the infant is pulled from a lying position into a sitting position. Head control develops rapidly, but by 3 months a typically developing infant can raise their head and shoulders from a prone position and use their arms to support this posture. By 4 months, head lag is minimal when the infant is pulled into a sitting position, and by 6 or 7 months, head and trunk control are strong enough to allow the infant to sit independently[10,15] (Figure 3.2).

Gross motor function continues to develop rapidly across the first year. By 7 months, most infants will start to crawl and will show an interest in exploring their environment. By 8 months, a typically developing infant can pull themselves into a standing position and stand while holding an object for support. Soon after, the infant begins to 'cruise'—walking upright while holding onto furniture or caregivers—and this leads to independent walking by about 12 months of age[10] (Figure 3.3).

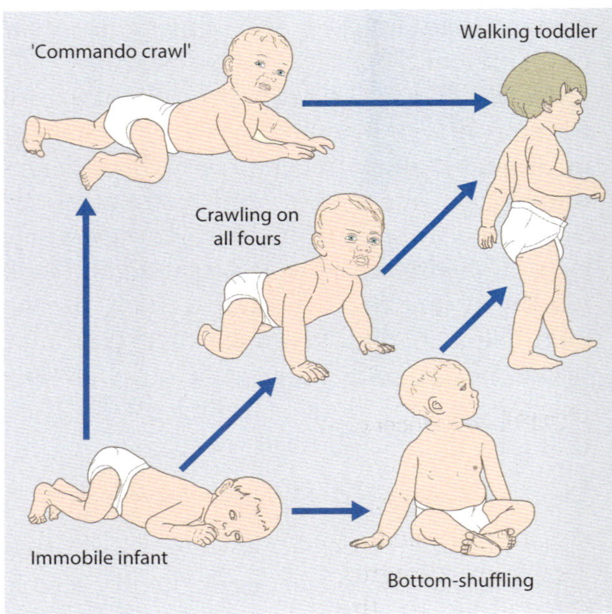

FIGURE 3.3 Crawling to walking

The development of **fine motor skills** involves using the hands and fingers for prehension, or the act of grasping. The infant is born with a grasp reflex that fades at 2 months of age and is absent at 3 months of age.[10] This extinction of the grasp reflex allows the infant to begin deliberately gripping and releasing objects. The voluntary two-handed grasp is present at 4 to 5 months. Further refinement of fine motor function occurs between 6 and 12 months, with a crude pincer grasp evident at around 7 or 8 months, followed by a neat pincer grasp at around 10 months (Figure 3.4). During this time, the infant is absorbed with picking up small items, and these are frequently conveyed straight to the child's mouth. By 11 months, the infant can place small objects into a container and remove them again, and by 13 months they can stack two blocks to build a tower.[10]

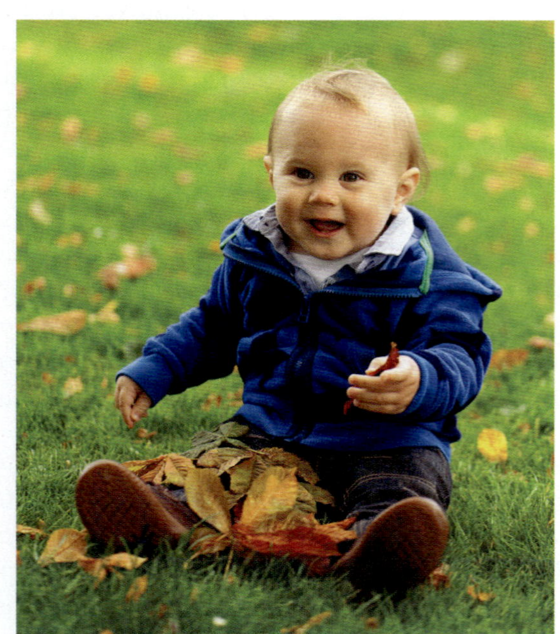
FIGURE 3.2 Toddler head and trunk control

Language skills

Newborns rely on crying as their primary form of verbal communication. Indeed, crying is an extremely adaptive behaviour,

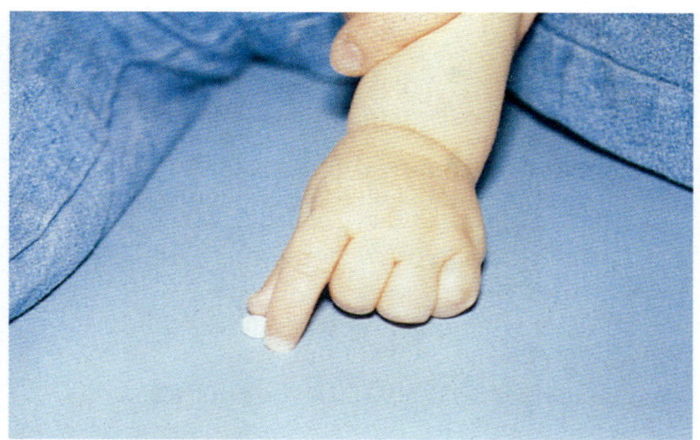

FIGURE 3.4 Pincer grip

creating physical and attentional arousal in caregivers designed to mobilise them into responding to the infant's needs.[16] From crying in early infancy, vocal sounds build rapidly: the infant coos when they awaken or when someone talks to them at 2 to 4 months and laughs out loud at 3 to 4 months; this progresses to babbling by 6 months. At 9 to 10 months, the infant can imitate the sounds of others. At 12 months, an infant usually can say the first recognisable word with meaning.

Language comprehension (our ability to understand others) is generally acquired more rapidly than expressive speech; between 6 and 9 months infants briefly pause when told 'no!' and between 9 and 12 months can follow simple commands in context. However, well before they develop the capacity to understand speech, infants pay close attention to the sound of language. Indeed, while still in utero, a fetus can respond to sound by 24 weeks' gestation and react differently to speech than other sounds by 35 weeks' gestation.[17]

Personal and social skills

From birth, infants steadily develop social skills that will allow them to interact with and relate to others. Early on, infants show a visual preference for the human face and, even in the first 30 to 60 minutes following birth, watches the mother intently. The **social smile** erupts at 6 to 8 weeks, providing a new and exciting means of interaction between parent and child. At 4 months, infants laugh and enjoy other people, and at 6 months they will extend their arms to the parent to be picked up.[10]

With development of the neurological system, an infant's imitations become increasingly complex; by 7 months infants can copy simple actions, at 9 months they imitate sounds and at 10 months they begin to engage in social behaviours such as waving or games such as peek-a-boo. At 11 months, infants can help with feeding and dressing and follow simple directions. Emotional expression develops across the first year, and by 12 months infants can give a hug or kiss and show jealousy, fear or anger.[10]

Another key aspect of social interaction that develops towards the end of the first year is called **joint attention**. Initially, infants can follow another person's pointing to look at an object in the environment. By 9 to 12 months, infants use pointing and gaze to direct the attention of others, a skill known as declarative (or protodeclarative) pointing. This behaviour represents a significant leap in social awareness. Declarative pointing indicates that an infant is gradually becoming aware that their view of the world is different from that of others; this will later serve as a basis for the child's **theory of mind**—an understanding that one's own thoughts and awareness are separate from that of other people.[18]

Periodic health check—infant

Tables 3.1 and 3.2 outline important aspects of well-child checks occurring in the neonatal period and the first 12 months of life. Note

TABLE 3.1 Periodic health check: neonate (0–28 days)

	Australia	Aotearoa New Zealand
Immunisations	Hepatitis B (usually offered within 24–48 hours after birth)	Hepatitis B (if mother is known to be hepatitis B-positive)
Areas for assessment	***Diagnostic testing:*** Metabolic screening (newborn screen) 48–72 hours of life ***Nutrition:*** Discuss method of infant feeding and provide breastfeeding support if applicable ***Hearing:*** Check that newborn hearing screen was conducted as per local guidelines ***Physical assessment:*** Complete the child health assessment as outlined in the child health record issued by the relevant state or territory, including but not limited to: • general appearance including skin colour and integrity • weight, length and head circumference • head shape, facial symmetry and formation of facial features; palpate fontanels, check that palate is intact, elicit red reflexes • examine neurological and developmental status, including responsiveness, posture and tone; examine spine for anomalies • assess cardiovascular status including auscultation of heart sounds and palpation of femoral pulse • examine umbilicus and ensure normal healing • examine hips, limbs for symmetry and length, joints for normal range of movement, hands (including presence of palmar creases and number of digits), feet (for talipes and number of digits)—see Chapter 20 for further information • examine perianal structures for congenital anomalies; check that testes are descended in males • at-risk children (exposed to alcohol prenatally)—screen for fetal alcohol syndrome.	
Psychosocial support	• Identify family strengths, elicit concerns and promote parental confidence, competence and mental health • Discuss any developmental questions or concerns that parents may have	
Safety and preventive care	***Discuss:*** • Non-accidental injury and reinforce that parents should never shake their infant • Risks to the infant from passive smoking • Using appropriate restraints in motor vehicles • Safe sleeping and recommendations for preventing sudden and unexplained death in infancy • Infant CPR	

Adapted from Ministry of Health 2023[19]; Department of Health and Aged Care 2023[20]; RACGP 2019[21]; National Aboriginal Community Controlled Health Organisation and The Royal Australian College of General Practitioners 2018[22]

TABLE 3.2 Periodic health check: infant (28 days to 12 months of age)

	Australia	Aotearoa New Zealand
Immunisations For up-to-date guidelines on COVID-19 vaccination see the additional resources section at the end of the chapter.	***2 and 4 months:*** Diphtheria, tetanus, pertussis (whooping cough), hepatitis B, polio, *Haemophilus influenzae* type b (Hib), pneumococcal, rotavirus (by 14 weeks of age), meningococcal B (Indigenous children) ***6 months:*** Diphtheria, tetanus, pertussis (whooping cough), hepatitis B, polio, *Haemophilus influenzae* type b (Hib), pneumococcal (Indigenous children in WA, SA, NT, Qld), meningococcal B (Indigenous children with specific medical conditions such as chronic respiratory disease or who are immunocompromised) ***6 months to < 5 years:*** Influenza vaccine annually ***12 months:*** Meningococcal ACWY measles, mumps, rubella pneumococcal, meningococcal B (Indigenous children)	***6 weeks:*** Rotavirus (by 15 weeks of age), diphtheria, tetanus, pertussis, polio, hepatitis B, *Haemophilus influenzae* type b (Hib), pneumococcal ***3 months:*** Rotavirus (by 25 weeks of age), diphtheria, tetanus, pertussis, polio, hepatitis B, *Haemophilus influenzae* type b (Hib), meningococcal B ***5 months:*** Diphtheria, tetanus, pertussis, polio, hepatitis B, *Haemophilus influenzae* type b (Hib), pneumococcal, meningococcal B ***12 months:*** Measles, mumps, rubella (MMR), pneumococcal, meningococcal B
Areas for assessment	***Nutrition:*** Discuss method of feeding and provide breastfeeding support if applicable; discuss introduction of solids from around 6 months. Indigenous children—check for anaemia (6–9 months and 18 months) ***Development:*** Explore developmental progress (e.g. parents' evaluation of developmental status (PEDS) assessment). Promote early interactive reading with the child At-risk children (exposed to alcohol prenatally)—screen for fetal alcohol syndrome ***Hearing and vision:*** Conduct hearing and vision screening ***2, 4 and 6 months:*** • Note general appearance including skin colour and integrity, head symmetry • Measure weight, length and head circumference and record on centile charts • Examine neurological and developmental status, including responsiveness and tone • Assess cardiovascular status including femoral pulse (for radio-femoral delay) • Examine umbilicus • Examine perianal structures and hips • Evaluate oral health/tooth eruption, palate and frenulum ***12 months:*** • Measure weight, length and head circumference and record on centile charts • Assess head symmetry • Check for visual fixing and following, test corneal light reflex • Evaluate oral health/tooth eruption	

Continued

TABLE 3.2 Periodic health check: infant (28 days to 12 months of age) cont'd

	Australia	Aotearoa New Zealand
Psychosocial support	• Assess quality of parent–child interactions • Identify family strengths, elicit concerns and promote parental confidence, competence and mental health	
Safety and preventive care	***Discuss:*** • Non-accidental injury and reinforce that parents should never shake their infant • Risks to the infant from passive smoking and UV exposure; promote sun protection • Risk to the infant from home environment (e.g. water temperature, bath safety, choking hazards, burns prevention) • Safe sleeping and SIDS prevention; strategies for settling the infant • Car restraints • Play and promotion of normal development (promote secure attachment and positive interaction) • Infant CPR	

Adapted from Ministry of Health 2023[19]; Department of Health and Aged Care 2023[20]; RACGP 2019[21]; National Aboriginal Community Controlled Health Organisation and The Royal Australian College of General Practitioners 2018[22]

the aspects of screening at birth, the Australian and the Aotearoa New Zealand immunisation schedules[19,20] and the health promotion messages about diet and injury prevention. Note also that these tables are not intended to be a complete list of all the steps that *should* be included in the periodic health assessment checkup. Instead, the tables list preventive interventions that have been studied and shown to be clinically effective.[21,22] People who are at high risk for specific health issues may need additional preventative health information and health assessment.

Early childhood—toddler (1 to 3 years)

Achieving milestones across the first year of life establishes a basis for future development. Gross and fine motor development enable interaction with the world (Figure 3.5), while the toddler's developing cognitive and social skills demand perpetual stimulation. Children of this age are constantly investigating their environment while using their caregivers as a secure base for exploration.[10]

Developmental tasks of this next stage include:

- differentiating self from others, particularly the mother
- tolerating separation from mother or parent
- withstanding delayed gratification
- controlling bodily functions
- acquiring socially acceptable behaviour

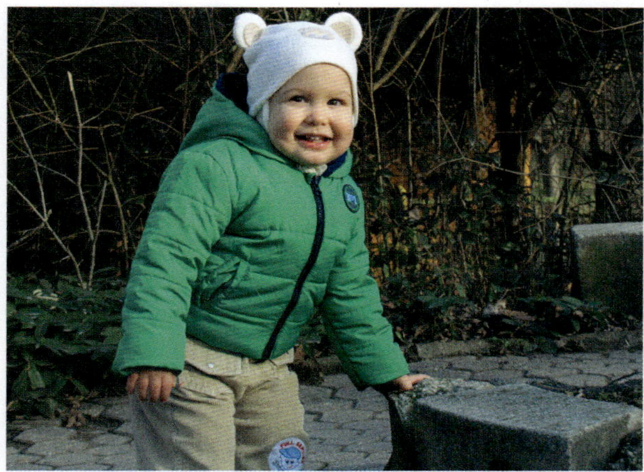

FIGURE 3.5 Developing independence in early childhood

- acquiring verbal communication
- interacting with others in a more empathic way (i.e. understanding another person's emotional state).

Physical development

The velocity of growth slows in toddlers, with children typically gaining 2.5 kg in weight and 12 cm in height across the second year of life.[3] Increases in head circumference also slow in the second and third years of life. Physical changes enable the child to master increasingly complex skills; for example, with the eruption of molars, the child can learn to chew. While maturation of physical systems will be discussed throughout this text, it is important to consider the interplay between neurological development and the achievement of developmental milestones. For example, increasing maturation of the cerebral cortex enables comprehensible speech and meaningful language to develop. Similarly, myelination of the spinal cord is almost complete by the end of the second year, facilitating motor development and resulting in increasingly coordinated movement.

Cognitive development

During their second year, toddlers are still considered to be in Piaget's **sensorimotor** period.[23] Between 12 and 18 months, children increasingly engage in experiments, using trial and error to reach a goal. For example, a toddler who is struggling to reach a desired toy at the bottom of their toybox may try numerous methods to reach it, including taking out all the toys one by one, overturning the box or climbing in to retrieve the toy. While this exploration is an important part of the child's learning, toddlers have limited awareness of risk, so careful supervision is important to ensure safety.

The concept of **object permanence** is now fully developed[23] and the toddler will seek objects even when they did not see them hidden and will search in multiple locations if the desired object is not discovered initially.

Between 18 and 24 months, children begin to develop **mental representation** for external events.[10] Mental representation allows toddlers to think through actions before undertaking them and to solve basic problems. While limited by egocentrism and rigidity of thought, these mental representations become increasingly organised and complex over time and will eventually form the basis of a child's understanding of cause and effect.

Psychosocial development

Autonomy is the aim of all activity for toddlers. Newly developed motor skills allow for independent actions such as walking and exploring, as well as involvement with self-care activities such as feeding and dressing. At the same time, the child is developing language that allows them to express needs and desires. As a result, toddlers will typically demand independence and will become frustrated if others try to do things for them. Between the ages of 12 and 18 months, toddlers begin to venture away from their parent to explore their environment but uses the parent as a 'secure base' to which they return for reassurance and protection.

AUTONOMY VERSUS SHAME AND DOUBT (1 TO 3 YEARS)

This quest for autonomy characterises the psychological conflict of Erikson's second stage.[11] Toddlers want to be autonomous and to govern their own body and experiences. They want to apply newly attained skills to explore the world. However, the toddler has not yet attained any sense of discrimination or judgement. Parents must attempt to balance the toddler's desire to explore with the need to protect them from danger, or from experiences that would overwhelm their available coping mechanisms. According to Erikson, overly permissive or controlling parenting can result in the child developing a sense of shame and doubt in their ability to act within the world.[11] Conversely, this conflict is resolved favourably when parents are patient, provide guidance and hold reasonable expectations about the child's current abilities and attention span.

Motor skills development

The primary motor skill acquired during toddlerhood is walking. By 12 to 15 months, most toddlers are walking independently, although they typically exhibit a wide-based gait that provides greater stability. By 18 months, toddlers can usually run but trip and stumble frequently. By 2 years of age, most toddlers can walk up and down stairs and run without falling, and by 30 months, they can balance briefly on one foot, or jump with both feet.[10]

Fine motor development progresses rapidly in toddlers. By 12 months of age, toddlers should exhibit a well-developed pincer grasp, enabling them to pick up and manipulate small objects. By 15 months, most toddlers can hold a pencil and scribble; by the age of 2 years, their dexterity allows them to reproduce a vertical line following a demonstration.

Language skills

A toddler's vocabulary expands rapidly from a few distinct words at around 1 year of age to an average of 200 words by their second birthday. Also, speech becomes increasingly complex, with a 2-year-old learning to combine words into simple two-word phrases such as 'we go' and 'all gone'. This **telegraphic speech** typically includes a noun and a verb and includes only words with concrete meaning.[10] By the age of 3 years, most children are consistently using three-word phrases. Receptive language skills remain more advanced than expressive skills; toddlers can typically comprehend a two-part command without cues, such as 'pick up your shoes and bring them here', by 18 to 24 months.

Personal and social skills

From around the age of 2 years, children begin to appreciate that certain actions are acceptable and others are not. At this age children develop a sense of right and wrong through punishment or praise; an action is good if the child is rewarded for it, and bad if the child is punished. This has been identified as a 'punishment/obedience' orientation.[23] Children of this age require firm and consistent boundaries to determine right from wrong.

Tantrums are a common form of expression in this age group and often stem from a frustrated urge to be independent. Because young children have not yet developed coping mechanisms to manage these frustrations, they find expression through physical resistance and aggression. Similarly, negativism is common in the toddler age group—all requests and suggestions are met with a firm and defiant 'NO!'. This is closely related to a toddler's growing need for independence and individuality. Providing limited choices, rather than asking open-ended questions, may help provide boundaries for toddlers while providing them with a sense of control that supports their growing autonomy.

Closely related to negativism in this age group is ritualism. Toddlers typically want things done in a consistent way, and any change in a routine or habit can be distressing. A consistent routine reassures the child that the world is predictable and orderly. Awareness of this developmental norm helps parents to anticipate and understand the toddler's strong reaction to anything that threatens an established routine, such as the arrival of a sibling or the need for hospitalisation.

Toddlers engage in parallel play with peers.[10] Parallel play occurs when toddlers play alongside another child; the two children may subtly observe each other but don't engage in shared activity. Imitation in play is apparent in this age group as well; in particular, toddlers frequently imitate parent activities such as sweeping the floor or cooking. As mental representations become more robust, play becomes increasingly imaginative.

Periodic health check—toddler

Table 3.3 (later) outlines key aspects of the periodic health examination for toddlers.

TABLE 3.3 Periodic health check: young child (12 months to 5 years of age)

	Australia	Aotearoa New Zealand
Immunisations For up-to-date guidelines on COVID-19 vaccination see the additional resources section at the end of the chapter	***18 months:*** *Haemophilus influenzae* type b (Hib) measles, mumps, rubella (MMR), varicella (chickenpox) diphtheria, tetanus, pertussis (whooping cough) hepatitis A (Indigenous children in WA, NT, SA, Qld) ***4 years:*** Diphtheria, tetanus, pertussis (whooping cough), polio pneumococcal (Indigenous children in WA, NT, SA, Qld), hepatitis A (Indigenous children in WA, NT, SA, Qld)	***15 months:*** *Haemophilus influenzae* type b (Hib), measles, mumps, rubella (MMR), varicella (chickenpox) ***4 years:*** Diphtheria, tetanus, pertussis, polio vaccine
Areas for assessment	***Nutrition:*** Discuss nutritional intake and needs; emphasise importance of physical activity; promote healthy eating habits ***Development:*** Explore developmental progress (e.g. PEDS assessment); evaluate communication; promote interactive reading with child; promote healthy sleep patterns At-risk children (exposed to alcohol prenatally)—screen for fetal alcohol syndrome	

Continued

TABLE 3.3 Periodic health check: young child (12 months to 5 years of age) cont'd

	Australia	Aotearoa New Zealand
	2 years: • Measure weight, length and head circumference and record on centile charts • Evaluate gait • Evaluate oral health and dentition • Evaluate vison and hearing ***3–4 years:*** • Measure height and weight (plot and interpret growth curve/calculate BMI) • Evaluate oral health (teeth and gums) • Discuss toileting • Discuss allergies • Conduct vision and hearing screening	
Psychosocial support	***Discuss:*** • Emerging behavioural or emotional problems • Identify family strengths, elicit concerns and promote parental confidence, competence and mental health	
Safety and preventive care	***Discuss:*** • Injury prevention (e.g. water safety, burns, falls, poisoning, car restraints, helmets) • Sun protection • Sleeping and eating • Regular dental visits • Social and emotional wellbeing • CPR in children • Promoting development (limit screen time < 1 hour a day, talking and reading to the child)	

Adapted from Ministry of Health 2023[19]; Department of Health and Aged Care 2023[20]; RACGP 2019[21]; National Aboriginal Community Controlled Health Organisation and The Royal Australian College of General Practitioners 2018[22]

Early childhood—preschooler (3 to 5 or 6 years)

Successfully achieving the developmental tasks of toddlerhood allows preschool children to build on their new-found autonomy to develop a sense of initiative. The social world of young children is also expanding, and preschoolers begin to develop relationships with people in addition to primary caregivers.[10] While still predominantly egocentric, preschoolers become increasingly aware of the needs, thoughts and feelings of others.

Developmental tasks for preschool-aged children include:

- realising separateness as an individual
- identifying gender role and its functions

- developing a conscience
- developing a sense of initiative
- interacting with others in socially acceptable ways
- growing use of language for social interaction
- developing readiness for school.

Physical development

While the major organ systems are relatively mature by 4 to 5 years of age, the musculoskeletal system is still rapidly developing throughout early childhood. To develop strength, coordination and balance, young children need space and time to engage in physical play. Similarly, refining fine motor skills requires practice through activities such as drawing or manipulation of small toys. During the preschool years, a child's proportions become more adult-like, with the limbs lengthening and the posture becoming more upright. The rate of growth continues at a slower pace, and the average child gains about 2 kg in weight and 7 cm in height per year.[3]

Cognitive development

The reoperational stage begins at around 2 years of age and extends until 7 or 8 years of age.[8] One of the distinguishing features of this stage is the use of **symbolic** thought; the child can now use symbols to represent people, objects and events. The symbolic function is revealed in the child's play as in delayed imitation. This means a child can witness an event, form a mental representation of it and imitate it later in the absence of the model. For example, a young child may see their mother talking on the phone and later mimic this conversation by talking into a remote control or other similarly shaped object. However, a preschooler's thought processes are still very concrete and literal, and they can only focus on one aspect of a problem at a time (this is known as **centration**). For example, a child in this stage of development may be able to correctly classify the family pet as a dog but will not recognise that their pet also fits into the broader category of 'animal'.

Also, thought during this period is often intuitive rather than logical, which can lead preschoolers to make faulty assumptions about cause and effect. Magical thinking is also common in this period of development, and preschoolers can have difficulty distinguishing wishes or stories from real-life events. Children of this age may believe they have caused events to occur by wishing for them or may connect two unrelated events because they occurred close together in time. Anthropomorphising is part of magical thinking—that is, attributing human characteristics such as thoughts, feelings and sensations to inanimate objects. This can be seen in a young child who packs a teddy into a bag for an outing and leaves its head sticking out 'so he can see'.

Children in the preoperational stage are egocentric.[9] Egocentric children cannot see another's point of view and assumes that others see things the way that they do. However, more recent research suggests that 4-year-olds can develop **theory of mind** (the understanding that others may have different thoughts or beliefs) and it is development of theory of mind that sets the stage for developing empathy later in childhood.[23]

Psychosocial development

Young children experience a crisis involving **initiative versus guilt**. Increasing physical and cognitive abilities give rise to new levels of energy and determination.[11] Young children 'attack' new tasks with enthusiasm and can not only plan their efforts but also persist in the face of frustrations. When a parent encourages and reassures a child (while protecting them from harm), the child learns self-assertion, spontaneity, self-sufficiency, direction and purpose. But if the parent ridicules, punishes or prevents the child from following through on tasks that could be done, the child feels guilty not only for their actions but also for their thoughts and plans, hindering creativity and initiative.

Another important aspect of psychosocial development in preschoolers is **identification of gender roles**. Around 3 years of age, children develop knowledge of their own gender (i.e. gender identity), although they may start using gender labels (i.e. 'boy' or 'girl') at an earlier age. Between 3 and 5 years, preschoolers develop stereotypes for acceptable activities (e.g. girls play with dolls), physical features (e.g. boys have short hair) and occupational roles (e.g. men are firefighters) connected to gender. These stereotypes tend to be inflexible until middle childhood, when the child develops an understanding that gender roles are socially dictated, but gender stereotypes tend to persist in some form into adulthood.[18]

Motor skills development

Skills such as running, jumping and climbing are well established by 3 years of age and continue to become increasingly well-coordinated.[10] Skills such as hopping on one foot show increasing control and balance; most children can accomplish this between 3 and 4 years of age. By 5 years, most children have enough gross motor control to enjoy games such as skipping and activities such as skating and swimming.

Fine motor control also becomes increasingly refined during this period. A toddler's scribbles are replaced by recognisable drawings by the age of 4 to 5 years.[10] A typically developing 5-year-old can string beads, use scissors proficiently and can manipulate buttons and zippers to dress and undress independently.

Language skills

Between 3 and 4 years of age, children use 3- to 4-word telegraphic sentences containing only essential words. Grammar in this age is developing, and children may use simplified grammatical forms. By 5 to 6 years, the sentences are 6 to 8 words long, and grammar is well developed. A typically developing 3-year-old has a vocabulary of around 1,000 words, and this will more than triple by the time they are ready to start primary school.

Preschoolers talk incessantly, often to themselves rather than to others. Piaget[8] described this pattern of speech as egocentric. However, it appears that this **private speech** is in fact a problem-solving tool that helps children to think through problems and manage their behaviour.[17] Children around the age of 4 chatter to themselves constantly; this fades to muttering in early school years but re-emerges as a coping strategy when the child encounters unfamiliar or stressful situations.

Personal and social skills

Socially, a preschooler's world is expanding (Figure 3.6). Fear of separation and anxiety

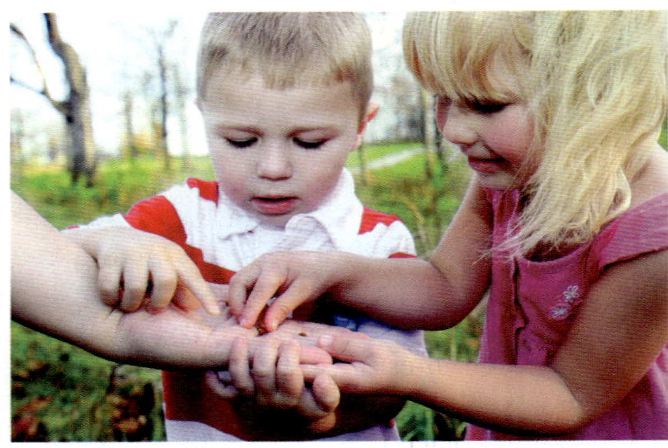

FIGURE 3.6 Social skills expand in preschoolers

around strangers diminishes, and children of this age can generally tolerate brief separations from parents to visit peers or attend preschool. With their growing social regard, preschoolers increasingly engage in **cooperative play** with each other.[24] This means they play the same game and interact with each other as part of their play. A child's imagination runs rampant, and this is evident in the games they choose. Preschoolers love to dress up and imitate the behaviours of their parents or other adult models such as nurses, doctors, media heroes, firefighters or police officers. This imaginative play has the potential to enhance learning but also acts as an emotional outlet through which children can work through conflicts or fears.[24]

In terms of moral development, children progress from a 'punishment/obedience' orientation in toddlerhood towards an individualistic orientation at around 4 years of age.[25] Children in the preconventional stage of moral development are motivated to follow rules to benefit themselves. They behave well towards others to ensure reciprocal gains rather than out of a sense of true 'right' or 'wrong'. For a child at this level of moral reasoning, it is right to behave nicely towards others so they will behave nicely towards you.

Periodic health check—young child

Table 3.3 outlines important aspects of well-child checks occurring in early childhood. In this age group, non-intentional injuries are a leading cause of morbidity and mortality, therefore health teaching with families focuses on identifying and managing possible risks.

Middle childhood—school-aged child (6 to 10 or 11 years)

Early development of trust and a sense of initiative enables the child to enter primary school and develop a sense of themselves as worthwhile people, as well as a part of a larger community.

Developmental tasks for school-aged children include:

- mastering skills that will be needed later as an adult
- winning approval from other adults and peers
- building self-esteem and a positive self-concept
- taking a place in a peer group
- adopting moral standards.

Physical development

The growth of school-aged children is typically steady, with most children gaining around 2 or 3 kg per year and growing around 6 cm per year. The physical appearance of school-aged children is relatively slimmer than that of younger children because of older children's proportionately longer legs, diminishing body fat and lower centre of gravity. Deciduous (or 'baby') teeth are lost at around 6 years of age, and new adult dentition erupts. Bones continue to ossify during these years, and bone replaces cartilage. Muscles are stronger and more developed, though not yet fully mature. Neuromuscular control is more refined. All these changes enable school-aged children to engage in complex physical tasks requiring strength, agility and coordination.

Cognitive development

The stage of middle childhood, ages 7 to 11 years, is described as the period of **concrete operations**.[8] At this age, children can use symbols (mental representations) of objects and events in more logical ways. This means a child can experience mentally what they would have had to do physically before. For example, rather than needing to show a manoeuvre in a video game, children can now articulate the steps without undertaking them.

Armed with the ability to use thinking to experience things or events, school-aged children can:

- Use numbers. Although counting with numbers begins in the preschool years, school-aged children have the combinational skill to add and subtract, multiply and divide.
- Read. By using printed symbols (words) for objects and events, children can process a significant amount of information. Also, reading fosters independence in learning.
- Serialise. While this begins in preschool years, school-aged children can order objects by an increasing or decreasing scale, such as according to number size (smallest to largest) or weight (lightest to heaviest).
- Classify. This is the ability to sort objects by something they have in common. While young children can do this, school-aged children can organise a hierarchy of classes and subclasses. This can be seen in a school-aged child's penchant for collections: rocks, shells, novelty cards, cars and dolls. Children spend many hours sorting the collections, and the logic of the classification system gets more complex as the child grows.
- Understand conservation principles. Understanding conservation of matter is the ability to see that mass or quantity stays constant even though shape or position is transformed. For example, a child who can conserve sees that two equal amounts of water remain the same even if one is poured into a glass with a different shape.

However, there are limitations to a school-aged child's cognitive abilities. While they can reason through problems that have a physical basis, they struggle to understand more abstract concepts. In this sense, school-aged children often learn best through practical demonstrations and hands-on experiences.

Psychosocial development

Erikson[11] labelled the psychosocial crisis facing school-aged children as **industry versus inferiority**. During this stage of development, a child's energy focuses on achievement and accomplishment. The approval and esteem of people outside the immediate family takes on greater importance, and children take pride in attempting new tasks and carrying them through to completion. Play and fantasy begin to give way to the mastery of tasks that the child will eventually need to compete in an adult world. Children learn to 'win recognition by producing things'.[24] Real achievement at this stage builds a feeling of confidence, competence and industry. Children are rewarded by their own inner sense of satisfaction in achieving a skill and, more importantly at this age, by external rewards such as approval from teachers, parents and peers in the form of marks, praise or gifts. Problems arise when children feel inferior. If a child believes they cannot measure up to society's expectations, they lose confidence in their abilities and may stop getting satisfaction from their efforts. While it is not possible for children to master every skill they encounter, it is important for caregivers to balance these weaker skills with opportunities for children to excel in other areas.

During middle childhood, it is important to belong to a peer group. The peer group is a key socialising agent, and group solidarity is enhanced by secret codes or strict rules. Children conform to group rules because acceptance is paramount. They eventually begin to prefer peer group activities to activities with their parents.

Motor skills development

Fine motor dexterity continues to improve in school-aged children.[24] Writing becomes smaller and more controlled, and hand–eye coordination reaches its peak at around 8 years of age for most children. Gross motor skills are well established, and movements become increasingly graceful. All these refinements ready school children to pursue activities requiring fine motor skills such as writing, drawing, needlework, small model building and playing instruments, and gross motor activities such as running, skipping, throwing, jumping, bike riding and swimming (Figure 3.7).

Language skills

Language development in school-aged children shifts in focus from language acquisition to more nuanced expression.[24] At around 8 years of age, children can give precise definitions to terms, and by age 10 they can articulate their thoughts and understand another person's perspective in conversation. School-aged children can appreciate increasingly subtle humour and may express sarcasm.

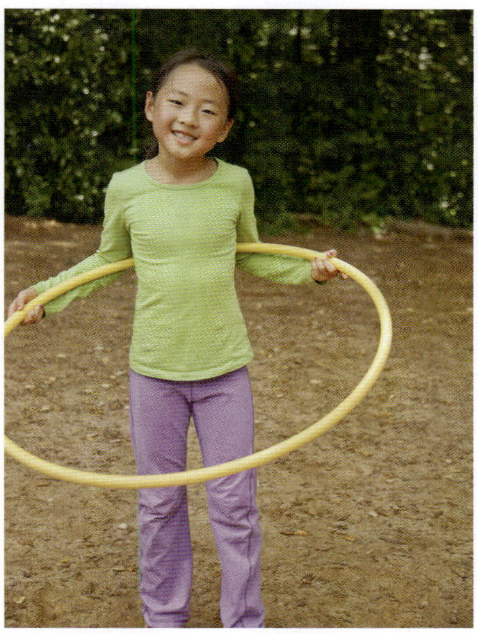

FIGURE 3.7 Gross motor skill development

Personal and social skills

School-aged children exhibit an increasing need to socialise with peers of the same gender, and peer acceptance is increasingly important as school-aged children move towards adolescence.[24] Initially, a child may have a large peer group, although by around 9 or 10 years of age, closer relationships have generally developed with one or more 'best friends'. More broadly, the value of social relationships emerges as children see the benefits of working in an organised group. Children learn to divide labour and to cooperate to achieve a common goal.

From a moral perspective, school-aged children are increasingly able to follow rules but are motivated to do the right thing to ensure others think well of them. Kolberg[25] termed this form of moral reasoning a 'nice girl' or 'nice boy' orientation. By the time a child is approaching preadolescence, they start to appreciate the need for social order and the need for rules to keep systems working effectively. This form of moral reasoning

TABLE 3.4 Periodic health check: older child (5 to 12 years of age)

Immunisations **For up-to-date guidelines on COVID-19 vaccination see the additional resources section at the end of the chapter**	Influenza (annually) (children with specified medical risk conditions such as chronic diseases or immunocompromised and Indigenous children)
Areas for assessment	• Measure weight and height (plot and interpret growth curve and calculate BMI) • Dental check—encourage regular dental screening • Evaluate vision and hearing • At-risk children (exposed to alcohol prenatally)—screen for fetal alcohol syndrome
Psychosocial support	• Anticipate and explore potential emotional and behavioural problems • Discuss school performance • Explore family functioning and family environment
Safety and preventive care	***Discuss:*** • Nutritional requirements and physical activity • Parent–child relationships and interaction • Injury prevention (e.g. car restraints, safe play, bicycle safety) • Sun protection

Adapted from Ministry of Health 2023[19]; Department of Health and Aged Care 2023[20]; RACGP 2019[21]; National Aboriginal Community Controlled Health Organisation and The Royal Australian College of General Practitioners 2018[22]

often depends on outside reinforcement, but school-aged children will typically follow the rules or do the 'right' thing if they know they are being monitored, but this may not persist if the child is left to their own devices.

Periodic health check—middle/school-aged child

Table 3.4 (later) outlines important aspects of well-child checks during middle childhood.

Preadolescence (10 or 11 to 12 or 13 years)

Preadolescence begins at 10 to 11 years of age and ends with puberty. Although this stage is still part of childhood, children in this group have common skills and interests that set them apart (Figure 3.8). A child may be at one level physically and intellectually but at another level socially. Also, development can differ significantly between children of the same age during preadolescence.

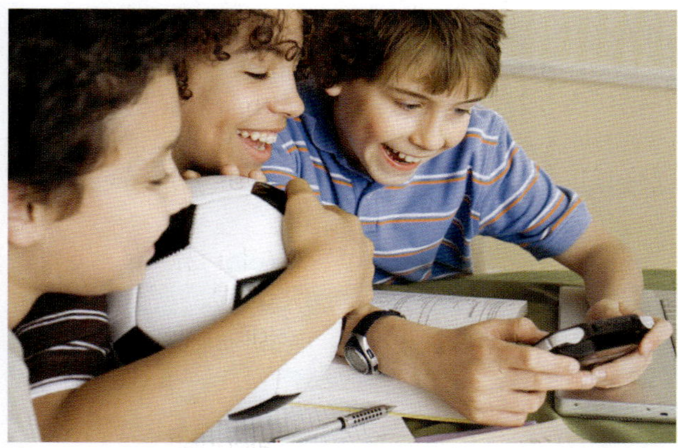

FIGURE 3.8 Preadolescents sharing common skills and interests

Physical development

Growth and development differ significantly between genders during this stage. On average, girls begin their growth spurt at around 10 years of age, and growth reaches its maximum velocity at around 12. Boys typically begin their growth spurt at around 12 and reach peak growth velocity at approximately 14 years of age. Weight gain during this period is predominantly caused by an increase in muscle mass, but care is needed to ensure the adolescent's diet provides enough energy and nutrients while maintaining weight within the healthy weight range. This is especially important because adolescents who are obese stand an 80% chance of being obese in adulthood.[27]

Attaining secondary sexual characteristics also varies widely between people of the same age. At the age of 10, some girls will still have the proportions and characteristics of children, while others have begun their growth spurt and show signs of early breast development and growth of pubic hair. Over time, the breasts enlarge, areolae darken and menarche occurs. Physical size among 11-year-old boys is uniform. At 12 years, boys show a wider range of growth. Most show the onset of secondary sex characteristics with initial genital growth, appearance of pubic hair and the occurrence of erections and nocturnal emissions.

Cognitive development

Children in this age group are beginning to transition from concrete operations, in which the focus is on what is occurring in the present and limited to what currently exists, to formal operations, in which the future can be considered and abstract thought becomes possible.[9]

Psychosocial development

Parent–child relationships frequently become strained during preadolescence as children begin to drift away from the family unit, placing increasing value on peer relationships. While parents continue to set standards and values, children begin to challenge authority and to reject these standards. This stage of development is marked by ambivalence towards one's family; there is an increasing desire for independence that conflicts with a continuing need for support and boundaries to feel secure.

Preadolescents show strong social interest outside of the family. There is strong identification with the peer group through a small clique or a larger, more loosely organised crowd formation. Girls and boys tend to stay within their own gender group. The clique has an exclusive membership, and one is privileged to belong; the code of the clique is important, with rules for dressing, speaking and behaving in common.[26] Children merge their own identity with that of the peer group. They begin to substitute conformity with the family to that with their peers because they need the security of a temporary identity before formulating a clear sense of self.

Even though peer groupings tend to comprise the same gender, some preadolescents show an emerging interest in mixed groups, an interest that will flourish in adolescence.

Periodic health check—older child

Table 3.4 outlines important aspects of well-child checks occurring in middle childhood and preadolescence. Unintentional injury remains a leading cause of morbidity and mortality throughout childhood and into adolescence, so harm minimisation strategies are an important part of health teaching.

Adolescence (12 or 13 to 19 years)

Adolescence is a transition stage between childhood and adulthood (Figure 3.9). Beginning at puberty and extending through the teenage years, the most important task of adolescence is the **search for identity**—now the adolescent must form a personal identity that is more than just the sum of childhood experiences. This search for identity is the motive behind all the other tasks of the period:

- searching for one's identity
- appreciating one's achievements
- growing independent from parents
- forming close relationships with peers
- developing analytical thinking
- evolving one's own value system
- developing a sexual identity
- beginning to choose a career.

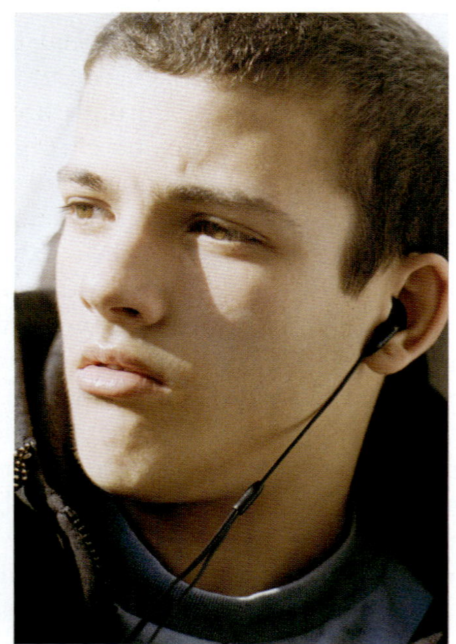

FIGURE 3.9 Adolescent developing relationships

Physical development

Adolescence begins with puberty. Puberty is a time of dramatic physiological change. It includes the growth spurt—rapid growth in height, weight and muscular development; developing primary and secondary sex characteristics; and maturation of the reproductive organs. Preoccupation with appearance and the body is characteristic during early adolescence. Young people are constantly comparing themselves with close friends and peers, as well as to standards of attractiveness gleaned through exposure to social media.

Physical health is typically good during adolescence; illnesses of childhood are behind them and illnesses associated with ageing are not yet a concern. However, adolescence is associated with an increase in risk-taking behaviours, which pose a threat to wellbeing. Poor decision making may result in accidental injury, injury through violence, abuse of alcohol and other drugs or unprotected sexual activity leading to sexually transmitted infections (STIs) or unplanned pregnancy. Early initiation of risk-taking behaviours has been linked with negative outcomes that persist into adulthood.[28,29] For example, an Australian study showed that weekly drinking in people younger than 17 was associated with a two- to threefold increase in high-risk behaviours in adulthood, including binge-drinking and alcohol dependence.[30]

Cognitive development

Adolescence corresponds to Piaget's fourth stage, in which the person develops the capacity for **formal operations**; this is the ability to develop abstract thinking, deal with hypothetical situations and make logical conclusions from reviewing evidence.[9] Once young people enter formal operations, thinking is no longer confined to the concrete or the real but encompasses all that is possible. Abstract thinking is liberating. Young people are no longer limited to the present but can consider the lessons of the past and the possibilities of the future. They can imagine hypotheses, then set up experiments to test them. They learn to use logic and solve problems by methodically eliminating each possibility one by one. This opens the doors to new academic achievements such as mastering advanced mathematical concepts.[9]

This analytical thinking extends to values. Developing personal values is a part of young people's search for identity. They no longer passively accept the values of parents or institutions but can reason through their inconsistencies and recognise injustices. Adolescents are sensitive to hypocrisy and note when an adult professes a value and then acts counter to it. According to Kohlberg,[25] some young people are capable of post-conventional reasoning, the mature form of moral thought. Young people who achieve this level of reasoning have an internalised moral code rather than relying on external definitions of right or wrong. However, it must be noted that not all people will reach this phase of moral development, and many continue to define right and wrong through rules and consequences throughout adulthood.

Psychosocial development

According to Erikson[11] adolescents experience a crisis of identity versus role confusion; young people focus on 'what they appear to be in the eyes of others as compared with what they feel they are'. In this search for identity, young people often form cliques, wear fad clothing and follow singers, movie stars or charismatic heroes to siphon identity from them. Falling in love also feeds the quest for personal identity. If young people successfully negotiate this crisis of identity, they are left with a stable sense of self, whereas young people who struggle to develop their sense of identity may be left feeling unsure about themselves and their place in the world, resulting in feelings of isolation and anxiety.

Risk taking is another way young people test their emerging identity. Risk-taking behaviours are argued to be a normative aspect of development, with large-scale international studies showing a consistent trend towards increased 'sensation-seeking' behaviours peaking at around 19 years of age and then declining. At the same time, young people develop increasing self-regulation, which reaches a steady state in the mid-20s.[31] While risk taking can be seen to be a typical part of adolescent psychosocial development, some risky behaviours, such as experimentation with alcohol and other drugs, high-risk sexual activity and unsafe driving practices, can have significant implications for health and wellbeing[29,30] (Figure 3.10).

Given the major psychosocial and physiological transitions associated with adolescence, young people are also particularly vulnerable to mental health problems. Young people with mental health disorders may experience stigma, isolation and discrimination and are at increased risk of self-harming behaviour and suicide. Indeed, suicide is the leading cause of death among Australians aged 15 to 24 years,[32] but this figure is somewhat misleading because people in this age group do not tend to die from other causes.[33] In addition to mental health conditions, social

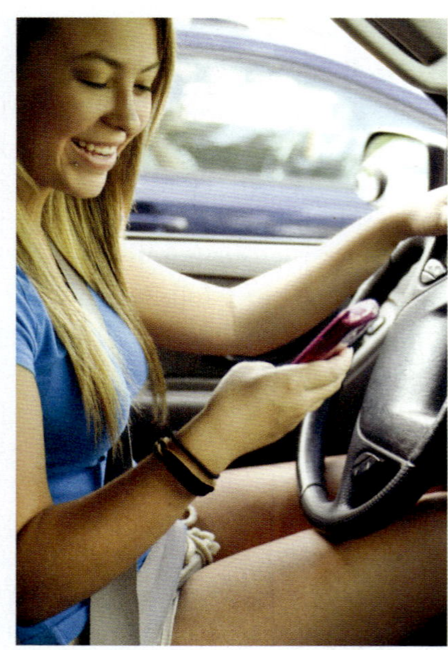

FIGURE 3.10 Risk taking (breaking the law)

and environmental factors may intensify or moderate risk for self-harm or suicide. Factors such as bullying or difficult family relationships increase risk, as does an unsupportive environment for young people who identify as lesbian, gay, bisexual or transgender.[34] Conversely, connections between young people and supports such as peers, school and their parents have been shown to be protective.[31]

Behavioural development

As previously discussed, the search for identity is all-consuming for young people, and this guides many of the behavioural changes that occur during adolescence. While young people may identify with their family less, they do not yet have a strong sense of their own identity. One strategy many adolescents use to cope with this transition is to immerse themselves in a peer group. Within their peer group, young people can test out a variety of social roles and receive validation and support from others.

While belonging to a peer group is vital to the psychosocial wellbeing of young people, developing close friendships is also important to personal identity. In preadolescence, experiencing a relationship with a best friend is valuable in teaching intimacy, trust and regard for another person. These lessons prepare young people to develop future close relationships. Finding a girlfriend or boyfriend enables the adolescent to learn their own sex role identity. In many settings, group dating (multiple couples sharing an activity) is the norm at first. This may represent a less intimidating situation than paired dating.

Gradual separation from the family unit and adopting personal responsibility is part of the transition from adolescent to adult. This is frequently a source of conflict between young people and parents; while young people outwardly express the need for freedom and control, they still need support from the family unit, both practically and emotionally. The struggle for parents is often in setting boundaries that respect young people's burgeoning autonomy while providing enough stability to maintain a sense of security.

Defining the end of adolescence is highly dependent on context and culture. In many cultures, there are rituals or rites of passage that mark the transition from child to adult, often coinciding with puberty and physical maturation. Conversely, in many Western cultures, traditional markers of the transition into adulthood such as moving away from home, forming intimate relationships and starting a family are steadily occurring later in the person's life span, for a variety of social and economic reasons.

Periodic health check—adolescent

Adolescents should undertake periodic general checks as well as health promotion. Health promotion information should include skin self-examination, breast self-examination or testicular self-examination, substance use, contraception and STI risk reduction. See Table 3.5 for a summary of the adolescent periodic health check.

TABLE 3.5 Periodic health check: adolescent

	Australia	Aotearoa New Zealand
Immunisations **For up-to-date guidelines on COVID-19 vaccination see the additional resources section at the end of the chapter**	***12–13 years (Year 7 or age equivalent)*** Human papillomavirus (HPV) Diphtheria, tetanus, pertussis (whooping cough), pneumococcal (Indigenous adolescents in WA, NT, SA, Qld), influenza (all Indigenous adolescents) ***14–16 years (Year 10 or age equivalent)*** Pneumococcal ACWY, pneumococcal (Indigenous children in WA, NT, SA, Qld), influenza (all Indigenous adolescents)	***11–12 years*** Tetanus/diphtheria/pertussis, human papillomavirus (HPV)
Areas for assessment	• Measure weight and height (plot and interpret growth curve and calculate BMI) • At-risk children (exposed to alcohol prenatally)—screen for fetal alcohol syndrome • STI screening if sexually active • Evaluate oral health	
Psychosocial support	• Screen for mental health disorders • Anticipate and explore potential emotional and behavioural problems • Discuss school performance • Explore family functioning and family environment	
Safety and preventive care	***Discuss:*** • Breast/testicular self-examination • Injury prevention—harm minimisation strategies and assess for risky behaviours • Possible effects of alcohol and other drug use—provide additional health information and support if illicit drug use is known or suspected • Promote oral health • Nutrition and physical activity • Sexual health education (consent, contraception and safe sex practices) • Promote strong anti-smoking and anti-vaping health messages • Sun protection	

Adapted from Ministry of Health 2023[19]; Department of Health and Aged Care 2023[20]; RACGP 2019[21]; National Aboriginal Community Controlled Health Organisation and The Royal Australian College of General Practitioners 2018[22]

Early adulthood (20 to 40 years)

Young adults are concerned with building an independent lifestyle. Developmental tasks during this phase of the life span include:

- growing independent from the parents' home and care
- establishing a career or vocation
- forming an intimate bond with another and choosing a mate
- learning to cooperate in an intimate relationship
- setting up and managing one's own household
- making friends and establishing a social group
- assuming civic responsibility and becoming a citizen in the community
- beginning a parenting role
- forming a meaningful philosophy of life.

Physical development

Physical growth, in terms of height, weight and maturation of organ systems, is generally complete by early adulthood. The epiphyses of the long bones typically fuse in the early 20s, and motor coordination and strength peak between the ages of 20 and 30.[35] Maximal bone mass is achieved by 35 years of age.[36] Since growth has finished, nutritional needs are dictated by maintenance and repair requirements and on activity levels. If activity decreases from its level during adolescence, kilojoules must be reduced. Sensible nutrition is a major problem for many adults; being overweight and obesity are at epidemic levels in Australia.[27] The diet should be high in fruits, vegetables and lean proteins, but all too often it is high in sugar, salt and fat. A sedentary lifestyle contributes to both increases in BMI and associated health risks. However, more adults are learning that frequent steady exercise maintains weight, muscle strength and joint flexibility. Exercise builds heart and lung capacity and reduces stress (Figure 3.11). Table 3.6 lists these and other preventive counselling measures to address during healthcare visits.

Cognitive development

Intellectual and cognitive skills reach a peak during early adulthood. During adolescence, young people achieve formal operations and develop the capacity for abstract thought.[9] While young adults retain this capability, their thinking is qualitatively different. Indeed, some theorists have proposed the term 'post-formal' operations to capture this subtle but important distinction.[37] These theorists claim that a young adult's growing experience allows them to view problems in a less egocentric way, integrating multiple perspectives to arrive at a solution. This gives

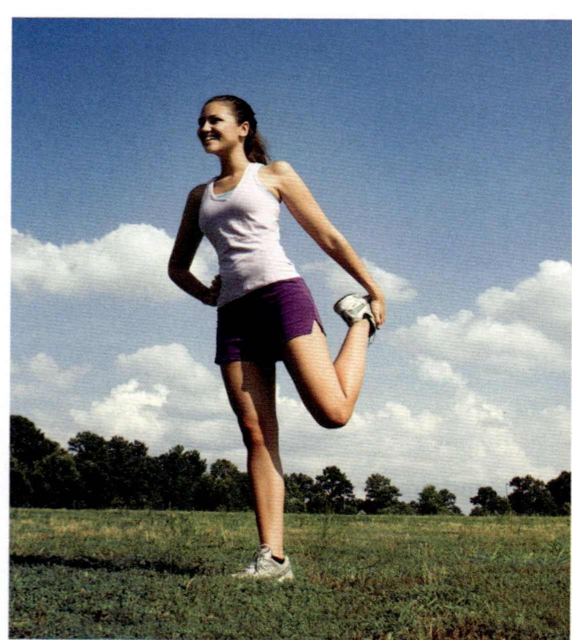

FIGURE 3.11 Maintaining fitness in early adulthood

TABLE 3.6 Periodic health check: young adult and middle adult

	Australia	Aotearoa New Zealand
Immunisations **For up-to-date guidelines on COVID-19 vaccination see the additional resources section at the end of the chapter**	***All ages:*** Influenza (especially those with specified medical conditions and Indigenous adults), pneumococcal (for adults with specified medical conditions and Indigenous adults) ***Pregnant women:*** Influenza, pertussis (whooping cough)	***45 years:*** diphtheria, tetanus, whooping cough vaccine ***Pregnant women:*** Influenza, pertussis (whooping cough)—tetanus, diphtheria and whooping cough vaccine
Areas for assessment	***20–40 years:*** • Measure BMI and waist circumference or waist-to-hip ratio • Record blood pressure • Measure fasting lipids (from 35 years in high-risk groups) • Evaluate risk factors relating to smoking, alcohol, nutrition and physical activity • Assess for type 2 diabetes (from 19 years in Aboriginal and Torres Strait Islander peoples) • Sexual health screening • Preconceptual care and breast cancer and cervical cancer screening for women ***40–65 years:*** • Measure BMI and waist circumference or waist-to-hip ratio • Record blood pressure • Measure fasting lipids • Evaluate risk factors relating to smoking, alcohol, nutrition and activity • Assess for type 2 diabetes • Calculate absolute cardiovascular risk (from 35 years in high-risk groups) • Pre-conceptual care, cervical screening test and breast cancer screening for women • Colorectal cancer screening (from 50 years) • Cervical screening test (from age 25 every 5 years until ages 70–74) and breast cancer screening for women (every 2 years from age 50 to ages 70–74) • Assess risk for osteoporosis (from 45 years in women and 50 in men)	
Psychosocial support	• Assess depression risk and other mental health issues	
Safety and preventive care	***Discuss:*** • Nutrition and physical activity guidelines • Sexual health and STI prevention • Substance use including alcohol, tobacco and illicit drugs • Sun protection	

Adapted from Ministry of Health 2023[19]; Department of Health and Aged Care 2023[20]; RACGP 2019[21]; National Aboriginal Community Controlled Health Organisation and The Royal Australian College of General Practitioners 2018[22]

young adults more sophisticated problem-solving capabilities and expands their potential for creative thinking.

Education continues for many young adults, from formal courses in a university or technical and further education (TAFE) environment to on-the-job training and continuing education classes. Usually, this education is designed to prepare the person for the workforce. Work is an important factor in a young adult's life because it is tied closely with a person's sense of identity.[38] Those who cannot find meaningful work are potentially vulnerable, not only to cognitive and psychosocial issues, but also to financial impacts on health and wellbeing more broadly.

Psychosocial development

Erikson's sixth stage covers the first years of early adulthood, from 20 to 24 years. He believed the major psychological conflict to be resolved is that of **intimacy versus isolation**.[11] Once self-identity is established after adolescence, it can be merged with another's in an intimate relationship. During the early 20s, many adults seek the love, commitment and intimacy of an intense, lasting relationship. This mature relationship includes mutual trust, cooperation, sharing of feelings and goals and complete acceptance of the other person. Although Erikson had a heterosexual union in mind, this intimacy could be satisfied through a same-sex relationship or through a bond with a cause or an institution.[11]

Erikson believed that without a secure personal identity, a person cannot form a love relationship. The result is that the person becomes isolated, withdrawn and lonely. Such issues with psychosocial development may result in attempts to fill the void with transient or casual sexual relationships. Erikson[11] proposes that these do not meet the needs of the person, worsening feelings of loneliness. However, not all young adults desire or seek marriage or family, finding fulfilment in their career or delaying childrearing until later in life.

It has been proposed that people in their 20s may be in a period of 'emerging adulthood', representing a newly defined stage of development.[37–39] As pressures such as housing affordability, limited employment opportunities for young people and the rising cost of education have come to bear, more young adults are choosing to stay in the family home for a prolonged period and therefore may adopt the responsibilities and independence central to early adulthood later than previous generations.

In contrast to the 20s, a person's 30s are typically characterised by 'settling down' and a search for order and stability. Part of this settling down may include having children. For those young adults who do choose to start a family, parenting raises a new series of developmental tasks to be accomplished. On discovering a pregnancy, both positive and negative emotions may be experienced. If this was a planned conception, there may be feelings of excitement and a strong desire to be the perfect parent, but this may be counterbalanced with concerns about one's parenting ability and the impact that childrearing will have on lifestyle, career and other commitments. Having children also results in a major readjustment to roles within an intimate relationship. Decisions about work and parenting leave may need to be made, and parental preferences about care at home may need to be weighed against financial and workplace obligations.

Periodic health check—young adult

Table 3.6 (earlier) outlines the periodic health check for a young adult.

Middle adulthood (40 to 65 years)

The primary focus of middle adulthood is developing meaningful life structures. Developmental tasks during this stage of the life span include:

- accepting and adjusting to the physical changes of middle age
- reviewing and redirecting career goals
- achieving desired performance in career
- developing hobby and leisure activities
- adjusting to ageing parents
- helping adolescent children in their search for identity
- accepting and relating to the spouse as a person
- coping with an empty nest at home.

Physical development

During middle adulthood, the function of organ systems is typically stable, with only a small reduction in respiratory reserve and cardiac function. There may be some changes to the person's vision, with presbyopia (decreasing near vision accommodation) becoming more prevalent.[36] Many of the physical changes occurring during this period are to do with appearance, with thinning and greying of hair and a loss of skin elasticity becoming increasingly evident. These physical signs of ageing, combined with occasional news of a peer's illness or death, may lead those in middle adulthood to contemplate their own mortality.

In their late 40s and early 50s, females experience menopause, the decreasing frequency and finally the cessation of menstruation. Decreased production of the female hormones estrogen and progesterone can cause troublesome symptoms such as vasomotor disturbances (hot flushes), sleep disturbance, vaginal dryness and mood swings (Chapter 26). Although men do not have such an abrupt halt to reproductive ability, they experience a decrease in the production of testosterone, which causes decreased sperm and semen production (Chapter 27).

During this stage of the life span, a decrease in lean muscle mass and bone density occurs, particularly if there is a decline in physical activity, while adipose tissue increases and tends to accumulate around the abdomen or hips.[36] This increase in adiposity is a risk factor for cardiovascular disease including hypertension, disorders of glucose metabolism and musculoskeletal dysfunction such as arthritis and back pain. Mortality in Australian people aged 45 to 64 is frequently a result of chronic disease. Cardiovascular and cerebrovascular disease, lung cancer, suicide, colorectal and liver cancers are the predominant causes of death for both men and women in this age group.[32,40]

Cognitive development

Intelligence levels remain generally constant during middle adulthood. Intelligence is further enhanced by the knowledge that comes with life experience, self-confidence, a sense of humour and flexibility. Middle-aged adults are interested in how new knowledge is applied, not just in learning for learning's sake. Cognitively, middle-aged adults may need more time to assimilate new knowledge, but once learnt, they have more accurate recall than younger age groups.

Psychosocial development

Erikson[11] argued that the most important task for personality development is resolving the conflict of generativity versus stagnation. Erikson believed that during the middle years, adults have an urge to contribute to the

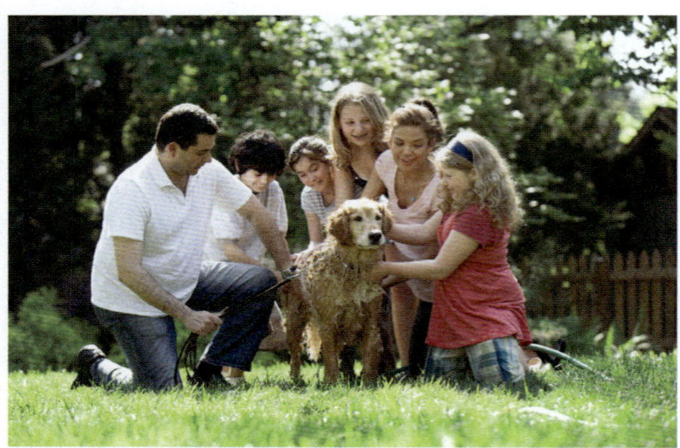

FIGURE 3.12 Middle adulthood—childrearing

next generation. This need can be fulfilled either by actively engaging in childrearing (Figure 3.12) or by producing something to pass on to the next generation. Middle-aged adults may therefore focus on childrearing or engage in other creative, socially useful work. Generativity may also include developing a career, managing a household or fostering close relationships.[11]

Middle-aged adults need to be needed, to leave something behind and to leave their mark on the world. Generativity is associated with sharing, giving and contributing to the growth of others. If this conflict is not successfully negotiated, the person experiences stagnation, turning their attention inwardly and becoming self-absorbed and potentially experiencing a loss of meaning and connectedness.

Midlife transition occurs between the ages of 40 and 45 years. As with the re-evaluation that occurs at around 30 years of age, this midlife appraisal includes questions about direction and purpose. The person may confront the reality that not all life goals will be met, while others require adjustment. For women, one aspect of the midlife transition is considering the approaching biological boundary of childbearing. For those who set aside childbearing in earlier adulthood, a review of options may occur at this point; indeed, this review occurs even in women who are satisfied with their family size and structure. The midlife transition often also incorporates a review of career goals and changes in career direction.

Another important aspect of psychosocial development in middle adulthood is maintaining a positive self-image. However, this can be difficult in cultures that place value on looking and acting young. When the person attempts to deny ageing or has trouble viewing themselves as middle-aged, they may have trouble making necessary lifestyle adjustments. Depression can result. Sometimes this denial of ageing can lead to a 'midlife crisis', in which the person engages in behaviours that are out of character.[36] Alternatively, the reflection associated with middle adulthood can bring about new insights into the person's past experiences and sense of self.

Family also contributes to this adjustment; a supportive intimate relationship or strong connections with children may promote adaptation, while challenges such as divorce or separation or caring for ageing parents may have a negative impact on psychosocial function. Middle-aged adults may also be supporting their own adolescent children as they strive for greater independence and control. Finally, once children leave home, middle-aged adults may experience a degree of isolation associated with the 'empty nest'. For parents who have focused vast amounts of time and energy on their children, this transition may challenge a parent's identity and sense of purpose. Parents may also experience a change to their intimate relationships once children have moved away from home. Some struggle to adjust to being a 'couple' again, while others revel in the increased freedom and intimacy that this phase of development can bring.

Periodic health check—middle adult

Table 3.6 (earlier) outlines the periodic health check for a middle adult.

Late adulthood (65+ years)

Developmental tasks during this stage of the life span include:

- adjusting to changes in physical strength and health
- forming a new family role as a parent-in-law and/or grandparent
- affiliating with one's age group
- adjusting to retirement and reduced income
- developing post-retirement activities that enhance self-worth and usefulness
- arranging satisfactory housing
- adjusting to the death of spouse, family members and friends
- conducting a life review
- preparing for the inevitability of one's own death.

Physical development

Ageing is a normal physiological process, although its mechanism is not fully understood. While ageing can be associated with an increase in health problems, each person ages differently. Indeed, differences in personal attitudes, health behaviours, physical activity, genetics and the occurrence of physical illness mean that one person at 80 years may be more vigorous and have a better subjective sense of wellbeing than another at the same age.[36]

Typical processes that occur as part of ageing include loss of total body water and bone mass. Within the cardiovascular system, structural changes over time may lead to thickening and stiffening of arterial walls, increasing blood pressure and compromising blood flow to the cardiac muscle. Hypertension is a common health issue in the Australian adults over 35 years (4.2%), rising steadily with age, peaking at around 41.5% for adults aged 75 years or older.[41] Older adults are generally living longer and healthier lives than those in previous generations. However, many older people live with chronic health conditions including cardiovascular disease, arthritis, other musculoskeletal conditions, chronic kidney disease and chronic respiratory diseases.[42] All these issues mean that older adults may be a more frequent consumer of health care than other age groups.

Cognitive development

Ageing does not have a predictable effect on intelligence. Intellectual function depends on various factors such as motivation, interest, sensory impairment, educational level, general health, social concerns and involvement in community activities or stimulating leisure activities. How we solve problems also tends to change with age.[43] While younger adults tend to rely primarily on 'fluid' reasoning ability (the ability to adapt mental operations to new tasks) to solve everyday problems, older adults retain and even build on their abilities (those formed from accumulated experiences and knowledge of the world). Older adults may experience a decline in memory function, especially in terms of storage and retrieval of short-term memories, but many older adults retain strong recall of long-term memories.[43]

Psychosocial development

In Australia and Aotearoa New Zealand there are increasing numbers of older adults remaining in the workforce after the age of 65 years. In Australia in 2021, 14.8% of older Australian remained in the workforce over the age of 65 years.[44] The improving health of older people, the desire to continue careers, changes in economic circumstances, availability of work and changes in family circumstances are common reasons for older adults to continue working.[44] The actual age of retirement is often tied to the availability of retirement income such as the age pension and superannuation benefits.

Retirement can be a difficult period for some older adults, particularly if their sense of identity is closely tied to their work. There is also a loss of social contact through co-workers and potentially a decrease in intellectual stimulation and activity if the job was relatively demanding.[45] For this reason, it is important to develop post-retirement activities that enhance self-worth and give a feeling of usefulness. These activities may include developing a new 'semi-retired' career, or a hobby, sport interest or community service activity (Figure 3.13). For other older adults, this may include assisting with caring for grandchildren and great grandchildren and greater involvement in work, whether paid or unpaid.[36] The transition to retirement is eased if these activities are well in place before the last formal day on the job. When financially and socially secure, older adults can pursue activities that hold personal significance for them.

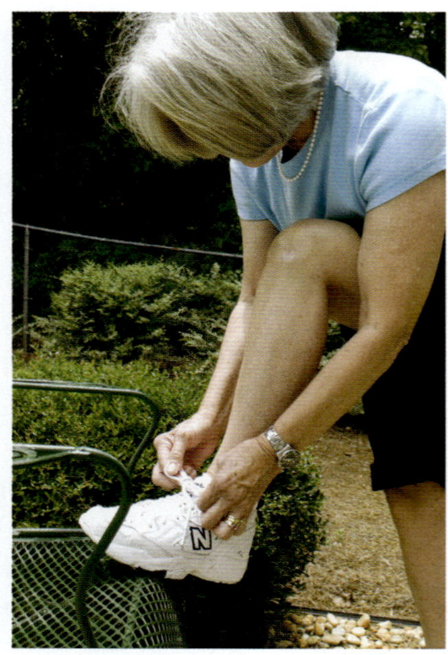

FIGURE 3.13 Late adulthood post-retirement activities

Loss of income associated with retirement and the potential for altered living arrangements may also impact on the psychosocial wellbeing of older adults. There may be a significant drop in income, and even those who own their own home may become overwhelmed with increasing costs of living on a fixed pension or superannuation benefit. Living arrangements may also need to change depending on financial circumstances and the need for support with day-to-day living. While some cultures incorporate their elders into the family home and view them as an active part of the family unit, this is less common in Western cultures. This may leave older adults with difficult choices to make about accommodation.

For some older adults, changes to their previous lives, loss of family members and friends and societal attitudes towards older people result in a sense of loneliness. Loneliness arises from a mismatch between a person's desired social interaction, and social connections with others can lead to a perception of poor-quality social connections and a sense of loneliness.[46] Loneliness can have significant impacts on general health and wellbeing including an increase in the risk of chronic health conditions, dementia, poor mental health (including depression and anxiety) and reduced capacity to manage activities of daily living. Loneliness, bereavement, poor physical and mental health and a dependence on others are all contributing factors to the high rate of suicide in older men,[47] especially those aged 85 or older.[33]

A typical task of late adulthood is reflecting on one's life. A life review is a cataloguing of life events—a considering of one's successes and failures with the perspective of age.[48]

According to Erikson,[11] the key psychological conflict for older adults is one of **ego integrity versus despair**. When older adults negotiate this conflict successfully, they can review life events, experiences and relationships. Engaging in life review can help older adults to find meaning and value in their life experiences, which has been found to improve subjective wellbeing.[36] Conversely, a person who struggles to find integration may be left with a sense of despair, resentment, futility, hopelessness and a fear of death. However, a successful outcome completes a cycle.

Periodic health check—adult over 65 years

Table 3.7 outlines the periodic health check for late adulthood.

TABLE 3.7 Periodic health check: late adulthood (65+)

	Australia	Aotearoa New Zealand
Immunisations **For up-to-date guidelines on COVID-19 vaccination see the additional resources section at the end of the chapter**	***65 years or older*** Influenza (annually), shingles (herpes zoster) ***70 years or older*** Pneumococcal	***65 years or older*** Influenza (annually), diphtheria, tetanus, whooping cough, shingles (herpes zoster)
Areas for assessment	• Measure BMI and waist circumference or waist-to-hip ratio • Record blood pressure • Measure fasting lipids • Evaluate risk factors relating to smoking, alcohol, nutrition and activity • Screen for type 2 diabetes • Calculate absolute cardiovascular risk • Cervical screening test (every 5 years until ages 70–74) and breast cancer screening for women (every 2 years to ages 70–74) • Colorectal cancer screening (ages 50–74) • Assess risk for osteoporosis • Assess vision and hearing • Assess falls risk • Assess risk for dementia	
Psychosocial support	• Discuss issues with memory • Discuss social supports and social activities • Assess for mood and depression	
Safety and preventive care	***Discuss:*** • Falls prevention strategies • Nutrition and physical activity guidelines • Medication safety • Sun protection	

Adapted from Ministry of Health 2023[19]; Department of Health and Aged Care 2023[20]; RACGP 2019[21]; National Aboriginal Community Controlled Health Organisation and The Royal Australian College of General Practitioners 2018[22]

Cultural and social considerations

Much of the developmental content of this chapter is informed by the findings of research and experience with people from cultures dominant in high-income countries. Given the rate of demographic change, it is imperative to consult with cultural brokers and/or patient advocates from the person's cultural heritage who have a deeper understanding of the expected norms of the various developmental tasks.[49,50]

The immunisation protocols from other nations may differ from those of Australia and Aotearoa New Zealand, and therefore immigrants may require 'catch-up' immunisation. Careful examination of health records must be undertaken when engaging with people who have received care outside of Australia. When assessments are conducted, competent interpreters must be used.[19,20]

Social factors also play a significant role in development and health across the life span. The role of socioeconomic status as a determinant for health and wellbeing has been well explored in infants and children[51] and extending from childhood into adult life.[52,53] Interventions that promote socioeconomic equity and limit childhood adversity achieve a host of health-related benefits including increased adult income, educational attainment and better health.[53]

Socioeconomic disadvantage experienced in adulthood may also have a significant effect on morbidity and mortality and on the rates of potentially harmful health behaviours.[54–56] Such information is helpful in designing effective health policy and providing valuable support to vulnerable populations.

Developmental screening tools

Parent's evaluation of developmental status (PEDS)

Age: Birth to 8 years
Time required: 2 to 5 minutes
Author: FP Glascoe[57]
Available from: www.pedstest.com

PEDS is a developmental screening tool designed to elicit parents' concerns about their child's development across a range of domains including fine and gross motor function, receptive and expressive language, behaviour and social and emotional skills.[57] The tool is designed to ensure early identification of developmental risk factors and signs of delay and to prompt further investigation where needed. As described by the Centre for Community Child Health (The Royal Children's Hospital Melbourne),[58] one of the potential weaknesses of traditional developmental screening tools is that they are typically performed in isolation, without due consideration of the child's sociocultural context, and without soliciting systematic input from parents who have extensive insight into their child's behaviour and abilities. The centre also highlights that involving parents actively in screening may improve accuracy as well as motivating families to follow the recommendations.[58]

The PEDS relies on responses from parents to 10 specific questions, which can be administered either as a written questionnaire or as an interview with the health provider. The tool includes suggested scoring, with a response algorithm that gives recommendations ranging from referral for detailed assessment, use of additional screening measures or education and reassurance depending on the concerns expressed and the age of the child.

The PEDS is a validated tool[59] that has shown strong sensitivity and specificity. A systematic review including 37 studies across 12 countries indicates that about 14% of parents identified concerns about their child's development when the PEDS tool was used and that these concerns were more likely in children experiencing biological and psychosocial adversity.[58] Benefits of this tool include its simplicity, meaning that providers require minimal training; the assessment package includes a reference guide, which is used to interpret results. Its brevity also means that it is feasible to include it in brief healthcare interactions. However, a 2018 study revealed some barriers to the tool including lack of awareness of the tool, access to referral pathways and time as contributors to the tool not being widely used.[60]

Adult life stress measures

Some tools are available that attempt to quantify the impact of life change on a person's health. They assume that a relationship exists between daily life stress and a person's susceptibility to physical and psychological problems. Many of the life change events are the developmental tasks discussed earlier in the chapter.

THE HASSLES AND UPLIFTS SCALE

Age range: Adult
Author: A DeLongis[61]
This is a 53-item self-administered questionnaire whose purpose is to assess day-to-day stress (Table 3.8). Take this test yourself just before you go to bed one day. Consider each item on the list and circle a number on the left-hand side regarding how much of a hassle the item was for you that day. On the right-hand side, circle a number representing how much of an uplift the same item was for you that day. Total scores are obtained by summing across ratings given to all items.

Relatively minor but frequently experienced stresses, termed *Hassles* in this tool, have been found to correlate strongly with negative health status. A significant relationship was found between daily stress and concurrent or later occurrence of physical health problems such as flu, sore throat, headaches and backaches. There was great individual variation, however, with one-third of the respondents reporting a somewhat improved health and mood with increased stress levels.[61] Regarding daily stress and psychological disturbance, they found that people with unsupportive social relationships and low self-esteem had a greater risk of psychological and somatic health problems, both on their stressful days and following their stressful days, than did people with positive social networks and high self-esteem.[61]

TABLE 3.8 The hassles and uplifts scale

HASSLES are irritants—things that annoy or bother you; they can make you upset or angry. UPLIFTS are events that make you feel good; they can make you joyful, glad or satisfied. Some hassles and uplifts occur on a regular basis and others are relatively rare. Some have only a slight effect; others have a strong effect.
This questionnaire lists things that can be hassles and uplifts in day-to-day life. You will find that during a day some of these things will have been only a hassle for you and some will have been only an uplift. *Others will have been both a hassle AND an uplift.*

Continued

TABLE 3.8 The hassles and uplifts scale cont'd

DIRECTIONS: Please think about how much of a hassle and how much of an uplift each item was for you today. Please indicate on the left-hand side of the page (under 'HASSLES') how much of a hassle the item was by circling the appropriate number. Then indicate on the right-hand side of the page (under 'UPLIFTS') how much of an uplift it was for you by circling the appropriate number.

Remember, circle one number on the left-hand side of the page *and* one number on the right-hand side of the page for *each* item.

PLEASE FILL OUT THIS QUESTIONNAIRE JUST BEFORE YOU GO TO BED.

After you complete the scale, you are encouraged to use the information as a baseline to consider how psychosocial and lifestyle factors influence your wellbeing over time.

HASSLES AND UPLIFTS SCALE

How much of a hassle was this item for you today?	**How much of an uplift was this item for you today?**
HASSLES	**UPLIFTS**
0 = None or not applicable	0 = None or not applicable
1 = Somewhat	1 = Somewhat
2 = Quite a bit	2 = Quite a bit
3 = A great deal	3 = A great deal

DIRECTIONS: Please circle one number on the left-hand side and one number on the right-hand side for each item.

0 1 2 3	1. Your child(ren)	0 1 2 3
0 1 2 3	2. Your parents or parents-in-law	0 1 2 3
0 1 2 3	3. Other relative(s)	0 1 2 3
0 1 2 3	4. Your spouse	0 1 2 3
0 1 2 3	5. Time spent with family	0 1 2 3
0 1 2 3	6. Health or wellbeing of a family member	0 1 2 3
0 1 2 3	7. Sex	0 1 2 3
0 1 2 3	8. Intimacy	0 1 2 3
0 1 2 3	9. Family-related obligations	0 1 2 3
0 1 2 3	10. Your friend(s)	0 1 2 3
0 1 2 3	11. Fellow workers	0 1 2 3
0 1 2 3	12. Clients, customers, patients, etc.	0 1 2 3
0 1 2 3	13. Your supervisor or employer	0 1 2 3
0 1 2 3	14. The nature of your work	0 1 2 3

TABLE 3.8 The hassles and uplifts scale cont'd

0 1 2 3	15. Your workload	0 1 2 3
0 1 2 3	16. Your job security	0 1 2 3
0 1 2 3	17. Meeting deadlines or goals on the job	0 1 2 3
0 1 2 3	18. Enough money for necessities (e.g. food, clothing, housing, health care, taxes, insurance)	0 1 2 3
0 1 2 3	19. Enough money for education	0 1 2 3
0 1 2 3	20. Enough money for emergencies	0 1 2 3
0 1 2 3	21. Enough money for extras (e.g. entertainment, recreation, holidays)	0 1 2 3
0 1 2 3	22. Financial care for someone who doesn't live with you	0 1 2 3
0 1 2 3	23. Investments	0 1 2 3
0 1 2 3	24. Your smoking	0 1 2 3
0 1 2 3	25. Your drinking	0 1 2 3
0 1 2 3	26. Mood-altering drugs	0 1 2 3
0 1 2 3	27. Your physical appearance	0 1 2 3
0 1 2 3	28. Contraception	0 1 2 3
0 1 2 3	29. Exercise(s)	0 1 2 3
0 1 2 3	30. Your medical care	0 1 2 3
0 1 2 3	31. Your health	0 1 2 3
0 1 2 3	32. Your physical abilities	0 1 2 3
0 1 2 3	33. The weather	0 1 2 3
0 1 2 3	34. News events	0 1 2 3
0 1 2 3	35. Your environment (e.g. quality of air, noise level, greenery)	0 1 2 3
0 1 2 3	36. Political or social issues	0 1 2 3
0 1 2 3	37. Your neighbourhood (e.g. neighbours, setting)	0 1 2 3
0 1 2 3	38. Conserving (gas, electricity, water, petrol, etc.)	0 1 2 3
0 1 2 3	39. Pets	0 1 2 3
0 1 2 3	40. Cooking	0 1 2 3

Continued

TABLE 3.8 The hassles and uplifts scale cont'd

0 1 2 3	41. Housework	0 1 2 3
0 1 2 3	42. Home repairs	0 1 2 3
0 1 2 3	43. Garden work	0 1 2 3
0 1 2 3	44. Car maintenance	0 1 2 3
0 1 2 3	45. Taking care of paperwork (e.g. paying bills, filling out forms)	0 1 2 3
0 1 2 3	46. Home entertainment (e.g. TV, music, reading)	0 1 2 3
0 1 2 3	47. Amount of free time	0 1 2 3
0 1 2 3	48. Recreation and entertainment outside the home (e.g. movies, sports, eating out, walking)	0 1 2 3
0 1 2 3	49. Eating (at home)	0 1 2 3
0 1 2 3	50. Religious or community organisations	0 1 2 3
0 1 2 3	51. Legal matters	0 1 2 3
0 1 2 3	52. Being organised	0 1 2 3
0 1 2 3	53. Social commitments	0 1 2 3

Source: DeLongis 1988[61]

ADDITIONAL RESOURCES

You can further develop your knowledge and skills relevant to developmental stages through the life span, related pathophysiology, common health issues and nursing interventions by:

- reading chapters of a fundamentals of nursing or medical-surgical nursing textbook
- reviewing Elsevier online resources. Log onto ClinicalKey Student. You can select various videos on a range of topics—focus on anatomy and physiology topics relevant to the chapter
- answering chapter multiple choice questions online. Log onto ClinicalKey Student and search for the text 'Health Assessment, 4th edition'. Choose the section titled 'Teaching material'. In this section you will find question and answer documents for each chapter.
- visiting websites

  UNICEF—Early childhood development: https://www.unicef.org/early-childhood-development

  World Health Organization

  Child health and development unit: https://www.who.int/teams/maternal-newborn-child-adolescent-health-and-ageing/child-health/healthy-growth-and-development

ADDITIONAL RESOURCES cont'd

Adolescent health: https://www.who.int/health-topics/adolescent-health#tab5tab_1

Additional information about COVID-19 immunisation

Australian Technical Advisory Group on Immunisation (ATAGI)—COVID-19 vaccination statements: https://www.health.gov.au/committees-and-groups/australian-technical-advisory-group-on-immunisation-atagi?language=und#covid19-updates

Ministry of Health New Zealand—COVID-19: Vaccine policy statements and clinical guidance: https://www.health.govt.nz/our-work/diseases-and-conditions/covid-19-novel-coronavirus/covid-19-vaccines/covid-19-vaccine-information-health-professionals/covid-19-vaccine-policy-statements-and-clinical-guidance

REFERENCES

1. Hamburger ER, Goethals ER, Choudhary A, Jaser SS. Sleep and depressive symptoms in adolescents with type 1 diabetes not meeting glycemic targets. Diabetes Research and Clinical Practice. 2020 Nov 1;169: 108442.
2. Eines TF, Kieczka EA, Klungnes SH, Johnsen TA, Grønvik CK. Adolescents' experiences living with type 1 diabetes mellitus: A scoping review. Nordic Journal of Nursing Research. 2022 Oct 19:20571585221132652.
3. World Health Organization (WHO). WHO child growth standards. Geneva, Switzerland: WHO; 2023. Available at: https://www.who.int/tools/child-growth-standards
4. Goyal S, Banerjee S. Fluid, electrolyte and early nutritional management in the preterm neonate with very low birth weight. Paediatrics and Child Health. 2021 Jan 1;31(1):7–17.
5. Derbyshire E, Obeid R. Choline, neurological development and brain function: a systematic review focusing on the first 1000 days. Nutrients. 2020 Jun 10;12(6):1731.
6. Dobson V, Teller DY. Visual acuity in human infants: a review and comparison of behavioral and electrophysiological studies. Vision Research 1978;18(11):1469–1483.
7. Bremner JG, Tham DS, Dunn K. Visual perception in infancy. The Encyclopedia of Child and Adolescent Development. 2020 Dec 20:1–9. https://doi.org/10.1002/9781119171492.wecad110
8. Piaget J. The stages of the intellectual development of the child. Educational psychology in context: Readings for future teachers. 1955;63(4):98–106.
9. Piaget J, Inhelder B. The psychology of the child. New York: Basic Books; 1969.
10. Sharma A, Cockerill H, Sanctuary L. Mary Sheridan's from Birth to Five Years Children's Developmental Progress [internet]. Milton: Taylor & Francis Group; 2021. (5th ed.). Routledge. Available from: https://doi.org/10.4324/9781003057154
11. Erikson EH. Childhood and society. London: Random House; 1963 & 1995.
12. Bowlby J (1982). Attachment and Loss (Vol. 1: Attachment) (2nd ed.). New York: Basic Books. ISBN 978-0465005437. LCCN 00266879. OCLC 11442968. *NLM 8412414.*
13. Bowlby EJM. Loss-Sadness and depression: attachment and loss, vol. 3. New York: Random House; 2008.
14. Lawrence M. The Theory of Educational Attachment. Journal of Organizational and Educational Leadership 2023;8(3):1–23.

15. Keenan T, Evans S, Crowley K. An introduction to child development. 3rd edition. Sage; 2016 Mar 17.
16. Gleason JB, Ratner NB. The development of language. Plural Publishing; 2022 Dec 20.
17. Feldman HM. The importance of language-learning environments to child language outcomes. Pediatrics. 2019 Oct 1;144(4).
18. Sodian B, Kristen-Antonow S, Kloo D. How does children's theory of mind become explicit? A review of longitudinal findings. Child Development Perspectives. 2020 Sep;14 (3):171–177.
19. Ministry of Health, New Zealand Government, National immunisation schedule; 2023. [internet]. Available from: https://www.health.govt.nz/our-work/preventative-health-wellness/vaccine-information-healthcare-professionals/new-zealand-immunisation-schedule
20. Australian Government Department of Health and Aged Care. National Immunisation Program schedule [Internet]. Australian Government Department of Health and Aged Care; 2023. Available from: https://www.health.gov.au/topics/immunisation/when-to-get-vaccinated/national-immunisation-program-schedule
21. Royal Australian College of General Practitioners (RACGP). Guidelines for preventive activities in general practice [Internet]. 9th ed. Melbourne, Australia: 2021. Available at: https://www.racgp.org.au/clinical-resources/clinical-guidelines/key-racgp-guidelines/red-book 2019 Dec 20:1-9.
22. National Aboriginal Community Controlled Health Organisation and The Royal Australian College of General Practitioners. National guide to a preventive health assessment for Aboriginal and Torres Strait Islander people. 3rd edn. East Melbourne, Vic: RACGP, 2018. Available at: https://www.racgp.org.au/clinical-resources/clinical-guidelines/key-racgp-guidelines/national-guide
23. Piaget J, Cook M. The development of object concept. In: The construction of reality in the child. New York, NY: Basic Books; 1954. pp. 3–96.
24. Crowley K. Child development: a practical introduction. 2nd ed. Thousand Oaks, CA: Sage Publications Inc; 2017.
25. Kohlberg L. The psychology of moral development. New York: Harper & Row; 1984.
26. Meadows S. Understanding Child Development: Psychological Perspectives and Applications. 2nd ed. New York: Routledge; 2018.
27. Australian Institute of Health and Welfare (AIHW). Overweight and obesity [Internet]. Canberra: Australian Institute of Health and Welfare, 2023. Available from: https://www.aihw.gov.au/reports/overweight-obesity/overweight-and-obesity
28. Tetering MV, Laan AV, Kogel CD, Groot RD, Jolles J. Sex differences in self-regulation in early, middle and late adolescence: A large-scale cross-sectional study. PLoS One. 2020 Jan 13;15(1):e0227607
29. Ciranka S, van den Bos W. Adolescent risk-taking in the context of exploration and social influence. Developmental Review. 2021 Sep 1;61:100979
30. Silins E, Horwood LJ, Najman JM, Patton GC, Toumbourou JW, Olsson CA, et al. Adverse adult consequences of different alcohol use patterns in adolescence: an integrative analysis of data to age 30 years from four Australasian cohorts. Addiction 2018;113(10):1811–1825.
31. Martinez JL, Hasty C, Morabito D, Maranges HM, Schmidt NB, Maner JK. Perceptions of childhood unpredictability, delay discounting, risk-taking, and adult externalizing behaviors: A life-history approach. Development and psychopathology. 2022 May;34(2):705–17.
32. Australian Institute of Health and Welfare. Deaths [Internet]. Canberra: Australian Institute of Health and Welfare, 2021. Available from: https://www.aihw.gov.au/reports/children-youth/deaths
33. Australian Institute of Health and Welfare. Suicide and Self-harm Monitoring [Internet]. Canberra: Australian Institute of Health and Welfare, 2023. Available from: https://www.aihw.gov.au/suicide-self-harm-monitoring
34. Madireddy S, Madireddy S. Supportive model for the improvement of mental health and prevention of suicide among LGBTQ+ youth. International Journal of Adolescence and Youth. 2022 Dec 31;27(1):85–101.
35. Beckett C, Taylor H. Human growth and development. Sage; 2019 Mar 18.

36. Polan E, Taylor D. Journey Across the Life Span: Human Development and Health Promotion. FA Davis; 2023 Feb 23.
37. Sinnott J, Hilton S, Wood M, Spanos E, Topel R. Does motivation affect emerging adults' intelligence and complex postformal problem solving? Journal of Adult Development 2016;23(2):69–78.
38. Haider ZF, von Stumm S. Predicting educational and social–emotional outcomes in emerging adulthood from intelligence, personality, and socioeconomic status. Journal of Personality and Social Psychology. 2022 May 12.
39. Arnett JJ, Robinson O, Lachman ME. Rethinking adult development: Introduction to the special issue. American Psychologist. 2020 May;75(4):425.
40. Ministry of Health, New Zealand. Major causes of death. 2018. Available at: https://www.health.govt.nz/our-work/populations/maori-health/tatau-kahukura-maori-health-statistics/nga-mana-hauora-tutohu-health-status-indicators/major-causes-death
41. Australian Bureau of Statistics. Hypertension and measured high blood pressure [Internet]. Canberra: ABS; 2017-18. Available from: https://www.abs.gov.au/statistics/health/health-conditions-and-risks/hypertension-and-measured-high-blood-pressure/2017-18
42. Australian Institute of Health and Welfare. Older Australians—Health status and functioning [Internet]. Canberra: Australian Institute of Health and Welfare, 2023. Available from: https://www.aihw.gov.au/reports/older-people/older-australians/contents/health/health-status-and-functioning
43. Marr C, Vaportzis E, Dewar M, Gow AJ. Investigating associations between personality and the efficacy of interventions for cognitive ageing: a systematic review. Archives of Gerontology and Geriatrics. 2020 Mar 1;87:103992
44. Australian Institute of Health and Welfare. Older Australians—Employment and work [Internet]. Canberra: Australian Institute of Health and Welfare, 2023. Available from: https://www.aihw.gov.au/reports/older-people/older-australians/contents/employment-and-work
45. La Rue CJ, Haslam C, Steffens NK. A meta-analysis of retirement adjustment predictors. Journal of Vocational Behavior. 2022 Aug 1;136:103723.
46. Ogrin R, Cyarto EV, Harrington KD, Haslam C, Lim MH, Golenko X, et al. Loneliness in older age: What is it, why is it happening and what should we do about it in Australia? Australas J Ageing. 2021;40:202–207. https://doi.org/10.1111/ajag.12929
47. De Leo D. Late-life suicide in an aging world. Nature Aging. 2022 Jan;2(1):7–12.
48. Van der Kaap-Deeder J, Soenens B, Van Petegem S, Neyrinck B, De Pauw S, Raemdonck E, et al. Live well and die with inner peace: The importance of retrospective need-based experiences, ego integrity and despair for late adults' death attitudes. Archives of Gerontology and Geriatrics. 2020 Nov 1;91:104184.
49. Schaaf M, Warthin C, Freedman L, Topp SM. The community health worker as service extender, cultural broker and social change agent: a critical interpretive synthesis of roles, intent and accountability. BMJ Global Health. 2020 Jun 1;5(6):e002296.
50. Lázaro Gutiérrez R, Álvaro Aranda C 2023, Introduction to New Trends in Healthcare Interpreting Studies. In: Lázaro Gutiérrez, R., Álvaro Aranda, C. (eds) New Trends in Healthcare Interpreting Studies. New Frontiers in Translation Studies. Springer, Singapore. https://doi.org/10.1007/978-981-99-2961-0_1
51. Booysen F, Botha F, Wouters E. Conceptual causal models of socioeconomic status, family structure, family functioning and their role in public health. BMC Public Health. 2021 Dec;21:1–6.
52. Green H, Fernandez R, MacPhail C. Well-being and social determinants of health among Australian adults: A national cross-sectional study. Health & Social Care in the Community. 2022 Nov;30(6): e4345–4354.
53. Wang J, Geng L. Effects of socioeconomic status on physical and psychological health: lifestyle as a mediator. International Journal of Environmental Research and Public Health. 2019 Jan;16(2):281.

54. Liu PY, Beck AF, Lindau ST, Holguin M, Kahn RS, Fleegler E, et al. A framework for cross-sector partnerships to address childhood adversity and improve life course health. Pediatrics. 2022 May 1;149(Supplement 5).
55. Green H, Fernandez R, MacPhail C. The social determinants of health and health outcomes among adults during the COVID-19 pandemic: a systematic review. Public Health Nursing. 2021 Nov;38(6):942–952.
56. McMaughan DJ, Oloruntoba O, Smith ML. Socioeconomic status and access to healthcare: interrelated drivers for healthy aging. Frontiers in Public Health. 2020 Jun 18;8:231.
57. Glascoe FP, Marks KP. Detecting children with developmental-behavioral problems: the value of collaborating with parents in early detection. Psychological Test and Assessment Modeling. 2011;53(2):258–279.
58. Royal Children's Hospital (RCH). Parents' Evaluation of Developmental Status (PEDS). [Internet]. Melbourne, Australia: Updated 2023. Available at: https://www.rch.org.au/ccch/peds/
59. Glascoe FP. Collaborating with parents: using parents' evaluation of developmental status (PEDS) to detect and address developmental and behavioral problems. 2nd ed. Nolensville, TN: PEDSTest.com, LLC; 2013.
60. Garg P, Ha MT, Eastwood J, Harvey S, Woolfenden S, Murphy E, et al. Health professional perceptions regarding screening tools for developmental surveillance for children in a multicultural part of Sydney, Australia. BMC Family Practice. 2018 Dec;19(1):1–2.
61. DeLongis A, Folkman S, Lazarus RS. The impact of daily stress on health and mood: psychological and social resources as mediators. Journal of Personality and Social Psychology 1988;54(3):486–495.

CHAPTER 4

Cultural safety

Written by Leonie Cox and Chris Taua

INTRODUCTION

Over the course of your nursing professional education, you will study human developmental tasks and much about human health across the life span. You will learn to conduct numerous assessments such as a health history, a physical health assessment and assessments of other functional areas including mental health, nutrition and metabolic, cardiovascular and pain. You will understand the many different factors that influence health and illness—for example, personal, social and political history, environment, government policy and practice, racism, gender, gender identity, age, class and other sociocultural circumstances (Figure 4.1). Importantly, your reactions to the person seeking your care can influence the information you gather in these assessments. It is imperative that you, as a health professional, come to understand how your personal culture and the cultures of your profession, ward, hospital, service or organisation in which you work influence health assessment findings and the health care you provide.[1] To summarise, you must understand the relationship between cultural dominance, power, privilege, oppression and health.[2]

There is considerable variation in how culture is defined and approached in health care, and terms such as race, ethnicity, cultural competence, cultural appropriateness, cultural responsiveness, cultural security, cultural diversity and cultural inclusion add to the complexity and confusion. To simplify, there are two major methods used in nurse education to address issues of culture and health, and these are transcultural approaches and cultural safety.

First, transcultural approaches tend to reduce culture to ethnicity and focus on the assumed personal 'culture' of health service users. This approach, which includes the notion of cultural competency based on cultural awareness training, was developed by Madeleine Leininger, who is generally considered the pioneer of 'transcultural nursing'. These approaches contend that to offer effective nursing care you need to have knowledge of the cultural heritage,

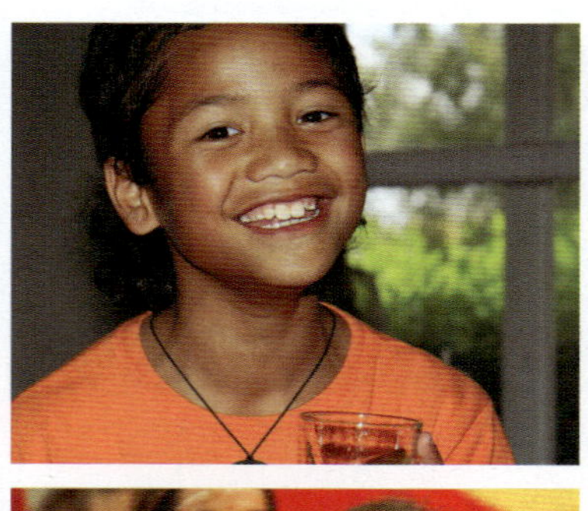
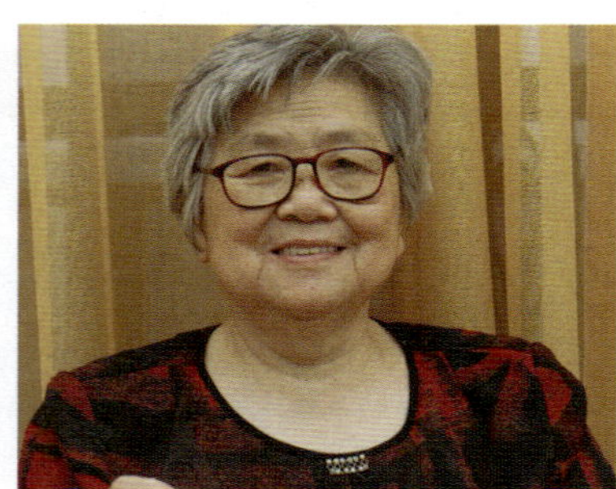
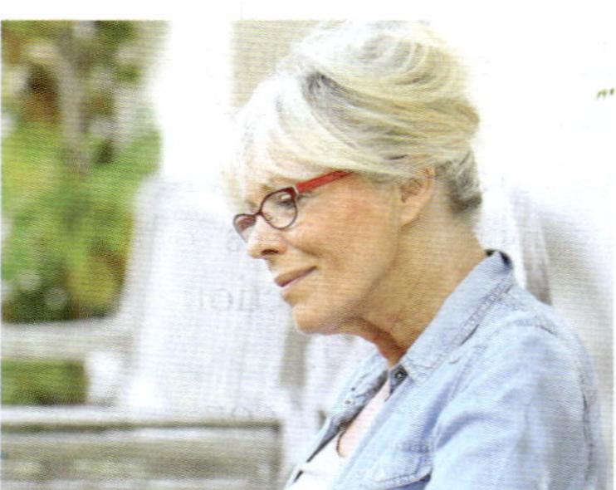
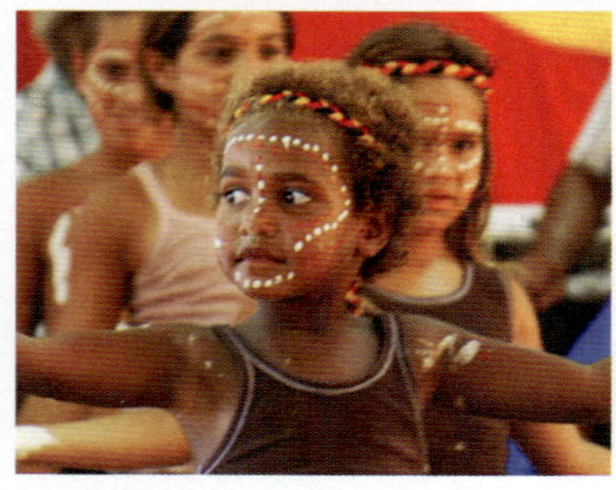
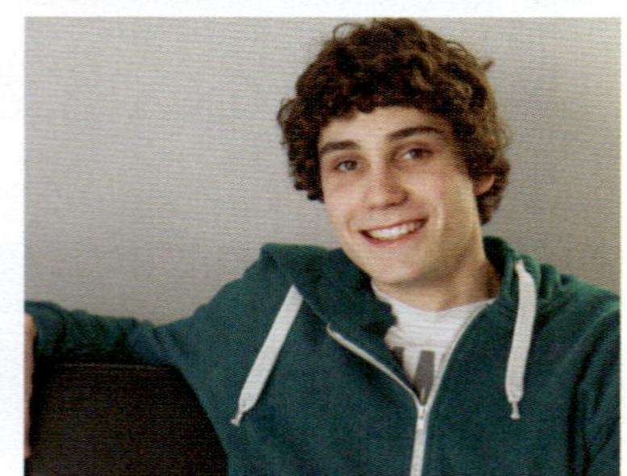
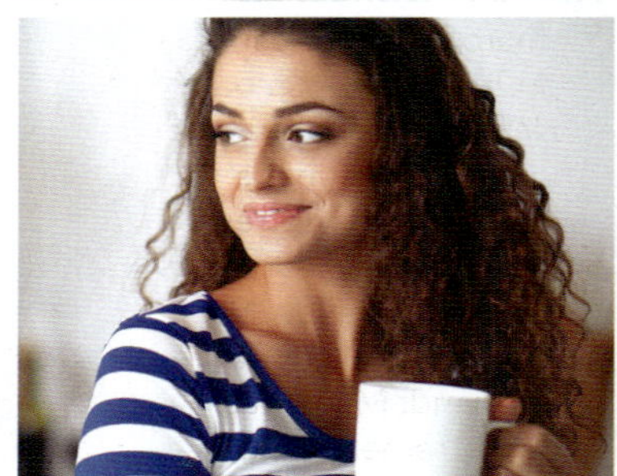

FIGURE 4.1 Factors that influence health and illness

language requirements and culturally based health and illness beliefs and practices of the people for whom you are caring. Cultural responsiveness also falls under this approach.[3]

In this chapter, our focus is not on the culture of others. We agree with the Australian national review of multicultural nurse education in 2001, which reported that Leininger's work was 'criticised as being too focused on the culture of the "other": presenting cultures as static and deterministic'.[4] Cultural capability, yet another framework, has aspects of a transcultural approach, but like cultural safety, it works with issues of power, discrimination and oppression.[5] Another related model is cultural security, which 'refers to the embedded structures, policies, workforce attributes and other elements required to enable health consumers to experience cultural security'.[3]

This text focuses on 'cultural safety', which is now embedded in the codes of conduct and registration standards for nurses and for midwives in Australia.[6–10] Cultural safety has long been a central facet of nursing practice and regulation in Aotearoa[i] New Zealand, where it was developed by Dr Irihapeti Ramsden in 1990. It centres on the cultures of health services and professions and on nurses' cultural self-awareness developed through ongoing processes of cultural self-reflection. So, during reflection you will ask:

- *Who am I?*
- *Where do I come from?*
- *What is my ethnicity and what is my social and cultural background?*
- *What are my beliefs and values?*
- *What prejudices, stereotypes and attitudes do I hold about those I consider different from myself?*
- *How might my cultural identity affect this person?*
- *Have I really listened to how this person experiences pain, or have I made assumptions about them, what they are saying or their behaviour?*

Culturally safe professions undertake reflection and ask such questions as:

- *Whose needs/priorities is this practice meeting?*
- *What role has this organisation/service/profession played in colonisation historically and in the present?*
- *How did the culture (values, power, priorities) of this organisation/service/profession, contribute to poor outcomes for individuals and families?*
- *What structures, processes and resources has this organisation/service/profession dedicated to addressing the impacts of history and current unsafe practices?*

So cultural safety is not about cultural practices of service users but is about how institutions and their staff treat people differently. A focus on the current social crisis in health care for groups such as immigrants and Indigenous[ii] people in political terms is a central feature of providing culturally safe

[i] 'Aotearoa' is the most widely known and accepted Māori name for New Zealand. It is used by both Māori and non-Māori. The word can be broken up as: ao = cloud, tea = white and roa = long, and it is therefore usually interpreted as 'the land of the long white cloud'.

[ii] The term 'Indigenous' is used in this chapter for brevity, but it should be noted that Indigenous people of mainland Australia and the Torres Strait Islands comprise many different groups with language group names and other terms that they use to refer to themselves. Indigenous people also use terms to refer to themselves that are roughly based on state boundaries: New South Wales: Koori, Goorie, Koorie, Coorie, Murri; Victoria: Koorie; South Australia: Nunga, Nyungar, Nyoongah; Western Australia: Nyungar, Nyoongar; Northern Territory: Yolngu (Top End); Anangu (Central); Queensland: Murri; Tasmania: Palawa, Koori. The term 'Aboriginal and Torres Strait Islanders' tends to be used most often but remember that both the Torres Strait Island context and the mainland context are informed by locally specific cultural and historical backgrounds and are extremely diverse. The term may also be used to refer to Māori who identify as Indigenous to Aotearoa New Zealand.

care. You will therefore also need to become knowledgeable about the history of your country and how it functions socially and politically to affect the health of those in your care. Sourced from the author's own experience, the following is a comment from an Australian Indigenous student after completing a unit on cultural safety in a Bachelor of Nursing program. The comment reveals these concerns:

> *The best aspect of this unit for me was having a subject that I understand and can relate to being Indigenous. We have come a long way from not being citizens in our own country and all the rest of it to have my people fight for rights and it is a huge thing for me as a Murri to see my people and culture be recognised and educating mainstream Australians about it because it obviously needs to be done.*

The purpose of this chapter is to:

- introduce the population contexts of Australia and Aotearoa New Zealand
- consider the relationship between health, history and cultures in Australian and Aotearoa New Zealand demographic contexts
- define culture, race, ethnicity and health
- consider ideas of cultural competence and cultural safety
- describe the position on Indigenous issues and cultural assessment of the Nursing and Midwifery Board of Australia and the Nursing Council of New Zealand
- provide comprehensive principles of cultural safety and discuss strategies to achieve it.

Cultural safety is urgently needed so the healthcare system and nursing as a part of that system can take its place as part of the solution to better life and social justice outcomes for Aboriginal and Torres Strait peoples. The Close the Gap campaign (a community-led and -driven social justice initiative) and the Closing the Gap strategy (a government initiative) give comprehensive detail on these matters that all professional nurses need to grasp.[11]

Resources available

You will find additional resources and the reference list at the end of this chapter.

Australia: colonisation and the current population context

Given the history of colonisation in Australia, the population comprises First Nations peoples, descendants of European colonisers and more recent migrants. Before discussing more fully how culture and health care interact, it is important for nurses planning to work in Australia to understand the context of their work in terms of the populations they will be serving. This is true for both international and domestic nurses. In Cox's experience,[12] the former often have little understanding of Australian populations and their histories and the latter have variable levels of historical knowledge and a mix of attitudes towards various population groups. Some people carry entrenched and unexamined attitudes towards Indigenous Australians, mainstream[iii] Australians or migrants. In the case of attitudes towards

[iii] 'Mainstream' is used to refer to members of the dominant culture in Australia.

Indigenous Australians, these may in part be due to their lack of experience and exposure to specific Indigenous contexts or to their lack of knowledge about Indigenous history, as reflected in this comment from a student:

> *I was surprised to see the number of students that had never had any interaction with Indigenous Australians or travelled outside their birth city. It was good to see them able to discuss their own culture and learn of the suffering still inflicted on Indigenous persons. I later saw it as a relevant topic to those students.*

Most people, however, are aware that Australia is now a multicultural society, but what is perhaps less well known is that before the British began the colonisation of Australia in 1788, some 500 Indigenous language groups had lived here for up to 80,000 years.[13,14] Also, Indigenous people were not the aimless wandering nomads so often depicted. Pascoe[15] wrote about:

> *... a much more complicated Aboriginal economy than the primitive hunter–gatherer lifestyle we had been told ... Hunter–gatherer societies forage and hunt for food and do not employ agricultural methods or build permanent dwellings; they are nomadic ... I came across repeated references to building dams and wells, planting, irrigating, and harvesting seed, preserving the surplus, and storing it in houses, sheds, or secure vessels, creating elaborate cemeteries and manipulating the landscape.*

Indigenous people lived in well-defined socioeconomic, political, land-owning units as Cox and Taua note.[14] From the perspective of Indigenous people then, the 200-odd years since colonisation is but a moment in their overall history. This point is important because it explains why it is that Indigenous Australians consider themselves to be First Nations or Status People; that is, it is why they have specific, unique and enduring rights in Australia.

Many non-Indigenous Australians lack knowledge of or refuse to accept Australia's history and either support or are unaware of the government's ongoing discriminatory approaches towards Indigenous people. Author Cox has, over 16 years, taught Australian history and contemporary issues in an undergraduate program to several thousand students. Countless discussions show that many see colonisation as a single event that occurred more than 200 years ago and find it difficult to understand why it is that 'historical' issues remain fresh for Indigenous people. In Australia, colonisation is an ongoing process, and it continues to be played out in government approaches to Indigenous people forming what is called neocolonialism.[iv] Unlike the situation in Aotearoa New Zealand (see below), the colonisation of Australia was enacted under the legal fiction of terra nullius (empty land) which, in the minds of the newcomers, morally justified the takeover of the land with its subsequent impact on Indigenous peoples. The war over land saw thousands of Indigenous people die in retaliatory massacres by the colonists, while restricted access to food sources and the imposition of an incoming population resulted in starvation, neglect and introduced diseases.

Many Indigenous people still see themselves in a state of war that continues to be unrecognised and undeclared by the government.[v] Reflect for a moment too on the Northern Territory Intervention and its clearly racist agenda.[16] To this day, Australian governments do not afford Indigenous people the dignity of truly recognising them as the

---

[iv] See, for example, the Northern Territory Emergency Response 2007 and the Stronger Futures Legislation that extended until 2022.[15]

[v] Listen to the 1988 song Secret War on the Warumpi Band Album *Go Bush*.

original owners with whom the negotiation of a treaty and reparation for war crimes should properly be held and finalised.

It would be hard to find more differing understandings of the world and humans' place in it than those held by the original owners and the newcomers. For Indigenous peoples, Country (place) was and is the source of identity and the basis of their cosmological understandings of the universe; for the newcomers, it was merely a resource to be exploited. The issues we see in Indigenous health today are profoundly related to dispossession and removal from kin and Country and related traditions, including language and ceremonial (religious) life, which often reduced Indigenous people to the status of slaves and fringe dwellers in their own land during the 19th and 20th centuries. Many were deterred from hunting and gathering traditional foods as they saw their countrymen and women shot, poisoned or harassed if they attempted to access lands that they had been using for thousands of years. Instead, Indigenous people were forced to live on poor-quality rations such as white flour, sugar and the fatty remains of meat unwanted by white people. Substances such as tea, tobacco and alcohol were introduced as a form of 'payment' for the menial work performed, entrapping the residents into cycles of addiction to sugar, alcohol and tobacco that we see today in the often-repeated poor population health status of Indigenous Australians.

The 20th century brought complex legislative frameworks in all states and territories that attempted to control every aspect of the lives of Indigenous people, first under the banner of 'protection' since the authorities assumed that Aboriginal people would 'die out'. As in Aotearoa New Zealand, the authorities were concerned about increasing numbers of those they conceived of as 'mixed-race'[vi] children, and they set about developing policies and practices to remove 'fair-skinned' children from their Aboriginal parents and kinship groups: those now generally known in Australia as 'the Stolen Generations' following a national enquiry into the removal of Indigenous children from their families.[17] When the government came to terms with the fact of continued Aboriginal existence, the policy changed to assimilation, where the goal was to train the Stolen Generations, and Indigenous people more generally, to live like white people. In these complex processes, families were fragmented by institutionalisation on government or mission reserves and reformatory schools and by marginalisation from the workforce, education and health services.[17–21] Indeed, health services were involved in some of these processes. The result is that since health services are largely run by governments, attending them is often resisted, as the experiences are bound up in fear and a lack of trust towards health services.[2,12,22] Historical processes, such as deeming petty misdemeanours a crime under the special laws on missions and reserves, also saw the widespread criminalisation of Indigenous populations that we still see today in the over-representation of Indigenous people at all levels of the criminal justice system.[23]

Although in the late 1970s the punitive discriminatory laws in the states and territories that applied only to Indigenous Australians began to be changed, the ideal of true self-determination cannot be achieved without a treaty or proper political representation. Space does not permit us to discuss native title and land rights here and the ongoing struggles for people to be recognised as Australia's original

[vi] The concept of race (a social construction) is discussed later in this chapter.

owners (see Ritter[24] for more information on the native title struggles). The deliberate attempted destruction of Indigenous societies, the many different situations in which Indigenous people now live, and the need for social justice in land/waters, health, education, welfare, housing, employment, language and inclusion are the result of these actions.

The federal government finally made a national apology for the Stolen Generations to Indigenous Australians in 2008, but adequate concrete compensation and proper representation was not established. Seeking constitutional change to address these matters, in 2015 a Referendum Council was established culminating in a National First Nations Constitutional Convention at Uluru in 2017. It issued the Uluru Statement from the Heart calling for Voice, Treaty and Truth, which was immediately rejected by the Turnbull government.[25] Led by Senator Pat Dodson, a Joint Select Committee of Parliament recommended that a proposal for The Indigenous Voice to Parliament be co-designed with Aboriginal and Torres Strait Islander people. In 2023 the Albanese government honored its election promise to hold a referendum where Australians were to vote on a constitutional change to enshrine the existence of an independent and permanent advisory body to parliament ('The Voice'), the first step towards treaty. The proposed constitutional change, supported by 83% of Indigenous people, would have helped ensure Indigenous people could advocate for locally specific needs and interests to parliament and that governments could not simply abolish these changes.

The 2023 referendum asked: 'A Proposed Law: to alter the Constitution to recognise the First Peoples of Australia by establishing an Aboriginal and Torres Strait Islander Voice. Do you approve this proposed alteration?' It was preceded by months of public debate from campaigners in support of the referendum (the 'Yes' campaign) and those against (the 'No' campaign), led by Opposition Leader Peter Dutton and prominent right-wing Indigenous politicians Warren Mundine and Senator Jacinta Nampijinpa Price.[26]

About 60% of Australians voted 'no' in a rejection of a possible way to begin to heal the deep rifts between Indigenous people, the State and the general population. Indigenous leaders declared a week of silence to mark their deep sense of rejection. Elder Geraldine Hogarth described the grief as being like 'A knife in your heart'.[27] So, to this day, Australian governments and most of the population do not afford Indigenous people the dignity of truly recognising them as the original owners with whom the negotiation of a treaty and reparation for war crimes can be finalised. Consider how that might feel for Indigenous people and how these matters will affect your relationships with people during your professional practice. The need for culturally safe practitioners is now more pressing than ever.

Indigenous identity and the Australian population

It is also important to understand that identifying as an Aboriginal or Torres Strait Islander person is not about skin colour but is about relationships. In his doctoral thesis, Drummond writes of the centrality of relationality for culturally safe nursing practice.[28] Because of the lack of trust and reciprocal relationships between mainstream health services and Indigenous Australians, the latter began to set up their own primary healthcare services from the 1970s. These are known as Aboriginal Community Controlled Health Services, and their peak body, the National Aboriginal Community Controlled Health Organisation (NACCHO), supports the nationally accepted means of determining Aboriginality. The means of determining has three parts and all are needed for Aboriginality to be recognised: descent (the person can prove that a parent is of Aboriginal or Torres Strait Islander descent); self-identification (the person identifies as an Aboriginal or Torres Strait Islander); and community recognition (the person is accepted as such by the Aboriginal or Torres Strait Islander community).[29]

According to the Australian Bureau of Statistics,[30] 812,728 people identified as Aboriginal and/or Torres Strait Islander in 2021, up from 649,171 in 2016. Aboriginal and Torres Strait Islander people represent 3.2% of the total population, up from 2.8% in 2016. Between 2016 and 2021:

- there were minor changes in the age distribution—all age groups reported very small changes (less than 0.8 percentage points)
- median age increased from 23 years to 24 years
- the ratio of males to females was steady—in 2016 there were 98.5 males per 100 females; in 2021 there were 98.7 males per 100 females.

In 2021, 41.1% of all Aboriginal and Torres Strait Islander people lived in major cities, 25.1% lived in inner regional areas and 14.5% lived in remote areas, while the proportion of Indigenous people rises the more remote the area.[30]

Another important factor for you as professional nurses is that 29.1% of Australians were born overseas. This means that you, your colleagues and those seeking your services will come from a range of ethnic, national and cultural backgrounds and have variable social positions as Australian-born, as migrants or as someone with experiences of seeking refuge or asylum. Those born in England continue to be the largest group of overseas-born residents, but those born in India is the population with the greatest increase since 2011.[31]

Since communication is central to nursing care, it is important that you understand that there is a multiplicity of languages in Australia. One in 10 spoke an Indigenous language at home and 150 Indigenous languages were spoken in 2021.[32] Sixteen per cent of the total Australian population did not speak English at home. In the 2021 Census[33] 72.4% of the Australian population were born in Australia. Nearly half (48.2%) of Australians had one or both parents that had been born overseas. In 2021, there were more than 300 separately identified languages spoken in Australian homes. More than one-fifth (22.8%) of Australians spoke a language other than English at home. Of these, 15.1% responded that spoke English not well or not at all. After English, the next most common languages spoken at home were Mandarin, Arabic, Vietnamese and Punjabi. The 2021 Census shows Australia's religious diversity with Christianity remaining the most reported religion (43.9% of the population), followed by no religion (38.9%). Islam, with 3.2% of responses, was the third most reported religion, closely followed by Hinduism (2.7%).[34]

Aotearoa New Zealand: colonisation and the current population context

Most people living in Aotearoa New Zealand[vii] know something of the history of the land, in as much as Māori settled Aotearoa New Zealand from the Pacific more than 1,000

[vii] Reportedly a cartographer from the Dutch East India Company bestowed the name Nieuw Zeeland after the coastal province Zeeland in the Netherlands. When James Cook arrived in 1769, he anglicised the name to New Zealand. This name was never one used by Māori. There is general agreement that Aotearoa—which is commonly translated to 'long white cloud' or 'long bright world'—is one used historically. In this textbook we forefront Aotearoa to respect the importance of te Reo (Māori language) terminology.

years before European explorers started arriving. Pre-European contact saw Māori as a people deeply connected to the land and natural world around them.[35] Their societal life structures were based on kinship and tribal affiliations; laws were based on custom. When the British began their antipodean colonising, they initially opted for the larger continent of Australia, and it was the sealers and whalers who set up temporary residence in Aotearoa New Zealand. Eventually, settlers arrived, and by the early 1800s the population of Europeans was believed to be around 2,000. The number of Māori at that time was estimated to be around 125,000.[36]

In 1838 the British sought to annex Aotearoa New Zealand due to numerous unscrupulous purchases of Māori land and the lawlessness that had arisen among the people. On 6 February 1840, a treaty was drafted (Te Tiriti O Waitangi hereinafter referred to as Te Tiriti / the Treaty of Waitangi). The English version is referred to as the Treaty of Waitangi and was signed by the English and approximately 45 Māori Rangatira (chiefs). In addition, the Māori text of the treaty was taken to northern parts of the country and copies were sent to other areas of the land to obtain additional Māori signatures. In signing Te Tiriti, the chiefs are believed to have yielded their sovereignty to the Queen of England in exchange for the Queen's protection and the granting to Māori the same citizenship rights, privileges and duties enjoyed by the citizens of England. Te Tiriti was meant to be a partnership between Māori and the British Crown. Although it was intended to create unity, different understandings of Te Tiriti, and breaches of it, have caused conflict. Te Tiriti guaranteed Māori possession of their land but with a stipulation they could sell their land only to the Crown. Te Tiriti was to recognise Aotearoa New Zealand at that time as one nation but two peoples: Māori and non-Māori, mainly European settlers and their descendants. There has been a great deal of debate over the ensuing years about translations between the two versions that were not fully correct and therefore interpreted differently by many of the Māori chiefs who originally signed Te Tiriti.[37]

Initial reading of Te Tiriti seemed to promise benefits for both sides, but when more and more settlers arrived, they wanted to buy land. If Māori did not wish to sell, conflict would eventuate. Many lost their lives in the wars that erupted. But it was not only the wars that eroded the Māori population, it was also the diseases introduced by the Europeans to which Māori had little or no natural immunity. Loss of land also saw many living in poor conditions in makeshift camps with poor sanitation. By 1900 the Māori population had dropped to an estimated 45,000,[35] and the settlers considered Māori to be a 'disappearing race'. Their tikanga (general behaviour guidelines for daily life and interaction in Māori culture, commonly based on experience and learning that has been handed down through generations) was also being eroded.

The intent and provisions of the Te Tiriti O Waitangi were largely ignored until the 1970s when legislation was introduced requiring statutory bodies and government to undertake their responsibilities in a manner consistent with the founding promises of the treaty. In 1975 the Waitangi Tribunal (see www.waitangi-tribunal.govt.nz/) was established to consider claims by Māori against the Crown over breaches of principles of the treaty and to make recommendations to the government to provide recompense. Since 1985 the tribunal has been able to consider acts and omissions by the Crown dating back to 1840. This has provided Māori with an important means to have their grievances against the actions of past governments investigated. Aside from these actions and grievances, attention and awareness is now also on the aforementioned health and social disparities, and there is a focus on improving the health and social status of Māori while recognising and respecting all aspects of cultural being. It is now openly acknowledged that Aotearoa New Zealand's constitution demands all public policy gives attention to Te Tiriti O Waitangi. All crown agencies must be wholly culturally responsive to the needs and aspirations of Māori and actively innovate solutions to reduce social disparities that have a negative impact on Māori.

The legacy from those early years is a society with 'major ethnic and cultural disparities in health status and most other markers of Indigenous wellbeing'.[38] As well as alienation from land, Māori experienced impacts on their language (te reo) as a first language and their cultural way of being, their tikanga. They are over-represented in nearly all negative social and health statistics—for example, unemployment, poverty, housing, income, education, youth suicide rates and general health and wellbeing. Kearns and colleagues[38] suggest that the processes of colonisation such as that which Māori experienced resulted in the 'denigration, marginalisation and alienation' of the very essence of their culture. Consedine and Consedine[35] suggest that because of this colonisation 'the infrastructure of New Zealand society is structured to deliver white privilege. Only the exotic features of Māori culture were encouraged, where they benefited the country in areas such as tourism and sport.'

While most early settlers were British, since that period people have arrived from Europe as well as Asia. In the second half of last century, following the world wars, a significant migration of people from the Pacific began.[39] The population of Pacific peoples in Aotearoa New Zealand grew quite rapidly during the late 1960s and early 1970s and caused a great deal of racial tension at times with both Māori and non-Māori groups. An important aspect of reducing this tension and ultimately accepting Pacific groups was the formation of partnerships with various community groups and activities as well as an increase in intermarriage. By the late 1990s, a large proportion of Pacific people were born in Aotearoa New Zealand and increasingly their children were also of Māori and other ethnic descent. The other major population group to appear was from Asia. Arrival of Asian groups predates the Pacific groups, although in much smaller numbers. Many arrived in the late 19th century during gold rush days. Later in the 20th century, the number of different Asian groups increased dramatically, and at the 2006 Census they had exceeded the Pacific groups in population numbers. Much more recently, refugees and other settlers from Africa and the Middle East have arrived.

The diverse generations born and arriving in Aotearoa New Zealand since the first colonial settlers have afforded opportunities for miscegenation (a very old term referring to the process by which children are born to parents who were assumed to be of different 'races') of Aotearoa New Zealand's population groups.[39] As suggested earlier, although colonial thinking was that Māori would eventually disappear or be absorbed into the European population, this assumption has been discredited. However, it is this thinking that firmly influenced the collection of official statistics for much of the 20th century. Khawaja and colleagues[39] refer to the routine assignment of 'ethnic grouping' based on ancestry (degree of blood), with little or no regard to lifestyle, culture or beliefs. As we discuss further below, these concerns also characterised the Australian situation.

The Census of 2023 states that the population is almost 5.2 million people.[40] The most available recent 2018 statistics show that 74% identified themselves as being of European ethnicity and 16.5% Māori, with the remainder being Asian (15.1%),

Pacific Islander (8.1%), Middle Eastern, Latin American, African (1.5%) and other (1.2%).[40] The apparent anomaly in these figures is caused by people identifying with more than one ethnic group. Because people can identify with more than one ethnicity, the total number of ethnic responses may be greater than the number of people. Consequently, understanding ethnicity is important, and having a mutual understanding of this might be even more important. This is, however, not so simple, and later in this chapter we explore the ideology of ethnicity.

Population context—conclusion

Suffice to say in summary that Indigenous groups have their own structural, institutional and interpersonal philosophies and practices from which they operate. Nonetheless, colonised societies such as Aotearoa New Zealand and Australia develop to fit the lifestyle, values, priorities and beliefs of the incoming dominant cultures and so the culture of the colonisers becomes the norm in society's main institutions such as health, education, welfare, corrections and the media. It is this kind of sometimes hidden but always present cultural dominance and unexamined privilege that the practice of cultural safety, discussed below, seeks to overcome. The Australian Institute of Health and Welfare[41] stated:

> *Access to appropriate, high-quality and timely health care throughout life is essential for improving health outcomes for Aboriginal and Torres Strait Islander people (Indigenous Australians). Barriers affecting their access, however, remain, as observed in their disparities in their level of access compared with non-Indigenous Australians.*

Given the preventable deaths and poor health outcomes Indigenous Australians continue to experience in the Australian healthcare system, there is no reason to think this has changed in the ensuing years.[42] Just consider the case of Ms Dhu,[43,44] who died in police custody after being taken in for unpaid fines, or that of Gurrumul Yunupingu,[45] an internationally renowned singer whose internal bleeding was neglected for 8 hours by health professionals who made misguided assumptions that alcohol was the cause of his ill health, or that of Naomi Williams,[46] who was pregnant and sent home 18 times after seeking help before dying from a treatable infection (also see Cox & Best 2022[1]).

Culture, ethnicity, race, racism and health

Before we can begin to consider cultural issues as they relate to professional nursing practice, we need to be clear about what we mean by the various terms used in this context. The common terms used include culture, ethnicity, race and health. While there are numerous definitions of these terms, we have taken a constructionist view referring to the notion that humans create ideas about culture, ethnicity, race and health. That is, such concepts do not just appear from nature but are constructed by humans to serve certain purposes at certain times, so cultural safety is underpinned by the theory of social constructionism.[47]

Culture

PERSONAL CULTURE

Some definitions of people's personal culture focus on material culture: art, dress, artifacts and so on; others focus on the capacity of humans to symbolise their world and experience through, for example, language, religion and kinship. Many definitions discuss cultures as 'bounded wholes' where members share systematised/patterned values and beliefs. We particularly like the definition in Kluckhohn and Kelly[48] because it indicates the **importance of history** for our cultural identity and it is clear that culture is created and acts as a **potential** guide to action: 'By culture we mean all those historically created designs for living, explicit and implicit, rational, irrational, and nonrational, which exist at any given time as potential guides for the behavior of men ... culture is constantly being created and lost'. Such definitions can be contrasted with other versions that suggest that cultures are unvarying, bounded canons of beliefs and practices that all members of a society embrace to an equal degree.

Our view of culture is grounded in the idea that cultures are dynamic and adapt to new circumstances and that they are learnt—that is, one is **born into a culture, not born with culture**. Further, we assume that culture is strategic since we emphasise or de-emphasise aspects of our culture depending on current needs and circumstances. So, we are less interested in *C*ulture (e.g. high art or classical artistic traditions) and more interested in *c*ulture (lower case 'c') as the everyday meanings and motivations in peoples' lived experience, how they make sense of life experiences such as illness and explain it to themselves. That is to say, in cultural safety, culture is in the interaction between **worldviews** (values, beliefs, etc.) and **lifeworlds** (everyday life and the context in which it is experienced).

Further, for our purposes, culture includes but is not just about ethnicity and customs such as food, dress and religion, beliefs and values; it addresses differences in socioeconomic status, age, gender, gender identity, sexual orientation, ethnic origin, citizenship/migrant/refugee status, religious beliefs, values, disability and power relations.[47]

So, it follows from the above, that each of us have multiple cultural identities where we might identify primarily as a woman, or as a mother, or as a feminist, or as a footballer, or as an LGBTIQ+ person, or as a nurse and as a working-class Australian with English or some other ethnicity. Our culture influences the many tiny and significant decisions we make in everyday life that then determine what actions we take. Part of your challenge is to bring your personal cultural assumptions to mind so you can understand why you act the way you do, particularly in your professional life as a nurse. We discuss cultural assumptions further below, but first we consider how culture operates at levels beyond the individual.

ORGANISATIONAL, INSTITUTIONAL AND PROFESSIONAL CULTURES

At the level of individual people, it is crucial that you can distinguish ethnicity from culture. To help you decipher the difference between ethnicity and culture, consider the culture of nursing or policing, which have nothing to do with ethnicity or particular foods. Organisational, institutional and professional cultures encompass histories, power hierarchies, knowledges such as language and technical know-how, values, priorities, assumptions, behaviours, attitudes and perhaps dress. Organisational cultures are about ways of doing things, thinking about things and understanding things. Does this mean all nurses do and think the same thing when faced with a particular situation or set of circumstances? Does it mean that all hospital wards or health services do things exactly the same way? No. And that's the point. Culture is always learnt, dynamic, changing and strategic. It is negotiated and expressed and understood differently by people who identify with a particular cultural group who make up an organisation such as a health service or hospital.

Ethnicity

In current usage, the term ethnicity is generally used to refer to the ethnic group or groups a person identifies with or feels they belong to. It is also now recognised that people may identify with more than one ethnic group. As indicated above, ethnicity can be part of culture but is not the same thing as culture. Ethnicity refers to socially constructed group identification or belonging based on familial descent (kinship) and history and traditions in language, food, dress and so on. In multicultural Australia—with Aboriginal people and Torres Strait Islander people being the Indigenous populations—non-Indigenous Australians are still reluctant to speak of ethnicity and ethnic differences in relation to their own identities. Many New Zealanders and Australians no longer feel any links to the cultures to which their ancestors belonged but do not have a well-established or well-recognised alternative ethnic identity either. An example of this is the term 'New Zealand European' often used on data collection sheets; there are now many generations of New Zealanders who feel no linkage to their European ancestors and express a reluctance to note this term in relation to their ethnicity.[49] People in this situation may say things like '*I don't have an ethnic identity*', '*I am a New Zealander*' or '*I'm just Australian*'. At the beginning of a unit on cultural safety, Bachelor of Nursing students were asked to tell the group about their cultural and ethnic identity. Consider this comment by a student of European descent in her reflection:

> *Learning about cultural safety was great! Never actually sat down and thought about my own personal culture before. Very rewarding!*

This way of thinking, that culture and ethnicity is only about 'others', stems from the fact that many non-Indigenous Australians come from generations of people born in Australia, a country with a long tradition of seeing ethnicity and culture as belonging solely to 'people of colour' or to 'the others from elsewhere', not realising that, ethnically speaking, that includes them. We only have to reflect on the term 'culturally and linguistically diverse', commonly rendered as CALD in government policies in Australia. It is a catch-all phrase to describe immigrants and implies that culture and diversity belong to immigrants, not to 'us'. An Australian internet search using CALD will yield many hits that make this point evident. Further, newcomers are expected to assimilate into the mainstream culture, as is particularly evident in the process of becoming an Australian citizen, when it is necessary to sit a citizenship test (see www.citizenship.gov.au/).

Early thinking in both Australia and Aotearoa New Zealand around ethnicity was related to biological lineage only. To take the Aotearoa New Zealand example, if your father was 'full Māori' and your mother non-Māori, you were considered by default ethnically 'half-Māori', regardless of your cultural beliefs, upbringing or cultural affiliations. Such statements are no longer acceptable. A similar concept used in Australia was 'half-caste' to refer to someone with a parent who the government deemed to be a 'full-blooded Aborigine' and a parent who the government deemed to be white; the term, along with related terms such as 'quarter-caste' and 'octoroon', are considered highly insulting to Indigenous Australians who recognise them as a form of identity policing that seeks to control who can and cannot identify as Aboriginal and to reduce cultural identity to biological ancestry.[50] Interestingly, these terms are never applied to white people, revealing an underlying assumption about the purity of white ancestral lines, which of course is nonsense, particularly because there is no such entity as different biological races, a point we turn to below.

Power, race, racialisation and racism

Identifying the roots of scientific racism, Baker[51] reminds us that, 'From its beginning, the field of biology was enmeshed with racist ideas. In the 18th century, Carl Linnaeus, founder of modern taxonomy, classified humans into what became a racial hierarchy.' Baker[51] continues: 'Race, as it is now generally accepted by scientists, is **not a biological reality** but rather reflects the cultural and social underpinnings originally used to justify slavery and that live on in a myriad of ways' (emphasis added). So historically, the concept of race was used to bolster the power and dominance of European cultures by supporting their claims of superiority to all other people. These strategies claimed the right to control other people and to take their land, as happened in Australia and Aotearoa New Zealand, so the emergence of race is closely related to power. The assumed superiority of some groups over others is also called 'social Darwinism', a theory advanced by Herbert Spencer, who applied biological evolutionary theory to social life (Box 4.1) and linked it to ideas such as the 'great chain of being'[52] (Box 4.2).

Because dominant cultures are so used to thinking in terms of race, it is hard for many to accept that the variation in how humans look can be understood in terms of genetic adaptation to environments and to familial descent and is not evidence of the existence of discrete races of humans. The persistence of the idea that race is a biological fact is striking because it is commonly used to understand differences not only in skin colour and physical attributes but also in health status. Believers in scientific racism see health inequality as natural and inevitable and engage in 'blame the victim' thinking that sufferers 'brought it all on themselves'. Such claims are then used to justify and perpetuate structural inequality when we know that social marginality is the result of specific

Box 4.1 Race overview

Historically, the concept of 'race' was used to say some people were inferior to others.

- At first, women were considered to be inferior to men, then 'people of colour' were placed lower than white women and so on. See Box 4.2.

'Social Darwinism' applies biological evolution to the evolution of societies. It is linked to the idea that white people are superior.

- Some 'whites' claim that they are destined or have the right to rule over others.
- At their worst, ideas of the superiority of white people led to Hitler's fanatical eugenics and justified all forms of imperialism, as happened in the European settlement of Australia and the accompanying concept of terra nullius.

Box 4.2 The so-called 'great chain of being' and its misguided social hierarchy

Great chain of being

- God
- Angels
- Demons
- Man
- Woman
- Animals
- Plants
- Minerals

Misguided racial hierarchy

- Anglo Saxons/Europeans
- Asians
- Africans
- Aborigines

policies, laws, historical events, social practices and cultural contexts.

Baker[51] writes that 'Brandon Mahal, a radiation oncologist at the University of Miami Health Center who studies prostate cancer, cautions that genetics should not be used to blame health disparities on African Americans being somehow innately more susceptible to ill health'.

The fact that race is a social construct is becoming more accepted, but that does not lessen the lived experience of racism today. Racist beliefs, anchored in the scientific racism of a bygone era, persist and are mostly hidden because it is socially and politically unacceptable to air them. Race categories are still used to justify the exploitation of one group by another. So, to summarise, racism is treating people based on assumed 'race' rather than on shared humanity; racism is the result of processes of racialisation.

There is one more issue concerning race that some readers may find confusing. In a strategic reversal and rejection of inferiorisation, belonging to an Australian Aboriginal 'race' is a source of pride among Indigenous Australians. These circumstances are hardly surprising given that Indigenous Australians have been distinguished, categorised and subordinated since colonisation because of notions that they were a separate (and inferior) race, and like many non-Indigenous Australians, many believe that there is a biological basis to race. When someone identifies as a particular race based on history, nationality and geography, their right to reclaim this social construct and use it in this way to identify and differentiate themselves can only be legitimate. Clearly, there are differences between people in terms of culture, ancestry, language and different nationalities depending on where one has full citizenship rights. There are differences, too, in opportunity and social experience, many of which are based on peoples' appearance including skin colour. Therefore, it is not helpful to claim one is not racist because one is 'colour blind'. As we saw above, society is not colour blind; many privileges and freedoms (such as being able to be in the world without attracting police attention) are afforded to white-skinned people. All these matters contribute to differences in health, which we turn to now.

Health

Willis and Shandell[53] discuss the development of notions such as 'health', showing that concepts we take as givens are constructed by humans. For our purposes, it is important that you understand that *health is not just about the absence of disease* as it may be defined in Western medical terms but is about the whole person within their life context. This contextual aspect is captured in the following definition, which was articulated in developing Aboriginal and Torres Strait Islander health policy:

> *[Health] means not just the physical wellbeing of a person but refers to the social, emotional and cultural wellbeing of the whole Community in which each person can achieve their full potential as a human being thereby bringing about the total wellbeing of their Community. It is a whole of life view and includes the cyclical concept of life–death–life.*[54]

For Māori, 'health' is also realised through an understanding of various holistic health models. One commonly used model, Te Whare Tapa Wha, is known as the 'four cornerstones of health'. This approach compares health to the four walls of a house (a Whare), in which all four walls are necessary to ensure strength and symmetry.[55] It can be applied to any health issue affecting Māori from physical to psychological wellbeing. Looking after all aspects of wellbeing (the four walls) are **taha wairua** (spiritual), **taha**

hinengaro (mental and emotional), **taha tinana** (physical) and **taha whānau** (family) considerations. Together all four are necessary and when in balance, they represent 'best health'. Accordingly, if any one of these components is deficient, this may have a negative impact on a person's health or, metaphorically speaking, affect the integrity of the house.[56] Interestingly, Ramsden clarified that the four walls symbolised in Durie's model do not constitute an ancient whakatauki (reference point or maxim) since the model was initially constructed for health care services to 'assist in healing the division between biomedicine and an integrated approach to human care'.[47] Ramsden argued that this individualistic model did not consider social determinants such as education, unemployment, racism and powerlessness, issues that are vitally connected to health. However, the model has prevailed and still informs Māori health policy and healthcare delivery, as well as being used to explore the importance of looking at and supporting a person in a holistic way. It is the framework for Māori and Iwi health and disability service providers and clinicians.[57] What is important is that, when using this model, nurses think beyond the individual and see them within the whole context of their life and the impacts that broader social issues have on health.

When health is understood from a traditional Western biological model, the attention is on treating disease and symptoms with drugs and/or surgery. Today, nurses are taught to care for people within a holistic model, in which the focus is on finding the underlying cause of the symptoms and making lifestyle changes that are conducive to health. Biomedicine is deeply moralistic, with its strong emphasis on personal responsibility. The person is considered the authority on their body and becomes the expert in caring for themselves. Mainstream holistic health care is similar to the Indigenous models previously discussed in acknowledging that all people have physical, intellectual, psychological, social, emotional and spiritual needs. The neglect of any of these areas may reduce the ability to withstand the effects of stress and ill health. However, when health care or health promotion is individualistic, it can result in blaming people in terms of their 'lifestyle'. Focusing solely on the behaviour of individuals denies the impact of social determinants and unhelpfully assumes that everyone has the same access to the conditions necessary to promote, create or maintain health.

Nevertheless, the relationship between a person and a health professional is cooperative and complementary today compared with previous eras where patients were just expected to do as they were told. Such shifts in the relationship between nurses and patients can be enhanced by the model of cultural safety, which also recognises that, not only might we all be culturally different, but also that society treats us differently, that there are social determinants of health. It is these dynamics that cultural safety seeks to address.

Cultural safety

In keeping with notions about race in the late 19th to early 20th century as already discussed, early nursing in Aotearoa New Zealand and Australia reduced culture to ethnicity and was therefore a racialised term, since ethnicity and culture were largely conceptualised as belonging to racialised others. The term 'culture' referred to superficial differences in appearance between the original inhabitants and colonisers, while the notion of civilisation denoted the superiority of colonisers' cultures. In their seminal paper Richardson[58] states: 'There is a tendency for colonising peoples to work from an ethic of beneficence, to presume that the dissemination of their cultural norms and beliefs will necessarily be to the benefit to the society affected', with an associated assumption that the knowledge of others was therefore inferior. As the century went on, nursing interest in culture generally declined, although some nurses chose to explore it further in university studies in the social sciences and humanities, such as in anthropology.

As indicated in the introduction to this chapter, from the 1970s, interest refocused on the relationships between nurses and patients and the term 'culture' became important to nurses and health service users. The new ideology, 'transcultural nursing', authored by Madeleine Leininger, was developed. In transcultural nursing, an essentialised idea of culture assumed the existence of culturally based healthcare needs of specific minority groups. These 'cultural needs' were to be learnt and used as a checklist to assess the needs of people who might identify with a specific culture. In this way, transcultural nursing positions nurses as the expert on the culture of 'others'. The consequence of such an approach is perhaps best summed up by bell hooks (the author chooses to not capitalise their name):

> *No need to hear your voice when I can talk about you better than you can speak about yourself … Only tell me about your pain. I want to know your story. And then I will tell it back to you in a new way. Tell it back to you in such a way that it becomes mine, my own. Re-writing you I write myself anew. I am still author, authority. I am still colonizer, the speaking subject and you are now the center of my talk.*[59]

The key point is that the unique experience of the person becomes cannibalised by the nurse. The person is expected to behave according to stereotypical attributes that outsiders have deemed as 'typical' of their particular group according to these idealist notions of the group's culture. The transcultural model was not fully embraced in Aotearoa New Zealand or Australia, although the second author of this text can recall her nursing student days in Aotearoa New Zealand when she was directed to visit various cultural (religious) sites to interview key leaders and ask them what their particular beliefs were around healthcare practices. She then had to write a report describing particular health preferences for these groups. An assumption was that having undertaken this exercise, the nurse would know how to work with any person from that group if they come into hospital.

However, we do not accept this argument. In this text, we focus on holism: students are facilitated to develop personal, professional and organisational cultural self-awareness and to assess and respond to the biological, psychological and social needs of specific people. The key is to avoid projecting dominant social assumptions on people as if groups are homogenous and a person is merely a representative of a specific cultural label or identity. The transition to culturally safe nursing from this point seems much simpler.

The Nursing and Midwifery Board of Australia[7] defines cultural safety as:

> *A philosophy of practice that is about how a health professional does something, not [just] what they do. It is about how people are treated in society, not about their diversity as such, so its focus is on systemic and structural issues and on the social determinants of health. Cultural safety represents a key philosophical shift from providing care regardless of difference, to care that takes account of people's unique needs. It*

requires nurses and midwives to undertake an ongoing process of self-reflection and cultural self-awareness, and an acknowledgment of how a nurse's/midwife's personal culture impacts on care. In relation to Aboriginal and Torres Strait Islander health, cultural safety provides a decolonising model of practice based on dialogue, communication, power sharing and negotiation, and the acknowledgement of white privilege. These actions are a means to challenge racism at personal and institutional levels, and to establish trust in healthcare encounters.

In contrast:

Unsafe cultural practice comprises any nursing practice which diminishes, demeans or disempowers the cultural identity and wellbeing of the individual.[60]

Cultural safety is a term initially unique to Aotearoa New Zealand and nursing education. The pioneer of the concept is Māori nurse Irihapeti Ramsden, so it is considered to form part of what is now known as Indigenous knowledges. The concept of **kawa whakaruruhau** (cultural safety) arose out of a nursing education leadership hui held in Christchurch, Aotearoa New Zealand in 1989 in response to recruitment and retention issues of Māori nurses. The National Health and Hospitals Reform Commission guidelines were initially written by Ramsden in 1991 and further developed by a council committee and Ramsden. By 1992 the Nursing Council of New Zealand had adopted the following definition of cultural safety:

The effective nursing practice of a person or family from another culture and is determined by that person or family. Culture includes, but is not restricted to, age or generation; gender; sexual orientation; occupation and socioeconomic status; ethnic origin or migrant experience; religious or spiritual belief; and disability. The nurse delivering the nursing service will have undertaken a process of reflection on his or her own cultural identity and will recognise the impact that his or her personal culture has on his or her professional practice. Unsafe cultural practice comprises any action which diminishes, demeans, or disempowers the cultural identity and wellbeing of an individual.[60]

Cultural safety relates to the experience of the recipient of a healthcare service. It gives health service users the power to resist or call out practices that demean, diminish and disempower them. It therefore contributes to achieving positive health outcomes and experiences. By this process, the meaning and experience of a person's illness is validated rather than challenged by biomedical understandings, and people retain the power to provide feedback on any negative experiences. Crucially services must undergo structural change to create and resource policy and processes and structures to support culturally safe practice and to challenge culturally unsafe practice.

Box 4.3 outlines the BE SAFE strategy towards cultural safety.

Box 4.3 The BE SAFE strategy towards cultural safety

Be curious to understand every person or family you work with.

Enquire and meet needs in ways that develop trust.

Self as a bearer of culture accepting that it influences our practice.

Acknowledge that our attitudes, values, beliefs, assumptions and unexamined prejudices about or towards others influence our practice and can be challenged.

Freedom of others to be themselves, assured by using clear, value free, open and respectful communication.

Ensure healthcare delivery constantly adheres to the principles of cultural safety and agitate for resourced structures and processes to interrogate and address culturally unsafe practice.

The process inherent in cultural safety education includes exploring the culture of nursing, recognising the impact that personal culture has on professional practice and the subsequent power relationship between nurses and the consumers of nursing care.[60] Cultural safety then 'contends that people are so diverse that teaching simple ritual and custom stereotypes rigidifies ideas of culture and does not allow for human diversity (nurse or patient), nor does it take into account historical effects and socio-economic status'.[61] See Ramsden's explanation in Box 4.4.

Following the model of 'cultural safety', we support the position that describing the practices, beliefs and values of diverse population groups in nurse education should not occur because this fosters an ideology of sameness and an erroneous assumption that culture is a simplistic concept that can be captured in lists of things to remember and do. It is this checklist mentality that is intrinsic to transcultural nursing.

Think about yourself being the recipient of nursing care. What do you need the nurse to know about you? Will that be the same as the person in the bed next to you who may share your cultural identity and come from the same ethnic group as you and be the same age and gender as you? What if there are two Vietnamese people in hospital? What if both identify as Vietnamese but one grew up in Australia and one in Vietnam? What if one happens to also identify as gay? What happens if one is a male and one a female? What happens if the male is 50 years old and very well off, but the woman is 16 years old and from a poor family? Are their needs the same because they both identify as Vietnamese? We stress that each person is an individual with many unique ways of being. Therefore, the underpinning philosophy of cultural safety is that each person should be nursed 'regardful of all that makes them unique', encompassing the cultural, emotional, social, economic and political contexts in which they live.[47,62] Ramsden talks about the nurse as a bearer of culture. She maintains that nurses must understand their own cultures to fully respond to the culture of others.

Cultural safety in contrast with transcultural nursing is summed up well by this newly graduated registered nurse in Aotearoa New Zealand reflecting on her own cultural safety education and initial puzzlement that she wasn't learning about specific cultures. She said in her summary of the course:

> *I can remember finding the concepts quite confusing initially. I think it was because I had trouble distinguishing them from a more transcultural perspective, as I thought it was concerned with learning about specific cultural differences and applying those in practice to various groups (i.e. Māori, Muslims, etc.). My understanding of cultural safety now is about knowing my own assumptions and being mindful about how this might impact on interactions. ... Overall though, cultural safety prevents us taking a one-size-fits-all approach to care.*[63]

Box 4.4 Ramsden's explanation

Cultural safety is based in a postmodern, transformed and multilayered meaning of culture as diffuse and individually subjective. It is concerned with power and resources, including information, its distribution in societies and the outcomes of information management. Cultural safety is deeply concerned with the effect of unequal resource distribution on nursing practice and patient wellbeing. Its primary concern is with the notion of the nurse as a bearer of his or her own culture and attitudes and consciously or unconsciously exercised power.

Source: Ramsden 2002[47]

Self-reflexivity and self-awareness

As indicated in the definition of cultural safety above, the first step of the process for people, professions and services is being committed to an ongoing practice of critical reflection. At the person level, self-reflection on one's own cultural identity and on social status, privilege and overall life experiences is crucial. As nurses we work in teams. It is by acknowledging and knowing our own beliefs, attitudes, assumptions, biases and values and respecting that the beliefs and values of others are equally legitimate that we minimise the impact of cultural dominance in health care. To truly understand how to relate to others, you must first understand yourself; this requires personal self-reflection and self-critique of the various personal, historical and social influences that impact on you. Students often find this process of self-awareness highly rewarding, as is shown in this student's comment: 'The personal reflection that was common in this unit opened a side of myself that I had never ventured to, made me really think where I had come from …'.

Box 4.5 has some guidelines for helping you to become culturally self-aware.

Box 4.5 Strategies for self-awareness

Think about the cultural group(s) that you identify with.

- List them.
- What is your way of living within your group(s)? (Think about age or generation, gender, gender identity, sexual orientation, occupation and socioeconomic status, ethnic origin or migrant experience, citizenship or refugee status, religious or spiritual belief and disability.)
- Are there different groups within these areas that you can identify with?

Think about the people, things and places that have socialised you.

- Who and what had impacts on you as you grew up (e.g. family, school, peers, environment, the mass media, popular culture, social media, politics, society in general, laws, policies, public health, national events/celebrations, international events, global events)?
- What did you learn from these areas regarding healthcare practices?
- What experiences shaped you?
- Did you grow up with enough (love, food, friends, money, etc.)?
- What values did you learn from your family?
- Were these the same as values held by your peers/teachers/friends/others?
- Do you hold the same values today as you did when you were growing up?
- Which values guide your decision making and how you see the world?
- Are values something that will affect your practice as a nurse?
- What customs/traditions do you and your families have around events such as births, birthdays, deaths, weddings, graduations?
- Are there certain cultural celebrations that your family participates in such as Chinese New Year, Christmas, Ramadan?
- What types of food do you eat?
- What are your beliefs about the big questions in life? For example: How did the world get here? How did I get here? What is my purpose?
- Where did these beliefs come from? Are they changeable?
- What attitudes do you hold about people you see as different from yourself?
- Are there particular groups of people that you hold prejudices towards?
- How do these prejudices make you feel?
- Do you feel these prejudices are justified? What values are these based on?
- What could you do to change your prejudices?

The misunderstandings of cultural safety and how racism leads to neglect and death

Many people when they first come across the term 'cultural safety' immediately think about 'race' and the ethnicity—of others! Common statements heard are '*When I nurse people, I don't see colour; we're all equal*'; and '*I treat everyone the same*'. The problem with this thinking is that treating everyone the same is a denial of inequality. As already indicated if colour does not matter, then why are there so many disadvantages or even entitlements that go with skin colour or with a family's cultural membership? A person's culture of origin and colour does matter in a culturally unsafe world as it brings different privileges, assumptions and varying levels of influence over health outcomes. Consider the experience of the young Indigenous woman described by Davey:[64]

> *The 19-year-old told emergency department doctors and nurses that her pain was 10 out of 10, and a test revealed her blood pressure was extremely low. She was given Mylanta and some morphine and told she had indigestion. No scan was performed to see if the pain had anything to do with her pregnancy. When Jane said she was still in severe pain, more Mylanta was given to her. Staff tried to send her home, but Jane collapsed back on to the bed while trying to get dressed ... In fact, Jane was bleeding internally, and her life was at risk. She was suffering from an ectopic pregnancy, a condition where a foetus develops outside the womb, usually in a fallopian tube.*

The power you have as a nurse in a healthcare relationship is well illustrated here and often is about your proximity to the dominant cultures of the country you are in. As relayed earlier, such issues have not gone away and Jane's is one case being examined in Australia by the National Justice Project[42] that is investigating instances of racial profiling, discrimination and negligence experienced in the Australian healthcare system by First Nations Australians and some other marginalised groups. Health inequality and what could be considered criminal neglect such as in the cases of Ms Dhu, Naomi Williams and Gurrumul Yunupingu cited earlier is directly related to the decisions nurses and other health professionals make when working with Aboriginal and Torres Strait Islander people. That is, these unnecessary and tragic outcomes result from the culture of health professionals, not from that of Aboriginal and Torres Strait Islander people or any other service user. In the case of Naomi Williams, the coroner found that her death was related to racialised preconceptions in the healthcare system.[65] **It is circumstances such as these that make cultural safety a necessary approach in nursing care.**

Biculturalism was a key element of the postcolonial theory of cultural safety; biculturalism originally referred to the relationship between Māori and the colonising state—the Crown—gesturing to the inherent imbalance of power involved.[47] The concept has evolved somewhat to refer to interpersonal encounters in clinical practice that always involve at least two cultures: the culture of the nurse and the culture of the person being served. These interactions of course take place within the cultures of professions, services and institutions. The recognition that these multifaceted cultural dimensions influence health care is in contrast to transcultural nursing that does not recognise the power differences inherent in its assumption that health service users are exotic, and that nurses and health systems are somehow free of culture. Furthermore, people have different abilities to exert control and influence in situations or relationships, especially in healthcare contexts that are inherently disempowering for service users who must rely on health service staff for their most intimate and basic needs. Imbalanced power relations also characterise our social, economic and political structures and institutions, with power and control usually being vested in members of dominant groups. See also Box 4.6. For a summary of the impacts of both cultural dominance and a change towards cultural safety see Figure 4.2.

Cultural safety education

The purpose of cultural safety in nursing education is not about the description of practices, beliefs and values of ethnic groups. As we now know, learning other peoples' rituals, customs and practices can be misleading and does not address the complexity of human behaviours and social realities. The assumption that cultures are simplistic can lead to a checklist approach by health professionals, which negates the contingent, strategic, contextual and dynamic nature of culture. Cultural safety education focuses on the knowledge and understanding of the self, professions, institutions, history and power structures of society. To practise cultural safety, nurses must understand their own culture, the sociopolitical context they are working in and the theory of power relations (Box 4.6 and Figure 4.3). Cultural safety education facilitates the ongoing process of reflection enabling clarification of values, beliefs and assumptions and how they sit with educational accreditation and with professional regulation, codes and standards. It gives a theoretical underpinning to professional nursing practice, introduces sociological approaches to health and health service, provides tools and a language to think with and so deepens the capacity for critical thinking on the part of nursing graduates.

In everyday work, cultural safety is underpinned by communication and recognition of the diversity in worldviews and lifeworlds (both within and between cultural groups including nurses' own). The impact of colonisation and ongoing marginalisation of minority groups or of those who choose to live differently to the expectations of the dominant culture creates diversity in lifeworlds—the context of life as it is experienced. As Ramsden put it: 'In the future it must be the patient who makes the final statement about the quality of care which they receive. Creating ways in which this commentary may happen is the next step in the cultural safety journey.'[47] This step remains a challenge in the implementation of cultural safety to date.

Box 4.6 Towards achieving cultural safety in your nursing practice

- Know your own story and its influences and accept that your way of knowing and doing things is not the only way.
- Practise cultural humility—never assume you know.
- Show respect—ask permission.
- Engage community accompaniment—find allies, contact cultural advisors.
- Always be respectful and collaborative.
- Remember that therapeutic nursing practice is grounded in relationships.
- Be aware of your timing. Ask yourself 'Is this the right time to be offering this particular form of service?'
- Focus on family-centred care when possible.
- Remember the best solutions are found through collaborative problem solving rather than expert/authority.
- Every situation should be reciprocal and mutual.
- Be aware that old and new forms of colonialism deplete cultures, communities and roles for families.
- Think about informed consent and what you may need to do to ensure it is understood.
- Do not demean, disempower or diminish others' choices.

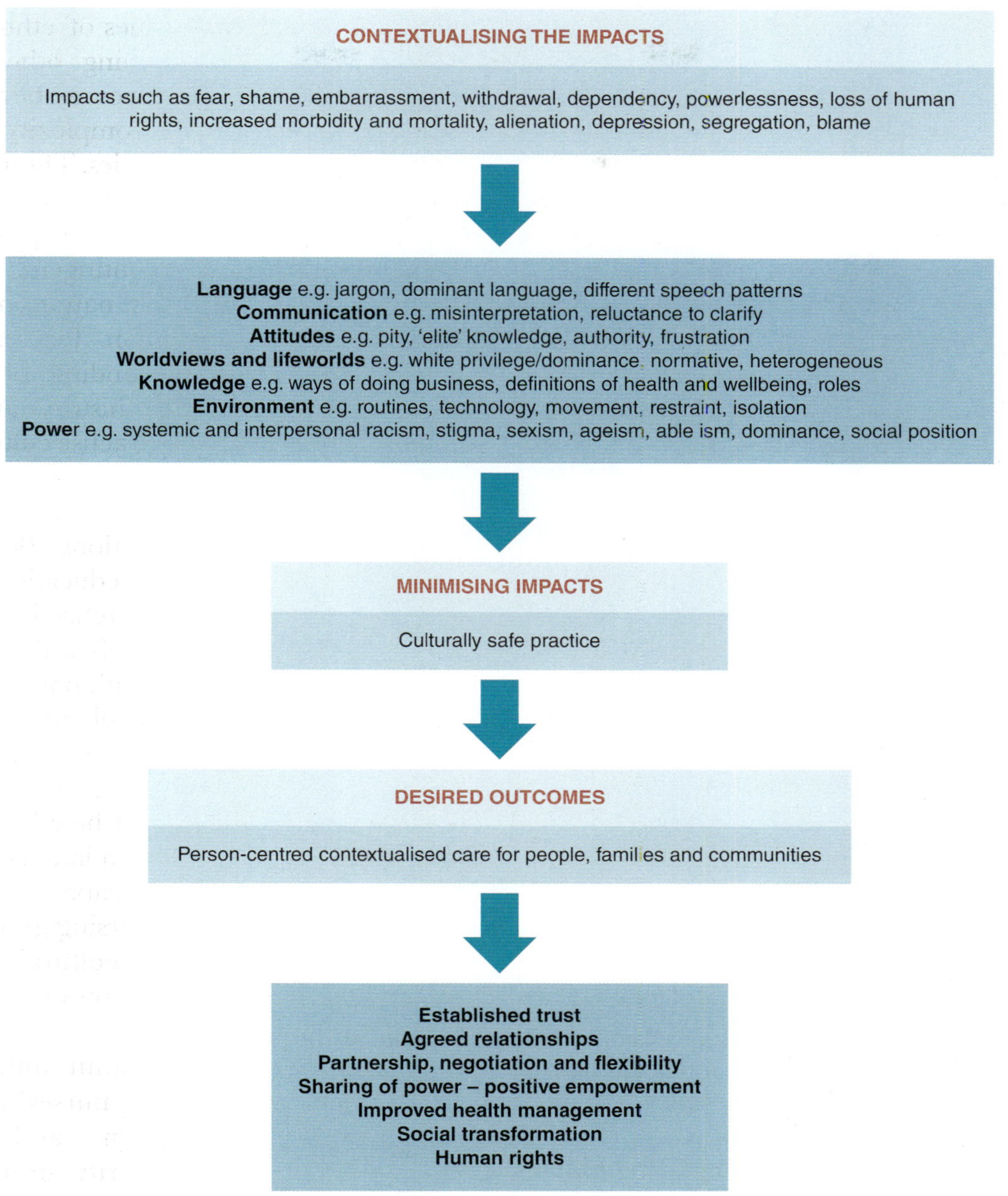

FIGURE 4.2 Cultural safety addressing the impacts of systemic cultural dominance. Source: Cox et al. 2021[14]

Cultural competence versus cultural safety

A new graduate nurse reflecting on her experience of learning about cultural safety as a student describes a clinical situation that helped her make sense of her learning and that nicely articulates the problem with the idea of cultural competency, the 'other'-centred approach of transculturalism discussed above.

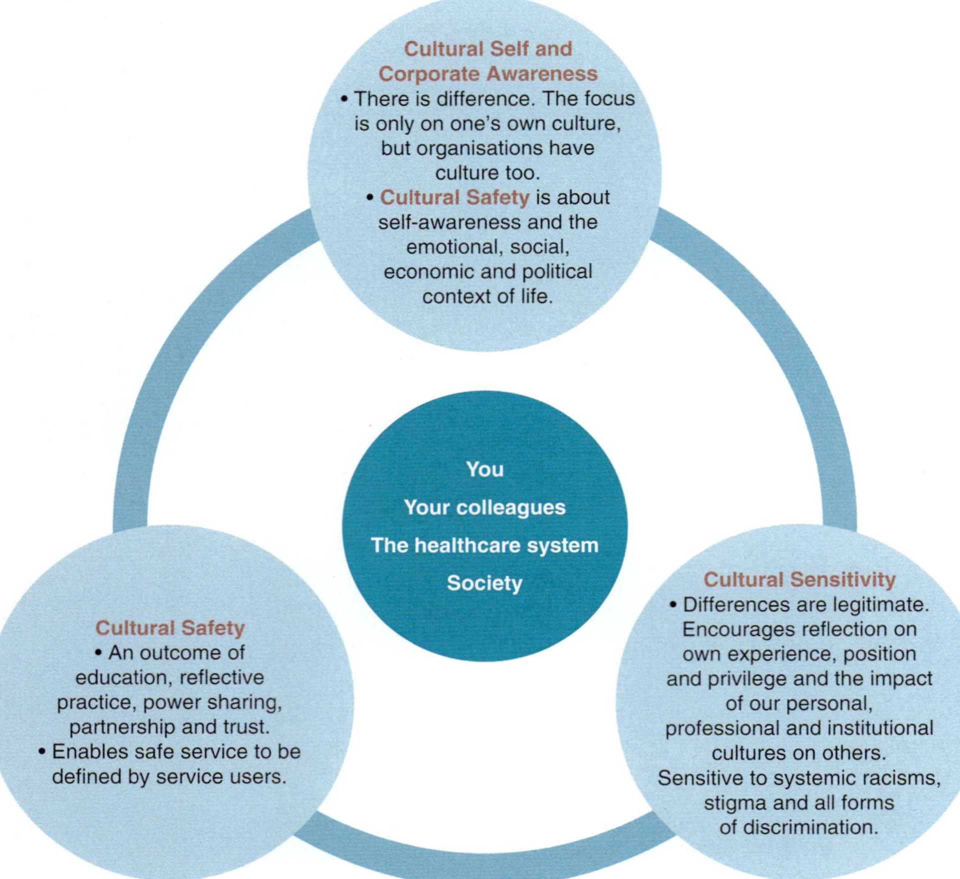

FIGURE 4.3 Cultural safety as an ongoing process Source: Cox et al. 2021[14]

Our cultural safety education was awesome; I just went to an in-service session at [hospital] a few weeks ago about cultural competency, and a lot of the stuff we were taught in nursing school was in there. Cultural awareness is a massive aspect of my nursing ... the best point I took from it all was to take cues from the patient/service user. If I'm not sure, I ask the service user directly ... they know their own culture best. I recently had a patient with a 'Buddhist outlook on life'; I offered to access some support for him, but he declined stating that he doesn't practise; he just shares some of the same views. So it would have been inappropriate to access that support for him, however it was appropriate to ask. Another person might have the same view AND want to access spiritual support ... I also think the biggest thing to cultural safety is being aware of my own culture. I'm working on this all the time and exploring it during my supervision.[66]

As indicated at the beginning of this chapter, there are many terms used to describe approaches to matters of culture and nursing care. Here we have focused on the approach of cultural safety. Many students come to courses on culture expecting to learn all about other cultures. The first author recalls a student who, after doing a unit of study on cultural safety, complained, '*I don't even know what that headdress that Muslims wear is called!*' This, of course, brings us to the very crux of the matter: there are various and complex dimensions to head, face and body coverings with different words, meanings and applications among the many cultural groups who wear them. With so many different cultures and so much variation within culture, it is quite impossible to expect students to learn about the diverse cultures that they will encounter in their work. As Warren[67] argues, generalising approaches to cultural competence conceptualises cultures as bounded wholes that exist out there to be learnt, rather than appreciating culture as a broad, dynamic, relational concept as used in cultural safety.

Becoming culturally safe is not a one-lesson program but rather a lifetime process of study and learning. There are several discrete areas in which you must have knowledge:

- your own cultural identity, social status, power and privilege
- the culture, power and privilege of the nursing profession
- the culture, power and privilege of the healthcare system
- the holistic needs of the person as they or their families/carers describe them to you.

Nursing students will notice that more and more institutions are mandating that those who practise must take cultural issues into account when providing health care. We turn to these requirements in Australia and Aotearoa New Zealand after first considering some crucial aspects of nursing care.

Communication

There are many forms of illegal discrimination based on ethnicity, skin colour, national origin, citizenship status, class, gender, gender identity and ability that frequently limit the opportunities of people to gain equal access to and good outcomes from healthcare services. Systemic racism is of particular concern.[68] A form of systemic racism is that the Australian and Aotearoa New Zealand healthcare systems assume strong English proficiency in healthcare encounters. However, for people who do not speak English or for whom it is a second or third language, seeking care in healthcare settings such as hospitals, nursing homes, clinics, day surgery centres and mental health facilities, language is a considerable barrier. As we saw in the section on population statistics, for each context there is a remarkable variety of languages used as a first language in Australia.

Those for whom English is not a first language experience barriers due to the system doing all its business in English. If there are challenges in speaking, reading, writing and understanding English, the result is limited access to critical public health, hospital and other medical and social services to which all Australians are legally entitled. Many health and social service programs provide information about their services in English only. When people whose first language is not English seek health care at hospitals or medical clinics in Australia and Aotearoa New Zealand, they are frequently faced with receptionists, nurses and doctors who speak English only. Inability to communicate with each other severely limits the ability to gain access to these services and to take part in programs and often results in delays in providing care and services based on inaccurate or incomplete information. For example, regarding medication, if a person with minimal understanding of English is not given clear, understandable instructions, adherence to or incorrect dosage may be a problem. Services denied, delayed or provided under such circumstances could have serious consequences for both users and providers of health care.

Chapter 7 describes in more detail how to communicate with people for whom English may be their second, third or fourth language or not in their lexicon at all, how to interact with interpreters and what services are available when no interpreter is available. It is vital that interpreters be present to not only serve to verbally translate the conversation but who are also able to assist you to conduct health assessments.

Family

Long ago, Laing[69] indicated that the concept of the family is a difficult one, and yet the term is invoked as if it is self-evident. Family means different things to different people, and it is very challenging to provide one definition of family. One of the biggest mistakes made in health care happens when the concept of family is considered from a mainstream understanding only or from rigid takes on Indigenous traditional kinship structures. In contemporary mainstream society, the concept of a nuclear family (a mum, dad and children) is most often assumed by health professionals to be the context that everyone lives within, when in fact this form of family is decreasingly the case, only making up around 43% of the total.[70] There are many occasions when someone's circumstances differ from the nuclear family type, when the people they designate as their family are not regarded as family at all by health services and, at times, such designations of next of kin by people can be considered deviant. For example, people in same-sex marriages/partnerships experience considerable difficulty in this regard.

It is crucial to think about how someone's family functions regarding healthcare decisions and hospital visiting preferences. This matter is especially important for Indigenous people who may designate next of kin and family relatedness in ways that are unfamiliar to nurses whose knowledge base is grounded in the assumptions made by the cultures of medicine and nursing. These nurses focus their care decisions on individuals and, for many, the idea of traditional marriage and the notion of blood relatedness as the only acceptable conditions to name someone as next of kin is entrenched.

Consider the following scenario: A young Indigenous man was admitted to a metropolitan intensive care unit (ICU) following a suicide attempt. His mother rang chapter author Leonie Cox (a non-Indigenous person) and requested that she go to the ICU to visit him. At the hospital ward, staff insisted that only close family could be allowed in to see the man. The problem was that the man's close family was several hundred kilometres away. An Indigenous health worker was at the ICU and knew of Leonie's long-term relationship with the family and convinced the nurses that she should be allowed to visit. When the young man was moved to a general ward, he introduced her to the doctor as 'my sister'.

We encourage you to bring to mind your assumptions about family and then to think very differently about family to encompass varied circumstances through a process of critical reflection. We know that in Australia and Aotearoa New Zealand families are diverse, so it is important we understand how to ensure family is considered in a person's health care, according to the context they describe. Historically, due to government policy of the day, many Indigenous people were raised in institutions or with white families, and so consider the people with whom they were reared as family.[17] Sadly, this is still true today due to the vast over-representation of Indigenous children in child removal practices. Aboriginal and Torres

Strait Islander children and young people are over-represented among those in out-of-home care. For those aged 10 to 14 years the rate was 63 per 1,000 Indigenous children—11 times the rate for non-Indigenous children. For those aged 15 to 17, it was 52 per 1,000 Indigenous children—9.3 times the rate for non-Indigenous children.[71] Think about who you include when you talk about your family. You might live with people you regard as family even though they are not blood relatives. Who can correctly say who someone's next of kin is? It might be the birth family or those who raised the person or perhaps the family they have created with a partner. There are numerous possibilities. How will you support same-sex relationships and struggles to have partners accepted as spouses and next of kin? How about those situations in which children have two mothers or two fathers? Think about people with longstanding estrangement from their families due to institutionalisation, imprisonment and other factors. There are times when the person may want staff members contacted because they are their significant others, rather than their birth families.

Making assumptions in this area of nursing care can bring significant distress for people. Culturally safe nurses and the profession as a whole are aware that our cultural assumptions are just that—they are not universal ways of being. We are alert to different ways of understanding the world and social institutions such as the family, or the support networks that constitute family for many. In sum, the concept of family and who is important and who can make decisions for someone can be decided only by service users themselves, in the context of their particular circumstances.

Cultural identity

Our identities as cultural beings are not only based on being born into a particular cultural milieu but are strongly related to our experiences as we go through life. Just as all members of a single family are not exactly the same and in fact may hold quite different beliefs and values from their parents and siblings, those who identify as belonging to a particular culture do not experience or express that cultural identity in the same way. In line with the broad definition of culture used in cultural safety, aspects of a person's cultural identity are influenced by their ethnicity, their gender and gender identity, their socioeconomic status, their ability or disability, their education and their status within society as members of either dominant or minority groups. Also, many people socialised in cultures in which traditional healthcare resources are used, such as in some Indigenous communities, may prefer to use this type of care even when living in a mainstream cultural setting with mainstream healthcare resources available. It is therefore not possible to teach you all the cultural dimensions that shape a person's worldview and create their lifeworld; these will be unique to each person. However, it is important that you understand that differences exist and are legitimate and that you know your own cultural identity and the assumptions that underlie it.

Spirituality and religion; philosophy and secularity

One possible component of a person's cultural identity is their religion or spirituality, but nurses must be mindful that many people hold an atheist or secularist philosophy and will not appreciate discussions of religion or spirituality.

This point is especially relevant for those nurses who hold strong religious or spiritual beliefs themselves, as at times they may not appreciate how distressing it is to non-religious people to have these issues raised. Nonetheless, spiritual or religious factors are important to many people, but these dimensions are often overlooked in health assessment, and this could be a particular problem for a secularist nurse who is indifferent to spiritual matters. If religion or spirituality is an integral part of a person's culture, their beliefs may influence their explanation of the cause(s) of illness, perception of its severity and choice of healer(s). In times of crisis, such as serious illness and impending death, religion and spirituality may be a source of consolation for the person and for their family. Religious or spiritual leaders may exert considerable influence on the person's decision making about acceptable medical and surgical treatment, choice of healer(s) and other aspects of the illness.

Religion and spirituality and a secular position play a most significant role in the ways people practise their health care. There are countless health-related behaviours promoted by nearly all religions or spiritualities and by rationalist secularity. The following list presents selected examples: ceremonies and rituals, meditating, exercising and maintaining physical fitness, getting enough sleep, being vaccinated, being willing to have the body examined, undertaking a pilgrimage for health reasons, telling the truth about how you feel, maintaining family viability, hoping for recovery, coping with stress, undergoing genetic screening and counselling, being able to live with a disability and caring for children.[72]

One's philosophy then, be it religious/spiritual or secular, gives a frame of reference and a perspective with which to organise information about health. Beliefs about health can constitute a system of health practices that are meaningful to the person. In healthcare settings, you will frequently encounter people who are searching for a spiritual meaning to help explain their illnesses or disabilities. Some healthcare providers find spiritual assessment difficult because of the abstract and personal nature of the topic, or due to their own secular position, whereas others feel quite comfortable discussing spiritual matters. Comfort with and mindfulness of your own beliefs is the foundation to effective assessment of the needs of others, including the ability to assess **whether or not a person requires a discussion of such matters**.

The concept and experience of time

Inherent in human socialisation and experience are approaches to time. Physicist Carlo Rovelli[73] notes that time is not what it seems to be and that it slows down and speeds up depending on where one is located. However, Western cultures' (including medicine and nursing) assumptions about time are based on notions of historical time, which conceives of it as linear with a past, a present and a future. The cultures of nursing and health systems are especially concerned with tasks and goals focused on 'now', and the future is perceived as vague or unpredictable. But there are alternative concepts of time such as that time is circular, as evident in various religious traditions, so that life and death are interdependent and constitute a never-ending cycle rather than the abrupt end in linear time. This idea is evident in the Indigenous definition of health quoted earlier.[74] Similarly in Māori perspectives of time, the past, the present and the future are intertwined, life is a continuous cosmic process and time has no restrictions.[75]

These circumstances have implications for nursing care. As Bruce[76] explains:

> *If time is primarily understood as a resource that is running out and must be managed effectively, then nursing actions may be guided by values of efficiency and management in assisting families to use their precious time in the best way possible. A role for nurses becomes one of assisting patients to better understand what they need to do in preparing to die and using the remaining time wisely and effectively.*

As this author argues, such an approach may prevent a person fully experiencing the now as they are rushed from one thing to the next. Bruce also clarifies that time is both a concept and an experience and that our perceptions of time shift depending on what is happening. We all know this from our own experience. As Bruce puts it, we are familiar with 'feeling the spaciousness of "free time" or the taut constriction of "running out" of time, the symmetry of "being timely", or the paradox of going beyond time'.[76] Thus, one of the major areas in which cultural conflicts between nursing culture and service users occur is the failure to understand that there is more than one way to perceive and experience time.

Further, the way people value time differently may impact on the way they assess priorities to do with their health care. There could be problems with keeping appointments, adhering to medication regimens, or differing priorities where family business may take precedence over appointments and the use of resources on personal health. It is important that nurses try to understand what is happening in people's lives [the lifeworld] to limit a sense of frustration and to prevent applying nurses' or services' culturally specific perceptions, values, assumptions and judgements to people's health and illness behaviours. See Figure 4.4 for a graphic depiction of how the nurses and broader levels of cultures interact with power dynamics in clinical decision making, such as those that led to the death of Naomi Williams and many others as indicated earlier.

Ideas about causes of illness and disease

Disease causation may be viewed in several ways including naturalistic or holistic, magico-religious biomedical and sociological perspectives or some combination of these.

Naturalistic

Some people explain the cause of illness from a **naturalistic** or **holistic** perspective: the belief that human life is only one aspect of nature and is a part of the general order of the cosmos. People with this perspective may believe that the forces of nature must be kept in natural balance or harmony. The naturalistic perspective posits that the laws of nature create imbalances, chaos and disease. People embracing the naturalistic view may use metaphors such as the 'healing power of nature', and they may call the earth 'Mother'.

Magico-religious

Another major way in which people explain the causation of illness is from a **magico-religious** perspective. The basic premise is that the world is seen as an arena in which supernatural forces dominate. The fate of the world and those in it depends on the action of supernatural forces for good or evil.

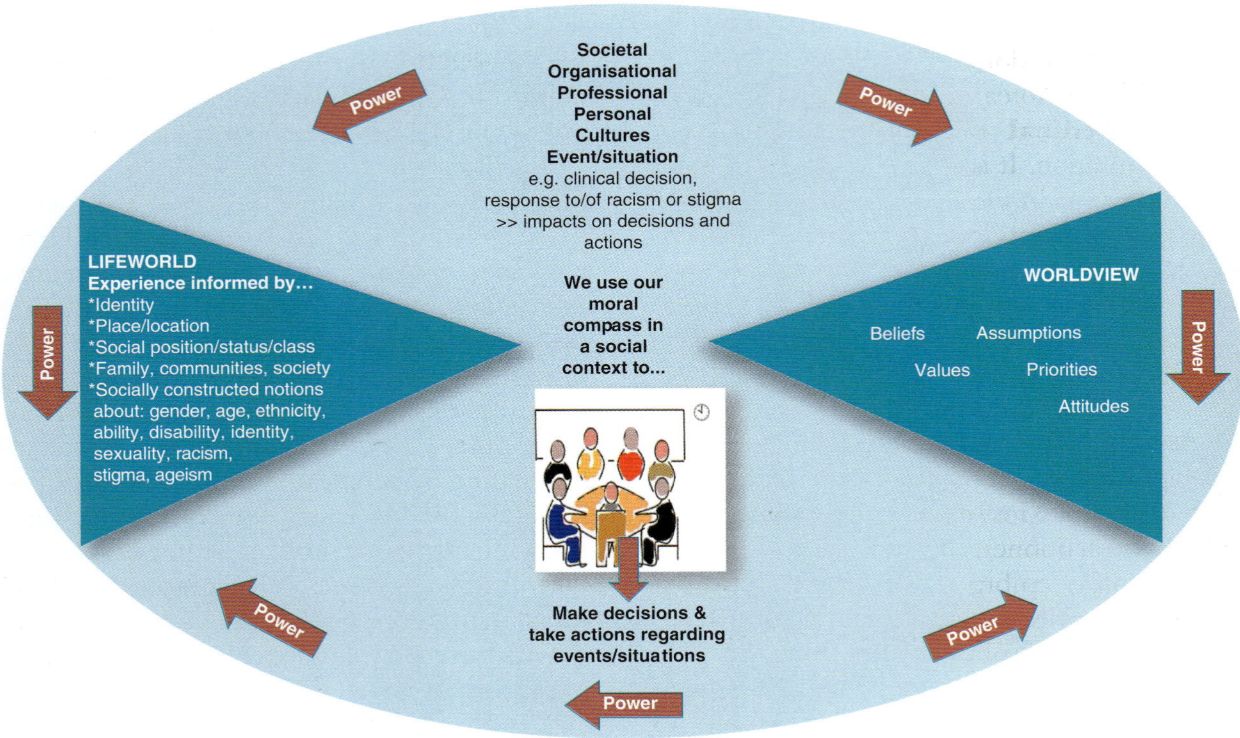

FIGURE 4.4 Culture: Worldview, lifeworld, organisational, professional and societal cultures interact and impact on practice

Social determinants of health and intersectionality

Sociological understandings of health and illness consider health and illness in their historical and social context and consider the social determinants of health beyond the capacity of single people to control—for example, patterned inequality affecting specific populations such as poverty, racism and other forms of discrimination, housing, employment, education and so on.[53] It is well known that neither health nor disease are distributed equally among segments of the population. For several generations, the mainstream population in Australia and Aotearoa New Zealand has enjoyed improved health status. There continues to be major disparity in deaths and illnesses experienced by Indigenous people and other minority groups and in how they experience health care.

Historically produced and currently reproduced social determinants of health include poverty, lack of employment opportunities, poor housing and low levels of education. Other socially marginalising issues such as scientific, institutional and personal racism on the part of health services and society also play a central role in health disparities. Racism is, however, just one aspect of a complex web of intersectional factors that affect a person's health and the way they may be treated by nurses and systems. Consider how sexism, ageism, hetero-dominance, ableism and stigma on the part of nurses and the profession might all intersect to produce poor outcomes for a gay, elderly, Indigenous woman who seeks help for severe pain. The latest National Aboriginal and Torres Strait Islander Health Plan (2021–2031) embraces place-based, person-centred health care based on cultural safety.[77]

Biomedical

The view that dominates health systems in Australia and Aotearoa New Zealand is called the **biomedical** or **scientific** theory of illness causation. It is based on the assumption that all events in life have a cause and effect, that the human body functions more or less mechanically (i.e. the functioning of the human body is analogous to the functioning of a car), that all life can be reduced or divided into smaller parts (e.g. the reduction of the human person into body, mind and spirit) and that all of reality can be observed and measured (e.g. intelligence tests and psychometric measures of behaviour). Most educational programs for medical practitioners, nurses and other health professionals embrace the biomedical or scientific theories and evidence that explain the causes of both physical and psychological illnesses. It is possible to do that without dismissing how service users see things and wish to have their needs met.

The variety of healing beliefs and practices used by the many populations found in Australia and Aotearoa New Zealand far exceeds the limitations of this chapter. It is important, however, that you are aware of the existence of various practices and recognise that, in addition to folk practices, traditional practices such as Rongoa Māori (Māori healing),[78] traditional Chinese medicine and Ayurveda are used along with many other complementary healing practices such as herbalism, homeopathy and acupuncture to name just a few.

Of course, it is possible to have a combination of worldviews, and many people are likely to offer more than one explanation for the cause of their illness and to take a biopsychosocial perspective that recognises the complex interaction of factors affecting health. As a profession, nursing largely embraces the scientific/biomedical worldview, but some other aspects are gaining popularity including techniques for managing chronic pain such as acupuncture, herbal therapies, hypnosis, therapeutic touch and biofeedback. For cultural safety it is imperative that nurses engage in power sharing and be prepared to both listen to and respect how people understand and choose to treat their own illnesses.

Expression of illness

Expression of pain

To illustrate the way in which symptom expression may reflect our cultural background, let's use an extensively studied symptom—pain. Pain is a universally recognised phenomenon, and it is an important aspect of assessment for people of various ages. Pain is a private, subjective experience influenced by our sociocultural background. Expectations, manifestations and management of pain are all embedded in sociocultural contexts. The definition of pain, like that of health or illness, is socially and culturally informed. The word 'pain' is derived from the Greek word for penalty, which helps explain the long association between pain and punishment in Judeo-Christian thought. The meaning of painful stimuli, the way we define our situation and the impact of personal experience all help determine the experience of pain.

Some cross-cultural research has been done on pain, with the acknowledgement that it may be perceived as a multidimensional experience. For example, Fenwick[79] conducted research on nursing assessments of pain in Central Australian Indigenous people that remains the only nursing research of its kind in Australia. Pain has been found to be a highly personal experience depending on cultural learning, the meaning of the situation and other factors unique to the person.[80] Sussex[81] observes that:

> *Many things contribute to how we experience and express pain. Gender, age, education, socioeconomic status, the relative power of the participants in the conversation, and whether the person in pain is speaking in their mother tongue or another language all affect a person's experience of pain. Each of these factors can have a crucial impact on how we communicate about pain, and how we understand pain communication from others.*

Therefore, pain should be explored in consideration of not only the physical or psychological experience but also its social, spiritual and cultural perceptions. Silent suffering has been identified as the most valued response to pain by health professionals, probably based on the stoicism of the English stiff upper lip since Western medicine and nursing arose from English culture. Most nurses are socialised to believe that in virtually any situation, self-control is better than open displays of strong feelings. These ideas lead to many poor outcomes and even death when assumptions are made by nurses and doctors about the veracity of someone's pain. They may be denied pain relief or treatment, as in some cases being investigated by the National Justice Project.[42]

Australian nursing standards

In 2016 the Nursing and Midwifery Board of Australia[6] released the updated Registered Nurse Standards. On page 1, it is stated:

> *Registered nurse (RN) practice is person-centred and evidence-based with preventative, curative, formative, supportive, restorative and palliative elements. RNs work in therapeutic and professional relationships with individuals, as well as with families, groups and communities. These people may be healthy and with a range of abilities or have health issues related to physical or mental illness and/or health challenges. These challenges may be posed by physical, psychiatric, developmental and/or intellectual disabilities.*

The Australian community has a rich mixture of cultural and linguistic diversity, and the Registered Nurse Standards for Practice are to be read in this context. Nurses recognise the importance of history and culture to health and wellbeing. This practice reflects understanding of the impact of colonisation on the cultural, social and spiritual lives of Aboriginal and Torres Strait Islander peoples, which has contributed to significant health inequity in Australia.

Of relevance are the following dimensions:[6]

> *A Registered Nurse:*
> *1.3 respects all cultures and experiences, which includes responding to the role of family and community that underpin the health of Aboriginal and Torres Strait Islander peoples and people of other cultures.*
> *2.2 communicates effectively, and is respectful of a person's dignity, culture, values, beliefs and rights.*

The Nursing and Midwifery Board of Australia Code of Conduct for Nurses[7] specifies cultural safety:

> ***3.1 Aboriginal and/or Torres Strait Islander peoples' health***
> *Australia has always been a culturally and linguistically diverse nation. Aboriginal and/or Torres Strait Islander peoples have inhabited and cared for the land as the first peoples of Australia for millennia, and their histories and cultures have uniquely shaped our nation. Understanding and acknowledging historic factors such as colonisation and its impact on*

Aboriginal and/or Torres Strait Islander peoples' health helps inform care. In particular, Aboriginal and/or Torres Strait Islander peoples bear the burden of gross social, cultural and health inequality. In supporting the health of Aboriginal and/or Torres Strait Islander peoples, nurses must:

a. provide care that is holistic, free of bias and racism, challenges belief based upon assumption and is culturally safe and respectful for Aboriginal and/or Torres Strait Islander peoples

b. advocate for an act to facilitate access to quality and culturally safe health services for Aboriginal and/or Torres Strait Islander peoples, and

c. recognise the importance of family, community, partnership and collaboration in the healthcare decision making of Aboriginal and/or Torres Strait Islander peoples, for both prevention strategies and care delivery.

See also Congress of Aboriginal and/or Torres Strait Islander Nurses and Midwives. https://catsinam.org.au

3.2 Culturally safe and respectful practice

Culturally safe and respectful practice requires having knowledge of how a nurse's own culture, values, attitudes, assumptions and beliefs influence their interactions with people and families, the community and colleagues. To ensure culturally safe and respectful practice, nurses must:

a. understand that only the person and/or their family can determine whether or not care is culturally safe and respectful

b. respect diverse cultures, beliefs, gender identities, sexualities and experiences of people, including among team members

c. acknowledge the social, economic, cultural, historic and behavioural factors influencing health, at the individual, community and population levels

d. adopt practices that respect diversity, avoid bias, discrimination and racism, and challenge belief based upon assumption (for example, based on gender, disability, race, ethnicity, religion, sexuality, age or political beliefs)

e. support an inclusive environment for the safety and security of the individual person and their family and/or significant others, and

f. create a positive, culturally safe work environment through role modelling, and supporting the rights, dignity and safety of others, including people and colleagues.

Aotearoa New Zealand guidelines for cultural safety

Registered nurses must prove competency specific to cultural safety to achieve initial registration and, later, to maintain a practising certificate from the Nursing Council of New Zealand. The council provides standards and guidelines for nurses. The following principles (see also Box 4.7) underpin cultural safety education.[60]

The Nursing Council of New Zealand[60] also stipulates the expected outcome of nursing education in Aotearoa New Zealand; that registered nurses are to 'practise in a culturally safe manner, as defined by the recipients of their care'. They require that a nurse will:

a. examine their own realities and the attitudes they bring to each new person they encounter in their practice;

b. evaluate the impact that historical, political and social processes have on the health of all people; and

c. demonstrate flexibility in their relationships with people who are different from themselves.

Box 4.7 Nursing Council of New Zealand

Principle one

Cultural safety aims to improve the health status of New Zealanders and applies to all relationships through:

1.1 an emphasis on health gains and positive health outcomes

1.2 nurses acknowledging the beliefs and practices of those who differ from them. For example, this may be by age or generation, gender, sexual orientation, occupation and socioeconomic status, ethnic origin or migrant experience, religious or spiritual belief, disability.

Principle two

Cultural safety aims to enhance the delivery of health and disability services through a culturally safe nursing workforce by:

2.1 identifying the power relationship between the service provider and the people who use the service. The nurse accepts and works alongside others after undergoing a careful process of institutional and personal analysis of power relationships.

2.2 empowering the users of the service. People should be able to express degrees of perceived risk or safety. For example, someone who feels unsafe may not be able to take full advantage of a primary healthcare service offered and may subsequently require expensive and possibly dramatic secondary or tertiary intervention.

2.3 preparing nurses to understand the diversity within their own cultural reality and the impact of that on any person who differs in any way from themselves.

2.4 applying social science concepts that underpin the art of nursing practice. Nursing practice is more than carrying out tasks. It is about relating and responding effectively to people with diverse needs in a way that the people who use the service can define as safe.

Principle three

Cultural safety is broad in its application:

3.1 recognising inequalities within healthcare interactions that represent the microcosm of inequalities in health that have prevailed throughout history and within our nation more generally.

3.2 addressing the cause-and-effect relationship of history, political, social, and employment status, housing, education, gender, and personal experience upon people who use nursing services.

3.3 accepting the legitimacy of difference and diversity in human behaviour and social structure.

3.4 accepting that the attitudes and beliefs, policies and practices of health and disability service providers can act as barriers to service access.

3.5 concerning quality improvement in service delivery and consumer rights.

Principle four

Cultural safety has a close focus on:

4.1 understanding the impact of the nurse as a bearer of his/her own culture, history, attitudes and life experiences and the response other people make to these factors.

4.2 challenging nurses to examine their practice carefully, recognising the power relationship in nursing is biased towards the provider of the health and disability service.

4.3 balancing the power relationships in the practice of nursing so that every consumer receives an effective service.

4.4 preparing nurses to resolve any tension between the cultures of nursing and the people using the services.

4.5 understanding that such power imbalances can be examined, negotiated, and changed to provide equitable, effective, efficient, and acceptable service delivery, which minimises risk to people who might otherwise be alienated from the service.

Source: Durie & Te Kingi 1997[56]

Strategies for collaborative assessment

The first author of this chapter was alerted to the difficulties students in Australian nursing contexts have when it comes to appreciating the need for holistic assessment. Students often marked 'not applicable' beside an item that asked whether cultural considerations had been included in their care on an assessment form used in a clinical practicum. This was because students do not appreciate that every encounter has cultural elements, even if the person has the same personal cultural identity as the nurse; they would include the item only if the person was seen as an 'ethnic' other. Cultural safety, however, teaches that all encounters are bicultural because they include the culture of the nurse (with aspects of their identity drawn from the culture of nursing and their personal cultural identity) and the culture of the person. As Warren[67] notes, 'information is not gained by specifically cultural questions, and this is also an important tenet of cultural safety'.

Box 4.8 outlines structures to support cultural safety.

Authors warn of the problem of trying to teach, learn or assess cultural generalities[67] and instead refer to the work of medical anthropologist Arthur Kleinman who, rather than focusing on cultural generalisations, offers questions to elicit what he calls the 'client's explanatory framework'. To help you elicit information of relevance to the person we suggest the questions in Box 4.9 designed by Kleinman.[82]

In Box 4.10 we offer some additional questions.

In Box 4.11 there is the basis for all care of people from any background.

Box 4.8 Practical steps towards culturally safe practice

- Management has a transparent process for reflection at the service level and aligns their values and priorities to those of service users.
- Management provides regular cultural safety education to all staff. The entire service including senior management are well educated in the model.
- Management establishes and advertises an open-door policy for any staff member to raise any concerns at any time that they have with their own or others, or the service's response to a person or family.
- Management resources and advertises a weekly cultural safety forum for all staff and pays off-duty staff to attend if they need to.
- Management provides and advertises to service users an evaluation process where they can safely communicate whether:
  - their needs were met
  - they and their family felt safe and were treated as equals
  - they felt their dignity and identity were respected and protected
  - they had the power to meaningfully communicate their wishes and have them respected.

Box 4.9 Kleinman's explanatory framework

1. What do you call your problem? What name does it have?
2. What do you think caused your problem?
3. Why do you think it started when it did?
4. What does your sickness do to you? How does it work?
5. How severe is it? Will it have a short or a long course?
6. What do you fear most about your sickness?
7. What are the chief problems your sickness has caused?
8. What kind of treatment do you think you should receive? What are the most important results you hope to receive from the treatment?

Source: Kleinman 1980[82]

Box 4.10 Health beliefs and practices assessment

1. How do you define health?
2. How do you rate your health?
3. Describe your illness to me.
4. What do you believe caused the illness?
5. How do you keep yourself from getting sick and what home remedies do you use?

Box 4.11 Guide for care

Preparing

Discover and understand your own social position, ethnicity, cultural values, biases, health beliefs and practices and those of the profession you belong to and the organisation/service you work for.

Respect

Realise that you *must* know and understand your heritage.

Evaluate people's holistic needs within the context of their sociocultural position.

Select open-ended questions and avoid questions where the person can give a yes/no response.

Pace questions throughout any health assessment or health service encounter—focus as much as possible on deeply listening. To achieve it, imagine it is you or your dearest loved one that you are working with.

Encourage people to express themselves without rush.

Check for people's understanding and acceptance of medical treatments and recommendations.

Touch can be therapeutic, but you must respect people's personal preferences and boundaries—manners are a vital component of the relationships in health care.

Conclusion: culturally safe nursing

In your professional nurse education, you are now learning the contemporary scientific meanings of health and illness, but such knowledge is just one part of the art of nursing care. There are several steps we must take in the lifelong practice of cultural safety. Integrating this knowledge into day-to-day practice will take time because many practitioners in the healthcare system are hesitant to adopt new ideas. Culturally safe nursing practice does not come instantly, certainly not after reading a chapter or several chapters or books on this specialised area. It is complex and multifaceted, and many facets change over time. It is confronting for many people to discuss issues such as racism, ageism, homophobia and various other biases, preconceptions and prejudices about specific ethnic, religious, sexual or socioeconomic groups. Please see Figure 4.2 (earlier) for a summary of historical impacts and how cultural safety minimises them. Culturally safe practice requires us to admit and challenge our socialisation into these damaging ways of perceiving people. It is hard and yet rewarding to practise deep self-reflection on our family's background, social position and traditional beliefs and practices. It can be harder still to contemplate systemic racism and marginalisation arising from systems that are set up ostensibly to help and serve the public. As Mills[68] says of systemic racism: 'For us [Indigenous people] to access mainstream health services, we are required to suspend our own beliefs and cultures and adopt or accept the western model of health'.

The first step in understanding the healthcare needs of others is to understand one's own social position and cultural values, beliefs, attitudes and practices. The second step is to identify the meaning of health to the other person, being open to their history and social experience, their interpretations, being flexible and aiming for the professional acquisition of trust.

Third, we must understand the culture of the healthcare delivery system, how it works, what it does, the meanings of various procedures and the costs and consequences to the public and to us as nurses. Fourth, we must be knowledgeable about the social backgrounds of people including experiences of immigration, racism, socioeconomic status and ageing. Fifth, we must be aware if English is not understood and of the resources available to help with interpreting.

This chapter is about developing a deep understanding that each person and nurse has their own reality, that these multiple realities are socially constructed and that they are informed by, but not reducible to, culture. **A central aim of this chapter is to consider the way you see yourself and the world around you so you can have a positive impact on the power relations between nurses and service users and between service users and health services.** Further, we aim to establish an appreciation that there is as much variation within cultures as there is between cultures. Health contexts such as hospitals and the health professions (nursing, medicine, etc.) also have their own cultures. Your challenge is to work within these systems without diminishing, demeaning or disempowering any person (Box 4.12).

We urge you to remember the many aspects of human experience connected to cultural safety: culture, ethnicity, religion, socialisation, population diversity, immigration, religion, demographic change, globalisation, health and illness, modern and traditional beliefs and practices, sociopolitical issues, education, sanitation, housing and infrastructure. The 'Additional resources' section includes selected websites to link you to further introductory material related to this content.

In concluding, we refer you to the reflections of eminent medical anthropologist Professor Arthur Kleinman, which arose from his own experience of caring for his wife of 40 years who developed a debilitating neurological disorder. He sums up perfectly the enduring need for self-awareness in caring professions such as nursing:

> *In my view, what is needed is reform of the very culture of contemporary biomedicine. We must train students and practitioners in critical self-reflection on that which limits their caregiving; in strategies and techniques aimed at opening a space for the moral acts of caregiving; and in the most concrete and practical acts of assistance, so that they never forget what caregiving actually means.*[83]

Box 4.12 Cultural safety summary

- Cultural safety involves recognising nurses as the bearers of our own personal and societal culture and that the cultures of nurses, the nursing profession, organisations/services impact on practice and outcomes.
- Cultural safety is applicable in any context since all people have culture(s) and workplaces and professions also have cultures; it is not only relevant to Indigenous populations, although it is a form of Indigenous knowledge.
- Cultural safety is achieved through a process of self-reflection and developing self-awareness on the part of nurses, other health professionals and organisations.
- Cultural safety sees culture as learnt, dynamic and strategic.
- The definition of personal culture used in cultural safety includes dimensions such as ethnicity, age, sex, gender identity, class, education, attitudes and political, philosophical and religious beliefs.
- Cultural safety requires that, as nurses, we are respectful of our colleagues' and service users' nationalities, histories and social experiences.
- Cultural safety is in contrast to transcultural nursing care; cultural safety encourages nurses to deliver service with respect to peoples' diverse experiences and needs.
- Culturally safe care empowers people because it reinforces the idea that each person's knowledge and reality is valid and valuable. It facilitates open communication and allows people to voice concerns about nursing care that they may deem unsafe.
- Cultural safety is political because it attempts to change health professionals' attitudes about their power relationships with service users and it actively promotes power sharing and negotiation. This is true also at organisational levels.
- Cultural safety does not focus on how people are different to dominant cultures and norms but how they are treated in society.
- Care may be deemed culturally unsafe if the person seeking service feels diminished, demeaned or disempowered or directly or indirectly dissuaded from accessing necessary care.

ADDITIONAL RESOURCES

You can further develop your knowledge relevant to cultural safety by:

- reading relevant chapters of a fundamentals of nursing or medical-surgical nursing textbook
- answering chapter multiple choice questions online. Log onto ClinicalKey Student and search for the text 'Health Assessment, 4th edition'. Choose the section titled 'Teaching material'. In this section you will find question and answer documents for each chapter.
- visiting websites

  Australian Nursing and Midwifery Accreditation Council: www.anmc.org.au

  Australian Government, Department of Health and Aged Care—National Aboriginal and Torres Strait Islander Health Plan 2013–2023: https://www.health.gov.au/resources/publications/national-aboriginal-and-torres-strait-islander-health-plan-2021-2031

ADDITIONAL RESOURCES cont'd

Congress of Aboriginal and Torres Strait Nurses and Midwives (CATSINaM): https://catsinam.org.au

Careers New Zealand for an interactive diagram of Te Whare Tapa Wha model: https://www.careers.govt.nz/resources/career-practice/career-theory-models/te-whare-tapa-wha/

National Aboriginal Community Controlled Health Organisation (NACCHO): www.naccho.org.au

National Council of Māori Nurses: www.Māorihealth.co.nz

Nursing Council of New Zealand—Guidelines for Cultural Safety, The Treaty of Waitangi, and Māori health in nursing education and practice: https://www.ngamanukura.nz/sites/default/files/basic_page_pdfs/Guidelines%20for%20cultural%20safety%2C%20the%20Treaty%20of%20Waitangi%2C%20and%20Maori%20health%20in%20nursing%20education%20and%20practice%282%29_0.pdf

New Zealand History: www.nzhistory.net.nz/politics/treaty- of-waitangi

REFERENCES

1. Cox L, Best O. Clarifying cultural safety: its focus and intent in an Australian context, Contemporary Nurse, 2022, 58 (1):71–81.
2. Best O, Fredericks B. Yatdjuligin: Aboriginal and Torres Strait Islander nursing and midwifery care. Melbourne: Cambridge University Press; 2021.
3. Northern Territory Government. Northern Territory Health Aboriginal Cultural Security Framework 2016–2026. Northern Territory. 2016. Available at: https://health.nt.gov.au/__data/assets/pdf_file/0010/1035496/aboriginal-cultural-security-framework-2016-2026.pdf
4. Department of Education, Science and Training. National review of nurse education: multicultural nursing education, 2001. Canberra: Commonwealth of Australia; 2001.
5. Bennett J. Training mental health professionals in cultural capability: sustainability of knowledge and skills. International Journal of Mental Health Systems, 2013;6(1):72–80.
6. Nursing and Midwifery Board of Australia. Registered nurse standards for practice. 2016. Available at: http://www.nursingmidwiferyboard.gov.au/Codes-Guidelines-Statements/Professional-standards.aspx
7. Nursing and Midwifery Board of Australia. Code of conduct for nurses. 2018. Available at: https://www.nursingmidwiferyboard.gov.au/Codes-Guidelines-Statements/Professional- standards.aspx
8. Nursing and Midwifery Board of Australia. Code of conduct for midwives. 2018. Available at: https://www.nursingmidwiferyboard.gov.au/Codes-Guidelines-Statements/Professional-standards.aspx
9. Nursing and Midwifery Board of Australia. Midwife Standards for Practice. 2018. Available at: https://www.nursingmidwiferyboard.gov.au/Codes-Guidelines-Statements/Position-Statements/leading-the-way.aspx
10. Nursing and Midwifery Board of Australia. Cultural safety: Nurses and midwives leading the way for safer healthcare. 2018. Available

at: https://www.nursingmidwiferyboard.gov.au/Codes-Guidelines-Statements/Position-Statements/leading-the-way.aspx
11. Australian Indigenous HealthInfoNet. n.d. Closing the Gap. https://healthinfonet.ecu.edu.au/learn/health-system/closing-the-gap/
12. Cox L. Fear, trust and Aborigines: the historical experience of state institutions and current encounters in the health system. Health History, 2007; 9(2):70–92.
13. Clarkson C, Jacobs Z, Marwick B, Fullagar R, Wallis L, Smith M, et al. Human occupation of northern Australia by 65,000 years ago. Nature 2017;547(7663):306–10. doi: 10.1038/nature22968.
14. Cox L, Taua C, Drummond, A, Kidd, J. Enabling Cultural Safety. In Crisp J, Douglas C, Rebeiro G, Waters D, editors. Potter and Perry's fundamentals of nursing. 6th ed. Chatswood, NSW: Elsevier; 2021.
15. Pascoe B. Dark Emu: Black seeds agriculture or accident? Broome, Australia: Magabala Books; 2014. ProQuest Ebook Central. Available at: https://ebookcentral.proquest.com/lib/qut/detail. action?docID=1675076
16. Perche D. Ten years on, it's time we learned the lessons from the failed Northern Territory Intervention. The Conversation; 2017. Available at: http://theconversation.com/ten-years-on-its-time-we-learned-the-lessons-from-the-failed-northern-territory-intervention-79198
17. Human Rights and Equal Opportunity Commission. Bringing them home: a guide to the findings and recommendations of the National Inquiry into the Separation of Aboriginal and Torres Strait Islander Children from their Families. Sydney: Commonwealth of Australia; 1997. https://humanrights.gov.au/our-work/bringing-them-home-report-1997
18. Human Rights and Equal Opportunity Commission. Indigenous deaths in custody 1989–1996. Sydney: Commonwealth of Australia; 1996.
19. Kidd R. The way we civilise: Aboriginal affairs—the untold story. St Lucia: University of Queensland Press; 1997.
20. Reynolds H. The other side of the frontier: aboriginal resistance to the European invasion of Australia. Ringwood, Vic: Pelican; 1982.
21. Rintoul S. The wailing: a national black oral history. Port Melbourne: William Heinemann; 1993.
22. Forsyth S. Telling stories: nurses, politics and Aboriginal Australians, c.1900–1980s. Contemporary Nurse 2007;24(1):33–44.
23. Russell S, Cuneen C. As Indigenous incarceration rates keep rising, justice reinvestment offers a solution. The Conversation; 2018. Available at: http://theconversation.com/as-indigenous-incarceration-rates-keep-rising-justice-reinvestment-offers-a- solution-107610.
24. Ritter D. Contesting native title: from controversy to consensus in the struggle over Indigenous land rights. Sydney: Allen & Unwin; 2009.
25. The Uluru Statement 2023. https://ulurustatement.org/history/the-journey-so-far/
26. Allam L 2023. Australia's Voice debate is being flooded with misinformation and lies. Here are some facts The Guardian 13 Sep 2023, https://www.theguardian.com/australia-news/2023/sep/13/indigenous-voice-to-parliament-referendum-fact-check-yes-campaign-no-campaign
27. Collard S 2023. 'A Knife in your heart': Indigenous Australians grapple with grief after Voice defeat. The Guardian 16 Oct 2023 https://www.theguardian.com/australia-news/2023/oct/16/a-knife-in-your-heart-indigenous-australians-grapple-with-grief-after-voice-defeat
28. Drummond A. 'It's about the humanity of nursing': Shifting Aboriginal and Torres Strait Islander health education beyond white possession and towards a relational approach. 2023. PhD thesis, Queensland University of Technology.
29. Australian Institute of Aboriginal and Torres Strait Islander Studies (AIATSIS). Proof of Aboriginality. 2022. https://aiatsis.gov.au/proof-aboriginality
30. Australian Bureau of Statistics. Census of Population and Housing – Counts of Aboriginal and Torres Strait Islander Australians, Canberra: ABS; 2021. Available from: https://www.abs.gov.au/statistics/people/aboriginal-and-torres-strait-islander-peoples/census-population-and-housing-counts-aboriginal-

and-torres-strait-islander-australians/latest-release

31. Australian Bureau of Statistics. Australia's Population by Country of Birth. Canberra: ABS; 2021. Available from: https://www.abs.gov.au/statistics/people/population/australias-population-country-birth/latest-release.
32. Australian Bureau of Statistics. Language Statistics for Aboriginal and Torres Strait Islander Peoples. Canberra: ABS; 2021. Available from: https://www.abs.gov.au/statistics/people/aboriginal-and-torres-strait-islander-peoples/language-statistics-aboriginal-and-torres-strait-islander-peoples/latest-release
33. Australian Bureau of Statistics. Cultural diversity: Census. Canberra: ABS; 2021. Available from: https://www.abs.gov.au/statistics/people/people-and-communities/cultural-diversity-census/2021
34. Australian Bureau of Statistics. Religious affiliation in Australia. Canberra: ABS; 2022. Available from: https://www.abs.gov.au/articles/religious-affiliation-australia
35. Consedine R, Consedine J. Healing our history: the challenge of the Treaty of Waitangi. Auckland: Penguin; 2001.
36. Waitangi Tribunal Te ropu whakamana I Te Tiriti O Waitangi. Treaty of Waitangi. n.d. Available at: www.justice.govt.nz/tribunals/waitangi-tribunal
37. Orange, C. 'Te Tiriti o Waitangi – the Treaty of Waitangi—Creating te Tiriti o Waitangi—the Treaty of Waitangi', Te Ara—the Encyclopedia of New Zealand. Available at: http://www.TeAra.govt.nz/en/te-tiriti-o-waitangi-the-treaty-of-waitangi/page-1
38. Kearns R, Moewaka-Barnes H, McCreanor T. Placing racism in public health: a perspective from Aotearoa New Zealand. GeoJournal 2009; 74:1239.
39. Khawaja M, Boddington B, Didham R. Growing ethnic diversity in New Zealand and its implications for measuring differentials in fertility and mortality. Wellington: Statistics New Zealand; 2007.
40. Statistics New Zealand Tatauranga Aotearoa 2023. Ethnicity. Available at: https://www.stats.govt.nz/topics/ethnicity
41. Australian Institute of Health and Welfare. Indigenous Australians and the Health System. 2022. Available at: https://www.aihw.gov.au/reports/australias-health/indigenous-australians-use-of-health-services
42. National Justice Project. Aboriginal Health Justice Project. 2023 Available at: https://justice.org.au/what-we-do/#aboriginal-health
43. Fogliani R. Record of investigation into death of Ms Dhu. Coroner's Court of Western Australia; 2016. Available at: http://www. coronerscourt.wa.gov.au/_files/dhu%20finding.pdf
44. Fogliani R. Inquest into the death of Ms Dhu. Coroner's Court of Western Australia; 2018. Available at: http://www.coronerscourt.wa.gov.au/I/inquest_into_the_death_of_ms_dhu.aspx?uid=1644-2151- 2753-9965
45. Davidson H. Gurrumul hospital row highlights Indigenous health obstacles. The Guardian 2016. Available at: https://www.theguardian. com/music/2016/apr/14/race-row-rages-on-over-gurrumul-hospi- tal-ordeal?CMP=share_btn_link
46. Zhou N. Naomi Williams's inquest: pregnant woman sent home too quickly, expert says. The Guardian 2019. Available at: https://www.theguardian.com/australia-news/2019/mar/13/naomi-williams-inquest-pregnant-woman-sent-home-too-quickly-expert-says
47. Ramsden I. Cultural safety and nursing education in Aotearoa and Te Waipounamu. Unpublished PhD thesis. Victoria University of Wellington, New Zealand; 2002.
48. Kluckhohn C, Kelly H. The concept of culture. In: Linton R, editor. The science of man in the world culture. New York: Columbia University Press; 1945.
49. Statistics New Zealand. 2018 European ethnic group. Available at: https://www.stats.govt.nz/tools/2018-census-ethnic-group-summaries/european
50. Bond C. Andrew Bolt isn't a racist, but ... The Drum, 25 March 2014. Available at: www.abc.net.au/news/2014-03-25/andrew-bolt-isnt-a-racist-but/5344286.
51. Baker B 2021. Race and biology. BioScience, 71(2):119–126. https://doi.org/10.1093/biosci/biaa157
52. Jeynes WH. Race, racism, and Darwinism. Education and Urban Society. 2011; 43:535.

53. Willis K, Shandell E. Society, culture and health: an introduction to sociology for nurses. 2nd ed. Melbourne, Vic: Oxford University Press; 2011.
54. National Aboriginal Community Controlled Health Organisation (NACCHO). Constitution. 2011. Available at: https://www.naccho.org.au/governance/
55. Durie M. Whaiora: Māori health development. New Zealand: Oxford University Press; 1994.
56. Durie MH, Te Kingi KR. A framework for measuring Māori mental health outcomes. A report prepared for the Ministry of Health. Palmerston North, New Zealand: Department of Māori Studies, Massey University; 1997.
57. Pitama S, Robertson P, Cram F, Gillies M, Huria T, Dallas-Katoa W 2007. Meihana model: a clinical assessment framework. New Zealand Journal of Psychology. Nov 1;36(3).
58. Richardson S. Aotearoa/New Zealand nursing: from eugenics to cultural safety. Nursing Inquiry. 2004;11(4):35–42.
59. hooks b. Choosing the margin as a space of radical openness. In: Yearning: race, gender, and cultural politics. Boston: South End Press; 1990, pp. 203–209.
60. Nursing Council of New Zealand. Guidelines for cultural safety, the Treaty of Waitangi, and Māori health in nursing education and practice. Te whakarite i ngā mahi tapuhi kia tiakina ai te haumaru ā-iwi. Regulating nursing practice to protect public safety. Wellington: Nursing Council of New Zealand; 2011. https://online.flippingbook.com/view/960779225/2/
61. Ramsden I. Kawa Whakaruruhau: guidelines for nursing and midwifery education. Wellington: Nursing Council of New Zealand; 1992.
62. Ramsden I. Kawa Whakaruruhau: cultural safety in nursing education in Aotearoa (New Zealand). Nursing Praxis in Aotearoa New Zealand. 1993;8(3):4–10.
63. Personal communication. Helen A. 2010.
64. Davey, M. How could this happen? Indigenous health tragedies spark search for answers. The Guardian, 12 August 2016. Available at: https://www.theguardian.com/australia-news/2016/aug/12/how-could-this-happen-indigenous-health-tragedies-spark-search-for-answers
65. Hayter, M, King, R. Naomi Williams's inquest concludes, with coroner calling for change at NSW hospital, 290719. ABC News. 2019 https://www.abc.net.au/news/2019-07-29/naomi-williams-tumut-sepsis-death-inquest-findings/11355244.
66. Personal communication. G. Yates. 2010.
67. Warren BJ. Teaching the fluid process of cultural competence at the graduate level: a constructionist approach. In: Bosher SD, Pharris MD, editors. Transforming nurse education: the culturally inclusive environment. New York: Springer; 2009.
68. Mills D. Systemic Racism in Health. Speech by NACCHO Chair at FECCA 2022 Conference, Melbourne. Available at: https://www.naccho.org.au/systemic-racism-in-health/
69. Laing RD. The politics of the family and other essays. Middlesex, UK: Penguin; 1969.
70. Australian Bureau of Statistics. Households and Families: Census. Canberra: ABS. 2021. Available from: https://www.abs.gov.au/statistics/people/people-and-communities/household-and-families-census/latest-release
71. Australian Institute of Health and Welfare. Young people in out-of-home care 2021. https://www.aihw.gov.au/reports/children-youth/young-people
72. Levin J. God, faith and health: exploring the spirituality-healing connection. New York: John Wiley; 2001.
73. Rovelli, C. The Order of Time, 2019. Penguin: Random House.
74. National Aboriginal Health Strategy Working Party. A national Aboriginal health strategy. Canberra. 1989.
75. Rameka L. 'Kia whakatōmuri te haere whakamua:' I walk backwards into the future with my eyes fixed on my past'. Contemporary Issues in Early Childhood. 2016 Dec;17(4):387–398. https://doi.org/10.1177/1463949116677923
76. Bruce A. Time(lessness): Buddhist perspectives and end-of-life. Nursing Philosophy 2007; 8(3):151–157.
77. Australian Government, Department of Health and Aged Care. National Aboriginal and Torres

Strait Islander Health Plan 2013–2023. Canberra. 2021. available https://www.health.gov.au/resources/publications/national-aboriginal-and-torres-strait-islander-health-plan-2021-2031
78. New Zealand, Ministry of Health. Rongoā Māori: Traditional Māori healing. 2018. Available at: https://www.health.govt.nz/our-work/populations/ maori-health/rongoa-maori-traditional-maori-healing.
79. Fenwick C. Assessing pain across the cultural gap: central Australian Indigenous peoples pain assessment. Contemporary Nurse, 2006;22(2): 218–227.
80. Free M.M. Cross-Cultural Conceptions of Pain and Pain Control, Proceedings (Baylor University. Medical Center) 15(2):143–145, 2022. DOI: 10.1080/08998280.2002.11927832
81. Sussex R. How different cultures experience and talk about pain. The Conversation; 2016. Available at: https://bodyinmind.org/cultures-pain/
82. Kleinman A. Patients and healers in the context of culture: an exploration of the borderland between anthropology, medicine, and psychiatry. Berkeley, CA, 1980, University of California Press.
83. Kleinman A. Caregiving and the moral impoverishment of medicine. Project Syndicate; 2009. Available at: www.project-syndicate.org/commentary/kleinman1/English.

CHAPTER 5

Screening for family violence

Adapted by Catina Adams

INTRODUCTION

Family violence is a serious public health issue with significant health consequences for women and children.[1] In Australia, police are called to a family violence incident every 2 minutes; 10 women per day are hospitalised due to violence; and every 7 days, a woman is killed by a current or ex-partner.[2] The violence often begins during pregnancy and may increase in severity into motherhood.[3] It is one of the leading causes of death and injury for childbearing women.[4] Risk factors for family violence include substance misuse, unemployment, financial problems, relationship issues, pregnancy, coercive controlling behaviours resulting in isolation and barriers to support, threats to harm/kill or suicide, mental illness, mood shifts and access to and/or use of weapons.

More than one million Australian children are affected by family violence.[5] Children exposed to violence are at higher risk for emotional and behavioural problems, poorer language development and impaired cognitive development.[6] Children do not have to witness family violence for there to be negative outcomes.[7]

Case study

The following case study provides an example of a typical situation involving screening for family violence and the initial clinical reasoning process. It will help you identify your learning needs.

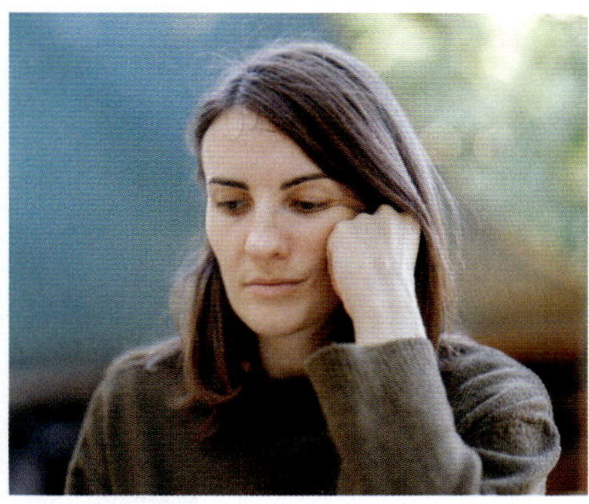

Context

You are working as a registered nurse in a primary healthcare clinic where you meet Ms King, who is there for a routine check-up.

Consider the patient's situation

Sarah King is a 35-year-old woman reporting chronic back pain, anxiety and difficulty sleeping. You notice that Ms King appears anxious and withdrawn during the consultation, exhibiting signs of emotional distress. Suspecting the possibility of family violence, you proceed to explore the woman's concerns.

Questions to further your learning

- What are the possible things that might be going on with Ms King?
- What knowledge do you need to be able to predict what might be going on?
- What approach to Ms King's health assessment will you take?
- What questions (subjective data) will you ask Ms King to extend the health history and why?
- What physical examination (objective data) will you conduct and why?
- What resources are available to help in your assessment of Ms King?
- Do you know where to refer Ms King to ensure she gets further help?

Assessment plan

Health professionals have an important role in identifying people and families in their care who may be affected. Major nursing and medical organisations support the need for health professionals to recognise, assess and respond to family violence. Assessing for family violence can help in identifying women, children and older people at risk, but any assessment must be done within the context of effective systems of support. There is increasing support for routine screening of all women presenting to health services. However, the efficacy of this practice remains contentious, particularly if health professionals do not fully appreciate the complexities of family violence and the consequences of disclosure for women and their children or their responsibilities as health professionals.

Nurses are often the first point of contact within the healthcare system for people and families affected by family violence. Not only is it important to confirm if the person is being abused, but assessment needs to also focus on the impact of the violence on the physical and psychological health and safety of the person and other family members. Nurses are in an ideal position to facilitate disclosure about abuse and to respond in a supportive, appropriate and timely manner while respecting privacy and the person's right to make their own decisions.[8] Even when health professionals have knowledge and screening skills, women may choose not to disclose the abuse for various reasons, including shame and fear of consequences.

The main areas for subjective assessment are:

- screening or routine inquiry
- risk assessment
- history of abuse
- validation of the person's experience.

Following subjective data collection, you will get a sense of the areas needed to be examined for objective data. Only the relevant areas should be examined. The main areas for physical examination when screening for family violence are:

- general inspection—hygiene, grooming, clothing
- inspection and palpation of skin, mouth and scalp
- inspection and palpation of muscles and joints
- mental status assessment.

Resources available

You will find additional resources and the reference list at the end of this chapter.

Types of violence

It is important that you understand the complexities of family violence in all its forms to sensitively conduct screening for domestic violence and undertake a sensitive and culturally appropriate assessment. The complexities include the types of violence, the drivers for violence towards family members, cultural and social considerations, the associated conditions related to family violence, the concept of intersectionality and the health and economic impacts of such violence.

Family violence

Family violence refers to violent behaviours directed towards a person, perpetrated by a family member, who may be a current or former intimate partner.[9] It includes acts of violence between an adult and a child, child to adult or between siblings. In Australia and Aotearoa New Zealand, 'family violence' is addressed in legislation and policy documents. In Australia, the *Family Law Legislation Amendment (Family Violence and Other Measures) Act 2011* amends the *Family Law*

Act 1975 and aims to protect children and families at risk of violence and abuse.[10] In Aotearoa New Zealand, the *Family Violence Act 2018*[11] updated the definition of family violence and provides a set of principles to guide decision making and timely responses. Aboriginal and Torres Strait Islander people in Australia prefer to use the term 'family violence' because it covers extended family and kinship relationships.[5] There are different categories of domestic and family violence (Table 5.1).

TABLE 5.1 Types of domestic and family violence

Form of violence	Description
Coercion and control	Coercive control is when an abuser repeatedly hurts, scares or isolates another person in order to scare them. Some examples of behaviour are belittling, demeaning, undermining, threats, intimidation, social isolation, financial abuse and monitoring movements online and offline. Coercive control is ongoing and cumulative. This is deliberate behaviour and is now against the law in some states in Australia.
Gaslighting	Gaslighting is a common form of coercive control. It is a psychological manipulation in which an offender sows seeds of doubt and confusion. It causes the person to question their memory, thoughts and sanity.
Psychological violence	Psychological violence behaviour includes intimidation, humiliation, emotional blackmail, abusing pets, gaslighting, threatening to 'out' someone's sexuality, transgender or intersex status and more. It also includes the impacts of financial, social and other non-physical forms of violence.
Sexual violence	Sexual violence is any form of coercion or unwanted sexual activity or sexual degradation. It includes child sexual abuse, rape, sexual assault, sexual harassment, human trafficking, image-based abuse and reproductive coercion (e.g. controlling contraception, preventing or forcing an abortion).
Financial abuse	Financial abuse includes controlling access to finances and/or making someone account for all their spending. Examples are welfare theft (taking money from Centrelink or other agencies), preventing someone from working or studying, and dowry-related abuse. Financial abuse can also continue after a separation where an abuser withholds child support and other payments that would allow someone to maintain a separate household.
Social violence	Social violence can include controlling or isolating a partner or family member from their family, friends or community. It might also include limiting social activities and relationships with friends and family and their partner or family member from accessing support.
Spiritual violence	Spiritual violence might include preventing someone from practising their faith or culture. An abuser might ridicule spiritual beliefs and manipulate religious and spiritual teachings or cultural traditions to excuse their violence.
Physical violence	Physical violence means any assault on the body including but not limited to slapping, hitting, punching, pushing, choking, sleep and food deprivation, burns and use of weapons.
Technology-facilitated violence	Technology facilitated abuse includes using text, email or phone to abuse, monitor, humiliate or punish. It also occurs when an abuser uses technology to track or monitor your movements and messages or emails. Abusers may also threaten or distribute private or sexual photos or videos.

Source: Full Stop Australia (2024). Types of domestic and family violence. Available at: https://fullstop.org.au[12]

Intimate partner violence

Intimate partner violence is any behaviour within a past or current intimate relationship that causes harm to those in that relationship. It can include physical, emotional or psychological harm.[13] Perpetrators of intimate partner violence may use controlling or dominating behaviour including emotional, sexual and physical abuse and harassment that can worsen over time. These behaviours may include:

- physical aggression such as hitting, kicking and beating
- psychological violence such as intimidation and constant humiliation
- forced intercourse and other sexual coercion
- various controlling behaviours such as isolation from family and friends, monitoring movements, financial control and restricting access to services.

Abuse during pregnancy is a significant health problem, with serious consequences for both the pregnant woman (e.g. depression and substance misuse) and the infant (e.g. low birthweight and increased risk of child abuse). Family violence significantly contributes to homelessness among Australian women.[13]

One-third of women and one-quarter of men have experienced physical violence by an intimate partner.[5] Nevertheless, repeated coercive, sexual or severe physical violence is perpetrated largely by men against women. Intimate partner violence also occurs in same-sex relationships, but most research has focused on heterosexual relationships.

For women, health conditions may include gynaecological problems such as sexually transmitted infections, pelvic pain, complaints of sexual dysfunction, antepartum haemorrhage, unwanted pregnancy and pregnancy in very young girls. Other health problems may include chronic irritable bowel syndrome, back pain, depression and symptoms of post-traumatic stress disorder, problems sleeping, anxiety and 'panic' attacks. A thorough and repeated assessment for family violence is needed when these problems occur, especially when they persist.[14]

Child abuse and neglect

Child abuse is also a significant global health issue with far-reaching consequences (Box 5.1). Child abuse is defined as abuse or maltreatment of children under the age of 18 years in the context of a relationship of responsibility, trust or power.[15] This includes all forms of physical or emotional ill-treatment, sexual abuse, neglect or negligent treatment, or commercial or other exploitation, resulting in actual or potential harm to the child's health, survival, development or dignity. Exposure to and witnessing intimate partner violence is also recognised as abuse. The abuse may be intentional or unintentional. For categories of child abuse, see Table 5.2.

In Australia, 1 in 6 women and 1 in 10 men had been sexually or physically assaulted before age 15 years.[16] Many factors contribute to child abuse and neglect. See Table 5.3 for the personal, family, community and societal risk factors.

Box 5.1 Health effects of child abuse

Disruption of early brain development:

- Extreme stress can impair the development of the nervous and immune systems.

Risk of behavioural, physical and mental health problems:

- depression
- smoking
- obesity
- alcohol and drug misuse
- high-risk sexual behaviour
- unintended pregnancy
- perpetrating or being a victim of violence

Sources: World Health Organization 2023[15] and Rivara et al 2019[17]

TABLE 5.2 Categories of child abuse

Category	Description
Physical abuse	Any non-accidental physical act inflicted upon a child by a person caring for the child that caused physical injury, including hitting, shaking, throwing, burning and biting.
Emotional abuse	A parent or caregiver's inappropriate verbal or symbolic acts towards a child or a pattern of failure over time to provide a child with adequate non-physical nurturing and emotional availability. Such acts of commission or omission will likely damage a child's self-esteem or social competence—for example, constant criticism, teasing, ignoring, yelling and rejection. It also includes the effects on children of exposure to family violence.
Neglect	A pattern of failure over time on the part of a parent or other family member to provide for the development and wellbeing of the child in one or more of the following areas: health, education, emotional development, nutrition, shelter and safe living conditions. This includes when a child's basic needs for food, housing, health care and warm clothing are unmet. Leaving children without adequate supervision for their age is also a form of neglect.
Sexual abuse	The child's involvement in sexual activity that they do not fully comprehend or is unable to give informed consent, or for which the child is not developmentally prepared, or else that violates society's laws or social taboos. Children can be sexually abused by adults and other children who are—by age or stage of development—in a position of responsibility, trust or power over the victim.
Exposure to family violence	Children exposed to violence are at an elevated risk for emotional, behavioural and cognitive problems. They are affected across all stages of child development, with a higher risk of poor language development and impaired cognitive development.

Adapted from Australian Government Institute of Family studies 2023.[18]

Of those referred to statutory child protection services in Australia, girls have a higher rate of sustained sexual abuse than boys (11% vs 7%), with boys having a slightly higher rate of sustained neglect and physical abuse. Aboriginal and Torres Strait Islander children were almost seven times as likely to be the subject of substantiated abuse and neglect as non-Indigenous children.[16,19] In Aotearoa New Zealand, 1 in 5 children are reported to have been sexually abused and rates of Māori involvement with child protection services were more than twice those of Pacific Islander children and more than three times those of European children.[20]

Estimating prevalence can be difficult because many cases of child abuse and neglect go unreported and may never be disclosed. The immediate consequences of child abuse can include a spectrum of physical injuries such as bruises, fractures and lacerations and can involve more severe injuries such as shaken baby syndrome. More severe abuse can lead to death or long-term physical and mental disability. Children experiencing violence or neglect may exhibit diminished

TABLE 5.3 Risk factors for child abuse and neglect

Risk Factor	Description
Child characteristics	• Being under 4 years old • Having special needs, crying persistently or having a physical disability • Being unwanted • Failing to fulfil the expectations of parents
Family characteristics	• Family breakdown • Violence between family members, including intimate partner abuse • Unstable family environment when the composition of the household changes frequently • A breakdown of support in childrearing from extended family members • Being isolated in the community or lacking a support network
Parental characteristics	• Having been mistreated as a child • Experiencing financial difficulties • Low self-esteem, poor control of impulses, difficulty coping with stress • Physical, developmental or mental health problems of a family member • Displays of antisocial behaviour • Misusing alcohol and drugs
Community and societal factors	• Gender and social inequality • Lack of adequate housing or family support services • High levels of unemployment • Inequities related to gender and income • Social and cultural norms that promote or glorify violence towards others • Beliefs that demand rigid gender roles or diminish the status of the child in parent–child relationships • Social, economic, health and education policies that lead to poor living standards or socioeconomic inequality

Adapted from World Health Organization 2023.[15]

executive functioning and cognitive skills, poor mental or emotional health, attachment and social difficulties, post-traumatic stress and behavioural consequences such as unhealthy sexual practices, substance misuse and future perpetration of maltreatment.[15]

Cultural values and beliefs define child maltreatment; what may be acceptable in one culture may not be in another. All states and territories in Australia have legislation to protect children from abuse and neglect. Australian nurses are mandated to report suspected child abuse to the appropriate authorities. However, legislative definitions of abuse or what constitutes abuse or maltreatment differ from state to state. Become familiar with the legislation in your local area.[10,11] Nurses are not mandated to report child abuse in Aotearoa New Zealand. A person *may* report the abuse or likely abuse to a social worker or police officer. However, you could be criminally liable if you do not take reasonable steps to protect a child or vulnerable adult.

Elder abuse and neglect

Elder abuse is a serious and complex problem that affects many older people and may occur in different settings including the privacy of the person's home, residential care or hospital. The World Health Organization defines elder abuse as a single or repeated act, or lack of appropriate action, occurring within any caring relationship with an expectation of trust.[21] The prevalence of elder abuse has been estimated to be 2 to 14%.[19] However, the extent of elder abuse is underestimated, remains largely invisible and is under-reported.

Elder abuse can have severe physical consequences including pain, discomfort and life-threatening injuries. Elder abuse is associated with an increased risk of premature morbidity and mortality and long-lasting psychological consequences.[21]

Caregivers may depend on the older person for emotional and financial support, whether sharing housing or struggling with their own mental health or substance abuse challenges and frailty.[22] Frailty can affect the carer's capacity and judgement as a carer. The carer's intentions may be good, but the older person in their care may experience profound unintentional neglect or other forms of abuse. While some older women have been in abusive relationships for decades, others are experiencing physical and sexual violence for the first time from normally non-abusive partners who are afflicted with behaviour-altering neurological illnesses such as Alzheimer's disease.

Older people are also vulnerable to abuse from other family members and caretakers. Assessing physical abuse or neglect in cognitively impaired people is much more complicated. Significant red flags of possible abuse and neglect are physical findings inconsistent with the history provided by the patient, family member or caregiver. Older people may be reluctant to disclose abuse or neglect because they fear being relocated to a different institution or nursing home. They may be dependent on or have a co-dependent relationship with their abuser and fear the abuse will get worse or that they will be abandoned.[22]

Elder abuse can occur within an intimate partner relationship, an adult child and parent relationship and other caregiving relationships including institutional care.[23] There are many forms of elder abuse including physical, sexual, psychological, emotional, harassment, financial/material, abandonment, neglect and serious loss of dignity and respect. See categories of elder abuse further defined in Table 5.4.

Financial abuse is among the most common types of elder abuse; women are twice as likely to be abused as men.[23] Financial abuse is used when the family member (or carer) deprives the older person of enough financial resources to fulfil their basic needs.[24] Another area of abuse is power of attorney abuse. This type of abuse occurs when a person given enduring power of attorney fails to operate in the best interests of an older person.

A power of attorney and an enduring power of attorney are legal documents that allow someone (the 'principal') to appoint another person (the 'attorney' or 'agent') to make certain decisions and act on their behalf. However, there are important differences between the two that relate to their scope and duration. A power of attorney can be limited and can be revoked by the principal. An enduring power of attorney remains valid even if the principal becomes mentally incapacitated. This ensures that someone is authorised to manage the principal's affairs and make decisions on their behalf, especially in situations where the principal can no longer make decisions independently. Power of attorney and enduring power of attorney are legislated in each state of Australia, but a mandatory national registration scheme for enduring powers of attorney relating to financial matters has been proposed as one way to reduce the financial abuse of older Australians.

Risk factors for elder abuse include functional dependence or physical disability,

TABLE 5.4 Categories of elder abuse

Category	Description
Physical abuse	When an older person is injured because of hitting, kicking, pushing, slapping, burning or other show of force, medication abuse and inappropriate use of restraint or confinement that causes pain or bodily harm
Neglect	Failure to meet older person's basic needs such as food, housing, clothing or medical care
Sexual abuse	Forcing an older person to take part in a sexual act when the elder does not or cannot consent
Psychological abuse	Any behaviour that causes anguish, stress, fear or embarrassment including verbal abuse, damaging/destroying property, not allowing the person to see friends/family, intimidation, harassment, threats of physical/sexual abuse or removal of decision-making powers
Financial/ material abuse	Illegally misusing an older person's money, property or assets; occurs when a person given ordinary or enduring power of attorney abuses their powers and fails to operate in the older person's best interests

Adapted from Yon et al. 2017[23]
Reprinted with permission from Elsevier (Yon Y, Mikton CR, Gassoumis ZD, Wilber KH. Elder abuse prevalence in community settings: a systematic review and meta-analysis. The Lancet Global Health. 2017;5(2):e147–e156.)

cognitive impairment including dementia, poor mental health, social isolation and low socioeconomic status. Elder neglect may be intentional (active neglect) or unintentional (passive neglect) caused by a carer's condition or inadequate knowledge. Neglect occurs when another person fails to meet an older person's physical and emotional needs.[21]

Drivers of family violence

The underlying drivers of family violence reflect inequalities in the distribution of power, resources and opportunity within family relationships, particularly between women and men and in intimate partner relationships.[25] Understanding the drivers of family violence can improve knowledge about what influences a perpetrator, as well as helping to identify risks and ways to respond to family violence.

Violence against women is a deeply gendered issue rooted in structural inequalities and an imbalance of power between men and women. As stated previously, the prevalence and experience of family violence disproportionately affects women and is overwhelmingly perpetrated by men who are their current or former intimate partners.[26,27] Although both men and women can be victims and perpetrators of family violence, most family violence is perpetrated by men against women. Most men who experience family violence are victim-survivors of other male family members' use of violence.

Communities with attitudes reflecting greater levels of gender inequality generally have higher rates of family and sexual violence.[28] In most cases, violent behaviour is part of the various tactics used to exercise power and control over women, children and older people.

Impact of family violence

Health effects

Intimate partner violence is a global health problem with serious public health consequences. A significant association exists between lifetime experience of partner violence and poor mental and physical health outcomes. Family violence can significantly negatively affect a person's physical and mental health. The effects can be immediate or long term and may persist even after the violence has stopped.[13] See some potential health effects of family violence in Table 5.5.

Economic impact

The economic burden of family violence includes the cost of pain and suffering, healthcare costs, productivity and administration related to violence against women. Intimate partner violence is a leading contributor to death, disability and illness in women aged between 15 and 44 years and is responsible for more disease burden than many well-known risk factors such as high tobacco use, high cholesterol and illicit drug use with wide-ranging and persistent effects on physical and mental health. Women who have been abused will

TABLE 5.5 Health effects of family violence

Effect	Potential Consequences
Physical injuries	Bruises and cuts, broken bones and head injuries; these injuries can lead to chronic pain, disability and even death (homicide/suicide)
Mental health problems	Anxiety, depression, post-traumatic stress disorder, substance abuse and suicide attempts
Functional health changes	Sleep difficulties, eating disorders, problems in relationships, work and school pain syndromes (back pain, abdominal pain, chronic pelvic pain), gastrointestinal disorders, limited mobility
Reproductive/ gynaecological problems	Worsening of menopausal symptoms, unintended pregnancies, induced abortions, miscarriage, stillbirth, preterm delivery and low-birthweight babies, sexually transmitted infections, HIV
Chronic health conditions	Heart disease, gastrointestinal problems and chronic pain
Intergenerational transmission	It can be a learnt behaviour that is passed down from one generation to the next; children who witness family violence may be more likely to perpetrate violence in their future adult relationships
Behavioural problems (children)	Children who witness or experience violence are more likely to develop behavioural problems like aggression, delinquency and substance misuse, smoking, risky sexual behaviours, perpetration of violence (for males) and being a victim of violence (for females)

Adapted from World Health Organization 2021[14]

most likely need to access health care. Physical injury is the most obvious and immediate health problem, including fractures, bruising and lacerations. Those women who have experienced severe physical violence are more likely to have told someone than those with less severe injuries.

Intimate partner violence causes more illness, disability and deaths than other risk factors for women aged 25 to 34.[29] It is estimated that the annual cost of domestic violence against women and children to the Australian national economy is $26 billion.[30]

Intersectionality

Intersectionality describes how inequality based on gender, race, ethnicity, sexual orientation, gender identity, disability, class and other forms of discrimination compound or 'intersect' to create unique dynamics and effects.[31] An intersectional lens focuses on a person's location in a social hierarchy based on age, sex, race, ethnicity, sexual orientation, gender identity, disability status, socioeconomic status and cultural experiences.[32]

Immigrant women in family violence situations have needs that differ from those of the mainstream population, particularly where the threat of deportation, including the potential loss of children, is used as a weapon against the woman.[33] Culturally diverse women experience systemic racism, language barriers and cultural beliefs that promote silencing of family violence. Culturally appropriate family violence responses must be mindful of these added complexities.[34] Culturally diverse women's experiences of family violence are often intertwined with experiences of racism, language barriers and inequitable access to health care and support services.[35]

Recent research has aimed to identify First Nations peoples' experiences and expectations of health professionals when experiencing family violence. First Nations peoples are reluctant to engage in help-seeking for support, despite experiencing higher rates of family violence than the non-Indigenous population.[34] This reluctance may be due to distrust of a system that is not culturally informed. Women of colour are less likely than white women to seek help formally from police and legal aid services and suffer disproportionately from family violence. They are more likely to seek informal support like family members or friends.[35]

Bisexual people are at increased risk of intimate partner violence compared with people of other sexualities and may face added barriers to seeking help.[36] There is a lack of research on the risk and protective factors for bisexual people, despite experiencing a disproportionate risk of intimate partner violence.[37]

With culturally appropriate knowledge, attitudes and behaviours, health practitioners may overcome some barriers created by generations of systemic racism and historical trauma experienced by people from marginalised communities.[38] System-wide interventions must be designed intentionally and consider the impact of cumulative harm and intersectionality and the structural aspects of trauma such as discriminatory systems, structural barriers, historical/current inequities and harmful institutional practices.[39]

Cultural and social considerations

Not all people of the same gender, sexuality, family, ethnicity or culture will share the same attitudes, values or beliefs. There may be different interpretations of what constitutes abuse in different cultures—for example, the right of parents to discipline their children using physical force such as slapping or hitting and rites of passage rituals that result in physical injury. Therefore, nurses must consider the person and family's cultural context and religious beliefs when assessing and responding to family violence.

The needs of people of culturally and linguistically diverse backgrounds will differ for a range of reasons including cultural and religious beliefs, level of education, language skills/fluency, family relationships, length of time since migration, prescribed gender roles, social networks, economic circumstance, lack of understanding of Australian laws/ beliefs and attitudes towards family violence. Differences across cultures may affect disclosure because of fear of religious beliefs, the need to protect the family name and fear of reprisal—for example, deportation and loss of children, social exclusion, death threats and honour killings.[40]

First Nations women are more likely to experience family violence and sustain a serious injury requiring hospitalisation and more likely to die due to family violence than non-Indigenous women.[12] In Aotearoa New Zealand, Māori women are twice as likely to experience current partner violence than the national average.[41]

Research has identified intimate partner violence rates in same-sex relationships are similar, if not higher, than in opposite-sex relationships and that the violence can be bidirectional.[42] According to the Australian Institute of Health and Welfare, the number of same-sex family violence reports to the police is rising.[13]

An interpreter should be considered if a person's first language is not English. However, it is important to be aware of the potential sensitivities associated with disclosure in the presence of a person from the same cultural or religious background.

Documenting family violence

Documentation in the health record of family/intimate partner violence, child and elder abuse must include:

- detailed, nonbiased documentation
- use of injury maps, diagrams and photographic documentation (taken by specialist photographers or healthcare staff) to show skin marks and injuries
- a description of injuries using forensic terminology (Table 5.6, Table 5.7 and Table 5.8)
- prior written consent before photographs can be taken—if the person is unconscious or cognitively impaired, taking photographs without consent is generally considered ethically sound since it is a noninvasive, painless intervention with a high potential to help a suspected abuse victim
- a victim statement that identifies the reported perpetrator
- a victim statement that includes severe threats of harm, with curses and

TABLE 5.6 Signs of trauma in adult victims

Form of Trauma		
Physical	• Bruising • Fractures • Chronic pain (neck, back) • Fresh scars or minor cuts • Terminations of pregnancy	• Complications during pregnancy • Gastrointestinal disorders • Sexually transmitted infections • Strangulation
Psychological	• Depression • Anxiety • Self-harming behaviour • Eating disorders • Phobias • Somatic disorders	• Sleep problems • Impaired concentration • Harmful alcohol use • Licit and illicit drug use • Physical exhaustion • Suicide attempts
Emotional	• Fear • Shame • Anger • No support networks	• Feelings of worthlessness and hopelessness • Feeling disassociated and emotionally numb
Social/financial	• Homelessness • Unemployment • Financial debt	• No friends or family support • Isolation • Parenting difficulties
Demeanour	• Unconvincing explanations of any injuries • Describing a partner as controlling or prone to anger • Being accompanied by their partner, who does most of the talking	• Anxiety in the presence of a partner • Recent separation or divorce • Needing to be back home by a certain time and becoming stressed about this • Reluctance to follow the advice

Adapted from Victorian Government 2023[43]

TABLE 5.7 Signs of trauma—from unborn children to adolescents

Observable signs of trauma that may indicate family violence for:

An unborn child	*A baby (under 18 months)*	*A toddler*
• Poor growth and neural development caused by rushes of maternal adrenalin and cortisol • Injuries sustained via injury to the mother or the perpetrator targeting the unborn child directly (such as inflicting blows to the mother's abdominal area)	• Excessive crying • Excessive passivity • Underweight for age • Significant sleep or feeding difficulties • Reactions to loud voices or noises • Extreme wariness of new people • No verbal 'play' (such as imitating sounds) • Frequent illness • Anxiety, overly clingy to the primary caregiver	As for babies (under 18 months) and also: • excessive irritability • excessive compliance • poor language development • delayed mobility • blood in nappy, underwear

TABLE 5.7 Signs of trauma—from unborn children to adolescents cont'd

Preschooler	*Primary school-aged child*	*Adolescent*
• Extreme clinginess • Significant sleep and eating difficulties • Poor concentration in play • Inability to empathise with other people • Frequent illness • Poor language development and significant use of 'baby talk' • Displaying maladaptive behaviour such as frequent rocking, sucking and biting • Aggression towards others • Adjustment problems (e.g. significant difficulties moving from kindergarten to school) • Antisocial play or lack of interest in engaging with others	• Rebelliousness, defiant behaviour • Limited tolerance and poor impulse control • Temper tantrums or irritability; being aggressive or demanding • Physical abuse or cruelty to others including pets • Avoidance of conflict • Showing low self-esteem • Extremely compliant behaviour; being passive, tearful or withdrawn • Excessively oppositional or argumentative behaviour • Risk-taking behaviours that have severe or life-threatening consequences • Lack of interest in social activities • Delayed/poor language skills • Experiencing problems with schoolwork • Poor social competence • Acting like a much younger child • Poor school performance • Poor coping skills • Sleep issues • Bed wetting • Excessive washing • Frequent illness • Complaining of headaches or stomach pains • Self-harm • Displaying maladaptive behaviour • Displaying sexual behaviour or knowledge unusual for the child's age • Telling someone sexual abuse has occurred • Complaining of pain going to the toilet • Enacting sexual behaviour with other children • Excessive masturbation	As for primary school-aged children and also: • school refusal/avoidance (absenteeism/disengagement) • criminal or antisocial behaviours, including using violence against others • eating disorders • substance abuse • depression • suicidal ideation • risk-taking behaviours • anxiety • pregnancy • controlling or manipulative behaviour • obsessive behaviour • homelessness or frequent changes in housing arrangements

Adapted from Family Safety Victoria 2018[25]

TABLE 5.8 Forensic terminology

Term	Definition
Abrasion	A wound caused by rubbing the skin or mucous membrane
Avulsion	The tearing away of a structure or part
Bruise	Superficial discolouration due to haemorrhage into the tissues from ruptured blood vessels beneath the skin surface, without the skin being broken; also called a contusion
Contusion	A bruise; injury to tissues without breakage of skin; blood from broken blood vessels accumulates, producing pain, swelling, tenderness
Cut	See 'incision'
Ecchymosis	A haemorrhagic spot or blotch larger than petechiae in the skin or mucous membrane forms a non-elevated, rounded or irregular, blue or purplish patch
Haematoma	A localised collection of extravasated blood is usually clotted in an organ, space or tissue
Haemorrhage	The escape of blood from a ruptured vessel, which can be external, internal or into the skin or other organ
Incision	A cut or wound made by a sharp instrument; the act of cutting
Laceration	The act of tearing or splitting; a wound produced by the tearing or splitting of body tissue, usually from blunt impact over a bony surface
Lesion	A broad term referring to any pathological or traumatic disruption of tissue
Patterned injury	An injury caused by an object that leaves a distinct pattern on the skin or organ (e.g. being whipped with an extension cord) or an injury caused by a unique mechanism of injury (e.g. immersion burns to the hands (glove burn) or feet (sock burns)
Pattern of injuries	Injuries, usually bruises and fractures, in various stages of healing
Petechiae	Minute, pinpoint, non-raised, perfectly round, purplish-red spots caused by intradermal or submucous haemorrhage later turn blue or yellow
Puncture	The act of piercing or penetrating with a pointed object or instrument
Stab wound	A penetrating, sharp, cutting injury that is deeper than it is wide
Traumatic alopecia	Loss of hair from pulling and yanking or by other traumatic means
Wound	A general term referring to a bodily injury caused by physical means

Sources: Sheridan & Nash 2007[44]; Miller-Keane 2003[45]

expletives made by the alleged perpetrator (can be extremely useful in future legal proceedings)
- a verbatim report using the person's words, but within reason (however, documenting every statement made by an abused person verbatim is unrealistic)
- use of words the child or older person has given to describe how their injury occurred
- reports of past abusive incidents, which can be paraphrased with partial direct quotations
- use of exact terms used by the victim to describe sexual organs or sexually assaultive behaviours
- statements from caregivers if the child or older person is nonverbal.

HEALTH EDUCATION

Preventing family violence

The Alma-Ata Declaration[46] and subsequently the Ottawa Charter for Health Promotion[47] were indicative of the increasing global recognition of the significance of primary health care and a change in emphasis towards promoting health. Health promotion encompasses an array of strategies that enhance the health prospects of individuals and communities.

Health promotion plays a crucial role in addressing and preventing family violence. While the primary focus is to improve overall health and wellbeing, it also encompasses efforts to prevent and address violence within families.

Health promotion initiatives aim to:

- raise awareness about the causes, consequences and dynamics of family violence
- provide education and information to individuals, families and communities
- foster understanding, challenge misconceptions and promote healthy relationships
- create supportive environments for survivors.

Health promotion strategies focus on:

- preventing family violence by addressing underlying risk factors and causes
- promoting positive family dynamics, healthy communication and conflict-resolution skills
- targeting root causes such as gender inequality, social norms that condone violence and substance abuse.

Nurse's role

A nurse's role in health promotion includes:

- recognising signs of trauma and responding sensitively
- providing support and resources to people and families affected by violence
- connecting survivors to support services, helplines, shelters, legal aid and other community resources
- reducing barriers to access services and ensuring they are inclusive and culturally appropriate.

Resources

For resources, see the 'Additional resources' section at the end of the chapter.

Subjective data

While there are similarities in assessment of family violence, child abuse and neglect and elder abuse there are important differences. For that reason, each of these groups will be treated separately in the subjective data section.

Preparation

The interview aims to identify what is most important to the person, respond to their needs and respect their wishes. As you are approaching the health assessment interview, it is important that you:

- Ensure privacy and confidentiality to establish trust.
- Conduct the interview away from public areas, partners, carers and family. This gives the woman a chance to say what she wants in a safe and private place to a caring person who wants to help.
- Assure the person that anything discussed will remain confidential, except in situations where safety or the safety of others is at risk.
- Listen actively and show empathy—this validates the person's concerns, experiences and emotions and helps the person feel comfortable and supported. Be aware of your feelings and reaction to the disclosure, abuse or violence.
- Demonstrate cultural awareness and sensitivity.
- Be prepared to initiate a referral to relevant support services. This step includes safety planning to remove, reduce or mitigate the risks, and to minimise harm and maximise safety.

Clinical alert

If sexual abuse or assault is suspected or reported, a specialist healthcare team will take over the person's assessment, collection of forensic evidence and care. The person must not change their clothes or wash any body part until seen by the specialist team. Check your local health service policies and procedures for details about expected processes.

ASSESSMENT GUIDELINES	CLINICAL SIGNIFICANCE AND CLINICAL ALERTS
Screening or routine enquiry	
This involves enquiring about personal history and history of family violence to identify people at risk who need further assessment or interventions. The questions that are provided in the subjective data collection can be augmented by referring to reference.[35]	If intimate partner violence is suspected, a risk assessment is undertaken.

ASSESSMENT GUIDELINES	CLINICAL SIGNIFICANCE AND CLINICAL ALERTS
Risk assessment	
A standard family violence screening tool may be used. Screening tools contain questions regarding physical, emotional and sexual abuse and controlling behaviours. Alert the person that questions about family violence and personal safety are asked of all women. The following opening statement is suggested: • *Because family violence is so common in our community, we ask all women the same questions.* If the woman is Indigenous, it is suggested that you start with the following statement: • *Tell me about your mob.* Examples of possible questions are provided below. • *Tell me about your relationships.* • *Do you feel safe at home?* • *Has anyone in your family done something that made you or your children feel unsafe or afraid?* • *Has this person controlled your day-to-day activities (e.g. who you see, where you go) or put you down?* • *Have they threatened to hurt you in any way?* • *Have they physically hurt you in any way? (hit, slapped, kicked or otherwise physically hurt you)* • *Do you have any immediate concerns about the safety of your children or someone else in your family?*	This is a longer and more detailed process to learn more about someone's views, behaviours, circumstances and interactions to determine the risk of harm to themselves and other family members. The nurse helps the person to assess their situation and plan for future safety. If the person answers yes to any of your questions, ask more detailed questions to understand the person's circumstances and better assess their and their children's safety. If the person minimises the level of abuse, such as '*only emotional*' or '*not that bad*' or '*we just fight a lot*', more may be revealed as you gently assess the situation. A person is not 'in denial' if they minimise the abuse; it is not uncommon for this response to accompany the experience of trauma from violence.
History of abuse	
It is important to assess and document prior abuse including: • intimate partner violence • childhood physical and sexual abuse • prior sexual assaults of all kinds (stranger, date, intimate partner) • traumatic injuries • the length of time of the abuse • whether it is still occurring • the severity of the abuse • knowledge of or experience with family violence services.	Understanding the person's history determines the impact of the past on the person's current health. For example, a person may have chronic but subtle neurological symptoms and problems that may be related to previous episodes of head trauma.
Validation of the person's experience	
Some possible ways to validate disclosure of abuse is to make statements such as: • *Everybody deserves to feel safe at home.* • *You don't deserve to be hit or hurt.* • *I am concerned about your safety and wellbeing.* • *Help is available, and I will help you.* • *You are not to blame. Abuse is common and happens in all kinds of relationships*	By showing concern about the degree of violence, you will convey the message that the abuse is not the woman's fault and that help is available. The person may not be ready to act, but having their experience validated and feelings acknowledged by a compassionate nurse can help facilitate the first steps towards change.

ASSESSMENT GUIDELINES	CLINICAL SIGNIFICANCE AND CLINICAL ALERTS
Additional history for infants and children (questions for parent/guardian)	
Assessing for child abuse and neglect	
	The questions that are provided in the subjective data collection can be augmented by referring to the Royal Children's Hospital Clinical Guidelines for Child Abuse.[48]
Screening or routine enquiry	
To identify if the child is at risk ask about the child's: • developmental stage • psychological function • social circumstances • personal history • history of family violence.	
Developmental stage	
Ask the parent or caregiver questions about the child's stage of development (Chapter 3). For example, for an infant: • *Is your child crawling, pulling to stand or walking?* • *How well is their speech developing?* • *Are they toilet trained?* For an older female child, ask about their menstrual history.	If there is an injury, consider if the child could have suffered the reported injury based on their developmental level. For example, the history that a 3-week-old child rolled off a bed (causing injury) is not developmentally plausible. Children experiencing violence or neglect may exhibit delays in reaching milestones.
Psychological function	
Assessment should include the child's: • past behaviour patterns • current behavioural problems (Chapter 3). Ask the parent or caregiver: • *What is it like caring for your child?* • *Are you experiencing any difficulties getting your child to bed?* • *Have you noticed any changes in behaviour or mood?* • *How is school/kindergarten going?*	When asking these questions, observe the interaction between the child and the parent or caregiver. Observation while collecting subjective data allows you to consider the caregiver's attachment to the child.
Social circumstances	
Ask questions about: • family relationships • current members of the household • arrangements when parents are separated • childcare arrangements • other children in the household.	Poverty, parent's gender, family structure, ethnicity and access to resources are inextricably tied to neglect. It is important to note, however, that children in poor circumstances are not always neglected.

ASSESSMENT GUIDELINES	CLINICAL SIGNIFICANCE AND CLINICAL ALERTS
If indicated, ask about: • parenting practices • family routines • parent's history • family history. For older children, ask about: • school attendance • extracurricular activities • friendships and peer relationships • drug and alcohol use • sexual relationships • about any prior contact with child protection agencies or police, and if there are any protective or court orders in place. For adolescents, see HEADSS assessment in Chapter 8.	 ***Clinical alert:*** Nurses who suspect child abuse or neglect should refer to other healthcare team members (medical practitioners, social workers, counsellors etc.) as screening and assessment processes are complex and have potentially serious implications for the child and their family. The healthcare team should gather and document the evidence carefully notifying child protection services.
Past health history	
• *Has the child had previous hospitalisations or injuries?* • *Do they suffer from any chronic medical conditions?* • *Is there a history of bleeding disorders, connective tissue disease or developmental disorders?* • *Does the child take any medication that may cause easy bruising?* • *Was there a delay in seeking care for anything other than a minor injury?* • *Are there any sleep problems?* • *Has your child experienced any mood changes?* • *Have there been any adjustment problems?*	Be alert to non-physical signs and symptoms and to adjustment problems.
Additional history for an adult over 65 years	
Screening for abuse in older people	
The questions that are provided in the subjective data collection can be augmented by referring to the Australian Elder Abuse Screening Instrument (DRAFT) (Figure 5.1).[49]	
Opening the discussion about elder abuse and neglect	
When assessing the older person, it is useful to start with indirect questions and then move to a more direct inquiry if abuse is suspected. A suggested beginning is: • *Can you tell me what happened?* • *What do you remember about how the injury occurred?*	Including caregivers in your assessment is important for those who rely on care from others in aged care facilities or their homes.
Screening or routine enquiry	
The opportunity for screening for family violence presents itself each time the nurse interacts with the person, but some presentations may strongly suggest an experience of violence.	

DRAFT

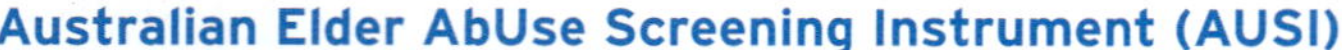

Australian Elder AbUse Screening Instrument (AUSI)

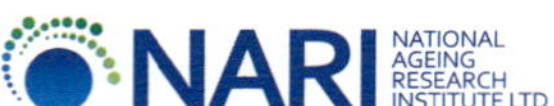

HOW TO USE THE AUSI

- Use the AUSI when elder abuse is suspected.
- Use the AUSI as part of a consultation AND to identify whether further assessment is required.
- Take time before asking questions. The older person will be more likely to disclose information when trust and rapport has been built.
- Use the AUSI in a private room. The older person should answer questions independently of any person who may be providing them with care.
- Seek an independent interpreter service if needed. Do not have a family member/friend translate.
- Explain that the conversation will be confidential, except where their safety is identified to be at risk (e.g. if they disclose that someone is someone is hurting or abusing them) you would need to notify your supervisor.
- Consider the client's ability to answer. Where possible, use the AUSI at a time and place when client capacity is maximised. If this is not possible, use the AUSI another time.

ASSESSOR TO NOTE:

Date:	Client Name:	DOB:	Gender:
Assessor Name:		Assessor Role:	

Place of screening: ☐ Hospital ☐ GP Clinic ☐ Private residence ☐ Aged Care ☐ Other: ....

Client's place of residence: *(note who else might live with the older person)* ....

SCREENING QUESTIONS:

1. Do you need help from another person with any of the following tasks?
☐ Social activities ☐ Dressing ☐ Bathing / showering
☐ Transportation ☐ Meals ☐ Medication
☐ Finances / bills / banking ☐ Shopping ☐ Toileting / personal care
☐ Other ....

2. Do all of the people helping you treat you with respect? ☐ Yes ☐ No ☐ Unsure

If YES, no further questions may be needed. However, the assessor should use professional judgement.
If NO or UNSURE answered, go to question 3.

3.	Do any of these people refuse to help you when you need help?	☐ Never	☐ Sometimes	☐ Often
4.	Do any of these people stop you from seeking help from others?	☐ Never	☐ Sometimes	☐ Often
5.	Do any of these people make you sign documents that you are not comfortable signing or do not understand?	☐ Never	☐ Sometimes	☐ Often
6.	Do any of these people take anything of yours without asking, such as your money (including accessing bank accounts) or valuables?	☐ Never	☐ Sometimes	☐ Often
7.	Do any of these people make you feel afraid?	☐ Never	☐ Sometimes	☐ Often
8.	Do any of these people speak to you in ways that make you feel upset?	☐ Never	☐ Sometimes	☐ Often

9. Would you like help with any of this now?
☐ **Yes** *(provide relevant referrals from overleaf then continue to question 10)*
☐ **No** *(respect client's wishes and provide them with information about help that is available if they decide to seek it in the future)*

IF THE OLDER PERSON IS IN IMMEDIATE DANGER OR RISK OF HARM CALL POLICE ON 000 (TRIPLE ZERO).
Regardless of the answer given to question 9, If SOMETIMES or OFTEN is given to questions 3-8 continue to question 10.

10.	Do any of these people threaten you? (E.g. threats with respect to money, property or access to grandchildren?)	☐ Never	☐ Sometimes	☐ Often
11.	Do any of these people touch you in ways that make you feel uncomfortable?	☐ Never	☐ Sometimes	☐ Often
12.	Do any of these people hurt you physically?	☐ Never	☐ Sometimes	☐ Often

If SOMETIMES or OFTEN is given to questions 10-12, notify your supervisor to decide on next steps regarding client safety.

FIGURE 5.1 Australian Elder Abuse Screening Instrument (DRAFT)
Source: National Ageing Research Institute 2023[49]

ASSESSMENT GUIDELINES	CLINICAL SIGNIFICANCE AND CLINICAL ALERTS
Screening for family violence in older people is the same as screening for younger people; similar questions can be used. Please review the previous sections titled '**Screening or routine enquiry**' and '**Risk assessment**' under 'Family violence'.	
Risk assessment	
Older people can present for health care with few or multiple health, physical and cognitive challenges. An opening statement might be: *Because family violence has such serious health consequences, we are asking people of all ages the following questions*: • *Are you afraid of anyone at home?* • *Has anyone ever locked you in a room or locked you in your house?* • *Has anyone at home ever pushed, hit or hurt you?* • *Has anyone demanded money from you?* • *Has anyone persuaded you to sign any documents?* • *Has anyone ever failed to help you take care of yourself when you needed help?* • *Does anyone scold or threaten you?* Questions that should be asked of the caregiver: • *How has your life changed since becoming the primary caregiver?* • *Have you been able to talk to someone about the changes in your life since becoming a caregiver?* • *Are you aware of what resources and practical help are available to help you?* If the caregiver is suspected to be the abuser, they should be interviewed alone. The following questions can be asked: • *Do you feel that (the older person receiving care) expects too much from you?* • *Do you feel that because of the time you spend with (older person receiving care), you don't have enough time to do things you want to do?* • *Are you tired of caring for (the older person receiving care)?* • *Have you ever felt like physically hurting (older person receiving care)?*	There is no mandatory reporting of elder abuse in either Australia or Aotearoa New Zealand. However, there are policies and systems set up so complaints about elder abuse can be investigated. For example, for those in residential care, in Australia, the *Aged Care Act 1997* was amended in 2007[50] and includes a Charter of Residents' Rights and Responsibilities,[51] which states that people living in aged care homes have the right to be treated with dignity and respect and to live without exploitation, abuse or neglect. Anyone who suspects elder abuse can report via an aged care complaints investigation scheme.
Past history	
The assessment should include a thorough medical and surgical history, current medications and psychosocial assessment. See Chapter 8.	

Objective data

Objective data collection for suspected abuse includes a general survey of the person, inspection and palpation of skin, mouth and teeth, hair and scalp, joints and muscles. Refer back to:

- Table 5.2 Categories of child abuse
- Table 5.6 Signs of trauma in adult victims
- Table 5.7 Signs of trauma—from unborn children to adolescents
- Table 5.8 Forensic terminology.

A structured process is undertaken when examining people who may have been abused. Objective data cited below is relevant to adults, older people, infants and children. See also Chapter 6, Chapter 21 and Chapter 22.

PROCEDURES AND NORMAL FINDINGS	ABNORMAL FINDINGS AND CLINICAL ALERTS
While collecting subjective data, you will have noticed the condition of the person's skin, lips, hair and mucous membranes, their breath odour, ease of breathing, height-to-weight ratio, body shape, level of hygiene and grooming and general demeanour. All these factors provide clues to the person's overall health.	
Inspect level of hygiene, grooming, clothing	
Inspect: • level of cleanliness • grooming • suitability of clothing.	Abuse and neglect may be evidenced by poor grooming and hygiene and a lack of adequate clothing, shelter or food.
Inspection and palpation of skin	
Inspect the skin for: • bruises • abrasions • burns • handprints from grabbing or slapping • bite marks • lacerations • black eyes • bruises on the arms • red or purple marks • pain/tenderness. It is common for **toddlers and children** to sustain bruising on the knees, anterior shins and forehead, but bruising on the feet, face, trunk, buttocks, posterior legs and arms is less likely to be accidental. They, therefore, should be viewed with suspicion because they are indicators of abuse.	Unexplained bruising, skin tears, long-bone and multiple fractures, chronic pain, anxiety and changes in behaviour align with potential abuse. ! ***Clinical alert:*** Any bruise that takes the shape of an object should be cause for concern such as belts, electric cords and kitchen utensils (wooden spoons, spatulas), which are common instruments of physical abuse. A new bruise is usually red and often develops a purple or purple-blue appearance 12 to 36 hours after blunt force trauma. The colour of bruises usually progresses from purple-blue to bluish-green to greenish-brown to brownish-yellow before fading away.

PROCEDURES AND NORMAL FINDINGS	ABNORMAL FINDINGS AND CLINICAL ALERTS
	Multiple factors contribute to bruising other than physical abuse. For example, **older people** may bruise more readily or severely than younger people. Medications and abnormal blood values related to medication side effects and underlying haematological disorders can result in bruising (ecchymoses). Common medications that increase the risk for bruising or bleeding include aspirin, clopidogrel, heparin, ibuprofen, any of the non-steroidal anti-inflammatory drugs, prednisone, valproic acid and warfarin. ! ***Clinical alert:*** Many inflicted injuries may not be reported by the person or their caregiver, making careful inspection necessary. The presence of bruises on an **infant** is significant and warrants further assessment for abuse. ! ***Clinical alert:*** Significant injuries can be hidden under clothing, nappies, socks and long hair. ! ***Clinical alert:*** Bruising found on **infants** who are not yet mobile should also raise concern and prompt further assessment for potential other injuries, including fractures and intracranial injury. It is important to document any bruising in children, whether there is a history of accidental trauma or not. The forensic terminology used to document **intimate partner** violence and **elder** abuse also applies to **children**. See Table 5.8.
Inspection and palpation of the mouth	
Inspect and palpate for: • damaged or missing teeth • bruising or split lip • tenderness on palpation of oral mucosa • chewing difficulties • abrasions or lacerations of the tongue, oral mucosa, hard and soft palate, frenulum.	Refer to Chapter 21.
Inspection and palpation of the scalp	
Inspect and palpate for: • pain and tenderness • bald spots from hair being pulled out.	Refer to Chapter 22.

PROCEDURES AND NORMAL FINDINGS	ABNORMAL FINDINGS AND CLINICAL ALERTS
Inspection and palpation of muscles and joints	
Inspect and palpate the muscles and joints for pain, swelling, bruising, decreased range of motion or lack of alignment. See Chapter 20.	Check for any suspicious areas that might indicate a fracture or dislocation of joints. Physical signs of abuse include fractures and dislocations.
Mental status assessment	
All survivors of violence should be given a mental status examination, with particular attention to the most frequent mental health problems associated with violence: depression, suicidality, post-traumatic stress disorder, substance abuse and anxiety.	Chapter 11 gives directions for conducting this part of the assessment.

Clinical reasoning and documentation

The following is a continuation of the case study provided at the beginning of this chapter and the clinical reasoning process including problem/issue identification. Consult a fundamentals of nursing or medical-surgical nursing text for information about goal setting, nursing interventions and evaluation.

Case study (continued)—Suspected family violence

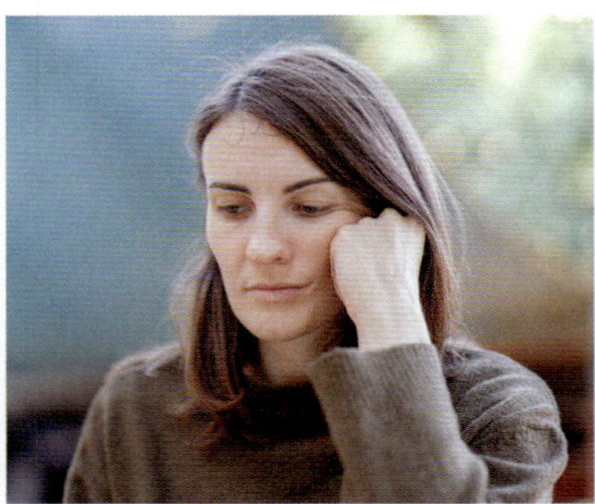

Context

You will recall from the case study described earlier in the chapter that you are the registered nurse working in a primary health care clinic.

Consider the patient's situation

You suspect that Ms King may be a victim of family violence given her mood, emotional distress and her reports of pain, anxiety and insomnia.

Collect cues/information

Your further assessment of Ms King reveals the following additional information.

Subjective data

Ms King has two children: Chad, 4 years and Sally, 2 years. Her partner Charley moved in with her and her elderly mother (Molly) 18 months ago. In recent months Ms King has been out with her girlfriends for drinks and came home late on some occasions. Charley got very angry with her. Last week, when she came home later than expected, he yelled again and knocked her backwards into the table and onto the floor. Ms King was stunned and says she has a bruise on her hip; she feels as if her finger is broken. Charley apologised, telling Ms King he loved her and that it wouldn't happen again. She states that she worries about her children and elderly mother and no longer feels safe. She is having trouble sleeping. Ms King has been assured that her concerns have been heard and she will be helped to get the assistance she needs.

Objective data

Ms King appears anxious and withdrawn during the consultation, exhibiting signs of emotional distress—agitation, crying.
Bruising is noted on her left hip.
Her mobility assessment showed her gait is within normal limits.
There is tenderness on palpation of the middle section of the thorax.

Clinical reasoning and documentation cont'd

Process information and identify problems/issues

Collaborative problems

Impaired mobility of ring finger (right hand)—for medical review.
Acute pain (hip, back, finger) related to physical abuse and physical injuries—for medical review.

Possible problem statement(s)/nursing diagnoses

Pain related to bruised hip, back and finger injury—for medical review.
Fear and anxiety related to the threat of punishment and other family members' safety.
Insomnia related to fear and anxiety.
Risk for injury related to physical trauma or abuse.
Impaired family functioning related to the family's pattern of abuse.
Ineffective decision making related to a lack of safety planning strategies.
Ineffective coping related to fear, stress and lack of support.
Hopelessness related to a feeling of wanting to escape from the violent situation.

The next step: referral and collaboration

Recognising the need for comprehensive care, you refer Ms King and her family to a multidisciplinary team including social workers, psychologists and legal professionals who specialise in supporting people affected by family violence.

ADDITIONAL RESOURCES

You can further develop your knowledge and skills relevant to screening for family violence, related pathophysiology, common health issues and nursing interventions by:

- reading chapters of a fundamentals of nursing or medical-surgical nursing textbook
- answering chapter multiple choice questions online. Log onto ClinicalKey Student and search for the text 'Health Assessment, 4th edition'. Choose the section titled 'Teaching material'. In this section you will find question and answer documents for each chapter.
- visiting websites

Australia

1800RESPECT—National sexual assault, domestic family violence, counselling service: https://www.1800respect.org.au

13 YARN—A National crisis support line for mob who are feeling overwhelmed or having difficulty coping. https://www.13yarn.org.au

Australian Government—Department of Human Services: https://www.humanservices.gov.au/individuals/subjects/family-and-domestic-violence

Kids Helpline: https://kidshelpline.com.au

Lifeline (Australia): https://www.lifeline.org.au/

MensLine Australia: https://mensline.org.au

Reach out.com (Australia): https://au.reachout.com/articles/sexual-assault-support

ADDITIONAL RESOURCES cont'd

White Ribbon Australia: https://www.whiteribbon.org.au

Aotearoa New Zealand

Family violence—It's not OK (NZ): http://www.areyouok.org.nz

Kidsline NZ: https://whatsup.co.nz//

New Zealand Government—Domestic or family violence: https://www.govt.nz/browse/law-crime-and-justice/abuse-harassment-domestic-violence/domestic-or-family-violence/

Victims Information—For people affected by sexual violence (NZ): https://sexualviolence.victimsinfo.govt.nz

White Ribbon New Zealand: https://whiteribbon.org.nz

REFERENCES

1. Brown SJ, Mensah F, Giallo R, Woolhouse H, Hegarty K, Nicholson JM, et al. Intimate partner violence and maternal mental health ten years after a first birth: an Australian prospective cohort study of first-time mothers. Journal of Affective Disorders. 2020;262:247–257.
2. Department of Social Services. Fourth action plan: National plan to reduce violence against women and their children 2010–2022. Canberra, Australia; 2019. Available from: https://www.dss.gov.au/women-publications-articles-reducing-violence/fourth-action-plan
3. Garcia-Moreno C, Hegarty K, d'Oliveira AFPL, Koziol-Mclain J, Colombini M, Feder G. The health-systems response to violence against women. The Lancet. 2015;385:1567–1579.
4. Our Watch. Quick Facts Melbourne, 2023. Available from: https://www.ourwatch.org.au/quick-facts/
5. Gartland D, Conway LJ, Giallo R, Mensah FK, Cook F, Hegarty K, et al. Intimate partner violence and child outcomes at age 10: a pregnancy cohort. Archives of Disease in Childhood. 2021;0(0):1–9.
6. Wathen CN, MacMillan HL. Children's exposure to intimate partner violence: impacts and interventions. Paediatrics and Child Health. 2013;18(8):419–422.
7. State of Victoria. Free from violence: Victoria's strategy to prevent family violence. Melbourne: State of Victoria; 2022. Available from: https://www.vic.gov.au/free-violence-victorias-strategy-prevent-family-violence
8. Adams C, Hooker L, Taft A. The characteristics of Australian maternal and child health home visiting nurses undertaking family violence work: an interpretive description study. Journal of Advanced Nursing. 2022; online(1):1–15.
9. Heyman RE, Mitnick DM, Smith Slep AM. Intimate Partner Violence: Terms, Forms, and Typologies. Springer International Publishing; 2022, pp. 2219–2247.
10. Australian Government. The Attorney General's Department. *Family Law Legislation Amendment (Family Violence and Other Measures) Act 2011*. Available at: https://www.ag.gov.au/families-and-marriage/families/family-violence/family-violence-act
11. Parliamentary Counsel Office. New Zealand Legislation. *Family Violence Act 2018*, Stat. 46 (2018). Available at: https://www.legislation.govt.nz/act/public/2018/0046/latest/whole.html
12. Full Stop Australia (2024).Types of domestic and family violence. Available at: https://fullstop.org.au
13. Australian Institute of Health and Welfare. Family, domestic and sexual violence data in Australia. Canberra: Government of Australia; 2023. Available at: https://www.aihw.gov.au/reports/domestic-violence/family-domestic-and-sexual-violence
14. World Health Organization. Violence against women. Geneva: World Health Organization; 2021. Available at: https://www.who.int/news-room/fact-sheets/detail/violence-against-women

15. World Health Organization. Child Maltreatment: World Health Organization; 2023. Available from: https://www.who.int/news-room/fact-sheets/detail/child-maltreatment
16. Australian Bureau of Statistics. Personal Safety, Australia [Internet]. Canberra: ABS; 2021–22. Available at: https://www.abs.gov.au/statistics/people/crime-and-justice/personal-safety-australia/latest-release
17. Rivara F, Adhia A, Lyons V, Massey A, Mills B, Morgan E, Simckes M, Rowhani-Rahbar A. The effects of violence on health. Health Affairs. 2019 Oct 1;38(10):1622–1629.
18. Australian Government Institute of Family studies. 2023. What is child abuse and neglect? Available at: https://aifs.gov.au/resources/policy-and-practice-papers/what-child-abuse-and-neglect
19. Australian Government Australian Institute of Family Studies. Child protection Aboriginal and Torres Strait Islander Children. CFCA Resource Sheet. 2020. Available at: https://aifs.gov.au/sites/default/files/publication-documents/2001_child_protection_and_atsi_children_0.pdf
20. Child Matters. New Zealand Child Abuse Statistics. New Zealand: Child Matters; 2021. Available at: https://www.childmatters.org.nz/insights/nz-statistics/#:~:text=Recorded%20violent%20offences%20against%20children,serious%20assault%20resulting%20in%20injury
21. World Health Organization. Abuse of older people. Geneva; 2022. Available at: https://www.who.int/news-room/fact-sheets/detail/abuse-of-older-people
22. Pillemer K, Burnes D, Riffin C, Lachs M. Elder abuse: global situation, risk factors, and prevention strategies. The Gerontologist. 2016;56:S194–S205.
23. Yon Y, Mikton CR, Gassoumis ZD, Wilber KH. Elder abuse prevalence in community settings: a systematic review and meta-analysis. The Lancet Global Health. 2017;5(2):e147–e156.
24. Australian Human Rights Commission. 5 Your right to be free of financial abuse. 2023. Available at: https://humanrights.gov.au/our-work/5-your-right-be-free-financial-abuse
25. Family Safety Victoria. (2018). Family violence multi-agency risk assessment and management framework: a shared responsibility for assessing and managing family violence risk. Melbourne, Australia: Victorian Government. Available at: https://www.vic.gov.au/family-violence-multi-agency-risk-assessment-and-management
26. Kearns MC, D'Inverno AS, Reidy DE. The association between gender inequality and sexual violence in the US. American Journal of Preventive Medicine. 2020;58(1):12–20.
27. Australian Government. Department of Prime Minister and Cabinet. National Strategy to Achieve Gender Equality, Discussion Paper. 2023. Available at: https://www.pmc.gov.au/resources/national-strategy-achieve-gender-equality-discussion-paper/current-state/gendered-violence
28. Flood M, Brown C, Dembele L, Mills K. Who uses domestic, family, and sexual violence, how, and why? The State of Knowledge Report on Violence Perpetration. Brisbane: Queensland University of Technology. 2022. Available at: https://research.qut.edu.au/centre-for-justice/wp-content/uploads/sites/304/2023/01/Who-uses-domestic-family-and-sexual-violence-how-and-why-The-State-of-Knowledge-Report-on-Violence-Perpetration-2023.pdf
29. Australian Institute of Family Studies. What is child abuse and neglect? 2018. Available at: https://aifs.gov.au/resources/policy-and-practice-papers/what-child-abuse-and-neglect
30. KPMG (2016) The Cost of Violence Against Women and Their Children in Australia: Final Report, Canberra: Department of Social Services.
31. Center for Intersectional Justice. What is intersectionality?; 2023. Available at: https://www.intersectionaljustice.org/what-is-intersectionality
32. White JW, Geffner R. Fundamentals of understanding interpersonal violence and abuse. In: Geffner R, White JW, Hamberger LK, Rosenbaum A, Vaughan-Eden V, Vieth VI, editors. Handbook of Interpersonal Violence and Abuse Across the Lifespan. Switzerland: Springer International Publishing; 2022, pp. 3–25.
33. Segrave M. Temporary migration and family violence: how perpetrators weaponise borders. International Journal for Crime, Justice and Social Democracy. 2021;10(4):26–38.

34. Pokharel B, Yelland J, Hooker L, Taft A. A systematic review of culturally competent family violence responses to women in primary care. Trauma, Violence, & Abuse. 2021;0(0): 1–18.
35. Fiolet R, Tarzia L, Hameed M, Hegarty K. Indigenous peoples' help-seeking behaviors for family violence: a scoping review. Trauma, Violence, & Abuse. 2021;22(2): 370–380.
36. Bagwell-Gray ME, Jen S, Schuetz N. How intimate partner violence and intersectional identities converge to influence women's sexual health across environmental contexts. Social Work. 2020 Oct 10;65(4):349–357.
37. Corey J, Duggan M, Travers Á. Risk and protective factors for intimate partner violence against bisexual victims: a systematic scoping review. Trauma, Violence, & Abuse. 2023 Oct;24(4):2130–2142.
38. Fiolet R, Cameron J, Tarzia L, Gallant D, Hameed M, Hooker L, et al. Indigenous people's experiences and expectations of health care professionals when accessing care for family violence: a qualitative evidence synthesis. Trauma, Violence, & Abuse. 2022 Apr;23(2):567–580.
39. Scott KL, Jenney A. Safe not soft: trauma- and violence-informed practice with perpetrators as a means of increasing safety. Journal of Aggression, Maltreatment & Trauma. 2022,32: 1088–1107.
40. Sawrikar P, Katz I. Barriers to disclosing child sexual abuse (CSA) in ethnic minority communities: a review of the literature and implications for practice in Australia. Child and Youth Services Review. 2017;83:302–315.
41. New Zealand Ministry of Justice. Family violence risk assessment and management framework: a common approach to screening, assessing and managing risk; 2017. Available at: https://www.justice.govt.nz/assets/family-violence-ramf.pdf
42. Longobardi C, Badenes-Ribera L. Intimate partner violence in same-sex relationships and the role of sexual minority stressors: a systematic review of the past 10 years. Journal of Child and Family Studies. 2017;26(8): 2039–2049.
43. Victorian Government 2023. Maram Practice Guides. Responsibility 2: identification of family violence risk. Available at: https://www.vic.gov.au/maram-practice-guides-and-resources
44. Sheridan DJ, Nash KR. Acute injury patterns of intimate partner violence victims. Trauma, Violence, & Abuse. 2007 Jul;8(3):281–289.
45. Miller-Keane, M. Miller-Keane Encyclopedia & Dictionary of Medicine, Nursing & Allied Health, 7th Edition, 2003. Retrieved June August 29, 2023 from https://www.elsevier.com/books/miller-keane-encyclopediaand-dictionary-of-medicine-+nursing-and-allied-health/millerkeane/978-0-7216-9791-8
46. World Health Organization. Regional Office for Europe. (1978). Declaration of Alma-Ata. World Health Organization. Regional Office for Europe. Available at: https://apps.who.int/iris/handle/10665/347879
47. World Health Organization. Ottawa Charter for Health Promotion. Geneva: World Health Organization; 1986. Available at: https://www.who.int/publications/i/item/WH-1987
48. The Royal Children's Hospital. Clinical Practice Guidelines. Child Abuse. 2023. Available at: https://www.rch.org.au/clinicalguide/guideline_index/Child_abuse/
49. National Ageing Research Institute (NARI). Australian Elder Abuse Screening Instrument (AUSI) DRAFT. (2023). Available at: https://www.nari.net.au/Handlers/Download.ashx?IDMF=b793ff77-d3ff-4440-91df-bd883a1ba86d
50. The Australian Government. Amendment (Security and Protection) Bill 2007. Available at: https://www.aph.gov.au/Parliamentary_Business/Bills_Legislation/Bills_Search_ResultsResult?bId=r2706#:~:text=Summary,the%20existing%20Commissioner%20for%20Complaints
51. The Australian Government. Aged Care Quality and Safety Commission. Charter of Aged Care Rights. 2023. Available at: https://www.agedcarequality.gov.au/consumers/consumer-rights

CHAPTER 6

Screening for substance misuse

Adapted by Catina Adams

INTRODUCTION

Tobacco smoking, harmful consumption of alcohol and illicit drug use are significant health issues and a disease burden in the Australian and Aotearoa New Zealand communities.[1] The potential harms of substance use affect not only the person but the community more broadly. Health, social and economic harms stem from substance misuse including disease and injury, road trauma, mental health conditions, family violence and crime.[1] Economically, tobacco, drug and alcohol use impose substantial financial burdens, encompassing healthcare costs, lost productivity and expenses related to law enforcement and rehabilitation programs. The harm from tobacco, alcohol and other drug use can disproportionately affect specific populations including Aboriginal and Torres Strait Islander people, people with mental health conditions and LGBTIQ+ people.[1]

Substance use encompasses the misuse of legal and illegal substances including tobacco, drugs and alcohol, leading to various negative consequences. Problematic use of a substance will involve two or more of the following over 12 months: daily use needed to function; craving for the substance; inability to stop despite the desire to; impaired social and occupational functioning; recurrent use when it is physically hazardous; substance-related legal problems; or significant time spent using or recovering from substance use.[2] Identifying substance misuse early on is crucial for effective intervention and support (Table 6.1). Screening tools and techniques play a vital role in the identification process, enabling health professionals to assess the presence and severity of substance misuse.

This chapter explores the various dimensions of harm and costs resulting from tobacco, drug and alcohol misuse. Adverse health effects, including physical and mental health consequences and the increased risks of addiction and overdose, will be identified and the nurse's role in assessment and health promotion will be explored.

TABLE 6.1 Misuse, abuse and addiction

Term	Definition
Drug misuse	It is generally associated with prescription medicines. Prescription medicines are meant to be taken as directed by doctors. Drug misuse happens when these substances are taken for a purpose inconsistent with legal or medical guidelines.
Drug use	It happens when drugs, including alcohol, illicit drugs or psychoactive substances, are misused to get 'high' or inflict self-harm. It is also known as substance use disorder (SUD) since people who abuse drugs experience significantly altered thinking, behaviour and body functions.
Drug addiction (substance use disorder)	It is a brain disorder that manifests as the uncontrollable use of a substance despite its consequences. People with drug addiction have a physical and psychological need to take a substance because they suffer intense or debilitating withdrawal symptoms when they go without that substance.

Source: Australian Institute of Health and Welfare 2020[1]

Case study

The following case study gives an example of a typical situation involving screening for substance misuse and the initial clinical reasoning process. It will help you identify your learning needs.

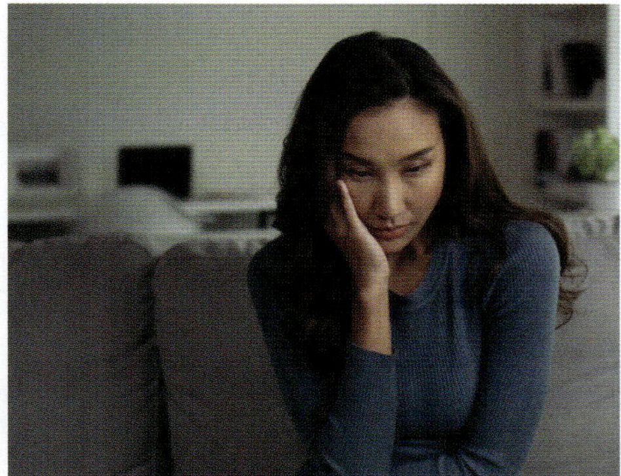

Context

You are a registered nurse working in the emergency department of a hospital. You are on your second rotation of your graduate year. You are asked to admit Ms Sharvi Sharma who has been in the department for several hours.

Consider the patient's situation

Ms Sharma is a 30-year-old woman reporting severe gastrointestinal pain. She tells you this is the fourth time she has been to this department with the same symptoms. She is very uncomfortable and rates her pain as 10/10. Ms Sharma tells you she has been using opioids for years to manage flare-ups of her symptoms. She has had many investigations, but no firm diagnosis has been provided.

Questions to further your learning

- What are the possible things that might be going on with Ms Sharma?
- What knowledge do you need to be able to predict what might be going on?
- What approach to Ms Sharma's health assessment will you undertake?
- What questions (subjective data) will you ask Ms Sharma to extend the health history and why?
- What physical examination (objective data) will you conduct and why?
- What resources are available to assist you in your assessment of Ms Sharma?

Assessment plan

The purpose of assessing a person with drug or alcohol addiction is to:

- identify severity of a person's alcohol and other drug use and impact on quality of life
- obtain a baseline measure against which outcomes can be mapped over time
- identify those at 'high risk' for whom immediate treatment is necessary
- identify those who need further treatment and support.

The multidisciplinary healthcare team includes specialist drug and alcohol nurses who provide expert knowledge and skills to assess, identify and respond to complex problems of people and families affected by alcohol- and drug-related health conditions, including dependence and mental and physical health comorbidities. The multidisciplinary healthcare team also includes clinical consultants, GPs, addiction medicine specialists, psychiatrists, psychologists, social workers, counsellors, peer workers and occupational therapists. The team monitors and assesses a person's treatment strategy and recovery process.

The main areas for subjective assessment are:

- presenting concern
- past history
- current medications
- activity and exercise
- nutrition and metabolism
- elimination
- sexuality and reproduction
- roles and relationships

- sleep
- alcohol history
- symptoms of alcohol withdrawal
- illicit drug history
- symptoms of drug withdrawal
- pain
- stress and coping.

Following subjective data collection, you will get a sense of the areas needed to be examined for objective data. Only the relevant areas should be examined. The main areas for physical examination are:

- general survey
- inspect and palpate the skin
- observe for signs of alcohol/drug withdrawal
- use of alcohol withdrawal tool
- vital signs
- neurological assessment
- abdominal assessment
- laboratory tests.

Resources available

You will find additional resources and the reference list at the end of this chapter.

Tobacco use

Tobacco use is the leading risk factor contributing to the burden of disease in Australia and New Aotearoa Zealand.[3,4] Exposure to tobacco smoke (second-hand smoking) also causes numerous health conditions among adults and children,[5] and smoking (first or second-hand) during pregnancy can affect the health of both mother and baby.[6]

Smoking rates—Australia (2021):[7]

- 10.7% of people aged 18 years or older were current daily smokers.
- 21.7% of people aged 18 to 24 years have used an e-cigarette or vaping device at least once.
- Those aged 14 or older smoking daily has more than halved (from 24% to 11.0%).
- Ex-smokers aged 14 years or older has since declined to 23% in 2019.

In Aotearoa New Zealand, in 2021–22, 8.0% of adults were daily smokers, reduced from 9.4% the previous year and 16.4% 10 years earlier.[8] Although smoking rates have decreased, large inequities between ethnicities remain. For example, daily smoking rates were as follows: Māori (19.9%), Pacific Islanders (18.2%) and European/Other (7.2%).[4]

E-cigarettes (vaping)

The use of e-cigarettes (vaping) is becoming more common. In Aotearoa New Zealand, 8.3% of adults were daily vapers/e-cigarette users in 2021–22, up from 6.2% the previous year. While e-cigarette use rose across most age groups, the rise among young adults was particularly notable.[8] Recent evidence suggests that vaping is highly addictive and poses a significant health risk to users with young people being most at risk.[9] Key findings include:

- E-cigarette use triples the risk of smoking uptake in never-smokers and non-smokers.
- Most e-cigarette users are young people.
- Most e-cigarette use is not related to quitting smoking.
- Most e-cigarette users vape and smoke in tandem.
- E-cigarette use by non-smokers results in dependence on e-cigarettes.
- Flavours and colourful packaging attract adolescents to e-cigarettes.

Alcohol use

Alcohol use is deeply ingrained in the social fabric of Australia, with a rich history of drinking culture. From celebratory to recreational consumption, alcohol plays a prominent role in various aspects of Australian society.[10] However, this widespread drinking culture also brings numerous challenges and consequences that demand careful examination and understanding. Research suggests widespread harmful alcohol and drug use and significant second-hand effects of alcohol or drug use in Aotearoa New Zealand.[11]

Alcohol increases the risk of oral, pharyngeal, laryngeal, oesophageal, liver, colorectal and (female) breast cancers.[12] There is evidence of a dose–response relationship, with the risk of developing these cancers increasing with higher alcohol consumption.[13] Notably, even small amounts of alcohol can increase cancer risk. Also, the joint effect of alcohol consumption and behavioural risk factors such as smoking and poor dietary practices further increases the risk of cancer.

Data on alcohol consumption have been regularly collected in Australia since 1960–61, providing trend data over a long period. These data indicate that per capita consumption increased throughout the 1960s and peaked in the mid-1970s when the annual consumption rate was 13.1 litres per capita. Since then, average annual alcohol consumption has declined to around 9.5 litres per capita with Australia ranking the fifth highest consumer of alcohol among 18 selected developed countries and Aotearoa New Zealand ranking the sixth highest, measuring 8.7 litres per capita.[14] Despite the high per capita consumption level, more Australians are giving up alcohol. Between 2016 and 2019, the proportion of ex-drinkers increased from 7.6% to 8.9%. In 2019, the proportion of people aged 18 or older abstaining from alcohol increased from 19.5% to 21%.[1]

In the most recent published survey, 74% of Aboriginal and Torres Strait Islander people aged 18 years or older reported consuming alcohol in the past year. The proportion of male-to-female alcohol consumption was 81% for males and 69% for females.[15] Although Aboriginal and Torres Strait Islander people aged 15 years or older are more likely than non-Indigenous people to have exceeded the alcohol consumption threshold for single occasion risk, the incidence is decreasing. In Aotearoa New Zealand 18.8% of adults had a hazardous drinking pattern in 2021–22: Māori (33.2%), Pacific Islander people (21.7%) and European/Other (20.1%).[8]

Although alcohol consumption is common, the risks include adverse health and social consequences related to its intoxicating, toxic and dependence-producing properties.[14] Approximately 3.3 million deaths each year (5.9% of all deaths worldwide) can be attributed to alcohol. It is considered the third leading risk factor for poor health globally. While there are numerous chronic and acute health effects, the harmful effects of alcohol use can be linked to many social, mental and emotional consequences.[16]

There is no safe drinking threshold for cancer risk. Compared with women who do not drink alcohol at all, women who have three alcoholic drinks per week have a 15% higher risk of breast cancer. Experts estimate that the risk of breast cancer goes up another 10% for each additional drink women regularly have each day. While the mechanism remains complex, the probable association is that alcohol interferes with estrogen levels, which affect breast tissue or estrogen receptors directly. The impact may vary depending on a woman's age—that is, whether they are adolescent, premenopausal or postmenopausal.[17]

What is a standard drink?

A standard drink in Australia and Aotearoa New Zealand is any drink that contains 10 g of alcohol. One standard drink always contains the same amount of alcohol regardless of container size or alcohol type—for example, beer, wine or spirits.[18] The number of standard drinks in alcoholic beverages is shown on the container's label. Figure 6.1 represents standard drink equivalents.

Drug misuse

The misuse of prescription drugs greatly affects health and safety and burdens the hospital emergency department system. High-risk medications have an increased risk of harm or death if not used correctly. These include opioids (e.g. oxycodone), benzodiazepines (e.g. diazepam) and others determined by each state or territory.

Pharmaceutical drug misuse in Australia ranks highly among other forms of illicit drug use. In 2016, approximately 3.1 million people (or 16%) in Australia aged 14 years or older had misused drugs in the previous 12 months. However, between 2016 and 2019, the proportion of people using pharmaceuticals for non-medical purposes in the previous 12 months fell from 4.8% to 4.2%, falling from the second to the fourth most used type of illicit drug in Australia.[1] In 2018–19 drug-related hospitalisations with a principal diagnosis of opioid poisoning were more likely to involve pharmaceutical opioids than heroin.

According to the Alcohol and Drug Foundation, more than 35,000 Australians have died from drug overdoses in the past 20 years, with most of these deaths involving prescription drugs such as opioids and benzodiazepines.[19] Of the 1,704 drug-induced deaths in Australia in 2021, 315 (18%) were due to heroin—a decrease from 462 deaths (or 25% of all drug-induced deaths) in 2020.[20] Every 2 minutes, one person in Australia is hospitalised because of prescription medications.

To address the growing problem of misuse of pharmaceuticals, real-time prescription monitoring (RTPM) has been introduced in Australia.[21] For example, SafeScript is available in one state of Australia as a clinical tool that provides real-time monitoring and additional information about a person's use of high-risk medications beyond a single pharmacy visit.[22] The prescription monitoring system identifies and alerts GPs and pharmacists to:

- patients on high daily doses of high-risk medications
- risky medication combinations
- high-risk medications prescribed by multiple providers.

Codeine

Codeine dependence warrants specific discussion due to its removal as an over-the-counter medication in Australia in 2018. While still available by prescription, the use of codeine for pain management has decreased since it became more difficult to access. Codeine has been shown to have limited effectiveness when taken in low doses for pain relief. Also, the risk of dependence is high with long-term use.[23,24]

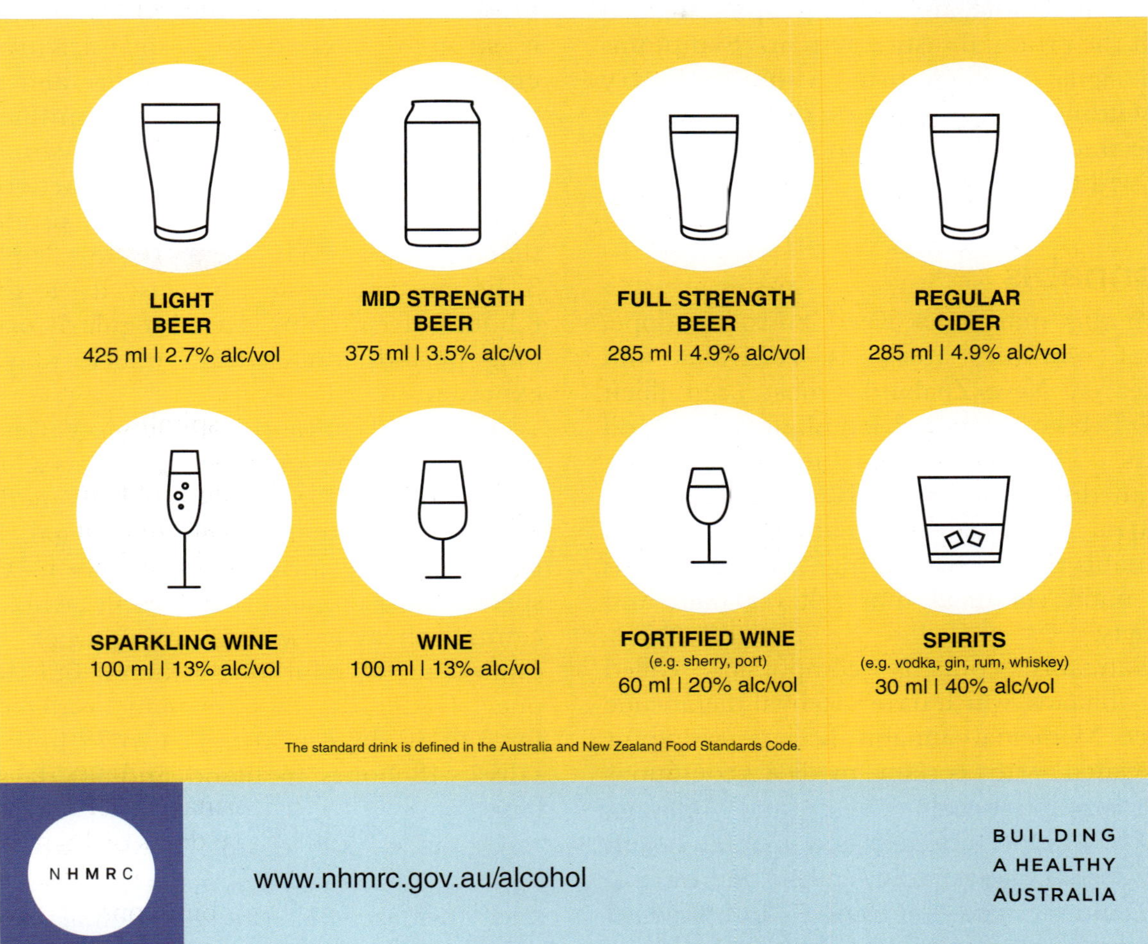

FIGURE 6.1 Standard drinks guide Source: Australian Government. National Health and Medical Research Council. 2020. What is a standard drink?[18]

Illicit drug use

Common illicit drugs in Australia include amphetamines, cannabis, cocaine, ecstasy, hallucinogens, heroin (and other opioids), inhalants, pharmaceuticals and steroids. The most recent Australian Institute of Health and Welfare survey reports cannabis was the most used illicit drug in 2019, with 11.6% of Australians using it in the preceding 12 months.[1] Cannabis was followed by cocaine (4.2%), ecstasy (3.0%)

and non-medical use of painkillers and opioids (2.7%). Vulnerable population groups identified as more likely to use illicit drugs are Indigenous Australians, people living in remote areas and people engaged with the criminal justice system.[1] Symptoms and signs of illicit drug withdrawal vary depending on the drug or drugs used, the time since use, the amount of the drug and the withdrawal stage.

Cannabis

Cannabis (marijuana, weed, buds, pot, dope, choof, chronic, trees) is Australia and Aotearoa New Zealand's most used illicit drug.[25] It comes in a dried plant, resin or oil form. The two main ingredients are tetrahydrocannabinol (THC) and cannabidiol (CBD). THC is the main chemical in cannabis that creates a 'high', while CBD is the main chemical that relieves pain and anxiety.

Cannabis contains compounds called cannabinoids, which have potential therapeutic effects. Medicinal cannabis alleviates symptoms associated with certain medical conditions such as chronic pain, nausea and vomiting, muscle spasms, epilepsy and mental health disorders. However, the specific indications, formulations and regulations for medical cannabis vary widely. In Australia, appropriately qualified medical practitioners can prescribe medicinal cannabis.

Cannabis use is associated with risks and side effects such as impaired memory, attention/coordination, altered perception and increased heart rate. Long-term or heavy use may lead to dependency, cognitive impairment, respiratory issues, mental health problems (particularly in vulnerable people) and other adverse effects. Cannabis can interact with certain medications including prescription drugs.

Cannabis use can impair cognitive and motor functions, affecting a person's ability to drive or operate machinery safely. It is strongly advised to avoid driving or engaging in activities that require alertness and coordination while under the influence of cannabis. Even at low doses, cannabis can affect performance of daily activities. The peak effects of cannabis products that contain THC usually last up to 3 hours, but some can last as long as 8 hours. If cannabis is used regularly over a long period, longer term effects may be experienced.

The legal status of cannabis varies by country and region. In some places, it is fully legalised for recreational or medical use, while in others it remains illegal. It is essential to be aware of the laws in your specific jurisdiction. For people who use cannabis heavily (several times a week), it is often detectable for longer than if only used once. Generally, cannabis can be detected for 3 to 30 days in urine, 24 to 72 hours in saliva, 48 hours in blood and 90 days in hair.[25]

Cannabis use during adolescence can significantly impact brain development and may increase the risk of mental health disorders. Pregnant women are generally advised to avoid cannabis use due to potential risks to fetal development.[26]

Methamphetamine

Methamphetamine is the second most frequently used illicit drug in Australia after cannabis. Data from national wastewater drug monitoring programs, which measure drug use within populations, show that of the 18 European countries with comparable reported data, Australia has the second-highest consumption of methamphetamine. Research indicates that many people who seek help for methamphetamine use have been chronic users for between 5 and 10 years, and relapses post-treatment are common.[27]

Rural communities in Australia have been especially hard hit by the use of amphetamine-type stimulants, specifically 'ice'. Consistent with Australia, the most frequently used amphetamine in Aotearoa New Zealand in the past year was methamphetamine in the form of 'ice'. In 2019–20, 1.1% of adults (16 years or older) used amphetamines. Men were more likely to use than women, and Māori people were 3.4 times more likely to use than non-Māori people.[28]

Heroin

Heroin is a highly addictive and illegal opioid drug derived from morphine, a naturally occurring substance extracted from the seed pod of certain poppy plants. Heroin abuse is a serious public health issue that can devastate people and communities. Heroin is known for its intense euphoric effects and rapid physical and psychological dependence. Regular use can lead to addiction, making it challenging for users to stop using the drug even when faced with negative consequences.[29]

Heroin misuse is associated with various health risks, including respiratory depression, overdose and the transmission of infectious diseases such as human immunodeficiency virus (HIV) and hepatitis through sharing needles. Heroin abuse can lead to changes in behaviour, strained relationships with family and friends, financial difficulties, legal issues and a decline in work or school performance.[29]

When someone becomes dependent on heroin and stops using it, they may experience withdrawal symptoms such as anxiety, muscle aches, nausea and intense cravings, making it challenging to quit without proper support. Treatment for heroin abuse typically involves a combination of behavioural therapies, counselling and, in some cases, medication-assisted treatment to manage withdrawal symptoms and cravings.[29]

Diagnosing substance use disorders

The American Psychiatric Association defines the gold standard of diagnosis in the Diagnostic and Statistical Manual of Mental Disorders, 5th edition (DSM-5).[2] Substance use disorder in DSM-5 combines the DSM-IV categories of substance use disorder and substance dependence into a single disorder measured from mild to severe. Each substance is addressed as a separate use disorder (e.g. alcohol use disorder, stimulant use disorder), but nearly all substances are diagnosed based on the same overarching criteria. The effects of a substance use disorder results in serious damage to the person and the way they live their life, necessitating accurate diagnosis so that appropriate advice, treatment and follow-up can be provided. Diagnosis of a substance use disorder requires the presence of at least two of 11 criteria within 12 months. The number of criteria determines the measure of severity. The criteria are clustered in four groupings: impaired control, social impairment, risky use and dependence.[2]

Developmental considerations

Adolescents

Adolescence is a critical phase of brain development, and the experiences encountered by adolescents during this period play a significant role in shaping their adult brains. The changes occurring in the brain during this time contribute to the hormonal shifts and the emotional, cognitive and behavioural characteristics observed during the teenage years. These changes foster a progression towards independence by developing more advanced reasoning skills, increased emphasis on social connections beyond the family and a desire to experiment and push boundaries.[30]

Alcohol and cannabis misuse are common in adolescence. The adolescent brain is sensitive to exposure to alcohol and cannabis, and researchers have found adolescent substance users showed abnormalities in measures of brain functioning, which is linked to changes in neurocognition over time.[30,31] Substance-using adolescents have been found to differ from non-users in neuropsychological performance, brain tissue volume, white matter integrity and functional brain response.

Pregnant women

Smoking during pregnancy can have serious health consequences for the mother and the developing baby (Table 6.2). Smoking during pregnancy increases the risk of various health issues for the expectant mother, such as ectopic pregnancy, placental abruption, premature rupture of membranes, preterm labour and gestational diabetes.[32]

Smoking during pregnancy exposes the developing baby to harmful substances like nicotine, carbon monoxide and other toxic chemicals. These substances can restrict the baby's oxygen supply and impair the delivery of essential nutrients, leading to potential health problems. Some risks include low birthweight, premature birth, stillbirth, SIDS, respiratory problems, developmental issues and an increased risk of certain congenital disabilities. Babies born to mothers who smoke during pregnancy have a higher risk of health issues

TABLE 6.2 Pregnancy-related health effects of smoking

Category	Health Effects
Fertility	• Delayed conception • Infertility—female and male • Assisted reproduction—less success
Obstetric	• Spontaneous miscarriage • Preterm birth (< 37 weeks) • Placenta praevia • Placental abruption • Ectopic pregnancy • Premature rupture of membranes • Pre-eclampsia • Reduced lactation
Fetal	• Growth restriction • Low birthweight (< 2,500 gm) • Small for gestational age • Congenital disabilities
Child and adult	• Sudden infant death syndrome (SIDS) • Type 2 diabetes • Obesity • Hypertension • High-density lipoprotein (HDL) • Nicotine dependence • Respiratory • Cognitive abilities • Behaviour–conduct disorder, ADHD • Psychiatric disorders

Source: Gould et al. 2014[32]

later in life; these include obesity, cardiovascular diseases, asthma and behavioural problems.

It is not only important for pregnant women to avoid smoking but also to stay away from second-hand smoke. Second-hand smoke contains many of the same harmful chemicals as directly inhaled smoke and can still harm the developing baby.[32]

The dangers of alcohol use to the growing fetus during pregnancy are well known. Alcohol easily crosses the placenta, which exposes the baby to similar concentrations of alcohol as the mother. There is no known safe amount of alcohol use during pregnancy or while trying to get pregnant. All types of alcohol are equally harmful, including all wines and beer.[33]

The harmful effects of alcohol on the fetus include impaired development of the fetal nervous system involving the brain and diminished nourishment of the growing baby. Problems that may occur in a fetus exposed to alcohol before birth[34] include:

- a range of lifelong physical, mental and behavioural disabilities known as fetal alcohol spectrum disorders (FASD)
- miscarriage
- stillbirth
- premature birth
- low birthweight.

FASD describes a range of permanent and lifelong conditions that can result from a baby being exposed to alcohol in utero.[34] A national strategic plan has been developed to reduce the incidence and impact of FASD in Australia. Alcohol is not the only substance harmful to a growing fetus. Illicit drug use can lead to neonatal abstinence syndrome, characterised by hyperactivity of the central and autonomic nervous systems.[26]

Older adults

Older adults have unique physiological changes and increased vulnerability associated with ageing. As people age, their bodies become more sensitive to the effects of alcohol. This increased sensitivity is due to changes in metabolism, decreased tolerance and a higher proportion of body fat, which can lead to higher blood alcohol levels and increased impairment even with lower alcohol consumption. Liver metabolism and kidney function may be decreased, which increases the bioavailability of alcohol in the blood for longer periods. Ageing people lose muscle mass; less tissue to which the alcohol can be distributed means an increased alcohol concentration in the blood.

The older person may be on multiple medications, which can interact adversely with alcohol. Alcohol use can exacerbate conditions commonly seen in older adults such as liver disease, cardiovascular disease, diabetes and cognitive impairment. It can also increase the risk of falls and injuries due to its impact on balance, coordination and cognitive function.

HEALTH EDUCATION

Harm minimisation

Tobacco, drug and alcohol harm minimisation is a public health approach that aims to reduce the negative consequences of tobacco, drug and alcohol use rather than focusing solely on prevention. The harm minimisation model recognises that tobacco, drug and alcohol use is a complex and multifaceted issue and acknowledges that complete abstinence may not be a realistic goal for everyone.[35] Instead, it seeks to minimise the potential harms caused by substance use to people and society[36] (Figure 6.2).

Harm minimisation does not condone or promote tobacco/vaping, drug or alcohol use. However, changes can be made in drug policies and laws to prioritise harm reduction over punitive measures, which can sometimes

Continued

HEALTH EDUCATION cont'd

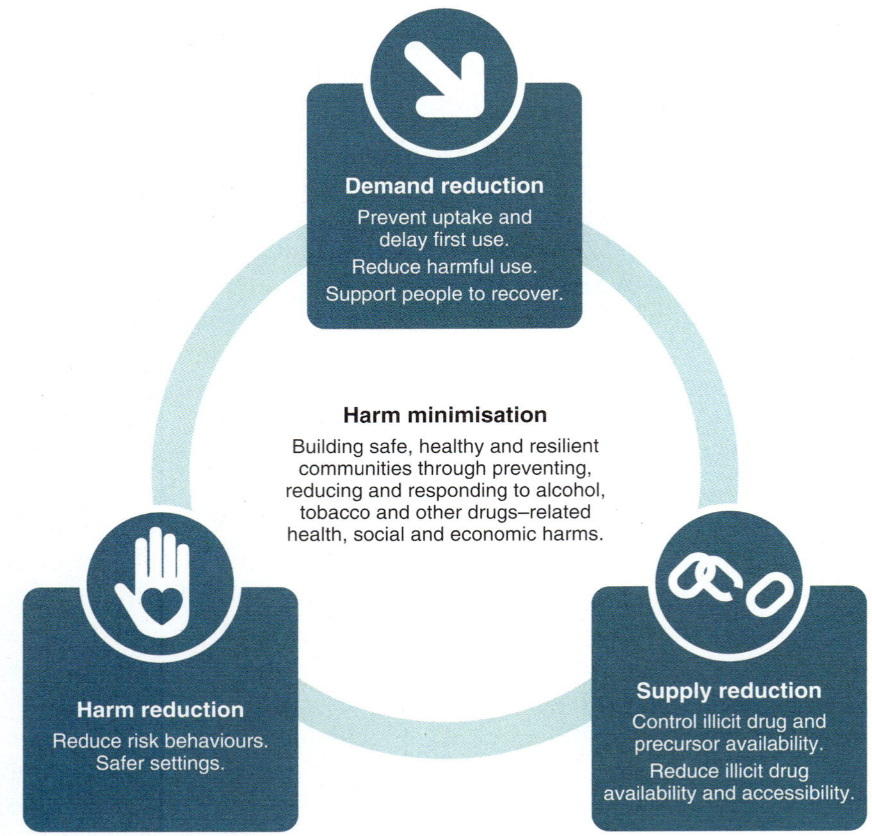

FIGURE 6.2 HARM1: the three pillars of harm minimisation Source: Australian Institute of Health and Welfare 2023[36]

exacerbate the negative consequences of substance use. By focusing on harm reduction, this approach aims to prevent illness, injury and death and reduce the social and economic impacts of substance misuse.

The nurse's role

The nurse's role in harm minimisation includes:

- providing accurate and evidence-based information about drugs and alcohol and their potential risks to people and communities such as HIV, hepatitis (transmission, symptoms, course of the illnesses, need for vaccines)
- promoting programs that aim to reduce adverse consequences of drug and alcohol use such as needle exchange programs, using clean equipment, supervised injection sites and opioid substitution therapy for people with opioid dependence
- providing information on overdose prevention and teaching how to use naloxone
- encouraging use of drug-checking services (where available) to allow substance testing
- teaching good hand hygiene, basic wound care, phlebotomy skills and equipment management
- providing information on health management such as on nutrition and sexual health
- passing on the location of supervised injection facilities
- giving information on support groups.

Screening tools

Including screening for alcohol and drug use within a general health assessment is important, even if problems are not suspected. Screening serves multiple purposes at the individual and population levels. At the individual level, screening for substance misuse is pivotal in identifying at-risk people and facilitating timely intervention thus preventing further progression of substance use disorders and associated harms. Screening also provides an opportunity to offer appropriate support and treatment to those in need, improving their chances of recovery and overall wellbeing. Many clients seeking health care may have underlying substance misuse and may not perceive there is any risk to their health.

Population-level screening helps identify trends and patterns of substance use within communities and societies. This information is crucial for public health planning, resource allocation and developing targeted prevention and intervention programs. By understanding the prevalence and nature of substance use, policymakers and health professionals can implement evidence-based strategies to address issues effectively.

Implementing effective screening programs for substance use faces several challenges. The stigma surrounding substance misuse can discourage people from seeking help or disclosing their substance use habits. Cultural and linguistic factors may also influence the validity and reliability of screening tools across diverse populations. Also, the availability of resources, such as trained personnel, time and funding, can affect the feasibility and sustainability of screening initiatives. Collaboration between healthcare providers, community organisations and relevant stakeholders is essential to develop comprehensive screening programs considering different populations' unique needs and contexts.

There are several screening tools in common use. They include the following:

1. The Alcohol Use Disorders Identification Test—**AUDIT Screening Tool**[37] (Table 6.3)
   - 10-item tool for detecting risky and harmful drinking patterns.
   - Questions 1 to 3 are on alcohol consumption; questions 4 to 6 on

TABLE 6.3 The alcohol use disorders identification test—AUDIT

Question	0	1	2	3	4
1. How often do you have a drink containing alcohol?	Never	Monthly or less	2–4 times a month	2–3 times a week	4 or more times a week
2. How many drinks containing alcohol do you have on a typical day when you are drinking?	1–2	3–4	5–6	7–9	10 or more
3. How often do you have six or more drinks on one occasion?	Never	Less than monthly	Monthly	Weekly	Daily or almost daily

Continued

TABLE 6.3 The alcohol use disorders identification test—AUDIT cont'd

Question	0	1	2	3	4
4. How often during the last year have you found that you could not stop drinking once you had started?	Never	Less than monthly	Monthly	Weekly	Daily or almost daily
5. How often during the last year have you failed to do what was normally expected of you because of drinking?	Never	Less than monthly	Monthly	Weekly	Daily or almost daily
6. How often during the last year have you needed a first drink in the morning to get yourself going after a heavy drinking session?	Never	Less than monthly	Monthly	Weekly	Daily or almost daily
7. How often during the last year have you felt guilt or remorse after drinking?	Never	Less than monthly	Monthly	Weekly	Daily or almost daily
8. How often during the last year have you been unable to remember what happened the night before because of your drinking?	Never	Less than monthly	Monthly	Weekly	Daily or almost daily
9. Have you or someone else been injured because of your drinking?	No		Yes, but not in the last year		Yes, during the last year
10. Has a relative, friend, doctor or other healthcare worker been concerned about your drinking or suggested that you cut it down?	No		Yes, but not in the last year		Yes, during the last year

Source: Babor et al. 2001[37]

drinking behaviour or dependence; questions 7 to 10 on adverse consequences from alcohol.

- An audit score of 8 points for men or 4 points for women, adolescents and those older than 60 indicates hazardous alcohol consumption, prompting a referral to a substance use disorder specialist.

2. Modified version of AUDIT Tool—**AUDIT-C Screening Tool**[38] (Table 6.4)
   - A three-item alcohol screen used to detect risky and harmful drinking patterns.
   - Used in various settings and applied to any age group.
   - Useful for women at risk of harmful alcohol or drug use during pregnancy.

TABLE 6.4 Modified version of audit tool—AUDIT-C

1. How often do you have a drink containing alcohol?
2. How many standard drinks of alcohol do you drink on a typical day when you are drinking?
3. How often do you have six or more drinks on one occasion?

AUDIT-C SCORE	0	1	2	3	4
Question 1	Never	Monthly or less	2–4 times per month	2–3 times per week	4+ times per week
Question 2	1–2	3–4	5–6	7–9	10+
Question 3	Never	Less than monthly	Monthly	Weekly	Daily or almost daily
SCORING GUIDE (Total points)					
3 or greater = increased risk					
					Total

Source: Van Gils et al. 2021[38]

3. Assessing alcohol consumption in adolescents using the **CRAFFT 2.1 Screening Tool**[39] (Table 6.5)
   - Administered to adolescents aged 12 to 21 to identify drug and alcohol use, riding/driving risk.
   - Six keywords represented by the acronym are **C**ar, **R**elax, **A**lone, **F**orget, **F**riends and **T**rouble.
   - Use the topic areas represented in the CRAFFT 2.1 screening tool as talking points to engage an adolescent in discussing substance use behaviours.
4. **Clinical Institute Withdrawal Assessment of Alcohol Scale**, Revised (CIWA-Ar)[40] (Table 6.6)
   - 10-item, validated scale designed for alcohol withdrawal.
   - Used by skilled nurses in inpatient settings.
   - Scores < 10 = mild withdrawal; between 10 and 20 = moderate withdrawal; and > 20 = severe withdrawal.
   - Enables early recognition of withdrawal and avoids overmedicating.
   - Those with CIWA-Ar scores > 10 at high risk of developing withdrawal complications if not medicated.[40]
5. **SMAST-G Alcohol Screening Tool for older adults**[41] (Table 6.7)
   - Alcohol Screening Test for older adults to detect alcohol or drug misuse/dependence.
   - Can be self-administered.
6. **DAST-10 Questionnaire—General screening for drug abuse**[42] (Table 6.8)
   - 10-item brief screening tool to assess drug use, not including alcohol or tobacco use, in the past 12 months.
   - Can be administered by a clinician or self-administered.
   - Each question requires a yes or no response.
   - Can be completed in less than 8 minutes.
   - Accompanied by a scoring guide that will assist in determining if further assessment or referral is needed.

TABLE 6.5 Assessing alcohol consumption in adolescents using CRAFFT-2.1 questionnaire

The CRAFFT Interview (version 2.1)

To be verbally administered by the clinician

Begin: *"I'm going to ask you a few questions that I ask all my patients. Please be honest. I will keep your answers confidential."*

Part A

During the PAST 12 MONTHS, on how many days did you:

1. Drink more than a few sips of beer, wine, or any drink containing **alcohol**? Say "0" if none. — ☐ # of days
2. Use any **marijuana** (cannabis, weed, oil, wax, or hash by smoking, vaping, dabbing, or in edibles) or **"synthetic marijuana"** (like "K2," "Spice")? Say "0" if none. — ☐ # of days
3. Use **anything else to get high** (like other illegal drugs, pills, prescription or over-the-counter medications, and things that you sniff, huff, vape, or inject)? Say "0" if none. — # of days

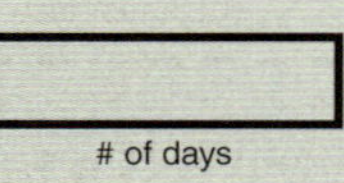

Did the patient answer "0" for all questions in Part A?

Yes ☐ ↓	No ☐ ↓
Ask 1st question only in Part B, then STOP	**Ask all 6 questions in Part B**

Part B		**Circle one**	
C	Have you ever ridden in a **CAR** driven by someone (including yourself) who was "high" or had been using alcohol or drugs?	No	Yes
R	Do you ever use alcohol or drugs to **RELAX**, feel better about yourself, or fit in?	No	Yes
A	Do you ever use alcohol or drugs while you are by yourself, or **ALONE**?	No	Yes
F	Do you ever **FORGET** things you did while using alcohol or drugs?	No	Yes
F	Do your **FAMILY** or **FRIENDS** ever tell you that you should cut down on your drinking or drug use?	No	Yes
T	Have you ever got into **TROUBLE** while you were using alcohol or drugs?	No	Yes

***Two or more YES answers in Part B suggests a serious problem that needs further assessment. See back for further instructions** ⟶

NOTICE TO CLINIC STAFF AND MEDICAL RECORDS:
The information on this page is protected by special federal confidentiality rules (42 CFR Part 2), which prohibit disclosure of this information unless authorised by specific written consent.

TABLE 6.5 Assessing alcohol consumption in adolescents using CRAFFT-2.1 questionnaire cont'd

CRAFFT Score Interpretation

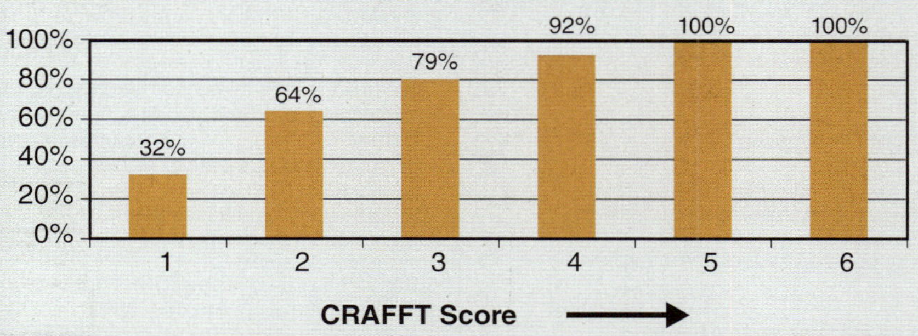

*Data source: Mitchell SG, Kelly SM, Gryczynski J, Myers CP, O'Grady KE, Kirk AS, & Schwartz RP. (2014). The CRAFFT cut-points and DSM-5 criteria for alcohol and other drugs: a reevaluation and reexamination. Substance Abuse, 35(4), 376–80.

Use the 5 R's talking points for brief counseling.

1. **REVIEW** screening results
   For each "yes" response: *"Can you tell me more about that?"*

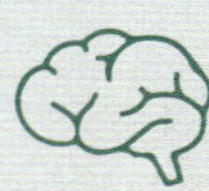

2. **RECOMMEND** not to use
   "As your doctor (nurse/health care provider), my recommendation is not to use any alcohol, marijuana or other drug because they can: 1) Harm your developing brain; 2) Interfere with learning and memory; and 3) Put you in embarrassing or dangerous situations."

3. **RIDING/DRIVING** risk counselling
   "Motor vehicle crashes are the leading cause of death for young people. I give all my patients the Contract for Life. Please take it home and discuss it with your parents/guardians to create a plan for safe rides home."

4. **RESPONSE** elicit self-motivational statements
   Non-users: *"If someone asked you why you don't drink or use drugs, what would you say?"* Users: *"What would be some of the benefits of not using?"*

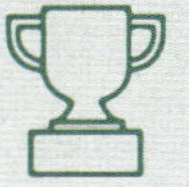

5. **REINFORCE** self-efficacy
   "I believe you have what it takes to keep alcohol and drugs from getting in the way of achieving your goals."

Give patient Contract for Life. Available at www.crafft.org/contract

crafft@childrens.harvard.edu www.crafft.org

For more information and versions in other languages, see www.crafft.org.

Source: Shenoi et al. 2019[39]

TABLE 6.6 The Clinical Institute Withdrawal Assessment For Alcohol–Revised Scale

Appendix: Addiction Research Foundation Clinical Institute Withdrawal Assessment for Alcohol (CIWA-Ar)

Patient ________ **Date** |__|__|__| y m d **Time** ___:___ **(24 hour clock, midnight = 00:00)**

Pulse or heart rate, taken for one minute: ________ **Blood pressure:** ____/____

NAUSEA AND VOMITING—As "Do you feel sick to your stomach? Have you vomited?" Observation.
0 no nausea and no vomiting
1 mild nausea with no vomiting
2
3
4 intermittent nausea with dry heaves
5
6
7 constant nausea, frequent dry heaves and vomiting

TREMOR—Arms extended and fingers spread apart. Observation.
0 no tremor
1 not visible, but can be felt fingertip to fingertip
2
3
4 moderate, with patient's arms extended
5
6
7 severe, even with arms not extended

PAROXYSMAL SWEATS—Observation.
0 no sweat visible
1 barely perceptible sweating, palms moist
2
3
4 beads of sweat obvious on forehead
5
6
7 drenching sweats

ANXIETY—Ask "Do you feel nervous?" Observation.
0 no anxiety, at ease
1 mildly anxious
2
3
4 moderately anxious, or guarded, so anxiety is inferred
5
6
7 equivalent to acute panic states as seen in severe delirium or acute schizophrenic reactions

AGITATION—Observation.
0 normal activity
1 somewhat more than normal activity
2
3
4 moderately fidgety and restless
5
6
7 paces back and forth during most of the interview, or constantly thrashes about

TACTILE DISTURBANCES—Ask "Have you any itching, pins and needles sensations, any burning, any numbness, or do you feel bugs crawling on or under your skin?" Observation.
0 none
1 very mild itching, pins and needles, burning or numbness
2 mild itching, pins and needles, burning or numbness
3 moderate itching, pins and needles, burning or numbness
4 moderately severe hallucinations
5 severe hallucinations
6 extremely severe hallucinations
7 continuous hallucinations

AUDITORY DISTURBANCES—Ask "Are you more aware of sounds around you? Are they harsh? Do they frighten you? Are you hearing anything that is disturbing to you? Are you hearing things you know are not there?" Observation.
0 not present
1 very mild harshness or ability to frighten
2 mild harshness or ability to frighten
3 moderate harshness or ability to frighten
4 moderately severe hallucinations
5 severe hallucinations
6 extremely severe hallucinations
7 continuous hallucinations

VISUAL DISTURBANCES—Ask "Does the light appear to be too bright? Is its colour different? Does it hurt your eyes? Are you seeing anything that is disturbing to you? Are you seeing things you know are not there?" Observation.
0 not present
1 very mild sensitivity
2 mild sensitivity
3 moderate sensitivity
4 moderately severe hallucinations
5 severe hallucinations
6 extremely severe hallucinations
7 continuous hallucinations

HEADACHE, FULLNESS IN HEAD—Ask "Does your head feel different? Does it feel like there is a band around your head?" Do not rate for dizziness or lightheadedness. Otherwise, rate severity.
0 not present
1 very mild
2 mild
3 moderate
4 moderately severe
5 severe
6 very severe
7 extremely severe

ORIENTATION AND CLOUDING OF SENSORIUM—Ask "What day is this? Where are you? Who am I?"
0 oriented and can do serial additions
1 cannot do serial additions or is uncertain about date
2 disoriented for date by no more than 2 calendar days
3 disoriented for date by more than 2 calendar days
4 disoriented for place/or person

Total CIWA-A Score ______
Rater's Initials ______
Maximum Possible Score 67

Source: Corniello & Skowronsky 2012[40]

TABLE 6.7 SMAST-G Alcohol screening tool for older adults

Questions are Answered with Yes (1) or No (0)
1. Do you ever underestimate how much you drink when talking with others?
2. After a few drinks, have you sometimes not eaten or skipped a meal because you didn't feel hungry?
3. Does having a few drinks help decrease your shakiness or tremors?
4. Does alcohol sometimes make it hard for you to remember parts of the day or night?
5. Do you usually take a drink to relax or calm your nerves?
6. Do you drink to take your mind off your problems?
7. Have you ever increased your drinking after experiencing a loss in your life?
8. Has a doctor or nurse ever said they were worried or concerned about your drinking?
9. Have you ever made rules to manage your drinking?
10. When you feel lonely, does having a drink help you?
TOTAL SMAST-G SCORE (0–10) ____________
SCORING: 2 OR MORE 'YES' RESPONSES ARE INDICATIVE OF AN ALCOHOL PROBLEM.

Source: The Regents of the University of Michigan 1991[41]

TABLE 6.8 General screening for drug abuse using DAST-10

These Questions Refer to the Past 12 Months.	No	Yes
1. Do you use drugs other than those required for medical reasons?	0	1
2. Do you abuse more than one drug at a time?	0	1
3. Can you always stop using drugs when you want to? (If you never use drugs, answer 'Yes'.)	1	0
4. Have you had 'blackouts' or 'flashbacks' due to drug use?	0	1
5. Do you ever feel bad or guilty about your drug use? (If you never use drugs, choose 'No'.)	0	1
6. Does your spouse (or parents) ever complain about your drug involvement?	0	1
7. Have you neglected your family because of your use of drugs?	0	1
8. Have you engaged in illegal activities to obtain drugs?	0	1
9. Have you ever experienced withdrawal symptoms (felt sick) when you stopped taking drugs?	0	1
10. Have you had medical problems due to drug use (e.g. memory loss, hepatitis, convulsions, bleeding, etc.)?	0	1

Continued

TABLE 6.8 General screening for drug abuse using DAST-10 cont'd

Dast-10 Score	*Degree of Problems Related to Drug Abuse*	*Suggested Action*
0	No problems reported	None at this time
1–2	Low level	Monitor and re-assess at a later date
3–5	Moderate level	Further investigation
6–8	Substantial level	Intensive assessment
9–10	Severe level	Intensive assessment

Source: Skinner 1982[42]

Subjective data

Screening and assessment should be approached sensitively, ensuring confidentiality, providing non-judgemental support and offering appropriate follow-up services. By maintaining an empathetic, non-judgemental attitude, you can highlight the importance of conducting an alcohol and drug assessment as part of a general health assessment for all people over the age of 14 years.

If the person is intoxicated or going through substance withdrawal, collecting any history data is difficult and unreliable. However, when sober, most people are willing and able to give reliable data, provided the setting is private, confidential and nonconfrontational.

Preparation: Before you start the assessment, introduce yourself to the person, confirm the person's identity, discuss the purpose and scope of the assessment, clarify any questions the person may have and get verbal consent from the person to perform the assessment. Careful and respectful use of language in describing substance misuse can improve engagement with clients[43] (Table 6.9).

TABLE 6.9 Terms to use, terms to avoid, and why

Use	Avoid	Why
• Drug addiction • Substance use disorder	• Habit	• 'Habit' implies that a person is *choosing* to use substances or can *choose* to stop. This implication is inaccurate. • Describing a substance use disorder as a habit makes the illness seem less serious than it is.
• Use (for illicit drugs) • Misuse (for prescription medications used other than prescribed)	• Abuse	• The term 'abuse' was found to have a high association with negative judgements and punishment. • Use outside of the parameters of how medications were prescribed is misuse.

TABLE 6.9 Terms to use, terms to avoid, and why cont'd

Use	Avoid	Why
• A person with a substance use disorder • A person with an opioid use disorder or a person with opioid addiction	• Addict • User • Drug abuser • Junkie	• Using person-first language shows that substance use disorder is an illness. • Using these words shows that a person with a substance use disorder 'has' a problem/illness rather than 'is' the problem. • The terms avoid eliciting negative associations, punitive attitudes and individual blame.
• A person with an alcohol use disorder • A person who misuses alcohol or engages in unhealthy/hazardous alcohol use	• Alcoholic • Drunk	
• Person in recovery or long-term recovery or person who previously used drugs	• Former addict • Reformed addict	

Source: National Institute on Drug Abuse 2021[43]

ASSESSMENT GUIDELINES	CLINICAL SIGNIFICANCE AND CLINICAL ALERTS
Presenting concern	
A person with a drug and/or alcohol addiction will present for care as a: • consequence of their addiction (e.g. accident, overdose, infection), or • planned admission surgery/medical management for treatment of medical complications related to use of substances, or • for pregnancy care or to give birth. Therefore, questions should initially focus on the reason the person has presented for health care. • *Can you tell me why you are here? What happened?* • *How long ago?* • *What is your main problem?*	

ASSESSMENT GUIDELINES	CLINICAL SIGNIFICANCE AND CLINICAL ALERTS
Past history	
• *Have you experienced any of the following?* – *head injury (with loss of consciousness due to assault, falls, accident)?* – *hypoxia (lack of oxygen to the brain due to overdose, carbon monoxide poisoning, near-drowning, cardiac arrest, strangulation, or attempted hanging)?* – *blackouts, seizures, or epilepsy?* – *brain—surgery, bleeding or tumour?* – *personality change?* – *chronic, heavy alcohol or other substance use greater than five years?* • *Have you been diagnosed with any of the following?* – *neurological disorder (e.g. stroke, multiple sclerosis, Parkinson's disease)?* – *learning difficulties?* – *mental illness (particularly with psychosis)?* • *When were you diagnosed?* • *How was the situation managed?*	
Current medications	
For each medication, record how often taken: • *What was the reason for taking the medication?* • *How long have you been taking it?* • *Does the medication seem to work?* • Have you had any side effects?	
Activity and exercise	
• *Describe a typical day for you* • *Can you do all your daily care activities?* • *Do you need any assistive devices?* • *Do you experience any breathing problems?* • *Do you have any mobility problems?* • Do you have any heart problems?	See also Chapters 16–20.
Nutrition and metabolism	
• *Have there been any changes to your eating patterns/appetite?* • *Have you lost/gained weight recently?* • *Describe your food and fluid intake for the past 24 hours.*	See Chapter 21.

ASSESSMENT GUIDELINES	CLINICAL SIGNIFICANCE AND CLINICAL ALERTS
Elimination	
• *Have you had any nausea, vomiting, constipation or diarrhoea?*	See Chapters 24 and 25.
Sexuality and reproduction	
• *Are you in a sexual relationship?* • *How many children do you have?* • *Do you use protection against sexually transmitted infections (STIs)?*	Substance misue may interfere with sexual function secondary to central nervous system depression, loss of libido and impotence—see Chapters 26 and 27.
Roles and relationships	
• *Where do you live?* • *Who do you live with?* • *Are you employed?* • *What work do you do?* • *How are those closest to you affected by your alcohol/drug use?*	Effects of substance misuse on social roles include: • failure to fulfil major obligations • important activities given up or reduced. Behaviour changes such as aggression, changes in mood, compromised judgement and inappropriate sexual decisions.[2]
Sleep	
Do you have any problems with sleep? Average per night?	
Alcohol history	
• *Do you sometimes drink beer, wine or other alcoholic beverages?* • *How many times in the past year have you had 5 or more drinks a day (for men) or 4 or more drinks a day? (for women)* • *On average, how many days a week do you have an alcoholic drink?* • *On a typical drinking day, how many drinks do you have?* Drinking patterns: for men ≤ 2 drinks/day; for women ≤ 1 drink/day. For women older than 65 years ≤ 1 drink/day. Use the **AUDIT Tool** to assess for risk alcohol consumption (Table 6.3). Or, use the AUDIT-C Tool (modified version of AUDIT tool)—useful for assessing alcohol consumption. Either tool will help identify problem drinking and those who may need further assessment (Table 6.4).	One or more heavy drinking days means that this person is an 'at-risk' drinker. At-risk drinking: • men ≥ 15 drinks/week = heavy or at-risk drinking • women ≥ 8 drinks. Recommend lower limits or abstinence for people who take medications that interact with alcohol, have a health condition exacerbated by alcohol, or are pregnant (advise abstinence here).

ASSESSMENT GUIDELINES	CLINICAL SIGNIFICANCE AND CLINICAL ALERTS
Symptoms of alcohol withdrawal	
• *Do you have any cravings for alcohol, irritability, anorexia, abdominal pain, fatigue, chills, muscle cramps or palpitations?* • *Are you experiencing any nausea, vomiting, anxiety, insomnia, visual or auditory, or visual disturbances?*	Alcohol withdrawal can develop within several hours or several days after a reduction or complete termination of alcohol consumption, provided such consumption has been heavy or prolonged.
Illicit drug history	
• *Are you taking any illicit drugs at the moment? What sort? How often?* • *When did you last use?* **Use The DAST-10 Questionnaire** to assess for drug misuse (Table 6.8).	
Symptoms of drug withdrawal	

• *Do you have any of the following symptoms?*
  • *irritability?*
  • *changing moods?*
  • *depression?*
  • *anxiety?*
  • *aches and pains?*
  • *cravings?*
  • *tiredness?*
	Withdrawal will occur after a reduction or termination after several weeks or more of opioid use. Withdrawal symptoms such as anxiety and agitation occur during withdrawal from illicit drugs.

Pain	
• *Do you have any pain?* • *How would you rate your pain?* • *Where is the pain?*	See Chapter 13.
Stress and coping	
• *How do your present circumstances interfere with your work/school?* • *Are you worried about anything now?* • *What frightens or annoys you?* • *How do you manage stress?* • *Where/who are your main supports?*	Use of drugs, alcohol or tobacco may be used to reduce stress or tension. Tolerance may occur when a person requires an increased amount of a substance to produce the same effect.[2]
Additional subjective data for pregnant women	
Use AUDIT Tool or AUDIT-C Tool (Tables 6.3 and 6.4).	A score of 3 or greater = increased risk. Advise abstinence.

ASSESSMENT GUIDELINES	CLINICAL SIGNIFICANCE AND CLINICAL ALERTS
Additional subjective data for adolescents	
Use of the CRAFFT tool to identify drug and alcohol use, riding/driving risk for those aged 12–21 years (Table 6.5).	Risky use of drugs and alcohol: • recurrent use in hazardous situations • continued use despite physical or psychological problems caused or exacerbated by substance use.
Additional subjective data for adults over 65 years	
Use SMAST-G tool to detect alcohol or drug misuse/ dependence (Table 6.7).	Dependence: physiological dependence on a substance.

Objective data

Preparation: Outline the process for assessing the person with drug or alcohol misuse and ask their consent to continue. The areas for assessment are detailed below.

PROCEDURES AND NORMAL FINDINGS	ABNORMAL FINDINGS AND CLINICAL ALERTS
General survey	
While collecting subjective data, you will have noticed the condition of the person's skin, lips, hair and mucous membranes, as well as any breath odour, ease of breathing, height-to-weight ratio, body shape, level of hygiene and grooming and general demeanour. All these factors offer clues to the person's overall health status but will differ depending on the substance being misused.	
Inspect and palpate skin	
See Chapter 22.	
Observe for signs of alcohol/drug withdrawal	
Observe for tachycardia, hypertension, fever, disorientation, slurred speech, staggered gait, poor dexterity.	Alcohol intoxication is characterised by recent consumption of alcohol and the presence of at least one of the following: • uncoordinated body movements • slurred or incoherent speech • reduced attention or memory difficulties • involuntary eye movements, stupor or coma.[2]

PROCEDURES AND NORMAL FINDINGS	ABNORMAL FINDINGS AND CLINICAL ALERTS
Use of alcohol withdrawal tool	
The Clinical Institute Withdrawal Assessment (CIWA) scale is the most sensitive scale for objective measurement of withdrawal from alcohol[40] (Table 6.6). It is quantified to measure the progress of withdrawal. • Assess and rate each of the 10 criteria of the CIWA scale. • Each criterion has a range from 0–7, except for 'Orientation', which is rated 0–4. • Add the scores for the total CIWA-Ar score. • A score of 0–7 means that you can reassess the person every 4 hours for 72 hours. • If all the scores are < 8 for 72 hours, you can safely discontinue use of the CIWA assessment.	Frequency of CIWA-Ar monitoring depends on treatment setting and clinical condition of the patient. Scores of: • 0–9 = absent or minimal withdrawal • 10–19 = mild-to-moderate withdrawal • ≥ 20 = severe withdrawal.
Vital signs	
Take the vital signs: blood pressure, pulse, respirations, oxygen saturation. Check for cardiac arrhythmias. If initial CIWA score is ≥ 8: • Take vital signs every hour for 8 hours. • A score of 8 may trigger a PRN prescribed medication requirement. • A score of ≥ 15 triggers scheduled prescribed medication.	Patients with CIWA-Ar scores > 10 need frequent monitoring (at least 4-hourly) and patients with severe withdrawal symptoms (CIWA-Ar score of more than 20) should be monitored every 1–2 hours.  ***Clinical alert:*** Tachycardia, hypertension, fever, nausea, vomiting, anxiety, agitation, visual or auditory hallucinations are signs of alcohol withdrawal.
Neurological assessment	
Observe level of alertness, behaviour, movements, gait—see Chapter 12.	Addiction can affect brain function such as memory, learning, motivation, motor activity and the ability to inhibit behaviour.  ***Clinical alert:*** It may be necessary to perform the Glasgow Coma Scale if there are any concerns about changing level of consciousness.
Abdominal assessment	
Assess for constipation.	See Chapters 23 and 25.

PROCEDURES AND NORMAL FINDINGS	ABNORMAL FINDINGS AND CLINICAL ALERTS
Laboratory tests	
Clinical laboratory findings (called biomarkers) give objective evidence of problem drinking. These are less sensitive than self-report questionnaires, but they are useful data to corroborate the subjective data and are unbiased.	
Serum protein gamma glutamyl transferase (GGT) is a commonly used biomarker of alcohol misuse. The GGT is helpful in detecting relapses for alcohol-dependent people who are in recovery. Normal: • Male: < 50 U/L • Female: < 30 U/L	Chronic alcohol drinking of ≥ 4 drinks/day for 4–8 weeks significantly raises GGT, but many chronic drinkers no longer have increased GGT. A person with non-alcoholic liver disease can show increase GGT levels in the absence of alcohol. A sudden elevated GGT after normal GGT levels may indicate relapse and prompts discussion with the person.
The **carbohydrate-deficient transferrin (CDT)** is used together with the GGT, which may increase detection of alcohol misuse. Healthy women have higher CDT levels than men; combining it with GGT may improve accuracy. CDT normalises during abstinence with a half-life of 15 days.	CDT is elevated after drinking 50–80 g alcohol/day for 1 week.
Serum aspartate aminotransferase (AST) is an enzyme found in high concentrations in the heart and liver. Normal: < 40 U/L	Chronic drinking for months increases AST.

From the **full blood count**, the **mean corpuscular volume (MCV)** is an index of red blood cell size. MCV is not sensitive enough to use as the only biomarker for problem drinking.
Normal:
• Child: 3 months (mean): 95 fL
  • 1 year: 70–86 fL; 3–6 years: 73–89 fL
  • 10–12 years: 77–91 fL
• Adult: 80–100 fL
	Heavy alcohol drinking for 4–8 weeks increases MCV.

Phosphatidylethanol (PEth). This is the only biomarker that can detect moderate alcohol intake. PEth is a phospholipid produced only in the presence of alcohol. PEth can be detected after only 1–2 standard drinks (14 gm of ethanol). A PEth level of 20 ng per mL or higher is often used as the threshold to identify moderate to heavy alcohol consumption.	

PROCEDURES AND NORMAL FINDINGS	ABNORMAL FINDINGS AND CLINICAL ALERTS
Breath analysis for alcohol detects any amount of ingested alcohol. This measure can be correlated with **blood alcohol concentration** and is the basis for legal interpretation of unsafe drinking. Normal values indicating no alcohol are 0.00.	A BAC ≥ 0.05% = legal intoxication in Australia.

Clinical reasoning and documentation

The case study provided at the beginning of this chapter is an example of a typical situation involving assessment of a person who may have a problem with addiction to opioid medication and the clinical reasoning process including problem/issue identification. Consult a fundamentals of nursing or medical-surgical nursing text for information about goal setting, nursing interventions and evaluation.

Case study (continued)

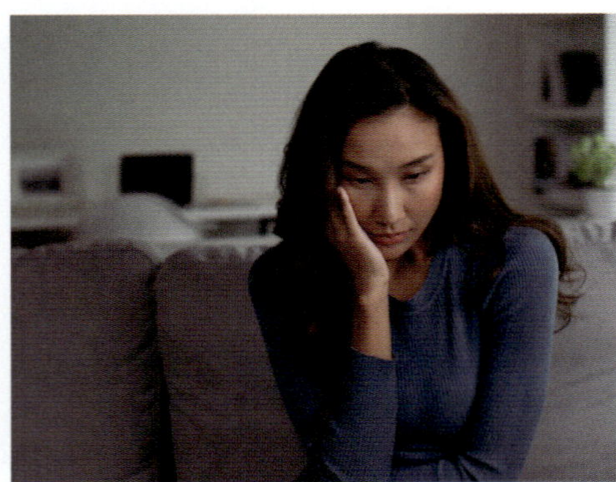

Context

You will recall from the case study described earlier in the chapter that you are a registered nurse working in an emergency department and you have been asked to assess Ms Sharvi Sharma.

Consider the patient's situation

Ms Sharma is a 30-year-old woman who has presented with severe abdominal symptoms. After initial medical assessment, she has been prescribed an opioid medication for the pain.

Collect cues/information

Subjective data

Ms Sharma reports flare-ups of severe abdo pain, nausea, vomiting, diarrhoea for several years. Ms Sharma has had several gastroscopies and colonoscopies with no abnormalities detected. The most recent colonoscopy was 3 months ago. States she has episodes of diarrhoea about 1 day per week, with multiple, watery bowel actions.

Sharvi came to the hospital because of severe abdominal pain (8/10) accompanied by nausea. She takes prescribed pain medication constantly and has found she needs higher doses to get any relief. She experiences heavy periods every 35 days. She has lost around 10 kg in the past 6 months and finds it hard to eat when nauseated. No specific food or drink appears to trigger nausea or diarrhoea.

Sharvi has run out of opioid medication and could not get another script. Ms Sharma tells you she gets very upset if staff suggest (as they have done in the past) that she may be addicted to these drugs. She states she wouldn't be on the medication if the doctors could figure out what is wrong with her. Ms Sharma has a history of anxiety and panic attacks. She feels the only relief for her emotional and physical pain is pain medication.

Objective data

Vital signs: – Temp 36.5, HR = 90, RR – 14, BP 130/85, BMI 17

General inspection: Thin (less than ideal body weight), appears less anxious than on initial presentation; Ms Sharma remains very insistent about the need to get another script for pain relief.

Abdo assessment: Scaphoid-shaped abdominal contour, bowel sounds heard, general guarding on light palpation, no masses identified.

Urine test: Urine light yellow coloured and clear; urine dipstick—pH 6 no abnormalities detected.

Continued

Clinical reasoning and documentation cont'd

Process information and identify problems/issues

Collaborative problem(s)

Abdominal pain and gastrointestinal symptoms related to unknown cause for further investigation.

Possible misuse of opioid pain medication for further investigation.

Problem statements/nursing diagnoses

Abdominal pain related to unknown cause.

Nutrition less than body requirements related to nausea.

Knowledge deficit related to long-term side effects of opioid medications.

Altered bowel elimination related to unknown cause.

Next steps

While the nurse conducts the initial substance use disorder assessment, it is not normally the nurse's responsibility to formulate a treatment plan if substance misuse is identified. Most hospitals or community settings will have identified alcohol and drug (or mental health) experts who can be contacted if a problem is suspected. Your assessment should provide enough information to determine if such a referral is needed.

ADDITIONAL RESOURCES

You can further develop your knowledge and skills relevant to screening for substance misuse, related pathophysiology, common health issues and nursing interventions by:

- reading chapters of a fundamentals of nursing or medical-surgical nursing textbook
- answering chapter multiple choice questions online. Log onto ClinicalKey Student and search for the text 'Health Assessment, 4th edition'. Choose the section titled 'Teaching material'. In this section you will find question and answer documents for each chapter.
- visiting websites

  Alcohol and Drug Foundation: https://adf.org.au/talking-about-drugs/having-conversation/

  Standard drinks guide: https://www.health.gov.au/topics/alcohol/about-alcohol/standard-drinks-guide

  The Right Mix: https://www.openarms.gov.au/right-mix-app

  Walking a tightrope: Alcohol and other drug use and violence—a guide for families: http://www.fds.org.au/images/FDS/NCETA_Walking_a_Tightrope.pdf

  Alcoholics Anonymous: https://aa.org.au/

  Beyond Blue: https://www.beyondblue.org.au/get-support/talk-to-a-counsellor

  Reach Out—Addiction: https://au.reachout.com/mental-health-issues/addiction

  Overcoming drug addiction: https://www.helpguide.org/articles/addictions/overcoming-drug-addiction.htm

  How to reduce or quit drug addiction: https://www.health.gov.au/topics/drugs/about-drugs/how-to-reduce-or-quit-drugs

  Narcotics Anonymous: https://www.na.org.au/multi/

REFERENCES

1. Australian Institute of Health and Welfare. National Drug Strategy Household Survey 2019. Canberra, Australia: 2020. Available at: https://www.aihw.gov.au/reports/illicit-use-of-drugs/national-drug-strategy-household-survey-2019/contents/summary
2. American Psychiatric Association, 2013. Diagnostic and Statistical Manual of Mental Disorders, 5th edn. APA, Virginia, United States.
3. Australian Institute of Health and Welfare. Australian Burden of Disease Study 2018: Interactive data on risk factor burden. Canberra, Australia: Government of Australia; 2021. Available at: https://www.aihw.gov.au/reports/burden-of-disease/abds-2018-interactive-data-risk-factors/contents/about
4. Ministry of Health New Zealand. New Zealand Health Survey. Government of New Zealand; 2022. Available at: https://www.health.govt.nz/nz-health-statistics/surveys/new-zealand-health-survey
5. Department of Health and Aged Care. About passive smoking. Canberra, Australia: Government of Australia; 2023. Available at: https://www.health.gov.au/topics/smoking-and-tobacco/about-smoking-and-tobacco/about-passive-smoking
6. Department of Health and Aged Care. Smoking and tobacco and pregnancy. Canberra, Australia: Government of Australia; 2023. Available at: https://www.health.gov.au/topics/smoking-and-tobacco/smoking-and-tobacco-throughout-life/smoking-and-tobacco-and-pregnancy
7. Australian Bureau of Statistics. Smoking. Canberra: ABS; 2020–21. Available at: https://www.abs.gov.au/statistics/health/health-conditions-and-risks/smoking/latest-release
8. Ministry of Health New Zealand. Annual Update of Key Results 2021–22: New Zealand Health Survey. Wellington; 2022. Available at: https://www.health.govt.nz/publication/annual-update-key-results-2021-22-new-zealand-health-survey
9. Banks E, Yazidjoglou A, Brown S, Nguyen M, Martin M, Beckwith K, et al. Electronic cigarettes and health outcomes: systematic review of global evidence. Report for the Australian Department of Health. National Centre for Epidemiology and Population Health, Canberra: April 2022. Available at: https://nceph.anu.edu.au/research/projects/health-impacts-electronic-cigarettes#health_outcomes
10. Chapman J, Harrison N, Kostadinov V, Skinner N, Roche A. Older Australians' perceptions of alcohol-related harms and low-risk alcohol guidelines. Drug and Alcohol Review. 2020 Jan;39(1):44–54.
11. Wamamili B, Stewart P, Wallace-Bell M. Factors associated with having family/whānau or close friends who used alcohol or other drugs in harmful ways among university students in New Zealand. International Journal of Environmental Research and Public Health. 2021;19(1). DOI: 10.3390/ijerph19010243
12. Australian Institute of Health and Welfare. Australian Burden of Disease Study 2022. Australian Institute of Health and Welfare; 2022. Available at: https://www.aihw.gov.au/reports/burden-of-disease/australian-burden-of-disease-study-2022/contents/summary
13. Yoo JE, Han K, Shin DW, Kim D, Kim B-S, Chun S, et al. Association between changes in alcohol consumption and cancer risk. JAMA Network Open. 2022;5(8):e2228544-e. DOI: 10.1001/jamanetworkopen.2022.28544
14. Cancer Australia. Apparent alcohol consumption. Canberra, Australia: Government of Australia; 2022. Available at: https://ncci.canceraustralia.gov.au/prevention/alcohol-consumption/apparent-alcohol-consumption.
15. Australian Bureau of Statistics. National Aboriginal and Torres Strait Islander Health Survey. Canberra, Australia: Government of Australia; 2019. Available at: https://www.abs.gov.au/statistics/people/aboriginal-and-torres-strait-islander-peoples/national-aboriginal-and-torres-strait-islander-health-survey/latest-release
16. World Health Organization. Alcohol. Geneva, Switzerland; 2022. Available at: https://www.who.int/news-room/fact-sheets/detail/alcohol

17. Freudenheim JL. Alcohol's effects on breast cancer in women. Alcohol Research – Current Reviews. 2020;40(2):1–12. DOI: 10.35946/arcr.v40.2.11
18. Australian Government. What is a standard drink? 2020. National Health and Medical Research Council. Available at: https://www.nhmrc.gov.au/file/16899/download?token=GyhhNeWg
19. Alcohol and Drug Foundation. Real-time prescription monitoring in Australia. Melbourne, Australia; 2023. Available at: https://www.health.gov.au/our-work/national-real-time-prescription-monitoring-rtpm
20. Australian Institute of Health and Welfare. Alcohol, tobacco & other drugs in Australia. Canberra, Australia. 2023. Available at: https://www.aihw.gov.au/reports/alcohol/alcohol-tobacco-other-drugs-australia/contents/drug-types/illicit-opioids-including-heroin#Deaths
21. Department of Health and Aged Care. National Real Time Prescription Monitoring (RTPM). 2023. Australian Government. Available at: https://www.health.gov.au/our-work/national-real-time-prescription-monitoring-rtpm
22. Department of Health, SafeScript. Melbourne, State of Victora; 2023. Available at: https://www.health.vic.gov.au/safescript
23. Alcohol and Drug Foundation. Codeine. 2023. Available at: https://adf.org.au/drug-facts/codeine/
24. Nielsen S, MacDonald T, Johnson JL. Identifying and treating codeine dependence: a systematic review. Medical Journal of Australia. 2018;208(10):451–461.
25. NZ Drug Foundation. Cannabis. Wellington: Government of New Zealand; 2023. Available at: https://www.drugfoundation.org.nz/info/drug-index/cannabis/
26. Safer Care Victoria. Substance use during pregnancy: care of the mother and newborn. Melbourne, Australia: Safer Care Victoria; 2021. Available at: https://www.safercare.vic.gov.au/clinical-guidance/maternity/substance-use-during-pregnancy-care-of-the-mother-and-newborn
27. Grigg J, Manning V, Arunogiri S, Volpe I, Frei M, Phan V, et al. Methamphetamine Treatment Guidelines: Practice Guidelines for Health Professionals. Melbourne, Australia: Turning Point; 2018. Available at: https://www.turningpoint.org.au/treatment/clinicians/methamphetamine-treatment-guidelines
28. New Zealand Parliament. Methamphetamine in New Zealand: A snapshot of recent trends. Government of New Zealand; 2021. Available at: https://www.parliament.nz/en/pb/library-research-papers/research-papers/methamphetamine-in-new-zealand-a-snapshot-of-recent-trends/
29. Volkow ND, Koob GF, McLellan AT. Neurobiologic advances from the brain disease model of addiction. New England Journal of Medicine. 2016;374(4):363–371. DOI: 10.1056/NEJMra1511480
30. Griffin A. Adolescent neurological development and implications for health and well-being. Healthcare (Basel). 2017;5(4). doi: 10.3390/healthcare5040062
31. Lees B, Debenham J, Squeglia LM. Alcohol and cannabis use and the developing brain. Alcohol Research – Current Reviews. 2021; 41(1):1–14. Available at: https://arcr.niaaa.nih.gov/volume/41/1/alcohol-and-cannabis-use-and-developing-brain
32. Gould GS, Oncken C, Medelsohn CP. Management of smoking in pregnant women. Australian Family Physician. 2014;43(1). Available at: https://www.racgp.org.au/afp/2014/january-february/smoking-in-pregnant-women
33. Centers for Disease Control and Prevention. Alcohol Use During Pregnancy. US Department of Health & Human Services; 2022. Available at: https://www.cdc.gov/ncbddd/fasd/alcohol-use.html
34. Department of Health and Aged Care. Reducing Fetal Alcohol Spectrum Disorder (FASD) in Australia. Canberra, Australia: Government of Australia; 2019. Available at: https://www.health.gov.au/news/reducing-fetal-alcohol-spectrum-disorder-fasd-in-australia
35. Bartlett R, Brown L, Shattell M, Wright T, Lewallen L. Harm reduction: compassionate care of persons with addictions. MEDSURG

Nursing. 2013 Nov–Dec;22(6):349–353, 358. PMID: 24600929; PMCID: PMC4070513

36. Australian Institute of Health and Welfare. Alcohol, tobacco & other drugs in Australia: Harm minimisation. 2023. Australian Government. Available at: https://www.aihw.gov.au/reports/alcohol/alcohol-tobacco-other-drugs-australia/contents/harm-minimisation
37. Babor TF, Higgins-Biddle JC, Saunders JB, Monteiro G. AUDIT: The Alcohol Use Disorders Identification Test Guidelines for Use in Primary Care, Second Edition, 2001. World Health Organization, Geneva.
38. Van Gils Y, Franck E, Dierckx E, Van Alphen SP, Saunders JB, Dom G. Validation of the AUDIT and AUDIT-C for hazardous drinking in community-dwelling older adults. International Journal of Environmental Research and Public Health. 2021 Sep 2;18(17):9266.
39. Shenoi RP, Linakis JG, Bromberg JR, Casper TC, Richards R, Mello MJ, et al. Predictive validity of the CRAFFT for substance use disorder. Pediatrics. 2019;144(2). DOI: 10.1542/peds.2018-3415
40. Corniello A, Skowronsky C. Clinical institute withdrawal assessment alcohol scale-revised (CIWA-Ar). Clinical Nurse Specialist. 2012; 26(2).
41. The Regents of the University of Michigan. Short Michigan Alcoholism Screening Test-Geriatric Version (SMAST-G). 1991. Available at: https://consultgeri.org/try-this/general-assessment/issue-17.pdf
42. Skinner HA (1982). The Drug Abuse Screening Test. Addictive Behaviour 7(4):363–371. DOI: 10.1016/0306-4603(82)90005-3
43. National Institute on Drug Abuse, 2021. Words matter: Preferred language for talking about addiction. Available at: https://nida.nih.gov/nidamed-medical-health-professionals/health-professions-education/words-matter-terms-to-use-avoid-when-talking-about-addiction

UNIT 2

Health assessment tools and techniques

CHAPTER 7

Person-centred communication in health assessment

Written by Carolyn Jarvis and Ann Eckhardt
Adapted by Elizabeth Pascoe

INTRODUCTION

In Australia, the National Safety and Quality in Health Service Standards were developed by the Australian Commission on Safety and Quality in Health Care (ACSQHC).[1] These standards aim to set a consistent standard of practice to protect patients from harm and to improve the quality of health service provision. There are eight standards including communicating for safety. High-quality health care occurs when the person is in control, has effective access to treatment, is safe and where illnesses are not just treated but prevented. The ACSQHC[1] emphasises the importance of effective communication for safe and quality health care. Communication failures and lack of interdisciplinary teamwork are major contributing factors for errors, misdiagnosis, inappropriate treatment and poor care outcomes.[1]

The first principle of quality and safety in health care is person-centred care. Person-centred care is complex and encompasses consideration of patients' values, needs and beliefs when planning and providing care. It includes empowering the person, empathy and respect; shared decision making; and a holistic approach to care where the focus is on the person rather than just on a health problem. Communication (verbal and nonverbal) between the healthcare provider and the person are fundamental elements of person-centred care.[2] Patient experiences of caring and person-centredness have an influential role in the extent to which patients experience the quality of nursing care.[3] Skilled communication is critical for forming effective relationships with the person and their family and facilitating person-centred care.[2]

As you have learnt in a previous chapter, collecting **subjective data** is important in beginning to identify the person's health strengths and health concerns and as a bridge to the next step in data collection, the physical examination. The process of collecting subjective data will sometimes involve a semiformal interview if comprehensive information is to be collected; at other times the interview will be more like a conversation that may be short as you focus on a particular health issue or concern. Successful communication in the context of health assessment involves your ability to:

- approach your interactions with the person and their family in a caring and person-centred way
- establish rapport and trust so the person feels accepted and therefore free to share all their relevant health history
- gather complete and accurate information about the person's health state, including the description and chronology of any past and present symptoms and illnesses
- provide health information to the person about their health state so they can take part in identifying potential and actual health issues and participate in decisions about their health care
- build rapport for a continuing therapeutic relationship; this rapport facilitates future diagnoses, planning and treatment
- begin educating for health promotion and disease prevention.

Effective communication skills are also important for documenting your health assessment findings and for effective interdisciplinary teamwork. Effective communication with other members of the healthcare team and teamwork involves:[1]

- undertaking structured communication
- using an agreed and common language
- using 'check back' communication to ensure the correct information is received
- having situational awareness
- documenting essential information.

Effective communication with other members of the healthcare team and accuracy of documentation are critical for safe and quality health care, but the focus of this chapter will be on developing knowledge and skill in communication for the purpose of establishing rapport and trust with the person and their family and for beginning the process of gathering subjective data through the systematic and purposeful collection of health information. This includes having awareness of the process and techniques of communication, developmental, social and cultural considerations, then being able to apply this to people with special needs or challenging behaviours and identifying strategies for overcoming communication barriers.

Case study

The following case study gives an example of a typical situation involving a ward admission assessment and the *initial clinical reasoning process*. It will help you identify your learning needs.

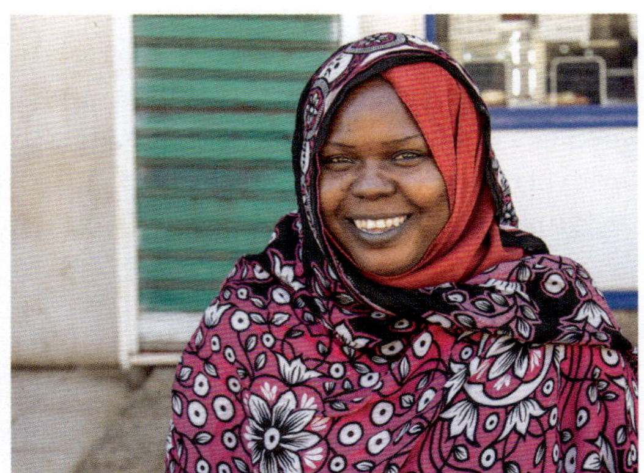

Context

You are on clinical placement in a subacute rehabilitation ward. Your preceptor (buddy) nurse tells you he is expecting a new patient admission to the ward shortly after the afternoon handover. He asks you to prepare to be involved in completing the ward admission assessment for this woman, who you will be meeting for the first time.

Consider the patient's situation

You have limited information about the new patient. Mrs Nyamal Bol is a 55-year-old woman who is undergoing rehabilitation following a car accident 3 days ago. She sustained a fractured right wrist, which has been internally fixed with a plate and screw, and she has a plaster cast from her fingers to her elbow. She also sustained a dislocated fractured ankle, which has been fixed with screws and plates, and she is now wearing an orthopaedic boot. She has extensive bruising and minor cuts. Mrs Bol is a South Sudanese–Australian who arrived in Australia as a refugee 8 years ago with her husband and five children. You are told that Mrs Bol speaks some English.

Questions to further your learning

- What do you need to consider before meeting Mrs Bol for the first time?
- How will you approach your first meeting with her?
- What are the possible things that might be going on with Mrs Bol?
- What knowledge do you need to be able to predict what might be going on?
- What approach to the admission health assessment will you take?
- What resources are available to assist in your assessment of Mrs Bol?

Resources available

You will find additional resources and the reference list at the end of this chapter.

The process of communication

In the context of health assessment, subjective data is obtained through an interview process that has two main goals. The first is to establish a positive therapeutic relationship between the nurse and the person and their family. The second is to gather health and personal information that will form the basis for identifying the person's strengths and planning goal-directed person-centred care. This is achieved by effective communication. Communication is exchanging information so that each person clearly understands the other—that is, mutual understanding.[4] If you do not understand each other, you have not conveyed a shared meaning and effective communication has *not* occurred. A lack of effective communication interferes with care and is a commonly reported patient complaint.[5]

It is challenging to teach the skill of interviewing in the context of health assessment because initially health professionals may think little needs to be learnt. They assume that if they can talk and hear, they can communicate. But much more than talking and hearing is necessary. Communication includes all behaviour, conscious and unconscious, verbal and nonverbal.[5] *All behaviour has meaning.*

The process of communication involves the way in which information is exchanged. It involves several components: **the sender**, the person who is communicating the information; **the receiver**, the person receiving the information; **the message**, the information that is being communicated; and the **channel of** communication.[1] You also need to consider the potential complexity of health communication because it may not be taking place face to face. In some contexts, the health assessment interview may be via phone, FaceTime, Skype, Zoom or another online platform.

Sending

It is likely that you are most aware of *verbal* communication—the words you speak, vocalisations and the tone of voice.[4] *Nonverbal* communication also occurs. This is your body language—posture, body gestures such as arms folded in front of you or sitting loosely by your side, physical responses such as blushing and sweating, facial expression, eye contact, touch, distance between you and the other person(s), even where you place your chair.[5] Since nonverbal communication is under less conscious control than verbal communication, nonverbal communication probably is more reflective of your true feelings. When verbal communication and nonverbal communication are incongruent, the nonverbal message tends to be the true one because it is under less conscious control.

Receiving

Being aware of the messages you send is only part of the process. Your words and gestures must be interpreted in a *specific context* to have meaning. You have a specific context in mind when you send your words. The receiver puts their own interpretation on them. The receiver attaches meaning determined by their past experiences, culture and self-concept, as well as their current physical and emotional state.[5] Sometimes, however, the contexts of the sender and receiver do not coincide. Remember how frustrating it may have been to try to communicate something to a friend, only to have your message totally misunderstood? Your message can be sabotaged by the listener's bias. It takes *mutual* understanding by the sender and receiver to have successful communication.[5]

Even greater risk for misunderstanding exists in the healthcare setting than in a social setting.

The person usually has a health problem, and this factor emotionally charges your professional relationship.[5] It *intensifies* the communication because the person feels dependent on you to correctly interpret their messages.

Communication is a *fundamental skill* that can be learnt, developed and improved with practice, experience, continuous learning, mentorship and support.[1] It is a tool, as intrinsic to quality health care as the tools and techniques of physical examination. To maximise your communication skills, first be aware of internal factors (personal qualities and abilities) and external factors (environmental and other issues) and their influence. Central to the ability to be aware of internal and external factors and their impact is self-awareness.[5] Self-awareness enables us to enhance self-understanding. Greater self-understanding leads to increased control of thought and behaviour—internal and external factors.[6] This then leads to positive interactions and effective communication.

Internal factors (personal qualities and abilities)

Internal factors are those particular to the nurse—that is, what you bring into the interview. Cultivate the three inner factors of liking others, empathy and the ability to listen.

LIKING OTHERS

One essential factor for a person's 'goodness of fit' into a helping profession is a genuine liking of other people. This means a generally optimistic view of people: an assumption of their strengths and a tolerance for their weaknesses. An atmosphere of warmth and caring is necessary. The person must feel that they are accepted unconditionally.

The respect for other people extends to respect for their own control over their health. Your goal is *not* to make the person dependent on you but to help them to be increasingly responsible for themselves. You wish to promote their growth. You have the healthcare resources to offer. The person must choose how to apply those resources to their own life.

EMPATHY

Empathy means viewing the world from the other person's inner frame of reference. Empathy means recognising and accepting the other person's feelings without criticism. It might be described as 'feeling with the person rather than feeling like the person'. It does not mean you become lost in the other person at the expense of your own self. If this occurred, you would cease to be helpful. Rather, it is to *understand with* the person how *they* perceive their world.

THE ABILITY TO LISTEN

Listening is not a passive role in the communication process; it is active and demanding. Listening requires your complete attention. You cannot be preoccupied with your own needs or the needs of other people or you will miss something important. At the time of the subjective data collection, no one is more important than the person you are talking with. This person's needs are your sole concern.

Active listening is the route to understanding. You cannot be thinking of what you are going to say as soon as the person stops for breath. Listen to *what* the person says. The story may not come out in the order you would ask it or will record it later. Let the person talk from their own outline; nearly everything that is said will be relevant. Listen to *the way* a person tells the story, such as difficulty with language, impaired memory, the tone of the person's voice and even to what the person is leaving out.

External factors (environmental and other issues)

Preparing the physical setting where the subjective data collection is to occur is essential. The setting may be in a hospital room, an examination room, in an office or clinic or in the person's home (where you will have less control). In any location, optimal conditions are important to have a smooth discussion. Therefore, preparing the physical setting must include attention to the following elements.

ENSURE PRIVACY

Aim for geographic privacy—a private room in the hospital, clinic, office or home. This may involve asking an ambulatory roommate to step out for a while or finding an unoccupied room or an empty lounge. If geographic privacy is not available, 'psychological privacy' by curtained partitions may suffice if the person feels sure no one can overhear the conversation or interrupt.

REFUSE INTERRUPTIONS

Most people resent interruptions except in cases of an emergency. Inform any support staff of the need for privacy and ask that they not interrupt you during this time. Discourage other health professionals from interrupting you with *their* need for access to the person. Concentrate and establish rapport. An interruption can destroy in seconds what you have spent many minutes building up.

PHYSICAL ENVIRONMENT

- Provide enough lighting so you can see each other clearly.
- Reduce noise. Multiple stimuli are confusing. Turn off the television, radio and any unnecessary equipment.
- Place the distance between you and the person at approximately 1 to 1.5 m (twice arm's length). If you place the person any closer, you may invade their private space and you may create anxiety. If you place the person further away, you seem distant and aloof. (See 'Cultural and social considerations' later in the chapter for more information.)
- Arrange equal-status seating. Both you and the person should be comfortably seated, at eye level. Avoid facing them across a desk or table because that feels like a barrier. Placing the chairs at 90 degrees is good because it allows the person either to face you or to look straight ahead from time to time (Figure 7.1). Most importantly, avoid standing. Standing does two things: (1) it communicates your haste; and (2) it assumes superiority. Standing makes you loom over the person as an authority figure. When you are sitting, the person feels some control in the setting.
- If the person is in bed they should not have to stare at the ceiling; this causes them to lose the visual message of your communication.

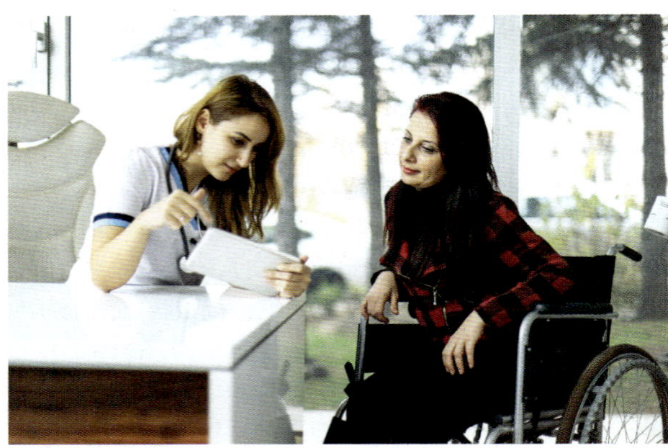

FIGURE 7.1 Equal-status seating

DRESS

- Your appearance and clothing should be appropriate to the setting and should meet conventional professional standards including conservative clothing, a name tag and neat hair. Avoid extremes.

NOTE TAKING

Some use of history forms and note taking may be unavoidable. When you sit down later to document the health history, you cannot rely completely on memory to furnish details of previous hospitalisations or the review of body systems, for example. But be aware that taking notes during the interview has disadvantages:

- It breaks eye contact too often.
- It shifts your attention away from the person, diminishing their sense of importance.
- It can interrupt the person's narrative flow. You may say '*Please slow down; I'm not getting it all*'. Or the person may see you recording furiously and, in an effort to please you, adjust their tempo to your writing. Either way, the person's natural mode of expression is lost.
- It impedes your observation of the person's nonverbal behaviour.
- It is threatening to the person during the discussion of sensitive issues (e.g. amount of alcohol and drug use, number of sexual partners or incidence of physical abuse).

So, keep note taking to a minimum, and try to focus your attention on the person. Any recording you do should be secondary to the dialogue and should not interfere with the person's spontaneity. With experience, you will not rely on note taking as much. Nevertheless, explain to the person that you may take a few moments to make notes and check with the person that your interpretation is correct.

ELECTRONIC MEDICAL RECORD

Many hospitals, clinics and other healthcare agencies will record all patient information in an electronic medical record. Admission, risk assessment, medication, fluid balance, vital signs and other charts can be located within the electronic record. Clinical progress notes are also documented in the electronic format. As with written note taking, typing into a computer while speaking with the person can affect your ability to establish rapport and to listen carefully to the person's responses. Try to keep your focus on the person. Use natural pauses in the conversation to take time to type in your notes. As with manual note taking, tell the person that you will take a few moments to make notes and check with the person that your interpretation is correct.

Techniques of communication

Introducing yourself

When you first meet the person, you may be nervous about how to begin collecting subjective data. The person may also be nervous, meeting a new nurse and feeling anxious about the environment and their health state. Address the person using their surname, and shake hands if that seems comfortable and is culturally appropriate. Start by **introducing yourself** and stating your role in the organisation (if you are a student, say so). *Hello, my name is ...* is the start of providing person-centred, compassionate care.[7] Request permission or a consent from the person before proceeding, and be aware of your ethical and legal obligations to protect the privacy of people. See the 'Additional resources' section for information on your responsibilities related to patient confidentiality and privacy.

If you are gathering a comprehensive health history, give the reason for this:

'Mrs Tran, I would like to talk about your illness that caused you to come to the hospital.'
'Ms Taft, I want to ask you some questions about your health so that we can identify what is keeping you healthy and explore any problems.'
'Mr Craig, I want to ask you some questions about your health and your usual daily activities so that we can plan your care here in the hospital.'

If the person is in the hospital, more than one health team member may be collecting a health history. Some people are apt to feel exasperated because they believe they are repeating the same thing unless you give a reason for asking these questions.

After this brief introduction, ask an open-ended question (see below) then let the person proceed. You do not need friendly small talk to build rapport. This is not a social visit; the person has some concern to talk about and wants to get on with it. You will build rapport best by letting them discuss the concern early.

The working phase

The working phase is the data-gathering phase. Verbal skills for this phase include your questions to the person and your responses to what they say. Two types of questions exist: open-ended and closed. Each type has a different place and function during data collection.

OPEN-ENDED QUESTIONS

An **open-ended** question asks for narrative information. It states the topic to be discussed but only in **general** terms. Use it to begin, to introduce a new section of questions and whenever the person introduces a new topic.

'Tell me how I can help you.'
'What brings you to the hospital?'
'Tell me why you have come here today.'
'How have you been getting along?'
'You mentioned shortness of breath. Tell me more about that.'
'How have you been feeling since your last appointment?'

An open-ended question is unbiased; it leaves the person free to answer in any way. This question encourages the person to respond in paragraphs and to give a spontaneous account in any order chosen. It lets the person express themself fully.

As the person answers, stop and *listen*. What usually happens is that they may answer with a short phrase or sentence, pause and then look at you expecting some direction as to how to go on. What you do next is the key. If you pose new questions on other topics, you may lose much of the initial story. Instead, respond to the first statement with '*Tell me about it*' or '*Anything else?*' or merely look acutely interested. The person will then tell the story.

CLOSED OR DIRECT QUESTIONS

Closed or **direct** questions ask for specific information. They elicit a short, one- or two-word answer, a yes or no or a forced choice. Where the open-ended question allows the person to have free rein, the direct question limits their answer (Table 7.1).

Use the direct questions after the person's opening narrative to fill in any details they may have left out. Also use direct questions when you need many specific facts such as when asking about past health problems or current health issues. You need direct questions to speed up the data collection. Asking all open-ended questions would be unwieldy and may take hours. But be careful

TABLE 7.1 Comparison of open-ended and closed questions

Open-ended	Direct, closed
Use for narrative information	Use for specific information
Calls for long paragraph answers	Calls for short one- or two-word answers
Elicits feelings, opinions, ideas	Elicits cold facts
Builds and enhances rapport	Limits rapport and leaves interaction neutral

not to overuse closed questions. Follow these guidelines:

1. Ask only one direct question at a time. Avoid bombarding the person with long lists: '*Have you ever had pain, double vision, watering or redness in the eyes?*' Avoid double-barrelled questions such as '*Do you exercise and drink enough water during the day?*' The person will not know which question to answer. And if the person answers '*yes*', you will not know which question the person has answered.
2. Choose language the person understands. Avoid using complicated medical terminology; for example, '*How many times do you void per day?*' may not be understood. Assess the person's level of understanding of medical terminology. For example, it might be more appropriate to ask, '*How many times a day do you pee?*'

RESPONSES—ASSISTING THE NARRATIVE

You have asked the first open-ended question and the person answers. As the person talks, your role is to encourage free expression but not let the person wander off course. Your responses help the teller amplify the story.

Some people seek health care for short-term or relatively simple needs. Their history is direct and uncomplicated; for these people, two responses (facilitation and silence) may be all you need to get a complete picture. Other people have a complex story, a long history of a chronic condition or accompanying emotions. Additional responses help you gather data without cutting the person off.

There are nine types of verbal responses in all. The first five responses (facilitation, silence, reflection, empathy, clarification) involve your *reactions* to the facts or feelings the person has communicated. Your response focuses on the person's frame of reference. Your own frame of reference should not enter into the response. In the remaining four responses (confrontation, interpretation, explanation, summary), you start to express *your own* thoughts and feelings. The frame of reference shifts from the person's perspective to yours. In the first five responses, the person leads; in the last four responses, you lead.

THE PERSON'S FRAME OF REFERENCE

Facilitation

These responses encourage the person to say more, to continue with the story ('*mm-hmm, go on, continue, uh-huh*'). Also called general leads, these responses show the person you are interested and will listen further. Simply maintaining eye contact, shifting forwards in your seat with increased attention, nodding or using your hand to gesture ('*Yes, go on, I'm with you*') encourages the person to continue talking.

Silence

Silence is golden after open-ended questions. Your silent attentiveness communicates that the person has time to think, to organise what they wish to say without interruption from you. This 'thinking silence' is the one health professionals interrupt most often. The interruption destroys the person's train of thought. The person is often interrupted because silence is uncomfortable for beginning nurses. They feel responsible for keeping the dialogue going and feel at fault if it stops. But silence has advantages. One advantage is letting the person collect their thoughts. Also, silence gives you a chance to observe the person unobtrusively and to note nonverbal cues. Finally, silence gives you time to plan your next approach.

Reflection

This response echoes the person's words. Reflection is repeating part of what the person has just said. In this example, it focuses further attention on a specific phrase and helps the person continue in their own way:

> Patient: *I'm here because of my water. It was cutting off.*
> Response: *It was cutting off?*
> Patient: *Yes, yesterday it took me 30 minutes to pass my water. Finally, I got a tiny stream, but then it just closed off.*

Reflection also can help express feeling behind a person's words. The feeling is already in the statement. You focus on it and encourage the person to elaborate:

> Patient: *It's so hard having to stay flat on my back in the hospital with this pregnancy. I have two more little ones at home. I'm so worried they are not getting the care they need.*
> Response: *You feel worried and anxious about your children?*

Think of yourself as a mirror reflecting the person's words or feelings. This helps the person to elaborate on the problem.

Empathy

A physical symptom, condition or illness often has accompanying emotions. Many people have trouble expressing these feelings, perhaps because of confusion or embarrassment. In the second reflecting example above, the person had already stated her feeling and you echoed it. But in the first example, he has not said it yet. An empathic response recognises a feeling and puts it into words. It names the feeling and allows the expression of it. When the empathic response is used, the person feels accepted and can deal with the feeling openly.

> Patient (sarcastically): *This is just great. I have my own business, I direct 20 employees every day, and now here I am having to call you for every little thing.*
> Response: *It must be hard—one day having so much control and now feeling dependent on someone else.*

Your response does not cut off further communication as would happen by giving false reassurance ('*Oh, you'll be back to work in no time*'). Also, it does deny the feeling and indicates that it is not justified ('*I don't do everything for you. You are feeding yourself*'). An empathic response recognises the feeling, accepts it and allows the person to express it without embarrassment. It strengthens rapport. The person feels understood, which in itself is therapeutic because it recognises the isolation of illness. Other empathic responses are, '*This must be very hard for you*' or placing your hand lightly on the person's forearm—if culturally appropriate (Figure 7.2).

Clarification

Clarify what a person means when their word choice is ambiguous or confusing—for example, '*Tell me what you mean by a heavy chest*'. You can also use clarification to summarise the person's words or simplify them to make them clearer. Confirm with the person that you are on the right track: you are asking for agreement, and the person can confirm or deny your understanding.

> Response: *Now as I understand you, this heaviness in your chest comes when you mow the lawn or climb stairs, and it goes away when you stop doing those things. Is that correct?*
> Patient: *Yes, that's pretty much it.*

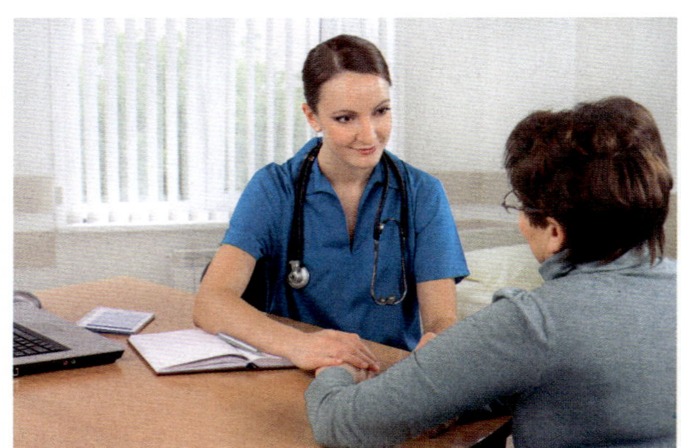

FIGURE 7.2 Empathetic response during a health assessment interview

YOUR FRAME OF REFERENCE

In these four responses, confrontation, interpretation, explanation and summary, the frame of reference shifts from the person's perspective to yours. These responses now include your own thoughts and feelings. Use these four responses judiciously. If you use them too often, you take over at the person's expense.

Confrontation

In the case of confrontation, you have noticed a certain action, feeling or statement and you now focus the person's attention on it. You give your honest feedback about what you see or feel. This may focus on a discrepancy: '*You say it doesn't hurt, but when I touch you here, you grimace*'. Or it may focus on the person's affect: '*You look sad*' or '*You sound angry*'. Or you may confront the person when you notice parts of the story are inconsistent: '*Earlier you said you were laying off alcohol and just now you said you had a few drinks after work yesterday*'.

Interpretation

Interpretation is based on your inference or conclusion. It links events, makes associations or implies cause: '*It seems that every time you feel stomach pain, you have had some kind of stress in your life*'. Interpretation also ascribes feelings and helps the person understand their own feelings in relation to the verbal message.

> Patient: *I have decided I don't want to have any more treatments. But I can't seem to tell my doctor that. Every time she comes in, I tighten up and can't say anything.*
> Response: *Could it be that you're afraid of her reaction?*

You do run a risk of making the wrong inference. If this is the case, the person will correct it. But even if the inference is corrected, interpretation helps to prompt further discussion of the topic.

Explanation

With these statements, you inform the person. You share factual and objective information. This may be for orientation to the agency setting: '*Your dinner comes at 5:30*'. Or it may be to explain cause: '*The reason you cannot eat or drink before your blood test is that the food will change the test results*'.

SUMMARY

This is a final review of what you understand the person has said. It condenses the facts and presents a summation of how you perceive the health problem, symptom or need. The summary provides an opportunity for the person to agree with or correct your understanding and perception. Both you and the person should take part. When the summary occurs at the end of the conversation, it signals that the end of the conversation is imminent.

Ten traps of interviewing

The verbal skills discussed above are productive and enhance the health assessment discussion. Now take time to consider nonproductive, defeating verbal messages or *traps*. It is easy to fall into these traps because you are anxious to help. The danger is that they restrict the person's response. The following traps are obstacles to obtaining complete data and to establishing rapport.

1. Providing false assurance or reassurance. A woman says, '*Oh, I just know this lump is going to turn out to be cancer*'. The automatic response of many clinicians is to say, '*Now don't worry; I'm sure you will be all right*'. This 'courage builder' relieves *your* anxiety and gives you the false sense of having provided comfort. But for the woman it actually closes off communication. It trivialises her anxiety and effectively denies any further talk of it. Also, it promises something that may not happen—

that is, she may *not* be all right. Consider instead these responses:

> *'You are really worried about the lump, aren't you?'*
> *'It must be hard to wait for the biopsy results.'*

These responses acknowledge the feeling and open the door for more communication. You *can* reassure the person that you are listening, that you understand, that you have hope for them and that you will take good care of them.

> Patient: *I feel so lost here since they transferred me to the medical centre. No one comes to see me. No one here cares what happens to me.*
> Response: *I care what happens to you. I am here today, and I will be caring for you. Is there anyone that you would like me to call?*

This type of reassurance makes a commitment to the person, and it can have a powerful impact.

2. Giving unwanted advice. Know when to give advice and when to avoid giving it. Often, people seek health care because they want your professional advice and information on the management of a health problem: '*My child has a sprained ankle; how should I take care of him?*' This is a straightforward request for information you have that the parent needs. You respond by assessing the situation, making a clinical judgement and providing a therapeutic plan based on your knowledge and experience.

In other situations, advice is different; it is based on a hunch or feeling. It is your personal opinion. Consider the woman who has just left a meeting with her consultant physician: '*Dr Kline just told me my only chance of getting pregnant is to have an operation. I just don't know. What would you do?*' Does the woman really want your advice? If you answer, '*If I were you, I'd ...*' then you would be making a mistake. You are not her. If you give your answer, you have shifted the accountability for decision making from her to you. She has not worked out her own solution.

Instead, a better response is reflection:

> Response: *Have an operation?*
> Woman: *Yes, and I'm terrified of being put to sleep. What if I don't wake up?*

Now you know her *real* concern and can help her deal with it. She will have grown in the process and may be better equipped to meet her next decision.

When asked for advice, other preferred responses are:

> *'What are the pros and cons of [this choice] for you?'*
> *'What concerns do you have?'*
> *'What is holding you back?'*

Although it is quicker just to give advice, take the time to involve the person in the problem-solving process. When a person takes part, they are more likely to learn and to change their behaviour.

3. Using authority. '*Your doctor/nurse knows best*' is a response that promotes dependency and inferiority. A better approach is to avoid using authority. Although you and the person cannot have equality of professional skill and experience, you do have equally worthy roles in the health process, each respecting the other. '*Based on the best evidence available ...*'

4. Using avoidance language. People use euphemisms such as 'passed on' to avoid reality or to hide their feelings. They think if they just say the word 'death', it might really happen. So, to protect themselves, they avoid the issue. Although it seems this will make them comfortable with potentially fearful topics, it does not. Not talking about the fear does not make it go away; it just suppresses the fear and makes it even more frightening. Using direct language is the best way to deal with frightening topics. '*I am very sorry to hear that your mother has died ...*'

5. Engaging in distancing. Distancing is the use of impersonal speech to put space between a threat and the self: '*My friend has a problem; she is afraid she ...*' or '*There is a* *lump in the left breast*'. By using 'the' instead of 'my', the woman can deny any association with her diseased breast and protect herself from it. Health professionals use distancing, too, to soften reality. This does not work because it communicates to the other person that you also are afraid of the procedure. The use of blunt specific terms is preferable to defuse anxiety.

6. Using professional jargon. What is called a myocardial infarction in the health profession is called a heart attack by most laypeople. Use of jargon sounds exclusionary and paternalistic. Adjust your vocabulary to the person, but avoid sounding condescending.

If a person uses medical jargon, do not assume they always know the correct meaning. For example, some people think 'hypertensive' means that they are very tense. As a result, they take their medication only when feeling stressed and not when they feel relaxed. This misinformation must be corrected. The person needs to understand that hypertension is a chronic condition that needs consistent medication to avoid side effects. On the other hand, you do not need to feel that it is a moral imperative to correct all misstatements (e.g. when a person says 'prostrate' for prostate gland).

7. Using leading or biased questions. Asking a man, '*You don't smoke, do you?*' implies that one answer is 'better' than another. If the person wants to please you, either he is forced to answer in a way corresponding to your values or he feels guilty when he must admit the other answer. He risks your disapproval. And if he feels dependent on you for care, the last thing he wants to do is alienate you.

8. Talking too much. Some nurses positively associate helpfulness with talking too much. If the air has been thick with their oratory and advice, these nurses leave thinking they have met the person's needs. Just the opposite is true. Anxious to please the nurse, the person lets the professional talk at the expense of their need to express themselves. A good rule for every health professional is to *listen more than you talk.*

9. Interrupting. Often, when you think you know what the person will say, you interrupt and cut the person off. This does not show that you are clever. Rather, it signals that you are impatient or bored with the discussion.

A related trap is preoccupation with yourself by thinking of your next remark while the person is talking. As the person speaks, you are thinking about what to say next, so you cannot fully understand what the person says. You are so preoccupied with your own role that you are not really listening. Aim for a second of silence between the person's statement and your next response.

10. Using 'why' questions. Consider your use of why questions in the healthcare setting. '*Why did you take so much medication?*' Or let's say you ask a man who has just come to the emergency department, '*Why did you wait so long before coming to the hospital?*' The only possible answer to a why question is '*because …*' and the man may not know the answer. He may not have worked it out. You sound whining, accusatory and judgemental. And the man now must produce an excuse to rationalise his own behaviour. To avoid this trap, say: '*I see you started to have chest pains early in the day. What was happening between the time the pains started and the time you came to the emergency department?*'

Nonverbal skills

There are five types of nonverbal behaviours that convey information about the person:

- *vocal cues* such as pitch, tone and quality of voice, including moaning, crying and groaning
- *action cues* such as posture, facial expression and gestures
- *object cues* such as clothes, jewellery and hair styles

- *use of personal and territorial space* in interpersonal transactions and care of belongings
- *touch*, which involves the use of personal space and action.[6]

Unless you try to understand the person's nonverbal behaviour, you may overlook important information such as that conveyed by facial expressions, silence, eye contact, touch and other body language. Communication patterns vary widely even for such conventional social behaviours as smiling and handshaking.

Learn to listen with your eyes as well as with your ears. Nonverbal messages are very important in establishing rapport and in conveying information, especially about feelings. Nonverbal messages provide clues to understanding feelings. When nonverbal and verbal messages are congruent, the verbal is reinforced. When they are incongruent, the nonverbal message tends to be the true one, because it is under less conscious control.

PHYSICAL APPEARANCE

In his seminal work, *The Stress of Life*, Hans Selye[8] reports his interest in the body's total response to stress began as a student. Unbiased as yet by medical knowledge, he noted that some patients just 'looked sick', even though they did not exhibit the specific characteristic signs that would lead to a precise medical diagnosis. Such people simply felt and looked ill or feverish. The same view can work for you. Inattention to dressing or grooming suggests the person is too sick to maintain self-care, has a mental illness such as depression or may be homeless and lack access to resources.

Your own appearance sends a message to the person. Professional dress varies among organisations and settings. Depending on the setting, the use of a professional uniform may create a positive stereotype (comfort, expertise or ease of identification) or a negative stereotype (distance, authority or formality). Whatever your personal choice in clothing or grooming, the aim should be to convey a competent, professional image.

POSTURE

Note the person's position. An open position with extension of large muscle groups shows relaxation, physical comfort and a willingness to share information. A closed position with arms and legs crossed looks defensive and anxious. Note any change in posture. If a person in a relaxed position suddenly tenses, it suggests discomfort with the new topic.

Your own calm, relaxed posture creates a feeling of warmth and trust and conveys an interest in the person. Standing and hastily filling out a history form with periodic peeks at your watch communicates that you are busy with many more important things than talking with this person. Even when your time is limited, appear calm and unhurried. Sit down, adopt an open and relaxed posture even if it is only for a few minutes and look as if nothing else matters except this person.

GESTURES

Gestures send messages. For example, nodding or an open turning out of the hand shows acceptance, attention or agreement. A wringing of the hands often indicates anxiety. Pointing a finger occurs with anger and vehemence. Also, hand gestures can reinforce a person's description of pain. When a crushing substernal chest pain is described, the person often holds the hand twisted into a fist in front of the sternum. Or pain that is acute and localised may be shown by pointing one finger to the exact spot: '*It hurts right here*'.

FACIAL EXPRESSION

The face reflects a wide variety of relevant emotions and conditions. The expression may look alert, relaxed and interested or it may look anxious, angry and suspicious. Physical conditions such as pain or shortness of breath also show in the expression.

Your own expression should reflect a professional who is attentive, sincere and interested in the person. Any expression of boredom, distraction, disgust, criticism or disbelief is picked up by the other person and rapport will dissolve.

EYE CONTACT

Lack of eye contact suggests that the person is shy, withdrawn, confused, bored, intimidated, apathetic or depressed. This applies to the nurse as well. Aim to maintain eye contact, but do not 'stare down' the person. Do not have a fixed, penetrating look but rather an easy gaze towards the person's eyes, with occasional glances away. Nevertheless, remember that in some cultures, little or no eye contact is a sign of respect.

VOICE

Beside the spoken words, meaning comes through the tone and volume of voice, the intensity and rate of speech, the pitch and any pauses. These are just as important as words in conveying meaning. For example, the tone of a person's voice may show sarcasm, disbelief, sympathy or hostility. An anxious person often speaks in a loud, fast voice. A whining voice is similar; it has a high-pitched wavering quality and long, drawn-out syllables. A soft voice may indicate shyness or fear. A hearing-impaired person may use a loud voice.

Even the use of pauses conveys meaning. When your question is easy and straightforward, a person's long, unexpected pause indicates the person is taking time to think of an answer. This may raise some doubt as to the integrity of the answer. However, it also may be that what you consider a straightforward question is not perceived as such. A long pause before a response may indicate that you need to check that your question has been understood.

TOUCH

Without doubt, touching is a necessary part of a health assessment. But from a cultural perspective, consider issues concerning touch. While recognising the benefits reported by many in establishing rapport through touch, physical contact conveys various meanings. The meaning of physical touch is influenced by the person's age, gender, cultural background, experience and current setting. The meaning of touch is easily misinterpreted. In most Western cultures, physical touch is reserved for expressions of love and affection or for rigidly defined acts of greeting. When appropriate, touch communicates effectively, such as a touch of the hand or arm to signal empathy.

In summary, an interviewer's nonverbal messages that are productive and enhancing to the relationship are those that show attentiveness and unconditional acceptance. Defeating, nonproductive nonverbal behaviours are those of inattentiveness, authority and superiority (Table 7.2).

Closing the interview

The discussion should end gracefully. An abrupt or awkward closing can destroy rapport and leave the person with a negative impression of the whole discussion. To ease into the closing, ask the person:

'Is there anything else you would like to mention?'
'Are there any questions you would like to ask?'
'Are there any other areas I should have asked about?'

This gives the person the final opportunity to add information. Then, to indicate that closing is imminent, say something like '*I am nearly finished with my questions. Is there anything you would like to add?*'. No new topic should be introduced now. This is a good time to give your summary of what you have learnt. It should include positive health aspects, any health problems that have been identified, any plans for action or an explanation of the following physical examination. If appropriate, as you part from the person, thank them for the time spent and for their cooperation.

TABLE 7.2 Nonverbal behaviours of the interviewer

Positive	Negative
Appropriate professional appearance	Appearance objectionable to person
Equal-status seating	Standing
Close proximity to person	Sitting behind desk, far away, turned away
Relaxed open posture	Tense posture
Leaning slightly towards person	Slouched back
Occasional facilitating gestures	Critical or distracting gestures: pointing finger, clenched fist, finger-tapping, foot-swinging, looking at watch
Facial animation, interest	Bland expression, yawning, tight mouth
Appropriate smiling	Frowning, lip biting
Appropriate eye contact	Shifty, avoiding eye contact, focusing on notes
Moderate tone of voice	Strident, high-pitched tone
Moderate rate of speech	Rate too slow or too fast
Appropriate touch	Too frequent or inappropriate touch

Developmental considerations

Family-centred practice

When your patient is a child, you have to build rapport with two people—the child and the accompanying parent or caregiver. Greet both by name, but with a younger child (1–6 years old), focus more on the caregiver. By ignoring the child temporarily, you allow the child to size you up from a safe distance. The child can observe your interaction with the caregiver, see that the caregiver accepts and likes you, and relax (Figure 7.3).

Begin by interviewing the caregiver and child together. Refer to the child by name—not as 'the baby'. Refer to the caregiver by name. Also, be clear when identifying the caregiver. The mother's present husband may not necessarily be the child's father. Instead of asking about 'your husband's health', ask '*Is Amber's father in good health?*'

If any sensitive topics arise (e.g. the caregiver's troubled relationship or the child's problems at school or with peers), explore them later when the caregiver is alone. Depending on the child's age, provide toys, picture books and colouring books to occupy them as you and the caregiver talk. This frees the caregiver to concentrate on the history. Also, it indicates the child's level of attention span or independent play. Through the discussion, be alert to ways the caregiver and child interact.

For younger children, the parent or caregiver will provide all or most of the history, so you are collecting the child's health data from the caregiver's frame of reference. Usually, this viewpoint is reliable because most caregivers have the child's wellbeing as a priority and see cooperation with you to enhance this wellbeing. But the possibilities exist for caregiver bias. Bias can occur when

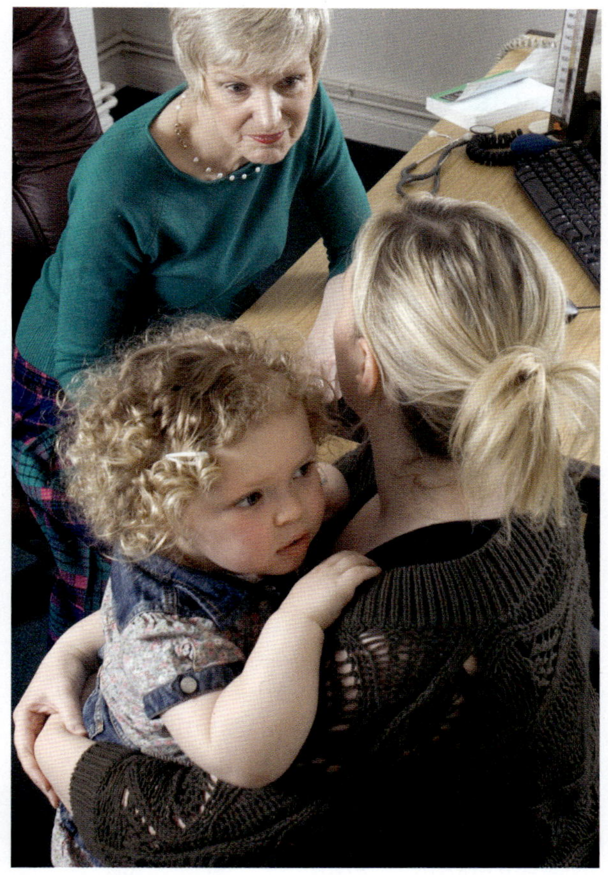

FIGURE 7.3 Gaining a child's trust by interacting with a parent

caregivers are asked to describe the child's achievements, or whenever their own parenting ability seems called into question. For example, if you say, '*His fever was 39.5°C and you didn't bring him in?*' you are implying a lack of parenting skill. This puts the caregiver on the defensive and increases anxiety. Instead, use open-ended questions that increase description and defuse threat, such as '*What happened when the fever went up?*'

A parent or caregiver with more than one child has more than one set of data to remember. Be patient as the caregiver sorts through their memory to pull out facts of developmental milestones or past history. A comprehensive history may be lacking if the child is accompanied by a family friend or day care provider instead of the parent.

In collecting developmental data, avoid being judgemental about the age of achievement of certain milestones. Parents are understandably proud of their child's achievements and are sensitive to inferences that these milestones may occur late.

Although most of your communication is with the caregiver, do not ignore the child completely. Make contact to ease into the physical examination later. Begin by asking about the toys the child is playing with or about a special doll or teddy bear brought from home: '*Does your doll have a name?*' or '*What can your truck do?*' Stoop down to meet the child at their eye level. Adult size can be overwhelming to young children and can emphasise their smallness.

Infants (1–12 months)

Because infants use the senses to receive information, nonverbal communication is the primary method.[5] Most infants look calm and relaxed when all their needs are met, and they cry when they are frightened, hungry, tired or uncomfortable. They respond best to firm, gentle handling and a quiet, calm voice. Your voice is comforting, even though they do not understand the words. Older infants have anxiety towards strangers. They are more cooperative when the caregiver is kept in view.[5]

Toddlers (12 months to 3 years)

Toddlers have not yet acquired the ability to effectively communicate verbally. They use expressive nonverbal and simple verbal communication.[8] When communicating with toddlers, use direct simple commands and familiar terms delivered with a soothing voice using age-appropriate vocabulary.[5] Explanations and descriptions need to be repeated several times.[5] Establish rapport through play. Use visual aids such as dolls to assist explanations. Where possible, either position yourself down to the child's level or raise them (if it is safe) to your level.[5] Toddlers and young children are frightened by quick or grandiose gestures. Do not try to maintain eye contact; this feels threatening to a small child. Use a quiet, measured voice and choose simple words in your speech.

Preschoolers (3–5 years)

A 3- to 5-year-old is egocentric. They see the world mostly from their own point of view. Everything revolves around them. It may not work to cite the example of another child's behaviour to get the child to cooperate. It has no meaning. Only the child's own experience is relevant.

Preschoolers' communication is direct, concrete, literal and set in the present. Avoid expressions such as 'climbing the walls' because they are easily misinterpreted by young children. Use short, simple sentences with a concrete explanation. Take time to give a short, simple explanation for any unfamiliar equipment that will be used on the child and allow them to handle the equipment. Attempt to decrease anxiety about being hurt; preschoolers can have *animistic* thinking about unfamiliar objects. They may imagine that unfamiliar inanimate objects can come alive and have human characteristics (e.g. that a blood pressure cuff can wake up and bite or pinch). Parental proximity is still important for this age group.[9] Use age-appropriate, simple vocabulary, distraction and play-therapy techniques to build a connection and to foster a therapeutic relationship with the child.[5]

School-age children (6–12 years)

A child 6 to 12 years old can tolerate and understand others' viewpoints. The child is more objective and realistic. They want to know functional aspects—how things work and why things are done.

Children of this age group have the verbal ability to add important data to the history. Talk with the parent and child together, but when a presenting symptom or sign exists ask the child about it first and then gather data from the parent. For a well child seeking a checkup, pose questions about school, friends or activities directly to the child.[5]

Preadolescent/adolescent (12–19 years)

Adolescents want to be adults, but they do not have the cognitive ability yet to achieve their goal. They are between two stages. Sometimes they are capable of mature actions, and other times they fall back on childhood response patterns, especially in times of stress. You cannot treat adolescents as children, yet you cannot overcompensate and assume that their communication style, learning ability and motivation are consistently at an adult level.

Adolescents value their peers. They crave acceptance and sameness with their peers. They may think no adult can understand them and will act with aloof contempt, answering only in monosyllables. Others make eye contact and tell you what they think you want to hear, but inside they are thinking, '*You'll never know the full story about me*'.

This knowledge about adolescents is apt to paralyse you in communicating with them. However, successful communication is possible and rewarding. The guidelines are simple.

The first consideration is your attitude, which must be one of respect. Respect is the most important thing you can communicate to the adolescent. The adolescent needs to feel validated as a human being, to be accepted and worthy.

Second, your communication must be totally honest. The adolescent's intuition is highly tuned and can detect phoniness or when information is withheld. Always give them the truth. Play it straight or you will lose them. They will cooperate if they understand your rationale.

Stay in character. Avoid using language that is absurd for your age or professional role. It is helpful to understand some of the jargon used by adolescents, but you cannot use those words yourself simply to try to bond with the adolescent. Do not try to be their peer. You are not, and they will not accept you as such.

Use icebreakers. Focus first on the adolescent, not on the problem. Although an adult just wants to get on with it and talk about the health concern immediately, adolescents respond best when the focus is on them as a person. Show an interest in them. Ask open, friendly questions about school, activities, hobbies and friends. Refrain from asking questions about parents and family for now—these issues can be emotionally charged during adolescence.

Do not assume adolescents know *anything* about a health assessment. Explain every step and give the rationale. They need direction. They will cooperate when they know the reason for the questions or actions. Encourage their questions. Adolescents are afraid they will sound 'dumb' if they ask a question to which they assume everybody else knows the answer. Keep your questions short and simple.

The communication responses described for the adult need to be reconsidered when talking with an adolescent. Silent periods are usually best avoided. Giving adolescents a little time to collect their thoughts is acceptable, but a silence for other reasons may be threatening.

Later in the discussion, after you have developed rapport with the adolescent, you can address the topics that are emotionally charged, including alcohol and drug use, sexual behaviours, suicidal thoughts and depression. Adolescents will assume that health professionals have similar values and standards of behaviour as most of the other authority figures in their lives, and they may be reluctant to share this information. You can assure them that your questions are not intended to be intrusive but cover topics that are important for most teens and on which you have relevant health information to share.

If confidential material is uncovered during the interview, consider what can remain confidential and what you feel you must share for the wellbeing of the adolescent. However, if the adolescent talks about an abusive home situation, state that you have to share this information with other health professionals for their own protection. Ask the adolescent, '*Do you have a problem with that?*' and then talk it through. Tell the adolescent, '*You will have to trust that I will handle this information professionally and in your best interest*'.

Finally, take every opportunity for positive reinforcement. Praise every action regarding healthy lifestyle choices: '*That's great that you don't vape. You get lots of gold stars in my book for staying off the vapes. It is great for your health*'.

People over 65 years

Older adults are often treated as if they represent a single cohort, but there are huge differences in their life experiences and capabilities. Because people are living longer, the term 'older adult' has been broken down into three age cohorts: young-old (65–74 years), middle-old (75–84 years) and oldest-old (85 years or older).[10]

Interviewing older people requires many of the same skills required for interviewing younger adults. Age-related changes to cognition in healthy older adults are minimal and should not require major modifications in communication, although mental processing and reaction time may be slowed.[10] However, if you have any concerns about a person's cognitive capacity, it is suggested that you perform a mental status assessment early in the interview to avoid obtaining questionable data.[5] The Mini-Mental State Examination[11] and the clock drawing test are useful assessment tools.[5] See Chapter 11.

Establish rapport by always addressing the person by their last name (e.g. '*Hello, Mr Choi*'; '*Good morning, Mrs Smith*'). Some older adults resent being called by their first name by younger people. To avoid undermining rapport, ask the older person what they would like to be called. Treat them as an equal.[5] Use open-ended questions first followed by focused questions. Ask one question at a time. Provide information in small segments. Acknowledge feelings and emotions. As with other adults, ensure congruency between verbal and nonverbal communication (words and body language), and use attentive and respectful behaviours. Pay attention to sensory deficits such as hearing and visual impairment.[5]

It is important to adjust the pace of the discussion to the age of the person. People over 65 have a great amount of background material to sort through, and this takes some time. Some older adults may need a longer response time to interpret the question and process their answer. Avoid trying to hurry them along.

Consider physical limitations when planning the interview. Frail older adults and sick people may fatigue earlier and may require the assessment to be broken up into shorter segments. When the person is hearing impaired, face them directly so that your mouth and face are fully visible. Do not shout; it does not help and distorts speech. Placing a hand on the arm or shoulder is an empathic message which communicates that you empathise with the person and want to understand their health issue.

Interviewing people with diverse needs

A person with hearing impairment

Although many people will tell you in advance that they have a hearing deficit, others must be recognised by clues such as staring at your mouth and face, not attending unless looking at you or speaking in a voice unusually loud or with guttural or garbled sounds. The deaf person may be familiar with some equipment in the hospital or clinic or may have had previous experience with healthcare settings. But without full communication, a hearing-impaired person is sure to feel isolated and anxious. Ask what their preferred way is to communicate—by hearing aid (check whether it is working properly), adjusting the volume of your voice, lip reading or writing. If lip reading is the preferred way to communicate, you may need to check whether wearing a mask is part of the healthcare agency protocol at the time. Choose a quiet, private place to communicate with the hearing-impaired person, and turn off radio or TV to decrease environmental noise. Tap the floor or table to get the patient's attention via vibration.[5]

A detailed health history requires a sign language (Auslan) interpreter. Since most health professionals are not proficient in signing, try to find an interpreter through a social service agency or the person's own social network. You may use family members but be aware that they sometimes edit for the person. Use the same guidelines as for the bilingual interpreter. If the person prefers lip reading, be sure to face them squarely and have good lighting on your face. Do not exaggerate your lip movements because this distorts your words. Similarly, shouting distorts the reception of a hearing aid the person may wear. Articulate clearly and speak in a steady pace using a moderate and even tone. Supplement your voice with appropriate hand gestures.[5] Nonverbal cues are important adjuncts because the lip reader understands at best only 50% of your speech when relying solely on vision. Be sure the person understands your questions. Many hearing-impaired people nod 'yes' just to be friendly and cooperative but really do not understand.[5]

A person with vision impairment

Because people with vision impairment have a limited or no ability to read information or see nonverbal gestures, posture and body language, they rely on the spoken word. There is a tendency for those communicating with a vision-impaired person to speak loudly and to over enunciate. Unless the person has a hearing impairment as well, tone of voice and speed of delivery should be the same as if you were talking to a non–vision impaired person.[5] Alert the person when you approach and when you are leaving. Remember to ask other personnel to introduce themselves to the vision-impaired person when they enter and leave a room. Continue to use everyday verbal and body language because they affect tone and meaning, which provides additional information to the visually impaired person.[5]

A person with aphasia

Because language is our basic way of communicating with the world, speech and language deficits can cause considerable distress to a person experiencing aphasia. Aphasia can manifest in several ways: (1) expressive or motor aphasia where words cannot be expressed or formed; (2) receptive or sensory aphasia where language is not understood; and (3) global aphasia, which includes both expressive and receptive deficits.[5] While communication strategies with a person with aphasia should attend to the type of presenting aphasia, it should be recognised that there is a high likelihood that the person's efforts to communicate will be frustrating for them. To minimise actual and potential distress experienced by the person in their efforts to communicate, allow ample time for them to formulate thoughts and receive information. Show patience and perseverance and keep trying to understand. Avoid responding with frustration.[5] Focus on their abilities and their communication preferences. Alternative communication methods such as picture boards and electronic devices can be used to supplement or replace verbal communication. Because of the effort involved in communicating, avoid prolonged conversations with a person with aphasia. Keep conversations short and to the point. Always remember to acknowledge the person's efforts.[5]

A person who is acutely ill

An acutely ill person may be anxious and fearful. They need to be reassured that the nurse is taking care of them. Subjective data are crucial to determine the cause and course of the episode of their illness. Abbreviate your questioning if necessary. Identify the main area of distress and direct your questions to them. Gather information from the person's progress notes rather than repeatedly asking the same questions. In an emergency, if you are unsure about the accuracy of information provided, ask for verification through nonverbal responses such as head or other body movements.[4] Family or friends can provide important data.

A hospitalised person with a critical or severe illness is usually too weak, too short of breath or in too much pain to talk. First attend to the comfort of the person. Then establish a priority; find out immediately what parts of the health history are the most relevant. Explore the first concern the person mentions. Begin to use closed, direct questions earlier.

A person who has decreased cognitive function

A person may be experiencing a mild, moderate or severe decrease in cognitive function related to, for example, dementia, delirium, intellectual disability or acquired brain injury.[4] A person with a mild cognitive dysfunction may be able to function independently, understand others, be able to express themselves and learn and remember with repetition and persistence.[4] A person with moderate cognitive dysfunction may have difficulty making choices, manage some self-care independently, may understand others but not always use words to communicate, learn tasks with repetition and visual cues. However a person with severe cognitive impairment may have inconsistent communication, have unpredictable behaviours and usually require constant supervision.[4]

A recent Australian study[12] found that in a health-related consultation situation, some people with an intellectual disability didn't feel that they were treated like a person, they 'felt more like an "it"'. Therefore, as with any other interpersonal communication situation, approach it from a person-centred perspective. Show respect, empathy and understanding and have a sense of humour.[4] In addition, O'Toole[4] suggests you invest time with the person to develop a therapeutic relationship and gain their trust, communicate gently and consistently. Don't take personally what the person says to you or about you, and maintain a feeling of safety and comfort for the person wherever possible. Make sure you focus on the person first, hear their story, then clarify with the support person or carer, although they may not always agree with each other's perspectives. Summarise the information frequently and check its accuracy by asking, '*Is this correct?*' The person may have trouble expressing themselves but are able to answer *yes* or *no* when asked. Use models and pictures where needed.

Responding to challenging behaviours

A PERSON UNDER THE INFLUENCE OF ILLICIT SUBSTANCES OR ALCOHOL

It is common for people under the influence of alcohol or other mood-altering drugs to be admitted to a hospital; all these drugs affect the central nervous system, increasing the risk for accidents and injuries. You may be faced with a wide range of problem behaviours due to substance misuse. When talking to a person currently under the influence of alcohol or illicit drugs, ask simple and direct questions. Take care to make your manner and questions nonthreatening. Avoid confrontation and any display of judgement because the person may become belligerent. For your own protection, be aware of hospital security or other personnel who could be called on for assistance. Once the person is no longer under the direct influence of alcohol or illicit substances, the person should be assessed for the extent of the problem. Further discussion related to assessment of people who have a substance misuse problem can be found in Chapter 6.

BEING ASKED PERSONAL QUESTIONS

Occasionally, people will ask you questions about *your* personal life or opinions such as '*Are you married?*', '*Do you have children?*'.

You do not need to answer every question. You may supply brief information when you feel it is appropriate but be sensitive to the possibility that there may be a motive behind the personal questions such as loneliness or anxiety. Try directing your response back to the person's frame of reference. You might say something like, '*No, I don't have children; I wonder if your question is related to how I can help you care for your child?*'

A PERSON WHO IS SEXUALLY AGGRESSIVE

Sometimes personal questions extend to flirtatious compliments, seductive innuendo or sexual advances. Your response must make it clear that you are a health professional who can best care for the person by maintaining a professional relationship. At the same time, communicate that you will not tolerate sexual advances. This may be difficult, considering that the person's words or gestures may have left you shocked, embarrassed or angry. Your feelings are normal. Set appropriate verbal boundaries by saying, '*I am uncomfortable when you talk to me that way; please stop*'. Always report such conduct and seek support from colleagues. If the person's behaviours are new, it could be an indication that their mental health is deteriorating and needs immediate intervention (see Chapter 30 for more information on acute mental health deterioration). Healthcare agencies will all have policies and procedures for dealing with sexual misconduct.

A PERSON WHO IS CRYING

Health professionals may feel overwhelmed when a person starts crying. But crying can be a big relief to a person. Health problems come with powerful emotions. Worries about illness, death or loss take a great amount of energy to keep bottled up inside. When you say something that 'makes the person cry', do not think you have hurt the person. You have just hit on a topic that is important. Do not go on to a new topic. Just let the person cry and express their feelings fully. You wait until the crying subsides to talk. The person will regain control soon. Ask them if they would like a tissue.

Sometimes the person looks as if they are on the verge of tears but is trying hard to suppress them. Again, instead of moving on to something new, acknowledge the expression by saying, '*You look sad*'. Do not worry that you will open an uncontrollable floodgate of tears. The person may cry but will be relieved, and you will have gained insight to a serious concern.

ANGER OR THREATS OF VIOLENCE

Occasionally you will try to communicate with a person who is already angry. Try not to personalise this anger; usually it does not relate to you. The person may be showing aggression in response to their own feelings of anxiety or helplessness. Do ask about the anger and hear the person out. Deal with the angry feelings before you ask anything else.

The healthcare setting is also not immune to violent behaviour. A person may act with such angry gestures that you feel a threat to your personal safety. Other red flag behaviours of a potentially disruptive person include fist clenching, pacing back and forth, a vacant stare, confusion, statements out of touch with reality, statements that do not make sense, a history of recent drug use (alcohol, recreational drugs) or perhaps even a recent history of intense bereavement (loss of spouse, loss of job). Trust your instincts. If you sense any suspicious or threatening behaviour, act immediately to defuse the situation. Show a sincere desire to help. Listen and offer to work with the threatening person to solve the problem. Do not raise your own voice or try to argue with them. Allow the person to set the pace to tell their story. Respond with patience and understanding. Empathise with the person but not necessarily their behaviour. Act calmly and talk to the person in a gentle voice.

Leave the room door open and position yourself between the person and the door. Seek assistance promptly if the situation is escalating. Within the hospital setting, there is usually a pre-established protocol for managing threats of violence. A prearranged sign or signal is used to alert colleagues to summon security for assistance. In the community setting, systems such as emergency pager or mobile alerts may be used to summon help. Remember that the most important goal is your personal safety, so avoid taking any risks.

ANXIETY

Finally, take it for granted that nearly all sick people have some anxiety. This is a normal response to being sick. It makes some people aggressive and others dependent. Remember that the person is not reacting as typically as when they are healthy. Acknowledging the person's situation, appearing unhurried and taking the time to listen to the person's concerns can help diffuse some of the anxiety. For further information on assessment of anxiety, refer to Chapter 11.

Cultural and social considerations

Chapter 4 provides a comprehensive overview on cultural safety in nursing practice. The issues identified in Box 4.5 should be used to inform and guide culturally appropriate communication. The following section examines specific cultural considerations around communication.

When two people come from different cultural backgrounds, the probability of miscommunication increases. Verbal and nonverbal communications are influenced by the cultural background of the health professional and the person (Figure 7.4). In Australia, information that assists in minimising the risk of miscommunication between the health professional and the person is freely available from the Centre for Culture, Ethnicity and Health. The information sheets 'Cultural considerations in health assessment' and 'Speaking with clients who have low English proficiency' are located on their website at www.ceh.org.au under 'Resources Hub'.[13–17] The documents highlight issues associated with a health assessment and ways to facilitate effective communication with people of limited English proficiency.[13,14]

Effective communication among Australia's Indigenous people is based on a community-centred model as opposed to a person-centred model.[4] Community leaders, community Elders and Indigenous health workers play an important role in facilitating culturally respectful communication.[4] There are also resources available to assist health professionals to communicate more effectively with Māori people in Aotearoa New Zealand.[19]

People with limited English proficiency must be provided with an interpreter who is *not* a family member or friend. It is essential to establish whether interpreter services are required. A simple way of establishing this need is to ask the question, '*Would you like an interpreter?*' A flash card, cue card or a translator on a mobile phone or computer can be used to ask the question in the person's preferred language. The Australian Institute of Interpreters and Translators Incorporated offers practical advice on communication

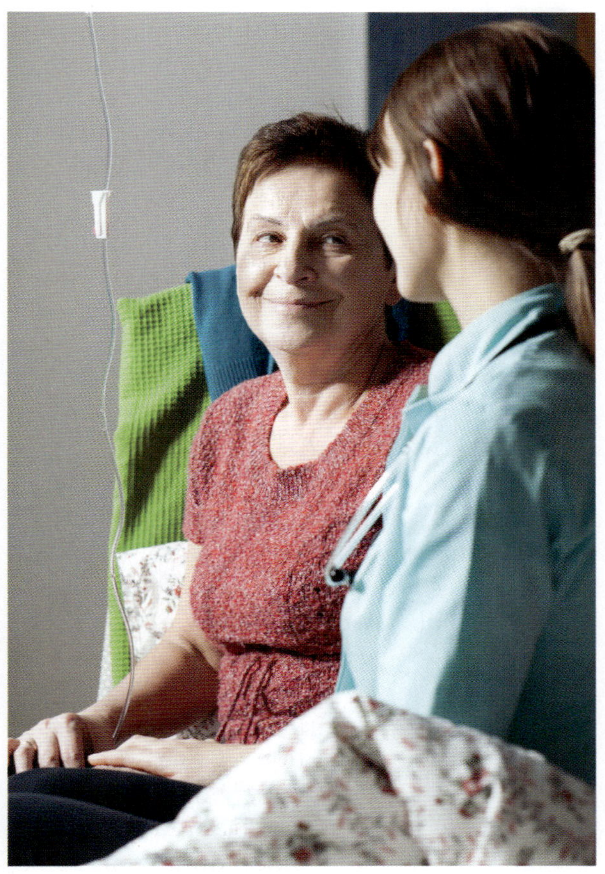

FIGURE 7.4 Position taking spatial relations into account.
Source: Hall 1963[18]

processes and working with interpreters.[20] In Aotearoa New Zealand, Te Tari Matawaki Ministry for Ethnic Communities offer culturally appropriate resources.[21]

At the end of a health assessment in which an interpreter is used, carefully document that the person and family fully understand what is happening to them in relation to their current health situation plan of care. The interpreter will also give nurses and other healthcare workers tools and advice on continuing communication with the person and their family.[15,16,22]

Etiquette

Etiquette refers to the conventional code of good manners that governs behaviour. When meeting a person for the first time, it is important to be professional in your approach. Everyone likes to be called by their correct name. Be certain that you know the person's name and pronounce it correctly. Avoid being unduly casual or familiar. For example, refrain from routinely using the person's first name before you have been invited to do so. The same guidelines should be followed when addressing the family members and other visitors. It is suggested to greet the person, '*Hello, Mr or Mrs or Ms ..., my name is ...*'. The common use of 'you guys' and other colloquialisms should not be used in a professional context. Among Chinese, Vietnamese and many other Asian groups, the family or surname is written and spoken first, followed by the first or given name. This is exactly the opposite of most European-Australian naming systems. If you are in doubt, be sure to ask the person or a significant other if they are unable to respond due to their condition.

Space and distance

Spatial distance is significant throughout the health assessment where appropriate distance zones vary. Summarised in Table 7.3 are the four distance zones identified for the functional use of space.

Cultural considerations on gender, sexuality and sexual orientation

If you determine that gender differences are important to the person, you might try strategies such as offering to have a third person present. If a family member or friend has accompanied the person, you might enquire whether they would like that person to be present during the history and/or physical examination. It is not unusual for a female to request examination by a female rather than a male and vice versa. Modesty is

TABLE 7.3 Functional use of space

Zone	Remarks
Intimate zone (0–0.5 m)	Visual distortion occurs Best for assessing breath and other body odours
Personal distance (0.5–1 m)	Perceived as an extension of the self; similar to a bubble Voice is moderate Body odours not apparent No visual distortion Much of the physical assessment occurs at this distance
Social distance (1–4 m)	Used for impersonal business transactions Perceptual information much less detailed Much of the interview occurs at this distance
Public distance (4 m+)	Interaction with others impersonal Speaker's voice must be projected Subtle facial expressions imperceptible

another issue, and it is imperative to ensure the person's body is carefully covered at all times, that curtains are closed and, when possible, doors are closed. A room must not be entered without knocking first and announcing yourself.

You also need to be aware of assuming that the person identifies as heterosexual, lesbian, gay, bisexual or a particular gender. Simple approaches can improve your communication with all people and help you avoid making inappropriate assumptions:

- Use the word 'partner' rather than 'husband' or 'wife' until you determine the person's preferences for these terms.
- Ask the same questions of a homosexual couple as a heterosexual couple.
- Don't make assumptions about a person's sexual orientation based on appearance.

Language is important in conveying acceptance of the person; therefore, it is important to understand commonly used terminology related to gender identity and sexuality. More information and guidelines about communicating effectively about sexuality and sexual function are available in Chapters 26 and 27.

Overcoming communication barriers

Working with an interpreter

In the most recent dataset, 72% of Australians aged 5 years or older spoke only English, while 3% did not speak English at all; this included both longer-standing migrants and recent arrivals.[23] Approximately five and a half million people in Australia did not speak the English language at home.[24] Among the Indigenous Australian population, 9.5% reported speaking an Aboriginal or Torres Strait Islander language, with Yumplatok (Torres Strait Creole) as the most spoken language, followed by Kriol and Djambarrpuyngu.[25] In Aotearoa New Zealand the official languages are English, Te reo Māori and New Zealand Sign Language. English is spoken by 97.8% of New Zealanders.[26] Te reo Māori is spoken by more than 1 in 6 Māori people.[27]

One of the greatest challenges in cross-cultural communication occurs when you and the person speak different languages

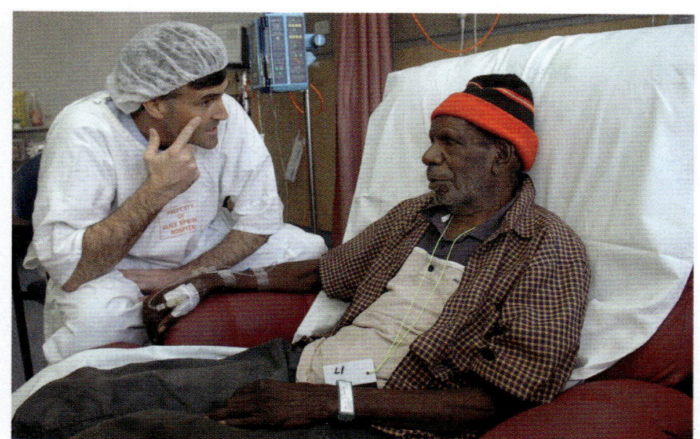

FIGURE 7.5 Communicating with someone who speaks a different language from you

(Figure 7.5). After assessing the English language skills of non–English speaking people, you may find yourself in one of two situations: trying to communicate effectively through an interpreter or trying to communicate effectively when there is no interpreter. Keep in mind however that the person may not speak English but may speak many languages fluently.

Interviewing a non–English speaking person requires a bilingual interpreter for full communication. Even the person from another culture or country who has some skill in speaking English may need an interpreter when faced with the anxiety-provoking situation of entering a hospital, describing a strange symptom or discussing sensitive topics such as those related to reproductive or urological concerns.

It is tempting to ask a relative, friend or even another person to interpret because they are readily available and probably would like to help. This is disadvantageous because it may violate confidentiality. Furthermore, the friend or relative, although fluent in ordinary language usage, is likely to be unfamiliar with medical terminology, hospital or clinic procedures and medical ethics.

Whenever possible, work with a bilingual team member or a trained medical interpreter. They know interpreting techniques, have a healthcare background and understand patients' rights. Although interpreters are trained to remain neutral, they can influence both the content of information exchanged and the nature of the interaction. Although acceptance of a code of ethics governing confidentiality and conflicts of interest is part of the training interpreters receive, discord may arise when they relate information that the person has not volunteered to the nurse.

Although you will oversee the focus and flow of the interview, view yourself and the interpreter as a team. Ask the interpreter to meet the person beforehand to establish rapport. Allow more time for this discussion. With the third person repeating everything, it can take considerably longer than interviewing English-speaking people. Focus on priority data.[15,17]

There are two styles of interpreting—line-by-line interpreting and summarising. Translating line by line takes more time, but it ensures accuracy. Use this style for most of the discussion. Both you and the person should speak only a sentence or two, and then allow the interpreter some time. Use simple language, not medical jargon that the interpreter must simplify before it can be translated. Summary translation progresses faster and is useful for teaching relatively simple health techniques with which the interpreter is already familiar. Be alert for nonverbal cues as the person talks. These cues can give valuable data. A good interpreter also notes nonverbal messages and passes them on to you. Summarised in Table 7.4 are suggestions for choosing and using an interpreter. Table 7.5 summarises some suggestions for overcoming language barriers.

Assessing a person's health literacy

The time you have with the person during a health assessment provides a perfect opportunity to identify areas where the person

TABLE 7.4 Using an interpreter

Choosing an interpreter

- Before locating an interpreter, identify the language the person speaks at home. Be aware that it may differ from the language spoken publicly.
- Whenever possible, use a *professional* interpreter, preferably one who knows medical terminology.
- Be aware of gender differences between interpreter and the person. In general, the same gender is preferred.
- Be aware of age differences between interpreter and the person.

Strategies for effective use of an interpreter

- Plan what you want to say ahead of time. Meet privately with the interpreter before the interview.
- Ask the interpreter to provide a line-by-line verbatim account of the conversation. Ask for a detailed interpretation when provided with brief summaries of longer exchanges between interpreter and the person.
- Be patient. When using an interpreter, interviews often take two to three times longer.
- Longer-than-expected explanatory exchanges are often required to convey the meaning of words such as *stress*, *depression*, *allergy*, *preventive medicine* and *physiotherapy* because there may not be comparable terms in the language the person understands.
- When discussing diagnostic tests such as mammograms, MRIs, CT scans or those involving body fluids such as blood, urine, stool, spinal fluid or saliva, be sure to clarify the nature of the test to the interpreter. Indicate the purpose of the test, exactly what will happen to the person, approximately how long the test will take, whether the procedure is invasive or noninvasive and what part(s) of the body will be tested.
- Avoid ambiguous statements and questions.
- Avoid abstract expressions, idioms, similes, metaphors and medical jargon.
- To ensure confidentiality and privacy, avoid using children or strangers as interpreters.

TABLE 7.5 Overcoming language barriers

1. Be polite and formal.
2. Pronounce names correctly. Use proper titles of respect, such as 'Mr', 'Mrs', 'Ms' and 'Dr'. Greet the person using the last or complete name. Gesture to yourself and say your name. Offer a handshake or nod. Smile.
3. Proceed in an unhurried manner. Pay attention to any effort by the person or family to communicate.
4. Speak in a low, moderate voice. Avoid talking loudly. Remember that there is a tendency to raise the volume and pitch of your voice when the listener appears not to understand. The listener may perceive that you are shouting and/or angry.
5. Use any words that you might know in the person's language. This indicates that you are aware of and respect their culture.
6. Use simple words such as 'pain' instead of 'discomfort'. Avoid medical jargon, idioms and slang. Avoid using contractions (e.g. don't, can't, won't). Use nouns repeatedly instead of pronouns. *Example:* Do not say: *He has been taking his medicine, hasn't he?* Do say: *Does Juan take medicine?*

TABLE 7.5 Overcoming language barriers cont'd
7. Mime words and simple actions while you verbalise them.
8. Give instructions in the proper sequence. *Example:* Do not say: *Before you rinse the bottle, sterilise it.* Do say: *First wash the bottle. Second, rinse the bottle.*
9. Discuss one topic at a time. Avoid using conjunctions. *Example:* Do not say: *Are you cold and in pain?* Do say: *Are you cold (while miming)? Are you in pain?*
10. Validate if the person understands by having them repeat instructions, demonstrate the procedure or act out the meaning.
11. Write out several short sentences in English and determine the person's ability to read them.
12. Get phrase books from a library or bookstore, make or buy flash cards, contact hospitals for a list of interpreters and use both a formal and an informal network to locate a suitable interpreter.

needs more information or where misconceptions need to be corrected. An important part of your assessment is determining if the person understands everything you say.

Health literacy is about how people understand information about health and health care and how they apply that information to their lives, use it to make decisions and act on it.[28] Health literacy is important because it shapes people's health and the safety and quality of health care.[29] The Australian Commission on Safety and Quality in Health Care also makes the point that another important component of health literacy is the health literacy environment—that is, the infrastructure, policies, materials, people and relationships within healthcare environments that affect the way in which a person can access, understand and apply health-related information and services. A person can have adequate literacy and not have adequate health literacy. For example, health literacy requires the person to understand how to read and interpret medical prescriptions, referrals, appointments and the concept of the need for follow-up of illness through further health-related appointments.[30] The nurse's role in in health literacy assessment is pivotal in checking the person's understanding of information provided and translating medical jargon to enable them to make informed choices in their care and take part in decision making.[31]

In Australia, several factors are linked to health literacy capability including personal health, country of birth, language first spoken and age.[28] It is estimated that 59% of Australians (15–74 years) have poor health literacy skills, which means that they may not be able to determine the correct amount of medicine to give a child or adult from information printed on the package.[28] People over 50 years of age are likely to have lower health literacy levels than those 49 years or younger.[28] In Aotearoa New Zealand, 36.7% of European older adults found it always easy to understand health information well enough to know what to do compared with less than 29% of Māori, Pacific and Asian adults.[32]

Health literacy encompasses a variety of factors beyond basic reading, including the ability to use quantitative (numeric) information and to understand and remember verbal instructions. People with low health literacy struggle to navigate the healthcare system and may not be able to understand or follow instructions because of a misunderstanding. Low health literacy has been associated with increased rates of hospitalisation and greater use of emergency care; lower use of health screening and influenza vaccination; poorer ability to take medications appropriately; poorer ability to interpret labels and health messages; poorer knowledge about personal health issues; poor overall health among older people; and higher risk of death in older people.[28] There are several factors that can impact on a person's health literacy including age, education level, disability, culture, their first language being other than English, gender, being Aboriginal or Torres Strait Islander[28] or Māori.[32] The Australian Government is currently developing the National Health Literacy Strategy as a priority area. The objective of the strategy is to provide an evidence-based health literacy environment, where health information is person-centred, accessible and culturally and linguistically appropriate, and to improve health literacy skills in Australians.[29]

TOOLS FOR DETERMINING LITERACY

As a clinician, you are in a good position to assess and improve the health literacy of your clients. There is a wide variety of tools to measure health literacy—some more challenging than others. Table 7.6 presents

TABLE 7.6 Tools for assessing health literacy

Tool	Description	Example questions
Test of Functional Health Literacy (TOFHLA) (Parker et al.)[34]	• Designed for use in research • Measures reading comprehension and numeracy • Uses actual client instructions and forms • Takes approximately 22 minutes to complete	Choose which is correct: Do not eat ___________ a. appointment b. walk-in c. breakfast d. clinic
Rapid Estimate of Adult Literacy in Medicine. Short Form Screening (REALM - SF) (Davis et al.)[35]	• Designed for clinical settings • Person reads 66 medical terms aloud • Score based on number of words read and pronounced correctly • Takes 2–3 minutes to administer	Words include: flu, smear, stress, gallbladder, inflammatory, diagnosis, potassium
Newest Vital Sign (NVS) (Weiss et al.)[36]	• Assesses numeracy and comprehension • Uses nutrition label that clients must read and interpret • Total of six questions related to label provided • Takes approximately 3 minutes to complete	Give client the nutrition label and ask: • *If you eat the entire container, how many calories will you eat?* • *If you usually eat 2,500 calories in a day, what percentage of your daily value of calories will you be eating if you eat one serving?*

three commonly used screening tools. Other validated health literacy tools are available from the online Health Literacy Tool Shed—a database of health literacy measures.[33]

Each of the tools can be used in the clinical setting. A single-item literacy screener has been suggested but with only marginal effectiveness. Some clinics simply ask standardised questions such as, '*Do you have any limitations in learning?*' or '*What is the highest grade level completed?*' instead of requiring a specific assessment tool.

HEALTH EDUCATION

As a clinician there are steps you can take to ensure your clients understand the information you are providing. Although completing a health literacy screener gives you objective data and can help you determine the appropriate level of information, most clients (regardless of literacy level) want to be provided with simple, easy-to-understand instructions; therefore, the practice of giving all clients simple instructions at a lower reading level is acceptable.

When discussing medical information with clients, keep it simple, use short sentences and choose words containing no more than two syllables (when possible). Limit the number of messages you are giving the client, be sure to tell the person what they will gain by following your instructions, present only needed information, focus on the client, use the active voice and avoid jargon.

Although you may think using complex terms and sentences makes you sound more professional or smarter, it can confuse them. You are better off speaking to them as you would to a friend, using a conversational structure that includes time for them to ask questions. A few examples follow:

Say: *Feel for lumps about the size of a pea.*
Don't say: *Feel for lumps about 5 to 6 millimetres.*
Say: *Birth control.*
Don't say: *Contraception.*
Say: *Place your hand palm up.*
Don't say: *Supinate your hand.*

Written materials

When preparing or using written materials, make sure to assess the appropriateness of the materials. Health education materials are often created at a reading level that is not suitable for most people. Written materials should be at the grade 5 reading level or below. Reading level can be determined with a variety of formulas that use several syllables per word and complexity of sentences to determine reading level. Materials should be in at least 12-point font, avoid all capital letters, use headings and subheadings, use bullet points and limit medical jargon. Pictures are often used in written materials, but be careful to select appropriate graphics.

Teach back

Although ensuring appropriate verbal and written communication is important, one of the easiest things you can do when teaching a person is to use the teach back approach. Teach back is simple and free. It allows you to assess whether the person understands and to immediately correct misconceptions. Many health professionals ask, '*Do you understand?*' or '*Do you have any questions?*' throughout the teaching sessions. Just because your client has no questions and indicates understanding with a nod does not mean that they understand the information. Using teach back encourages the client to repeat in their own words what you have just said. For example, '*Can you explain to me in your own words what you can do to prevent having another bladder infection?*' This verbal discussion allows you to assess the person's understanding and may open the door for them to ask questions.

Clinical reasoning and documentation

The following is a continuation of the case study provided at the beginning of this chapter.

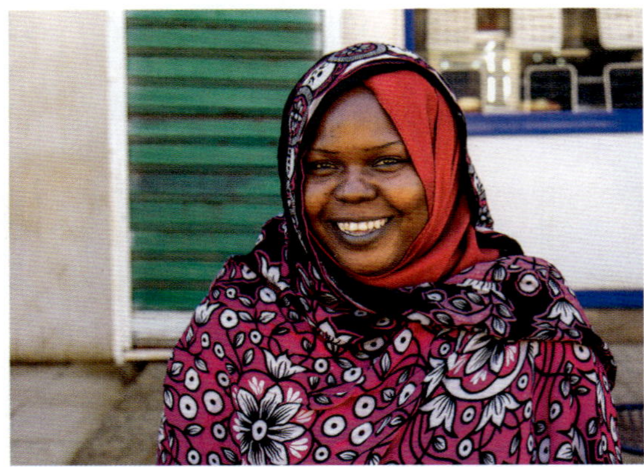

Case study (continued)—Approach to person-centred communication

Context

You will recall from the case study described earlier in the chapter that you are on clinical placement in a subacute rehabilitation ward. Your preceptor (buddy) nurse tells you he is expecting a new patient admission to the ward shortly after the afternoon handover. He asks you to prepare to be involved in completing the ward admission assessment for this person, who you will be meeting for the first time.

Consider the patient's situation

You have limited information about the new patient. Mrs Nyamal Bol is a 55-year-old woman who is undergoing rehabilitation following a car accident 3 days ago. She sustained a fractured right wrist, which has been internally fixed with a plate and screw, and she has a plaster cast from her fingers to her elbow. She also sustained a dislocated fractured ankle, which has been fixed with screws and plates, and she is now wearing an orthopaedic boot. She has extensive bruising and minor cuts. Mrs Bol is a South Sudanese-Australian who arrived in Australia as a refugee 8 years ago with her husband and five children. You are told that Mrs Bol speaks some English.

Collect cues/information

Consider the following:

- How has your approach to your first meeting with Mrs Bol changed after reading the chapter and accessing the additional resources or references?
- How has your approach to the admission health assessment changed after reading the chapter and accessing the additional resources or references?
- What further information would you want to collect before progressing with the admission health assessment?
- How would your approach to the admission health assessment change if:
  - the person was hearing impaired?
  - the person was very upset about being in hospital?
  - the person had an intellectual disability?
  - the person was very confused or had dementia?
  - the person's partner died in the car accident?

ADDITIONAL RESOURCES

You can further develop your knowledge and skills relevant to communication in health assessment by:

- reading chapters of a fundamentals of nursing or medical-surgical nursing textbook
- answering chapter multiple choice questions online. Log onto ClinicalKey Student and search for the text 'Health Assessment, 4th edition'. Choose the section titled 'Teaching material'. In this section you will find question and answer documents for each chapter.

ADDITIONAL RESOURCES cont'd

- visiting websites

Auslan signbank: https://auslan.org.au

Clinical Excellence Commission—Safety fundamentals for person-centred communication: https://www.cec.health.nsw.gov.au/__data/assets/pdf_file/0003/618384/Hello-My-Name-Is.PDF

Australian Commission for Safety and Quality in Health Care—Communicating for safety standard: https://www.safetyandquality.gov.au/standards/nsqhs-standards/communicating-safety-standard

Centre for Culture, Ethnicity and Health: https://www.ceh.org.au

Australian Federation of Disability Organisations—Communication with people with disabilities: https://www.afdo.org.au/resource-communication-with-people-with-disabilities/

Dementia Australia—Communication: https://www.dementia.org.au/national/support-and-services/carers/managing-changes-in-communication

National Disability Insurance Service Quality and Safeguards Commission—Supporting effective communication: https://www.ndiscommission.gov.au/workers/worker-training-modules-and-resources/supporting-effective-communication

Nursing and Midwifery Board of Australia. Code of conduct for nurses—Informed consent (section 2.3) and Confidentiality (section 3.5): https://www.nursingmidwiferyboard.gov.au/Codes-Guidelines-Statements/Professional-standards.aspx

Nursing Council of New Zealand. Code of conduct for nurses: https://www.nursingcouncil.org.nz/Public/Nursing/Standards_and_guidelines/NCNZ/nursing-section/Standards_and_guidelines_for_nurses.aspx?hkey=9fc06ae7-a853-4d10-b5fe-992cd44ba3de

REFERENCES

1. Australian Commission for Safety and Quality in Health Care. Communicating with patients and colleagues; 2023. Available at: https://c4sportal.safetyandquality.gov.au/communicating-with-patients-and-colleagues
2. Grover S, Fitzpatrick A, Azim FT, Ariza-Vega P, Bellwood P, Burns J, et al. Defining and implementing patient-centered care: an umbrella review. Patient Education and Counseling. 2022 Jul 1;105(7):1679–1688.
3. Edvardsson D, Watt E, Pearce F. Patient experiences of caring and person-centredness are associated with perceived nursing care quality. Journal of Advanced Nursing. 2017 Jan;73(1):217–227.
4. O'Toole G. Communication—core interpersonal skills for health professionals. 4th ed. Chatswood: Elsevier; 2020.
5. Underman Boggs K. Interpersonal relationships: professional communication skills for nurses.9th ed. St Louis: Elsevier. 2023.
6. Stein-Parbury J. Patient and person: interpersonal skills in nursing. 7th ed. Chatswood, NSW: Elsevier Australia; 2021.
7. #hello my name is. A campaign for more compassionate care. United Kingdom. 2023. Available at: https://www.hellomynameis.org.uk
8. Selye H. The stress of life. Revised ed. New York: McGraw-Hill; 1984.
9. Forster E, Fraser J. Paediatric nursing skills for Australian nurses. Sydney, Australia: Cambridge University Press; 2018.

10. Moody HR, Sasser JR. Aging: concepts and controversies. 10th ed. Sage Publication Inc.; 2020.
11. Folstein MF, Folstein SE, McHugh PR. Mini-mental state: a practical method for grading the cognitive states of patients for the clinician. Journal of Psychiatric Research 1975;12(3): 189–198.
12. Strnadová I, Loblinzk J, Scully JL, Danker J, Tso M, Jackaman K-M, et al. 'I am not a number!' Opinions and preferences of people with intellectual disability about genetic healthcare. European Journal of Human Genetics. 31, 1057–1065 (2023). https://doi.org/10.1038/s41431-023-01282-
13. Centre for Culture, Ethnicity and Health. Speaking with clients who have a low English proficiency. 2020. Available at: http://www.ceh.org.au/wp-content/uploads/2016/03/CEH_ClientsLowEnglish_Tipsheet.pdf
14. Centre for Culture, Ethnicity and Health. Assessing the need for an interpreter. 2020. Available at: https://www.ceh.org.au/resource-hub/assessing-the-need-for-an-interpreter/
15. Centre for Culture, Ethnicity and Health. Communication via an interpreter. 2020. Available at: https://www.ceh.org.au/resource-hub/communicating-via-an-interpreter/
16. Centre for Culture, Ethnicity and Health. Debriefing with an interpreter. 2020. Available at: https://www.ceh.org.au/resource-hub/debriefing-with-an-interpreter/
17. Centre for Culture, Ethnicity and Health. Cultural considerations in health assessment. 2020. Available at: https://www.ceh.org.au/resource-hub/cultural-considerations-in-health-assessment-tip-sheet/
18. Hall E: Proxemics: the study of man's spatial relations. In Galdston I (ed.): *Man's image in medicine and anthropology*. New York, 1963, International University Press, pp. 109–120.
19. Ministry of Health. Manatū Hauora: Māori health models – Te Whare Tapa Whā. Wellington: Ministry of Health. 2017. Available at: https://www.health.govt.nz/our-work/populations/maori-health/maori-health-models/maori-health-models-te-whare-tapa-wha
20. Australian Institute of Interpreters and Translators Incorporated (AUSIT). Guide for clinicians working with interpreters in healthcare settings. 2019. Available at: https://ausit.org/wp-content/uploads/2020/02/Guide-for-clinicians-working-with-interpreters-in-healthcare-settings-Jan2019-1.pdf
21. Ministry for Ethnic Communities. Te Tari Mātāwaki, 2023. Available at: https://www.ethniccommunities.govt.nz/resources/
22. Raising Children Network. The Australian parenting website. Professionals working with Interpreters and parents. Australian Government Department of Social Services. 2023. Available at: https://raisingchildren.net.au/for-professionals/working-with-parents/cultural-diversity/working-with-interpreters
23. Australian Bureau of Statistics. Language used at home (LANP). 2021. Available at: https://www.abs.gov.au/census/guide-census-data/census-dictionary/2021/variables-topic/cultural-diversity/language-used-home-lanp
24. Australian Bureau of Statistics. Program for the international assessment of adult competencies, Australia, 2016–2021. 2021. Available at: https://profile.id.com.au/australia/speaks-english
25. Australian Bureau of Statistics. Language statistics for Aboriginal and Torres Strait Islander peoples. 2021. Available at: https://www.abs.gov.au/statistics/people/aboriginal-and-torres-strait-islander-peoples/language-statistics-aboriginal-and-torres-strait-islander-peoples/latest-release
26. Statistics New Zealand, Tatauranga Aotearoa. 2018 Census. Language, 2018. Available at: https://www.stats.govt.nz/tools/2018-census-ethnic-group-summaries#Statistics%20New%20Zealand%202018%20Census%20ethnic%20group%20summaries
27. Statistics New Zealand, Tatauranga Aotearoa. Ngā reo/Languages, 2020. Available at: https://www.stats.govt.nz/topics/nga-reo-languages
28. Australian Institute of Health and Welfare (AIHW). Health literacy. AIHW; 2022. Available at: https://www.aihw.gov.au/reports/australias-health/health-literacy
29. Australian Government. Department of Health and Aged Care. National health literacy strategy framework consultation. AIHW; 2022. Available at: https://consultations.health.gov.

au/national-preventive-health-taskforce/national-health-literacy-strategy-framework-consul/
30. Van Servellen G. Communication skills for the healthcare professional: context, concepts, practice and evidence. 3rd ed. Burlington MA: Jones and Bartlett; 2020.
31. Hogan A, Hughes L, Coyne E. Understanding nursing assessment of health literacy in a hospital context: a qualitative study. Journal of Clinical Nursing 2023; Oct;32(19–20):7495–7508.
32. Ministry of Health. Manatū Hauora. 2022 Understanding health and healthcare 2017/18: New Zealand health survey. Available at: https://www.health.govt.nz/nz-health-statistics/surveys/new-zealand-health-survey/understanding-health-and-healthcare-2017-18-new-zealand-health-survey
33. Boston University. Health Literacy Tool Shed. 2023. Available at: https://healthliteracy.bu.edu
34. Parker RM, Baker DW, Williams MV, Nurss JR. The test of functional health literacy in adults: a new instrument for measuring patients' health literacy skills. In: Van Servellen G. Communication skills for health care professionals: context, concepts, practice and evidence. 3rd ed. Burlington MA: Jones and Bartlett; 2020.
35. Davis TC, Long SW, Jackson RH, Mayeaux EJ, George RB, Murphy PW, et al. Rapid estimate of adult literacy in medicine: a shortened screening instrument. In: Van Servellen G. Communication skills for health care professionals: context, concepts, practice and evidence. 3rd ed. Burlington MA: Jones and Bartlett; 2020.
36. Weiss BD, Mays MZ, Martz W, Castro KM, DeWalt DA, Pignone MP, et al. Quick assessment of literacy in primary care. The newest vital sign. In: Van Servellen G. Communication skills for health care professionals: context, concepts, practice and evidence. 3rd ed. Burlington MA: Jones and Bartlett; 2020.

CHAPTER 8

The health history

Written by Carolyn Jarvis
Adapted by Helen Forbes and Elizabeth Watt

INTRODUCTION

The purpose of collecting the health history is to gather information from the person, their carer or significant other's point of view (subjective data). The health history provides a guide for the nurse for what to focus on when collecting objective data. The data from the health history are combined with the **objective data** from the physical examination, measurement and specimen screening and reviewing of any other testing done by other health professionals to describe the person's current health situation. This information is used to make a clinical judgement to identify the person's health strengths or a health problem/nursing diagnosis about the state of health of the person.

This chapter overviews the health history including biographical data, the reasons for seeking care, past history, the history of the present illness and a review of symptoms (including analysis of symptoms), function and risk.

Case study

The following case study gives an example of a typical situation involving collecting data for a health history. It will help you identify your learning needs.

In the previous chapter you considered your approach to meeting the patient for the first time before starting a health assessment. In this chapter you will be considering and planning the type and extent of subjective data you will be collecting.

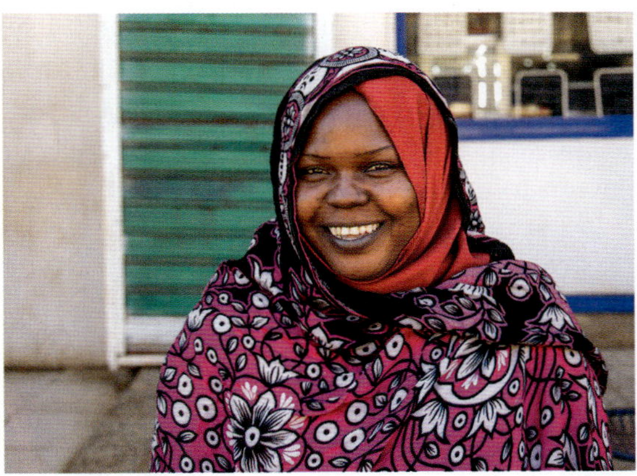

Context

You will recall from the previous chapter that you are on clinical placement in a subacute rehabilitation ward. Your preceptor (buddy) nurse tells you he is expecting a new patient admission to the ward shortly after the afternoon handover. He asks you to prepare to be involved in completing the ward admission assessment for this woman, who you will be meeting for the first time.

Consider the patient's situation

You have limited information about the new patient. Mrs Nyamal Bol is a 55-year-old woman who is undergoing rehabilitation following a car accident 3 days ago. She sustained a fractured right wrist, which has been internally fixed with a plate and screw, and she has a plaster cast from her fingers to her elbow. She also sustained a dislocated fractured ankle, which has been fixed with screws and plates, and she is now wearing an orthopaedic boot. She has extensive bruising and minor cuts. Mrs Bol is a South Sudanese–Australian who arrived in Australia as a refugee 8 years ago with her husband and five children. You are told that Mrs Bol speaks some English.

Questions to further your learning

- What are the possible things that might be going on with Mrs Bol?
- What knowledge do you need to be able to predict what might be going on?
- What questions (subjective data) will you ask Mrs Bol to extend the health history and why?
- What resources are available to assist in your assessment of Mrs Bol?

Assessment plan

The following health history framework provides a complete picture of the person's past and present health. It describes the person as a whole and how the person interacts with the environment. It also records health strengths and coping skills. The health history should recognise and affirm what the person is doing to help stay well.

For a well person, the history is used to assess their lifestyle including such factors as exercise, diet, risk reduction and health promotion behaviours. For an unwell person, the health history includes a detailed and chronological record of the health problem(s). For all, the health history is a screening tool for abnormal symptoms, health problems and concerns, and it records ways of responding to the health problems.

In many settings the person fills out an admission history form or checklist. This allows the person enough time to recall and consider such items as key health events and relevant family history. However, these forms assume the person has a good understanding of written English and adequate health literacy. You may become aware that the person has poor health literacy or may not have the capacity of the English language to complete the forms. In that case a nurse will need to help the person to complete the forms using information provided by the person and/or family (see Chapter 7 for more information on health literacy).

In some situations, a nurse completes the health history at the time the person is admitted to the ward or unit. However, the health history may also be completed before the person arrives at the hospital at a formal preadmission interview or by the person completing the printed or online history form themselves before admission. At the time of admission to the hospital the nurse should always check through the information with the person and clarify the details to ensure the information is accurate and complete. It is important to note that the health history data collection is conducted in such a way as to ensure the person's privacy.

Although history forms vary, most contain information in this sequence of categories:

- biographical data
- reason for seeking care
- present health or history of present illness
- past history
- family history
- review of symptoms, function and risks.

The health history discussed in the following section follows this format and presents a generic database for all clinicians. Those in primary care settings may use all of it, whereas those in a hospital may focus primarily on the history of the present illness, effect on function and possible risks related to the reason for admission and its treatment. Each chapter in this textbook details specific areas for subjective data collection relevant to the area being assessed.

Resources available

You will find additional resources and the reference list at the end of this chapter.

The health history—adults and adults aged 65 years or older

Before you begin any health assessment, it is important for safety reasons that approved patient identifiers are used to confirm the identity of the person.[1] The approved identifiers include: the person's name (family and given names), date of birth, gender, address (including postcode) and health record number or individual healthcare identifier such as a Medicare number. It is recommended that at least three identifiers are used prior to any procedure, service or care activity.[1] Avoid using the person's bed or room number as an identifier because they are not unique to one person and are likely to change.

Biographical data

The biographical data includes the person's name, address and phone number, age and birth date, gender, marital status, religion, first language spoken (and other languages) including Indigenous status, occupation, both usual and present (an illness or disability may have prompted change in occupation), and next of kin name and contact details. In some circumstances, the person's nominated medical power of attorney (if any) is also recorded. The name and address of the person's usual GP or medical clinic is recorded. Often this information is collected and prepared on an admission form by an administrator before the person arrives at the ward or unit. The nurse should recheck the validity of the recorded information.

Source of history

1. Record who provides the information—usually the person themselves, although the source may be a relative or friend.
2. Judge how reliable the informant seems and how willing they are to communicate. A reliable person always gives the same answers, even when questions are rephrased or are repeated later in the interview.
3. Note any special circumstances such as the need for an interpreter or the need for a nominated spokesperson to speak for a person who is unable to speak for themselves—for example, a person with dementia. Another possibility to consider is that, in some circumstances, a person may have nominated a specific spokesperson through substitute decision-maker or medical power of attorney (see links in the 'Additional resources' section about appointing a substitute or medical decision-maker and advance care planning).

Reason for seeking care

This is a brief spontaneous statement in the person's own words that describes the reason for seeking health care. The reason(s) is often a symptom(s) or change in function that the person considers to be troublesome. A **symptom** is a subjective abnormal sensation that the person is experiencing such as nausea or pain. Whatever the person says as the reason for seeking care is recorded, either stating clearly what the person or carer has stated or enclosed in quotation marks to indicate the person's exact words. For example:

- 'Mr Johnson reports experiencing chest pain for 2 hours' or '*Chest pain for 2 hours*'.
- 'Ms Chan says that her son had an earache and was unsettled all night' or '*Earache and unsettled all night*'.
- 'Cheyne reports that he has had abdominal pain for the past 2 days and it is getting worse' or '*Pain in abdomen for 2 days. It is getting worse.*'

A **sign** is an objective abnormality that the examiner identifies on physical examination or in laboratory reports—for example, crackles on auscultation of the person's lungs.

The reason for seeking care is not a diagnostic statement. Avoid translating it into the terms of a medical diagnosis. Even if the person is known to have emphysema or asthma from previous visits, it is not the chronic emphysema or asthma that prompted *this visit* to the hospital or clinic but the '*increasing shortness of breath*' for 4 hours.

Some people try to self-diagnose based on similar signs and symptoms in their relatives or friends, the internet or based on conditions they know they have. Rather than record a person's statement that they have a '*strep throat*', ask them what symptoms they have that make them think this is present and record those symptoms.

Occasionally, a person may list many reasons for seeking care. The most important reason to the person may not necessarily be the one stated first. Try to focus on which is the most pressing concern by asking the person which one prompted them to seek help now.

Person's perception of present state of health or health concern

In this section you are trying to ascertain how the person perceives or describes their usual level of health. For people seeking health care for illness, this section is a chronological record of the reason for seeking care, from the time the symptom first started until now. Isolate each reason for care identified by the person and say, for example, '*Please tell me all about your headache, from the time it started until the time you came to the hospital*'. If the concern started months or years ago, record what occurred during that time and find out why the person is seeking care now.

As the person talks, avoid jumping to conclusions or biasing the story by adding your opinion. Collect all the data by asking the person what the problem is and what they think is the reason for the problem.

Healthcare workers often use a mnemonic to organise questions. A mnemonic ensures you remember all the points when analysing symptoms such as nausea, constipation or incontinence. These are some examples:

COLDSPA

The COLDSPA mnemonic is commonly used and includes these seven critical characteristics.

C: Character. This calls for specific description of the symptom using terms such as burning, sharp, dull, aching, gnawing, throbbing, shooting, vice-like.
Use similes: *Does the blood in the stool look like sticky tar?*; *Does the blood in the vomit look like coffee grounds?*
Find out the meaning of the symptom by asking how it affects daily activities and quality of life. Also ask directly, *What do you think it means?* This is crucial because it alerts you to potential anxiety if the person thinks the symptom may be ominous.

O: Onset/timing. *When did the symptom first appear?* Give the specific date and time, or state specifically how long ago the symptom started before arriving at the hospital. 'The pain started yesterday' will not mean much when you return to read the record in the future. If intermittent, *What is the frequency? Was it steady (constant) or did it come and go during that time?*

L: Location. Be specific; ask the person to point to the location. If the problem is pain, note the precise site. 'Head pain' is vague, whereas descriptions such as 'pain behind the eyes', 'jaw pain' and 'occipital pain' are more precise and are diagnostically significant. *Is the pain localised to this site or radiating?*; *Is the pain superficial or deep?*

D: Duration. *How long did the symptom last?*; *Was it constant or intermittent?*; *Did it resolve completely and reappear later?*

S: Severity. Attempt to quantify the symptom such as 'profuse menstrual flow soaking five pads per hour'. *How bad is it (on a scale of 1 to 10)?*; *What impact has the symptom had on your daily activities?* Then the person might say, *I was so sick I was doubled up and couldn't move* or *I was able to go to work, but then I came home and went to bed.*

P: Pattern. *What makes the symptom worse?*; *Is it aggravated by weather, activity, food, medication, standing, bent over, fatigue, time of day, season and so on?*; *What relieves* *it? Rest? Medication? An ice pack?*; *What is the effect of any treatment?* Ask, *What have you tried?* or *What seems to help?*; *Where were you or what were you doing when the symptom started?*; *What brings it on?* For example: *Did you notice the chest pain after mowing the lawn, or did the pain start by itself ?*

A: Associated factors. Is this primary symptom associated with any others (e.g. urinary frequency and burning associated with fever and chills)? Review the body system related to this symptom now rather than wait for the physical assessment.

PQRSTU

PQRSTU is another example of a mnemonic that is useful for analysing a person's experience of pain:

P: Provocative or Palliative. *What brings it on? What were you doing when you first noticed it? What makes it better? Worse?*

Q: Quality or Quantity. *How does it look, feel, sound? How intense/severe is it?*

R: Region or Radiation. *Where is it? Does it spread anywhere?*

S: Severity scale. *How bad is it (on a scale of 1 to 10)? Is it getting better, worse or staying the same?*

T: Timing. Onset—*Exactly when did it first occur?* Duration—*How long did it last?* Frequency—*How often does it occur?*

U: Understand patient's perception of the problem. *What do you think it means?*

Symptom measurement and screening tools

There are validated tools available to assess symptoms in detail—for example, assessing pain (Chapter 13), depression (Chapter 11) and distress. The distress thermometer,[2] for example, is a self-report screening tool for measuring psychological distress in cancer patients. There is an 11-point scale ranging from 0 (no distress) to 10 (extreme distress). See Figure 8.1. The distress thermometer has been validated internationally in different age groups, settings and cancer types. It is quick and easy to implement and has become a useful screening tool for distress. You will be referred to other symptom assessment tools throughout the text.

Past health history

The extent of the information about the person's past health history will depend on the situation and the context. See the following list of key aspects for example of typical information that may be relevant. Keep in mind that past health events may have residual effects on the person's current health state. Also, the previous experience with illness may give clues as to how the person responds to illness and to the significance of illness for the person.

CHILDHOOD ILLNESSES/ HEALTH ISSUES

Ask about serious childhood illnesses that may have consequences for the person in later years—for example, childhood infectious diseases such as measles, mumps, rubella, chickenpox, pertussis, poliomyelitis (all uncommon in Australia and Aotearoa New Zealand currently because of immunisation but may be an issue for some migrants or refugees), rheumatic fever and scarlet fever.

OTHER DISEASES OR HEALTH ISSUES EXPERIENCED IN CHILDHOOD

Examples include a congenital health issue such as a cardiac, urinary tract, gastrointestinal tract problem or mental health issue. Note if the person has a history of learning difficulties, is neurodiverse or has any other disability. The impact that this may have on the person will be explored further in other sections of the health history.

NCCN Clinical Practice Guidelines in Oncology (NCCN Guidelines®)
Distress Management V.2.2024.

NCCN DISTRESS THERMOMETER

Distress is an unpleasant experience of a mental, physical, social, or spiritual nature. It can affect the way you think, feel, or act. Distress may make it harder to cope with having cancer, its symptoms, or its treatment.

Instructions: Please circle the number (0–10) that best describes how much distress you have been experiencing in the past week, including today.

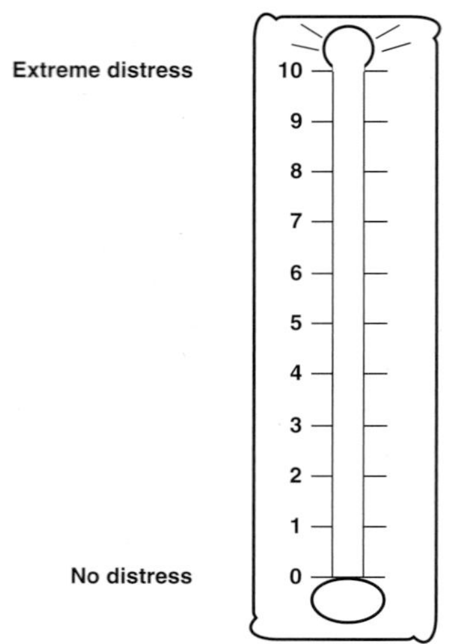

PROBLEM LIST

Have you had concerns about any of the items below in the past week, including today? (Mark all that apply)

Physical Concerns
- ❑ Pain
- ❑ Sleep
- ❑ Fatigue
- ❑ Tobacco use
- ❑ Substance use
- ❑ Memory or concentration
- ❑ Sexual health
- ❑ Changes in eating
- ❑ Loss or change of physical abilities

Emotional Concerns
- ❑ Worry or anxiety
- ❑ Sadness or depression
- ❑ Loss of interest or enjoyment
- ❑ Grief or loss
- ❑ Fear
- ❑ Loneliness
- ❑ Anger
- ❑ Changes in appearance
- ❑ Feelings of worthlessness or being a burden

Social Concerns
- ❑ Relationship with spouse or partner
- ❑ Relationship with children
- ❑ Relationship with family members
- ❑ Relationship with friends or coworkers
- ❑ Communication with health care team
- ❑ Ability to have children
- ❑ Prejudice or discrimination

Practical Concerns
- ❑ Taking care of myself
- ❑ Taking care of others
- ❑ Work
- ❑ School
- ❑ Housing
- ❑ Finances
- ❑ Insurance
- ❑ Transportation
- ❑ Child care
- ❑ Having enough food
- ❑ Access to medicine
- ❑ Treatment decisions

Spiritual or Religious Concerns
- ❑ Sense of meaning or purpose
- ❑ Changes in faith or beliefs
- ❑ Death, dying, or afterlife
- ❑ Conflict between beliefs and cancer treatments
- ❑ Relationship with the sacred
- ❑ Ritual or dietary needs

Other Concerns:

____

____

____

Note: All recommendations are category 2A unless otherwise indicated.
Clinical Trials: NCCN believes that the best management of any patient with cancer is in a clinical trial. Participation in clinical trials is especially encouraged.

DIS-A

FIGURE 8.1 Distress thermometer
©National Comprehensive Cancer Network 2020, All Rights Reserved. There is a 2023 edition available – https://www.nccn.org/docs/default-source/patient-resources/nccn_distress_thermometer.pdf?sfvrsn=ef1df1a2_4

ACCIDENTS OR INJURIES

Ask about motor vehicle accidents, fractures, joint injuries, penetrating wounds, head injuries (including concussion) and burns.

SERIOUS OR CHRONIC ILLNESSES

Examples include diabetes, hypertension, heart disease, heart irregularities (arrhythmias), vascular disease, Crohn's disease, ulcerative colitis, cancer and seizure disorder. If the person has one or more of these conditions, ask them about their current treatment, including medications, rather than waiting until later in the conversation: *Have you ever experienced a blood clot in your legs or lungs?*

HOSPITALISATIONS

Note the reason for past hospitalisations, the names of the hospitals, how the condition was treated, how long the person was hospitalised and names of the medical practitioners (if known).

SURGICAL PROCEDURES

Note the type of surgery, date, name of the surgeon, name of the hospital and how the person recovered.

OBSTETRIC HISTORY

Record the number of pregnancies, number of deliveries in which the fetus reached full term, number of preterm pregnancies (preterm), number of incomplete pregnancies (miscarriage or termination of pregnancy) and number of children (living). For each complete pregnancy, note the mother's health during the pregnancy; labour and birthing; sex, weight and condition of each infant; and postpartum health.

IMMUNISATIONS

The following immunisations are on the Australian and Aotearoa New Zealand National Immunisation program schedules. Note the immunisations that have been completed including the most recent flu and COVID-19 shots (Chapter 3).

ALLERGIES AND ADVERSE REACTIONS

Note both the allergen (medication, food or contact agent, such as fabric or environmental agent, including latex/rubber) and the reaction (rash, itching, runny nose, watery eyes, difficulty breathing) and, if food, what foods are excluded from their diet. Note any previous adverse reactions to an anaesthetic or if a family member has had an adverse reaction.

Family history

Ask about the age and health or the age and cause of death of blood relatives such as parents, grandparents and siblings. This information may have genetic significance for the person. Also ask about close family members such as spouse and children. You need to know about the person's prolonged contact with any communicable disease or the effect of a family member's illness on this person.

Specifically ask for any family history of heart disease, high blood pressure, stroke, diabetes, blood disorders, cancer, arthritis, allergies, obesity, alcoholism, mental illness, seizure disorder and kidney disease. Construct an accurate family tree or genogram to show this information clearly and concisely (Figure 8.2).

Review of symptoms, function and risks

The purposes of this section of the health history are to:

- evaluate the past and present health state of the person
- re-check in case any significant data were omitted in the present illness section
- gain insight into the person's health promotion and health maintenance practices
- identify symptoms and potential health risks.

The items listed in each section are not exhaustive, and only the most common symptoms are included. If the 'present illness' section covered one body system, you do not need to repeat all the data. For example, if the reason for seeking care is earache, the present illness section describes most of the symptoms listed for the auditory system. Just ask anything that was not asked in the present illness section.

Another area of review is to determine the effect of illness and symptoms on the person's functional ability. Functional assessment measures a person's self-care ability in the areas of general health; activities of daily living, such as bathing, dressing, toileting, eating and walking, or those needed for independent living such as housekeeping, shopping, cooking, doing laundry, using the telephone and managing finances; nutrition; social relationships and resources; self-concept and coping; and home environment. For example, alterations in cardiovascular, respiratory and/or musculoskeletal health

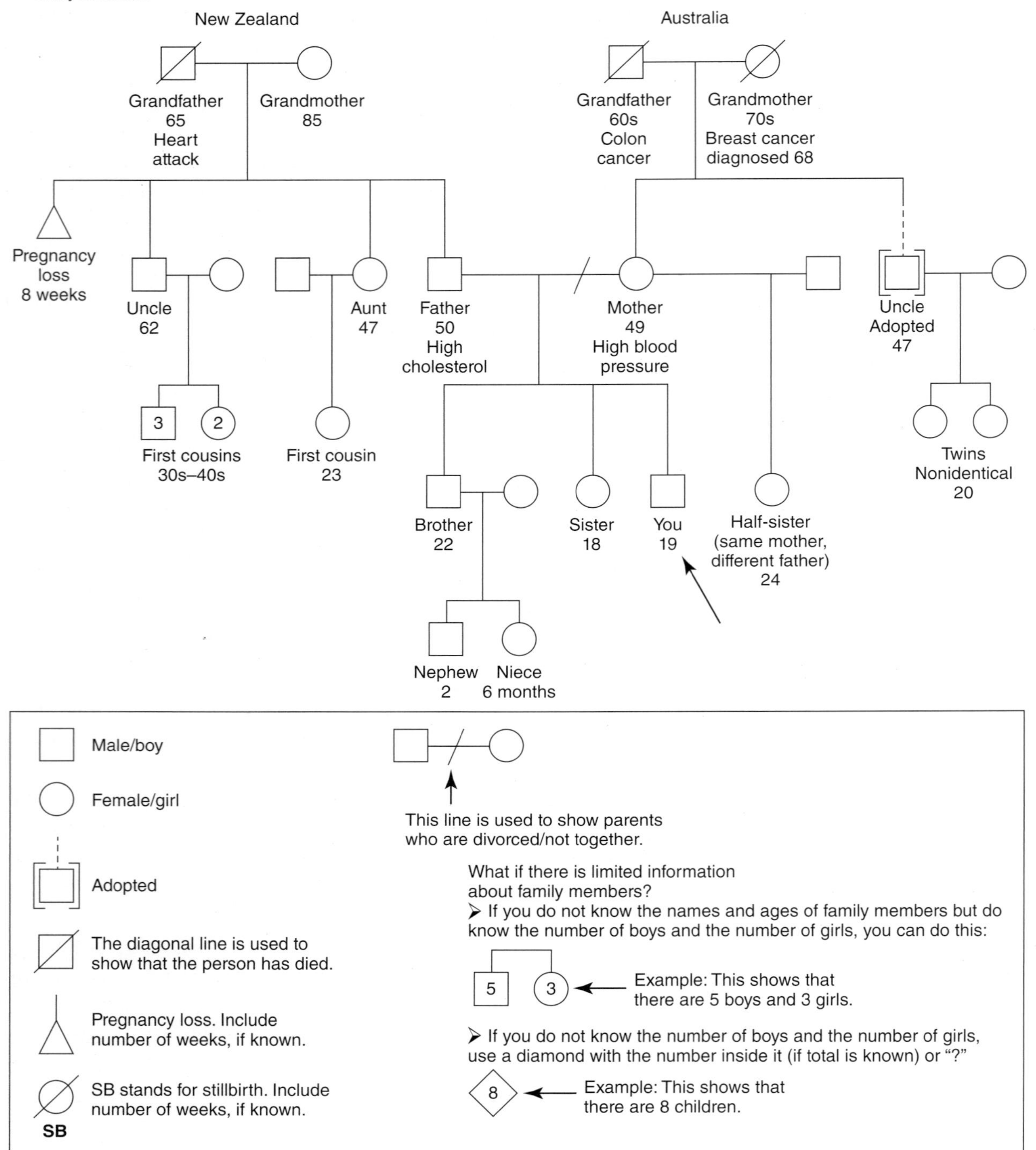

FIGURE 8.2 Genogram or family tree

may affect a person's ability to be active and participate in daily living activities. (See Units 4–6 for details.) Similarly, alterations in mental status, neurological and sensory function (Unit 3), nutrition and metabolic function (Unit 7), urinary and bowel elimination (Unit 8), sexuality and reproductive function (Unit 9) can also have an impact on the person's ability to perform their daily activities and take part in exercise and leisure activities. Within each of these areas, the focus is on eliciting the nature of the effect and how it relates to the person's quality of life.

To assess functional ability, questions focus on the person's lifestyle and how they manage daily living and whether they need assistance to manage everyday life activities. Functional assessment may also mean that the health history may be supplemented by a standardised functional assessment tool (Figure 8.3). These instruments objectively measure a person's present functional status and monitor any changes over time.[3,4] Whether or not you use

Katz Activities of Daily Living

Activities

Points (1 or 0)

Independence
(1 Point)
NO supervision, direction, or personal assistance

Dependence
(0 Points)
WITH supervision, direction, personal assistance, or total care

Bathing
Points ______
(1 Point) Bathes self completely or needs help in bathing only a single part of the body such as the back, genital area or disabled extremity
(0 Point) Needs help with bathing more than one part of the body or with getting in or out of the bath or shower; requires total bathing

Dressing
Points ______
(1 Point) Gets clothes from closet and drawers and puts on clothes and outer garments complete with fasteners; may have help tying shoes
(0 Point) Needs help with dressing self or needs to be completely dressed

Toileting
Points ______
(1 Point) Gets to toilet, gets on and off, arranges clothes, cleans genital area without help
(0 Point) Needs help transferring to the toilet or cleaning self, or uses bedpan or commode

Transferring
Points ______
(1 Point) Moves into and out of bed or chair unassisted; mechanical transferring aids are acceptable
(0 Point) Needs help in moving from bed to chair or requires a complete transfer

Continence
Points ______
(1 Point) Exercises complete self-control over urination and defecation
(0 Point) Is partially or totally incontinent of bowel or bladder

Feeding
Points ______
(1 Point) Gets food from plate into mouth without help; preparation of food may be done by another person
(0 Point) Needs partial or total help with feeding or requires parenteral feeding

Total Points = ______
6 = High (patient independent)
0 = Low (patient very dependent)

FIGURE 8.3 Katz' activities of daily living
Source: Katz et al. 1963[3]

any of these formalised instruments, functional assessment questions such as those listed in each of the chapters should be included in the standard health history.

Admission to a health facility provides an opportunity to identify areas for further health education or to pass on health information and to identify factors that could put the person at risk during their hospitalisation or admission to the health service. For example, known areas of potential risk include skin breakdown, unrelieved pain, falls, confusion and effects of alcohol or drug abuse.

When recording information, record the presence or absence of all symptoms, otherwise another health professional does not know about which factors you asked. A common mistake made by beginning clinicians is to record some physical finding or objective data here, such as 'skin warm and dry'. Remember that the history should be limited to the person's statements or subjective data—factors that the person says were or were not present.

General overall health and wellbeing

PERCEPTION OF HEALTH

Ask the person questions such as: '*How do you define health?*' '*How do you view your health situation now?*' '*What are your health concerns?*' '*What are your health goals?*' If relevant, '*How do your health issues effect your daily life?*'

INTERPERSONAL RELATIONSHIPS/ RESOURCES

Education level achieved and current employment or other activities. For example: '*How would you describe your role in the family?*', '*How would you say you get along with family, friends and co-workers?*' Ask about support systems composed of family and significant others: '*Who could you go to for support with a problem at work, with your health or a personal problem?*' Include contact with spouse, siblings, parents, children, extended family and friends, organisations and workplace: '*What hobbies do you have?*', '*What effect will your current illness/hospitalisation have on your relationships and roles?*'

VALUES AND BELIEFS/SPIRITUAL RESOURCES

Cultural and ethnic background and practices, as well as religious/spiritual beliefs, values and practices. For example: '*Do you identify with any specific cultural group?*', '*In your culture are there some health practices that are important to you?*', '*Does religious faith or spirituality play an important part in your life?*', '*Do you consider yourself to be a religious or spiritual person?*', '*How does your religious faith or spirituality influence the way you think about your health or the way you care for yourself?*', '*Are you a part of any religious or spiritual community or congregation?*', '*Would you like me to address any religious or spiritual issues or concerns with you?*', '*What effect will your current illness/hospitalisation have on your capacity to practise your religion?*'

COPING AND STRESS MANAGEMENT

Ask about stresses in the person's life, especially in the past year. Note down any change in lifestyle or any current stress, methods tried to relieve stress and if these have been helpful. For example: '*Have there been any significant changes in your life in the past year?*', '*How do you think this has affected your health?*', '*How do you relieve tension or stress?*'

SELF-CONCEPT

Find out about the person's perception of personal strengths, social identity (perception of the sort of person they believe they are), life values and beliefs and body image. For example: '*What is it about your present situation that is most worrying for you?*'

SLEEP/REST

Sleep patterns, daytime naps, any sleep aids used. For example: '*What time do you usually go to sleep?*', '*When do you normally wake up?*', '*Do you have difficulty getting to sleep?*', '*If so, how do you manage that?*'

Health and lifestyle management

As you progress through each chapter you will be prompted to ask questions related to the person's usual health and lifestyle management. This may be an opportunity for beginning health education.

CURRENT HEALTH SCREENING

Undertake a current health screening if relevant to the person's age and gender. For example, ask the person about their participation in screening such as bowel cancer screening, blood pressure checking, cervical screening test, breast cancer screening, blood lipids, blood pressure, prostate check, dental check, vision and hearing.

CURRENT MEDICATIONS

Nurses have an important role in medication reconciliation. This is a process where an accurate list of the person's medications must be obtained and verified as part of the admission process. Medications include all over-the-counter medicines and complementary or traditional therapies. Ask specifically about vitamins, oral contraceptives, aspirin, sedatives and antacids because many people do not consider these to be medications. Also include a question about the use of prescribed (or acquired) medicinal cannabis preparations. Efforts are made to match the medicines that have been prescribed to those that are actually being taken. Explanations for any changes are documented. Care must be taken when a person is transferred from one healthcare environment to another.

For each medication, record the name, purpose and daily schedule and ask: '*How often do you take it each day?*', '*What is it for?*' and '*How long have you been taking it?*' Does the person have a system to remember to take the medicine? Does medicine seem to work? Are there any side effects? If so, does the person feel like skipping medicine because of them? Also consider the following issues:

- Some people take many medications prescribed by different medical practitioners or obtained from family or friends.
- Is cost a problem? When the person is unable to afford a medication, they may decrease the dosage, take one pill instead of two or not refill the empty bottle immediately.
- Is travelling to the pharmacy to refill a prescription a problem?
- Has the person ever shared medications with family members, neighbours or friends? Some establish 'lay referral' networks by comparing symptoms and thus medications.

TOBACCO, ALCOHOL AND ILLICIT DRUGS

Ask questions directly: '*Do you smoke cigarettes or vape?*', '*At what age did you start?*', '*How many packs do you smoke per day?*', '*How many years have you smoked?*' Record the number of packs smoked per day (PPD) and duration—for example, 1 PPD × 5 years. Then ask, '*Have you ever tried to quit?*' and '*How did it go?*' to introduce plans about smoking cessation. '*How long since you quit smoking?*'

Health professionals often fail to question about alcohol unless problems are obvious. Be alert, then, to early signs of hazardous alcohol use. Ask whether the person drinks alcohol. If yes, ask specific questions about the amount and frequency of alcohol use: '*When was your last drink of alcohol?*', '*How much did you drink that time?*', '*What do you drink?*', '*Out of the past 7 days, about how many days would you say that you drank alcohol?*', '*Have you ever had a drinking problem?*', '*Any history of alcohol treatment?*', '*Involvement in recovery activities?*', '*Any history of a family member with a problem drinking?*'

Ask specifically about illicit drugs such as heroin, cocaine, amphetamines and methamphetamines. Indicate frequency of use and how usage has affected work or family. Refer to Chapter 6 for more information about screening for substance misuse.

ENVIRONMENT/HAZARDS

Ask about the person's housing and neighbourhood—living alone, knowledge of neighbours, security of housing (renting/purchasing), safety of the neighbourhood, adequate heat and utilities, access to transportation and involvement in community services. Note environmental health, including hazards in workplace, hazards at home (e.g. mould on walls, difficult to use stairs), use of seatbelts, geographical or occupational exposures and travel or residence in other countries, including time spent overseas.

OCCUPATIONAL HEALTH

Ask the person to describe their job. '*Have you ever worked with any health hazard, such as excessive noise, asbestos or silica dust, inhalants, chemicals or repetitive motion?*', '*Do you wear any protective equipment while working?*', '*Are there work programs in place that monitor exposure?*', '*Are you aware of any health problems now that may be related to work exposure?*' Note the timing of the reason for seeking care and whether it may be related to work or home activities such as hobbies, job titles or exposure history. Finally, ask the person what they like or dislike about the job.

The health history—children

The health history needs to be adapted to include information specific for the age and developmental stage of the child (e.g. the mother's health during pregnancy, labour and birthing and the perinatal period). Note that the developmental history and nutritional data are listed as separate sections because of their importance for current health. See also Chapter 3 for a detailed discussion of developmental tasks.

Biographical data

Include the child's name, nickname, address and phone number, parents' names and work numbers, family situation (e.g. parents living in same house or not living together), the child's age and birth date, birthplace, gender and information on other children and family members at home. If parents are living apart, ask about the parenting arrangements and who is authorised to have access to the child or speak on their behalf.

Source of history

1. Person providing information and relation to child
2. Your impression of reliability of information
3. Any special circumstances such as the use of an interpreter

Reason for seeking care

Record the parent's spontaneous statement. Reasons for health problems may be initiated by the child, parent or by a third party such as the schoolteacher or grandparent. Parent concerns about the health of their child must be taken seriously and thoroughly investigated. A parent's intuitive sense of a problem is often accurate.

Even if proved otherwise, this factor gives you an idea of the parent's area of concern.

Present health or history of present illness

Include a statement about the usual health of the child and any common health problems or major health concerns. Describe any presenting symptom or sign, using the same format as for the adult. Some additional considerations include:

- Severity of pain: '*How do you know the child is in pain?*' (e.g. pulling at ears alerts parent to ear pain). Note the effect of pain on usual behaviour (e.g. '*Does it stop the child from playing?*').
- Associated factors such as relation to activity, eating and body position.
- Parent's coping ability and reaction of other family members to child's symptoms or illness.

Past health

PRENATAL STATUS (IF RELEVANT)

What was the mother's health during pregnancy? Were there any complications? (bleeding, excessive nausea and vomiting, unusual weight gain, high blood pressure, swelling of hands and feet, falls, infections—rubella or sexually transmitted infections). Were medications prescribed and/or taken during pregnancy? (What medications, when were they taken, dose and duration?) Record the mother's use of alcohol, illicit drugs, cigarettes or vaping.

Start with an open-ended question: '*Tell me about your pregnancy*'. If she questions the relevancy of the statement, mention that these questions are important to gain a complete picture of the child's health.

LABOUR AND BIRTHING (IF RELEVANT)

Ask about gravidity (number of times a female is or has been pregnant) and parity (viable pregnancies over 20 weeks' gestation), duration of the pregnancy, name of the hospital, course and duration of labour, use of anaesthesia, type of birth (vertex, breech, caesarean section), birthweight, Apgar scores, need for resuscitation and use of special equipment or procedures after birth.

POSTNATAL STATUS

In the neonatal stage, were there any health problems requiring hospitalisation? Record the length of the hospital stay, neonatal jaundice, whether the baby was discharged with the mother, whether the baby was breast or bottle fed, weight gain, any feeding problems, colic, diarrhoea, patterns of crying and sleeping and the mother's perception of her physical and mental health postpartum.

CHILDHOOD ILLNESSES

Ask the child's age at the time of any illnesses such as tonsil or ear infections or any infectious diseases.

SERIOUS ACCIDENTS OR INJURIES

Check the age of occurrence, extent of injury, how the child was treated and complications of motor vehicle accidents, falls, head injuries, fractures, burns and poisonings.

SERIOUS OR CHRONIC ILLNESS, SURGERY OR HOSPITALISATIONS

Illnesses such as seizure disorders, asthma, pneumonia, diabetes, renal disorders, allergies (see section below), rheumatic fever, scarlet fever (especially for rural and remote communities), age of onset, reason for hospitalisation, age at admission, name of surgeon or primary care providers, name of hospital, duration of stay, how child reacted to hospitalisation and any complications are all relevant. If the child reacted poorly, they may be afraid now and will need special preparation for the examination that is to follow.

IMMUNISATIONS

For immunisations, record the age when administered, date administered and any reactions. See Chapter 3 for immunisation schedules.

ALLERGIES OR FOOD INTOLERANCES

Write down any medications, foods, contact agents and environmental agents to which the child is allergic and reaction to allergen. Note allergic reactions particularly common in childhood such as hay fever, insect hypersensitivity, eczema and urticaria. Note if the child has had a past anaphylactic reaction and whether they carry an EpiPen. Ask the parent for a copy of the child's asthma or anaphylaxis plan.

DEVELOPMENTAL HISTORY

The child's growth and development may need to be assessed in detail. See Chapter 3.

PSYCHOSOCIAL HISTORY

It is important to get a sense of the child as a person, their usual home environment and the people who care for them. This will provide a baseline for assessing that the child is coping with the current health situation and will assist in person-centred care planning for the child and their family. Talley and O'Connor[5] outline the following areas:

- behavioural history includes unusual behaviours, altered patterns of sleep and toileting problems such as bedwetting
- social development and interactions—for example, for a school-aged child, consider school performance in the context of vision, hearing, speech, gross and fine motor function and social interactions
- describe a typical day in the life of this child including physical activity, food and diet, living conditions and family life
- relationships within the family including communication, family support, alternative care arrangements—for example, childcare or foster care (Does the child spend time between family members?)
- effect of illness on the child and family.

Family history

In some circumstances, a detailed family history may be required. Drawing a family tree for the child, including siblings, parents and grandparents, may be a useful strategy. See the information detailed previously in the adult section and Figure 8.2 about drawing a family genogram. Avoid making assumptions about the structure of the family. Rather than assume, be sure to ask a parent to clarify the family structure.

General overall health and wellbeing

As with the adult, changes in any of the areas of the body will have an impact on function and give rise to symptoms and risks, which need to be investigated in detail. For details of assessing each of the areas of the body see the relevant chapters in the text.

The health history—adolescents

As with children, the health history for adolescents is adapted to include information specific for the age and developmental stage of the adolescent, which is aimed to maximise communication. The **HEEADSSS**[6] (Figure 8.4) method of interviewing focuses on assessment of the:

Home environment
Education and employment
Eating

The HEEADSSS Psychosocial Interview for Adolescents

Home
Who lives with you? Where do you live? Do you have your own room?
What are relationships like at home?
To whom are you closest at home?
To whom can you talk at home?
Is there anyone new at home? Has someone left recently?
Have you moved recently?
Have you ever had to live away from home? (Why?)
Have you ever run away? (Why?)
Is there any physical violence at home?

Education and Employment
What are your favourite subjects at school? Your least favourite subjects?
How are your grades? Any recent changes? Any dramatic changes in the past?
Have you changed schools in the past few years?
What are your future education/employment plans/goals?
Are you working? Where? How much?
Tell me about your friends at school.
Is your school a safe place? (Why?)
Have you ever had to repeat a class? Have you ever had to repeat a grade?
Have you ever been suspended? Expelled? Have you ever considered dropping out?
How well do you get along with the people at school? Work?
Have your responsibilities at work increased?
Do you feel connected to your school? Do you feel as if you belong?
Are there adults at school you feel you could talk to about something important? (Who?)

Eating
What do you like and not like about your body?
Have there been any recent changes in your weight?
Have you dieted in the past year? How? How often?
Have you done anything else to try to manage your weight?
How much exercise do you get in an average day? Week?
What do you think would be a healthy diet? How does that compare with your current eating patterns?
Do you worry about your weight? How often?
Do you eat in front of the TV? Computer?
Does it ever seem as though your eating is out of control?
Have you ever made yourself throw up on purpose to control your weight?
Have you ever taken diet pills?
What would it be like if you gained (lost) 5 kilos?

Activities
What do you and your friends do for fun? (with whom, where, and when?)
What do you and your family do for fun? (with whom, where, and when?)
Do you participate in any sports or other activities?
Do you regularly attend a church group, club or other organised activity?
Do you have any hobbies?
Do you read for fun? (What?)
How much TV do you watch in a week? How about video games?
What music do you like to listen to?

Drugs
Do any of your friends use tobacco? Alcohol? Other drugs?
Does anyone in your family use tobacco? Alcohol? Other drugs?
Do you use tobacco? Alcohol? Other drugs?
Is there any history of alcohol or drug problems in your family?
Do you ever drink or use drugs when you're alone?
(Assess frequency, intensity, patterns of use or abuse, and how youth obtains or pays for drugs, alcohol or tobacco.)

Sexuality
Have you ever been in a romantic relationship?
Tell me about the people that you've dated. *OR* Tell me about your sex life.
Have any of your relationships ever been sexual relationships?
Are your sexual activities enjoyable?
What does the term 'safer sex' mean to you?
Are you interested in boys? Girls? Both?
Have you ever been forced or pressured into doing something sexual that you didn't want to do?
Have you ever been touched sexually in a way that you didn't want?
Have you ever been raped, on a date or any other time?
How many sexual partners have you had altogether?
Have you ever been pregnant or worried that you may be pregnant? (females)
Have you ever made someone pregnant or worried that that might have happened? (males)
What are you using for birth control? Are you satisfied with your method?
Do you use condoms every time you have intercourse?
Does anything ever get in the way of always using a condom?
Have you ever had a sexually transmitted infection (STI) or worried that you had an STI?

Suicide and Depression
Do you feel sad or down more than usual? Do you find yourself crying more than usual?
Are you 'bored' all the time?
Are you having trouble getting to sleep?
Have you thought a lot about hurting yourself or someone else?
Does it seem that you've lost interest in things that you used to really enjoy?
Do you find yourself spending less and less time with friends?
Would you rather just be by yourself most of the time?
Have you ever tried to kill yourself?
Have you ever had to hurt yourself (by cutting yourself, for example) to calm down or feel better?
Have you started using alcohol or drugs to help you relax, calm down or feel better?

Safety (Savagery)
Have you ever been seriously injured? (How?) How about anyone else you know?
Do you always wear a seatbelt in the car?
Have you ever ridden with a driver who was drunk or high? When? How often?
Do you use safety equipment for sports and/or other physical activities (e.g. helmets for biking or skateboarding)?
Is there any violence in your home? Does the violence ever get physical?
Is there a lot of violence at your school? In your neighbourhood? Among your friends?
Have you ever been physically or sexually abused? Have you ever been raped, on a date or at any other time? (If not asked previously)
Have you ever been in a car or motorcycle accident? (What happened?)
Have you ever been picked on or bullied? Is that still a problem?
Have you been in physical fights in school or your neighbourhood? Are you still getting into fights?
Have you ever felt that you had to carry a knife, gun or other weapon to protect yourself? Do you still feel that way?

Green = essential questions
Blue = as time permits
Red = optional or when situation requires

FIGURE 8.4 The HEEADSSS psychosocial interview for adolescents
Source: Royal Children's Hospital 2019[6]

peer-related **A**ctivities
Drugs
Sexuality
Suicide/depression
Safety from injury and violence.

The tool minimises adolescent stress because it moves from expected and less threatening questions to those that are more personal. The tool presents the questions in three colours:

- **Green questions** are considered essential to explore with every adolescent.
- **Blue questions** are important for you to ask if time permits.
- **Red questions** delve more deeply if the situation demands it.

Parents do not need to be present during a HEEADSSS assessment. Ask the young person if they would prefer to be assessed without a parent present. The other areas for health history can be adapted from the adult section described above.

Clinical reasoning and documentation

The following is a continuation of the case study provided at the beginning of this chapter.

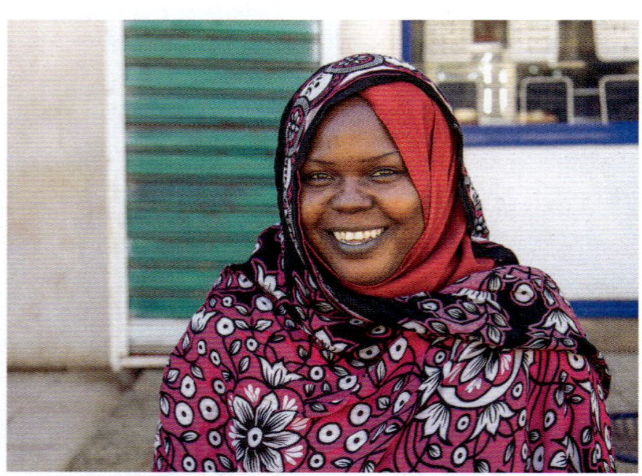

Case study (continued)—Approach to collecting a health history

Context

You will recall from the case study described earlier in the chapter that you are on clinical placement in a subacute rehabilitation ward. Your preceptor (buddy) nurse tells you he is expecting a new patient admission to the ward shortly after the afternoon handover. He asks you to prepare to be involved in completing the ward admission assessment for this woman, who you will be meeting for the first time.

Consider the patient's situation

You have limited information about the new patient. Mrs Nyamal Bol is a 55-year-old woman who is undergoing rehabilitation following a car accident 3 days ago. She sustained a fractured right wrist, which has been internally fixed with a plate and screw, and she has a plaster cast from her fingers to her elbow. She also sustained a dislocated fractured ankle, which has been fixed with screws and plates, and she is now wearing an orthopaedic boot. She has extensive bruising and minor cuts. Mrs Bol is a South Sudanese–Australian who arrived in Australia as a refugee 8 years ago with her husband and five children. You are told that Mrs Bol speaks some English.

Collect cues/information

Consider the following:

- How has your plan for collecting subjective data (the health history) with Mrs Bol changed after reading the chapter and accessing the additional resources or references?
- How would your plan for collecting the health history change if the person was:
  - a child?
  - deaf?
  - unable to answer your questions?
  - unable to cooperate?
  - very fatigued?

ADDITIONAL RESOURCES

You can further develop your knowledge and skills relevant to collecting a health history by:

- reading chapters of a fundamentals of nursing or medical-surgical nursing textbook
- answering chapter multiple choice questions online. Log onto ClinicalKey Student and search for the text 'Health Assessment, 4th edition'. Choose the section titled 'Teaching material'. In this section you will find question and answer documents for each chapter.
- visiting websites

  Advance Care Planning Australia—Appointing a substitute or medical treatment decision-maker (medical power of attorney): https://www.advancecareplanning.org.au/law-and-ethics/state-and-territory-laws

  HEEADSSS Assessment learning video resource—NSW Health: https://www.health.nsw.gov.au/kidsfamilies/youth/Pages/heeadsss-videos.aspx

  Royal Australian College of General Practitioners—Resources to support health checks for Aboriginal and Torres Straight Islander people: https://www.racgp.org.au/the-racgp/faculties/aboriginal-and-torres-strait-islander-health/guides/2019-mbs-item-715-health-check-templates

REFERENCES

1. Australian Commission on Safety and Quality in Health Care. Correct identification and procedure matching. Available at: https://www.safetyandquality.gov.au/standards/nsqhs-standards/communicating-safety-standard/correct-identification-and-procedure-matching/action-605
2. National Comprehensive Cancer Network. NCCN Distress thermometer. Version 2.2023. Available at: https://www.nccn.org/docs/default-source/patient-resources/nccn_distress_thermometer.pdf?sfvrsn=ef1df1a2_4
3. Katz S, Ford AB, Moskowitz RW, Jackson BA, Jaffe MW. Studies of illness in the aged. The index of ADL; a standardized measure of biological and psychosocial function. JAMA 1963;185:914–919.
4. Mahoney FI, Barthel DW. Functional evaluation: the Barthel Index. Maryland State Medical Journal 1965;14:61–65.
5. Talley NJ, O'Connor S, editors. Talley and O'Connor's clinical examination: a guide to specialty examinations. 9th ed. Chatswood: Elsevier; 2021.
6. Royal Children's Hospital. Engaging with and assessing the adolescent patient. 2019. Available at: https://www.rch.org.au/clinicalguide/guideline_index/engaging_with_and_assessing_the_adolescent_patient/

CHAPTER 9

Physical examination techniques

Written by Carolyn Jarvis
Adapted by Elizabeth Watt

INTRODUCTION

The health history described in the preceding chapter provides **subjective** data for health assessment, the person's perception of their current health state and their past health history. The next part of data collection involves using your senses—sight, smell, touch and hearing—to gather health assessment data during a physical examination—inspection, palpation, percussion and auscultation. Because you need to be in close physical contact with the person being examined, a fundamental part of physical examinations is preventing healthcare-associated infections.

Case study

In the previous chapter you considered your approach to collecting subjective data (the health history) from Mrs Bol. In this chapter you will be considering and planning the techniques you will use to undertake a physical examination (objective data).

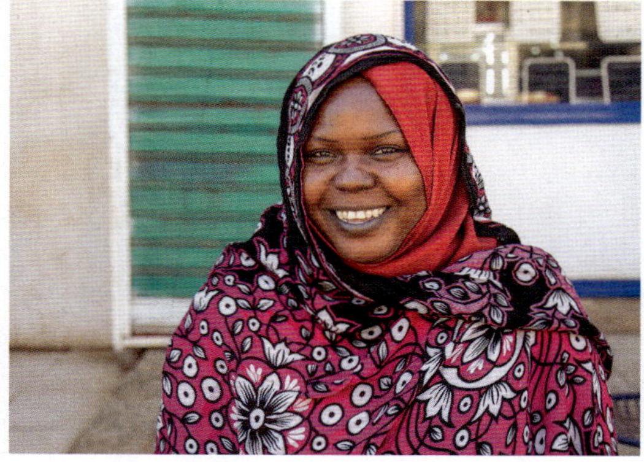

Context

You will recall from the previous chapter that you are on clinical placement in a subacute rehabilitation ward. Your preceptor (buddy) nurse tells you he is expecting a new patient admission to the ward shortly after the afternoon handover. He asks you to prepare to be involved in completing the ward admission assessment for this woman, who you will be meeting for the first time.

Consider the patient's situation

You have limited information about the new patient. Mrs Nyamal Bol is a 55-year-old woman who is undergoing rehabilitation following a car accident 3 days ago. She sustained a fractured right wrist, which has been internally fixed with a plate and screw, and she has a plaster cast from her fingers to her elbow. She also sustained a dislocated fractured ankle, which has been fixed with screws and plates, and she is now wearing an orthopaedic boot. She has extensive bruising and minor cuts. Mrs Bol is a South Sudanese–Australian who arrived in Australia as a refugee 8 years ago with her husband and five children. You are told that Mrs Bol speaks some English.

Questions to further your learning

- What are the possible things that might be going on with Mrs Bol?
- What physical examination techniques (objective data) will you use?
- What preparation would you make to undertake a physical examination?
- What resources are available to you to assist you in your physical examination of Mrs Bol?

Assessment plan

The data you obtain from physical examination includes specimen screening and assessment findings obtained from other healthcare team members. Also, findings from blood tests and diagnostic imaging will add to the **objective** dataset. The techniques used in physical examination are **inspection** (looking), **palpation** (feeling), **percussion** (tapping) and **auscultation** (listening). They are performed systematically, one at a time, and usually in this order except for abdominal assessment—see Chapter 23. In most cases, the subjective data you collect will guide your plan for gathering objective data.

Resources available

You will find additional resources and a reference list at the end of this chapter. There is a series of videos that accompany this text that show physical examination techniques applied to specific assessments. These are vital sign measurement, neurological assessment, cardiac assessment, respiratory assessment and abdominal assessment. You will find a QR code in each relevant chapter that will enable you to access the particular video easily on your device.

Preventing healthcare-associated infections

Physical examination requires the examiner to touch the person's skin and to use equipment to assist in hearing sounds or measuring body processes. Any direct contact with the person or their immediate environment requires healthcare workers to take deliberate steps to avoid possible transmission of infection between people or between the person and the nurse. A **nosocomial** infection (an infection acquired in a healthcare facility) is a hazard because healthcare facilities such as hospitals have sites that are possible reservoirs for virulent microorganisms. Some of these microorganisms have become resistant to most antibiotics (multi-resistant organisms) such as methicillin-resistant *Staphylococcus aureus* and vancomycin-resistant *Enterococcus*.

The single most important step to decrease risk of healthcare-associated infection is **hand hygiene**. Hospitals, clinics and other healthcare facilities have dispensers mounted on walls outside every person's room or bed area and at each person's bedside (Figure 9.1). Healthcare workers working in the community will carry a container of hand hygiene solution with their other clinical equipment. Following the COVID-19 epidemic, most people will be aware of using a waterless, quick-drying, alcohol-based solution for hand cleansing. In healthcare settings, it is used before you have any contact with the person, their bed linen or belongings; before a procedure, after touching a person or their surroundings (including curtains surrounding a bed); and after a procedure or where there is any risk that you were exposed to body fluids.[1] You can use an alcohol-based hand rub in most situations where your hands are not visibly soiled.

You will need to wash hands with soap and water after inadvertent contact with blood, body fluids, secretions and excretions; after contact with any equipment contaminated with body fluid; or when gloves have not been worn when caring for a patient who has *Clostridioides difficile* because the bacterium's spores are not killed by the hand hygiene solutions.[1] There are several other organisms that are not killed by alcohol-based hand rubs including some viruses such as rotavirus and

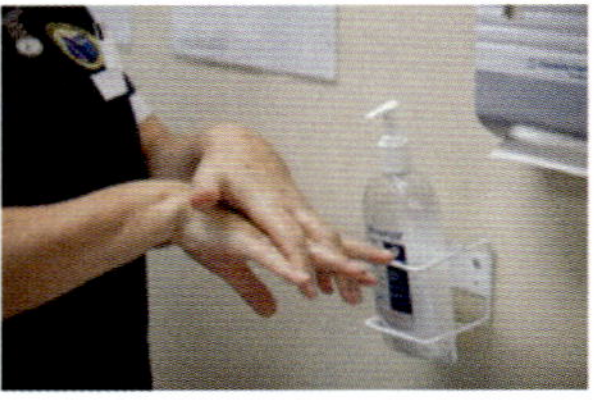

FIGURE 9.1 Hand hygiene
Reproduced from: https://healthywa.wa.gov.au/Articles/F_I/Facts-about-hand-hygiene

norovirus (non-enveloped viruses), tropical parasites and protozoan oocysts, and therefore handwashing with soap and water is preferred.[1] See the websites of the Australian Commission on Safety and Quality in Health Care and Hand Hygiene Australia for up-to-date information about hand hygiene practices and an online learning package (in resources section at the end of the chapter).

Wear disposable gloves when the potential exists for contact with any body fluids (e.g. blood, urine, faeces, mucous membranes, drainage, open skin lesions). However, routine hand hygiene should always be performed before putting on gloves and after removing gloves.[1]

The Australian Guidelines for the Prevention and Control of Infection in Health Care[2] describe important aspects of infection prevention and control. A significant part of the guidelines describes a two-tiered approach involving effective work practices that minimise the risk of selection and transmission of infectious agents.[2]

Standard precautions (Table 9.1) relate to the routine application of basic infection control strategies to minimise risk to patients and healthcare workers such as hand

TABLE 9.1 Standard and transmission-based infection control precautions relevant to health assessment

Please note: The information in this table has been adapted from the Australian Guidelines for the Prevention and Control of Infection in Healthcare.[2] Only the information specifically relevant to health assessment has been included. For the complete guidelines document see the bibliography at the end of the chapter. Similar information is available on the Health Quality and Safety Commission New Zealand.[3]

Standard precautions

Standard precautions are applied regardless of known or suspected pathogens being transmitted via the contact, droplet or airborne route.

It is recommended that healthcare workers have short nails, do not wear rings and other jewellery on their hands or wrists and do not wear artificial fingernails or nail polish. These factors decrease the effectiveness of hand hygiene and increase the incidence of infectious agents on the skin, nails and under jewellery. Cuts on the hands should be covered with waterproof dressings.

Hand hygiene

1. It is recommended that routine hand hygiene is performed before and after every episode of contact. This includes the '5 moments of hand hygiene':
    - before touching a person
    - before a procedure
    - after a procedure or body substance exposure risk
    - after touching a person
    - after touching the person's surroundings.
2. Hand hygiene should also be performed:
    - when arriving at or leaving the clinical environment
    - before and after eating/handling food/drinks
    - before and after using a computer keyboard, tablet or mobile device in a clinical area
    - being in patient-care areas during outbreaks of infection
    - before putting on gloves and after the removal of gloves
    - after visiting the toilet
    - after blowing/wiping/touching the nose or mouth
    - after handling laundry/equipment/waste.

Continued

TABLE 9.1 Standard and transmission-based infection control precautions relevant to health assessment cont'd

3. Use alcohol-based hand rubs that contain between 60% and 80% v/v ethanol or equivalent for routine hand hygiene.
4. If hands are visibly soiled, hand hygiene should be performed using soap and water.
   - Wet hands under warm running water and apply the recommended amount of liquid soap.
   - Rub hands together for a minimum of 20 seconds so the solution comes into contact with all surfaces of the hand, paying particular attention to the tips of the fingers, the thumbs and the areas between the fingers.
   - Rinse hands thoroughly under running water, then pat dry with single-use towels.
5. Hand hygiene for known or suspected *Clostridioides difficile* and non-enveloped viruses such as norovirus should be performed as follows:
   - If gloves have not been worn, if gloves have been breached or if there is visible contamination of the hands despite glove use, use soap and water to facilitate the mechanical removal of spores. After washing, hands should be dried thoroughly with a single-use towel.
   - If gloves have been worn, a lower density of contamination of the hands would be expected and alcohol-based hand rub remains the agent of choice for hand hygiene.

Personal protective equipment

When personal protective equipment is used as part of standard precautions, it protects against the risk of anticipated blood and body fluid exposure.
Note: Follow the current additional guidelines and organisational policy for using personal protective equipment for protecting against COVID-19 or other airborne diseases. In addition, the following apply.

1. Masks/face shields and eye protection should be worn during procedures that generate splashes or sprays of blood and body substances into the face and eyes.
2. Aprons or gowns should:
   - be appropriate to the task being undertaken
   - be worn for a single procedure or episode of care and removed in the area where the episode of care takes place
   - should be removed after use in the area where the episode of care takes place.
3. Single-use, fit-for-purpose gloves are worn for:
   - each invasive procedure
   - contact with sterile sites and non-intact skin or mucous membranes
   - any activity that has been assessed as carrying a risk of exposure to blood and body substances.
4. Hand hygiene should be performed before putting on gloves and after removing gloves.
5. Gloves must be changed between patients and after every episode of individual patient care.

Use and management of sharps, safety engineered devices and medication vials

1. Appropriate use of devices (single-use items such as blood glucose monitoring lancets/needles)
   - Use safety engineered devices with built-in safety features where available (e.g. a retractable safety device on sharps).
   - Use for one patient only and for one occasion only.
   - Immediately dispose of the item into an approved sharps container at the point of use.
   - Sharps containers must not be filled above the mark that indicates the maximum fill level.

TABLE 9.1 Standard and transmission-based infection control precautions relevant to health assessment cont'd

Routine environmental cleaning

1. Cleaning of shared clinical equipment (trolleys, stethoscopes, axillary temperature monitoring probes, blood pressure cuffs, etc.)
   - Shared clinical equipment should be cleaned with detergent solution after each use.
   - Disposable equipment, including thermometers and blood pressure cuffs, should be used when caring for people requiring contact precautions (e.g. those with *Clostridioides difficile*).
2. Management of blood or other body substance spills

   Strategies for decontaminating spills of blood and other body substances (e.g. vomit, urine) differ based on the setting in which they occur and the volume of the spill (a spill kit should be available in the clinical area). In general:
   - use personal protective equipment
   - healthcare workers can manage small spills by cleaning with detergent solution
   - for spills containing large amounts of blood or other body substances, workers should contain and confine the spill by:
     - removing visible organic matter with absorbent material (e.g. disposable paper towels)
     - removing any broken glass or sharp material with forceps
     - soaking up excess liquid using an absorbent clumping agent (e.g. absorbent granules).
   - Hand hygiene should be performed after the clean-up.

Respiratory hygiene and cough etiquette

1. Anyone with signs and symptoms of a respiratory infection, regardless of the cause, should follow or be instructed to follow respiratory hygiene and cough etiquette as follows:
   - cover the nose/mouth with disposable single-use tissues when coughing, sneezing, wiping and blowing noses
   - use tissues to contain respiratory secretions
   - dispose of tissues in the nearest waste receptacle or bin after use
   - if no tissues are available, cough or sneeze into the inner elbow rather than the hand
   - practise hand hygiene after contact with respiratory secretions and contaminated objects/materials
   - keep contaminated hands away from the mucous membranes of the mouth, eyes and nose
   - in healthcare facilities, patients with symptoms of respiratory infections should sit as far away from others as possible; if available, healthcare facilities may place these patients in a separate area while waiting for care
   - healthcare workers with viral respiratory tract infections should remain at home until their symptoms have resolved.

Transmission-based precautions

Transmission-based precautions are used **in addition** to standard precautions, where the suspected or confirmed presence of infectious agents represents an increased risk of transmission by the contact, droplet or airborne routes. **Note:** Follow the current additional guidelines and organisational policy for using personal protective equipment for protecting against COVID-19 or other airborne diseases.

Contact precautions

Direct transmission—infectious agents are transferred from one person to another person without a contaminated intermediate object or person. For example, blood or other body substances from an infectious person may come into contact with a mucous membrane or breaks in the skin of another person.

Continued

TABLE 9.1 Standard and transmission-based infection control precautions relevant to health assessment cont'd

Indirect transmission—involves the transfer of an infectious agent through a contaminated intermediate object (fomite) or person. Examples include contaminated hands of healthcare workers, contaminated clothing or environmental surfaces.

1. When working with people who require contact precautions:
   Before going to the patient's bedside:
   - perform hand hygiene
   - put on gown/plastic apron (if required)
   - put on a mask
   - put on protective eye wear and/or face shield
   - put on gloves
   - take care to ensure clothing and skin do not contact potentially contaminated environmental surfaces.

   After leaving the patient's bedside (as close as possible to the patient care area):
   - remove gloves
   - perform hand hygiene
   - remove gown/plastic apron (if worn)
   - remove protective eyewear or face shield—perform hand hygiene if mask or eyewear is contaminated
   - remove mask—without touching the front of the mask; discard in waste container
   - perform hand hygiene using alcohol hand rub
   - keep patient room doors closed where safe to do so (this may not be possible for patients requiring high visualisation)
   - make sure rooms are clearly signed with appropriate directions for the level of potential infection risk
   - patient-dedicated equipment or single-use patient-care equipment to be used for patients on contact precautions.

Droplet precautions

In addition to standard precautions, implement droplet precautions for patients known or suspected to be infected with agents transmitted by respiratory droplets that are generated by a person when coughing, sneezing or talking.

1. Hand hygiene as described in the standard precautions section above.
2. Use personal protective equipment (including a mask) when entering a patient-care environment (and hand hygiene before putting on the mask and following removal of the mask). Follow local guidelines on the type of mask that is required.
3. Where possible, patients who require droplet precautions should be placed in a single-occupancy room.

Airborne precautions

In addition to standard precautions, implement airborne precautions for patients known or suspected to be infected with infectious agents transmitted person-to-person by the airborne route (e.g. COVID-19, measles, chickenpox [varicella] and *Mycobacterium tuberculosis*). **Note:** In certain circumstances, patients may need to wear personal protective equipment to protect themselves or protect healthcare staff.

1. Standard precautions, including respiratory hygiene and cough etiquette.
2. Wear a correctly fitted P2/N95 respirator when entering the patient-care area when an airborne-transmissible infectious agent is known or suspected to be present.
3. Minimise exposure of other patients and staff members to the infectious agent.

TABLE 9.1 Standard and transmission-based infection control precautions relevant to health assessment cont'd

Multi-resistant organisms and outbreak situations
Multi-resistant organisms include methicillin-resistant *Staphylococcus aureus*, vancomycin-resistant *Enterococcus* and multi-resistant Gram-negative bacteria.
1. Applying standard precautions, including hand hygiene, is the most effective measure to prevent and control the spread of multi-resistant organisms. 2. Applying transmission-based and contact-based precautions should be considered for all patients colonised or infected with a multi-resistant organism including: • performing hand hygiene and putting on gloves and gowns before entering the patient-care area • using patient-dedicated or single-use non-critical patient-care equipment • using a single-patient room or, if unavailable, cohorting patients with the same strain of multi-resistant organism in designated patient-care areas (upon approval from the healthcare facility's infection control team) • ensuring consistent cleaning and disinfection of surfaces in close proximity to the patient and those likely to be touched by the patient and healthcare workers.

hygiene, personal protective equipment, cleaning and appropriate handling of equipment and disposal of sharps.[2]

The second-tier infection control strategy involves extra work practices in situations where standard precautions alone are not enough to prevent transmission. These are known as **transmission-based precautions**. These involve interventions that interrupt the mode of transmission of infections—droplet precautions, airborne precautions depending on the infective agent. Examples of such precautions include isolation of a person, wearing specific personal protective equipment and having specific equipment for that person only.[2]

Performing a physical examination

Context

Often nurses are conducting health assessments in busy ward or clinic situations, which are noisy and lack privacy. However, where possible, the setting for the physical examination should be warm and comfortable, quiet, private and well lit. Try to eliminate any distracting noises—such as humming machinery, radio or television or people talking—that could make it difficult to hear body sounds. If the assessment is to take place in a multi-bed ward area, pull the curtains around the bed to minimise interruptions from other healthcare personnel or visitors and to ensure privacy. In the home environment, you may need to ask the person to lie down on their bed or a couch, but still ensure their privacy from other household members unless they particularly ask for another person to be present. Lighting with natural daylight is best, although it is often not available; try to position an artificial light source to prevent silhouettes.

Where possible, position the bed or examination table so both sides of the person are easily accessible. In the hospital setting, the bed should be at a height at which you can stand without stooping and should be equipped to raise the person's upper body up to 45 degrees. If the examination is being conducted in the person's home, you may need to kneel beside a bed or couch to be in a position that protects your neck and back from being in a bent or stooped position for any length of time.

Equipment

You need to plan what equipment you are likely to need to perform the physical examination. The equipment used will depend on the purpose of the examination—for example, complete health assessment of all body systems or the focus of a specific area for assessment (e.g. focused neurological assessment). Each chapter outlines the specific equipment required for the areas being assessed and it is described as it comes into use throughout the text.

In a situation where you will be using several pieces of equipment during the physical examination, designate a 'clean' versus a 'used' area for handling of your equipment. In a ward or clinic setting, use a metal dressing trolley, the top surface for the clean equipment and the bottom shelf for the used equipment surface. A waste bag or container can be attached for disposal of single use equipment such as tongue blades and gloves. In a home situation, it can be challenging finding an uncluttered surface nearby the person at an appropriate height. Whatever surface is chosen, it needs to be free of clutter and cleaned with an appropriate surface disinfectant before putting any equipment on it. All equipment that is suitable to be reused must be cleaned according to infection control guidelines after use.

Establishing rapport and gaining consent

You need to make every contact with the person effective because it can set the tone for the relationship you have with the person in the future and the person's experience of health care. Effective communication between healthcare workers and the recipient of care is fundamental to person-centred care, quality care and patient safety. Good communication fosters positive relationships and trust, encourages a two-way exchange of information, engages the person and their family in shared decision making, as well as reducing errors, misdiagnosis and inappropriate treatment.[4] An important start to effective communication is introducing yourself to the person with your name and your position (clinical nurse, nursing student, etc.). For a more detailed discussion about the importance of communication, see Chapter 7.

Hopefully you have established rapport with the person while you are collecting subjective data—the health history. As you progress to objective data collection, you need to make sure the person understands the purpose of the physical examination and the types and extent of examination that will be performed. Be detailed about what you are going to be doing and that you will stop if they ask you to. Make sure you express yourself in a way that the person understands. If English is not their first language, ensure an appropriate interpreter is available if needed. Inform yourself of their specific cultural needs related to physical examination.

The person cannot give you informed consent unless they understand the purpose and extent of the examination. In some circumstances, the person may prefer to have another person (another health professional, a friend or family member) present during the examination. Note this in the person's medical record. In all other cases, additional family or friends should be asked to wait outside until the examination is completed.

There are many people for whom physical examination and health screening may be a confronting experience. For example, a person who has experienced sexual or any other kind of abuse, a person who is neurodiverse, a person with a cognitive, neurological, sensory or physical disability, an Indigenous person, a refugee newly arrived in the country, or a transgender or gender diverse person. Many trans and gender diverse people have had previous experience of discrimination, misgendering and disrespectful communication, often avoiding contact with health professionals and missing important health screening.[5,6] Your approach to the person is critical in gaining their trust, including asking the person if there are any terms they prefer for their body parts, ensure they understand what is going to happen and why, and continuously reconfirming consent to touch them in a new location.[7]

General approach

People in a hospital environment probably expect nurses and other health professionals to 'assess' their health. However, as stated previously, before you start you need to make sure they understand the extent and purpose of any physical examination. The person may be anxious; therefore, you need to approach the assessment with this in mind, telling them what you are doing, giving them feedback on your findings as you go and frequently checking with them that they are comfortable.

You need to feel comfortable with your physical assessment skills before you can absorb what you are seeing, feeling or hearing in a 'real' clinical situation. Confidence comes with practice under the guidance of an experienced mentor in a simulated situation, in an atmosphere in which it is acceptable to make mistakes and to ask questions. Using simulation with a mannequin or a fellow student or colleague can help you learn to deal with the 'real' clinical situation while still in a safe setting. To reinforce your learning, the skills need repeated practice.

After you feel more confident performing the skills in the simulation/skills laboratory setting, you will be ready to undertake a health assessment on a person who is seeking health care. Don't be afraid to ask your preceptor, buddy nurse or clinical facilitator for feedback so you can improve the accuracy of your physical examination skills and your interpretation of the findings. Always seek clarification if you are unsure about a finding in the clinical setting or if you are concerned about the person's health state.

Techniques of a physical examination

As stated previously, the techniques required for physical examination are **inspection** (looking), **palpation** (feeling), **percussion** (tapping) and **auscultation** (listening). They are performed systematically, one at a time and usually in this order except for abdominal assessment—see Chapter 23. Table 9.2 (later in the chapter) summarises the four physical examination techniques.

Inspection

Inspection is close, careful scrutiny, first of the whole person (**general inspection**) and then of each body area/system (**detailed inspection**). Inspection begins the moment you first meet the person and develop a 'general survey' (specific data to consider for the general survey are presented in the following chapter). Inspection is always the

TABLE 9.2 Summary of commonly used physical assessment techniques

Technique	Approach	Assessment focus	Notes
Inspection: Detailed and purposive observation	• General inspection or general survey • Detailed inspection of each body part/area—see each chapter for full description	• Physical appearance (age, sex, level of consciousness, skin colour, face, overall appearance, body odour) • Body structure (stature, nutrition, symmetry, posture) • Mobility (gait, range of motion) • Behaviour (facial expression, mood and affect, speech, speech pattern, personal hygiene)	Compare each side of the body, determine symmetry
Palpation: Use of touch Compare both sides of the body Use of slow and systematic movements	• Surface palpation (e.g. a joint)	• Texture • Temperature • Moisture Presence of: • tenderness or pain • crepitation of joints • swelling	The dorsa (backs) of hands and fingers Fingertips
	• Light palpation (only used in abdominal examination)	Presence of: • tenderness or pain • lumps or masses (e.g. faecal loading, distended urinary bladder) • swelling • vibration or pulsation	Base of fingers (metacarpophalangeal joints) Ulnar surface of the hand—best for vibration
Percussion: Tapping the person's skin and underlying structures with short, sharp strokes	• Indirect (most commonly used in abdominal examination)	• Signaling the density (air, fluid or solid) of a structure by a characteristic note • Detecting a mass or structure if it is fairly superficial (e.g. a distended bladder above the symphysis pubis)	The striking hand contacts the stationary hand fixed on the person's skin Sound described as: resonant, hyper-resonant, tympany, dull or flat (Table 9.3)
Auscultation: Listening to sounds produced by the body usually with a stethoscope	• Systematic sequence • Compare both sides of the body	• Bowel sounds • Breath sounds • Heart sounds	Use diaphragm of the stethoscope Avoid listening over clothing

first assessment technique you will use during physical examination. You can begin your general survey when you first meet the person and continue while you are talking with them about their health history. Then, as you move through each relevant body area/system you will also begin with a detailed inspection (an outline of the areas for inspection will be presented in each chapter). A detailed inspection takes time and yields a surprising amount of data.

Learn to use each person as their own control and compare the right and left sides of the body. The two sides are nearly symmetrical. Inspection requires good lighting and adequate exposure of the body part being assessed. In some circumstances, you need to use equipment (an otoscope, penlight torch, etc.) to enhance your own sense of vision.

Palpation

Palpation involves using touch during physical examination and usually follows detailed inspection of the specific body part or area. Palpation is used to assess texture, temperature, moisture, organ location and size, as well as any swelling, vibration or pulsation, rigidity, crepitation of joints, presence of lumps or masses and presence of tenderness or pain. Different parts of the hands are best suited for assessing different factors. See Table 9.2.

Practice note

You should always attend to hand hygiene before touching the person and at the end of the physical examination,[2] but it is not necessary to use gloves every time you perform palpation. Throughout the subsequent chapters you will be prompted about when it is necessary to use gloves. You should be guided by standard infection control precautions (Table 9.1) and hospital or healthcare agency policy.

Your palpation technique should be slow and systematic. A person may stiffen when touched suddenly, making it difficult for you to feel very much. Use a calm, gentle approach and inform the person about what you are going to do to them and why. Warm your hands by rubbing them together or rinsing them under warm water. Identify any tender areas and palpate them last.

There are three palpation techniques: surface palpation, light palpation and bimanual palpation.

- **Surface palpation** involves using the gentle pressure from the finger pads of your dominant hand. You need to place the flattened finger pads onto the skin surface (keeping the fingers together) and apply gentle pressure to the body surface (approximately 1–2 cm deep, depending on the part of the body being assessed) while moving the fingers in a gentle, slow, circular motion. Move the hand and cover the entire surface to be examined, noting the findings as you progress. Always start with surface palpation to detect surface characteristics. For example, you would use surface palpation to assess swelling, crepitation, range of movement and pain in an injured joint.
- **Light palpation** follows surface palpation and is usually only performed as part of abdominal assessment. The technique for light palpation is like surface palpation, but the skin surface is more deeply depressed with the fingers. The actual depth of light palpation largely depends on the amount of abdominal fat the person has. For a person with a normal body mass index, you may only need to palpate to a depth of 2.5 cm to evaluate abdominal contents, whereas for a person who is obese you may have to palpate to a depth of 5 cm to be able to evaluate abdominal contents. When light palpation is needed (as for

abdominal examination), intermittent pressure is better than one long continuous palpation. You should not progress from surface to light palpation when the person complains of pain or when traumatic abdominal injury is suspected, as you could cause further pain or even injury to the person. You should always refer the person to a medical practitioner when you detect significant abdominal pain or discomfort on light palpation.

- **Bimanual palpation** requires using both of your hands to envelop or capture certain body parts or organs—such as the spleen, liver, kidneys, uterus, ovaries—for more precise examination of the size and shape. This technique is usually only performed by nurses working in advanced practice roles.

Percussion

Percussion involves tapping the person's skin with short, sharp strokes to assess underlying structures. The strokes yield a palpable vibration and a characteristic sound that depicts the location, size and density of the underlying structure or organ.

Percussion has the following uses:

- mapping out the **location** and **size** of an organ or structure by exploring where the percussion note changes between the borders of an organ and the adjacent structures—for example, location of a distended (overfilled) bladder in the lower abdomen or the presence of faecal loading in the colon
- signalling the **density** (air, fluid or solid) of a structure by a characteristic note
- eliciting pain if the underlying structure is inflamed, as with maxillary sinus areas or over a kidney
- eliciting a deep tendon reflex using the percussion hammer.

Two methods of percussion can be used—**direct** and **indirect**. The technique of direct percussion involves the striking hand directly contacting the body wall, producing a sound. However, indirect percussion is the technique most used in a nursing health assessment and involves using both hands, most commonly in abdominal assessment. The striking hand contacts the stationary hand fixed on the person's skin. This yields a sound and a subtle vibration. The procedure of indirect percussion is as follows.

THE STATIONARY HAND

Hyperextend the middle finger and/or index finger of your non-dominant hand and place the distal portion, the phalanx and distal interphalangeal joint *firmly* against the person's skin—for example, over the abdominal skin. Avoid the person's ribs and scapulae. Percussing over a bone yields no data because it always sounds 'dull'. Lift the rest of the stationary hand (fingertips, other fingers, thumb and heel of the hand) off the person's skin (Figure 9.2), otherwise the resting hand will dampen off the produced vibrations, just as a drummer uses the hand to halt a drum roll.

THE STRIKING HAND

Use the middle finger of your dominant hand as the *striking finger* (Figure 9.3). Hold your forearm close to the skin surface, with your upper arm and shoulder steady. Scan your muscles to make sure they are steady but not rigid. The action is all in the wrist, and it *must* be relaxed. Spread your fingers, move from the wrist in a hammer-like motion and bounce your middle finger off the stationary one. Aim for just behind the nail bed or at the distal interphalangeal joint; the goal is to hit the portion of the finger that is pushing the hardest into the skin surface. Flex the striking finger so its tip, not the finger pad, makes contact. It hits directly at right angles to the stationary finger.

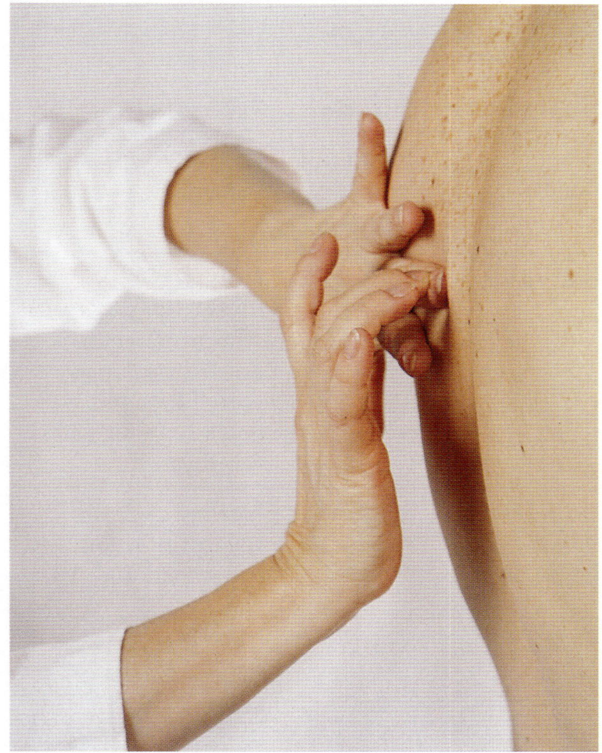

FIGURE 9.2 Percussion technique.

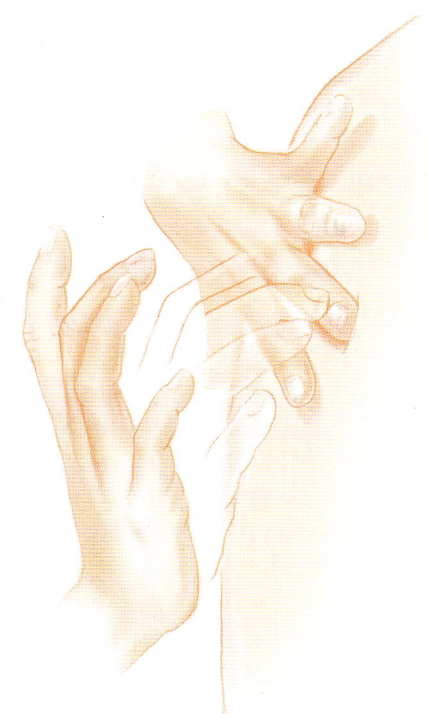

FIGURE 9.3 Percussion technique showing the striking finger

Percuss two times in this location using even, staccato blows. Lift the striking finger off quickly; a resting finger damps off vibrations. Then move to a new body location and repeat, keeping your technique even. The force of the blow determines the loudness of the note. You do not need a very loud sound; use just enough force to achieve a clear note. The thickness of the person's body wall will be a factor. You will need a stronger percussion stroke for people with obese or very muscular body walls.

Percussion can be an awkward technique for beginning examiners. You may feel surprised and embarrassed if your striking finger misses your stationary hand completely. It will hurt if your nails are too long. As with all new skills, refinement follows practice. After a few weeks your hand placement becomes precise and feels natural, and your ears learn to perceive the subtle difference in percussion notes.

PRODUCTION OF SOUND

All sound results from vibration of some structure (Figure 9.4). Percussing over a body structure causes vibrations that produce characteristic waves and are heard as 'notes' (Table 9.3). Each of the five percussion notes is differentiated by the following components:

- **Amplitude** (or intensity), a loud or soft sound. The louder the sound, the greater the amplitude. Loudness depends on the force of the blow and the structure's ability to vibrate.
- **Pitch** (or frequency), the number of vibrations per second, written as 'cps' or cycles per second. More rapid vibrations

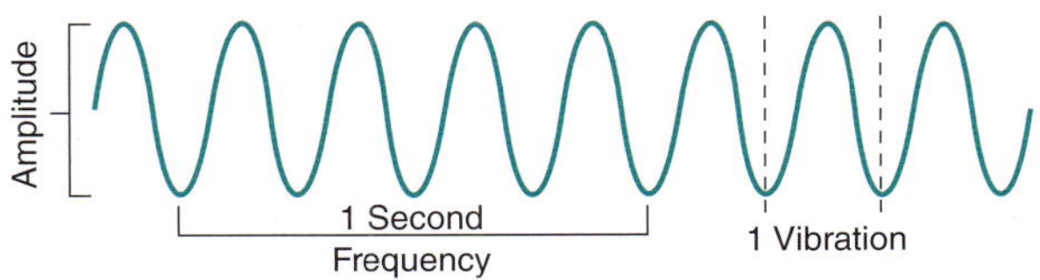

FIGURE 9.4 Percussion sound wave

TABLE 9.3 Characteristics of percussion sounds

Sound	Amplitude/ intensity	Pitch	Quality	Duration	Example location
Resonant	Medium–loud	Low	Clear, hollow	Moderate	Over normal lung tissue
Hyperresonant	Louder than resonant	Lower than resonant	Booming	Longer than resonant	Normal over child's lung Abnormal in the adult, over lungs with increased amount of air, as in emphysema
Tympany	Loud	High	Drum-like (like the kettle drum)	Sustained longest	Normal over the gastric air bubble or the intestine
Dull	Soft	High	Muffled thud	Short	Relatively dense organ, as liver or spleen

produce a high-pitched tone; slower vibrations yield a low-pitched tone.

- **Quality** (timbre), a subjective difference due to a sound's distinctive overtones. A pure tone is a sound of one frequency. Variations within a sound wave produce overtones. Overtones allow you to distinguish a C on a piano from a C on a violin.
- **Duration**, the length of time the note lingers.

A basic principle is that a structure with relatively more air (e.g. the lungs) produces a louder, deeper and longer sound because it vibrates freely, whereas a denser, more solid structure (e.g. the liver) gives a softer, higher, shorter sound because it does not vibrate as easily. Although Table 9.3 describes four 'normal' percussion notes, variations occur in clinical practice. The sound you hear will be affected by the thickness of the body wall, the nature of the underlying structure and your technique. The skill of recognising the various percussion sounds takes repeated practice. The percussion technique is used infrequently by nurses. Throughout the chapters you will be guided to when percussion needs to be performed, what percussion note you can expect to hear and how to interpret what you are hearing.

Auscultation

Auscultation is listening to sounds produced by the body such as the heart, the lungs and large bowel. You have probably already heard certain body sounds with your ear alone—for example, your stomach gurgling when you are hungry. Most body sounds are soft, and the stethoscope assists health professionals to listen to body sounds by blocking out extraneous ambient sounds.

The fit and quality of the stethoscope are important, and you are advised to purchase a quality instrument for your own personal use.

The slope of the earpiece should point forwards towards your nose. This matches the natural slope of your ear canal and efficiently blocks out environmental sound. If necessary, twist the earpieces to parallel the slope of your ear canals. The earpieces should fit snugly, but if they hurt, they are inserted too far. Adjust the tension and experiment with different rubber or plastic earplugs to achieve the most comfort. The tubing should be of thick material, with an internal diameter of 4 mm and about 36 to 46 cm long. Longer tubing may distort the sound.

The most common type of stethoscope used by nurses and other health professionals is one with two endpieces—a diaphragm and a bell (Figure 9.5). You will use the **diaphragm** most often because its flat edge is best for high-pitched sounds—breath, bowel and normal heart sounds. Hold the diaphragm firmly against the person's skin—firm enough to leave a slight ring afterwards.

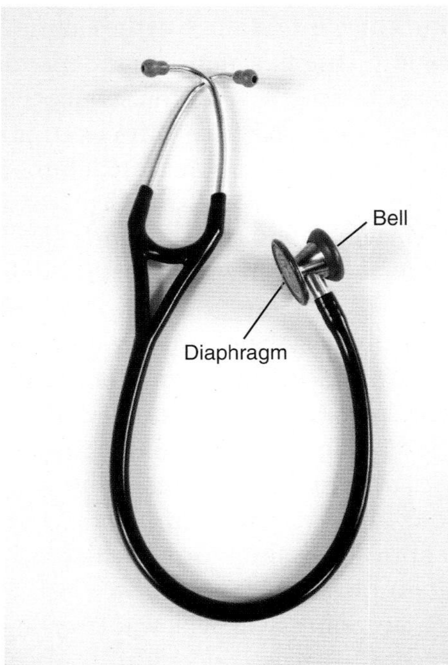

FIGURE 9.5 Stethoscope diaphragm (front) and bell (back)

The **bell** endpiece has a deep, hollow cup-like shape. It is best for soft, low-pitched sounds such as extra heart sounds or murmurs. Hold it lightly against the person's skin—just enough that it forms a perfect seal. Any harder causes the person's skin to act as a diaphragm, obliterating the low-pitched sounds.

Some stethoscopes have one endpiece with a 'tunable diaphragm'. This allows you to listen to both low- and high-frequency sounds without rotation of the endpiece. For low-frequency sounds (traditional bell mode), hold the endpiece very lightly on the skin; for high-frequency sounds (traditional diaphragm mode), press the diaphragm or bell firmly on the skin. This type of stethoscope is used in cardiac care settings to listen to heart sounds.

Before you can evaluate body sounds, you should attempt to eliminate or reduce ambient noise from the environment:

- Any extra room noise can produce a 'roaring' in your stethoscope, so the room should be as quiet as possible.
- When the diaphragm is placed on, for example, a man's hairy chest, you may hear a crackling sound that mimics an abnormal breath sound called *crackles*. Try to avoid the hairy areas as much as possible to reduce these sounds caused by friction.
- Never listen through clothing. Where possible ask the person to remove clothing. In situations where this is not possible you will need to place the stethoscope under the clothing to listen but take care that no clothing rubs on the stethoscope.
- Finally, avoid creating your own artifact sounds such as breathing on the tubing or the 'thump' from bumping the tubing together.

Practice note:

The diaphragm and bell of the stethoscope must be cleaned before and after use with a disposable alcohol-based disposable wipe or with a suitable detergent solution if the cuff or tubing needs cleansing.[2]

Warm the stethoscope by rubbing it in your palm (after hand hygiene has been performed) before placing it on the person's skin.

Auscultation is a skill that is difficult to master. First you must learn to recognise the wide range of normal sounds. Once you can recognise normal sounds, you can distinguish the abnormal sounds and 'extra' sounds. Be aware that in some body locations you may hear more than one sound; this can be confusing. You will need to listen selectively to only one thing at a time. As you listen, ask yourself: '*What am I actually hearing*?' and '*What should I be hearing at this spot*?' Throughout the chapters you will be guided as to where to place your stethoscope, what you can expect to hear through auscultation and how to interpret what you hear.

Beginning objective data collection

The extent and focus of a physical examination depends on the purpose and context of the assessment. In most situations, the extent and focus of the physical examination is directed by the person's presenting signs and symptoms and what they have already told you about their health concerns. Regardless of the purpose of the assessment, begin by measuring the person's temperature, heart rate, respirations, oxygen saturation and blood pressure (Chapter 10) and pain (Chapter 13). All of these are familiar, relatively nonthreatening actions; they will gradually accustom the person to the examination process. Make sure you perform hand hygiene in the person's presence before you start the examination. Explain each step in the examination and how the person can cooperate and confirm their consent to allow you to undertake the physical examination. Encourage the person to ask questions. Keep your own movements slow, methodical and deliberate.

The sequence of the steps may differ depending on the extent of the assessment, the age of the person and your own preference. Organise the steps so the person does not change positions too often and watch out for the person tiring—for example, listening to heart sounds and breath sounds one after the other. Providing rest breaks might be necessary for very sick, easily fatigued or frail older people. Although proper exposure is necessary, use additional drapes (e.g. a clean towel or bed sheet) to maintain the person's privacy and to prevent chilling.

Do not hesitate to write out the examination sequence and refer to it as you proceed. The person will accept this as quite natural if you explain you are making brief notations to ensure accuracy. Many healthcare organisations use a printed or digital form. You will find that you will glance at the form less and less as you gain experience. Even with a form, you sometimes may forget a step in the examination. When you realise this, perform the manoeuvre in the next logical place in the sequence.

As you proceed through the examination, occasionally offer some brief teaching about the person's body. For example, you might say, '*Everyone has two sounds for each heartbeat, something like this—lub-dub. Your own heart beats sound normal*'. Don't do this with every single step, or you will be hard pressed to make a comment when you do come across an abnormality. But some sharing of information builds rapport and increases the person's confidence in you as an examiner. It also gives the person a little more control in a situation in which it is easy to feel completely helpless.

At some point, you will want to linger in one location to concentrate on some complicated findings. To avoid anxiety, tell the person, for example, '*I always listen to bowel sounds on a few places on the abdomen. Just because I am listening for a long time does not necessarily mean anything is wrong with you*'. And it follows that sometimes you *will* discover a finding that may be abnormal and you want another examiner to double-check. You need to give the person some information, yet you should not alarm the person unnecessarily. Say something like, '*I do not have a complete assessment of your abdomen. I will ask another nurse to listen, too*'.

At the end of the examination, summarise your findings and share the necessary information with the person. Thank the person for the time spent. In a hospital setting, advise the person of what is scheduled next. Before you leave a hospitalised person, lower the bed; make the person comfortable and safe; put the call bell within reach; and return the bedside table, television or any equipment to the way it was originally. Perform hand hygiene before leaving the person's bed area.

Developmental considerations

Children are different from adults. Their difference in size is obvious. Their bodies grow in a predictable pattern that can be assessed during a physical examination. However, their behaviour is also different. Behaviour grows and develops through predictable stages, just as the body does. Each examiner needs to know the expected emotional and cognitive features of these stages and to perform the physical examination based on developmental principles.[8]

With all children, the goal is to increase their comfort in the setting. This approach reveals their natural state as much as possible and will give them a more positive memory of healthcare providers. Remember that a 'routine' examination is anything but routine to the child. You can increase their comfort by attending to the following developmental principles and approaches. The *order* of the developmental stages is more meaningful than the exact chronological age. Each child is an individual and will not fit exactly into one category. For example, if your efforts to 'play games' with a preschooler are rebuffed, modify your approach to the security measures used with a toddler.

Parents are an important part of the assessment process. Listening carefully to parents' concerns can alert you to possible health issues and they may identify early clinical deterioration sooner than you will.[8] Establishing rapport with parents is also important because they can help in the examination process (e.g. comforting and holding the child) and in gaining the trust of the child. You are also observing the interaction between the child and the parent, including eye contact, verbal communication, family dynamics, family connectedness and approach to problem solving.[9]

Infants (birth to 1 year)

Erikson[9] defines the major task of infancy as establishing trust. An infant is completely dependent on the parent for their basic needs. If these needs are met promptly and consistently, the infant feels secure and learns to trust others.

POSITION

- The parent/guardian should always be present for the child's feeling of security.
- Place the neonate or young infant flat on a padded examination table (Figure 9.6).

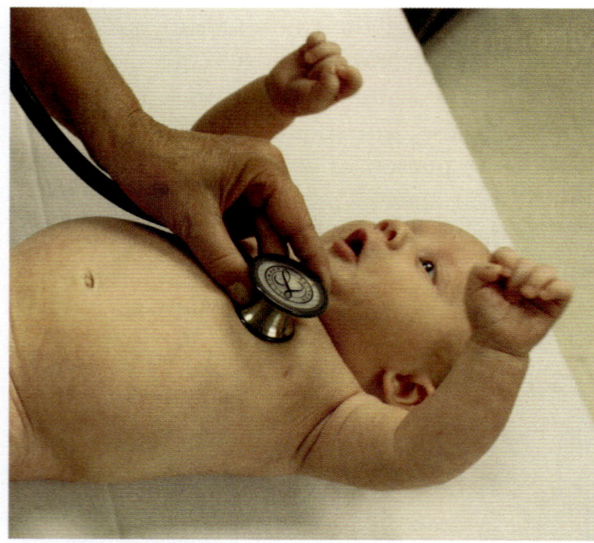

FIGURE 9.6 Baby and stethoscope.

The infant may also be held against the parent's chest if necessary.

- Once the baby can sit without support (around 6 months), as much of the examination as possible should be performed while the infant is in the parent's lap.
- By 9 to 12 months, the infant is acutely aware of the surroundings. Anything outside the infant's range of vision is 'lost', so the parent must be in full view.

PREPARATION

- Timing should be 1 to 2 hours after feeding, when the baby is not too drowsy or too hungry.
- Maintain a warm environment. A neonate may require an overhead radiant heater.
- Have the parent remove the child's outer clothing when necessary.
- Perform hand hygiene before touching the infant.
- Infants do not mind being touched, but make sure your hands and stethoscope endpiece are warm.
- Use a soft, crooning voice during the examination; babies respond more to the feeling in the tone of the voice than to what is said.
- Infants like eye contact; lock eyes from time to time.
- Smile; babies prefer a smiling face to a frowning one. Take time to play.
- Keep movements smooth and deliberate, not jerky.
- Offer brightly coloured toys for a distraction.

SEQUENCE (DEPENDS ON THE PURPOSE OF THE EXAMINATION)

- Seize the opportunity with a sleeping baby to listen to heart, lung and abdomen sounds first.
- Perform least distressing steps first. Save the invasive steps of examination of the eyes, ears, nose and throat until last.
- Elicit the Moro or 'startle' reflex at the *end* of the examination because it may cause the baby to cry.

Early childhood: toddlers (1–3 years)

This is Erikson's stage of developing autonomy.[10] However, the need to explore the world and be independent conflicts with the basic dependency on the parent. This often results in frustration and negativism. The toddler may be difficult to examine; do not take this personally. Since they are acutely aware of the new environment, the toddler may be frightened and cling to their parent. Also, toddlers are likely to be afraid of invasive procedures and dislike being restrained (Figure 9.7).

POSITION

- The toddler should be sitting up on the parent's lap for all the examination. When the toddler must be supine (as in the abdominal examination), move chairs to sit knee-to-knee with the parent. Have the toddler lie in the parent's lap with the toddler's legs in your lap.

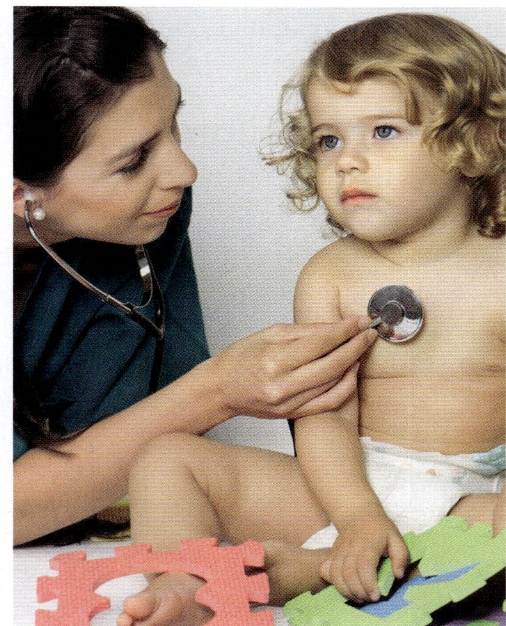

FIGURE 9.7 Toddler and stethoscope

- Gain the aid of a cooperative parent to help position the toddler during invasive procedures. The child's legs can be captured between the parent's. An arm of the parent can encircle the child's head, holding it against the chest, and the other arm can hold the child's arms.

PREPARATION

- Children 1 or 2 years of age can understand symbols, so a security object, such as a special blanket or teddy bear, is helpful.
- Begin by greeting the child and the accompanying parent by name, but with a child 1 to 6 years old, focus more on the parent. By essentially 'ignoring' the child at first, you allow the child to adjust gradually and to size you up from a safe distance. Then turn your attention gradually to the child, at first to a toy or object the child is holding or perhaps to compliment clothing or the hair. If the child is ready, you will note these signals: eye contact with you, smiling, talking with you or accepting a toy or a piece of equipment.
- Two-year-old children do not like to take off their clothes; have the parent undress the child one part at a time.
- Children 1 or 2 years of age like to say 'No'. Do not offer a choice when there really is none. Avoid saying, '*May I listen to your heart now?*' When the 1- or 2-year-old child says 'No' and you go ahead and do it anyway, you lose trust. Instead, use clear firm instructions, in a tone that expects cooperation, '*Now it's time for you to lie down so I can check your tummy*'.
- Also, 1- or 2-year-old children like to make choices. When possible, enhance autonomy by offering the *limited option*: '*Shall I listen to your heart next or your tummy?*'
- Demonstrate the procedures on the parent, a teddy or doll if needed.
- Praise the child when they are cooperative.

Up until approximately 18 months, toddlers explore the world through the mouth, so take caution when familiarising with the equipment by letting them touch the stethoscope or tongue blade.

SEQUENCE (DEPENDS ON THE PURPOSE OF THE EXAMINATION)

- Collect some objective data during the history, which is a less stressful time for the child. While you are focusing on the parent, note the child's gross motor and fine motor skills and gait.
- Start with nonthreatening areas. Save potentially distressing procedures—such as examining the head, ears, nose or throat—for last.

Early childhood: preschool children (3–5 or 6 years)

Child at this stage display developing initiative. Preschoolers take on tasks independently, plan the task and see it through. A child of this age is often cooperative, helpful and easy to involve. The concept of body image is limited.

POSITION

- With a 3-year-old child, the parent should be present and may hold the child on their lap.
- A 4- or 5-year-old child usually feels comfortable on the examination table or bed, with the parent present.

PREPARATION

- A preschooler can talk. Verbal communication becomes helpful now, but remember that the child's understanding is still limited. Use short, simple explanations.
- Talk to the child and explain the steps in the examination exactly.
- Do not give the child a choice when there is none. However, as with toddlers, enhance the autonomy of preschoolers by offering choice when possible.
- Allow the child to play with equipment to reduce fears.
- A preschooler likes to help; have the child hold the stethoscope for you.
- Use games. Have the child 'blow out' the light on the penlight as you listen to the breath sounds. Or pretend to listen to the heart sounds of the child's teddy bear first.
- Use a slow, deliberate approach. Do not rush.
- During the examination, give preschoolers needed feedback and reassurance: '*Your tummy feels just fine*'.
- Compliment the child on their cooperation.

SEQUENCE (DEPENDS ON THE PURPOSE OF THE EXAMINATION)

- Examine the thorax, abdomen and extremities first. Although preschoolers are usually cooperative, continue to assess the head, eyes, ears, nose and throat last.

School-age children (6–12 years)

During the school-age period, the major task of the child is developing industry. The child is developing basic competency in school and in social networks and desires the approval of parents, teachers and friends. When successful, the child has a feeling of accomplishment. During the examination, children of this age are usually cooperative and interested in learning about the body. Language is more sophisticated now, but do not overestimate and treat a school-age child as a small adult. The child's level of understanding does not match that of their speech.

POSITION

- A school-age child should sit on the examination table or bed.

PREPARATION

- A child in this age group is likely to be shy and modest, so you need to be sensitive to their need for privacy and independence. Break the ice with small talk about family, school, friends, music or sports.
- The child should undress themselves, leave underpants on and use a gown and drape.
- Demonstrate equipment—a school-age child is curious to know how equipment works.
- Comment on the body and how it works (Figure 9.8). An 8- or 9-year-old child has some understanding of the body and is interested to learn more. It is rewarding to see the child's eyes light up when they hear the heart sounds.

SEQUENCE (DEPENDS ON THE PURPOSE OF THE EXAMINATION)

- As with adults, start with an examination relevant to the presenting health concern

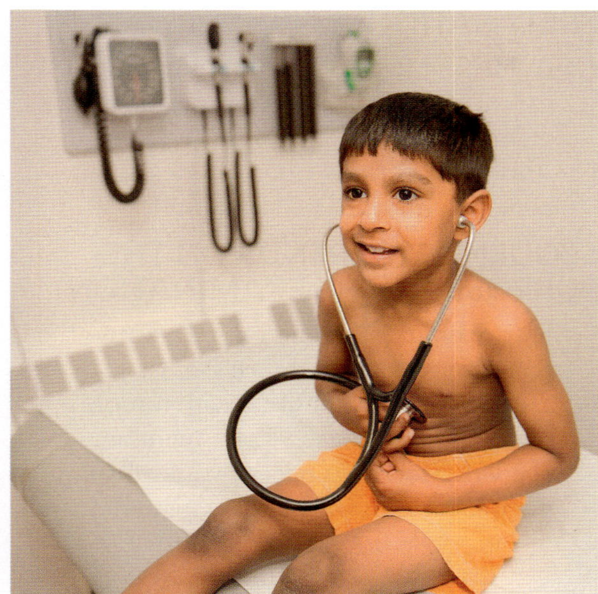

FIGURE 9.8 Involving a school-aged child in a physical examination

(focused assessment) and continue with a more comprehensive health assessment as needed.

Preadolescents/adolescents (10–19 years)

The major task of adolescence is developing a self-identity. This takes shape from various sets of values and different social roles (son or daughter, sibling and student). In the end, each person needs to feel satisfied and comfortable with who they are. In the process, adolescents are increasingly self-conscious and introspective. Peer group values and acceptance are important. It is important to gain the adolescent's consent before beginning the assessment and to ensure confidentiality. While establishing rapport and trust is important, care needs to be taken to maintain professional boundaries.[11]

POSITION

- Adolescents should sit on the examination table or bed.
- Examine the adolescent alone, without parent or sibling present.

PREPARATION

- The body is changing rapidly. During the examination, adolescents need feedback that their own body is healthy and developing normally.
- Adolescents have a keen awareness of body image, often comparing themself to peers. Advise adolescents of the wide variation among teenagers on the rate of growth and development.
- Communicate with some care. Do not treat teenagers like children, but do not overestimate and treat them like an adult either.
- Adolescents are usually interested in finding out more about their health. Positive attitudes developed now may last through adult life. Focus your teaching on ways the adolescent can promote wellness.

SEQUENCE (DEPENDS ON THE PURPOSE OF THE EXAMINATION)

- As with adults, start with an examination relevant to the presenting health concern (focused assessment) and continue with a more comprehensive health assessment as needed.

Adults

Developmentally, the adult stage spans from young adulthood (20–40 years of age) to older adulthood (85+ years). You will need to adjust your approach depending on the age and state of health of the person you are examining.

POSITION

- Adults should sit on a chair, bed or examination table (Figure 9.9); a frail older adult may need to lie down.
- Arrange the sequence to allow as few position changes as possible.

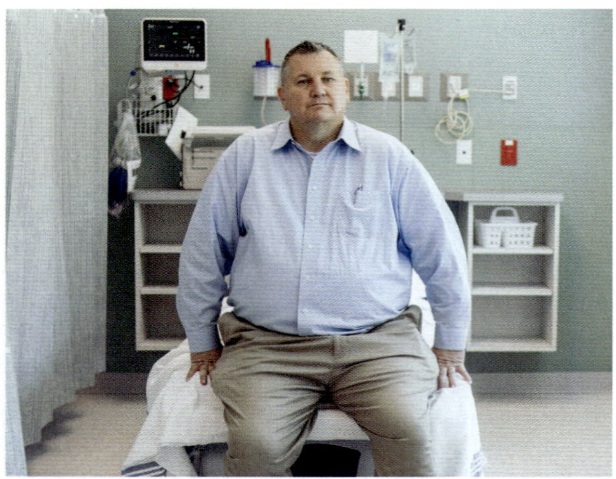

FIGURE 9.9 Positioning of an adult for a physical examination.

PREPARATION

- Adjust the pace of the examination to meet the possible slowed pace of a frail older person.
- Allow rest periods when needed if the person is unwell.

SEQUENCE (DEPENDS ON THE PURPOSE OF THE EXAMINATION)

- Start with an examination relevant to the presenting health concern (focused assessment) and continue with a more comprehensive health assessment as needed. Modify as necessary, particularly if the person is unwell, easily fatigued or frail.

Clinical reasoning and documentation

The following is a continuation of the case study provided at the beginning of this chapter. You should consult a fundamentals of nursing or medical-surgical nursing text for information about goal setting, nursing interventions and evaluation.

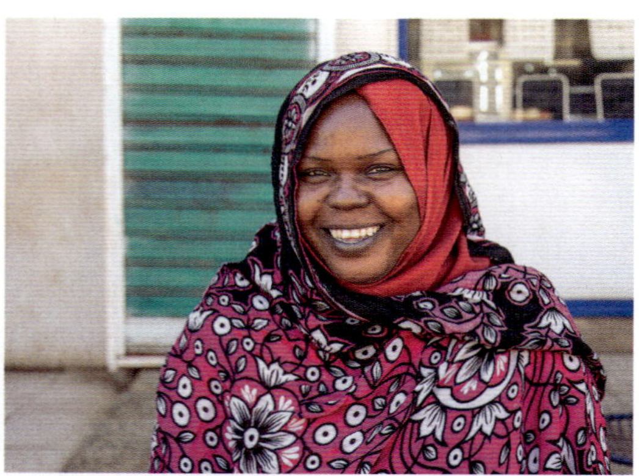

Case study (continued)—Approach to physical examination

Context

You will recall from the case study described earlier in the chapter that you are on clinical placement in a subacute rehabilitation ward. Your preceptor (buddy) nurse tells you he is expecting a new patient admission to the ward shortly after the afternoon handover. He asks you to prepare to be involved in completing the ward admission assessment for this woman, who you will be meeting for the first time.

Consider the patient's situation

You have limited information about the new patient. Mrs Nyamal Bol is a 55-year-old woman who is undergoing rehabilitation following a car accident 3 days ago. She sustained a fractured right wrist, which has been internally fixed with a plate and screw, and she has a plaster cast from her fingers to her elbow. She also sustained a dislocated fractured ankle, which has been fixed with screws and plates, and she is now wearing an orthopaedic boot. She has extensive bruising and minor cuts. Mrs Bol is a South Sudanese–Australian who arrived in Australia as a refugee 8 years ago with her husband and five children. You are told that Mrs Bol speaks some English.

Collect cues/information

Consider the following:

- How has your plan for collecting objective data (physical examination) with Mrs Bol changed after reading the chapter and accessing the additional resources or references?
- How has your plan for the physical examination change if the person was:
  - a child?
  - in pain?
  - unable to cooperate?
  - very fatigued?

ADDITIONAL RESOURCES

You can further develop your knowledge and skills relevant to physical examination techniques by:

- reading chapters of a fundamentals of nursing or medical-surgical nursing textbook
- answering chapter multiple choice questions online. Log onto ClinicalKey Student and search for the text 'Health Assessment, 4th edition'. Choose the section titled 'Teaching material'. In this section you will find question and answer documents for each chapter.
- visiting websites

  Hand Hygiene Australia: https://www.hha.org.au

  Hand Hygiene New Zealand: https://www.hqsc.govt.nz/our-work/infection-prevention-and-control/our-work/hand-hygiene/

  Trans Hub—Health and gender affirmation in New South Wales. Downloads for clinicians: https://www.transhub.org.au/downloads-health

REFERENCES

1. Australian Commission on Safety and Quality in Health Care (ACSQHC). Alcohol-based hand rubs. 2023. Available at: https://www.safetyandquality.gov.au/our-work/infection-prevention-and-control/national-hand-hygiene-initiative-nhhi/what-hand-hygiene/alcohol-based-handrubs
2. Australian Commission on Quality and Safety in Health Care & National Health & Medical Research Council. The Australian guidelines for the prevention and control of infection in healthcare. V11.13. 2022. Available at: https://www.safetyandquality.gov.au/publications-and-resources/resource-library/australian-guidelines-prevention-and-control-infection-healthcare
3. New Zealand Health Quality & Safety Commission. Infection prevention and control. Available at: https://www.hqsc.govt.nz/our-work/infection-prevention-and-control/
4. Australian Commission on Safety and Quality in Health Care. Communicating for safety portal. 2023. Available at: https://c4sportal.safetyandquality.gov.au
5. Haire BG, Brook E, Stoddart R, Simpson P. Trans and gender diverse people's experiences of healthcare access in Australia: s qualitative study in people with complex needs. PloS ONE. 2021 Jan 28;16(1): e0245889.
6. Hill AO, Bourne A, McNair R, Carman M, Lyons A 20201. Private Lives 3: The health and wellbeing of LGBTIQ people in Australia. ARCSHS Monograph Series No. 122. Melbourne, Australia: Australian Research Centre in Sex, Health and Society, La Trobe University.
7. Vermeir E, Jackson LA, Marshall EG. Improving healthcare providers' interactions with trans patients: recommendations to promote cultural competence. Healthcare Policy 2018 Aug;14(1):11.
8. Safer Care Victoria. Lessons learned from paediatric sentinel events. 2022. Victorian State Government. Available at: https://www.safercare.vic.gov.au/news/lessons-learned-from-paediatric-sentinel-events#:,:text=Parents%2Fcarers%20know%20their%20child,worse%20in%20any%20clinical%20setting
9. Wilson SF, Giddens JF. Developmental tasks across the lifespan. In: Wilson SF, Giddens JF. Health assessment for nursing practice—e-book. Elsevier Health Sciences; 2020. pp. 396–411.
10. Erikson E. The life cycle completed (extended version). New York: WW Norton & Company; 1998.
11. Royal Children's Hospital. Engaging with and assessing the adolescent patient. Clinical Practice Guidelines, Melbourne: Royal Children's Hospital; 2019. Available: https://www.rch.org.au/clinicalguide/guideline_index/Engaging_with_and_assessing_the_adolescent_patient/

CHAPTER 10

General survey and vital signs

Written by Carolyn Jarvis and Ann Eckhardt
Adapted by Helen Forbes

INTRODUCTION

The data you obtain from your general inspection of the person and measurement of their vital signs are important components of the **objective** dataset. These assessments will be measured and recorded multiple times during a person's illness trajectory or as part of health screening. They reflect interrelationships between body systems—for example, the cardiovascular, respiratory, neurological, endocrine and immune systems—and the psychological state of the person.

Assessment plan

You will use your observational skills as you take note of the person's general appearance, paying attention to the following characteristics: **physical appearance**, **body structure**, **mobility**, **skin colour**, **ease of breathing** and **behaviour**. Following the general survey, you will proceed through the health history (Chapter 7), physical examination (Chapter 9) and measurement of vital signs.

Measuring vital signs includes taking measurements of **temperature**, **blood pressure (BP)**, **heart** and **respiratory rates** which, as such, are critical indicators of health status, in particular deterioration (Chapter 30).

Resources available

You will find additional resources and a list of references at the end of this chapter. Also, there are two videos that accompany this chapter where measurement of vital signs is demonstrated. One video includes taking a BP manually. The other video includes taking a BP using an automatic device. You will find a QR code in this chapter that will enable you to access the relevant video easily on your device.

Objective data—general survey

The general survey (**physical appearance**, **body structure**, **mobility**, **skin colour**, **ease of breathing** and **behaviour**) assists in getting an impression of the person and includes the general health state and any obvious physical characteristics of the person. A general survey begins from the moment you first meet the person (Figure 10.1). What leaves an immediate impression? Does the person look sick, are they moving slowly or with effort, are the shoulders slumped and eyes without lustre or downcast? Is a hospitalised person conversing with visitors, involved in reading or television or lying perfectly still? Even as you introduce yourself you begin to collect data. Does the person make eye contact or smile? Does the person look relaxed or anxious?

Conducting a general survey each time you encounter the person will alert you to changes that may have taken place that need further assessment. In an emergency, the primary survey is used to assess a seriously ill or injured person and is conducted at the same time as

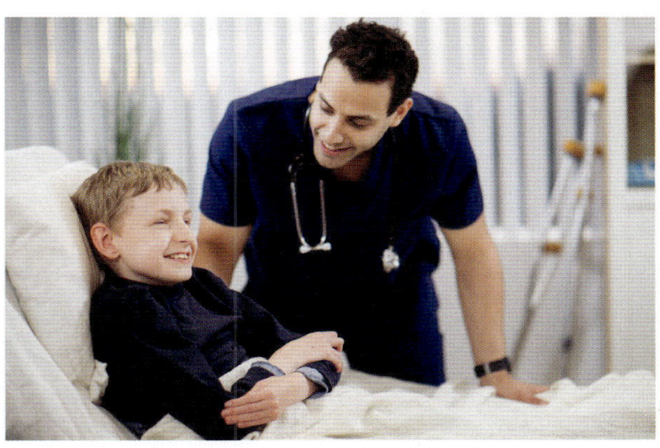

FIGURE 10.1 A general survey starts on meeting the person

management. A primary survey is used to identify priorities based on the person's condition, injuries, vital signs and/or mechanism of injury (Chapter 1). In emergency situations speed and accuracy are essential for patient safety. The primary survey includes assessment of life-threatening conditions such as airway, breathing, circulation, disability (neurological assessment) and exposure (person is undressed and the nurse examines them for injury). A more focused assessment is conducted following the primary survey.

PROCEDURES AND NORMAL FINDINGS	ABNORMAL FINDINGS AND CLINICAL ALERTS
The general survey – detailed inspection	
The aim is to determine the general state of health and whether the person appears well, chronically unwell or acutely ill.	
Physical appearance	
Observe physical appearance of the person on meeting, then throughout the collection of history information and the physical assessment and throughout the episode of care.	
Age. The person appears their stated age.	Appears older than stated age, as can occur with chronic illness, alcoholism and smoking.
Sex. Sexual development is appropriate for gender and age.	Delayed or precocious puberty. Be aware of assuming that the person identifies as a particular gender or sexual orientation. See Chapters 26 and 27 for more information and guidelines about communicating effectively about sexuality.
Level of consciousness. The person is alert and oriented, attends to your questions and responds appropriately.	Confused, drowsy, lethargic (Chapter 12).  ***Clinical alert:*** Change in conscious state requires **immediate** further assessment. Consider the need for urgent medical referral.

PROCEDURES AND NORMAL FINDINGS	ABNORMAL FINDINGS AND CLINICAL ALERTS
Skin. Skin is intact. Colour tone is even, pigmentation varying with genetic background; skin is intact with no obvious lesions.	 ***Clinical alert:*** Bleeding or other signs of trauma must be investigated immediately. **Pallor**: unnaturally pale skin. **Jaundice**: yellow discolouration. **Erythema**: redness of the skin. **Lesions**: refer to Chapter 22. **Central cyanosis**: bluish discolouration of tongue and mucous membranes due to decreased arterial oxygen saturation.[1]  ***Clinical alert:*** Presence of central cyanosis requires immediate further assessment. Consider the need for urgent medical attention. **Peripheral cyanosis**: bluish discolouration of peripheral tissues.
Facial features. Facial features are symmetrical with movement, appropriate smiling, frowning.	Immobile, mask-like, asymmetrical, drooping (Table 12.7).
No signs of acute distress are present.	Respiratory signs such as the following: • **dyspnoea**—shortness of breath, rapid breathing • **tachypnoea**—rapid breathing • **use of accessory muscles**—sternocleidomastoid, scalene, pectoral, latissimus, serratus, posterior superior, abdominal, external and internal intercostal muscles • **wheezing**—high-pitched, coarse, whistling sound on expiration or inspiration • **stridor**—noisy breathing on inspiration, expiration or both • **pain**, indicated by facial grimace, holding body part, crying, moaning, sweating • **mental state** such as acute anxiety, agitation (Chapter 19). 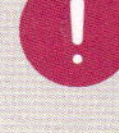 ***Clinical alert:*** Presence of any of these signs of distress requires immediate attention. Consider the need for urgent medical referral.
Body structure	
Stature. The height appears within normal range for age, genetic heritage (see 'Measurement' below).	Excessively short or tall for age.

PROCEDURES AND NORMAL FINDINGS	ABNORMAL FINDINGS AND CLINICAL ALERTS
Nutrition. The weight appears within normal range for height and body build; body fat distribution is even.	**Cachectic**—emaciated. Impression of **cachexia** or obesity is verified by objective measurement. **Obesity**, with even fat distribution. **Centripetal (truncal) obesity**—fat concentrated in face, neck, trunk, with thin extremities, as in **Cushing's syndrome**.
Symmetry. Body parts look equal bilaterally and are in relative proportion to each other.	**Unilateral atrophy**—wasting of muscle(s) on one side of the body. **Hypertrophy**—increased size of a body part. Asymmetrical location of a body part.
Posture. The person stands comfortably erect as appropriate for age. Note the normal 'plumb line' through anterior ear, shoulder, hip, patella, ankle.	**Abnormal posture** may be associated with neurological, bone or muscle disorders. **Rigid spine and neck**; moves as one unit (e.g. **arthritis**). **Lordosis**—inward curving of the spine in the lower part of the back. **Kyphosis**—a permanent curvature of the spine as can be seen in the older person giving a stooped or hunched-over appearance. **Scoliosis**—an excessive sideways curvature of the spine. Shoulders look slumped (Chapter 20).
Position. The person sits comfortably in a chair or on the bed or examination table, arms relaxed at sides, head turned to examiner.	Stiff and tense, ready to spring from chair, fidgety movements. **Tripod**—leaning forwards with arms braced on chair arms; occurs with chronic pulmonary disease. Sitting straight up and resists lying down (e.g. heart failure). Curled up in fetal position (e.g. acute abdominal pain) (Chapters 17 and 19).
Body build, contour. Proportions are: • Arm span (fingertip to fingertip) equals height. • Body length from crown to pubis roughly equal to length from pubis to sole of foot.	Elongated arm span, arm span greater than height (e.g. **Marfan's syndrome**, **hypogonadism**).
Obvious physical deformities—note any congenital or acquired defects.	Missing extremities or digits; webbed digits; shortened limb.
Mobility	
Observe the person sit, walk and change positions.	

PROCEDURES AND NORMAL FINDINGS	ABNORMAL FINDINGS AND CLINICAL ALERTS
Gait. Normally, the base is as wide as the shoulder width; foot placement is accurate; the walk is smooth, coordinated, even and well-balanced; and associated movements, such as symmetrical arm swing, are present.	Exceptionally wide base. Staggering, stumbling. Shuffling, dragging, nonfunctional leg. Limping with injury. Propulsion—difficulty stopping (Table 12.10).
Range of motion. Note full mobility for each joint and that movement is deliberate, accurate, smooth and coordinated. (See Chapter 20 for information on more detailed testing of joint range of motion.)	Limited joint range of motion. **Paralysis**—absent movement. Movement jerky, uncoordinated.
No involuntary movement.	Tics, tremors, seizures (Table 12.9).
Behaviour	
Observation of the facial expression, mood and affect and quality of speech are performed at the same time as observing behaviour.	
Facial expression. The person maintains eye contact (unless a cultural taboo exists), expressions are appropriate to the situation such as thoughtful, serious or smiling. (Note expressions both while the face is at rest and while the person is talking.)	Flat, depressed, angry, sad, anxious. However, note that anxiety is common in ill people. Be aware also that some people smile when they are anxious.
Mood and affect. The person is comfortable and cooperative with the examiner and interacts pleasantly.	Agitated, hostile, distrustful, suspicious, crying.
Speech. Articulation (the ability to form words) is clear and understandable.	Alterations in quality of speech such as: • **dysarthria**—slowed or slurred speech caused by disturbed muscular control • **expressive dysphasia**—garbled speech (Table 12.6) • **aphasia**—inability to form speech. Speech disorders may occur as a result of neurological disorders (Chapter 12).
The stream of talking is fluent, with an even pace. The person conveys ideas clearly. Word choice is appropriate to context. The person communicates in prevailing language easily or with an interpreter.	Extremes of few words or of constant talking. Inappropriate use of words needs to be further evaluated in a mental status and/or neurological assessment.

PROCEDURES AND NORMAL FINDINGS	ABNORMAL FINDINGS AND CLINICAL ALERTS
Dress. Clothing is appropriate to the climate, looks clean and fits the body and is appropriate to the context and age.	Trousers too large and held up by belt suggest weight loss, as does the addition of new holes in belt. If the belt is moved to a looser fit, it may indicate obesity or ascites. Inappropriate clothing may be related to heat/cold intolerance, mental illness or poverty.
Personal hygiene. The person appears clean and groomed appropriately for their age, occupation and socioeconomic group. (Note that a wide variation of dress and hygiene is 'normal'.)	Abnormal body odours (perspiration, urine, faeces) may be related to inadequate personal hygiene. Abnormal breath odours may be observed such as alcohol, acetone or ammonia.
Hair is groomed, brushed. Women's make-up, if used, is appropriate for age and culture.	In a previously carefully groomed woman, unkempt hair and absent make-up may indicate malaise or illness.

Measurement

Weight

Use a standardised *balance* or electronic standing scale. Ask the person to remove their shoes and heavy outer clothing if not in a hospital context before standing on the scale (Figure 10.2). When a sequence of repeated weights is necessary, aim for approximately the same time of day and the same type of clothing worn each time. Record the weight in kilograms.

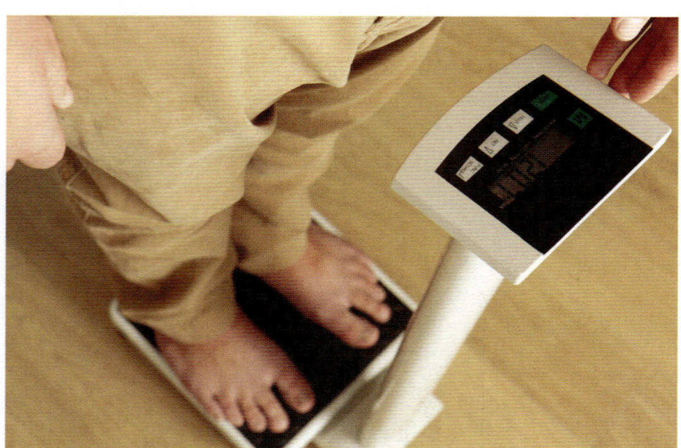

FIGURE 10.2 Weighing the person with shoes removed.

An **unexplained weight loss** may be a sign of a short-term illness (e.g. fever, infection, disease of the mouth or throat), chronic illness (endocrine disease, malignancy, mental health dysfunction) or successful dieting and/or exercise program.

Unexplained weight gain may indicate fluid retention such as in heart failure, overabundant kilojoule intake, unhealthy eating habits and sedentary lifestyle or changes in health status.

PROCEDURES AND NORMAL FINDINGS	ABNORMAL FINDINGS AND CLINICAL ALERTS
Height	
Use a wall-mounted device or the measuring pole on the balance scale. Align the extended headpiece with the top of the head. The person should be shoeless, standing straight with gentle traction under the jaw and looking straight ahead. Feet, shoulders and buttocks should be in contact with the hard surface. For bed-bound patients, length can be assessed using a pliable measuring tape to measure the body in sections. Measurements should be taken from the heel to knee, knee to hip, hip to shoulder and shoulder to top of the head. These measurements are then totalled to determine height.	
Body mass index is a standard measure of weight for height and an indicator of obesity or protein-calorie malnutrition. BMI formula.[1] $$\text{BMI} = \frac{\text{mass in kg}}{\text{height in m}^2}$$ A healthy BMI is a level of 19 or greater to less than 25. Show the person how his or her own weight matches up to the national guidelines for optimal BMI. Compare the person's current weight with that from the previous health visit. Note that BMI overestimates body fat in people who are very muscular and underestimates body fat in older adults who have lost muscle mass.[3]	The cause of weight gain is usually excess kilojoule intake; occasionally it is endocrine disorders, drug therapy (e.g. corticosteroids) or depression. BMI interpretation for adults:[2] • < 18.5—Underweight • $18.5 \leq 25$—Normal weight • $25.0 \leq 30$—Overweight • $30.0 \leq 35$—Obesity class I • $35 \leq 40$—Obesity class II • 40–45—Obesity class III. Caution needs to be taken in interpreting BMI since it was validated on a particular population group and it may not be relevant to all groups—for example, an elite athlete is likely to have a high BMI because of increased muscle mass but would not be considered unhealthy. BMI interpretation for children aged under 5 years:[1] • Overweight is weight-for-height over 2 standard deviations above WHO Child Growth Standards median. • Obesity is weight-for-height over 3 standard deviations above the WHO Child Growth Standards median. BMI interpretation for children aged 5–19 years[2]: overweight is defined as a BMI for age value over +1 SD. Obesity is defined as a BMI for age value over +2 SD. Refer to percentile charts for boys and girls.[1]

PROCEDURES AND NORMAL FINDINGS	ABNORMAL FINDINGS AND CLINICAL ALERTS

Waist circumference

Waist circumference alone can be used to predict greater health risk. Excess abdominal fat is an important independent risk factor for disease, over and above that of BMI. If most of the weight is carried around the waist instead of around the hips, the person is at higher risk for heart disease and type 2 diabetes.

With the person standing, locate the hip bone—the very top is the iliac crest. Place a measuring tape around the waist, parallel to the floor, at the level of the iliac crest. The tape should be snug but not pinching in the skin. Note the measurement at the end of a normal expiration (Figure 10.3).

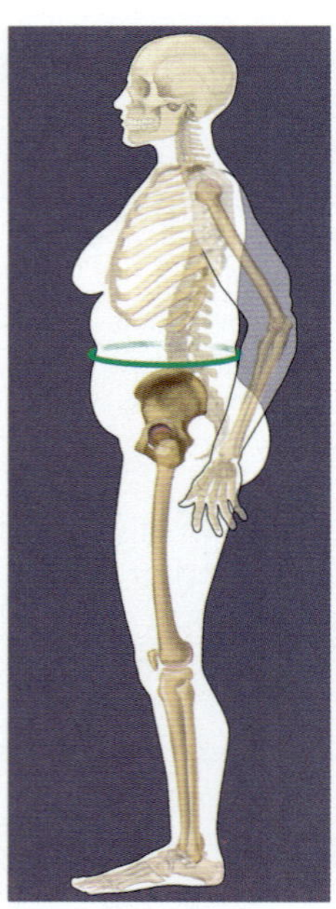

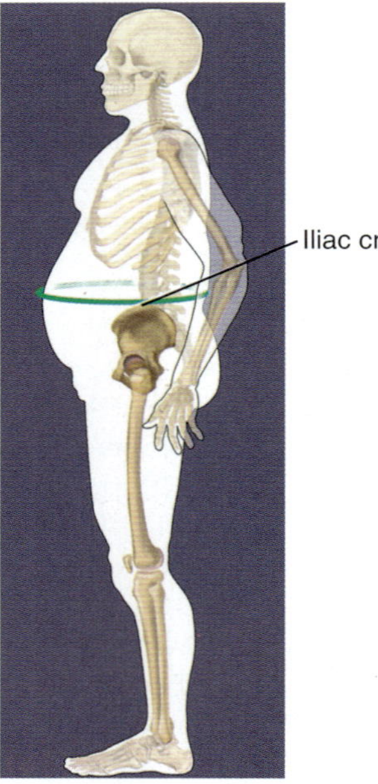

FIGURE 10.3 Measuring tape position for waist circumference

A waist circumference over 80 cm in women and over 94 cm in men increases risk of cardiovascular and metabolic diseases.

More than 88 cm for women and over 102 cm for males indicates greatly increased health risk. These measurements can be recorded at each health visit.[2,3]

Waist-to-hip ratio

The waist-to-hip ratio assesses body fat distribution as an indicator of health risk. Obese people with a greater proportion of fat in the upper body, especially in the abdomen, have android obesity; obese people with most of their fat in the hips and thighs have gynoid obesity. The equation is:

$$\text{Waist-to-hip ratio} = \frac{\text{waist circumference}}{\text{hip circumference}}$$

A waist-to-hip ratio of ≥ 1.0 in men or ≥ 0.8 in women is indicative of android (upper body) obesity and increasing risk for obesity-related diseases and early mortality. Increased risk occurs when the measure exceeds 1.0 for men and 0.85 for women.[1,2]

PROCEDURES AND NORMAL FINDINGS	ABNORMAL FINDINGS AND CLINICAL ALERTS
For example: If a woman has a 112 cm waist and 101 cm hips, the calculation would be as follows: 112 cm/101 cm = 1.1 waist-to-hip ratio The desired waist-to-hip ratio for women is 0.8 or less and for men is 1.0 or less.	
Additional objective data for infants and children	
General survey	
Physical appearance, body structure, mobility. Note the same basic elements as with adults, with consideration to age and development. Exceptions are the standing toddler who normally has a protuberant abdomen ('toddler lordosis').	
Behaviour. Note the response to stimuli and level of alertness appropriate for age.	
Parental bonding. Note the child's interactions with parents, that parent and child show a mutual response and are warm and affectionate, appropriate to the child's condition.	Some signs of child abuse are that the child avoids eye contact; the child exhibits no separation anxiety when you would expect it for age; the parent is disgusted by child's odour, sounds, drooling or stools. Deprivation of physical or emotional care (Chapter 5).
Measurement	
Weight. Weigh infants on an electronic scale. Guard the baby so they do not fall (Figure 10.4). Weigh to the nearest 10 g for infants and 100 g for toddlers. 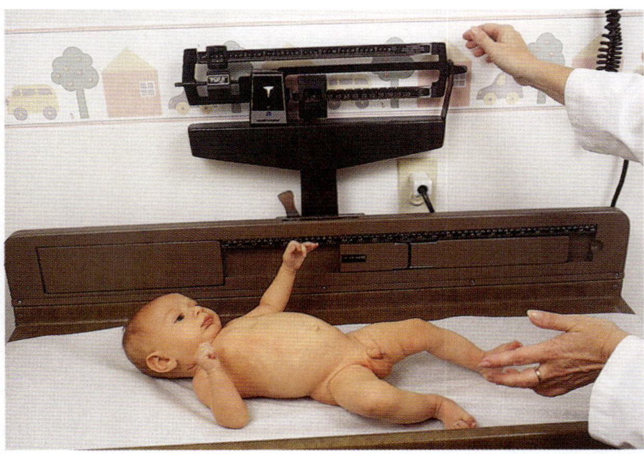 **FIGURE 10.4** Measuring an infant's weight using an electronic scale	

PROCEDURES AND NORMAL FINDINGS	ABNORMAL FINDINGS AND CLINICAL ALERTS

By age 2 or 3 years, use the upright scale. Leave underpants on the child. Use the upright scale with preschoolers and school-age children, maintaining modesty with light clothing (Figure 10.5).

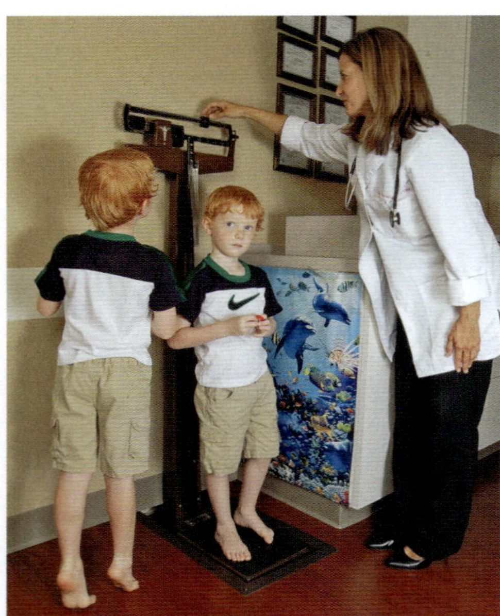

FIGURE 10.5 Using upright scale to measure child's weight

Length. Until age 2 years, measure an infant's body length supine by using a horizontal measuring board (Figure 10.6). Hold the head in the midline. Because infants normally have flexed legs, extend them momentarily by holding the knees together and pushing them down until the legs are flat on the table. Avoid using a tape measure along the infant's length because this is inaccurate.

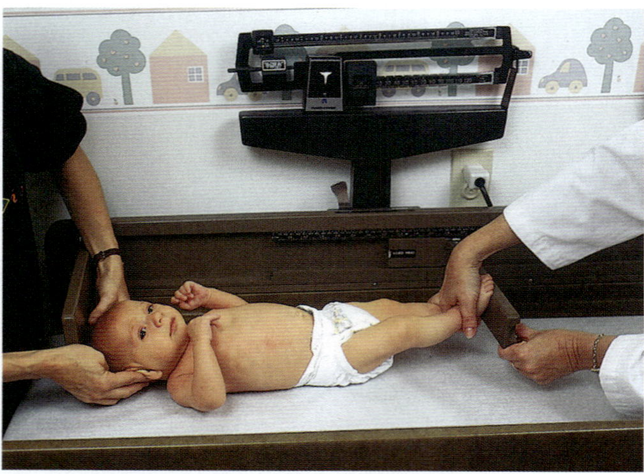

FIGURE 10.6 Using a horizontal measuring board to measure infant's length

PROCEDURES AND NORMAL FINDINGS	ABNORMAL FINDINGS AND CLINICAL ALERTS

For age 2 or 3 years, measure the child's height by standing the child against the pole on the platform scale (Figure 10.7) or back against a flat ruler taped to the wall. (Sometimes a child will stand more erect against the solid wall than against the narrow measuring pole on the scale.) Encourage the child to stand straight and tall and to look straight ahead without tilting the head. The shoulders, buttocks and heels should touch the wall. Hold a book or flat board on the child's head at a right angle to the wall. Mark just under the book, noting the measure to the nearest 1 mm.

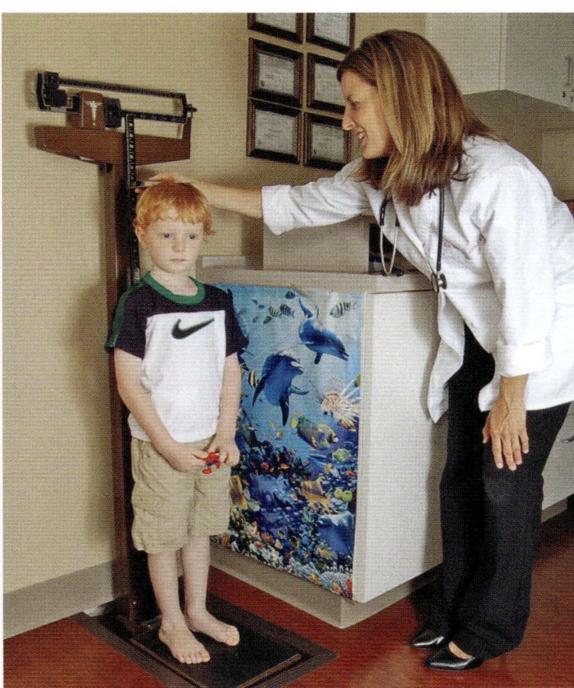

FIGURE 10.7 Measuring a child's height

Physical growth is perhaps the best index of a child's general health. The child's height and weight are recorded at every healthcare visit to determine normal growth patterns. The results are plotted on growth charts.

Healthy childhood growth is continuous but uneven, with rapid growth spurts occurring during infancy and adolescence. Results are more reliable when comparing numerous growth measures over a long time. These charts also compare an individual child's measurements against the general population. Normal limits range from the 5th to the 95th percentile on the standardised charts.

PROCEDURES AND NORMAL FINDINGS	ABNORMAL FINDINGS AND CLINICAL ALERTS
Use your judgement and consider the ethnic background of the small-for-age child. Explore the growth patterns of the parents and siblings. Be aware that the statistical averages for Australia are based on American charts, which are based on norms for Caucasian children and may not necessarily generalise to other ethnic groups.	Further explore any growth measure that: • falls below the 5th or above the 95th percentile • shows a wide percentile difference between height and weight—such as a 10th percentile height with a 95th percentile weight • shows that growth has suddenly stopped when it had been steady • fails to show normal growth spurts during infancy and adolescence.
Head circumference. Measure the infant's head circumference at birth and at each well child visit up to age 2 years and then yearly up to 6 years (Figure 10.8). Circle the tape around the head at the prominent frontal and occipital bones; the widest span is correct. Plot the measurement on standardised growth charts. Compare the infant's head size with that expected for age. A series of measurements is more valuable than a single figure to show the *rate* of head growth. 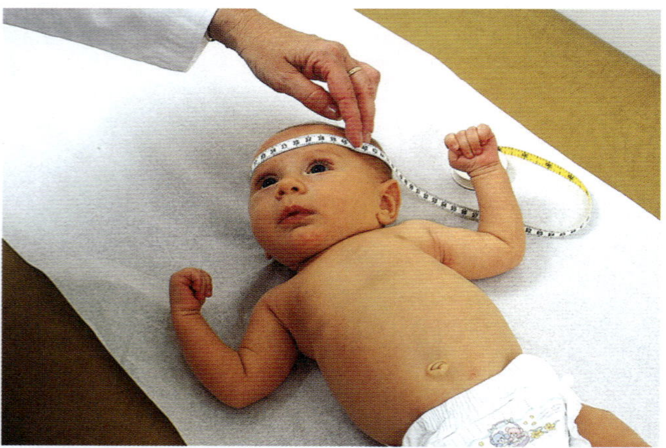 **FIGURE 10.8** Measuring infant's head circumference	
A newborn's head measures 32 to 38 cm (average about 34 cm) and is about 2 cm larger than the chest circumference. The chest grows at a faster rate than the cranium; at some time between 6 months and 2 years, both measurements are about the same, and after age 2 years the chest circumference is greater than the head circumference.	Enlarged head circumference occurs with increased intracranial pressure (Chapter 12).

PROCEDURES AND NORMAL FINDINGS	ABNORMAL FINDINGS AND CLINICAL ALERTS
Measurement of the chest circumference is valuable in comparison with the head circumference but not necessarily by itself. Encircle the tape around the chest at the nipple line. It should be snug, but not so tight that it leaves a mark (Figure 10.9).	

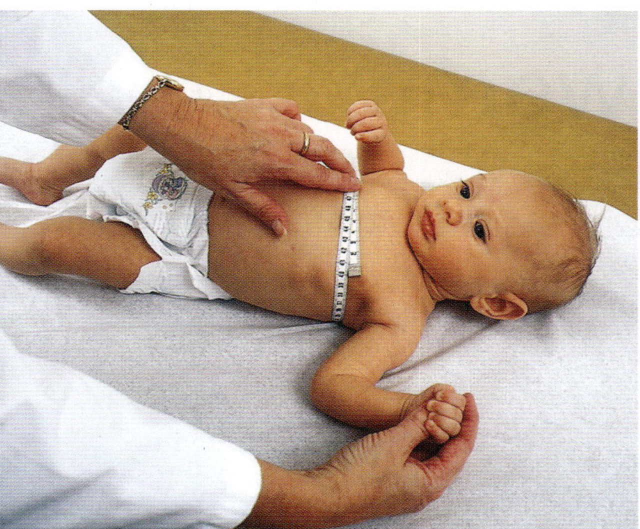

FIGURE 10.9 Measuring an infant's chest circumference

Additional objective data for an adult over 65 years

General survey

Physical appearance. By the 8th and 9th decades, body contour is sharper, with more angular facial features and body proportions are redistributed. (See measuring weight and height, above.)

Posture. A general flexion occurs by the 8th or 9th decade.

Gait. Older adults often use a wider base to compensate for diminished balance; arms may be held out to help balance and steps may be shorter or uneven.

Measurement

PROCEDURES AND NORMAL FINDINGS	ABNORMAL FINDINGS AND CLINICAL ALERTS
Weight. People over 65 years often appear sharper in contour, with more prominent bony landmarks than younger adults. Bodyweight decreases during the 80s and 90s. This factor is more evident in males, perhaps because of greater muscle shrinkage. The distribution of fat also changes during the 80s and 90s. Even with good nutrition, subcutaneous fat is lost from the face and periphery (especially the forearms), whereas additional fat is deposited on the abdomen and hips.	Obesity can continue into later adult life.

PROCEDURES AND NORMAL FINDINGS	ABNORMAL FINDINGS AND CLINICAL ALERTS
Height. By the 80s and 90s, many people are shorter than they were in their 70s. This results from shortening in the spinal column from thinning of the vertebral discs and shortening of the individual vertebrae and from the postural changes of kyphosis and slight flexion in the knees and hips. Because long bones do not shorten with age, the overall body proportion looks different—a shorter trunk with relatively long extremities.	

Objective data—vital signs

Changes in vital signs reflect the body's response to illness, treatment and/or stress. The vital signs chart is a standardised chart that enables visualisation of trends in the vital signs and specifies the physiological parameters and other factors that trigger the escalation of care. The chart was developed by the Australian Commission on Safety and Quality in Health Care for use across Australian hospitals.[4] See Figure 10.10 for the standardised adult general observation chart 'The Adult Deterioration Detection System' (ADDS).[4] A similar chart is used in Aotearoa New Zealand healthcare settings.[5]

Your approach to measuring vital signs should include informing the person about the procedure, gaining their consent, measuring the vital signs accurately, documenting your findings and reporting changes of concern. Always remember to perform hand hygiene before and after the procedure.

Position

Vital signs can be performed with the person in bed or in a chair but should be performed while the person is at rest.

Equipment

Vital signs chart (electronic or paper)
Wristwatch with a second hand
Digital vital signs machine (including oral or aural thermometer, oxygen saturation probe and relevant sized BP cuff)
A pillow may be necessary to support the person's arm when measuring BP

DRAFT

DO NOT WRITE IN THIS BINDING MARGIN

UR Number: ______		
Family name: ______		
Given names: ______		
Date of birth: ___/___/___	Sex: ☐ M ☐ F	

(Affix patient identification label here)

Date / Time		
Respiratory Rate (breaths / min)	Write ≥ 35	Write ≥ 35
	30–34	30–34
	25–29	25–29
	20–24	20–24
	15–19	15–19
	10–14	10–14
	5–9	5–9
If respiratory rate ≥ 35 or ≤4, write value in box	Write ≤ 4	Write ≤ 4
O_2 Saturation (%)	98–100	98–100
	95–97	95–97
	93–94	93–94
	90–92	90–92
	87–89	87–89
	85–86	85–86
If O_2 saturation ≤ 84, write value in box	Write ≤ 84	Write ≤ 84
O_2 Flow Rate (L / min)	≥ 13	≥ 13
	10–12	10–12
	7–9	7–9
	4–6	4–6
	≤ 3	≤ 3
Blood Pressure (mmHg)	Write ≥ 200	Write ≥ 200
	190s	190s
	180s	180s
	170s	170s
	160s	160s
	150s	150s
	140s	140s
	130s	130s
	120s	120s
	110s	110s
	100s	100s
	90s	90s
	80s	80s
	70s	70s
	60s	60s
	50s	50s
If systolic BP ≥ 200, write value in box	40s	40s
Heart Rate (beats / min)	Write ≥ 140	Write ≥ 140
	130s	130s
	120s	120s
	110s	110s
	100s	100s
	90s	90s
	80s	80s
	70s	70s
	60s	60s
	50s	50s
	40s	40s
If heart rate ≥ 140 or ≤ 30, write value in box	Write ≤ 30s	Write ≤ 30s
Temperature (°C)	Write ≥ 39.1	Write ≥ 39.1
	38.5–39.0	38.5–39.0
	38.0–38.4	38.0–38.4
	37.5–37.9	37.5–37.9
	37.0–37.4	37.0–37.4
	36.5–36.9	36.5–36.9
	36.0–36.4	36.0–36.4
	35.5–35.9	35.5–35.9
If temperature ≥ 39.1 or ≤ 35.4, write value in box	Write ≤ 35.4	Write ≤ 35.4
Consciousness	Alert	Alert
If clinically necessary, wake patient to assess and score	To Voice	To Voice
	To Pain	To Pain
	Unresp.	Unresp.
ADDS Scores	Respiratory Rate	**ADDS Scores**
	O_2 Saturation	
	O_2 Flow Rate	
	Systolic BP	
	Heart Rate	
	Temperature	
	Consciousness	
	TOTAL ADDS	
Intervention	E.g. 'a'	E.g. 'a'

Usual/target systolic BP:	Signature:
mmHg	

Circle the column showing the patient's usual systolic BP

Score current systolic BP using circled column

	190s	180s	170s	160s	150s	140s	130s	120s	110s	100s	90s	80s
Write ≥ 200	0	0	1	1	2	2	2	3	3	4	5	5
190s	0	0	0	1	1	1	2	2	3	3	4	4
180s	0	0	0	0	0	1	1	2	2	3	3	4
170s	1	0	0	0	0	1	1	2	2	3	3	3
160s	1	1	0	0	0	0	0	1	1	2	2	2
150s	1	1	1	0	0	0	0	0	1	1	2	2
140s	2	1	1	1	0	0	0	0	0	1	1	1
130s	2	2	1	1	0	0	0	0	0	0	0	1
120s	2	2	2	1	1	0	0	0	0	0	0	0
110s	3	2	2	2	1	1	0	0	0	0	0	0
100s	3	3	3	2	2	2	1	1	0	0	0	0
90s	4	3	3	3	2	2	2	2	1	1	0	0
80s	Emergency call										1	0
70s–40s	Emergency call											

Adult Deterioration Detection System (ADDS)

If any observation is in a shaded area, add up the Total ADDS Score and take the action required for that score.

- Score 0
- Score 1
- Score 2
- Score 3
- Score 4
- Score 5
- **Emergency call**

Actions Required

Total ADDS Score 1–3

- Increase frequency of observations *[specify frequency]*
- Inform senior nurse and/or Team Leader

Total ADDS Score 4 – 5

- Senior nurse and/or junior medical officer review within 30 minutes

Total ADDS Score 6 – 7

- Senior medical officer review (registrar or above) within 30 minutes
- Request review, and note on the back of this form

Total ADDS Score ≥ 8

- Place Emergency call
- Begin initial life support interventions (support airway, breathing, circulation)
- Advanced life support provider to attend patient immediately

Emergency call if:

- Any observation is in a purple area
- Airway threat
- Respiratory or cardiac arrest
- New drop in O_2 saturation < 90%
- Sudden fall in level of consciousness
- Seizure
- You are seriously worried about the patient but they do not fit the above criteria

<INSERT SITE LOGO>

Adult Deterioration Detection System (ADDS) Chart

UR Number: ______

Family name: ______

Given names: ______

Date of birth: ___/___/___ Sex: ☐ M ☐ F

(Affix patient identification label here)

Other Observation Charts In Use

☐ Alcohol Withdrawal ☐ Insulin Infusion ☐ Pain/Epidural/Patient Controlled Analgesia

☐ Anticoagulant ☐ Neurology ☐ ______

☐ Fluid Balance ☐ Neurovascular ☐ ______

General Instructions

» You must record appropriate observations:
- On admission
- At a frequency appropriate for the patient's clinical state.

» You must calculate a Total ADDS Score:
- If the patient is deteriorating or an observation is in a shaded area
- Whenever you are concerned about the patient.

» When graphing observations, place a dot (•) in the centre of the box which includes the current observation in its range of values and connect it to the previous dot with a straight line. For blood pressure, use the symbols indicated on the chart.

» Whenever an observation falls within a shaded area, you must enter the ADDS Score for that vital sign in the appropriate row of the ADDS Scores table, unless a modification has been made (see below).

Modifications

- If abnormal observations are to be tolerated for the patient's clinical condition, write the acceptable ranges below (where the ADDS Score will be 0).
- Modifications must be reviewed at least every 72 hours.
- If **any** vital sign needs further modifying, draw two diagonal lines through the entire Modification record in use and write the new acceptable ranges in the next Modification record.

	Modification 1	Modification 2	Modification 3	Modification 4
Respiratory Rate	- breaths / min	- breaths / min	- breaths / min	- breaths / min
O_2 Saturation	- %	- %	- %	- %
O_2 Flow Rate	- L / min	- L / min	- L / min	- L / min
Systolic BP	- mmHg	- mmHg	- mmHg	- mmHg
Heart Rate	- beats / min	- beats / min	- beats / min	- beats / min
Temperature	- °C	- °C	- °C	- °C
Consciousness	-	-	-	-
Doctor's name				
Signature				
Date	/ /	/ /	/ /	/ /
Time	:	:	:	:

ADDS CHART WITH BP TABLE

DRAFT

DO NOT WRITE IN THIS BINDING MARGIN

DRAFT

UR Number: ______

Family name: ______

Given names: ______

Date of birth: ___/___/___ Sex: ☐ M ☐ F

(Affix patient identification label here)

Interventions Associated With Abnormal Vital Signs

If you administer an intervention, record here and note letter in Intervention row over page in appropriate time column.

Reference Letter	Intervention (initial if required)
a	
b	
c	
d	
e	
f	
g	
h	

Clinical Review Requests

Review requested Date / / Time : ☐ Ward doctor ☐ ☐ Emergency

Specify reason:

Review requested Date / / Time : ☐ Ward doctor ☐ ☐ Emergency

Specify reason:

Review requested Date / / Time : ☐ Ward doctor ☐ ☐ Emergency

Specify reason:

Additional Observations

Date		
Time		
Blood Glucose Level (mmol / L)		
Weight (kg)		
Bowels		
Urinalysis	Specific gravity	
	pH	
	Leukocytes	
	Blood	
	Nitrite	
	Ketones	
	Bilirubin	
	Urobilinogen	
	Protein	
	Glucose	

FIGURE 10.10 Adult Deterioration Detection System (ADDS) chart

PROCEDURES AND NORMAL FINDINGS

ABNORMAL FINDINGS AND CLINICAL ALERTS

Vital signs

Manual

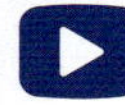

Digital

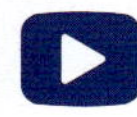

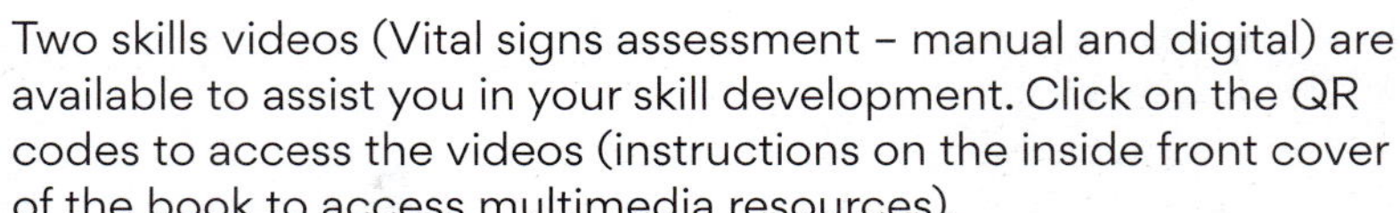

Two skills videos (Vital signs assessment – manual and digital) are available to assist you in your skill development. Click on the QR codes to access the videos (instructions on the inside front cover of the book to access multimedia resources).

This collection of measurements is used as part of **baseline assessment** of people, **routine monitoring** of response to treatments and to **detect deterioration**.

Pulse oximetry, neurological observations (Chapter 12), wound (Chapter 22) or circulation checks (Chapter 16) and/or pain assessment (Chapter 13) may also supplement vital signs and are done according to the person's needs.

A consistent, systematic method for measuring vital signs is necessary for accuracy. The order in which the various components of vital signs are taken varies according to need. The frequency of vital sign measurements will also depend on need, and care should be taken so vital sign measurements are not done unnecessarily.

Interpretation of vital sign measurements is always considered in the context of the broader assessment of the person. Document vital signs on the Australian ADDS chart[4] (NZEWS chart in New Zealand hospitals[5]) and note the variation of results from previous recordings. If any result falls outside normal parameters, follow instructions on the chart as to further actions (Figure 10.10).

Abnormal findings and clinical alerts:

It is important that vital signs are correlated with other physical assessment findings. Trends in vital signs are evaluated over time to enable accurate decision making and planning of treatment and/or referral.

Vital signs should be taken when the person is at rest and not immediately after ambulating.

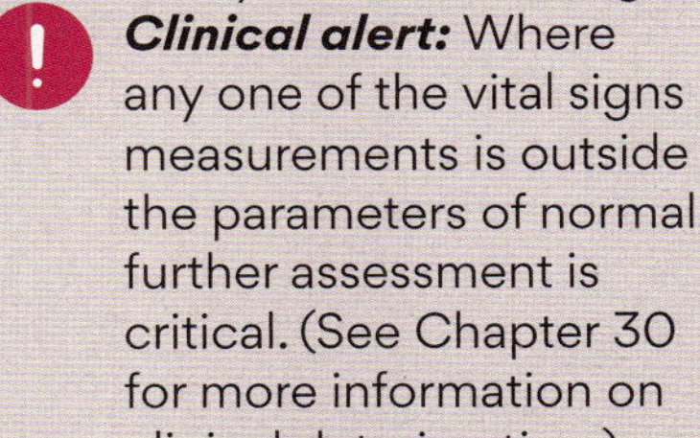

Clinical alert: Where any one of the vital signs measurements is outside the parameters of normal, further assessment is critical. (See Chapter 30 for more information on clinical deterioration.)

Temperature

Body temperature is the difference between heat produced by metabolism, exercise and activity and heat lost through radiation, evaporation of sweat, convection and conduction. Cellular metabolism requires a stable core temperature ranging between 35.8 and 37.5°C. Constant core temperature is maintained through homeostasis and is regulated by the hypothalamus.

The hypothalamus works in conjunction with autonomic and sympathetic mechanisms such as muscle tone, activity of the thyroid and adrenal glands as well as basal metabolic rate and vasoconstriction or vasodilation of peripheral vessels.[6]

Abnormal findings and clinical alerts:

Body temperature above or below the normal range (35.8–37.5°C) may occur due to illness, medical treatment or central nervous systems disorders.

Normothermia or afebrile: Body temperature ranges between 35.8 and 37.5°C, but this depends on which site is used for measurement.

Among healthy people, the average daily temperature can differ by 0.5°C.

PROCEDURES AND NORMAL FINDINGS	ABNORMAL FINDINGS AND CLINICAL ALERTS

Body temperature is influenced by the following:

- **Circadian rhythms.** Body temperature normally fluctuates over the day, with the lowest levels around 4 am and the highest in the late afternoon, between 4 and 6 pm.
- **Ovulation.** The menstruation cycle, progesterone secretion occurs with ovulation, creating a 0.15 to 0.45°C rise in temperature—caused by sharply elevated levels of progesterone—that continues until menses occurs.
- **Exercise and stress.** Moderate-to-hard exercise and stress increases body temperature.
- **Digestion** causes an elevation in body temperature.
- **Extremes of age.** Thermoregulation is less effective in infants, young children and very old people.

Hypothermia occurs when the body temperature registers between 25.0 and 35.0°C. Additional physical changes include skin (cool to touch) and cardiovascular changes (capillary endothelium becomes 'leaky' due to prolonged exposure to cold).

Body temperature can be measured at different body sites using various equipment (Table 10.1). Sites include the mouth, axilla, external auditory canal and rectum. Temperatures will differ according to selected body site. For example:

- Rectal temperatures are usually 0.4°C higher than oral temperatures.
- Axillary temperatures are 0.6°C lower than oral temperatures.

Site selection depends on conscious state, age and ability to cooperate. Use of the oral route is contraindicated for young children or people who have had facial or nasal surgery.[7]

Elevated body temperature is described in a variety of ways.

Pyrexia is an elevated temperature due to an increase in the body's temperature set point. Pyrexia is also known as fever or febrile response.

Hyperthermia or **hyperpyrexia** are terms used to describe a temperature exceeding 39.0°C.

Pyrogens (substances that produce a fever) cause the thermostat in the hypothalamus to reset to a higher level.

Hyperthermia occurs following myocardial infarction, trauma, surgery, malignancy, sepsis and neurological disorders (e.g. stroke, cerebral oedema, brain tumour).

! ***Clinical alert:*** Sudden increase in temperature usually indicates infection and as such requires further investigation. Report to a medical practitioner if the temperature exceeds 39.0°C.

A febrile person will usually demonstrate pale, cool skin and shiver to generate body heat. This may be followed by vasodilation of the skin and sweating.

PROCEDURES AND NORMAL FINDINGS | ABNORMAL FINDINGS AND CLINICAL ALERTS

TABLE 10.1 Summary of approaches to temperature measurement

Site	Type of thermometer	Use	Advantages/Disadvantages
Mouth	Digital probe thermometer Strip thermometer	• Older children • Adults	• Reading affected by ingestion of food, fluid or smoking before measurement the temperature • Normal range 35.8 to 37.5°C • Strip thermometer less accurate than other methods
External auditory canal (tympanic membrane)	Electronic tympanic thermometer	• Commonly used • Minimally invasive • Provides rapid results • Children over 3 months • Adults	• Unsuitable for babies under 3 months • Change probe cover each time temperature taken • Moderate correlation with core temperature • Risk of tympanic membrane perforation • Not reliable in critically ill adults • Presence of cerumen (wax) may affect accuracy
Axilla	Digital probe thermometer	Site may be used for people with mouth injuries and/or cannot breathe through their nose	• Less accurate than other methods • Affected by local blood flow, sweat • Moderate concordance with core temperature • Lower than oral temperature • Normal range 34.8 to 36.3°C • Not recommended for a critically ill person
Forehead	Strip thermometer	Can be used for children, adults	• Less accurate than other methods
Forehead/ temple	Infrared thermometer	• Can be used for any person providing forehead is visible • Portable, handheld • Noninvasive • Provides rapid results	• Does not reliably reflect core temperature

Continued

PROCEDURES AND NORMAL FINDINGS	ABNORMAL FINDINGS AND CLINICAL ALERTS

TABLE 10.1 Summary of approaches to temperature measurement cont'd

Site	Type of thermometer	Use	Advantages/Disadvantages
Rectal	Rectal thermometer	• May be used for people who are critically ill or undergoing complex surgery • Traditionally used to measure core temperature • Rarely used	• Discomfort and risk of rectal perforation • Higher than oral temperature • Found to not be an accurate predictor of core temperature
Invasive temperature measurement	Pulmonary artery, oesophageal, nasopharyngeal and bladder temperature monitors use thermistors, which are thermally sensitive	• Accurate • Cost-effective • Used for critically ill people	• Invasive • Risk of infection/perforation

Body temperature can be measured in a variety of ways.

A. The **electronic thermometer** is a thermo-resistive device in which the electrical resistance changes in response to temperature changes. This type of thermometer has the advantages of swift and accurate measurement (usually in a few seconds) using safe, unbreakable, disposable probe covers.

This type of thermometer can be used in the mouth, axilla, tympanic membrane or rectum.

The instrument must be fully charged and correctly calibrated.

Regardless of the body site used to measure temperature, a disposable probe cover is put on the electronic probe before use on each person. The device produces a digital reading which is read and recorded on the vital signs chart. After the measurement has been taken, the probe cover is removed and disposed into a suitable waste receptacle (Figure 10.11).

Using an electronic thermometer to measure rectal temperature is rarely used but, if used, gloves are worn, add a lubricated rectal probe cover on an electronic thermometer, insert only 2 to 3 cm into an adult rectum, directed towards the umbilicus.

Extreme care should be taken if the temperature is taken via the rectum. Complications such as rectal perforation have occurred.

PROCEDURES AND NORMAL FINDINGS	ABNORMAL FINDINGS AND CLINICAL ALERTS

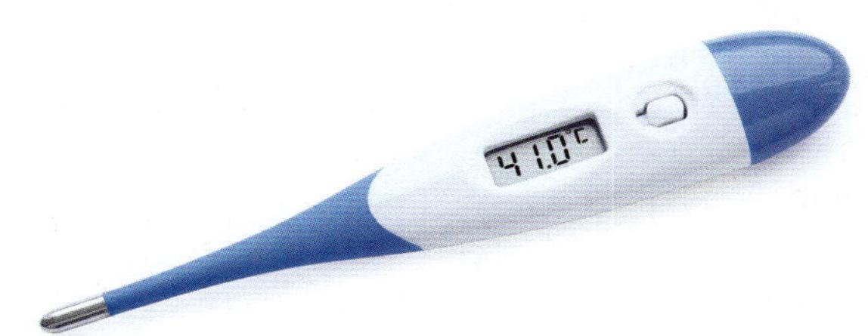

FIGURE 10.11 An electronic thermometer.

B. The **tympanic membrane thermometer** is another example of an infrared device. This type of thermometer directly reflects core temperature. The tympanic membrane and the hypothalamus share an arterial blood supply originating from the carotid artery.
It is a noninvasive, non-traumatic device that is extremely quick and efficient. The probe tip has the shape of an otoscope (instrument used to inspect the ear).
Gently pull the pinna of the ear upwards and backwards and place the covered probe tip in the person's ear canal (Figure 10.12). Do not force it and do not occlude the canal. Activate the device and you can read the temperature in 2 to 3 seconds.

The tympanic membrane thermometer is not suitable for use in babies under 3 months of age.

Incorrect placement of the probe tip or earwax buildup could account for a low temperature reading.[8]

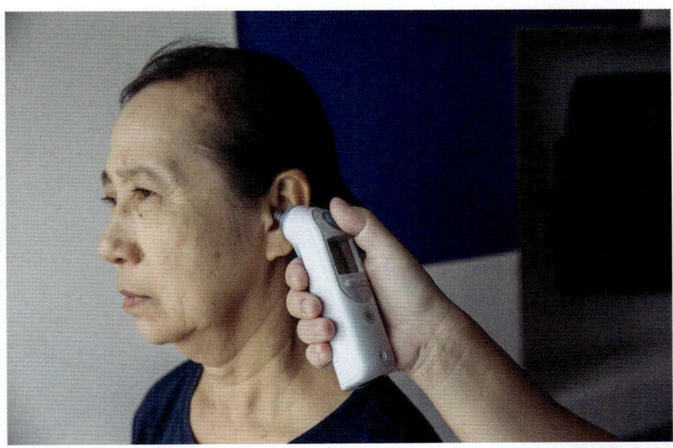

FIGURE 10.12 Measuring tympanic temperature.

PROCEDURES AND NORMAL FINDINGS	ABNORMAL FINDINGS AND CLINICAL ALERTS

Temporal artery thermometer The temporal artery thermometer (Figure 10.13) is used by sliding the probe across the forehead and behind the ear. The thermometer works by taking multiple readings using infrared emissions and providing an average. The reading takes approximately 6 seconds. Although well tolerated by patients, these thermometers have questionable reliability and are likely not to be as accurate as other methods.

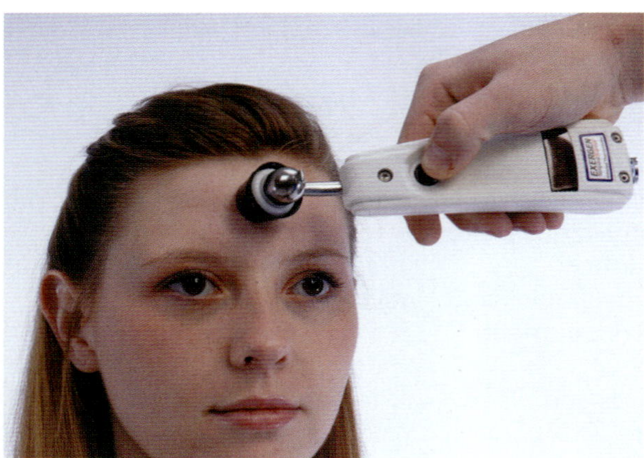

FIGURE 10.13 Temporal artery thermometer

The **handheld infrared thermometer** (Figure 10.14) is another example of an infrared thermometer. It is a noninvasive device that works on the principle that heat is converted into an electrical signal. This type of thermometer measures the temperature of the skin. It is held 3 to 15 cm away from the person's forehead. Activate the device and you can read the temperature in 2 to 3 seconds.

Abnormal findings and clinical alerts:

Skin should be dry.

Less accurate than other measures and are not sensitive to temperatures above 37.5°C

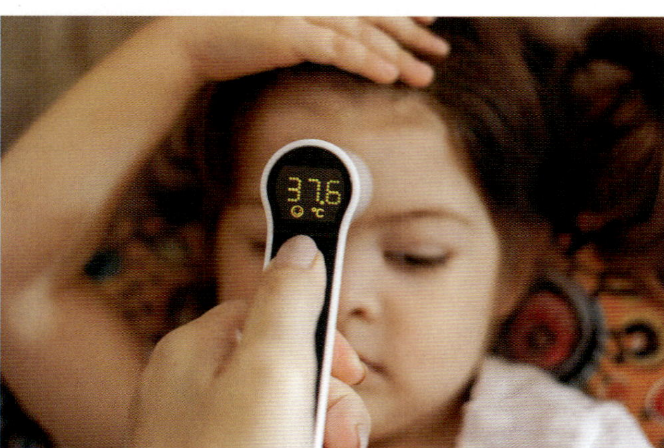

FIGURE 10.14 Handheld infrared thermometer

PROCEDURES AND NORMAL FINDINGS	ABNORMAL FINDINGS AND CLINICAL ALERTS

C. Strip thermometers are plastic strips, which can be placed on the forehead and change colour to indicate the temperature. The strip is placed on the forehead and read after 1 minute. Read it while the strip is in place (Figure 10.15).

This method is the least accurate of all methods.

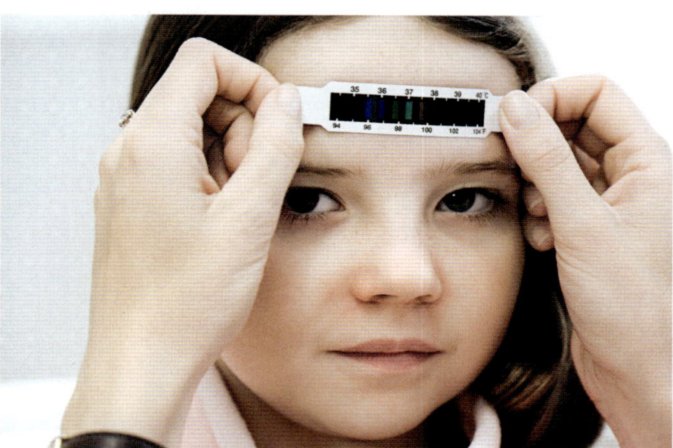

FIGURE 10.15 Measuring temperature using a strip thermometer.

Document the temperature in degrees Celsius onto the vital signs chart (ADDS chart).[4,5] Make sure to note the route used to get the temperature reading.

Pulse

With every beat, the heart pumps an amount of blood—the **stroke volume**—into the aorta. This is about 70 mL in an adult. The force flares the arterial walls and generates a pressure wave, which is felt in the periphery as the **pulse.** Palpating the peripheral pulse gives the rate and rhythm of the heartbeat, as well as local data on the condition of the artery. The radial pulse is usually palpated when measuring vital signs.

Using the pads of your first three fingers, palpate the radial pulse at the flexor aspect of the wrist laterally along the radius bone (Figure 10.16). Push until you feel the strongest pulsation. Press firmly but not so hard as to obliterate the pulse. While it is recommended to count for 60 seconds, if the rhythm is regular, count the number of beats in 30 seconds and multiply by 2. The 30-second interval is the most accurate and efficient when heart rates are normal or rapid and when rhythms are regular.
Assess the pulse for (1) rate, (2) rhythm, (3) force/strength (strong, weak or thready).
Document the heart rate on the vital signs chart.[4,5]

Should difficulty be encountered with taking a peripheral pulse (e.g. faint or irregular rhythm), then an apical heart rate should be taken (Chapter 17).

Pulse force (strength) reflects the volume of blood ejected against the arterial wall with each heart contraction.

If the rhythm is **irregular**, count the pulse for a full minute.

PROCEDURES AND NORMAL FINDINGS	ABNORMAL FINDINGS AND CLINICAL ALERTS

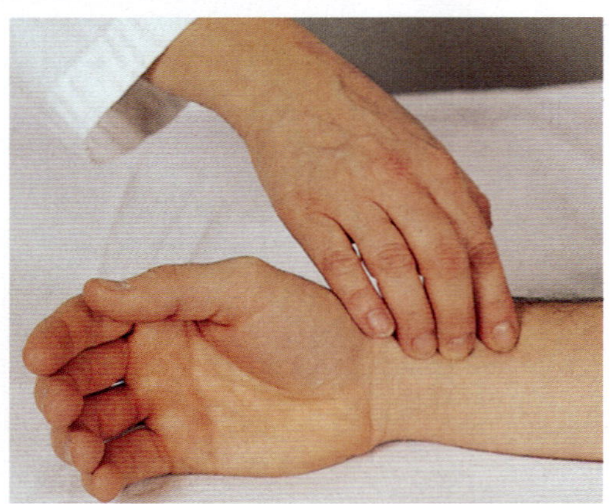

FIGURE 10.16 Palpating a radial pulse.

Heart rate

In a resting adult, the normal heart rate range is 60 to 100 beats per minute (bpm). The rate normally varies with age, being more rapid in infancy and childhood and more moderate during the adult and older years. The rate also varies with gender; after puberty, females have a slightly faster rate than males (Table 10.2).

TABLE 10.2 Normal resting heart rates across age groups

Age	Average (Beats per minute)	Normal limits
Newborn	120	70–190
1 year	120	80–160
2 years	110	80–130
4 years	100	80–120
6 years	100	75–115
8 years	90	70–110
10 years	90	70–110
12 years		
Female	90	70–110
Male	85	65–105

Bradycardia—heart rate < 60 bpm in an adult. However, a low pulse rate occurs normally in well-trained athletes whose heart muscle develops along with the skeletal muscles. A stronger, more efficient heart muscle pushes out a larger stroke volume with each beat, therefore requiring fewer beats per minute to maintain a stable cardiac output.

Tachycardia (rate > 120 beats per minute) occurs with fever, sepsis, hypovolaemia, pneumonia, myocardial infarction and pancreatitis.

Many medications affect the heart rate, with nearly all people with heart disease taking at least one medication that slows the heart rate.

! ***Clinical alert:*** If **tachycardia or bradycardia** occur, auscultate the apical pulse (Chapter 17). Report tachycardia or bradycardia to a medical practitioner.

PROCEDURES AND NORMAL FINDINGS

ABNORMAL FINDINGS AND CLINICAL ALERTS

TABLE 10.2 Normal resting heart rates across age groups cont'd

Age	Average (Beats per minute)	Normal limits
14 years		
Female	85	65–105
Male	80	60–100
16 years		
Female	80	60–100
Male	75	55–95
18 years		
Female	75	55–95
Male	70	50–90
Well-conditioned athlete	May be 50–60	50–100
Adult	74–76	60–100
Over 65 years	74–76	60–100

For descriptions of abnormal rates and rhythms, see Table 16.1.

Rhythm

The rhythm of the heart rate normally has an even tempo.

An irregular rhythm indicates a **cardiac arrhythmia.**

One irregularity that is commonly found in children and young adults is **sinus arrhythmia.** Here the heart rate varies with the respiratory cycle, speeding up at the peak of inspiration and slowing to normal with expiration. Inspiration momentarily causes a decreased stroke volume from the left side of the heart; to compensate, the heart rate increases.[1] (See Chapter 17 for a full discussion of sinus arrhythmia.) If any other irregularities are felt, auscultate heart sounds for a more complete assessment (Chapter 17).

PROCEDURES AND NORMAL FINDINGS	ABNORMAL FINDINGS AND CLINICAL ALERTS

Force (strength)

The force of the pulse shows the strength of the heart's stroke volume. The pulse force is recorded using a three-point scale:

- 3+ —Full, bounding
- 2+ —Normal
- 1+ —Weak, thready
- 0 —Absent.

Make sure your documentation of pulse force (strength) is consistent with that used by your health agency.

A **'weak, thready' pulse** reflects a decreased stroke volume (e.g. as occurs with haemorrhagic shock).

A **'full, bounding' pulse** denotes an increased stroke volume, as with anxiety, exercise or a number of medical conditions.

Respirations

Normally, a person's breathing is relaxed, regular, automatic and silent. Because most people are unaware of their breathing, do not mention you will be counting the respirations because sudden awareness may alter the normal pattern. Instead, maintain your position of counting the radial pulse and unobtrusively count the respirations by placing the person's arm in a relaxed position across the abdomen or lower chest.

Count for 30 seconds or for a full minute if you suspect an abnormality. If you are having difficulty observing the rise and fall of the person's chest wall place your hand on the person's hand.

Document the respiratory rate on the vital signs chart.[4, 5]

The optimal method of respiratory rate count involves counting for a full minute using a stethoscope against the chest when respiratory rate is rapid to ensure all breaths are counted and counting respiratory rate when the person is at rest.

Clinical alert:

Abnormalities in respiration rates are a very important early indicator of patient deterioration and must be reported and managed immediately. (See Chapter 30 for further discussion of clinical deterioration.)

Respiratory rates presented in Table 10.3 show normal respiratory rates across age groups. More detailed assessment on respiratory status is presented in Chapter 19.

TABLE 10.3 Normal respiratory rates

Age	Breaths per minute
Neonate	30–40
1 year	20–40
2 years	25–32
8–10 years	20–26
12–14 years	18–22
16 years	12–20
Adult	10–19

PROCEDURES AND NORMAL FINDINGS	ABNORMAL FINDINGS AND CLINICAL ALERTS

Blood pressure

BP is the force of the blood pushing against the side of the arterial wall. The strength of the push changes with the stage in the cardiac cycle. The **systolic** pressure is the maximum pressure exerted on the arterial wall during left ventricular contraction or systole. The **diastolic** pressure is the resting pressure exerted by blood on the arterial wall between each contraction or diastole. The **pulse pressure** is the difference between the systolic and diastolic pressures and reflects the stroke volume (Figure 10.17).

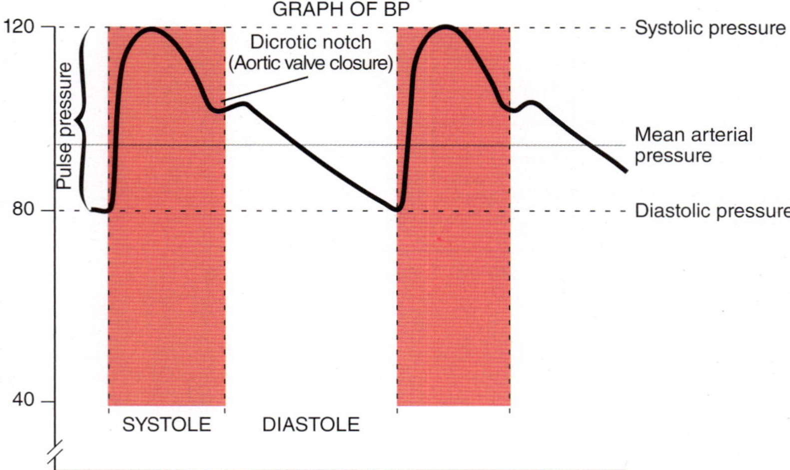

FIGURE 10.17 Blood pressure changes over the cardiac cycle

The average BP in a young adult is 120/80 mmHg, although this varies normally with many factors, as listed below.

Age. Normally, a gradual rise occurs through childhood and into the adult years (Figure 10.18).

PROCEDURES AND NORMAL FINDINGS	ABNORMAL FINDINGS AND CLINICAL ALERTS

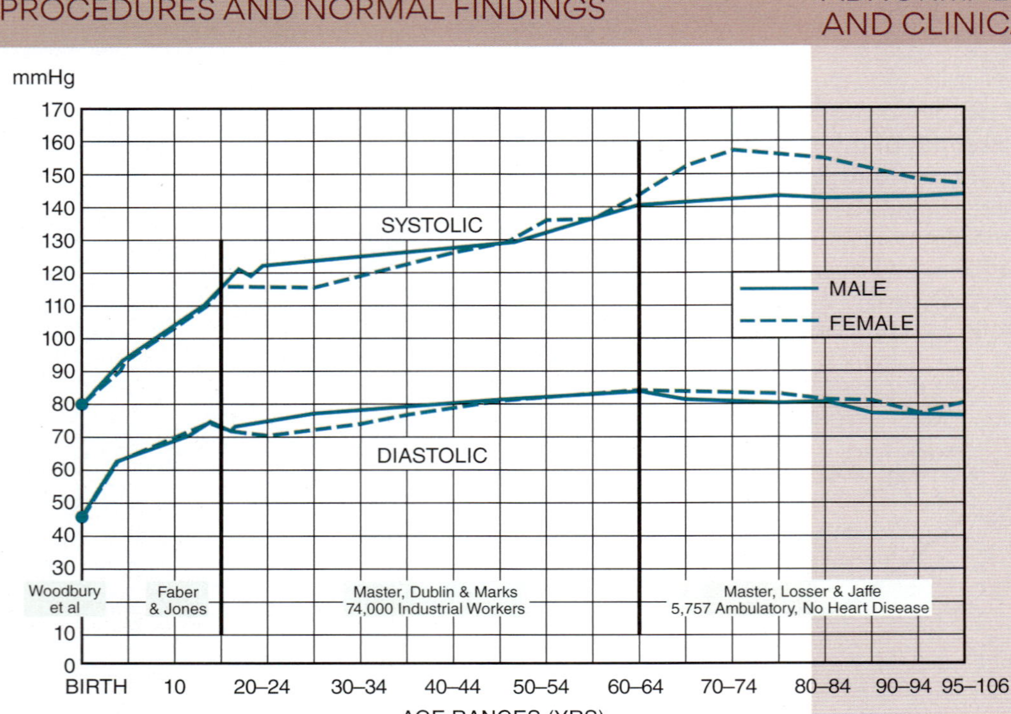

FIGURE 10.18 Blood pressure changes from birth to adulthood

Sex. Before puberty, no difference exists between males and females. After puberty, females usually show a lower BP reading than do males. After menopause, BP in females is higher than in males.

Diurnal rhythm. A daily cycle of a peak and a trough occurs: the BP climbs to a high in late afternoon or early evening and then declines to an early morning low.

Weight. BP is higher in obese people than in people of normal weight of the same age (including adolescents).

Exercise. Increasing activity yields a proportionate increase in BP. Within 5 minutes of terminating the exercise, the BP normally returns to baseline.

Emotions. The BP momentarily rises with fear, anger and pain because of stimulation of the sympathetic nervous system.

Stress. The BP is elevated in people feeling continual tension because of lifestyle, occupational stress or life problems.

The level of **BP** is determined by 5 factors as depicted in Figure 10.19.

PROCEDURES AND NORMAL FINDINGS | ABNORMAL FINDINGS AND CLINICAL ALERTS

FACTORS CONTROLLING BLOOD PRESSURE

FACTOR	CONDITION	RESULT
Cardiac output	↑ with heavy exercise to meet body demand for increased metabolism	↑ BP
	↓ with pump failure (weak pumping action after myocardial infarction, or in shock)	↓ BP
Vascular resistance	↑ resistance (vasoconstriction)	↑ BP
	↓ resistance (vasodilation)	↓ BP
Volume	↓ volume (haemorrhage)	↓ BP
	↑ volume (increased sodium and water retention, intravenous fluid overload)	↑ BP
Viscosity	↑ viscosity (increased haematocrit in polycythaemia)	↑ BP
Elasticity of arterial walls	↑ rigidity, hardening as in arteriosclerosis (heart pumping against greater resistance)	↑ BP

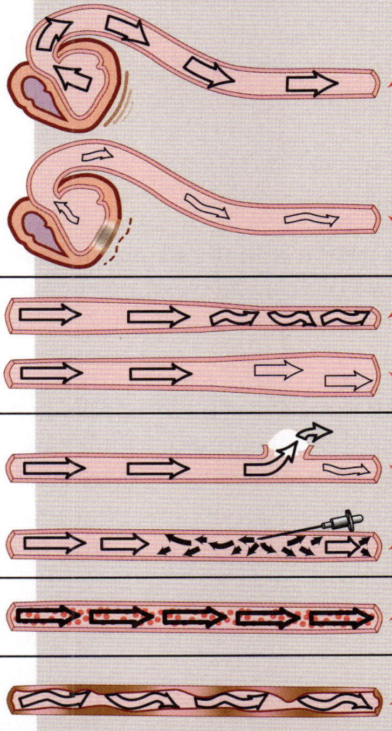

FIGURE 10.19 Factors affecting blood pressure

1. **Cardiac output.** The more blood the heart pumps into the blood vessels, the higher the pressure on the arterial walls.
2. **Peripheral vascular resistance.** Peripheral vascular resistance is the opposition to blood flow through the arteries. When the arteries become smaller (e.g. with constricted vessels), the pressure needed to push the blood volume becomes greater.

Many medications used in the treatment of critically ill people affect peripheral vascular resistance.

3. **Volume of circulating blood.** A high circulating blood volume increases the pressure in the arteries.

Blood volume is increased, for example by blood transfusions or volume expanders or by fluid retention, and decreased, for example through haemorrhage or dehydration.

4. **Viscosity.** The 'thickness' of blood is determined by the number of blood cells. When the blood is thicker, the pressure within the circulator system increases.

PROCEDURES AND NORMAL FINDINGS	ABNORMAL FINDINGS AND CLINICAL ALERTS
5. **Elasticity of vessel walls.** When the arterial walls are stiff and rigid, the pressure needed by the heart to push the blood increases.	
BP is measured with a stethoscope and an anaeroid sphygmomanometer or an electronic BP monitor.	Regular maintenance and calibration of anaeroid manometers or electronic devices is required to ensure accuracy of readings.
Taking a BP manually using an anaeroid sphygmomanometer The anaeroid gauge must be recalibrated at least once each year and it must rest at zero.	
The cuff consists of an inflatable bladder inside a fabric cover. The width of the cuff should equal 40% of the circumference of the person's arm. The length of the bladder should equal 80% of this circumference. Available cuffs include sizes that fit newborn infants to the extra-large adult (Figure 10.20).	Ill-fitting or wider cuffs deliver false low readings and narrow cuffs give a false high reading.[3]

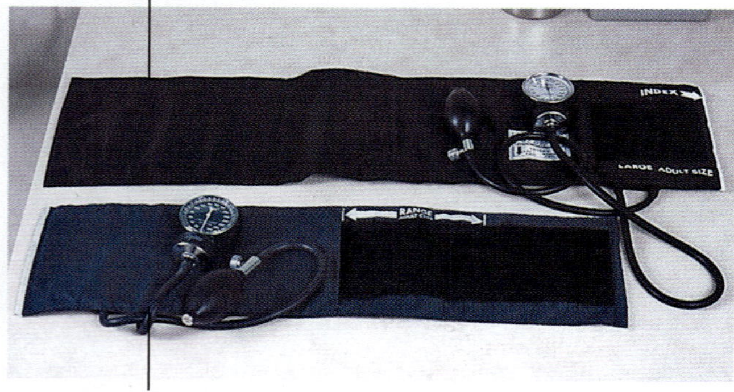

FIGURE 10.20 Adult blood pressure cuffs (thigh and standard)

PROCEDURES AND NORMAL FINDINGS	ABNORMAL FINDINGS AND CLINICAL ALERTS
Match the appropriate size cuff to the person's arm size and shape.	
Many people are anxious at the beginning of an examination; allow at least a 5-minute rest before measuring the BP. Then take two or more BP measurements separated by 2 minutes.	The BP is more likely to be valid if the person is comfortable and relaxed.

PROCEDURES AND NORMAL FINDINGS	ABNORMAL FINDINGS AND CLINICAL ALERTS
For each person, verify BP in both arms once, either on admission or for the first complete physical examination. It is not necessary to continue to check both arms for screening or monitoring.	Occasionally, a 5 to 10 mmHg difference may occur in BP in the two arms (if values are different, use the higher value).[3]  ***Clinical alert:*** If there is a significant discrepancy in the BP between the two arms, report this finding to a medical practitioner for further assessment because this may be a sign of aortic aneurysm.
The person may be sitting or lying, with the bare arm supported at heart level.	Wait up to 5 minutes before taking a BP measurement following exertion or position change.
Palpate the brachial artery, which is located just above the antecubital fossa, medial to the biceps tendon. With the cuff deflated, centre it about 2.5 cm above the brachial artery and wrap it evenly and firmly around the arm.	
Now palpate the brachial or the radial artery (Figure 10.21). Inflate the cuff until the artery pulsation is obliterated and then 20–30 mmHg beyond. This will avoid missing an auscultatory gap, which is a period when Korotkoff sounds disappear during auscultation (Table 10.3).	An **auscultatory gap** occurs in about 5% of people, most often in hypertension caused by a noncompliant arterial system.

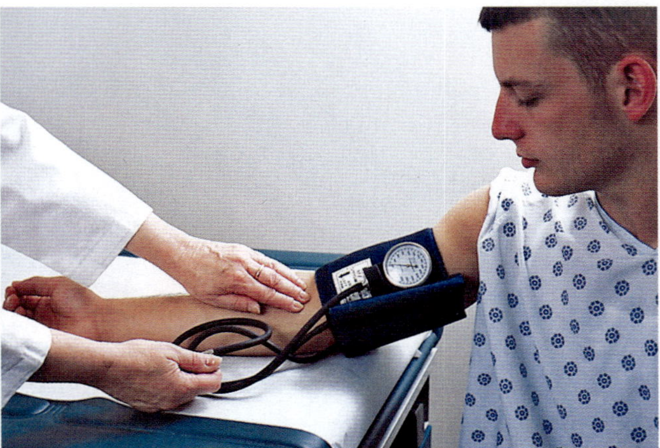

FIGURE 10.21 Palpating the brachial artery

PROCEDURES AND NORMAL FINDINGS	ABNORMAL FINDINGS AND CLINICAL ALERTS
Deflate the cuff quickly and completely; then wait 15 to 30 seconds before reinflating so the blood trapped in the veins can dissipate. Place the bell of the stethoscope over the site of the brachial artery, making a light but airtight seal (Figure 10.22). The diaphragm endpiece is usually adequate, but the bell is designed to pick up low-pitched sounds such as the sounds of a BP reading. So if you have a bell, use it.	Blood pressure measurement is more accurate when using the bell rather than the diaphragm of the stethoscope.

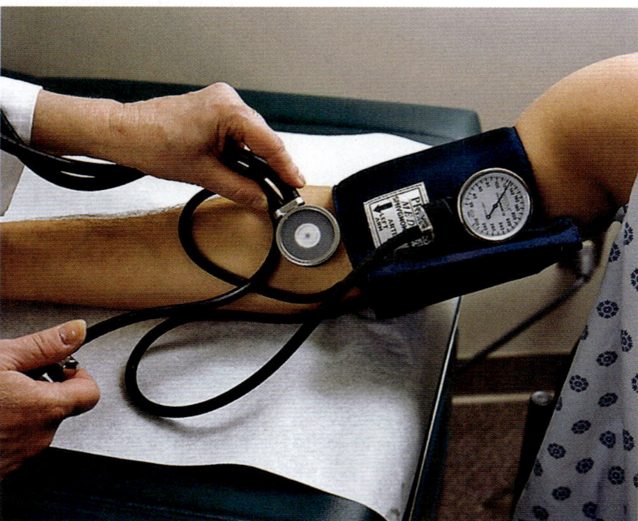

FIGURE 10.22 Placing the bell of the stethoscope over the brachial artery

Rapidly inflate the cuff to the maximal inflation level you determined via previous palpation. Then deflate the cuff slowly and evenly, about 2 mmHg per heartbeat. Note the points at which you hear the first appearance of sound, the muffling of sound and the final disappearance of sound. These are phases I, IV and V of **Korotkoff sounds**, which are the components of a BP reading first described by a Russian surgeon in 1905 (Table 10.4).

PROCEDURES AND NORMAL FINDINGS | ABNORMAL FINDINGS AND CLINICAL ALERTS

TABLE 10.4 Korotkoff sounds

Phase	Quality	Description	Rationale
Cuff correctly inflated	No sound		Cuff inflation compresses brachial artery. Cuff pressure exceeds heart systolic pressure, occluding brachial artery blood flow.
I	Tapping	Soft, clear tapping, increasing in intensity	**Systolic pressure.** As cuff pressure lowers to reach intraluminal systolic pressure, artery opens and blood first spurts into the brachial artery. Blood is at very high velocity because of the small opening of the artery and large pressure difference across the opening. This creates turbulent flow, which is audible.
Auscultatory gap	No sound	Silence for 30–40 mmHg during deflation; an abnormal finding	Sounds temporarily disappear during the end of phase I and reappear in phase II. Common with hypertension. If undetected, results in falsely low systolic or falsely high diastolic reading.
II	Swooshing	Softer murmur follows tapping	Turbulent blood flow through still partially occluded artery.
III	Knocking	Crisp, high-pitched sounds	Longer duration of blood flow through the artery. Artery closes just briefly during late diastole.
IV	Abrupt muffling	Sound mutes to a low-pitched, cushioned murmur; blowing quality	Artery no longer closes in any part of cardiac cycle. Change in quality, not intensity.
V	Silence		Decreased velocity of blood flow. Streamlined blood flow is silent. The last audible sound (marking the disappearance of sounds) is **diastolic** pressure. The fifth Korotkoff sound is now used to define diastolic pressure in all age groups.

For all age-groups, the fifth Korotkoff phase is used to define diastolic pressure. However, when a variance greater than 10 to 12 mmHg exists between phases IV and V, record both phases along with the systolic reading (e.g. 142/98/80).

Clear communication is important because the results significantly affect diagnosis and planning of care. See Table 10.5 for a list of common errors in BP measurement.

Document the BP reading on the vital signs chart.[4,5]

Hypotension, abnormally low BP; **hypertension**, abnormally high BP (see parameters in Table 10.6 below).

PROCEDURES AND NORMAL FINDINGS | ABNORMAL FINDINGS AND CLINICAL ALERTS

TABLE 10.5 Common errors in blood pressure measurement

Common error	Result	Rationale
Taking BP reading when person is anxious or angry or has just been active	Falsely high	Sympathetic nervous system stimulation
Faulty arm position		
Above level of heart	Falsely low	Eliminates effect of hydrostatic pressure
Below level of heart	Falsely high	Additional force of gravity added to brachial artery pressure
Person supports own arm	Falsely high diastolic	Sustained isometric muscular contraction
Faulty leg position (e.g. person's legs are crossed)	Falsely high systolic and diastolic	Translocation of blood volume from dependent legs to thoracic area
Inaccurate cuff size (most common error)		
Cuff too narrow for extremity	Falsely high	Needs excessive pressure to occlude brachial artery
Cuff wrap is too loose or uneven or bladder balloons out of wrap	Falsely high	Needs excessive pressure to occlude brachial artery
Failure to palpate radial artery while inflating cuff		
Inflating cuff not high enough	Falsely low systolic	Misses initial systolic tapping or may tune in during auscultatory gap (tapping sounds disappear for 10 to 40 mmHg and then return; common with hypertension)
Inflating cuff too high	Pain	
Pushing stethoscope too hard on brachial artery	Falsely low diastolic	Excessive pressure distorts artery, and sounds continue
Deflating cuff		
Too quickly	Falsely low systolic or falsely high diastolic	Insufficient time to hear tapping
Too slowly	Falsely high diastolic	Venous congestion in forearm makes sounds less audible
Halting during descent and reinflating cuff to recheck systolic	Falsely high diastolic	Venous congestion in forearm

PROCEDURES AND NORMAL FINDINGS	ABNORMAL FINDINGS AND CLINICAL ALERTS

TABLE 10.5 Common errors in blood pressure measurement cont'd

Common error	Result	Rationale
Failure to wait 1 to 2 minutes before repeating entire reading	Falsely high diastolic	Venous congestion in forearm
Any observer error		
Examiner's 'subconscious bias'; a preconceived idea of what BP reading should be because of person's age, race, gender, weight, history or condition	Error anywhere	Never assume that, because a person appears healthy, their BP will be within normal limits
Examiner's haste		
Faulty technique		
Examiner's digit preference; 'hears' more results that end in zero than would occur by chance alone (e.g. 130/80) Diminished hearing acuity Defective or inaccurately calibrated equipment	Error anywhere	

TABLE 10.6 Abnormalities in blood pressure

Hypotension

In normotensive adults: < 95/60
In children: less than expected value for age

Occurs with	*Rationale*
Acute myocardial infarction	Decreased cardiac output
Shock	Decreased cardiac output
Haemorrhage	Decrease in total blood volume
Vasodilatation	Decrease in peripheral vascular resistance
Addison's disease (hypofunction of adrenal glands)	
As a side effect of treatment for hypertension	

Associated symptoms and signs

In conditions of decreased cardiac output, a low BP is accompanied by an increased pulse, dizziness, diaphoresis, confusion and blurred vision. The skin feels cool and clammy because the superficial blood vessels constrict to shunt blood to the vital organs.

Continued

PROCEDURES AND NORMAL FINDINGS | ABNORMAL FINDINGS AND CLINICAL ALERTS

TABLE 10.6 Abnormalities in blood pressure cont'd

Hypotension

Orthostatic hypotension (postural hypotension) occurs when a normotensive person develops symptoms of low BP when changing from lying or sitting to a standing position. In this case, the BP should be measured in both positions.

Hypertension

Essential or primary hypertension

Essential or primary hypertension accounts for 95% of people with high BP. Obesity, smoking, high salt and alcohol intake and sedentary lifestyle and continued exposure to high levels of stress are known contributing factors.

Secondary hypertension

Secondary hypertension has known causes such as renal disease, endocrine disorders, coarctation of the aorta and others such as use of oral contraceptives, amphetamines, increased intracranial pressure and pre-eclampsia in pregnancy.

National Heart Foundation of Australia[10] classification of blood pressure in adults*

Diagnostic category	*Systolic (mmHg)*		*Diastolic (mmHg)*
Optimal	< 120	and	< 80
Normal	120–129	and/or	80–84
High normal	130–139	and/or	85–89
Grade 1 (mild) hypertension	140–159	and/or	90–99
Grade 2 (moderate) hypertension	160–179	and/or	100–109
Grade 3 (severe) hypertension	≥ 180	and/or	≥ 110
Isolated systolic hypertension	> 140	And	< 90

* When a person's systolic and diastolic BP falls into different categories the higher diagnostic category applies.

PROCEDURES AND NORMAL FINDINGS	ABNORMAL FINDINGS AND CLINICAL ALERTS

Electronic vital signs monitor

An automated vital signs monitor is commonly used in hospital and clinic settings. The artery pulsations create vibrations that are detected by an electronic sensor. The BP mode is noninvasive and fast and has automatic measurement intervals and a bright numeric display. As with manual BP equipment, accuracy depends on correct cuff selection and placement. A stethoscope is not required when using an electronic BP device.

Most electronic BP devices also have probes for thermometry and pulse oximetry (Figure 10.23).

Electronic BP devices are not capable of evaluating the quality of the pulse, i.e. force (strength) or rhythm.

The device can be programmed to alarm should the BP vary from desired limits.

! ***Clinical alert:*** Electronic BP monitors cannot sense vibrations of low BP; do not use them with a person who has a systolic BP of < 90 mmHg or conditions of an irregular heart rate, shivering, tremors or seizures.

If the numeric display does not fit with the person's clinical picture, always validate the measurement with a manual sphygmomanometer and your own stethoscope.

Digital and aneroid devices have been found to be similarly accurate.[11]

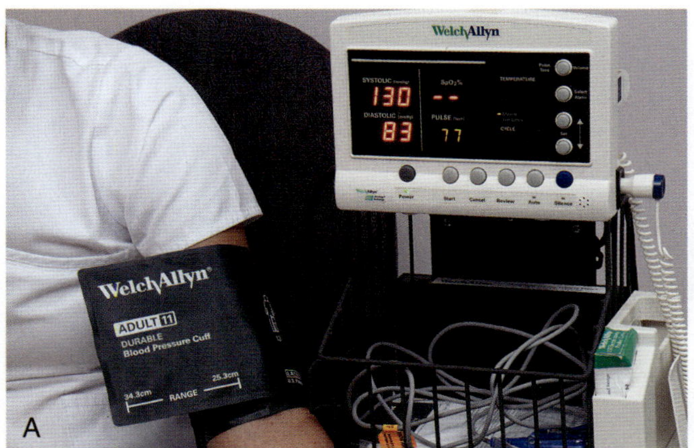

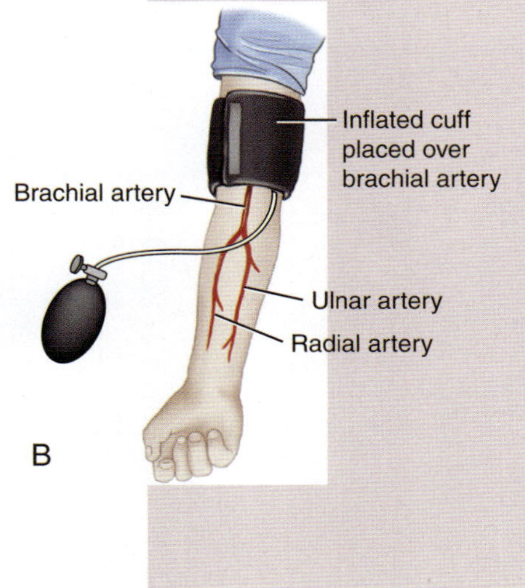

FIGURE 10.23 Electronic vital signs monitor

PROCEDURES AND NORMAL FINDINGS	ABNORMAL FINDINGS AND CLINICAL ALERTS

Orthostatic (or postural) blood pressure measurement

Take serial measurements of BP when you suspect:

- volume depletion
- when the person is known to have hypertension or is taking antihypertensive medications, or
- when the person reports fainting (syncope).

Have the person rest supine for 2 to 3 minutes, take baseline readings of BP, then repeat the measurements with the person sitting, then standing.

For a person who is too weak or dizzy to stand, assess supine and then sitting with the legs dangling. When the position is changed from supine to standing, a slight decrease (less than 10 mmHg) in systolic pressure may occur.

Document the BP on the vital signs chart.[4,5] Also record the person's position and the arm used.

Orthostatic hypotension is a drop in systolic pressure of more than 20 mmHg. These changes are due to abrupt peripheral vasodilatation without a compensatory increase in cardiac output. Orthostatic changes also occur with prolonged bed rest, older age, hypovolaemia and some medications.

Thigh pressure

Thigh pressures are used when there are no other alternatives.

If possible, turn the person into the prone position. (If the person must remain in the supine position, bend the knee slightly.) Wrap a large cuff, 18 to 20 cm, around the lower third of the thigh, centred over the popliteal artery on the back of the knee. Auscultate the popliteal artery for the reading (Figure 10.24). Normally, the systolic value is 10 to 40 mmHg higher in the thigh than in the arm, and the diastolic pressure ambiguous: 'is the same as normal' or 'is also 10 to 40 mmHg higher'.

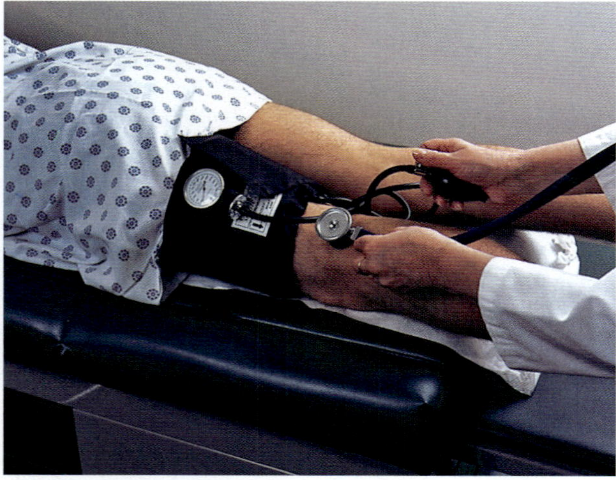

FIGURE 10.24 Measuring blood pressure at the thigh

PROCEDURES AND NORMAL FINDINGS	ABNORMAL FINDINGS AND CLINICAL ALERTS

Measurement of oxygen saturation

The **pulse oximeter** is a noninvasive method to assess arterial oxygen saturation (SpO_2). A sensor attached to the person's finger or earlobe has a diode that emits light and a detector that measures the relative amount of light absorbed by oxyhaemoglobin (HbO_2) and deoxygenated (reduced) haemoglobin. The pulse oximeter compares the ratio of light emitted to light absorbed and converts this ratio into the percentage of oxygen saturation. Because it only measures light absorption of pulsatile flow, the result is arterial oxygen saturation. A healthy person with no lung disease and no anaemia normally has an SpO_2 of 95 to 100%.

Oxygen saturation measurement commonly accompanies measurement of vital signs and is done according to the person's need.

Clinical alert: SpO_2 reading less than 95% requires immediate further investigation and the measurement repeated.

SpO_2 readings are an approximation of the person's oxygen saturation, which can only be accurately measured by arterial blood gas.

Select the appropriate pulse oximeter probe. The finger probe is spring loaded and feels like a clothespin attached to the finger but does not hurt (Figure 10.25)

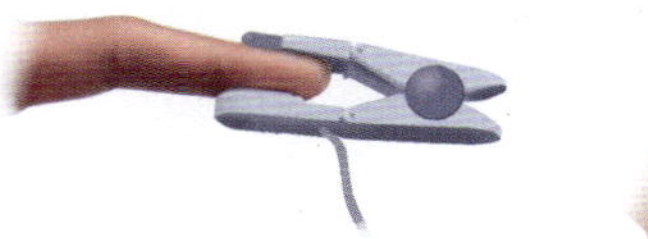
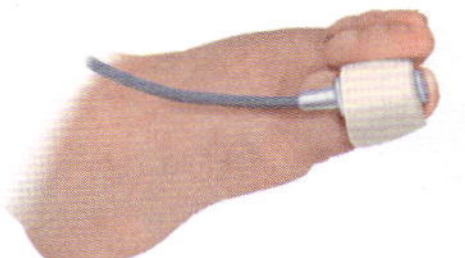
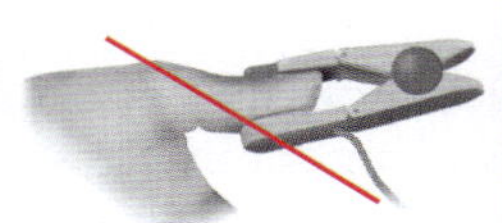

FIGURE 10.25 Placement of pulse oximeter

SpO_2 readings may be minimally affected with dark nail polish.[11]

Pulse oximetry readings are less accurate in patients with low perfusion (e.g. hypothermia, vasoconstriction), low haemoglobin.[3]

Additional objective data for infants and children

Vital signs

When taking a child or infant's vital signs ask the parent to assist, where appropriate. The infant or child should be positioned correctly and comfortably prior to and during the procedure.

Measure vital signs with the same purpose and frequency as you would in an adult. With an infant, reverse the order of vital sign measurement to respiration, pulse and temperature. For infants under 3 months of age, take the temperature using a digital thermometer at sites such as inguinal, axilla and rarely rectal.

For older children take a tympanic, inguinal or axillary temperature. The tympanic temperature measurement is so rapid that it is usually over before the child realises it.

Promote the cooperation of school-age children by explaining the procedure completely and encouraging the child to handle the equipment. Your approach to measuring vital signs with an adolescent is much the same as with an adult.

Infants must be more than 3 months of age to use tympanic temperature measurements.[12]

PROCEDURES AND NORMAL FINDINGS	ABNORMAL FINDINGS AND CLINICAL ALERTS
Temperature	
Tympanic. Temperature measurements are commonly used for children > 3 months of age (Figure 10.26). 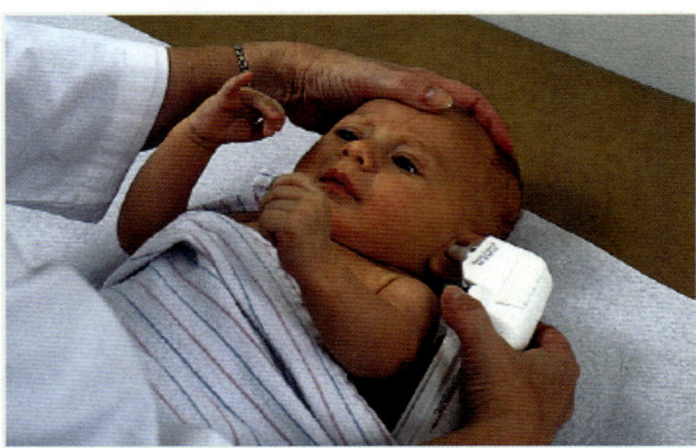 **FIGURE 10.26** Tympanic temperature on infant	Up to ages 6 to 8 years, children have higher fevers with illness than adults do. Even with minor infections, fevers may elevate the temperature to 39.5 to 40.5°C.
Axillary. The axillary route is safe and accessible and is used for infants < 3 months of age. When cold receptors are stimulated, brown fat tissue in the area releases heat through chemical energy, which artificially raises skin temperature. When the axillary route is used: • Place the thermometer tip in the centre of the armpit over the axillary artery, ensuring the skin is dry and intact prior to probe placement. • Hold the child's arm securely against their body. • Turn the thermometer on. For a more accurate reading, wait more than 3 minutes with the thermometer in situ before obtaining a measurement.[12]	Oral and rectal routes should not be routinely used to measure the body temperature in children aged from 0 to 5 years.
Inguinal. The inguinal route is also safe for measuring a child's body temperature. Its results may be closer to core temperature than the axillary site because the inguinal area has a rich supply of blood vessels, it lacks the brown fat tissue that interferes with axillary temperatures, and you can form a tight skin-to-skin seal. Abduct the infant's leg and locate the femoral pulse. Place the thermometer probe lateral to the pulse site and adduct the leg to create a seal.	
Oral. This route may also be used for a child who is old enough to keep their mouth closed. This is usually at age 5 or 6 years, although some 4-year-old children can cooperate.	Whenever possible use a tympanic or temporal artery thermometer.

PROCEDURES AND NORMAL FINDINGS	ABNORMAL FINDINGS AND CLINICAL ALERTS
Rectal. Use this route with neonates only if a fever is firstly demonstrated by axillary temperature.[12] Check with your organisation as a medical order may be required. An infant may be supine or side lying, with the examiner's hand flexing the knees up onto the abdomen. An infant also may lie prone across an adult's lap. Separate the buttocks with one hand, and insert the lubricated electronic rectal probe no further than 2.5 cm. Any deeper insertion risks rectal perforation because the colon curves posteriorly at 3 cm. Normally, rectal temperatures measure higher in infants and young children than in adults, with an average of 37.8°C at 18 months.	Rectal site should be avoided for those who have cancer, low platelets, coagulopathy, perineal trauma and pelvic area surgery, due to the increased risk of bowel perforation.[12]
Heart rate	
Palpate or auscultate an apical heart rate with infants and toddlers (see Chapter 17 for the location of the apex and technique). In children older than 2 years, use the radial site. Count the heart rate for a full minute to take into account normal irregularities such as sinus arrhythmia. The heart rate normally fluctuates more with infants and children than with adults in response to exercise, emotion and illness.	
Respirations	
Infants and children under 6 or 7 years are predominantly abdominal breathers. Watch the abdomen for movement because the respirations are normally more diaphragmatic than thoracic (Figure 10.27). Count a full minute because the pattern varies significantly from rapid breaths to short periods of apnoea. Note the normal rate in Table 10.3.	

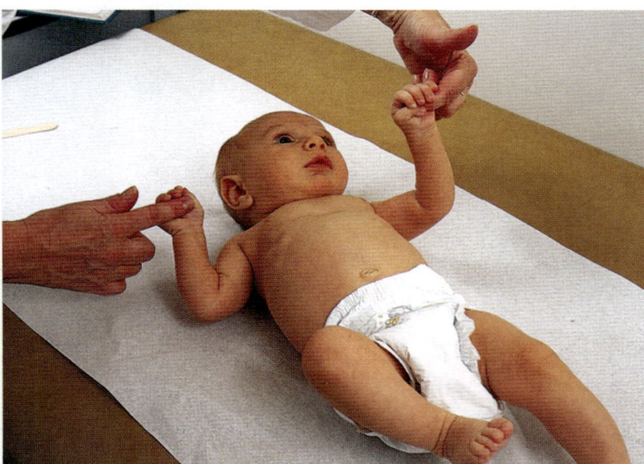

FIGURE 10.27 Observing respiratory rate

PROCEDURES AND NORMAL FINDINGS	ABNORMAL FINDINGS AND CLINICAL ALERTS
Blood pressure	
In children aged 3 years and older and in younger children at risk, measure a routine BP at least annually. For an accurate measurement in children, adjust the choice of equipment and technique. The correct size cuff width must cover two-thirds of the upper arm, and the cuff bladder must completely encircle it.	When it is not possible to use the arm for BP measurement in infants, the lower leg can be used. Crying, eating or sucking can influence BP measurements and should be noted at the time of measurement.
Use a paediatric-sized endpiece on the stethoscope to locate the Koritkoff sounds. If possible, allow a crying infant to become quiet for 5 to 10 minutes before measuring the BP; crying may elevate the systolic pressure by 30 to 50 mmHg. Use the disappearance of sound (phase V Korotkoff) for the diastolic reading in children. Note the guidelines for BP standards based on sex, age and height. These standards give a more precise classification of BP according to body size and avoid misclassifying children who are very tall or very short. (See Figure 10.1 for mean BP readings in apparently healthy people from birth to old age.) Children under 3 years of age have such small arm vessels that it is difficult to hear Korotkoff sounds with a stethoscope. Instead, use an electronic BP device that gives a digital readout for systolic and diastolic BP and heart rate. A Doppler can also be used to amplify the sounds. This instrument is easy to use and can be used by one examiner. (Note the technique for using the Doppler device; see Figure 10.28.) **FIGURE 10.28** Using a Doppler to locate peripheral pulses	Further explore any BP that is greater than the 95th percentile and refer for diagnostic evaluation.
Measurement of oxygen saturation—pulse oximeter	
An infant has a probe taped to the large toe. Some clinics use single-use probes that stick to the finger or ear instead of the multipatient-use spring-loaded model. If you are using a finger, make sure your hand is warm to prevent false low readings caused by vasoconstriction. At lower oxygen saturations, the earlobe probe is more accurate. The probe will show both the oxygen saturation and the heart rate. Make sure the heart rate reading you see on the pulse oximeter matches the palpated heart rate.	If the heart rate on the oximeter does not correlate with the palpated heart rate, reposition the probe and repeat (Figure 10.25).

PROCEDURES AND NORMAL FINDINGS	ABNORMAL FINDINGS AND CLINICAL ALERTS

Additional objective data for an adult over 65 years

Vital signs

Temperature. Changes in the body's temperature regulatory mechanism leave a person over 65 less likely to have fever but at a greater risk for hypothermia and hyperthermia. Thus, the temperature is a less reliable indicator of the older person's true health state. Sweat gland activity is also diminished.

Heart rate. The normal range of heart rate is 60 to 100 bpm, but the rhythm may be slightly irregular. The radial artery may feel stiff, rigid and tortuous in an older person, although this condition does not necessarily imply vascular disease in the heart or brain. The increasingly rigid arterial wall needs a faster upstroke of blood, so the pulse is easier to palpate.

Respirations. Ageing causes a decrease in vital capacity (the maximum amount of air the person can expel from the lungs after a maximum inhalation) and a decreased inspiratory reserve volume (the additional amount of air that can be inhaled after a normal inspiration). You may note a shallower inspiratory phase and an increased respiratory rate.

Blood pressure. The aorta and major arteries tend to harden with age. As the heart pumps against a stiffer aorta, the systolic pressure increases, leading to a widened pulse pressure (see Figure 10.18 for mean BP readings in apparently healthy people from birth to old age).

Additional measurement techniques

The Doppler technique

In many situations, pulse and BP measurement are enhanced by using an electronic device, the Doppler ultrasonic flowmeter. Sound varies in pitch in relation to the distance between the sound source and the listener; the pitch is higher when the distance is small, and the pitch lowers as the distance increases. Think of a railway train speeding towards you; its train whistle sounds higher the closer it gets, and the pitch of the whistle lowers as the train fades away.

In this case, the sound source is the blood pumping through the artery in a rhythmic manner. A handheld transducer picks up changes in sound frequency as the blood flows and ebbs and it amplifies them. The listener hears a whooshing pulsatile beat.

PROCEDURES AND NORMAL FINDINGS	ABNORMAL FINDINGS AND CLINICAL ALERTS
The Doppler technique is used to locate the peripheral pulse sites (see Chapter 16 for further discussion of this technique). For BP measurement, the Doppler technique will augment Korotkoff sounds (Figure 10.28). Through this technique, you can evaluate sounds that are hard to hear with a stethoscope, such as those in critically ill people with a low BP, in infants with small arms and in obese people in whom the sounds are muffled by layers of fat. Also, proper cuff placement is difficult on an obese person's cone-shaped upper arm. In this situation, you can place the cuff on the more even forearm and hold the Doppler probe over the radial artery. For either location, use the following procedure: • Apply coupling gel to the transducer probe. • Turn the Doppler flowmeter on. • Touch the probe to the skin, holding the probe perpendicular to the artery. • A pulsatile whooshing sound indicates location of the artery. You may need to rotate the probe and maintain contact with the skin. Do not push the probe too hard or you will obliterate the pulse. • Inflate the cuff until the sounds disappear; then proceed another 20 to 30 mmHg beyond that point. • Slowly deflate the cuff, noting the point at which the first whooshing sounds appear. This is the systolic pressure. • It is difficult to hear the muffling of sounds or a reliable disappearance of sounds indicating the diastolic pressure (phases IV and V of Korotkoff sounds). However, the systolic pressure alone gives valuable data on the level of tissue perfusion and on blood flow through patent vessels.	

ADDITIONAL RESOURCES

You can further develop your knowledge and skills relevant to general survey and assessing vital signs, related pathophysiology, common health issues and nursing interventions by:

- reading chapters of a fundamentals of nursing or medical/surgical nursing textbook.
- answering chapter multiple choice questions online. Log onto ClinicalKey Student and search for the text 'Health Assessment, 4th edition'. Choose the section titled 'Teaching material'. In this section you will find question and answer documents for each chapter.
- visiting websites

Australian Commission on Safety and Quality in Healthcare. Vital Signs: The state of safety and quality in Australian health care. https://www.safetyandquality.gov.au/publications-and-resources/state-patient-safety-and-quality-australian-hospitals-2019/vital-signs-state-safety-and-quality-australian-health-care

REFERENCES

1. World Health Organization (WHO) 2023. Obesity and Overweight. Available at: https://www.who.int/data/gho/data/themes/topics/topic-details/GHO/body-mass-index
2. Australian Institute of Health and Welfare (AIHW). 2023. Obesity and Overweight. Available at: https://www.aihw.gov.au/reports/overweight-obesity/overweight-and-obesity/contents/summary
3. Talley NJ, O'Connor S. Clinical examination. 9th ed. Elsevier; 2021.
4. Australian Commission on Safety and Quality in Health Care (ACSQHC). Observation and response charts. 2012. Available at: https://www.safetyandquality.gov.au/publications-and-resources/resource-library/adult-deterioration-detection-system-adds-chart-blood-pressure-table
5. Health Quality and Safety Commission New Zealand. 2017. New Zealand Early Warning Score Vital Sign Chart User Guide. Available at: https://www.hqsc.govt.nz/assets/Our-work/Improved-service-delivery/Patient-deterioration/Publications-resources/Vital_sign_chart_user_guide_July_2017_.pdf
6. Hymczak H, Gołąb A, Mendrala K, Plicner D, Darocha T, Podsiadło P, et al. 'Core temperature measurement—principles of correct measurement, problems, and complications.' International Journal of Environmental Research and Public Health, 18, no. 20 (2021): 10606.
7. Geneva II, Cuzzo B, Fazili T, Javaid W. 2019, April. Normal body temperature: a systematic review. Open Forum Infectious Diseases (Vol. 6, No. 4, p. ofz032): Oxford University Press.
8. Crossley, Becky. 'Troubleshoot it: accuracy of various thermometer types is important to consider during the COVID-19 pandemic.' Biomedical Instrumentation & Technology 54, no. 3 (2020): 228–229.
9. Pandarbale SS, Fernandes C. 'A comparative study of automated vs manual measurement of blood pressure.' Journal of Evolution of Medical and Dental Sciences, 9, no. 35 (2020): 2511–2515.
10. National Heart Foundation of Australia. Guideline for the diagnosis and management of hypertension in adults. 2016. Available at: https://www.heartfoundation.org.au/getmedia/f06f795d-1c77-4122-a4ae-54be2238916b/Hypertension_Guidelines-2016_Presentation_.pdf
11. Aggarwal AN, Agarwal R, Dhooria S, Prasad KT, Sehgal IS, Muthu V. 'Impact of fingernail polish on pulse oximetry measurements: a systematic review.' Respiratory Care (2023), 68 (9): 1271–1280.
12. Royal Children's Hospital 2019. Temperature management. Available at: https://www.rch.org.au/rchcpg/hospital_clinical_guideline_index/Temperature_management/

CHAPTER 11

UNIT 3

Assessing mental health, neurological and sensory function

Mental health assessment

Adapted by Rebecca Corbett

INTRODUCTION

To be mentally healthy means having life satisfaction through the achievement of one's potential in work, in caring relationships, in society and within one's self.[1] According to the World Health Organization (WHO)[2] the determinants of mental health include access to education, work, justice, transport, environment, housing and welfare assistance. Mental health is relative and ongoing and is affected by internal and external stressors. Exposure to unfavourable circumstances such as poverty, deprivation or violence increases the risk of experiencing a mental health condition. While everyone has 'good' and 'bad' days, mentally well people display resilience in the face of adversity, having the capacity to attribute meaning to difficult life events and restore a sense of balance to their life. Coping strategies, emotional regulation, connectedness to others, help seeking and meaningful engagement in work/study and community all contribute to psychological resilience.[3]

Contemporary approaches to mental health care worldwide now include the people with lived experience of mental illness in all levels of service design and delivery. Previous service systems and treatments have often breached human rights by being coercive (forced treatment), disempowering and stigmatising. Co-design and co-production of any services (or projects) that include mental health service users is now considered the gold standard to improve the experience and outcomes of people with mental illness, as well as that of their carers.[4] The consumer movement, which is a social and political movement representing the rights and views of those with mental illness, has demanded that treatment approaches change to reflect inclusive, respectful, person-centred care.[5]

Case study

The following case study gives an example of a typical situation involving mental health assessment and the initial clinical reasoning process. It will help you identify your learning needs.

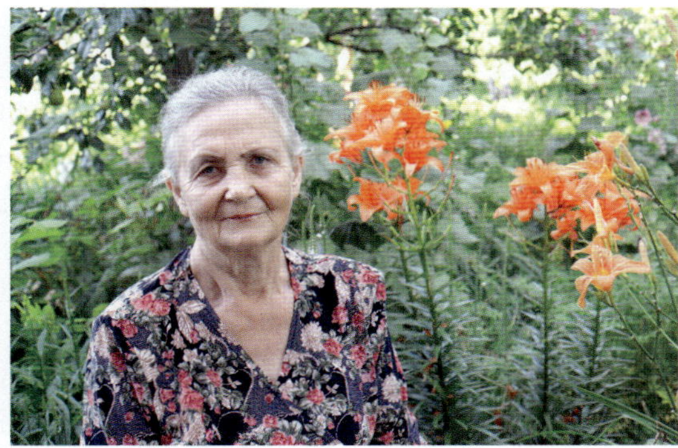

Context

You are a practice nurse working in a general practice clinic. One part of your role is to conduct annual health checks for clients over 75 years of age.

Consider the patient's situation

Mrs Lola Peters is a 79-year-old woman accompanied by her husband, Ray. Her last annual check showed that while she had no physical health problems at that time, she was having some issues with memory. Ray tells you that Lola now has increasing memory loss, confusion and is exhibiting socially inappropriate behaviour.

Questions to further your learning

- What are the possible things that might be going on with Mrs Peters?
- What knowledge do you need to be able to predict what might be going on?
- What approach to Mrs Peters' health assessment will you take?
- What questions (subjective data) will you ask Ray and Lola Peters to extend the health history and why?
- What physical examination (objective data) will you conduct and why?
- What resources are available to assist in your assessment of Mrs Peters?

Assessment plan

The full Mental Status Examination is an objective systematic assessment of a person's psychological, emotional and behavioural functioning at a particular time. This assessment identifies dysfunction and determines how that dysfunction affects self-care and engagement in everyday life. The aim of mental health assessment therefore is to identify cognitive, behavioural, mental and physical conditions, issues and risks of harm to the person as well as the identifying circumstances that may have an impact on these risks.

A person's mental state is a description of a general 'internal' state of mind; it is not a momentary state but one that endures for some time. Onset of mental illness usually develops over time (days or weeks/months), whereas organic causes such as delirium or drug-induced psychosis have a more sudden onset (hours to days). As with any assessment, it is always important to determine the previous level of functioning and the length of time the disruption has been experienced. All diagnostic parameters for mental disorders require a length of time during which the cluster of symptoms has been experienced.[6]

A full Mental Status Examination is conducted when you observe any abnormality in affect, thinking or behaviour, and in the following situations:

- **Family members are concerned** about a person's recent behavioural changes, such as memory loss, strange or unusual/out of character behaviour, sleep and appetite disturbance or social withdrawal.
- **Brain lesions** (trauma, tumour and cerebrovascular accident/stroke). A mental status assessment documents any emotional or cognitive change associated with the lesion. Not recognising these changes hinders care planning and creates problems with social readjustment. It can be helpful in planning interventions to have a snapshot of a person's mental status.
- **Aphasia** (the impairment of language ability secondary to brain damage, substance intoxication or withdrawal or other psychiatric presentations). A Mental Status Examination assesses language dysfunction as well as any emotional problems associated with it, such as depression or agitation.
- **Symptoms of psychiatric illness** such as responding to stimuli not visible to the assessor, expressions of hopelessness, self-neglect or disruption to usual functioning (care of children, attendance at work).

Mental illness increases the likelihood of physical illness, which in turn can contribute to poor mental health.[7,8] A person with a mental illness will often present with physical symptoms such as tiredness, palpitations, gastrointestinal upset or lack of appetite—this is because the mind and body are interrelated and function in unison.

It is essential that you employ a caring, respectful, non-judgemental approach so a therapeutic relationship can be formed.[9] It is also important that you honour each person as an expert in their own health experience; this means working collaboratively and respectfully alongside the person. This approach will enable you to enquire about the very personal domains of mental health assessment with warmth and respect.[9]

When collecting subjective information, keep in mind the main domains of the Mental Status Examination (see below). The language and categories described in the Mental Status Examination can help you to formulate your observations and provides you with a common language for your documentation. Knowledge of the language of mental health assessment facilitates communication with other health professionals should you be concerned about clinical deterioration of mental state (Table 11.1). The Mental Status Examination domains can also help you think about the types of questions you may ask the person.

The main areas for subjective data collection are:

- presenting concern
- history of present illness
- mental health history
- current and past health history
- family history
- interpersonal relationships/resources
- values, beliefs or spiritual resources
- coping and stress management
- sleep and rest
- health and lifestyle management
- activity and exercise
- nutrition and metabolic pattern
- elimination pattern
- risk of harm to self or others.

Physical examination requires assessing all aspects of the person in comparison with what would be in the normal range for their age, gender, education, social position, cultural norms and the current environment. You should not expect the person to perform at a higher level on the Mental Status Examination than their usual educational and behavioural level. You are looking for congruence between what the person says, what you see and what you know. The main areas of the Mental Status Examination are:

- appearance
- posture
- body movements
- dress
- grooming and hygiene
- behaviour
- level of consciousness
- facial expression
- mood and affect
- speech (quality, pace, articulation, word choice)
- cognitive functions
- orientation
- attention span
- recent and remote memory
- new learning—the 'Four unrelated words' test
- judgement and insight
- Mini-Mental State Examination.

Resources available

You will find additional resources and a reference list at the end of this chapter.

Key concepts and terminology

A **mental health disorder** is apparent when a person's response is much greater than the expected reaction to a traumatic life event such as being diagnosed with a serious illness, or when the person does not begin to show signs of recovery/return to normal functioning following a traumatic event. A mental health disorder is defined as a significant behavioural or psychological *pattern* that is associated with distress such as a painful symptom or disability affecting function, and which has a significant risk of pain, disability, death, or a loss of freedom.[6]

Poverty, exposure to violence, sexual abuse, problematic substance use, lack of social support, parental mental illness, rurality, chronic health issues, trauma, grief and lack of education all have an impact on mental health and recovery. The stress surrounding a traumatic life event such as the death of a loved one or serious illness can disrupt the balance of one's mental state, causing transient dysfunction. This is a normal response. Most people will begin to recover their previously experienced levels of functioning from trauma within approximately

TABLE 11.1 The language of mental health assessment

Term	Description
Consciousness	• Describes the level of wakefulness in the individual. • Awareness of one's own existence, feelings, thoughts and the environment. • Is the most elementary of mental status functions that can be objectively assessed using the Glasgow Coma Scale (Chapter 12).
Language	• Is the direct medium through which the voice is used to communicate one's thoughts and feelings. • A basic tool of humans. Its loss has a heavy social impact on the individual. • Language formation is also a highly complex cognitive function. Its impairment is a key early indicator of many neurological as well as psychiatric conditions. • The absence or delay of language development in children is a strong indicator of an underlying condition or may be due to trauma in the child's environment.
Mood and affect	• Both of these elements deal with the prevailing emotions: Affect is a temporary expression of feelings—it is visible to the assessor in the form of facial expressions and expressed emotion. • Mood is pervasive over time (weeks rather than days)—how the person feels internally—and is not always visible to the assessor.
Orientation	• Awareness of the objective world in relation to the self, specifically time, place and person.
Attention	• The power of concentration, the ability to focus on one specific thing without being distracted by many environmental or internal stimuli.
Memory	• The ability to lay down and store experiences and perceptions for later recall. • *Recent* memory evokes day-to-day events. • *Remote* memory stores years' worth of experiences.
Abstract reasoning	• Pondering a deeper meaning beyond the concrete and literal. • Abstract reasoning ability will give some cues to level of intelligence.
Thought process	• The *way* a person thinks. • The formation, sequence, relatedness, speed, availability and logic of thinking.
Thought content	• *What* the person thinks—specific ideas, beliefs, fears, preoccupations and the use of words.
Perceptions	• What the person perceives in the environment through the senses and through their body as a whole.

4 weeks and grief within a period of 12 months (6 months for children).[6]

Mental disorders also include organic conditions due to brain disease of *known* causes—delirium, dementia, depression (Table 11.2) and substance withdrawal (Table 6.2).

Psychiatric mental illness on the other hand is where aetiology has not yet been established—anxiety disorders (Table 11.3), schizophrenia (Table 11.4) and depressive and bipolar disorder (Table 11.5).

One in five (20%) Australians aged 16 to 85 years meet the diagnostic criteria for a high prevalence (common) mental disorder such as anxiety disorder, depression or substance use disorder in any given year.[10] In Aotearoa New Zealand, one in five people aged 15 years or older are diagnosed with a mood and/or anxiety disorder.[11] Approximately 5% of the Australian population (over and above the one in five) meet the criteria for a less common but high-impact mental disorder such as **schizophrenia**, **severe depression, bipolar disorder** or **schizo-affective disorder** (symptoms of bipolar disorder and schizophrenia).[10] Mental ill health presents as one of the five greatest burdens of disease worldwide, with some authors more recently arguing that the global cost of mental illness may have been grossly underestimated and may be up to three times greater than previously thought.[12]

People with severe mental illnesses experience a 30% reduction in life expectancy (14–23 years) as compared with the general population. Most of these early deaths (close to 80%) are from treatable and preventable diseases such as cardiovascular disease, respiratory disease and cancer, rather than the mental illness itself. People with mental illnesses are over-represented in the healthcare system, as co-occurring physical and mental health disorders are common.[7] People with severe mental illness are more likely to smoke tobacco, have a poor diet, live a sedentary lifestyle, live in poverty and are less likely than the general population to seek out health services.[13] This lack of help-seeking is often due to stigma experienced from healthcare providers resulting in those with mental illness being treated differently and experiencing shame and embarrassment if they do seek help.

Diagnostic overshadowing is when a health practitioner makes assumptions about a person and their state of health that affects their clinical judgement regarding co-existing disorders. This diagnostic bias is likely to contribute to increased mortality.[14] Diagnostic overshadowing frequently occurs in emergency departments and primary health settings, where the person with a diagnosed mental illness will be assessed and treated for their mental health issues but not the physical health issues they may have presented with.[5,15] Health professionals are also less likely to offer basic, lifesaving screening (e.g. cardiovascular risk screening) to those with mental illness and those with serious mental illness are less likely to take part in national screening programs (e.g. mammogram or bowel screening).

Developmental considerations

Infants and children

Age of onset for mental illness is usually between 15 and 25 years, and one in seven (14%) of children aged 4 to 17 years meet the diagnostic criteria for a mental disorder.[10] This has significant developmental and functional implications for study, work, relationships and the emerging sense of self.

The maturation of emotional and cognitive functioning is described in detail in Chapter 3. It is difficult to separate and trace the development of just one aspect of mental status. All aspects are interdependent. For example, consciousness is rudimentary at birth because the cerebral cortex is not yet developed; the infant cannot distinguish the self from the mother's body.

Consciousness gradually develops along with language, so by 18 to 24 months the child learns that it is separate from objects in the environment and has words to express this. Language development can also be traced from the differentiated crying at 4 weeks, the cooing at 6 weeks, through one-word sentences at 1 year to multi-word sentences at 2 years. Yet the concept of language as a social tool of communication occurs at around 4 to 5 years of age, coinciding with the child's readiness to play cooperatively with other children.

Attention span gradually increases through preschool years so, by school age, most children can sit and concentrate on their work for a period of time. However, some children are late in developing concentration. School readiness coincides with the development of the thought process; around age 7 years, thinking becomes more logical and systematic, and the child can reason and understand. Abstract thinking is the ability to consider a hypothetical situation and usually develops between ages 12 and 15 years. Healthy physical, psychological, emotional and social development all depend on forming trusting attachments with parents or caregivers.[16]

Where there has been trauma, physical or sexual abuse or neglect in the child's environment there will be a disruption to development. Prolonged physical illness can also affect a child's mental health. This may present itself in many ways in the healthcare setting—possibly in regressed, sexualised or angry behaviour, developmental delay, excessive fear, passivity or clinginess. Should you observe any unusual behaviour while assessing children and young people, further assessment is warranted.

Childhood trauma is a strong precursor to developing a mental health disorder. Perinatal issues such as physical illness, mental illness, birth trauma and stress can also affect the mental health and psychological development of a child. It is pertinent to ask some basic screening questions of parents about pregnancy, childbirth and maternal and paternal mental health after birth when assessing a child.

Family history of mental illness and the nature and disposition of the child are important factors to assess for and document. Shy, sensitive, easily distressed children are more likely to develop depression and anxiety. Most childhood mental illness will first manifest as anxiety. Mood and anxiety disorders also commonly co-occur with other health and medical conditions including asthma, insulin resistance and other chronic medical conditions and might affect treatment adherence for these conditions.[17]

Neurodiversity is a term coined in the 1990s to describe variability of human nervous systems in which no two systems can ever be exactly alike. This term is used to acknowledge that our brains work differently from each other and incorporates differences in thinking and ways of operating. The emphasis is on difference rather than deficit or disability.[18] Neurodiversity is briefly covered in this text because the medical model views cognitive differences as deficits or faults to be corrected.[6] Syndromes such as **autism spectrum disorder**, **attention deficit hyperactivity disorder** (ADHD), **dyslexia** and **dyspraxia** each have characteristics that may include social and communication issues, restricted and repetitive habits, actions and routines to some degree or other, which are thought to require management. The neurodiversity movement believes that neurodiverse people ought instead to be respected in the way other human differences are valued such as sexuality, race and gender.[19] It is argued that syndromes such as those identified should not be seen as mental illnesses since they do not just appear in adulthood or following a traumatic event. Since management of associated behaviours of the syndromes may include medications, it is important that nurses are familiar with these syndromes and the surrounding politics.

Adolescents and young adults

The National Study of Mental Health and Wellbeing[20] found that 38.8% of young people in Australia aged 16 to 24 years had experienced a mental disorder in the previous 12 months. Suicide remains the leading cause of death for young people aged 15 to 24 years. Other recent studies confirm that up to 50% of young people in Australia (and internationally) are experiencing very high levels of psychological distress.[10] Anxiety disorders and depression are more common for females, whereas substance use disorders are more common for males. In Aotearoa New Zealand, 23.6% of young people aged 15 to 24 years had experienced high or very high levels of psychological distress.[21]

An **eating disorder** is a complex mental illness characterised by disturbance to thoughts, behaviours and attitudes to food and eating and may extend to obsession with body weight/shape and exercise.[4] Eating disorders include **anorexia nervosa**, **bulimia**, **avoidant/restrictive food intake disorder** and **binge eating**. Eating disorders affect both men and women of all ages and from all socioeconomic groups and cultural backgrounds. The onset for an eating disorder such as anorexia nervosa is during adolescence or early adulthood, although more and more younger children are becoming affected.[22]

While there is no single identifiable cause for an eating disorder to develop, biological, psychological and social risk factors may increase the likelihood of an eating disorder developing. While eating disorders can take many different forms, essentially the disorder interferes with a person's emotional, physical and social health. Behaviours associated with an eating disorder result in notable risk or damage to health, significant distress or significant physical dysfunction.[23] In Australia, of those with an eating disorder, 12.8% were male, 32.9% female.[24] Lifetime prevalence is 8.4% (3.3–18.6%) for women and 2.2% (0.8–6.5%) for men. Mortality rates are alarmingly high; the highest for any mental health disorder.[25] The most common causes of death are from cardiovascular impairment or suicide.[26] See Table 11.6 for more about the characteristics of eating disorders.[27]

GENDER AND SEXUAL DIVERSITY

Identity formation is a crucial adolescent developmental milestone that can have an impact on mental illness and psychological distress. For many young people, determining their gender identity, sexual preferences and forming relationships can also significantly affect mental health and wellbeing. LGBTIQ+ young people are more likely to develop a mental disorder, attempt suicide and die by suicide than the cis-gendered population. These unacceptable outcomes are directly correlated to experiences of prejudice, discrimination, stigma and homophobic abuse.[28] Health services are increasingly adopting a welcoming, non-judgemental stance so LGBTIQ+ people feel accepted and invited to seek care. See further information in Chapters 26 and 27 related to sexual and reproductive health.

THE IMPACT OF THE COVID-19 PANDEMIC

The global COVID-19 pandemic has had a significant impact on mental health for young people, people with disabilities and Aboriginal or Torres Strait Islander peoples.

Separation from peers, place and culture during lockdowns meant that many people experienced isolation, loneliness and financial insecurity. Fear of infection and contagion also added to the worries of young people with a propensity towards anxiety. Rural, disadvantaged, diverse and isolated young people experienced increased disadvantage and increased mental health issues such as anxiety and depression during COVID-19 lockdowns. The full impact of the global pandemic on the mental health of young people is yet to be determined longitudinally.[10]

Late adulthood (65+ years)

The ageing process leaves the parameters of mental status mostly intact. There is no decrease in general knowledge and little or no loss in vocabulary. Response time is slower than in youth; it takes a bit longer for the brain to process information and react to it. Performance on timed intelligence tests may therefore be lower for older people—not because intelligence has declined but because it takes longer to respond to the questions. The slower response time may affect new learning; if new information is rapidly paced, there may not be time for the older person to grasp and integrate this new information.

Recent memory, which requires some processing (e.g. medication instructions, 24-hour diet recall, names of new acquaintances), is somewhat decreased with ageing. Remote memory is not affected (Chapter 12).

Age-related changes in sensory perception can affect mental status. For example, vision loss may result in apathy, social isolation and depression (Chapter 14). Hearing changes are common in older adults (see the discussion of presbycusis in Chapter 15). Age-related hearing loss involves high frequencies of sound. Consonants are high-frequency sounds, so older people who have difficulty hearing them have problems with normal conversation. This problem may produce frustration, suspicion and social isolation and makes the person look confused.

Older adults, if physically well, are generally happy and satisfied with their lives compared with the general population. It should not be assumed that it is normal for older adults to be depressed. Mental health concerns in older people should be assessed and treated. The era of older adulthood contains more potential for loss than do earlier eras. These include the loss of loved ones, loss of work roles and identity, loss of income and the loss of an energetic and resilient body. The grief and despair surrounding these losses can affect mental health. These losses can result in disorientation, disability or depression. Depression is highly treatable in all ages. If detected in older people, nurses may need to take a strong advocacy position for the condition to be correctly treated. Adults over the age of 85 years have a higher suicide rate than the general population; this is particularly so for males. While the prevalence of depression occurring in older adults is decreasing, aetiology can be attributed to many complex reasons including loneliness, social isolation and physical health issues—in particular chronic disease and pain.[29]

While for most people older age presents a time of significant life changes and some sense of loss, previously resilient people will cope and adjust to these life changes with appropriate support. Most older Australians are happy and resilient. Social inclusion, meaningful engagement in life, physical activity and effective treatment of health issues will assist older people to maintain good mental health. Health screening, early detection and health education are crucial nursing roles that can prevent mental illness developing or worsening in older people. People in this age group experiencing mental illness often get missed by health professionals because no one asks the question: '*Is this the best health this person can obtain?*' Older people are often left to suffer with mental health issues unnecessarily for longer than younger people because as a society we assume mental decline and depression are normal in older age. Nurses need to advocate for the highest level of attainable health for all their patients, regardless of age.[30] It is therefore important that as a registered nurse you screen for mental illness in older adults because there may not be a previous history of mental ill health. The impact of ageism and discrimination on mental health is significant and contributes to the experiences of grief and loss in older people.

Cultural and social considerations

There is a significant correlation with the development of mental health issues with specific cultural groups and social circumstances within the Australian and Aotearoa New Zealand communities. Refer to Chapter 4 for in-depth discussion of these issues. Different cultural groups have their own explanatory models of health and illness and their own accepted cultural practices when interacting with health professionals.

Mental illness can be poorly understood and stigmatised in many cultural groups, which in turn may have a negative impact on the help-seeking behaviours of those suffering distressing symptoms. Aboriginal and Torres Strait Islander Australians are in a very high-risk group for suicide (twice the rate for the general population) and are often over-represented in the health system in general due to multiple overlapping vulnerabilities. Similar concerns are held for Māori people. Careful consideration of cultural issues must be incorporated into assessment of Aboriginal and Torres Strait Islander and Māori people. It is important for all healthcare staff to train in cultural sensitivity and competence, as this skill set applies across healthcare settings and can help guide the nurse in how to ask sensitive and difficult questions.

People who have arrived in Australia or Aotearoa New Zealand as either asylum seekers awaiting refugee status or refugees (confirmed status) will have endured significant hardship and suffering throughout the various stages of their journey. This may include exposure to torture, violence (at a personal, family or community level), sexual assault, persecution, extreme deprivation and loss of loved ones in the pre-migration period. The migration period also involves great hardship and uncertainty with people waiting many years in camps or detention centres before finding refuge. Families are often separated during the migration phase, and it is quite normal for mental health and wellbeing of refugees/asylum seekers to be profoundly affected.

Depression, **anxiety**, **substance use disorder** and **post-traumatic stress disorder** are commonly associated with prolonged migration experiences.[29,31] Each person is unique in their resilience and capacity to manage change, and it is therefore important to always use a strengths-based approach in mental health assessment, whereby a person's courage and survival is acknowledged and respected and existing skills are built on (Table 11.3). The main risks for people from culturally and linguistically diverse backgrounds relate to social exclusion due to language and cultural barriers and to lack of understanding of the healthcare system.[32]

The most significant strategy a nurse can employ when assessing people with languages other than English is to use a properly trained interpreter whenever possible. Using family members to interpret may seem convenient, but issues of privacy may mean the person is not honest about stressors, suicide and other risks in the presence of family. Also, when using untrained or personally involved family/friends, incorrect explanation of medical information and filtering or misunderstanding of assessment data may occur. Mental health concerns are fraught with fear, lack of understanding and high levels of emotion for most people. In many cultures, there is great stigma and shame associated with mental illness, and healthcare workers may be viewed as authority figures that are not trustworthy. To properly understand the cultural impact/sensitivities around mental illness for each person, and to decrease exclusion and fear, skillful communication needs to occur via an interpreter.[31] See Chapter 7 for information on working effectively with interpreters (see also Figure 11.1).

Nurses are in a key position to screen for mental illness and to offer holistic assessment, support and referral to specialist services for further assessment and treatment. Nurses routinely conduct mental status assessments across a variety of clinical settings including emergency departments, surgical and medical wards, GP clinics, community health settings, aged persons services, midwifery settings or in the person's home.

The nurse's role as advocate is very important for those experiencing psychological distress because mental illness can invoke feelings of fear, helplessness and powerlessness. Empathic, caring support at the point of entry to any health setting can play a significant role in positive mental health outcomes. Assuring patients in our care that mental illness is treatable, and that treatment is available, promotes help seeking and hope. This can be a lifesaving intervention for many because the nature of emotional distress is all consuming and many people suffer believing they cannot be helped.

HEALTH EDUCATION

Are you ok? (R U OK?)

More than 3,000 people die by suicide in Australia each year (rate of 12.3 per 100,000 population in 2022). Males are more likely to commit suicide than females. Almost 19 per 100,000 male population in Australia took their own lives in 2022 as compared with 5.9 per 100,000 female population. There were more suicide deaths in the mid-life population (30–59 years) compared with other age groups. The suicide rate for First Nations people aged 0 to 24 years is 3.1 times higher than equivalent age group of non-Indigenous people.[33] In 2018 the age-standardised rate of confirmed suicide deaths for Aotearoa New Zealand was 12.1 per 100,000 population. Males were more highly represented (17.4 per 100,000 males) than females (6.9 per 100,000 females). The age group with the highest suicide rate in 2018 was the 20 to 24 age group, with a rate of 23.5 per 100,000 people. Suicide rates for Māori people are higher than those for non-

HEALTH EDUCATION cont'd

Māori people—24.8 per 100,000 Māori male population.[34,35]

There is a relationship between social disconnection, mental health and suicide risk.[36,37] Suicide is considered a preventable death and most people who are feeling suicidal do not necessarily want to die. They may want the pain of their suffering to stop or feel they have no other options. If a person is depressed or in acute emotional distress, they may not be able to problem solve or feel any hope for the future. Should you become aware that a person is experiencing suicidal thoughts when you are performing a routine screening and assessment this can be pivotal in preventing suicide.

R U OK? day was founded as a national day of action to prevent suicide. The mission of the R U OK? Foundation is to encourage people to connect meaningfully and support each other, in particular those who are undergoing significant life problems.

The goals of the R U OK? Foundation are to:

- boost confidence to meaningfully connect and ask about life's ups and downs
- nurture our sense of responsibility to regularly connect and support others
- strengthen our sense of belonging because we know people are there for us
- be relevant, strong and dynamic.

The R U OK? Foundation has developed four simple steps to encourage connection when someone you know or care about is not behaving as they normally would:

1. **Ask**—are you OK?
2. **Listen**—without judgement
3. **Encourage action**
   For example, you could ask:
   - *What have you done to manage a similar situation in the past?*
   - *How would you like me to support you?*
   - *What is something you could do for yourself right now?*
4. **Check in**—put a reminder in your diary to follow up in a couple of days/weeks. If the person is really struggling, follow up sooner. Stay in touch and be there for the person.

Nurse's role

Nurses can contribute significantly to mental health management of people in their care by:

- embedding promotion and prevention efforts within health services
- advocating, initiating and, where appropriate, facilitating collaboration and coordination.

There are many resources for any person who may be thinking about suicide. If someone in your care is suicidal, seek immediate professional mental health support to manage the situation.

Websites

The following websites provide resources to help people ask questions and support a person who is having difficulties:

- Aboriginal and Torres Strait Islander suicide prevention: https://cbpatsisp.com.au
- Beyond Blue (Australia): https://www.beyondblue.org.au/mental-health/suicide-prevention
- Orygen (Australia)—Youth mental health: https://www.orygen.org.au/Research/Research-Areas/Suicide-Prevention
- R U OK?: https://www.ruok.org.au/about-us
- Suicide prevention Australia: https://www.suicidepreventionaust.org
- TIACS (for tradies, truckies, rural and blue-collar workers): https://www.tiacs.org

Suicide First Aid Guidelines for People from Immigrant and Refugee Backgrounds

SUICIDE CAN BE PREVENTED

Most suicidal people do not want to die, they just do not want to live with the pain they are feeling. Helping a suicidal person talk about their thoughts and feelings can help save a life.

HOW DO I KNOW?

A suicidal person may not ask for help directly, but they are likely to show certain warning signs.

WATCH FOR

WITHDRAWING from friends, family or the community

Suddenly becoming **VERY SAD**

Expressing in words or actions:

- a big change in **MOOD, BEHAVIOUR** or **APPEARANCE**
- **FEELINGS OF HOPELESSNESS**
- Having **NO REASON TO LIVE** or **NO PURPOSE IN LIFE**
- **NO INTEREST** in or **PLANS FOR THE FUTURE**
- **FEAR OF BEING INVOLUNTARILY REMOVED** or returned to home country, especially if there is a risk of torture or death
- **FEELING TRAPPED**, like there is no way out
- **DISTRESS ABOUT INTRUSIVE MEMORIES** of past traumatic events
- **STRONG SENSE OF FEELING ALONE** and cut off, even if surrounded by family or friends
- feeling that **DEATH IS AN HONOURABLE SOLUTION** to their situation
- **FEELINGS OF GUILT OR SHAME**, or belief of being a burden to others
- Feeling that their **LIFE HAS BEEN A FAILURE**

OTHER WARNING SIGNS

A person may threaten to hurt or kill themselves, or say that they wish to die, verbally (speaking) or in writing.

A person may behave in ways that are life-threatening or dangerous.

A person may try to set their affairs and relationships in order.

If you have noticed some of these warning signs and you are concerned a person may be at risk of suicide, you need to talk to them about your concerns. Warning signs for suicide may also be different among cultures or their expressions might vary.

HOW CAN I HELP?

Act quickly if you think someone is considering suicide, even if you have only a mild suspicion. Choose a private place to talk with the person and allow time to talk about your concerns.

ASK ABOUT THOUGHTS OF SUICIDE

"Are you having thoughts of suicide?" or "Are you thinking about killing yourself?"

Be mindful of how you ask.

~ Asking the person about suicidal thoughts will give them the chance to talk about their problems and show them that somebody cares. ~

Be supportive and understanding of the person, and listen to them with all your attention, encouraging them to do most of the talking.

~

If the person is having trouble communicating in your language, you should speak slowly, use simple words, check for understanding and, if necessary, repeat what you have said.

~

Do not let the fear of saying the wrong words or of not saying the perfect words stop you from encouraging the person to talk.

Once you have established that a suicide risk is present, you need to take action to keep the person safe.

The suicidal person should not be left on their own. Make sure that potentially harmful items are not available to them.

Remind the person that suicidal thoughts don't have to be acted on, and that even though these thoughts may feel like they will never go away, they are usually temporary.

Assure the person that there is support available . Ask the person if they would like you to contact someone for them such as a friend, family member or trusted religious, spiritual or community leader.

Encourage the person to get suitable professional help as soon as possible.

Find out about local services for people from immigrant and refugee backgrounds, including gender-specific services.

TAKE ALL THOUGHTS OF SUICIDE SERIOUSLY AND TAKE ACTION!

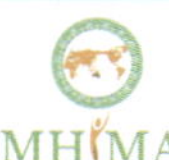

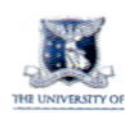

MELBOURNE SCHOOL OF POPULATION & GLOBAL HEALTH

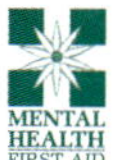

The complete guidelines can be downloaded from MHiMA (www.mhima.org.au) and GCMHU websites (cimh.unimelb.edu.au). All Mental Health First Aid guidelines can be downloaded from www.mhfa.com.au.

FIGURE 11.1 Suicide first aid guidelines for people from immigrant and refugee backgrounds

Subjective data

It is important that your approach to mental health assessment includes understanding that the person is an expert in their own recovery and that symptom control is no longer the primary treatment goal of mental health care. People living with mental illness or psychological distress wish to live full lives, contributing to their respective communities and cultures.[38] In collecting subjective data it is important to familiarise yourself with the language of mental health assessment (Table 11.1).

Practice note

Choose a quiet, private and welcoming space and ensure the person is comfortable. Before you start the assessment, introduce yourself to the person, confirm the person's identity and their preferred pronouns, discuss the purpose and scope of the assessment, clarify any questions the person may have and get the person's verbal consent to perform the assessment. Advise the person how long the assessment might take and offer breaks if the person needs them. If a family member or friend is with the person, ask if they prefer that person to stay for the assessment. This is important in situations where the person may wish to disclose private or distressing information (e.g. where there is family violence). Give the person your full attention, sit at the same level, use a warm and confident approach and open body language.[9]

ASSESSMENT GUIDELINES	CLINICAL SIGNIFICANCE AND CLINICAL ALERTS
Presenting concern	
The presenting concern, told in the person's own words, provides the assessor with some insight into subjective symptoms and other healthcare concerns. Responses to these questions will guide the sequence to the rest of the subjective data collection. Take cues from the person and what they say. The more you 'tune in' to the person the more natural and confident you will feel in guiding the assessment. A suggested approach: • *I would like to ask you some questions about why you are here today. Some of the questions may seem personal and intrusive but they'll help me work out what might be happening and how we can help you. Is that OK?* • *Everything we discuss will remain confidential and will only be shared to help you and keep you safe.* Mental status assessment during a traumatic life event can identify remaining strengths and help the person mobilise resources and use their coping skills (Table 11.2).	The person may present for treatment following a traumatic event or with new symptoms/ behaviours or an exacerbation of a current diagnosis. Often people feel extremely vulnerable and may have told their personal story many times. It can be very exposing and thus is important that the nurse assures discretion. How the person responds to questions is just as important as what the person says. Taking note of both will help you to develop insight into the person's problems and their perception of the problems.

ASSESSMENT GUIDELINES	CLINICAL SIGNIFICANCE AND CLINICAL ALERTS
History of present illness (if relevant)	
• *Can you tell me how you have been feeling?* • *What symptoms have you been experiencing?* • *Have you been feeling down/depressed/hopeless?* • *When did the symptoms start? Have you been feeling like this for weeks? Months?* • *How frequent are the symptoms? Are these feelings there first thing in the morning? Do they last all day? Have they changed over time?* • *What level of distress have you been feeling? (scale of 1 to 10)* • *What factors make them worse? Is there anything that helps? What have you tried?* • *Are you experiencing any other associated symptoms? (e.g. insomnia, reduced or increased appetite)* Should there be any hesitancy to answer questions, you could use statements such as: • *You were talking about ... Can you tell me more about that?*	It is important to note that mental illness and medical problems may be interlinked. ! ***Clinical alert:*** If the person answers yes (to feeling down/hopeless), then depression should be explored in detail. (Tables 11.3 and 11.7). The person should be referred to a mental health nurse or medical practitioner. ! ***Clinical alert:*** It is important to note that the person experiencing a mental health crisis may not believe a mental health problem exists. In situations like this it is important to get further information from relevant people such as parents, children, spouse, best friend, teacher, police officers and/or other healthcare providers.
Mental health history (if relevant)	
• *Have you ever seen a doctor or been admitted to hospital for mental or emotional concerns?* • *Were you given a diagnosis?* • *What treatment/s did you receive?* Treatments may include counselling or talking therapy with a psychologist, medications or other types of treatment such as electroconvulsive therapy. • *How effective was the treatment?* • *Did you feel better after having this treatment?*	Many people may not have received a formal diagnosis or if they did may not recall what it is. Only psychiatrists and psychologists are formally trained in mental health diagnosis.
Current and past health history	
• *Have you had any accidents/injuries?* • *Have you had any serious or chronic medical illnesses or surgery?* If relevant, ask about pregnancy, health during and after.	Known illnesses, such as **substance use disorder**, **hyperthyroidism**, **chronic renal disease** or **head injury** could affect your interpretation of the findings.
Family history	
• *Is there any family history of mental illness?* • *Has anyone in your family attempted suicide or died by suicide?*	Family history of mental illness is clinically relevant, especially with low prevalence disorders such as **schizophrenia**, **drug-induced psychosis** and **affective psychosis** (a state where the person finds it difficult to know what's real or imagined)/ ! ***Clinical alert:*** History of familial suicide may be an indicator of increased risk.

ASSESSMENT GUIDELINES	CLINICAL SIGNIFICANCE AND CLINICAL ALERTS
Interpersonal relationships/resources	
• *Where do you live?* • *Who do you live with?* • *Are you renting or are you buying your own home?* • *Do you work or study? How do you support yourself?* • *How would you describe your role in your family?* • *Can you please describe your relationships with family, friends and co-workers? Do you get along with them?* • *Who can you go to for support if you have a problem with work, your health, or personal problems?* • *How do you fill in your time?* • *What year level did you finish in school?* If any of this information has already been obtained by another health professional, there is no need to ask for this information again; instead confirm the details with the person. It is normal for the person to become emotional when describing their situation and appropriate for the nurse to offer comfort, validation and reassurance. People often feel a lot of shame that they aren't coping as they normally would.	Homelessness, including temporary accommodation and couch surfing, can have a significant impact on mental health and wellbeing. Older people are at risk of social isolation and loss of access to social support and health care, which may lead to poor mental health and wellbeing that in turn may be associated with cognitive decline. **! *Clinical alert:*** These questions are sensitive and should be asked compassionately and kindly. As mental health deteriorates, so too do relationships, and this will often be the tipping point for presentation. If you suspect that the person is experiencing family violence, refer to Chapter 5 for specific questions and an approach to assessment.
Values, beliefs or spiritual resources	
• *What is important to you?* • *Does your religious faith or spirituality play an important part in your life?* • *Do you identify with any specific cultural group?* • *Are there some cultural health practices that are important to you?*	Spiritual and religious faith and practices are known protective factors. Encouraging and supporting the person to maintain their practices or linking them to cultural or spiritual supports increases wellbeing.
Coping and stress management	
• *What do you consider to be the most significant stressors in your life, especially in the past year?* • *How has that affected you?* • *What is it about your present situation that is most worrying for you?* • *What methods have you tried to relieve stress and were these helpful?*	If this information has already been revealed, then use clinical judgement to leave out questions and avoid repetition of painful information. When people are overwhelmed, they can forget to do the things that make them feel better.

ASSESSMENT GUIDELINES	CLINICAL SIGNIFICANCE AND CLINICAL ALERTS
Sleep and rest	
• *What time do you usually go to sleep?* • *Do you have difficulty getting to sleep? If so, how do you manage it?* • *Do you have difficulty staying asleep?* • *What time do you usually get up?* • *Do you feel refreshed in the morning after sleep?*	Often insomnia will either be initial (difficulty getting to sleep) or early morning waking (3 or 4 am and ruminating). Insomnia is associated with depression, anxiety disorders and bipolar disorder.
Health and lifestyle management	
• *What treatment have you received for your physical and/or mental health problem?* • *What are your current medications? Have you had any side effects?* • *Do you smoke cigarettes/vape? At what age did you start? How many packs do you smoke per day? How many years have you smoked? Have you ever tried to quit?* • *How much and how often do you drink alcohol?* • *When was your last drink?* • *How much did you drink at that time?* • *What do you drink?* • *In the past week, how many days would you say you drank alcohol?* • *Do you use illicit drugs? How often?* • *What type of drug?*	Classes of psychotropic medications include: • antianxiety—benzodiazepines, beta-blockers • antipsychotics—atypical antipsychotics, phenothiazines, butyrophenones, major tranquillisers (used for schizophrenia, mania, delirium) • antidepressants—tricyclics, selective serotonin reuptake inhibitors (SSRIs) and serotonin-noradrenaline reuptake inhibitors (SNRIs) (used for depression, anxiety disorders, obsessive compulsive disorder) • mood-stabilising—lithium, anticonvulsants such as carbamazepine and sodium valproate (used for prevention of manic depression or mania). ! ***Clinical alert:*** Psychotropic medications increase the likelihood of obesity and metabolic disorders, as well as other physical complications such as sexual dysfunction.[13,15] Side effects of current prescribed medications such as contraceptives or corticosteroids may cause confusion or depression. Refer to Chapter 6 for screening for substance misuse.
Activity and exercise	
• *Can you describe a typical day?* • *Can you perform your activities of daily living?*	Changes in levels of energy may occur in those with depressive disorders resulting in less attention paid to activities of daily living. Refer to Chapters 17, 19 and 20 for specific questions about activity and exercise.
Nutrition and metabolic pattern	
• *Can you describe your usual eating habits?*	Reduced appetite may be seen in depression. Refer to Chapter 21 for specific questions about nutrition and metabolism.

ASSESSMENT GUIDELINES	CLINICAL SIGNIFICANCE AND CLINICAL ALERTS
Elimination pattern	
• *Can you describe your usual bowel and urinary elimination patterns?*	Irritable bowel syndrome may be associated with some psychological disorders. Refer to Chapters 24 and 25 for specific questions about urinary and bowel elimination.
Risk of harm to self or others	
This information is elicited in the thought content component of the Mental Status Examination in the objective data section	
Additional subjective data for infants, children and adolescents (parents or guardians)	
If relevant: • *Did you have a normal pregnancy and labour?* • *How did you and your partner manage with a newborn baby?* • *Did you breast feed or bottle feed? Did you experience any difficulties?* • *Has the child lost weight in recent days/months?*	
Children should gain weight as they grow. • *Has the child had poor weight gain over the past few months?* • *Has the child been eating/feeding less in the last few weeks?* If so, ask: • *How does this compare with the child's usual nutritional intake?* • *Does the child have an underlying neurodevelopmental syndrome? (e.g. autism, ADHD, receptive or expressive language delay, intellectual disability or any mental health issues such as anxiety or depression?)* If so, ask: • *Are there supports already in place, like communication tools/aids, behaviour management plans, sensory considerations? What has worked in the past? Are they still suitable?* • *Is there a history of adverse childhood experiences or psychosocial difficulties?*	Weight gain of children depends on their age. Refer to growth standards to determine if weight gain is appropriate.

ASSESSMENT GUIDELINES	CLINICAL SIGNIFICANCE AND CLINICAL ALERTS
Additional subjective data for adults over 65 years	
In addition to the previous questions for collecting subjective data ask the following: • *Do you have any problems with your memory?* • *Do you think you are more forgetful than most people?* • *Are you worried about being forgetful?* • *Have you experienced changes in your mood?* • *Are you wanting to stay home rather than getting outside and being with people?*	
Additional subjective data for pregnant women	
Identifying symptoms of depression and anxiety in pregnant women enables referral for more formal mental health assessment and follow-up. Ask the following questions: • *Do you have anxiety, depression or any other mental illness?* If so: • *How long has it been a problem? How is it being managed?* For serious mental illnesses such as bipolar, schizophrenia or other disorders, ask: • *Are you seeing a medical professional? How often?*	See Chapter 29 The pregnant woman.

Objective data

Use the categories below to assess the person's mental state at that moment in time, then enquire whether this is different from their usual way of being. It is not necessary to formally ask all the questions in the Mental State Examination each shift or episode of care. However, observe the person's behaviour at each interaction. If you observe unusual or significant change in the person's behaviour, complete the full Mental State Examination.

When a person is mentally unwell, their mental state may change frequently, often because of the effects of the person's environment and current stressors.

Equipment needed

Pencil, paper, reading material
A Mini-Mental Status Examination prompter card is very helpful (available from your organisation)

PROCEDURES AND NORMAL FINDINGS	ABNORMAL FINDINGS AND CLINICAL ALERTS
General survey	
While collecting subjective data, you will have noticed the condition of the person's skin, lips, hair and mucous membranes, as well as any breath odour, ease of breathing, height-to-weight ratio, body shape, level of hygiene and grooming and general demeanour. All these factors provide clues to the person's overall health status. More detailed information is provided below. When assessing mental status in a person's own environment, take note of whether they are attending to their home, family, hygiene and commitments as observed in their environment. This will give you an indication of how the person is managing life's demands each day.	Significant functional decline (not being able to perform one's previous duties in life) is an indicator of severity and will help to inform your clinical decision making.
Behaviour	
The assessment of appearance and behaviour begins the moment you meet the person. Be careful to use clear, non-judgemental descriptors that also consider the person's culture. Is the person acting appropriately for their current situation?	Impassive, restless, agitated, aggressive.
Level of consciousness. Is the person awake, alert and attentive?	Drowsy, sedated, obtunded, lethargic, yawning, hypervigilant, hyper-aroused, distracted, easily startled. Clouding occurs with delirium.
Physical characteristics. Gender, age, appears stated age, race, physical build, gait, distinguishing features, injuries, physical disabilities, sounds or odours emanating from the person.	When a person appears older or younger than their stated age this has clinical significance regarding past history of the person. Ideally a written/verbal physical description is thorough enough that another staff member could recognise the person based on your description (Table 11.1).
Posture and engagement. Is the person's sitting/standing posture erect, relaxed? Is the person lying in bed or standing? Does the person face you? Are they engaged in the process?	Sitting on the edge of the chair or curled in bed, tense muscles, folded arms, turned away. Restless pacing occurs with anxiety and paranoia. Agitation can occur with depression, delirium and hyperthyroidism. Sitting slumped in chair, psychomotor retardation (slowing down or hampering of mental or physical activities) occurs with depression and some organic brain diseases. Unusual posturing or gesturing **(catatonia, schizophrenia**), unusual gait or rigidity of movement (**autism spectrum disorder**, antipsychotic side effects).

PROCEDURES AND NORMAL FINDINGS	ABNORMAL FINDINGS AND CLINICAL ALERTS
Body movements. Are body movements voluntary, deliberate, coordinated, smooth and even?	Restless, fidgety movements or hyperkinetic appearance occur with anxiety or medication side effects. **Apathy and psychomotor slowing** occur with depression and organic brain disease, including delirium. **Stereotypical movement disorder** is a condition in which a person makes repetitive, purposeless movements such as hand waving, body rocking or head banging. Occurs in autism spectrum disorder. **Tics** are sudden twitches, movements or sounds that people do repeatedly. People who have tics cannot stop their body from doing these things. Occurs with psychotic disorders, severe depression and some brain disorders. **Abnormal posturing and bizarre gestures** occur with schizophrenia.
Dress. Is the person's dress appropriate for setting, season, age, gender identity and social group? Is their clothing clean? Does it fit? Is the clothing put on appropriately? You need to be mindful about making assumptions based on a person's dress because this can be affected by personal choice, access to resources (e.g. secure housing and money). Describe what you see rather than making a judgement.	Inappropriate dress can occur with organic brain syndrome. Dress that appears suited to the opposite sex may indicate gender role confusion or gender identity issues. Eccentric dress combination and bizarre make-up occurs with schizophrenia or manic phase of bipolar affective disorder. Soiled, torn clothing and lack of footwear may indicate disorganisation, homelessness or self-neglect due to depression.
Grooming and hygiene. The person is clean and well groomed; hair is neat and clean; women/transgender and non-binary people may have moderate or no make-up; men are shaved, or their beard or moustache is well groomed. Nails are clean (though some jobs leave nails chronically dirty). Whatever you notice, check the congruence to lifestyle for that individual such as if a person who identifies as male is wearing make-up, ask if this is usual for that person. Be aware of your own cultural and generational biases.	**Unilateral neglect** (total inattention to one side of body) occurs following some strokes. Inappropriate dress, poor hygiene and lack of concern with appearance may occur with depression, schizophrenia and advanced Alzheimer's disease. Meticulously dressed and groomed appearance and fastidious manner may occur with obsessive-compulsive disorders. ! ***Clinical alert:*** A disheveled appearance in a previously well-groomed person is significant. Use care in interpreting clothing that is dishevelled, bizarre or in poor repair, piercings and tattoos because these sometimes reflect the person's economic status or a deliberate fashion trend (especially among adolescents).

PROCEDURES AND NORMAL FINDINGS	ABNORMAL FINDINGS AND CLINICAL ALERTS
Facial expression. The expression is appropriate to the situation and responds to the topic. There is comfortable eye contact unless precluded by cultural norms.	A flat, mask-like expression can occur with: • **parkinsonism** (brain condition that causes slowed movements, stiffness and tremors) • **depression** (feelings of sadness and/or a loss of interest in activities) • **psychosis** (thought disorder where person experiences delusions) • **hyperthyroidism** (where the thyroid gland makes too much thyroid hormone and speeds up metabolism) • **myasthenia gravis** (chronic autoimmune disorder in which antibodies destroy the communication between nerves and muscle, resulting in weakness of the skeletal muscles). Grimacing, frowning and grinning that are incongruent may occur with **psychosis**. Perplexed, confused expression may occur with **dementia** and **psychosis**. Suspicious, fearful expression and darting eyes suggest **paranoia**. Responses to hallucinations can affect facial expressions (e.g. preoccupation, smiling).
Mood and affect	
Mood is the internal feeling state. It usually persists over time: hours, days, weeks. It is the subjective way the person feels. Affect is the external expressed emotion and can be observed by others in facial expression, tone and expressed emotion. **Mood.** Mood is the subjective and pervasive emotional state, affecting functioning and relationships. Euthymic (normal mood) may fluctuate mildly throughout the day or over time, with good and bad days, but generally is manageable, consistent with life events, able to be improved through enjoyable activities/social supports/meaningful activities. **Affect.** The way a person shows their emotional state. A normal affect is emotional expression that can be observed by the assessor. It is congruent with the situation, responsive and reactive. It has a range from happy to sad and is visible.	Depressed, anxious/irritable (Table 11.7) If depressed, one feels down and sad all the time—nothing is enjoyable, nothing is easy. Depression can range from mild to severe and can also manifest in irritability and anger. Rating the mood from 1 to 10 can be useful. Deterioration in mood can be very gradual and the person may not realise their mood has become depressed. If mood is elevated, the person feels elated, speedy, irritable, powerful, energetic and often does not feel they need to sleep. Elevated mood ranges from hypomanic to hypermanic. A person who has an anxiety disorder may describe feeling worried, tense, frightened and nervous most of the time. Anxiety has many physical symptoms and people may often feel they have a bodily disorder, not a mental disorder (Table 11.7). Affect: flat, blunted, expressionless to exaggerated and dramatic, mask-like without reactivity. Mood may not be congruent with the topic and stated mood (grinning when talking about their mother's death) or inappropriate to topic. Congruence of mood and affect are very important clinical indicators of psychosis.

PROCEDURES AND NORMAL FINDINGS	ABNORMAL FINDINGS AND CLINICAL ALERTS
Other measures affected by mood. Normal mood fluctuations will generally not affect sleep, appetite, enjoyment, libido and memory for long periods of time. One may have 1 or 2 nights of poor sleep, but balance is quickly recovered. Asking about these factors are excellent objective measures of mood overall.	Sleep will often be disturbed (hypo- or hypersomnia) with a pattern of difficulty falling asleep, staying asleep or early morning waking. Appetite will be reduced or increased, with marked weight loss. **Anhedonia** (lack of pleasure in previously enjoyable activities) is common. Decreased libido or increased with **mania**.
Speech	
Speech reveals the content, order, speed of thought as well as possible organic concerns or intoxication.	Disruptions to the normal structure, flow and formations of speech reveal a great deal about cognitive function, education and mental state.
Volume and comprehensiveness of speech. Note appropriateness. In people without disability, speech will be spontaneous, audible, clear, expressive, at the correct volume, pitch, rate and rhythm and be age appropriate. **Pace of conversation** is moderate, in keeping with the other person and stream of talking is fluent. **Articulation** (ability to form words) is clear and understandable. **Word choice** is effortless and appropriate to educational level. The person completes sentences, occasionally pausing to think.	Physical or cognitive difficulties with speaking such as after a stroke or oral surgery or slurring with intoxication, or with the formation of language due to mood or thought disorder. **Depression** may cause mutism, slow or quiet speech. **Psychosis** may cause nonsensical, jumbled speech of a strange pace or pitch. Elevated mood may cause rapid, pressured speech or grandiose tones. **Paranoia** may cause hushed, secretive speech. Anger will often be loud in volume, sarcastic in tone and pressured or interrupting others. Slow, monotonous speech with **parkinsonism**, **depression**. Rapid-fire, pressured and loud talking occurs with **manic or hypomanic episodes**. **Dysarthria** is distorted speech (Table 12.6). Misuse of words; omits letters, syllables or words; transposes words—occurs with aphasia. Circumlocution or repetitious abnormal patterns: • **neologism** (using made-up words). • **echolalia** (when someone meaninglessly repeats what another person says) (Table 11.8). Unduly long word-finding or failure in word search occurs with **aphasia** (Chapter 12). Thought blocking occurs with depression and psychosis.

PROCEDURES AND NORMAL FINDINGS	ABNORMAL FINDINGS AND CLINICAL ALERTS
Thought processes and content	
Thought processes cannot be objectively observed because they are internal and personal but can be inferred through language and observation of behaviour. Thought processes have a usual, logical and coordinated profile; when thought processes are disrupted, this can be observed in several ways. Ask yourself: *Does this person make sense? Can I follow what the person is saying?* The *way* a person thinks should be logical, goal-directed, coherent and relevant. The person should complete a thought. **Thought content.** What is the person thinking about? You may need to enquire quite specifically here and follow a line of enquiry to reveal the content of thoughts. This is a very important part of the assessment. Is the person aware that their thoughts are unusual?	Flight of ideas. Poverty of ideas. Illogical, unrealistic thought processes. Digression from initial thought. Ideas run together. Evidence of blocking (person stops in middle of thought) (Table 11.8 and Table 11.9). Delusions, obsessions, compulsions. Suicidal thoughts, homicidal thoughts (violent ideation), preoccupation with guilt or hopelessness, paranoia, phobias.
Screen for suicidal thoughts	
It is very difficult to question people about possible suicidal ideas, especially for beginning nurses. Examiners fear invading privacy and may have their own normal denial of death and suicide. However, the risk is far greater if you skip these questions. You may be the only health professional to pick up clues of suicide risk. You are responsible for encouraging the person to talk about suicidal thoughts (see Table 11.10 for screening questions).	**Additional content on mental disorders** is listed in Tables 11.2, 11.3, 11.4 and 11.5. See also Figure 11.1 for suicide first aid guidelines for people from immigrant and refugee backgrounds.  ***Clinical alert:*** Decide about the level of suicide risk based on your screening. If the answer is 'yes' to many of the risk alerts, the risk is higher. If you feel the risk is moderate or above, do not leave the person alone and seek specialist mental health support.
Perception	
Perception is the way something is regarded, interpreted or understood.	Hallucinations, illusions, derealisation (things not seeming real), déjà vu or depersonalisation (one's person, body or self does not feel real). Auditory, tactile, visual, gustatory, olfactory hallucinations occur in the absence of external stimuli: • Auditory and visual hallucinations occur with psychiatric and organic brain disease and with psychedelic drugs. • Tactile hallucinations occur with alcohol withdrawal. • Gustatory and olfactory hallucinations are more common with organic brain issues or severe psychotic depression (smelling and tasting foul things like faeces). (Table 11.11).

PROCEDURES AND NORMAL FINDINGS	ABNORMAL FINDINGS AND CLINICAL ALERTS
Cognitive function	
Cognition is the ability to think, reason, know, understand and remember. It is dependent on brain function and should be formally tested if there is a suspected deficit, so later testing can compare with previous scores/results. If you think there is something unusual in a person's cognition, it is worth exploring with the family/carer as well as the person. A family will often adjust to changes without noticing because cognitive decline can be gradual. By making enquiries as to whether anything has changed in the person's behaviour, you are prompting the family to reflect. Again, you may be the first person to screen for these changes.	Abnormal findings are more likely to occur with organic disorders and less likely to occur with mental illness such as psychosis. Where a person has a pre-existing mental illness, cognitive decline may be less obvious. Medication interactions and side effects can cause significant cognitive disturbances, such as serotonergic syndrome (from SSRIs) and may cause sudden racing, suicidal thoughts. ! ***Clinical alert:*** Where a person exhibits altered cognition a Mini-Mental Status Examination should be conducted to determine orientation, memory and concentration.
Orientation	
You can discern orientation through the course of the interview, or ask for it directly, using tact: *Some people have trouble keeping up with the dates while in the hospital. Do you know today's date?* • Time: day of week, date, year, season • Place: where person lives, present location, type of building, name of city and state • Person: own name, age, who examiner is, type of worker. Many hospitalised people normally have trouble with the exact date but are fully oriented on the remaining items. It is unusual for a person with psychosis to be disoriented, other than to perhaps the date.	Disorientation occurs with organic brain disorders such as delirium and dementia. Orientation is usually lost in this order—first to time, then to place and rarely to person. A severely depressed person may be disoriented to time/date due to withdrawal from functioning and psychomotor slowing. **Anorexia nervosa** (fear of gaining weight along with a distorted body image) causing an electrolyte imbalance may cause disruption to cognition (thinking, decision making), but this will not usually affect orientation.
Attention and concentration	
Attention is the ability to focus on someone or something (e.g. the assessment) and concentration being the ability to sustain that attention over time. Check the person's ability to concentrate by noting whether they complete a thought without wandering. Note any distractibility or difficulty attending to you. Or give a series of directions to follow and note the correct sequence of behaviours such as: *Please take this glass of water with your left hand, drink from it, shift it to your right hand, and place it on the table.* Note that attention span commonly is impaired in people who are anxious, fatigued or intoxicated.	Digression from initial thought. Irrelevant replies to questions. Easily distracted, 'stimulus bound'—any new stimulus quickly draws attention. Confusion, negativism. Disturbance in attention is common with most acute psychiatric presentations such as psychosis, moderate-to-severe depression, mania, severe anxiety. This occurs because of disruption to thought processes and preoccupations with thought content. Confusion, rather than distractibility, is more evident with dementia or delirium (e.g. trying to urinate in a cupboard, thinking it is a toilet, or putting clothes on incorrectly).

PROCEDURES AND NORMAL FINDINGS	ABNORMAL FINDINGS AND CLINICAL ALERTS
Memory	
Recent memory. Assess by asking for a 24-hour diet recall or by asking the time the person arrived at the health service. Ask questions you can corroborate. This screens for the occasional person who confabulates or makes up answers to fill in the gaps of memory loss. For people who appear depressed or anxious, ask if they are forgetting things like appointments, where they left their keys and so on. Ask if they have a favourite television program and, if so, can they still watch from beginning to end?	Recent memory deficit occurs with organic disorders such as: • **delirium** (alteration of attention, consciousness and cognition, with a reduced ability to focus, sustain or shift attention; it develops over a short period and fluctuates during the day) • **dementia** (loss of cognitive functioning—thinking, remembering and reasoning) • **amnestic syndrome** (group of neurological disorders characterised by a dense global amnesia) • **Korsakoff's syndrome** (memory disorder that results from a vitamin B1 deficiency and is associated with chronic alcoholism).
Remote memory. In the context of the interview, ask the person verifiable past events—for example, ask them to describe past health, their first job, birthday and anniversary dates, and historical events that are relevant for that person. There should be no effect on remote memory with psychiatric illness.	Short-term memory issues are common in depression and anxiety; this occurs because of internal distraction rather than organic issues. The person will often be aware of their difficulty and may feel quite distressed by it. If there is reduced capacity to concentrate on previously enjoyed activities, this can help you ascertain a timeline of deterioration. Remote memory is lost when cortical storage area for that memory is damaged such as in Alzheimer's dementia or any disease that damages the cerebral cortex. Memory may be partially affected due to episodes of hospitalisation (medications) or traumatic events (fight-or-flight mechanism interfering with the laying down of long-term memories).
New learning	
Four unrelated words test. This tests the person's ability to lay down new memories. It is a highly sensitive and valid memory test. It requires more effort than does recalling personal or historic events. It also avoids the danger of unverifiable material. To the person, say: *I am going to say four words. I want you to remember them. In a few minutes I will ask you to recall them.* To be sure the person has understood, have the words repeated. Pick four words with semantic and phonetic diversity. Examples are:	People with Alzheimer's dementia score a zero- or one-word recall. Impaired new learning ability also occurs with anxiety (due to inattention and distractibility) and depression (due to lack of effort mobilised to remember).

PROCEDURES AND NORMAL FINDINGS	ABNORMAL FINDINGS AND CLINICAL ALERTS
1. brown 2. honesty 3. tulip 4. eyedropper — 1. fun 2. carrot 3. ankle 4. loyalty After 5 minutes, ask the person to recall the four words. To test the duration of memory, ask for a recall at 10 minutes and at 30 minutes. The normal response for people under 60 years is an accurate three- or four-word recall after a 5-, 10- and 30-minute delay.	
Insight and judgement	
Insight is a person's ability to reflect on their current situation, including their illness, with a level of self-awareness and self-understanding. Insight affects a person's judgement, which in turn affects the decisions that they make. A person with well-developed insight and judgement will generally make decisions about their health, work, family and recreation that consider risks and benefits. This does not mean people will not take risks, as dignity of risk is afforded to all people in life. This is part of free will and learning by mistakes. **Judgement.** A person exercises judgement when they can compare and evaluate the alternatives in a situation and reach an appropriate course of action. Ask about the person's daily or long-term life goals, the likelihood of acting in response to delusions or hallucinations and the capacity for violent or suicidal behaviour. Note what the person says about job plans, social or family obligations and other plans. Are plans realistic considering the person's health situation? Ask the person to describe the rationale for personal healthcare, and how they decided about whether to comply with prescribed health regimens. The person's actions and decisions should be realistic.	A person with limited insight may not agree that they have an illness or that they have any problems. They therefore may make risky or impulsive decisions (e.g. driving after having no sleep, not taking medications that keep them alive, leaving children unattended to go out or frequent unprotected sexual encounters). Judgement can be impaired when a person takes excessive, ill-thought-out and out-of-character risks. Impaired judgement can be a helpful indicator of overall coping and is often seen in: • depression (doesn't care, self-neglect, taking risks) • anxiety (can't decide, paralysed by fear) • elevated mood (promiscuity, spending), pain (impulsivity) • psychosis (acting on paranoia, impulsive risk taking). Sometimes people who have very high risk factors and poor insight and judgement will be treated against their will under mental health legislation in their state. This will only occur if they meet strict legal criteria, and there are many oversight and checking mechanisms built into each mental health Act to ensure treatment is appropriate and cannot be delivered in a less restrictive manner. **Impaired judgement** (unrealistic or impulsive decisions, wish fulfilment) occurs with intellectual disability, emotional dysfunction, schizophrenia, mood disorders, substance use disorders, anxiety disorders, personality disorders and organic brain disease.  ***Clinical alert:*** If you are worried about the person's safety now or soon, it is important to seek senior/specialist assessment. A person who presents a high level of risk will often be rapidly changing and unpredictable in their behaviour.

PROCEDURES AND NORMAL FINDINGS	ABNORMAL FINDINGS AND CLINICAL ALERTS
Mini-Mental State Examination	
The Mini-Mental State Examination[39] is a test of cognitive function (memory, orientation to time and place, naming, reading, copying or visuospatial orientation, writing and the ability to follow a three-stage command). It is useful for both initial and serial measurement; therefore, you can demonstrate worsening or improvement of cognition over time and with treatment. It concentrates only on cognitive functioning, not on mood, thought processes or executive function. It is a valid detector of organic disease but lacks sensitivity for mild cognitive impairment. The Mini-Mental State Examination is quick and easy, includes a standard set of only 11 questions, and requires only 5 to 10 minutes to administer. The examination is copyrighted but is widely available in healthcare settings and from the internet.	The Mini-Mental State Examination is used with caution for people with low education or those for whom English is not their first language. The exam lacks sensitivity for mild cognitive impairment. The maximum score on the test is 30; people with normal mental status average a score of 27. Scores between 24 and 30 indicate no cognitive impairment.
Additional objective data for infants and children	
The mental status assessment of infants and children covers behavioural, cognitive and psychosocial development and examines how the child is coping with their environment. Follow the same guidelines as for the adult, with special consideration for developmental milestones. Your best examination 'technique' arises from thorough knowledge of developmental milestones described in Chapter 3. The parent's health history, especially the sections on the developmental history and personal history, yields most of the mental status data. The Parent's Evaluation of Developmental Status Screening Tool (Chapter 3) provides an opportunity to interact directly with the young child to assess mental status. The tool is designed to identify children who may be slow in development in behaviour, language, cognitive and psychosocial areas. For children aged 7 to 11, who have grown beyond the age when developmental milestones are very useful, the 'Behavioural checklist' (Table 11.12) is an additional tool that can be given to the parent. It covers five major areas: mood, play, school, friends and family relations. It is easy to administer and takes about 5 minutes.	Abnormalities are often problems of *omission*—for example, the child does not achieve a milestone you would expect. Most mental illness in children will manifest as anxiety, depression, withdrawal and social conduct problems initially. Anxiety can manifest in repetitive and stereotypical behaviours such as tics, rocking and rituals. Persistent toileting problems may occur as a sign of mental illness in children. Children experiencing abuse or neglect will often come to the attention of schoolteachers and healthcare services. They may exhibit developmental delay, emotional dysregulation (anger, distress and withdrawal), aggression, sexualised behaviours or regression. Abused children may disassociate (have periods when they seem absent/blank or frozen) as a means of self-protection.[40] Aggressive, abusive, destructive, isolative behaviours, extreme clinginess, fear, distress or bizarre behaviour warrant further assessment. Self-injury (cutting, scratching, hair tearing, self-punching, head banging, burning, swallowing objects or inserting objects) is a very clear indicator of emotional distress and must be further investigated.

PROCEDURES AND NORMAL FINDINGS	ABNORMAL FINDINGS AND CLINICAL ALERTS
Additional objective data for adolescents	
Follow the same guidelines as described for adults. Assess the adolescent away from, as well as with, parents to allow for confidential material to be discussed. This will allow you to screen for health risks such as sexual risk taking or substance use.	Excessive risk-taking behaviour, excessive substance use, school refusal, promiscuity, self-injury, eating disorders.
Additional objective data for adults over 65 years	
It is important to conduct even a brief Mental Status Examination of all older people when admitted to hospital.	Between a third and a half of older adults admitted to acute care medical and surgical services show varying degrees of confusion on admission. In the community, about 5% of adults over 65 and almost 20% of those over 75 have some degree of clinically detectable impaired cognitive function.[42] ! ***Clinical alert:*** Depression and anxiety in older adults is not normal. Older adults may become depressed, anxious or confused when there is a co-occurring physical issue that is not being managed (pain, constipation, infection), affecting their cognition, independence and/or mobility. Conduct a relevant assessment.
Assess vision and hearing	
Check sensory status before assessing any aspect of mental status.	Vision and hearing changes due to ageing may alter alertness and leave the person looking confused. When older people cannot hear your questions, the results of the test may be inaccurate.
Mental status	
Follow the previous guidelines for conducting a Mental Status Examination—appearance, behaviour, mood and affect, cognitive functions, judgement and insight and Mini-Mental State Examination.	Uncooperative behaviour, abnormal mannerisms, stereotyped movements, agitation, retardation. ! ***Clinical alert:*** Developing an acute confusional state in an older person characterised by disorientation, disordered thinking and perceptions (illusions and hallucinations), agitation and inattention is a medical emergency. Refer to a medical practitioner for immediate assessment and management. See Table 11.2 and Chapter 30 for a detailed discussion of assessing for delirium.

PROCEDURES AND NORMAL FINDINGS	ABNORMAL FINDINGS AND CLINICAL ALERTS
Supplemental mental status examination	
There are two predominant supplemental mental status examination scales used in Australia. 1. The Geriatric Depression Scale[43,44] indicates the level of depression an older person may be experiencing. It is used for cognitively intact older people. It is not used to determine cognitive impairment. 2. The Psychogeriatric Assessment Scale is administered to assess for clinical changes in dementia, depression and cognitive impairment.[45] See additional resources section for link to this tool.	See Table 11.13.
Additional objective data for pregnant women	
Follow the previous guidelines for conducting a mental status examination—appearance, behaviour, mood and affect, cognitive functions, judgement and insight and Mini-Mental State Examination. The **Edinburgh Postnatal Depression Scale** is a useful screening tool for identifying symptoms that suggest anxiety and depression. This tool can be used in the antenatal period as well as the postnatal period (ideally 6–9 months after the birth). Using a screening tool will provide guidance as to whether a referral to a medical practitioner is required (Table 11.14).	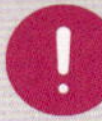 ***Clinical alert:*** A score of 13 or more may indicate possible depression requiring further assessment and follow-up by a medical practitioner.

Abnormal findings

TABLE 11.2 Delirium dementia and depression

Delirium is an acute confusional state, potentially preventable in hospitalised people. Characterised by disorientation, disordered thinking and perceptions (illusions and hallucinations), defective memory, agitation and inattention.

Dementia is a chronic progressive loss of cognitive and intellectual functions, although perception and consciousness are intact. Characterised by disorientation, impaired judgement and memory loss.

Depression is a long-term depressed mood (≥ 2 weeks) with lack of pleasure; disturbed sleep and appetite; feelings of hopelessness, guilt, worthlessness, sadness, loneliness and despair; and suicide ideation.

Continued

TABLE 11.2 Delirium dementia and depression cont'd

See the following comparisons.

	Delirium	Dementia	Depression
Onset	Sudden, over hours to days	Slowly, over months	May be gradual, with exacerbation during crisis or stress
Cause or contributing factors	Hypoglycaemia, fever, dehydration, hypotension; infection, other conditions that disrupt body homeostasis; adverse drug reaction; head injury; change in environment (e.g. hospitalisation); pain; emotional stress; substance abuse	Alzheimer's disease, vascular disease, human immunodeficiency virus infection, neurological disease, chronic alcoholism, head trauma	Lifelong history, losses, loneliness, crises, declining health, medical conditions
Cognition	Impaired memory, judgement, calculations, attention span; can fluctuate through the day	Impaired memory, judgement, calculations, attention span, abstract thinking; agnosia	Difficulty concentrating, forgetfulness, inattention
Level of consciousness	Altered	Not altered	Not altered
Activity level	Can be increased or reduced; restlessness; behaviours may worsen in evening (sundowning); sleep–wake cycle may be reversed	Not altered; behaviours may worsen in evening (sundowning)	Usually decreased; lethargy, fatigue, lack of motivation; may sleep poorly and awaken in early morning
Emotional state	Rapid swings; can be fearful, anxious, suspicious, aggressive, have hallucinations and/or delusions	Flat; agitation	Extreme sadness, apathy, irritability, anxiety, paranoid ideation
Speech and language	Rapid, inappropriate, incoherent, rambling	Incoherent, slow (sometimes due to effort to find the right word), inappropriate, rambling, repetitious	Slow, flat, low
Prognosis	Reversible with proper and timely treatment	Not reversible; progressive	Reversible with proper and timely treatment

Adapted from Halter 2022[27]

TABLE 11.3 Anxiety disorders

Anxiety disorders occur where the person experiences excessive levels of anxiety. Symptoms include palpitations, difficulty breathing, nausea, dry mouth, muscle tension, frequency of urination, sweating, abdominal pain, feelings of dread, irritability.

Panic attack[6] An abrupt surge of intense fear or intense discomfort in situations where most people would not be afraid. The attack will reach a peak within minutes. The person will change their behaviour related to the attacks and will avoid situations that may trigger panic attacks. Individuals will also show persistent concern about future panic attacks and the consequences. Can occur in the presence of other disorders such as major depressive disorder or medical conditions including vestibular disorders.	**Symptoms** Four or more of the following symptoms will occur: • sweating, palpitations or an accelerated heart rate, chest pain • shortness of breath, shaking or trembling, light-headedness, feeling dizzy • abdominal discomfort, nausea, sensation of choking • feeling detached from oneself or from reality • fear of losing control or a fear of dying • numbness or tingling and a feeling of heat or chills. **Impact** Disruption to occupational, social and interpersonal functioning.
Agoraphobia[6] Occurs when there is an increased anxiety or fear of two or more of the following situations: • open spaces—parks, bridges, markets • enclosed spaces such as cinemas or elevators • using public transport • being alone outside of the home and being in a crowd or standing in line. **Risk factors:** • Having panic disorder or other excessive fear reactions, called phobias • Responding to panic attacks with fear and avoidance • Experiencing stressful life events such as abuse, death of a parent or being attacked	**Symptoms** • Anxiety or fear out of proportion to the actual danger and sociocultural context • Avoiding situation(s) either entirely or needing the assistance of a companion Fear, anxiety and avoidance will be exacerbated if another medical condition is present such as Parkinson's disease or inflammatory bowel disease. **Impact** Occupational, social and interpersonal functioning are severely affected.
Panic disorder[6] This is when a person has persistent panic attacks and is constantly worried about future panic attacks.	**Symptoms** Changes in behaviour, like avoiding unfamiliar locations, are common, and people suffering panic disorder will often predict a catastrophic outcome from a minor physical symptom or medication side effect. **Impact** Persistent, full-symptom panic attacks as part of panic disorder lead to increased risk of disability and a poorer quality of life, absence from work or school and disruption to social and interpersonal functioning.

Continued

TABLE 11.3 Anxiety disorders cont'd

Social anxiety disorder (social phobia)[6] A persistent and irrational fear of being in social situations. **Risk factors** • Fear of being judged socially • Bullying by peers (children) • Obesity (teens)	**Symptoms** • Fear of being judged or criticised, feeling or looking foolish • Embarrassment • Being unable to answer questions, or being unable to remember the lines or notes • Avoidance of social situations or endures with intense anxiety Children will present differently (crying, throwing tantrums, being clingy, freezing or failing to speak in social situations with their peers as well as with adults).[6] **Impact** Occupational, social and interpersonal functioning are severely affected.
Generalised anxiety disorder[6] A chronic condition whereby the person worries excessively about everyday things. The person finds it difficult to control their excessive anxiety and worry about occasions, activities or performance (e.g. related to work) over a period of 6 months or more.	The apprehensive expectation will be associated with three or more of the following symptoms: • difficulty concentrating and directing thoughts • feeling on edge and restless, interrupted sleep, issues falling asleep • fatigue, muscle aches and pains and irritability, hypervigilance • muscle tension, diarrhoea, palpitations, tachypnoea • fatigue or sleep disturbance. • difficulty making decisions • avoidance • no apparent trigger for symptoms. **Impact** Occupational, social and interpersonal functioning are severely affected.
Post-traumatic stress disorder[6] May occur when there has been exposure to serious injury, sexual violence or threatened or actual death. **Cause:** The person will have directly experienced the traumatic event, witnessed in person the event as it happened to another person or learnt of the traumatic event as it occurred to a close family member or friend. In the case of death, threatened or actual, the event must have been either accidental or violent. Changes in arousal and reactions associated with the traumatic event will last for longer than 1 month.	**Symptoms** Negative changes in mood, emotional state and cognition will be present with two or more of the following symptoms over a period of 1 month or more: • consistent distorted thoughts about the cause of the traumatic event leading to the individual blaming themselves or others • an inability to remember a key part of the traumatic event, usually due to dissociative amnesia • noticeably diminished interest and participation in everyday activities • inability to feel happy and feelings of detachment from others

Continued

TABLE 11.3 Anxiety disorders cont'd

	• altered sleep, concentration and memory may be affected • re-enactments of the traumatic event via images, dreams or flashbacks • reckless or self-destructive behaviour • verbal or physical aggression towards other people or inanimate objects • hypervigilance, lack of concentration. **Impact** Occupational, social and interpersonal functioning are severely affected.
Obsessive-compulsive disorder[6] Occurs where there is a pattern of recurrent obsessions (intrusive, uncontrollable thoughts) and compulsions (repetitive ritualistic actions) that are done to decrease anxiety and prevent a catastrophe (e.g. fear of germs, violence, perfectionism and superstitions).	**Symptoms** • Repetitive behaviours (handwashing, checking) • Intrusive thoughts and actions are time consuming, interfering with daily activities • Attempts to ignore or suppress such thoughts, urges • Feels humiliated or ashamed for giving in to thoughts, urges • Insight varies as to whether the person thinks their beliefs are definitely or probably not true or that they may or may not be true **Impact** Functioning such as self-care, relationships and occupation may be affected.

TABLE 11.4 Schizophrenia

Schizophrenia is a mental illness that becomes apparent in adolescence or young adulthood. The disturbance will persist for 6 months or more. The person will experience two or more of:

- disorganised thinking and speech (formal thought disorder)
- unusual experiences such as hearing unpleasant voices
- hallucinations
- delusions
- disorganised or catatonic behaviour
- difficulty planning tasks, problem solving, focusing attention, remembering information and interacting with others
- lack of emotional expression and motivation.[6]

Cause: Unknown. There may be a genetic link, and certain stressors, circumstances and lifestyle factors can put someone at greater risk if they are already vulnerable to the illness.
Risk factors: Extreme stress, trauma, abuse and harmful alcohol or other drug use.
Impact: Will have a significant impact on functioning such as self-care and relationships and occupational functioning.

TABLE 11.5 Depressive disorder and bipolar disorder

Bipolar disorder[6]

Bipolar disorder has three different conditions:

Bipolar I is a recurrent illness where the person experiences episodes of mania and depression with and without psychotic episodes.

Bipolar II consists of depressive and manic episodes which alternate and are typically less severe and do not inhibit function.

Cyclothymic disorder is a cyclic disorder that causes brief episodes of hypomania and depression.[6]

Major depressive episode[6]

Symptoms

Loss of interest or pleasure in daily life and activities and/or a depressed mood with at least three of the following symptoms consistently over a 2-week period:

- fatigue
- psychomotor retardation or agitation
- excessive sleepiness or insomnia almost every day
- noticeable weight loss or weight gain with the accompanying decrease or increase in appetite or, in children, a failure to meet expected weight gains
- recurring suicidal thoughts or an obsession with death without a specific plan for how to commit suicide
- indecisiveness, lack of concentration, interrupted thought processes and feelings of worthlessness.

Impact

Functioning such as self-care, relationships and occupation are severely affected.

Manic episode[6]

The person experiences a defined change in mood, activity or energy lasting at least 1 week, with continually elevated or irritable moods or amplified purpose-driven activity present for most of the day. Noticeable changes in behaviour will be obvious with *three or more* of the following symptoms present, four if the mood is only irritable:

- decreased need for sleep, grandiosity or inflated self-esteem
- excessive talking or a feeling that the person must keep talking
- racing thoughts, flight of ideas, easily distracted
- excessive risk taking in pleasurable activities that could lead to negative consequences such as unwise business decisions, unsafe sexual encounters and unrestrained shopping binges.

Impact

Significant impact on functioning such as self-care, relationships and occupational. Hospitalisation may be necessary if there are psychotic features or the person or those around the person are at risk of harm.

TABLE 11.6 Characteristics of eating disorders

Anorexia nervosa	Bulimia nervosa	Binge eating

• Intense fear of weight gain
• Restricted calories, with significantly low body mass index
• Distorted body image
• Subtypes:
  ◦ Restricting (no consistent bulimic features)
  ◦ Binge eating/purging type (primarily restriction, some bulimic behaviours)
	• Recurrent episodes of uncontrollable bingeing
	• Inappropriate compensatory behaviours: vomiting, laxatives, diuretics or exercise
	• Self-image largely influenced by body image
		• Recurrent episodes of uncontrollable bingeing without compensatory behaviours
		• Bingeing episodes induce guilt, depression, embarrassment or disgust

Adapted from Halter 2022[27]

TABLE 11.7 Abnormalities of mood and affect

Type of mood or affect	Definition	Clinical example
Flat affect (blunted affect)	Lack of emotional response; no expression of feelings; voice monotonous and face immobile	No emotional response when telling a sad story about the death of their dog; face and voice remain expressionless
Depression	Sad, gloomy, dejected; symptoms have a physical dimension of tiredness, no energy, no appetite	'*I feel so empty, I just don't want to see anyone. I just don't enjoy anything anymore ...*'
Depersonalisation (lack of ego boundaries)	Loss of identity, feels estranged, perplexed about own identity and meaning of existence	'*I don't feel real. I feel like I'm not really* here.'
Elation	Joy and optimism, overconfidence, increased motor activity, not necessarily pathological	'*Wow, this is so exciting, I'm so happy, I just can't sit still ...*'
Euphoria	Excessive wellbeing, unusually cheerful or elated, which is inappropriate considering physical and mental condition, implies a pathological mood	'*I am high.*' '*I feel like I'm flying.*' '*I feel on top of the world.*'
Anxiety	Worried, uneasy, apprehensive from the anticipation of a danger whose source is unknown Physical symptoms such as butterflies, dizziness, jelly legs and palpitations are very common	'*I just know that something bad is going to happen, please don't leave me alone ...*'
Fear	Worried, uneasy, apprehensive; external danger is known and identified	Scared about coming into hospital, shaking and pale
Irritability	Annoyed, easily provoked, impatient, often presents as sarcastic and hostile	Person internalises a feeling of tension, and a seemingly mild stimulus 'sets them off' '*I told you I hate carrots ... you are so stupid, you never listen!*'
Rage	Furious, loss of control	Person has expressed violent behaviour towards self or others
Ambivalence	The existence of opposing emotions towards an idea, object or person; common with depression and anxiety, which causes indecision and emotional distress/paralysis.	'*I just can't decide whether to go to work or call in sick ... I can't decide about anything ...*'
Lability	Rapid shift of emotions	Person expresses euphoric, tearful, angry feelings in rapid succession
Incongruent affect	Affect clearly discordant with the content of the person's speech	Laughs while discussing admission for liver biopsy

TABLE 11.8 Abnormalities of thought process (formal thought disorder)

Type of process	Definition	Clinical example
Blocking	Sudden interruption in train of thought, unable to complete sentence, usually occurs with psychosis	The person will stop mid-sentence and when they resume talking are not aware what happened or of the previous topic
Confabulation	Fabricates events to fill in memory gaps; frequently occurs with dementia	Gives detailed description of their long walk around the hospital although you know they stayed in their room all afternoon
Neologism	Coining a new word—an invented word has no real meaning except for the person; may condense several words	'*I'll have to turn on my thinkilator.*'
Circumlocution	Roundabout expression, substituting a phrase when cannot think of the name of an object	Says 'the thing you open the door with' instead of 'key'
Circumstantiality	Talks with excessive and unnecessary detail, talks around a topic, but eventually reaches the point	'*When was my surgery? Well, I was 27, I was living with my aunt, she's the one with psoriasis, she had it bad that year because of the heat, the heat was worse then than it was in the summer of 2009 ...*'
Tangentiality	The topic of conversation repeatedly goes off on a tangent and does not return to the original topic without frequent redirection	When asked about a family member's health, the person diverts on to describing their choice of clothing and does not mention their health
Loosening associations	Shifting from one topic to an unrelated topic; person seems unaware that topics are unconnected There may be some connection between topics, but there is no logic to their connection	'*My boss is angry with me and it wasn't even my fault.* (pause) *I saw that movie too, Lord of the Rings. I felt really bad about it. But she kept trying to land the aeroplane and she never knew what was going on.*'
Flight of ideas	Abrupt change, rapid skipping from topic to topic, practically continuous flow of accelerated speech; topics usually have recognisable associations or are plays on words	'*Take this pill? The pill is blue. I feel blue.* (sings) *She wore blue velvet.*'
Word salad	Incoherent mixture of words, phrases and sentences; illogical, disconnected, includes neologisms	'*Beauty, red-based five, pigeon, the street corner, sort-of.*'
Perseveration	Persistent repeating of verbal or motor response, even with varied stimuli; the person seems stuck on a topic	'*I'm going to lock the door, lock the door. I walk every day and I lock the door. I usually take the dog and I lock the door.*'

TABLE 11.8 Abnormalities of thought process (formal thought disorder) cont'd

Type of process	Definition	Clinical example
Echolalia	Imitation, repeats others' words or phrases, often with a mumbling, mocking or mechanical tone	Nurse: '*I would like you to take your pill.*' Patient (mocking): '*Take your pill. Take your pill.*'
Clanging	Word choice based on sound, not meaning, includes nonsense rhymes and puns	'*My feet are cold. Cold, bold, told. The bell tolled for me.*'

TABLE 11.9 Abnormalities of thought content

Type of content	Definition	Clinical example
Phobia	Strong, persistent, irrational fear of an object or situation; feels driven to avoid it	Birds, spiders, snakes, heights, enclosed spaces, flying
Preoccupations such as hypochondriasis	Morbid worrying about their own health; feels sick with no actual basis for that assumption	Preoccupied with the fear of having cancer; any symptom or physical sign means cancer
Obsession	Unwanted, persistent thoughts or impulses; logic will not purge them from consciousness; experienced as intrusive and senseless	Violence (parent having repeated impulse to kill a loved child); contamination (becoming infected by water from the shower)
Compulsion	Unwanted repetitive, purposeful act; driven to do it; the ritualistic behaviour reduces anxiety and discomfort or prevents some dreaded event	Handwashing, counting, checking, and rechecking, touching. '*If I clean my hands with bleach every time I touch a door handle my mother won't die in an accident ...*'
Delusions	Firm, fixed, false beliefs; irrational; the delusional belief does not alter despite objective evidence to the contrary	Grandiose: the person believes they are God, famous or that they have a special mission to complete to save the human race Paranoid/persecutory: the person feels they are being followed, harassed, poisoned or people are trying to harm them
Violent ideation (suicidal and homicidal)	Intrusive preoccupation with ideas of one's own death, plans to suicide, thoughts of harming others, thoughts of revenge	'*I just don't feel like my life is worth living anymore. I wish I was dead, I'm in so much pain.*'

TABLE 11.10 Screen for suicidal thoughts

While not all suicide deaths can be prevented, the very effort of asking questions kindly and confidently can have a profound protective impact on a person. For people who are ambivalent about dying, and they are the majority, you can buy time so the person can be helped to find an alternative route through the situation. Most people who think about suicide do not go on to attempt it.
Share any concerns you have about a person's suicidal ideation with a mental health professional. Questions need to be specific and direct; saying 'hurt yourself' is too ambiguous because it could mean self-injury only. A person who has suicidal thoughts will often feel very relieved to be able to tell someone.

When the person expresses feelings of sadness, hopelessness, despair or grief, it is important to assess for any possible risk of physical harm to themselves. Begin with more general questions. If you hear affirmative answers, continue with more specific questions:

- *Have you ever felt so down you thought of suicide?*
- *Are you thinking about suicide now, or have you been thinking about it today?*

If the person says yes here, slow down and try to reflect on how sad and painful this must be for them. Validate their experiences and suffering before asking more questions.

- *Do you have a plan of how you might kill yourself?*
- *Have you tried to kill yourself before?*

If so:
What did you do last time to recover from what happened?

A precise suicide plan (which includes a specific method with materials already collected, such as a rope for hanging) to take place in the next 24 to 48 hours using a lethal method constitutes a very high risk.

Clinical alert:
Important clues and warning signs of suicide include:

- previous suicide attempts
- having a family member or close friend who has suicided
- feelings of pain and desperation (physical and mental)
- depression, hopelessness
- social withdrawal, running away
- self-injury
- hypersomnia or insomnia
- slowed psychomotor activity
- anorexia
- a mental disorder
- increased risk taking
- minimal supports, being alone
- verbal suicide messages (defeat, failure, worthlessness, loss, giving up, desire to kill self)
- death themes in art, jokes, writing, behaviours
- saying goodbye (giving away prized possessions).

TABLE 11.11 Abnormalities of perception

Type of perception	Definition	Clinical example
Hallucination	Sensory perceptions for which there are no external stimuli; may strike any sense: visual, auditory, tactile, olfactory, gustatory, somatic	Visual: seeing an image (ghost) of a person who is not there; auditory: hearing voices (one or many, even hundreds) or music/sounds
Illusion	Misperception of an actual stimulus, by any sense	Folds of bedsheets appear to be animated, jumper on end of bed appears to be a cat
Depersonalisation (lack of ego boundaries)	Loss of identity, feels estranged, perplexed about own identity and meaning of existence	'*I don't feel real.*' '*I feel like I'm not really here.*'

TABLE 11.12 Behavioural checklist[41]

1. Prefers to play alone	15. Seems afraid of someone or something
2. Gets hurt in major accidents	16. Is nervous and jumpy
3. Do they ever play with fire?	17. Has a nervous habit
4. Has difficulties with teachers	18. Does not show feelings
5. Gets poor grades in school	19. Fights with other children
6. Is absent from school	20. Is understanding of other people's feelings
7. Becomes angry easily	21. Refuses to share
8. Daydreams	22. Shows jealousy
9. Feels unhappy	23. Takes things that are not theirs
10. Acts younger than other children their age	24. Blames others for their troubles
11. Does not listen to parents	25. Prefers to play with children not their age
12. Does not tell the truth	26. Gets along well with grownups
13. Unsure of themselves	27. Teases others
14. Has trouble sleeping	

Scoring is a point system: 0—never; 1—sometimes; 2—often. Scoring is reversed for items 20 and 26. Scores between 15 and 22 indicate closer following; scores above 22 warrant psychiatric evaluation.
Source: Jellinek et al. 1979[41]

TABLE 11.13 The Geriatric Depression Scale (short form)

Used to screen for depression in older adults. Consists of 15 questions requiring 'yes' or 'no' answers.

Directions: Choose the best answer for how you have felt over the past week:

1. Are you basically satisfied with your life? YES/**NO**
2. Have you dropped many of your activities and interests? **YES**/NO
3. Do you feel that your life is empty? **YES**/NO
4. Do you often get bored? **YES**/NO
5. Are you in good spirits most of the time? YES/**NO**
6. Are you afraid that something bad is going to happen to you? **YES**/NO
7. Do you feel happy most of the time? YES/**NO**
8. Do you often feel helpless? **YES**/NO
9. Do you prefer to stay at home, rather than going out and doing new things? **YES**/NO
10. Do you feel you have more problems with memory than most? **YES**/NO
11. Do you think it is wonderful to be alive now? YES/**NO**
12. Do you feel pretty worthless the way you are now? **YES**/NO
13. Do you feel full of energy? YES/**NO**
14. Do you feel that your situation is hopeless? **YES**/NO
15. Do you think that most people are better off than you are? **YES**/NO

Score 1 point for each bolded answer.
A score > 5 points is suggestive of depression.
A score > 10 points is almost always indicative of depression.
A score > 5 points should warrant a follow-up comprehensive assessment.

Source: Stanford University: http://www.stanford.edu/~yesavage/GDS.html

TABLE 11.14 The Edinburgh Postnatal Depression Scale

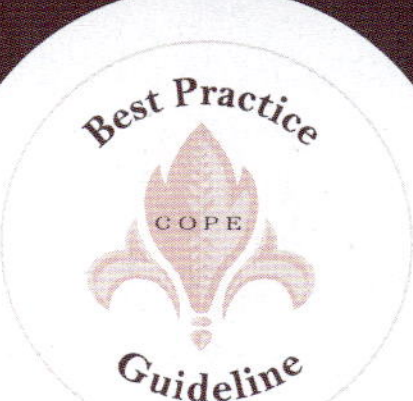

Edinburgh Postnatal Depression Scale (EPDS)

Cox JL, Holden JM Sagovsky R (1987) Detection of postnatal depression: development of the 10-item Edinburgh postnatal depression scale. Brit J Psychiatry 150 782-86. Reproduced with permission.

Name: ______________________ **Date:** ____________

We would like to know how you have been feeling in the past week. Please indicate which of the following comes closest to how you have been feeling over the past seven days, not just how you feel today. Please tick one circle for each question that comes closest to how you have felt in the **last seven days.**

Here is an example already completed.

I have felt happy:

- ☐ Yes, all of the time
- ■ Yes, most of the time
- ☐ No, not very often
- ☐ No, not at all

This would mean: 'I have felt happy most of the time during the past week'.

Please complete the other questions in the same way.

1. I have been able to laugh and see the funny side of things

0 As much as I always could
1 Not quite so much now
2 Definitely not so much now
3 Not at all

2. I have looked forward with enjoyment to things

0 As much as I ever did
1 Rather less than I used to
2 Definitely less than I used to
3 Hardly at all

3. I have blamed myself unnecessarily when things went wrong

3 Yes, most of the time
2 Yes, some of the time
1 Not very often
0 No, never

4. I have been anxious or worried for no good reason

0 No, not at all
1 Hardly ever
2 Yes, sometimes
3 Yes, very often

5. I have felt scared or panicky for no very good reason

3 Yes, quite a lot
2 Yes, sometimes
1 No, not much
0 No, not at all

6. Things have been getting on top of me

3 Yes, most of the time I haven't been able to cope at all
2 Yes, sometimes I haven't been coping as well as usual
1 No, most of the time I have coped quite well
0 No, I have been coping as well as ever

7. I have been so unhappy that I have had difficulty sleeping

3 Yes, most of the time
2 Yes, sometimes
1 Not very often
0 No, not at all

8. I have felt sad or miserable

3 Yes, most of the time
2 Yes, quite often
1 Not very often
0 No, not at all

9. I have been so unhappy that I have been crying

3 Yes, most of the time
2 Yes, quite often
1 Only occasionally
0 No, never

10. The thought of harming myself has occurred to me

3 Yes, quite often
2 Sometimes
1 Hardly ever
0 Never

cope.org.au

Available at: https://www.cope.org.au/health-professionals/health-professionals-3/calculating-score-epds/

Interpreting Edinburgh Postnatal Depression Scale scoring

Clinical judgement is integral to interpreting EPDS scores because in some cases the score may not accurately represent a woman's mental health. For example, a woman may have a low score, even though there is good reason to believe that she is experiencing depressive symptoms. A very high EPDS score could suggest a crisis, other mental health issues or unresolved trauma.

Scores may be influenced by several factors including the patient's understanding of the language used, their fear of the consequences if depression is identified and differences in emotional reserve and perceived degree of stigma that is associated with depression.

When follow-up care is required

A total score of 13 or more is considered a flag for the need to follow up possible depressive symptoms. In the antenatal period, repeat the EPDS in 2 to 4 weeks if a woman's score is 13 or more in line with clinical judgement. If the second EPDS score is 13 or more, refer to an appropriate health professional, ideally the woman's usual GP. In the postnatal period, arrange referral or ongoing care if a woman's score is 13 or more in line with clinical judgement.

Follow-up may also be needed if scores on questions 3, 4 and 5 suggest possible symptoms of anxiety.

For scores of 1, 2 or 3 on question 10, the safety of the woman and children in her care should be assessed and, according to clinical judgement, advice sought and/or mental health assessment arranged.

Clinical reasoning and documentation

Case study (continued)

The following is a continuation of the case study provided at the beginning of this chapter and the initial clinical reasoning process including problem/issue identification and documentation of clinical data. Consult a fundamentals of nursing or medical-surgical nursing text for information about goal setting, nursing interventions and evaluation.

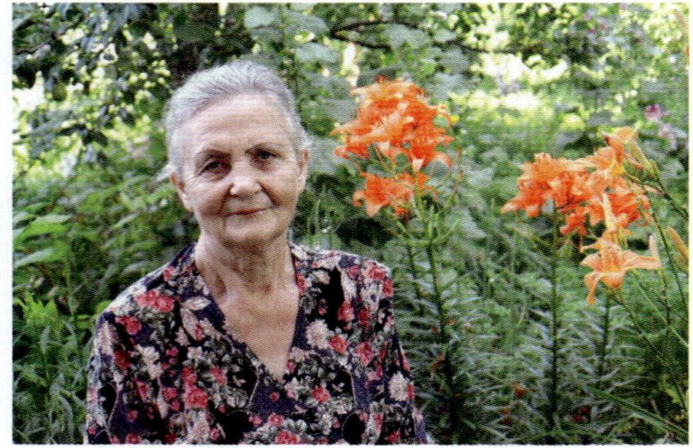

Context

You will recall from the case study described earlier in the chapter that you are a practice nurse working in a general practice clinic. One part of your role is to conduct annual health checks for clients over 75 years of age.

Consider the patient's situation (altered cognitive state)

Mrs Lola Peters is a 79-year-old woman accompanied by her husband, Ray. Her last annual check showed that while she had no physical health problems at that time, she was having some issues with memory. Ray tells you that Lola has increasing memory loss, confusion and is now exhibiting socially inappropriate behaviour.

Collect cues/information

Your further assessment reveals the following information.

Clinical reasoning and documentation cont'd

Subjective data

Lola is oriented to person and place. She says it's a hot day but cannot state the day of the week. When I asked Lola how she was feeling, she said 'good', and she looked to her husband. She had difficulty finding words for my questions. According to Ray, his wife has been irritable with her friends and family and recently left a supermarket with items she did not pay for. Her hygiene and grooming standards have decreased; she eats very little and appears to have lost weight. She does not sleep through the night, has angry emotional outbursts that are unlike her former demeanour and does not recognise her younger grandchildren. Her husband reports that she has drifted away from the stove while cooking, allowing food to burn on the stovetop. He has found her wandering through the house in the middle of the night, unsure of where she is. She used to 'talk on the phone for hours', but now he has to push her into having conversations. Ray describes her mood as angry and irritable, with some social withdrawal.

Objective data

Appearance: Sitting quietly, somewhat slumped, picking on loose threads on her dress. Hair is gathered in loose ponytail with stray wisps. No make-up.
Behaviour: Awake and gazing at hands and lap. Expression is flat and vacant. Will make eye contact when called by name, although gaze quickly shifts back to lap. Speech is a bit slow but articulate; some trouble with word choice.
Mood and affect: Appears distracted and sad during interview.
Thought processes and content: Experiences blocking in train of thought, needs prompting to answer questions.
Cognitive functions: Oriented to person and place. Can state the day of the week. Is not able to repeat the correct sequence of complex directions involving lifting and shifting glass of water to the other hand. Scores a one-word recall on the 'Four unrelated words' test. Cannot tell me how she would plan a grocery shopping trip.

Process information and identify problems/issues

Collaborative problem(s)

Slow change cognitive state—probable dementia; needs referral for further assessment

Problem statements/nursing diagnoses

Chronic confusion related to slow change cognitive state
Impaired social interaction related to slow change cognitive state
Impaired memory related to slow change cognitive state
Risk for injury related to wandering and poor concentration
Self-care deficit (hygiene, dressing, grooming) related to confusion and memory loss
Increased family stressors related to change in health status

ADDITIONAL RESOURCES

You can further develop your knowledge and skills relevant to conducting mental health assessments by:

- reading chapters of a fundamentals of nursing or medical-surgical nursing textbook
- answering chapter multiple choice questions online. Log onto ClinicalKey Student and search for the text 'Health Assessment, 4th edition'. Choose the section titled 'Teaching material'. In this section you will find question and answer documents for each chapter.
- visiting websites

  Black Dog Institute: https://www.blackdoginstitute.org.au/

ADDITIONAL RESOURCES cont'd

Butterfly Foundation: https://butterfly.org.au/get-support/helpline/

Eating Disorders Victoria: https://www.eatingdisorders.org.au/about-us/

Mental Health and Wellbeing Act 2022 in your language: https://www.health.vic.gov.au/mental-health/mental-health-and-wellbeing-act-2022-in-your-language

Mental Health First Aid Australia (schizophrenia): https://www.mhfa.com.au/schizophrenia-offering-support-and-overcoming-barriers/

Psychogeriatric assessment scale—Australian Government, Department of Health and Aged Care: https://www.health.gov.au/resources/publications/cognitive-impairment-scale-pas

World Health Organization (suicide prevention): https://www.who.int/publications/i/item/9789240026629

REFERENCES

1. World Health Organization. Intention to action series: people power. Perspectives from individuals with lived experience of noncommunicable diseases, mental health conditions and neurological conditions. Geneva; 2023 (Intention to action series). Licence: CC BY-NC-SA 3.0 IGO. Available at: https://iris.who.int/bitstream/handle/10665/366666/9789240069725-eng.pdf?sequence=1
2. World Health Organization. Mental Health. 2022. Available at: https://www.who.int/news-room/fact-sheets/detail/mental-health-strengthening-our-response#:,:text=Determinants%20of%20mental%20health&text=Exposure%20to%20unfavourable%20social%2C%20economic,of%20experiencing%20mental%20health%20conditions
3. Afek A, Ben-Avraham R, Davidov A, Berezin Cohen N, Ben Yehuda A, Gilboa et al. Psychological resilience, mental health, and inhibitory control among youth and young adults under stress. Front. Psychiatry, 2021 11:608588. doi: 10.3389/fpsyt.2020.608588
4. Roper C, Grey F, Cadogan C. 2018. Co-production: Putting principles into practice in mental health contexts. Available at: https://healthsciences.unimelb.edu.au/__data/assets/pdf_file/0007/3392215/Coproduction_putting-principles-into-practice.pdf
5. Australian Commission on Safety and Quality in Health Care. National Safety and Quality Health Service standards user guide for health services providing care for people with mental health issues. Sydney: ACSQHC; 2018. Available at: https://www.safetyandquality.gov.au/sites/default/files/2019-05/nsqhs-standards-user-guide-for-health-services-providing-care-for-people-with-mental-health-issues_0.pdf
6. American Psychiatric Association (APA). Diagnostic and statistical manual of mental disorders, fifth edition, text revision. Washington: American Psychiatric Association, 2022.
7. Harris B, Duggan M, Batterham P, Bartlem K, Clinton-McHarg T, Dunbar JA, et al. Australia's Mental and Physical Health Tracker: Background Paper, Australian Health Policy Collaboration issues paper no. 2018-02. Melbourne: AHPC; 2018. Available at: https://www.vu.edu.au/sites/default/files/australias-mental-and-physical-health-tracker-background-paper.pdf.
8. Australian Institute of Health and Welfare. Physical health of people with mental illness [Internet]. Canberra: Australian Institute of Health and Welfare, 2023. Available from: https://www.aihw.gov.au/reports/mental-health/physical-health-of-people-with-mental-illness

9. Sommers-Flanagan, J. Conversations about suicide: strategies for detecting and assessing suicide risk. Journal of Health Service Psychology 44, 33–45 (2018). https://doi.org/10.1007/BF0354466
10. Australian Institute of Health and Welfare. Australian Burden of Disease Study 2022. Catalogue number. BOD 37, AIHW, 2022 Australian Government. Available at: https://www.aihw.gov.au/getmedia/d9ae4bfa-df27-4e3c-9846-ba452bef6ac5/aihw-bod-37.pdf?v=20230605164222&inline=true
11. Ministry of Health New Zealand. Mental Health in Aotearoa Results from the 2018 Mental Health Monitor and the 2018/19 New Zealand Health Survey. 2020. Available at: https://www.hpa.org.nz/sites/default/files/Mental_Health_Aotearoa_Insight_2020.pdf
12. Arias D, Saxena S, Verguet S. Quantifying the global burden of mental disorders and their economic value. EClinicalMedicine; 2022;54: 101675
13. Australian Institute of Health and Welfare. Mental health services—in brief 2018. Cat. no. HSE 211. Canberra: AIHW; 2018b. Available at: https://www.aihw.gov.au/reports/mental-health-services/mental-health-services-in-australia-in-brief-2018/contents/table-of-contents
14. Hallyburton A. Diagnostic overshadowing: an evolutionary concept analysis on the misattribution of physical symptoms to pre-existing psychological illnesses. International Journal of Mental Health Nursing. 2022 Dec;31(6):1360–1372.
15. Morgan M, Peters D, Hopwood M, Castle D, Moy C, Fehily C, et al. Better physical health care and longer lives for people living with serious mental illness. Mitchell Institute, Victoria University, 2021, Melbourne.
16. Fearon RMP, Roisman GI. Attachment theory: progress and future directions. Current Opinion in Psychology. 2017 Jun;15:131–136. doi: 10.1016/j.copsyc.2017.03.002. Epub 2017 Mar 8. PMID: 28813253
17. Butler A, Van Lieshout RJ, Lipman EL, MacMillan HL, Gonzalez A, Willem Gorter J, et al Mental disorder in children with physical conditions: a pilot study. BMJ Open 2018;8:e019011. doi: 10.1136/bmjopen-2017-019011
18. Ne'eman A, Pellicano E. Neurodiversity as politics. Human Development. 2022;66(2):149–157.
19. Nelson RH. A critique of the neurodiversity view. Journal of Applied Philosophy. 2021 May;38(2):335–347.
20. Australian Bureau of Statistics. (2020–2022). National Study of Mental Health and Wellbeing methodology. ABS. https://www.abs.gov.au/methodologies/national-study-mental-health-and-wellbeing-methodology/2020-2022.
21. Ministry of Health New Zealand Annual update of key results 2021/22: New Zealand Health Survey. 2023. Available at: https://www.health.govt.nz/nz-health-statistics/health-statistics-and-data-sets/mental-health-data-and-stats
22. Keski-Rahkonen A, Raevuori A, Hoek HW. Epidemiology of eating disorders: an update. Annual Review of Eating Disorders. 2018 Apr 19:66–76.
23. World Health Organization. Mental disorders. 2022. Available at: https://www.who.int/news-room/fact-sheets/detail/mental-disorders
24. Mitchison D, Mond J, Bussey K, Griffiths S, Trompeter N, Lonergan A, et al. (2020). DSM-5 full syndrome, other specified, and unspecified eating disorders in Australian adolescents: prevalence and clinical significance. Psychological Medicine 50, 981–990.
25. van Hoeken, Daphne, Hoek, Hans W. Review of the burden of eating disorders: mortality, disability, costs, quality of life, and family burden. Current Opinion in Psychiatry 33(6): 521–527, November 2020.
26. Mehler PS, Watters A, Joiner T, Krantz MJ. What accounts for the high mortality of anorexia nervosa? International Journal of Eating Disorders. 2022 May;55(5):633–636.
27. Halter, M J. (2022). Varcarolis' foundations of psychiatric mental health nursing (9th ed.). St Louis: Elsevier.
28. Productivity Commission 2020, Mental Health, Report no. 95, Australian Government. Canberra. Available at: https://www.pc.gov.au/inquiries/completed/mental-health/report/mental-health.pdf
29. Australian Institute of Health and Welfare (2022)

Australia's health 2022: data insights, catalogue number AUS 240, Australia's health series number 18, AIHW, Australian Government.
30. Wand APF, Peisah C, Draper B, Brodaty H. Carer insights into self-harm in the very old: a qualitative study. International Journal of Geriatric Psychiatry 2019;34(4):594–600.
31. Australian Commission on Safety and Quality in Health Care. National Safety and Quality Health Service Standards User Guide for Health Service Organisations Providing Care for Patients from Migrant and Refugee Backgrounds. Sydney: ACSQHC; 2021.
32. Au M, Anandakumar AD, Preston R, Davis M. A model explaining refugee experiences of the Australian healthcare system: a systematic review of refugee perceptions. BMC International Health and Human Rights, 2019, 19(22), doi: org/10.1186/s12914-019-0206-
33. Australian Institute of Health and Welfare. Suicide & self-harm monitoring. 2023. Available at: https://www.aihw.gov.au/suicide-self-harm-monitoring
34. Ministry of Health New Zealand Annual update of key results 2021/22: New Zealand Health Survey. 2023. Available at: https://www.health.govt.nz/nz-health-statistics/health-statistics-and-data-sets/mental-health-data-and-stats
35. Te Whatu Health New Zealand. 2023. Suicide web tool. Available at: https://www.tewhatuora.govt.nz/our-health-system/data-and-statistics/suicide-web-tool/
36. Aran N, Card KG, Lee K, Hogg RS. Patterns of suicide and suicidal ideation in relation to social isolation and loneliness in newcomer populations: a review. Journal of Immigrant and Minority Health. 2023 Apr;25(2):415–426.
37. Motillon-Toudic C, Walter M, Séguin M, Carrier J, Berrouiguet S, Lemey C. 2022, Social isolation and suicide risk: literature review and perspectives. European Psychiatry, 65(1), E65. doi: 10.1192/j.eurpsy.2022.2320
38. National Mental Health Commission (2023). Monitoring mental health and suicide prevention reform: National Report 2022—reflections on a journey of change. National Mental Health Commission, Sydney. Available at: https://www.mentalhealthcommission.gov.au/getmedia/14ed263e-41dd-4b2e-92b5-a31b2637ab60/NMHC_Reflections_Report_2022_MK3_Accessible
39. Folstein M, Folstein S. Copyright 1975, 1998, 2001 by Mini-Mental LLC, Inc. Published 2001 by Psychological Assessment Resources, Inc.
40. Sadock B, Sadock V, Ruiz P. Kaplan and Sadock's Comprehensive Textbook of Psychiatry. 10th ed. Philadelphia: Lippincott, Williams & Wilkins; 2017.
41. Jellinek M, Evans N, Knight RB. Use of a behavior checklist on a pediatric inpatient unit. The Journal of Pediatrics. 1979 Jan 1;94(1):156–158.
42. Draper BM. Suicidal behaviour and suicide prevention in later life. Maturitas 2014;79(2): 179–183.
43. American Psychological Association. Geriatric Depression Scale (GDS) construct: depressive symptoms. 2017. Available at: https://www.apa.org/pi/about/publications/caregivers/practice-settings/assessment/tools/geriatric-depression
44. Yesavage J.A. Geriatric Depression Scale. Psychopharmacology Bulletin. 1988 Jan 1;24(4):709–711.
45. Jorm A, Mackinnon A. 2016. Psychogeriatric Assessment Scales: User's Guide, 4th edition. Available at: https://www.dementiaresearch.org.au/wp-content/uploads/2016/06/PAS-User-Guide-4th-Edition-May-2016.pdf

CHAPTER 12

Neurological assessment

Written by Carolyn Jarvis
Adapted by Josh Allen

INTRODUCTION

The nervous system can be divided into two parts—central and peripheral. The **central nervous system** (CNS) includes the brain and spinal cord. The **peripheral nervous system** (PNS) includes the 12 pairs of cranial nerves, the 31 pairs of spinal nerves and all their branches. The PNS carries (afferent) messages *to* the CNS from sensory receptors, motor (efferent) messages *from* the CNS out to muscles and glands, as well as autonomic messages that govern the internal organs and blood vessels. This chapter focuses on assessing core neurological functions. Specific assessment of pain (Chapter 13), vision (Chapter 14) and hearing (Chapter 15) is covered in the following chapters. It is important to note that assessment of neurological function is often conducted concurrently with assessment of the peripheral vascular system (Chapter 16).

To be able to perform a neurological assessment, identify potential or actual problems and plan care, detailed knowledge of structure and function, developmental and cultural considerations are necessary.

Case study 1

The following case study gives an example of a typical situation involving ongoing neurological assessment and the clinical reasoning process including problem/issue identification.

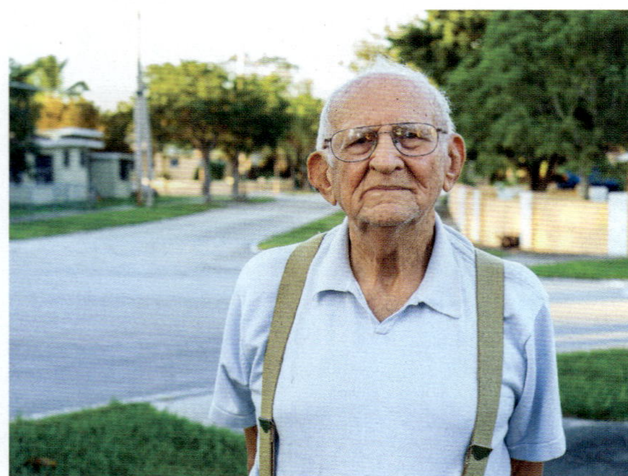

Context

It is bedside handover at change of shift. You are the registered nurse undertaking a baseline assessment of Mr Stanislaw Adamik's neurological status in conjunction with the nurse who has been caring for him on the morning shift.

Consider the patient's situation

Mr Adamik is 80 years old, a retired builder who lives with his son in a single-storey house. He was previously living independently performing his activities of daily living without assistance. He was referred to the hospital neurosurgery department after a 2-month history of increasing confusion and generalised malaise. A CT scan showed a left-sided cerebral lesion. He is scheduled to undergo a craniotomy and removal of the left temporal parietal lesion later today.

Questions to further your learning

- What are the possible things that might be going on with Mr Adamik?
- What knowledge do you need to be able to predict what might be going on?
- What approach to Mr Adamik's health assessment will you take?
- What questions (subjective data) will you ask Mr Adamik to extend the health history and why?
- What physical examination (objective data) will you conduct and why?
- What resources are available to assist in your assessment of Mr Adamik?

Assessment plan

Assessing neurological function is important for nurses in a variety of healthcare settings and is part of the primary survey undertaken when first meeting a person, particularly in an emergency. The extent of the questioning and examination will depend on the person's main health concern.

Subjective assessment of neurological function investigates a variety of symptoms such as headache, dizziness, seizures, tremors, weakness, lack of coordination, numbness or tingling, dysphagia and dysphasia. Symptoms such as these can affect the person's safety and capacity to perform their activities of daily living. There may also be effects on the nutritional state of the person, their relationships and capacity to work. Also, significant past history and environmental/ occupational hazards are also explored. Neurological subjective assessment is performed in conjunction with assessing the person's mental state, vision, hearing, ability to smell, taste and touch and their position sense. Subjective data collection aims to clarify any presenting symptoms in the person's own words, after which you will need to carefully question the person to get more details. The main areas for subjective assessment are:

- presenting concern
- headache
- neck pain, limitation of motion
- pain
- head injury
- dizziness/vertigo
- seizures
- tremors and involuntary movements
- weakness
- lack of coordination
- numbness or tingling
- visual disturbances and deafness
- difficulty swallowing (dysphagia)
- difficulty speaking
- relevant health and family history
- health and lifestyle management
- environmental/occupational hazards.

Following subjective data collection, you will get a sense of the areas needed to be examined for objective data. Only the relevant areas should be examined.

There are three main types of objective neurological assessments—ongoing neurological observations, a screening assessment and a complete assessment.

Ongoing neurological observations ('neuro obs') is conducted on people with neurological deficits who need periodic or ongoing assessments or those at risk of a changed neurological state. Most hospitals have specific charts to guide you in this assessment and for ease in recording the data (commonly referred to as a 'neuro obs chart'). The assessment data is presented in graphic form and usually includes the Glasgow Coma Scale (Table 12.1), pupillary response and vital signs.

Routine neurological screening assessment is conducted on seemingly well people with no significant subjective findings from the history.

Complete neurological assessment is conducted on people with neurological symptoms (e.g. change in conscious state, headache, weakness, loss of coordination) or who have shown signs of neurological dysfunction. The complete neurological assessment sequence is described in the advanced practice section.

The main areas for objective assessment are:

- general inspection
- level of consciousness
- using the Glasgow Coma Scale
- pupillary response
- vital signs
- limb movement and strength
- assessing delirium.

Resources available

You will find additional resources at the end of this chapter. This chapter also has a video available demonstrating objective data collection related to a neurological screening assessment. You will find a QR code in the objective data section, which enables you to access the video easily on your device.

Structure and function

The head and neck are important structures to consider when assessing neurological function. These structures support and protect parts of the nervous system.

The head

The **skull** is a rigid bony box that protects the brain and special sense organs, and it includes the bones of the cranium and the face (Figure 12.1). Note the location of these **cranial bones**: frontal, parietal, occipital and temporal. Use these names to describe any of your findings in the corresponding areas.

The adjacent cranial bones unite at meshed immovable joints called the **sutures**. The bones are not firmly joined at birth; this allows for the mobility and change in shape needed for the birth process. The sutures gradually ossify during early childhood. The **coronal** suture crowns the head from ear to ear at the union of the frontal and parietal bones. The **sagittal** suture separates the head lengthwise

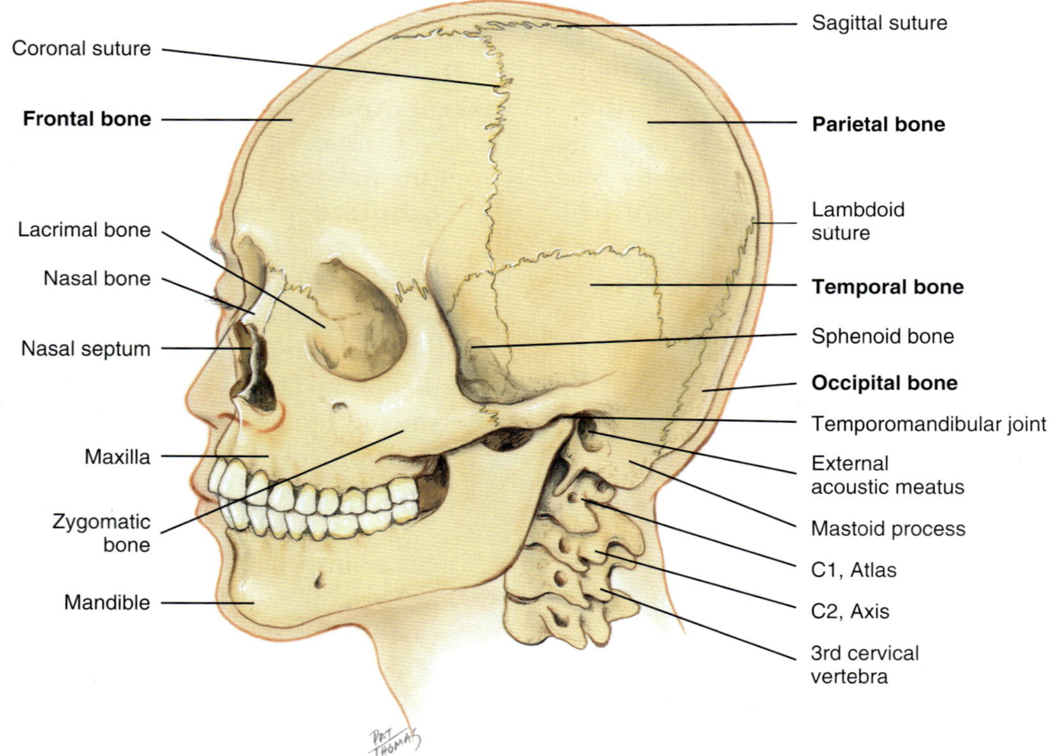

FIGURE 12.1 The skull

between the two parietal bones. The **lambdoid** suture separates the parietal bones crosswise from the occipital bone.

The 14 **facial bones** also articulate at sutures (note the nasal bone, zygomatic bone and maxilla), except for the mandible (the lower jaw). It moves up, down and sideways from the temporomandibular joint, which is anterior to each ear.

The cranium is supported by the cervical vertebra: C1, the 'atlas'; C2, the 'axis'; and down to C7. The C7 vertebra has a long spinous process that is palpable when the head is flexed. Feel this useful landmark, the **vertebra prominens**, on your own neck.

The human **face** has myriad appearances and a large array of facial expressions that reflect mood. The expressions are formed by the facial muscles (Figure 12.2), which are mediated by cranial nerve VII, the facial nerve. Facial muscle function is symmetrical bilaterally, except for an occasional quirk or wry expression.

Facial structures also are symmetrical; the eyebrows, eyes, ears, nose and mouth appear about the same on both sides. The palpebral fissures—the openings between the eyelids—are equal bilaterally. Also, the nasolabial folds, the creases extending from the nose to each corner of the mouth, should look symmetrical. Facial sensations of pain or touch are mediated by the three sensory branches of cranial nerve V, the trigeminal nerve.

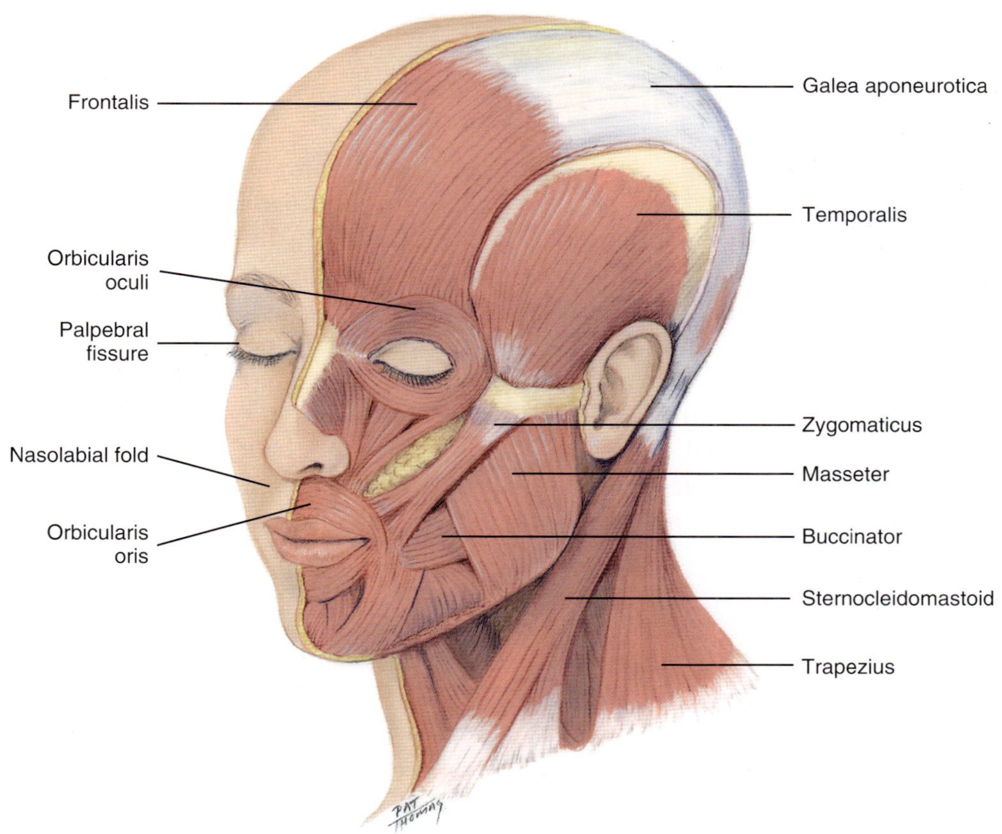

FIGURE 12.2 Facial muscles

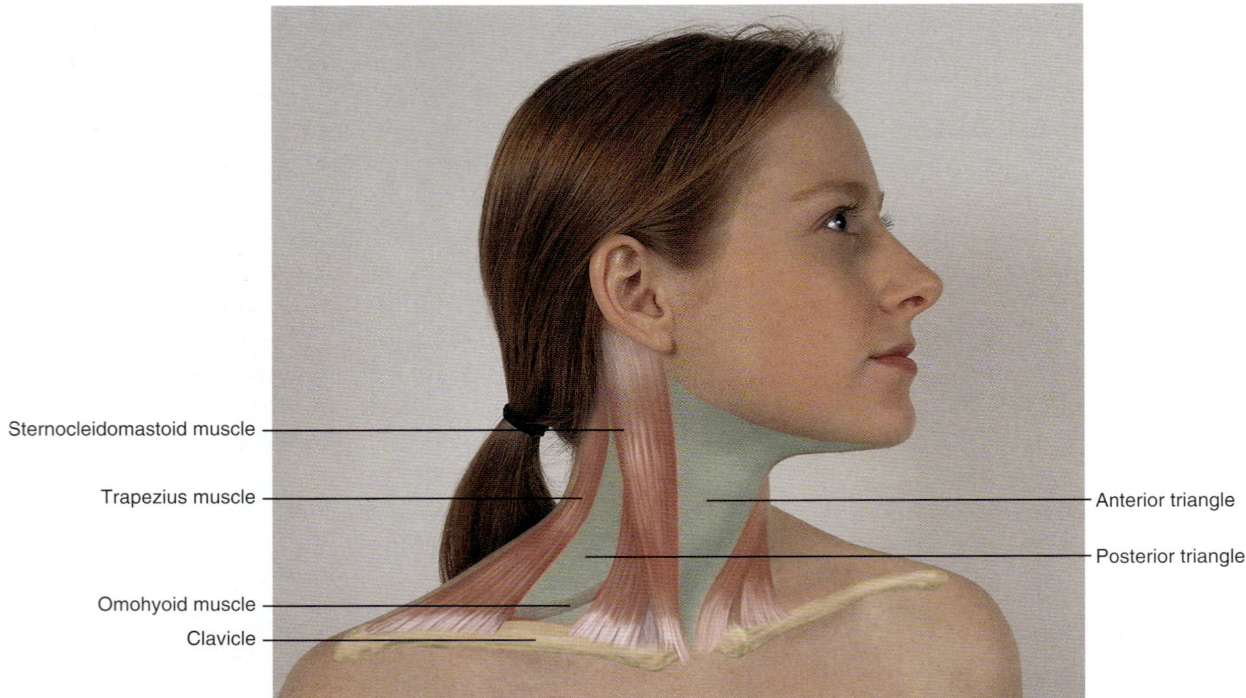

FIGURE 12.3 Neck muscles

The neck

The **neck** is delimited by the base of the skull and inferior border of the mandible above and by the manubrium sterni, the clavicle, the first rib and the first thoracic vertebra below. Think of the neck as a *conduit* for the passage of many structures, which are lying in close proximity: vessels, muscles, nerves, lymphatics and viscera of the respiratory and digestive systems. Blood vessels include the common and internal carotid arteries and their associated veins. The internal carotid branches off the common carotid and runs inwards and upwards to supply the brain; the external carotid supplies the face, salivary glands and superficial temporal area. The carotid artery and internal jugular vein lie beneath the sternocleidomastoid muscle. The external jugular vein runs diagonally across the sternomastoid muscle.

The major **neck muscles** are the **sternocleidomastoid** and the **trapezius** (Figure 12.3); they are innervated by cranial nerve XI, the spinal accessory nerves. The sternocleidomastoid muscle arises from the sternum and the medial part of the clavicle and extends diagonally across the neck to the mastoid process behind the ear. It accomplishes head rotation and head flexion. The two trapezius muscles form a trapezoid shape on the upper back. Each arises from the occipital bone and the vertebrae and extends, fanning out to the scapula and clavicle. The trapezius muscles move the shoulders and extend and turn the head.

The sternocleidomastoid muscle divides each side of the neck into two triangles. The **anterior triangle** lies in front, between the sternocleidomastoid and the midline of the body, with its base up along the lower border of the mandible and its apex down at the suprasternal notch. The **posterior triangle** is behind the sternocleidomastoid muscle, with the trapezius muscle on the other side and with its base along the clavicle below. It contains the posterior belly of the omohyoid muscle. These triangles are helpful guidelines when describing findings in the neck.

The central nervous system

The brain is made up of three main parts: prosencephalon (or forebrain), consisting of the cerebrum, thalamus, hypothalamus and limbic system; mesencephalon (or midbrain), consisting of the tectum and tegmentum; and rhombencephalon (or hindbrain), consisting of the cerebellum, pons and medulla.

PARTS OF THE CENTRAL NERVOUS SYSTEM

Cerebral cortex

The cerebral cortex is the cerebrum's outer layer of nerve cell bodies, which looks like 'grey matter' because it lacks myelin. Myelin is the white insulation on the axon that increases the conduction velocity of nerve impulses.

The cerebral cortex is the centre for humans' highest functions, governing thought, memory, reasoning, sensation, language and voluntary movement (Figure 12.4). Each half of the cerebrum is a **hemisphere**; the left hemisphere is dominant in most people (95%), including those who are left-handed.

Each hemisphere is divided into four main **lobes**: frontal, parietal, temporal and occipital. The lobes have certain areas that mediate specific functions.

- The **frontal** lobe has areas concerned with reasoning, concentration, personality, behaviour, emotions and intellectual function. The frontal lobe also contains the frontal eye fields, responsible for vision.
- The precentral gyrus of the frontal lobe is the primary centre involved in voluntary contralateral movement.

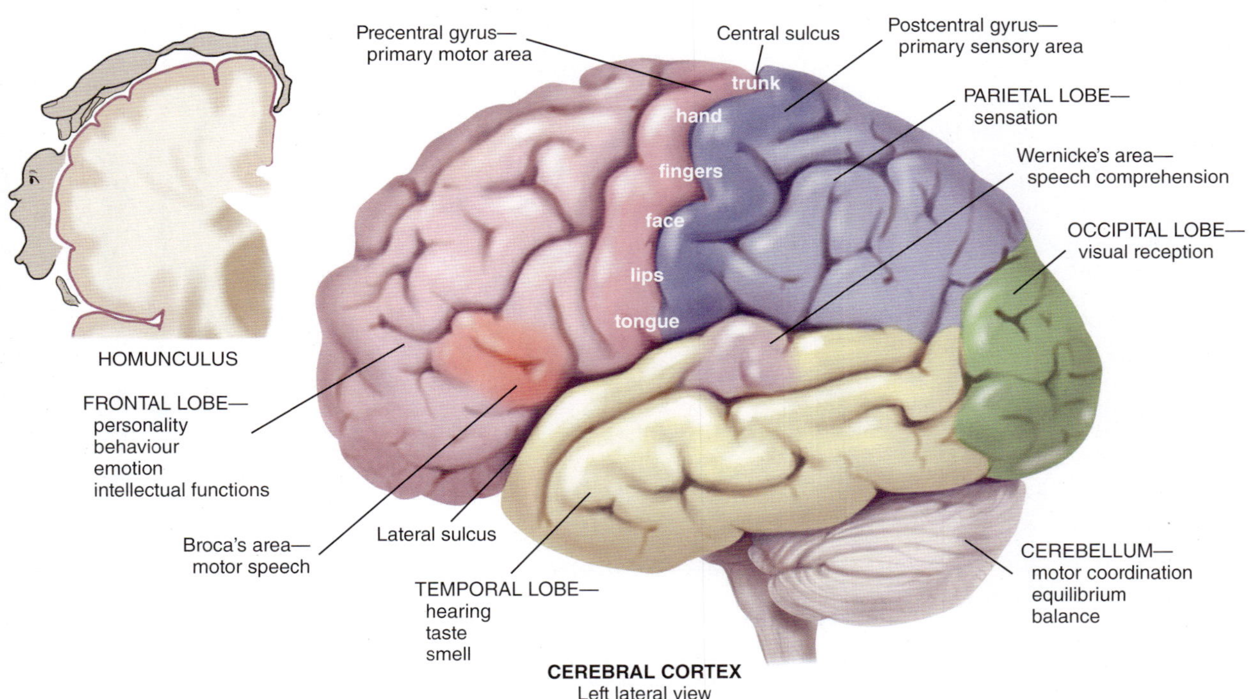

FIGURE 12.4 Cerebral cortex—left lateral view

- The **parietal** lobe's postcentral gyrus is the primary centre for the interpretation of contralateral sensation. Also, in the non-dominant hemisphere it is important in visual/proprioception and in the dominant hemisphere it is important in calculation.
- The **occipital** lobe is the primary visual receptor centre, some visual reflexes and involuntary smooth eye movements.
- The **temporal** lobe behind the ear has the primary auditory reception centre, language function, learning and memory.
- **Wernicke's area** in the temporal lobe is associated with language comprehension. When damaged in the person's dominant hemisphere, *receptive* or *Wernicke's aphasia* results. The person hears sound but it has no meaning, like hearing a foreign language.
- **Broca's area** (inferior part of the dominant frontal lobe) in the frontal lobe mediates motor speech. When injured in the dominant hemisphere the person may experience *expressive aphasia* (cannot talk at all) or *expressive dysphasia* (difficulty in communicating). The person can understand language and knows what they want to say but cannot express what they want to say.

Damage to any of these specific cortical areas produces a corresponding loss of (usually contralateral) function: motor weakness, paralysis, loss of sensation or impaired ability to understand and process language. Damage occurs when the highly specialised neurological cells are affected by trauma or deprived of their blood supply, such as when a cerebral artery becomes occluded or when vascular bleeding or vasospasm occurs.

Basal ganglia

The basal ganglia are large bands of grey matter buried deep within the two cerebral hemispheres that form the subcortical associated motor system (the extrapyramidal system) (Figure 12.5). They help to initiate

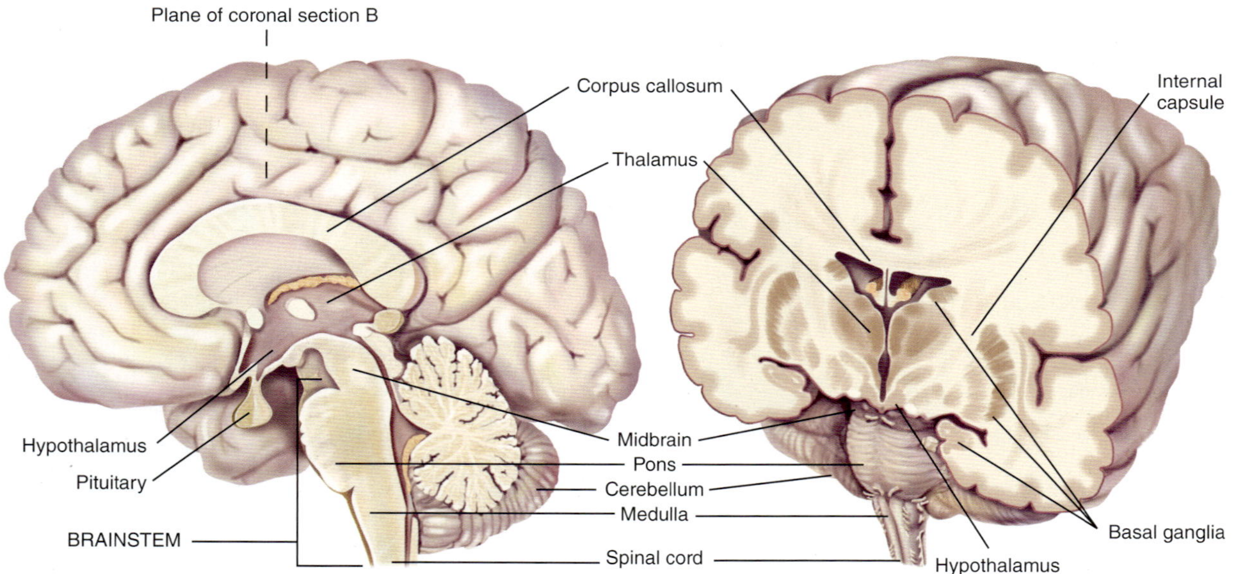

FIGURE 12.5 Components of the central nervous system

and coordinate movement and control—for example, the arm-swing alternating with the legs during walking.

Thalamus

The thalamus is the main relay station for the nervous system where sensory pathways of the spinal cord and brainstem form *synapses* (sites of contact between two neurons) on their way to the cerebral cortex. It is an integrating centre with connections that are crucial to emotion and creativity.

Hypothalamus

The hypothalamus is a major respiratory control centre with basic vital functions: temperature, heart rate and blood pressure control, water metabolism, appetite, sleep centre, sexual arousal, anterior and posterior pituitary gland regulator and coordinator of autonomic nervous system activity and emotional status.

Limbic system

The limbic system (also known as the paleomammalian cortex) is a set of structures (amygdala, mammalian bodies, stria medullaris, central grey, dorsal and ventral nuclei of Gudden) responsible for emotion, behaviour, motivation, olfaction and aiding the formation of memories.

Cerebellum

The cerebellum is a coiled structure located under the occipital lobe that is concerned with motor coordination of voluntary movements, equilibrium (i.e. the postural balance of the body) and muscle tone. It does not initiate movement but coordinates and smooths it—for example, the complex and quick coordination of many different muscles needed in playing the piano, swimming or juggling. It is like the 'automatic pilot' on an aeroplane in that it adjusts and corrects the voluntary movements but operates entirely below the conscious level.

Brainstem

The brainstem is the central core of the brain consisting of mostly nerve fibres. It has three areas:

1. **Midbrain**—the most anterior part of the brainstem that still has the basic tubular structure of the spinal cord. It merges into the thalamus and hypothalamus. It contains many motor neurons and tracts. Cranial nerves III and IV nuclei are in the midbrain.
2. **Pons**—the enlarged area containing ascending and descending fibre tracts. Also, cranial nerves V through to VIII have nuclei in the pons.
3. **Medulla**—the continuation of the spinal cord in the brain that contains all ascending and descending fibre tracts connecting the brain and spinal cord. It has vital autonomic centres (respiration, heart, gastrointestinal function), as well as nuclei for cranial nerves IX through to XII. Pyramidal decussation (crossing of the motor fibres) occurs here (see below).

Spinal cord

The spinal cord is the long cylindrical structure of nervous tissue with a circumference about as big as that of the little finger. It occupies the upper two-thirds of the vertebral canal from the medulla to lumbar vertebrae L1 to L2. It is the main highway for ascending and descending fibre tracts that connect the brain to the spinal nerves, and it mediates reflexes. Its nerve cell bodies, or grey matter, are arranged in a butterfly shape with anterior and posterior 'horns'.

PATHWAYS OF THE CENTRAL NERVOUS SYSTEM

Crossed representation is a notable feature of the nerve tracts: the *left* cerebral cortex receives sensory information from and controls motor function to the *right* side of the body, while the *right* cerebral cortex

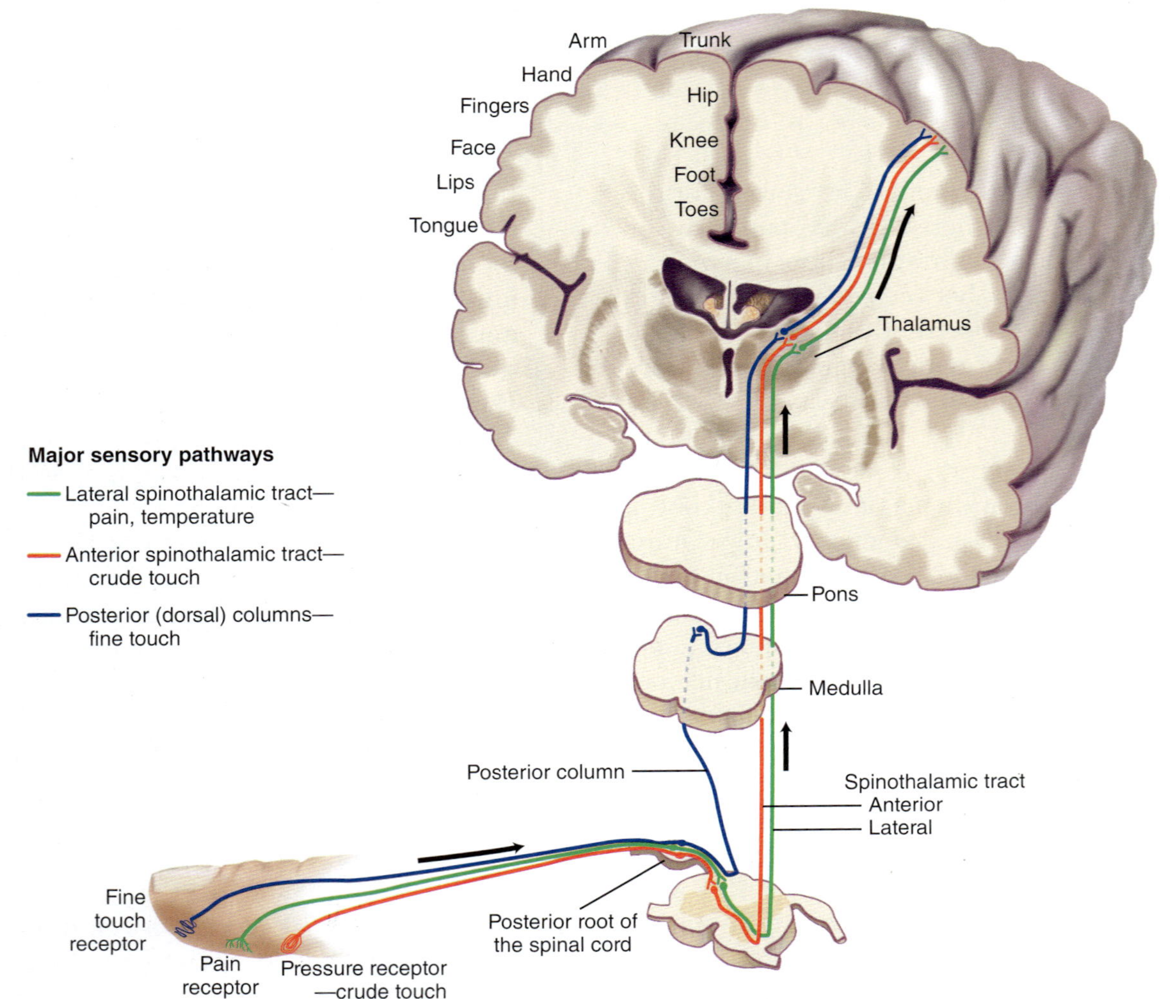

FIGURE 12.6 Major sensory pathways

likewise interacts with the *left* side of the body. Knowledge of where the fibres cross the midline will help you interpret clinical findings.

Sensory pathways

Millions of sensory receptors are embroidered into the skin, mucous membranes, muscles, tendons and viscera. They monitor conscious sensation, internal organ functions, body position and reflexes. Sensation travels in the afferent fibres in the peripheral nerve, then through the posterior (dorsal) root, then into the spinal cord. There, it may take one of two routes—the spinothalamic tract or the posterior (dorsal) columns (Figure 12.6).

Spinothalamic tract

The spinothalamic tract contains sensory fibres that transmit the sensations of pain, temperature and crude or light touch (i.e. not precisely localised). The fibres enter the dorsal root of the spinal cord and synapse with a second sensory neuron. The second-order neuron fibres cross to the opposite side and ascend up the spinothalamic tract to the thalamus. Fibres carrying pain and temperature sensations ascend the *lateral* spinothalamic tract, whereas those of crude touch form the *anterior* spinothalamic tract. At the thalamus, the fibres synapse with a third sensory neuron, which carries the message to the sensory cortex for full interpretation.

Posterior (dorsal) columns

These fibres conduct the sensations of position, vibration and finely localised touch:

- **position** (proprioception)—without looking, you know where your body parts are in space and in relation to each other
- **vibration**—feeling vibrating objects
- **finely localised touch** (stereognosis)—without looking, you can identify familiar objects by touch.

These fibres enter the dorsal root and proceed immediately up the same side of the spinal cord to the brainstem. At the medulla, they synapse with a second sensory neuron and then cross. They travel to the **thalamus**, synapse again and proceed to the sensory cortex (the postcentral gyrus, Figure 12.4), which localises the sensation and makes full discrimination.

The sensory cortex is arranged in a specific pattern forming a corresponding 'map' of the body (see the homunculus in Figure 12.4). Pain in the right hand is perceived at its specific spot on the left cortex map. Some organs are absent from the brain map, such as the heart, liver or spleen.

You know you have one, but you have no 'felt image' of it. Pain originating in these organs is referred, because no felt image exists in which to have pain. Pain is felt 'by proxy' by another body part that does have a felt image. For example, pain in the heart is referred to the chest, shoulder and left arm, which were its neighbours in fetal development. Pain originating in the spleen is felt on the top of the left shoulder.

Motor pathways

Corticospinal or pyramidal tract

The area has been named 'pyramidal' because it originates in pyramid-shaped cells in the motor cortex (Figure 12.7). Motor nerve fibres originate in the motor cortex (precentral gyrus, Figure 12.4) and travel to the brainstem, where they cross to the opposite or contralateral side (*pyramidal decussation*) and then pass down in the lateral column of the spinal cord. At each cord level, they synapse with a lower motor neuron contained in the anterior horn of the spinal cord. Ten per cent of corticospinal fibres do *not* cross, and these descend in the anterior column of the spinal cord. Corticospinal fibres mediate voluntary movement, particularly very skilled, discrete, purposeful movements, such as writing.

The corticospinal tract is a newer, 'higher' motor system that permits very skilled and purposeful movements. The tract's origin in the motor cortex is arranged in a specific pattern called *somatotopic organisation*. It is another body map, this one of a person or *homunculus*, hanging 'upside down' (Figure 12.4). Body parts are not equally represented on the map, and the homunculus looks distorted. To use political terms, it is more like an electoral map than a geographic map. That is, body parts whose movements are relatively more important to humans (e.g. the hand) occupy proportionally more space on the brain map.

Extrapyramidal tracts

The extrapyramidal tracts include all the motor nerve fibres originating in the motor cortex, basal ganglia, brainstem and spinal cord that are *outside* the pyramidal tract. This is a phylogenetically older, 'lower', more primitive motor system. These subcortical motor fibres maintain muscle tone and control body movements, especially gross automatic movements such as walking.

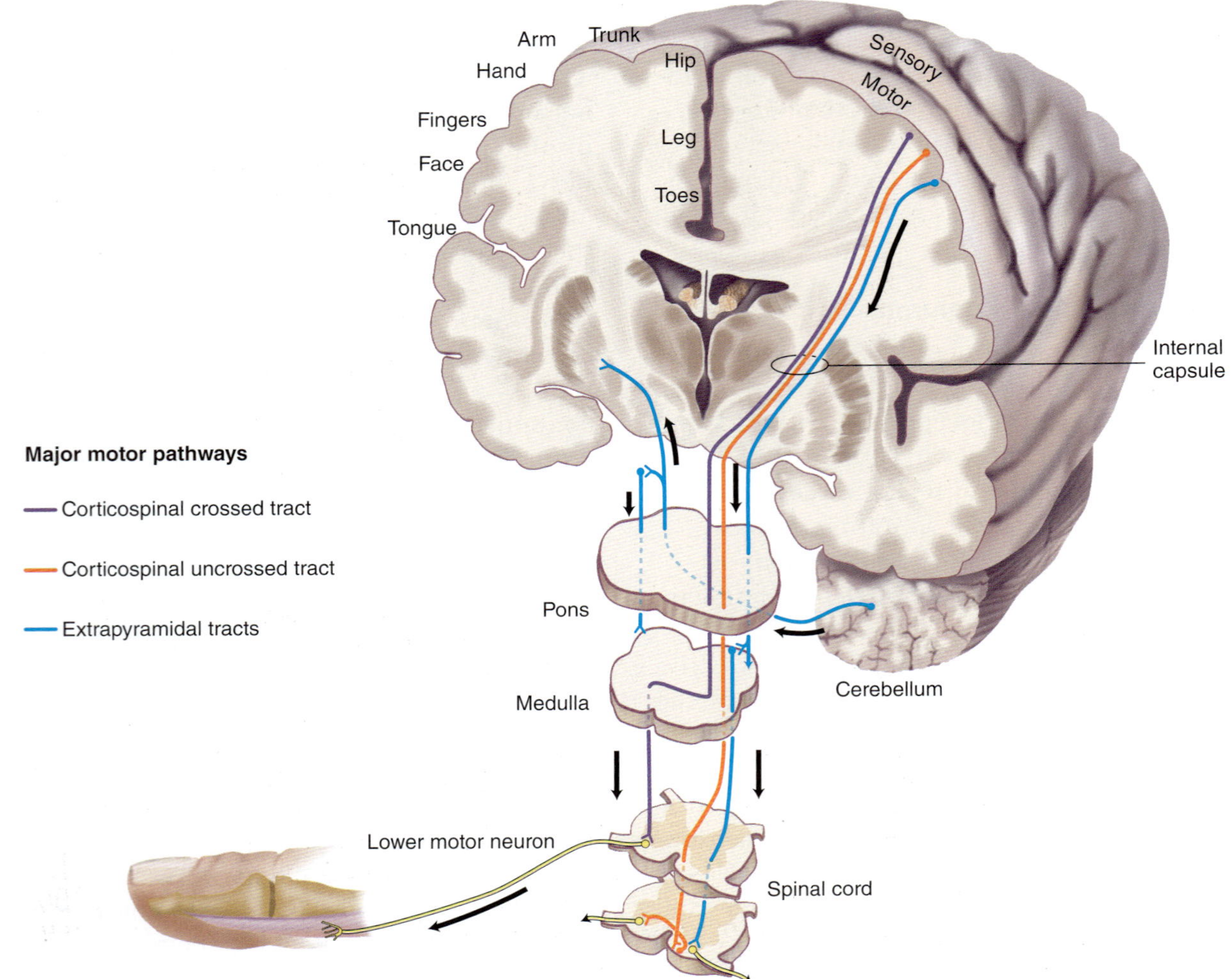

FIGURE 12.7 Major motor pathways

Cerebellar system

This complex motor system coordinates movement, maintains equilibrium and helps maintain posture. The cerebellum receives information about the position of muscles and joints, the body's equilibrium and what kind of motor messages are being sent from the cortex to the muscles. The information is integrated and the cerebellum uses feedback pathways to exert its control back on the cortex or down to lower motor neurons in the spinal cord. This entire process occurs on a subconscious level.

Upper and lower motor neurons

Upper motor neurons are a complex of all the descending motor fibres that can influence or modify the lower motor neurons. Upper motor neurons are located completely within the CNS. The neurons convey impulses from motor areas of the cerebral cortex to the lower motor neurons in the anterior horn cells of the spinal cord (Figure 12.8). Examples of upper motor neurons are corticospinal, corticobulbar and extrapyramidal tracts. Examples of upper motor neuron diseases are stroke, cerebral palsy and multiple sclerosis.

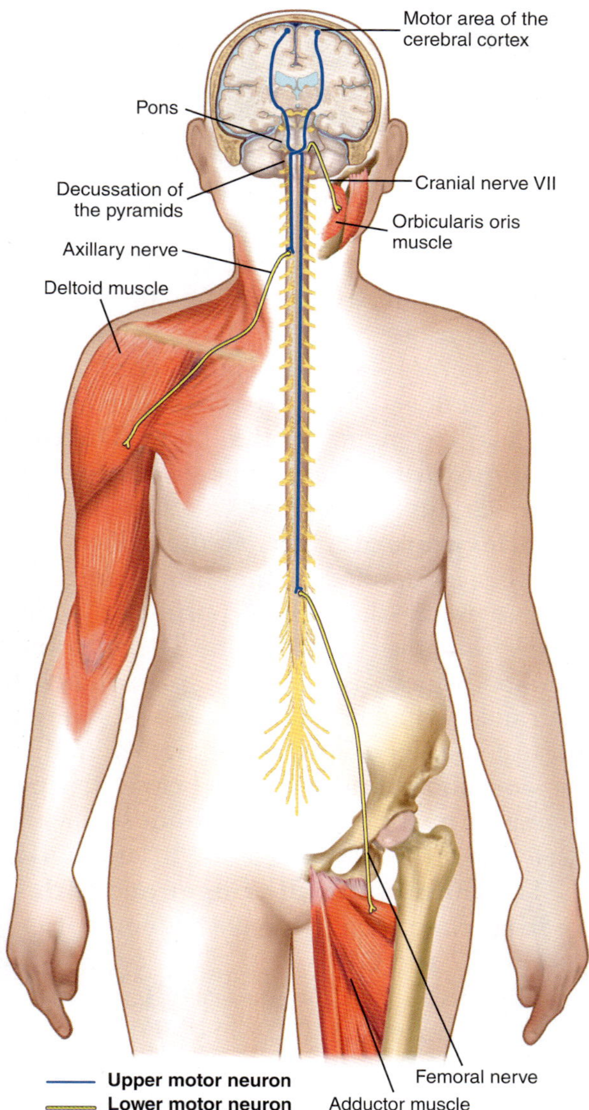

FIGURE 12.8 Upper and lower motor neurons

Lower motor neurons are located mostly in the PNS. The cell body of the lower motor neuron is in the anterior grey column of the spinal cord, but the nerve fibres extend from here to the muscle. The lower motor neuron is the 'final common pathway' because it funnels many neural signals here and it provides the final direct contact with the muscles. Any movement must be translated into action by lower motor neuron fibres. Examples of lower motor neurons are cranial nerves and spinal nerves of the PNS. Examples of lower motor neuron diseases are Bell's palsy in cranial nerve lesions and in spinal cord lesions, poliomyelitis and motor neuron disease.

The peripheral nervous system

A **nerve** is a bundle of neurons *outside* the CNS. The peripheral nerves carry input to the CNS via their sensory afferent fibres and deliver output from the CNS via the efferent fibres.

REFLEX ARC

Reflexes are basic defence mechanisms of the nervous system. They are involuntary, operating below the level of conscious control and permitting a quick reaction to potentially painful or damaging situations. Reflexes also help the body maintain balance and appropriate muscle tone. There are four types of reflexes: (1) deep tendon reflexes (myotatic), for example, patellar or knee jerk; (2) superficial, for example, corneal reflex, abdominal reflex; (3) visceral (organic), for example, pupillary response to light and accommodation; and (4) pathological (abnormal), for example, Babinski's or extensor plantar reflex.

The fibres that mediate the reflex are carried by a specific spinal nerve. In the simplest reflex, tapping the tendon stretches the muscle spindles in the muscle, which activates the sensory afferent nerve. The sensory afferent fibres carry the message from the receptor and travel through the dorsal root into the spinal cord (Figure 12.9). They synapse directly in the cord with the motor neuron in the anterior horn. Motor efferent fibres leave via the ventral root and travel to the muscle, stimulating a sudden contraction.

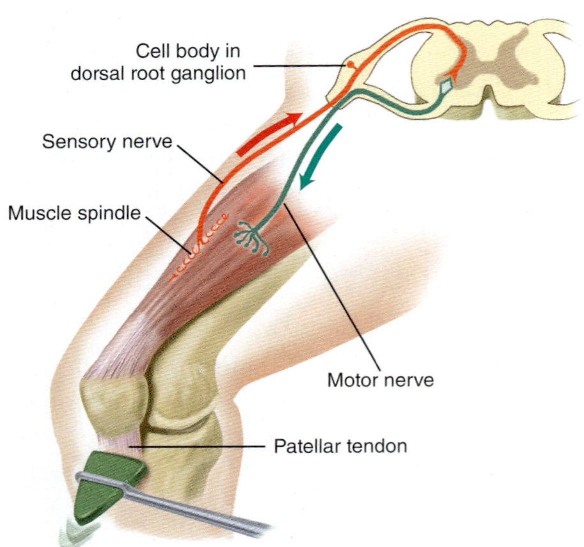

FIGURE 12.9 Reflex arc

The deep tendon (myotatic or stretch) reflex has five components: (1) an intact sensory nerve (afferent); (2) a functional synapse in the cord; (3) an intact motor nerve fibre (efferent); (4) the neuromuscular junction; and (5) a competent muscle.

Cranial nerves are formed by lower motor neurons that enter and exit directly from the brain rather than the spinal cord (Figure 12.10). Cranial nerves I and II extend from the cerebrum; cranial nerves III–XII extend from the lower diencephalon and brainstem. The 12 pairs of cranial nerves supply primarily the head and neck, except the vagus nerve (Lat. *vagus* or wanderer, as in 'vagabond') that, apart from supplying some sensory (tympanic membrane, external auditory canal, external ear and pharynx) and motor function (muscles of the palate, pharynx and larynx) in the head and neck, also travels to the heart, respiratory muscles, stomach and gall bladder.

SPINAL NERVES

The 31 pairs of spinal nerves arise from the length of the spinal cord and supply the rest of the body. They are named for the region of the spine from which they exit: eight cervical, twelve thoracic, five lumbar, five sacral and one coccygeal. They are 'mixed' nerves because they contain both sensory and motor fibres. The nerves enter and exit the cord through roots—sensory afferent fibres through the posterior or dorsal roots and motor efferent fibres through the anterior or ventral roots.

The nerves exit the spinal cord in an orderly ladder. Each nerve innervates a particular segment of the body. **Dermal segmentation** is the cutaneous distribution of the various spinal nerves.

A **dermatome** is a circumscribed skin area that is supplied mainly from one spinal cord segment through a particular spinal nerve (Figure 12.11). The dermatomes overlap, which is a form of biological insurance. That is, if one nerve is severed, most of the sensations can be transmitted by the one above and the one below. Do not attempt to memorise all dermatome segments; just focus on the following as useful landmarks:

- The **thumb**, **middle finger** and **fifth finger** are each in the dermatomes of **C6**, **C7** and **C8**.
- The **axilla** is at the level of **T1**.
- The **nipple** is at the level of **T4**.
- The **umbilicus** is at the level of **T10**.
- The **groin** is in the region of **L1**.
- The **knee** is at the level of **L4**.

Somatic and autonomic nervous system

The PNS is composed of cranial nerves and spinal nerves. These nerves carry fibres that can be divided functionally into two parts—somatic and autonomic. The somatic fibres innervate the skeletal (voluntary) muscles; the autonomic fibres innervate smooth (involuntary) muscles, cardiac muscle and glands. The autonomic system mediates

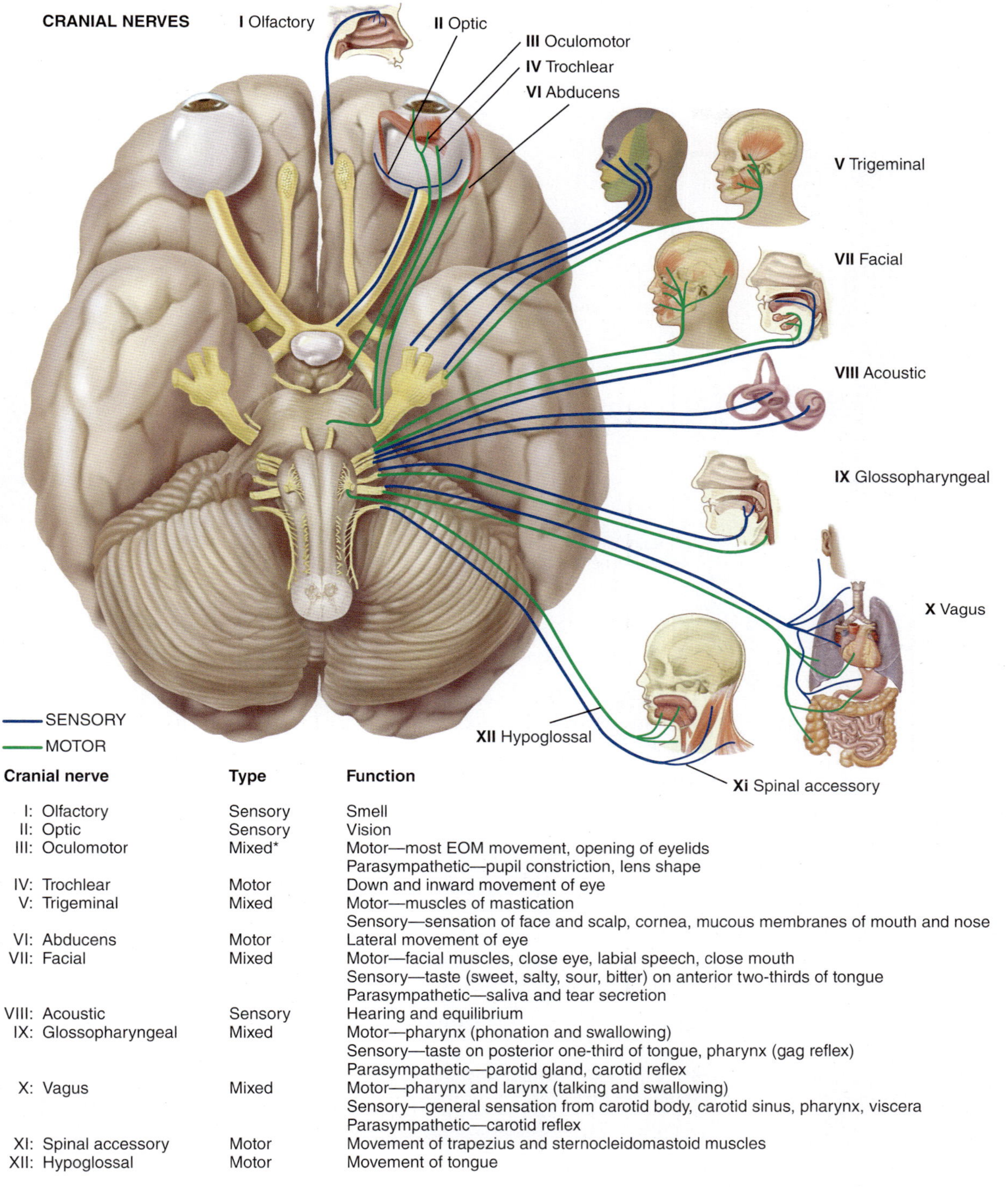

Cranial nerve	Type	Function
I: Olfactory	Sensory	Smell
II: Optic	Sensory	Vision
III: Oculomotor	Mixed*	Motor—most EOM movement, opening of eyelids Parasympathetic—pupil constriction, lens shape
IV: Trochlear	Motor	Down and inward movement of eye
V: Trigeminal	Mixed	Motor—muscles of mastication Sensory—sensation of face and scalp, cornea, mucous membranes of mouth and nose
VI: Abducens	Motor	Lateral movement of eye
VII: Facial	Mixed	Motor—facial muscles, close eye, labial speech, close mouth Sensory—taste (sweet, salty, sour, bitter) on anterior two-thirds of tongue Parasympathetic—saliva and tear secretion
VIII: Acoustic	Sensory	Hearing and equilibrium
IX: Glossopharyngeal	Mixed	Motor—pharynx (phonation and swallowing) Sensory—taste on posterior one-third of tongue, pharynx (gag reflex) Parasympathetic—parotid gland, carotid reflex
X: Vagus	Mixed	Motor—pharynx and larynx (talking and swallowing) Sensory—general sensation from carotid body, carotid sinus, pharynx, viscera Parasympathetic—carotid reflex
XI: Spinal accessory	Motor	Movement of trapezius and sternocleidomastoid muscles
XII: Hypoglossal	Motor	Movement of tongue

**Mixed* refers to a nerve carrying a combination of fibres: motor + sensory; motor + parasympathetic; or motor + sensory + parasympathetic.

FIGURE 12.10 Cranial nerves

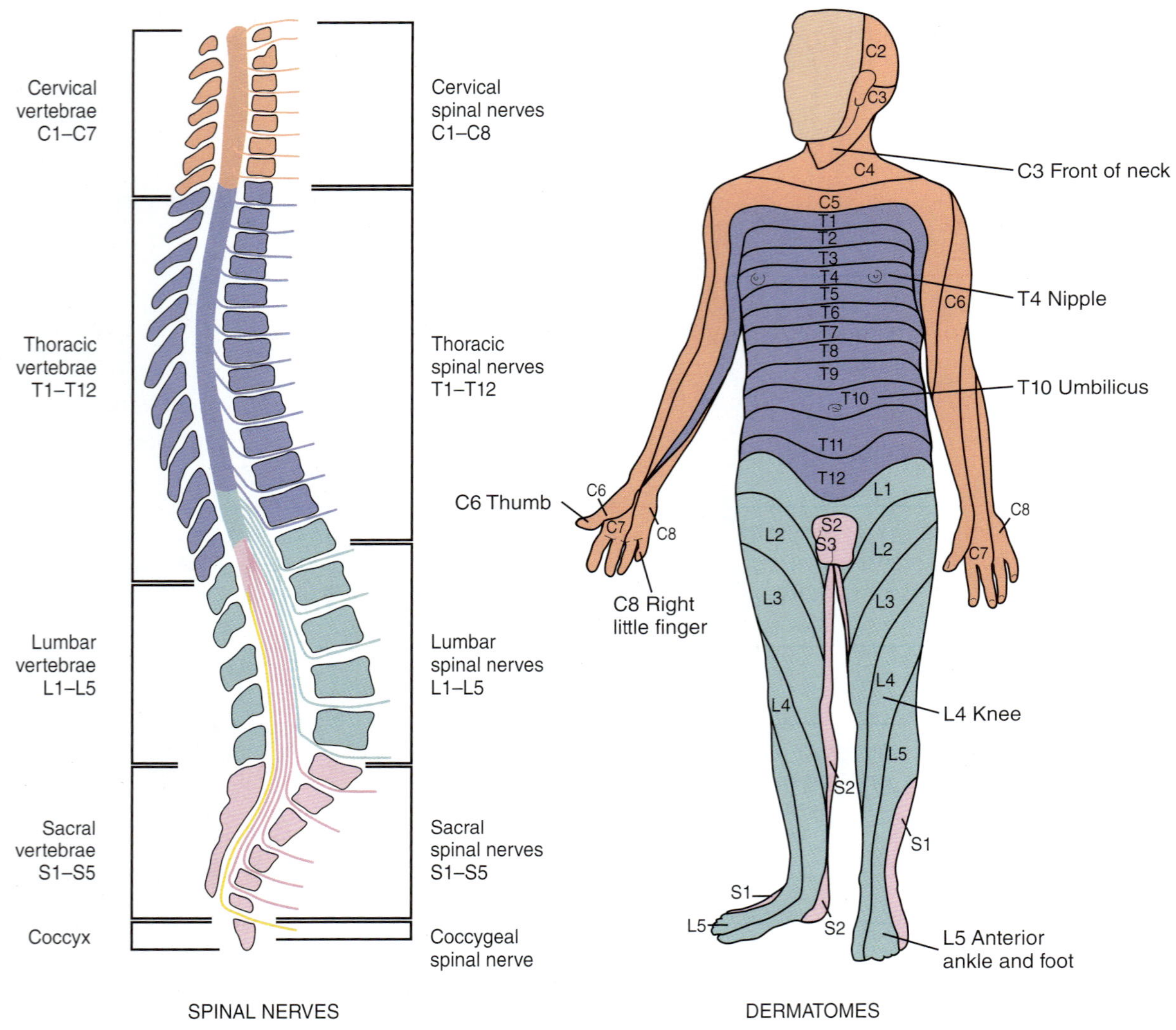

FIGURE 12.11 Spinal nerves dermatomes

unconscious activity. Although a description of the autonomic system is beyond the scope of this book, its overall function is to maintain homeostasis of the body.

Developmental considerations

Infants and children

The bones of the neonatal skull are separated by sutures and by **fontanels**, the spaces where the sutures intersect (Figure 12.12). These membrane-covered 'soft spots' allow for growth of the brain during the first year. They gradually ossify; the triangle-shaped posterior fontanel is closed by 1 to 2 months and the diamond-shaped anterior fontanel closes between 9 months and 2 years.

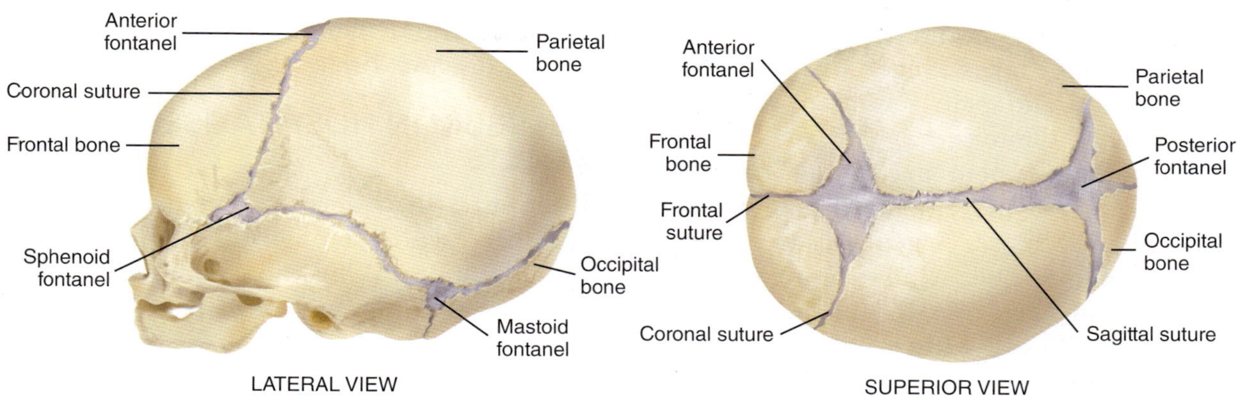

FIGURE 12.12 Bones of the neonatal skull

During the fetal period, head growth predominates. Head size is greater than chest circumference at birth. The head size grows during childhood, reaching 90% of its final size when the child is 6 years old. But during infancy, trunk growth predominates so that head size changes in proportion to body height. Facial bones grow at varying rates, especially nasal and jaw bones. In toddlers, the mandible and maxilla are small, and the nasal bridge is low so the whole face seems small compared with the skull.

The infant's sensory and motor development proceeds along with the gradual acquisition of myelin because myelin is needed to conduct most impulses. The process of myelinisation follows a cephalocaudal and proximodistal order (head, neck, trunk and extremities). This is just the order we observe the infant gaining motor control (lifts head, lifts head and shoulders, rolls over, moves whole arm, uses hands, walks). As the milestones are achieved, each is more complex and coordinated. Milestones occur in an orderly sequence, although the exact age of occurrence may vary.

The ability to localise sensation is also rudimentary at birth. Newborns need a strong stimulus and then respond by crying and with whole body movements. As myelinisation develops, the infant can localise the stimulus more precisely and make a more accurate motor response.

Late adulthood (65+ years)

As a person ages, the facial bones and orbits may appear more prominent, and the facial skin sags because of decreased elasticity, decreased subcutaneous fat and decreased moisture in the skin. The normal ageing process causes neurons to undergo changes that make them more vulnerable to degeneration,[1] leading to a steady loss of neurons in the brain and spinal cord. The loss of neurons causes a decrease in weight and volume of the brain. Neuron loss leads many older people to show signs that, in a younger adult, would be considered abnormal, such as general loss of muscle bulk, loss of muscle tone in the face, in the neck and around the spine, decreased muscle strength, impaired fine coordination and agility, loss of vibratory sense at the ankle, decreased or absent Achilles reflex, loss of position sense at the big toe, pupillary miosis, irregular pupil shape and decreased pupillary reflexes.

The velocity of nerve conduction decreases between 5 and 10% with ageing, making the reaction time slower in some older people.

An increased delay at the synapse also occurs, so the impulse takes longer to travel. As a result, touch and pain sensation, taste and smell may be diminished.

The motor system may show a general slowing down of movement. Muscle strength and agility decrease. A generalised decrease occurs in muscle bulk, which is most apparent in the dorsal hand muscles. In the older-old (75–84 years) and oldest old (85+ years) muscle tremors may occur in the hands, head and jaw, along with possible repetitive facial grimacing (dyskinesias).

Ageing is accompanied by a progressive decrease in cerebral blood flow and oxygen consumption. In some people this causes dizziness and a loss of balance with position change, which needs to be considered—for example, when standing from a sitting position. When they are in good health, older people walk about as well as they did during their middle and younger years, but they tend to have slower and more deliberate movements.

ALZHEIMER'S DISEASE AND OTHER DEMENTIAS

Dementia is the term used to describe the symptoms of a large group of illnesses that cause a progressive decline in a person's functioning. It is a broad term used to describe a loss of memory, intellect, rationality, social skills and physical functioning. There are many types of dementia, including Alzheimer's disease, vascular dementia and Lewy body disease. Dementia is the second leading cause of death of Australians (and the leading cause of death among Australian females). It is also the leading cause of disability for older Australians (over age 65) and the third leading cause of disability burden overall. In 2019 there were approximately 447,115 Australians living with dementia and more 1.5 million Australians involved in the care of someone with dementia.[2] Currently, there is no cure for the disease (Table 12.2).

DELIRIUM IN HOSPITALISED OLDER ADULTS

Delirium is an acute alteration in mental state associated with acute illness, surgery, trauma or medications. While more common in older patients, delirium can affect patients of any age and is especially prevalent in critical care, palliative care and residential aged-care settings. There are several predisposing (baseline) or precipitating (contributing) factors that increase the risk of a patient developing delirium, including age, sensory impairment, infection, urinary catheterisation and hip fracture among others.[3] Delirium is associated with poor short-term and long-term outcomes including increased length of stay, risk of falls, developing dementia and death, and so care focused on prevention, early diagnosis and appropriate management of delirium is essential (including addressing any reversible causes and providing interventions to reduce the incidence, severity and duration of delirium). However, studies show that only 12 to 35% of delirium cases are recognised. This is perhaps partly because historically the condition has been variably described and there was not a well-defined criterion for diagnosis, but also because delirium is associated with many complex underlying medical conditions and can be hard to recognise.[4]

In recent years there have been significant advances in the recognition and management of delirium in Australia. The Australian Commission on Safety and Quality in Health Care identifies a range of assessment tools that can be used to assess for delirium, including the Confusion Assessment Method (CAM), Confusion Assessment Method ICU (CAM-ICU), Delirium Observation Screening (DOS) scales and the 4AT Assessment test for delirium and cognitive impairment.[3] The current Diagnostic Statistical Manual of Mental Disorders (DSM-5) requires all the following criteria to be present for delirium to be diagnosed:[5]

- disturbance in attention and awareness
- disturbance develops acutely and tends to fluctuate in severity
- at least one additional disturbance in cognition
- disturbances are not better explained by a pre-existing dementia
- disturbances do not occur in the context of a severely reduced level of arousal or coma
- evidence of an underlying organic cause or causes.

See Chapter 11 and Chapter 30 for more information.

Cultural and social considerations

Many neurological health issues have profound impact on the person and their family. Some will be progressive and chronic (e.g. Parkinson's disease and multiple sclerosis); others have acute onset such as head or spinal cord injury or stroke. Many people will have ongoing cognitive and functional difficulties that will affect their ability to live a full and active life.

Stroke is a serious health problem in the Australian and Aotearoa New Zealand community. Stroke occurs when an artery supplying blood to the brain either suddenly becomes blocked or begins to bleed.

Stroke has a high prevalence and incidence and is a leading cause of death and disability worldwide. The prevalence of stroke is higher in Australian males (1.6%) than females (1.1%). Australians living in regional areas are up to 17% more likely to suffer a stroke than those living in metropolitan areas.[6] The incidence of stroke among Australia's Aboriginal and Torres Strait Islander population is reported to be between 1.7 and 3.0 times as high as the non-Indigenous population.[6] The incidence of new stroke in Australia equates to one stroke every 19 minutes[6] and one every 55 minutes in Aotearoa New Zealand, where stroke is the second biggest cause of mortality.[7]

Stroke is more common in older age groups; 71% of people who had a stroke were aged 65 years or older.[8] However, stroke is not just a disease of older people; young people are also at risk. While the median age for stroke in Australia is around 75 years, one in every four strokes occurs in a person aged 54 or younger.[6] Compared with older people, young people with stroke tend to take longer to seek medical attention, are less likely to receive rehabilitation and have more unmet needs in relation to psychosocial functioning and return to work. Though there is a lack of solid local trend evidence, rates of stroke in young people are increasing worldwide due to an increase in modifiable risk factors such as obesity, hypertension and diabetes.

Stroke is largely a preventable health problem with modifiable risk factors such as high blood pressure, atrial fibrillation, hyperlipidaemia and smoking.[9] It is the high prevalence of these risk factors in Aboriginal and Torres Strait Islander people and Māori and Pacific Islander people that accounts for the high incidence of stroke in these groups.[7] For further discussion of stroke risk factors, symptoms and prevention see the 'Health education' section (and Table 12.3).

HEALTH EDUCATION

Stroke prevention

Stroke is a leading cause of long-term disability and death. A stroke occurs when the blood flow is interrupted to a part of the brain. The most common type is an ischaemic stroke, occurring when a blood clot blocks a blood vessel in the brain. Less common is a haemorrhagic stroke, which occurs when a blood vessel in the brain ruptures and causes bleeding.

Symptoms

The symptoms and after-effects of a stroke depend on which area of the brain is affected and to what extent. This can make a stroke difficult to diagnose. However, early recognition of symptoms and prompt treatment are essential.

The **most common** symptoms of stroke include sudden:

- weakness or numbness in the face, arms or legs, especially when it is on one side of the body
- confusion, trouble speaking or understanding speech
- changes in vision, such as blurry vision or partial or complete loss of vision in one or both eyes
- trouble walking, dizziness and/or loss of balance or coordination
- severe headache with no reason or explanation.

Less common symptoms of stroke include:

- sudden nausea and/or vomiting
- brief loss of consciousness, including fainting.

Stroke symptoms usually do not cause pain, which is why many people ignore them or delay seeking medical attention. Sometimes, people can have a 'mini-stroke' or transient ischaemic attack (TIA). In these cases, the stroke symptoms last only temporarily and then disappear, often within an hour. Because the symptoms 'go away', people too often do not report them or seek medical attention. However, a TIA is a warning sign that should not be ignored. When people experience chest pain, they seek medical attention, to rule out a heart attack. Having a TIA should also prompt people to seek medical attention to rule out the possibility of a future stroke.

The Stroke Foundation Australia[10] has devised an easy-to-remember acronym to assist the public in recognising the signs and symptoms of stroke quickly and calling for an ambulance. The acronym is FAST:

- **F**ace—Check the person's face—has their mouth drooped?
- **A**rm—Can they lift both arms?
- **S**peech—Is their speech slurred? Do they understand you?
- **T**ime is critical—if you see any of these signs call the emergency number (Triple Zero [000] in Australia; 111 in Aotearoa New Zealand).

Stroke can strike anyone without warning. People need to be aware of their stroke risk and take steps to change the risk factors they can control.

Modifiable risk factors for stroke include:

- history of cardiovascular disease including hypertension, atrial fibrillation, dyslipidaemia and asymptomatic carotid stenosis
- cigarette smoking
- type 1 and type 2 diabetes
- sickle cell disease
- postmenopausal hormone therapy
- diet and nutrition
- physical inactivity
- obesity.

Non-modifiable risk factors for stroke include:[11]

- age
- gender—strokes are generally more prevalent in men than in women; however, exceptions are in 35- to 44-year-olds and those 85 years of age or older—groups in which women have slightly greater age-specific stroke incidence than do men
- low birthweight
- ethnicity—Aboriginal and Torres Strait Islander people have higher stroke incidence and mortality rates than other Australians
- genetic factor disorders (e.g. Marfan's syndrome, Fabry's disease, cerebral autosomal dominant arteriopathy with sub-cortical infarcts and leucoencephalopathy (CADASIL)).

Non-modifiable risk factors for stroke may help to identify those who, in conjunction with well-documented modifiable risks, are at highest risk of stroke and who may benefit from more rigorous treatment of modifiable risk factors.

HEALTH EDUCATION cont'd

Nurse's role

- Assess the person's health literacy and readiness to learn about stroke prevention.
- Teach the signs of stroke using the FAST acronym.
- Encourage adoption of a healthy lifestyle such as not smoking, eating a healthy diet, drinking alcohol in moderation, exercising daily and losing weight where necessary.
- Provide information in ways that is understandable and timely and with the appropriate amount of content.
- Encourage those at risk to take preventive medications (e.g. lipid-lowering, anticoagulant and antihypertensive drugs).[12]

Subjective data

Practice note

Before you start the assessment, introduce yourself to the person, confirm the person's identity, discuss the purpose and scope of the assessment, clarify any questions the person may have and get verbal consent from the person to perform the assessment.

ASSESSMENT GUIDELINES	CLINICAL SIGNIFICANCE AND CLINICAL ALERTS
Presenting concern	
• *Do you have any problems concerning your ability to think, your memory, hearing, vision, sensation or with movement and coordination?* It is important to ascertain the person's perception of their presenting health concern. If they do perceive a problem, ask: *How does this affect your quality of life?*	
Headache	
• *Have you experienced any unusually frequent or severe headaches?* • *When did this start? How often does this occur? Gradual, over hours or a day? Or, suddenly, over minutes or less than 1 hour?* • *Have you ever had this kind of headache before?* • *Where in your head do you feel the headaches? In the front, side, over the temple area, behind your eyes, like a band around the head, in the sinus area or in the back of the head?* • *Do the headaches seem to be associated with anything?*	***Clinical alert:*** If a person reports any sudden onset of headache of increasing severity, they should be referred to a medical practitioner for urgent further assessment. For location, character, duration, timing triggers of headaches, see Table 12.4.

ASSESSMENT GUIDELINES	CLINICAL SIGNIFICANCE AND CLINICAL ALERTS
• *Is the headache localised on one side or all over?*	Unilateral or bilateral (e.g. with cluster headaches pain is always unilateral and always on the same side of the head).
• *Can you describe the character (how the headache feels)? Throbbing (pounding, shooting) or aching (vice-like, constant pressure, dull)?*	Character is typically vice-like with tension headache, throbbing with migraine or temporal arteritis.
• *Is it mild, moderate or severe?*	Quality—often severe with migraine or excruciating with cluster headache.
Course and duration • *What time of day do the headaches occur: morning, evening, awaken you from sleep?* • *How long do they last? Hours, days?* • *Have you noted any daily headaches or several within a time period?*	Migraines occur about two per month, each lasting 1 to 3 days; one to two cluster headaches occur per day, each lasting 30 minutes to 2 hours for 1 or 2 months; then complete remission may last for months or years.
Precipitating factors • *Is there anything that brings it on: activity or exercise, work environment, emotional upset, anxiety, alcohol?*	Alcohol ingestion and daytime napping typically precipitate cluster headaches, whereas alcohol, let down after stress, menstruation and eating chocolate or cheese may precipitate migraines.
Associated factors • *Is there any relation to other symptoms: any nausea and vomiting?* (Note which came first: headache or nausea.) • *Any vision changes, pain with bright lights, neck pain or stiffness, fever, weakness, moodiness, stomach problems?*	Nausea, vomiting and visual disturbances are associated with migraines; eye reddening and tearing, eyelid drooping, **rhinorrhoea** (runny nose) and nasal congestion are associated with cluster headaches; anxiety and stress are associated with tension headaches; neck rigidity and fever are associated with **meningitis** or **encephalitis** (brain inflammation disorders).
• *Do you have any other illness?*	**Hypertension**, **fever**, **hypothyroidism** and **vasculitis** produce headaches.
• *Is there anything that makes it worse: movement, coughing, straining, exercise?*	
• *Is there any family history of headache?*	Migraines are associated with family history of migraine.
• *What is the frequency of your headaches: once a week? Are your headaches occurring more frequently?* • *Are they getting worse? Or are they getting better?* • (For females) *When do they occur in relation to your menstrual periods?*	
Relieving factors • *What seems to help: going to sleep, medications, positions, rubbing the area?*	With migraines, people lie down to feel better, whereas with cluster headaches they need to move—even to pace the floor—to feel better.

ASSESSMENT GUIDELINES	CLINICAL SIGNIFICANCE AND CLINICAL ALERTS
Coping strategies • *How have these headaches affected your self-care or your ability to function at work, home and socially?*	
Neck pain	
• *Have you experienced any neck pain?*	
Onset • *How did the pain start: injury, car accident, after lifting, from a fall? Or with a fever? Or did it have a gradual onset?*	Acute onset of stiffness with headache and fever occurs with meningeal inflammation.
Location • *Does the pain radiate? To the shoulders, arms?*	
Associated symptoms • *Do you have any limitations to range of motion, numbness or tingling in shoulders, arms or hands?*	
Precipitating factors • *What movements cause pain? Do you need to lift or bend at work or home?* • *Does stress seem to bring it on?*	
Coping strategies • *Are you able to do your work, to sleep?*	Pain creates a vicious circle. Tension increases pain and disability, which produces more anxiety.
Other pain	
• *Do you have any pain in any other part of the body?* • Intensity (using a numerical rating scale): *How would you rate your pain at the moment? At its worst, it is ... what? At its best, it is ... what?* • Quality: *Is it dull, sharp pressure, burning?* • Onset/duration: *When does it occur and for how long?* • Relief of pain: *Do you use medication or other strategies for relief of pain?* • Effect of pain: *How does the pain affect your work, any functional limitations, emotional status, concentration, appetite and relationship with others?*	Refer to Chapter 13 for discussion of pain assessment.

ASSESSMENT GUIDELINES	CLINICAL SIGNIFICANCE AND CLINICAL ALERTS
Head injury	
• *Have you ever had any head injury? Or have you sought health care because of a head injury? Please describe.* • *How did this occur?* (Describe the mechanism.) *Can you show me where on your head the injury occurred?* • *Did you have a loss of consciousness? For how long?* • *Were there any other effects such as nausea, vomiting, drowsiness, amnesia or confusion?*	In some circumstances you might be obtaining this information from another person if the person is unable to respond or remember. While non-specific, any report of the following symptoms should prompt consideration of the diagnosis of concussion and warrants further investigation and follow-up: • **somatic** (e.g. headache), cognitive (e.g. feeling like in a fog) and/or emotional symptoms (e.g. lability) • **physical signs** (e.g. loss of consciousness, amnesia, neurological deficit) • **balance impairment** (e.g. gait unsteadiness) • behavioural changes (e.g. irritability) • **cognitive impairment** (e.g. slowed reaction times) • **sleep–wake disturbance** (e.g. somnolence, drowsiness). ***Clinical alert:*** Any change in conscious state should be referred to the responsible medical or nurse practitioner. The presence of nausea, vomiting, drowsiness or confusion can indicate rising intracranial pressure. Urgently refer the person to the responsible medical or nurse practitioner for further assessment.
Dizziness/vertigo	
• *Do you ever feel lightheaded, experience a swimming sensation or feel faint?* • *When have you noticed this? How often does it occur? Does it occur with activity, change in position?*	**Dizziness:** Often described as a period of light-headedness and may be associated with a drop in blood pressure. **Syncope:** Sudden loss of strength, a temporary loss of consciousness (a faint) due to lack of cerebral blood flow such as low blood pressure.
• *Do you ever feel a sensation called vertigo, a rotational spinning sensation? Do you feel as if the room is spinning or that your head is spinning? Did this come on suddenly or gradually?*	People often find it difficult to discriminate between dizziness and vertigo. **Vertigo** is a sense of rotational spinning caused by neurological disease in the vestibular apparatus in the ear or in the vestibular nuclei in the brainstem.
Seizures	
• *Have you ever had any seizures (sometimes referred to as convulsions or fits)? When did they start? How often do they occur?*	**Seizures** occur with **epilepsy**, a paroxysmal disease characterised by altered or loss of consciousness, involuntary muscle movements and sensory disturbances. However, an isolated seizure does not mean the person has epilepsy.

ASSESSMENT GUIDELINES	CLINICAL SIGNIFICANCE AND CLINICAL ALERTS
Course and duration • *When a seizure starts, do you have any warning sign? What type of sign?* **Motor activity** • *Where in your body do the seizures begin? Do the seizures travel through your body? On one side or both? Does your muscle tone seem tense or limp?* **Associated signs** • *Have you noticed a colour change in the face or lips, loss of consciousness (for how long?), automatisms (eyelid fluttering, eye rolling, lip smacking, vocalisation), incontinence?* **Postictal (phase—after the seizure)** • *Are you told you spend time sleeping? Do you have any confusion, weakness, headache or muscle ache?* **Precipitating factors** • *Does anything seem to bring on the seizures: activity, discontinuing medication, flashing lights, fatigue and stress?* • *Are you on any medication? If so, what is the medication?* **Coping strategies** • *How have the seizures affected daily life, occupation?*	**Aura** is a subjective sensation that precedes a seizure; it could be auditory, visual or motor.
Tremors and involuntary movements	
• *Do you ever experience shakes or tremors in the hands or face? When did these start?* • *Do they seem to grow worse with anxiety, intention or rest?* • *Are they relieved with rest, activity, alcohol? Do they affect daily activities?* • *Are you on any medication? If so, what is the medication?*	**Tremor** is an involuntary shaking, vibrating or trembling. Often people will not report shakes or tremors without being directly asked about them. However, these may be signs that you observe during an assessment. You can use these questions to explore this observation. See Table 12.5 for more information.
Weakness	
• *Do you experience any weakness or problem moving any part of the body?* • *Is this generalised or local?* • *Does weakness occur with any movement?* (e.g. with proximal or large muscle weakness, it may be hard to get up out of a chair or reach for an object; with distal or small muscle weakness, it is hard to open a jar, write, use scissors or walk without tripping) • *Is there a fatiguable element? In other words, does the weakness get worse with repeated actions or is it worst at the end of the day?*	**Paresis** is a partial or incomplete paralysis. **Paralysis** is a loss of motor function due to a lesion in the neurological or muscular system or loss of sensory innervation (Tables 12.5 and 12.6).

ASSESSMENT GUIDELINES	CLINICAL SIGNIFICANCE AND CLINICAL ALERTS
Lack of coordination	
• *Do you experience any problems with coordination?* • *Any problems with balance when walking?* • *Do you lean to one side?* • *Any falling?* • *Which way?* • *Do your legs seem to give way?* • *Any clumsy movement?*	**Dysmetria** is the inability to control the range of motion of muscles.
Numbness or tingling	
• *Do you have any numbness or tingling in any part of the body?* • *Does it feel like pins and needles?* • *When did this start?* • *Where do you feel it?* • *Does it occur with activity?*	**Paraesthesia** is an abnormal sensation such as burning or tingling. ***Clinical alert:*** If the person is experiencing dizziness, tremor, paralysis, lack of coordination or paraesthesia, report to a medical or nurse practitioner. Note there will be an impact of these symptoms on the person's ability to manage activities of daily living.
Visual disturbances and deafness	
• *Have you experienced any periods of visual disturbances—double vision **(diplopia)**, blurred vision **(amblyopia)**, light intolerance **(photophobia)**—or visual loss?* • *When did this occur? In one eye or both eyes?* • *Sudden or gradual onset?* • *How long did it last?* • *What did you do about it?* See Chapter 14 for further assessment of vision. • *Have you experienced any periods of deafness or changes in your hearing (such as ringing sound)?* • *When did this occur?* • *Was it on one side or both?* • *Sudden or gradual onset?* • *How long did it last?* • *Have you been exposed to loud noise in your workplace or recreationally?* • *What did you do about it?* See Chapter 15 for further assessment of hearing.	***Clinical alert:*** Visual disturbances can be signs of a problem within the eye or symptoms of other neurological health issues. A person with a sudden change in vision should be referred for urgent medical assessment. **Unilateral deafness** is likely to be the result of a nerve lesion (e.g. acoustic neuroma or trauma). The person should be referred for an assessment by a medical practitioner.[9]
Difficulty swallowing (dysphagia)	
• *Have you experienced a problem with swallowing?* • *Does this occur with solids or liquids?* • *Have you experienced excessive saliva, drooling?*	***Dysphagia*** is difficulty with swallowing. See Chapter 21 for further discussion of swallow assessment.  ***Clinical alert:*** Difficulty with swallowing can pose serious risk to a person's airway and requires further detailed assessment. Report to a medical or nurse practitioner.

ASSESSMENT GUIDELINES	CLINICAL SIGNIFICANCE AND CLINICAL ALERTS
Difficulty speaking	
• *Have you experienced any problem speaking—for example, with forming words or with saying what you intended to say?* • *When did you first notice this?* • *How long did it last?*	**Dysarthria** is difficulty forming words. **Dysphasia** is difficulty with language comprehension or expression (Table 12.7).
Relevant health and family history	
• *Have you or a family member ever been diagnosed with a stroke, head injury, spinal cord injury, hypertension, meningitis or encephalitis, mental health problems, neurological or degenerative neurological conditions?*	
Health and lifestyle management	
• Ask about current medications. • Ask about smoking history (predisposition to cerebrovascular disease), alcohol use and illegal drug use.	Many common medications can cause neurological symptoms. For example, antipsychotic medications can have the side effect of sedation, parkinsonian tremor and ataxia; antihypertensive drugs can cause postural dizziness and fainting.[9]
Environmental/occupational hazards	
• *Are you exposed to any environmental/occupational hazards—for example, pesticides, organic solvents, lead, excessively loud noise?*	
Additional history for infants and children	
Pregnancy • *Did you* (the mother) *have any health problems during the pregnancy—for example, any infections or illnesses, medications taken, preeclampsia, hypertension, alcohol or drug use, type 1 and type 2 diabetes?* • Also ask the parent whether the infant or child has undergone regular assessment with a maternal and child health nurse.	Prenatal history may affect infant's neurological development.
Birth • *Please tell me about this baby's birth. Was the baby at term or premature? Birthweight?* • *Any birth trauma? Did the baby breathe immediately?* • *Were you told the baby's Apgar scores?* • *Any congenital defects?*	**Apgar** is a test performed on a newborn at 1 minute and 5 minutes after delivery to see how well the baby tolerated the birthing process. Aspects assessed are breathing effort, heart rate, muscle tone, reflexes and skin colour. Each category is scored as 0, 1 or 2. A score of 7–10 is normal.

ASSESSMENT GUIDELINES	CLINICAL SIGNIFICANCE AND CLINICAL ALERTS
Reflexes • *What have you noticed about the baby's behaviour?* • *Does the baby's sucking and swallowing seem coordinated?* • *When you touch the cheek, does the baby turn their head towards the touch?* • *Does the baby startle with a loud noise or shake of crib? Does the baby grasp your finger?*	
Balance • *Does the child seem to have any problem with balance?* • *Have you noted any unexplained falling, clumsy or unsteady gait, progressive muscular weakness, problem with going up or down stairs, problem with getting up from lying position?*	If occurs, may not be noticed until starts to walk in late infancy.
Seizures • *Has this child had any seizures? Please describe.* • *Did the seizure occur with a high fever?* • *Was there any loss of consciousness—how long?* • *How many seizures occurred with this same illness (if occurred with high fever)?*	Seizures may occur with high fever in infants and toddlers. Or seizures may be a sign of neurological disease.
Developmental milestones • *Did this child's motor or developmental milestones seem to come at about the right age?* • *Does this child seem to be growing and maturing normally to you?* • *How does this child's development compare to siblings or to age mates?*	
Environmental exposure • *Do you know if your child has had any environmental exposure to lead?*	Chronically elevated lead levels may cause a developmental delay, a loss of a newly acquired skill or no clinical signs may be present.
Learning difficulties • *Have you been told about any learning problems in school: any problems with attention span, cannot concentrate, hyperactive?*	
Family history • *Does the child or any other family member have a seizure disorder, cerebral palsy or muscular dystrophy?*	See Table 12.8.

ASSESSMENT GUIDELINES	CLINICAL SIGNIFICANCE AND CLINICAL ALERTS
Additional history for adults over 65 years	
Dizziness • *Do you experience any problem with dizziness?* • *Does this occur when you first sit or stand up, when you move your head, when you get up and walk just after eating?* • *Does this occur with any of your medications?*	Diminished cerebral blood flow and diminished vestibular response may produce staggering with position change, which increases risk of falls.
• *Do you ever get up at night and then feel faint while standing to urinate* (for men)? • *How does dizziness affect your daily activities?* • *Are you able to drive safely and to manoeuvre within your house safely?* • *What safety modifications have you applied at home?*	Micturition syncope is a temporary loss of consciousness while urinating and is thought to be caused by a sudden positional drop in blood pressure.
Memory • *Have you noticed any decrease in memory, change in mental function?* • *Have you felt any sense of confusion? Did this seem to come on suddenly or gradually?* • *Has a family member expressed concern about your memory or ability to make decisions?*	
Tremor • *Have you ever noticed any tremor? Is this in your hands or face?* • *Is this worse with anxiety, activity or rest?* • *Does the tremor seem to be relieved with alcohol, activity or rest?* • *Does the tremor interfere with daily or social activities?*	Tremor is relieved by alcohol, although this is not a recommended treatment. Assess if the person is abusing alcohol to relieve tremor.
Visual changes • *Have you ever had any sudden vision change or fleeting blindness?* • *Did this occur along with weakness? Did you have any loss of consciousness?* • Refer to Chapter 14 for further assessment of vision.	! ***Clinical alert:*** These symptoms can be characteristic of decreased blood flow to the brain and require more detailed medical investigation.
Hearing • *Have you ever had any sudden changes to your hearing?* Refer to Chapter 15 for further assessment of hearing.	

Objective data

You will recall from the beginning of this chapter that there are three main types of objective neurological assessments—ongoing neurological observations, a screening assessment and a complete assessment. The sequence for ongoing neurological observations and a screening assessment are described in the section below. In the event of a disorientated or uncooperative person, some parts of the assessment may need to be modified or omitted. You will also note that the initial stage of an objective neurological assessment shares many features with a mental health assessment.

Preparation

Outline the process for neurological assessment for the client and ask their consent for you to continue. On some occasions, it may be necessary to have a support person (usually another nurse) present during the examination. Ensure privacy by closing the door or pulling the screens. Adequate lighting is essential, as is the ability to reduce lighting when assessing the pupils.

People who have recent head trauma, neurological surgery, stroke or a neurological deficit due to a systemic disease process must be monitored closely for any improvement or deterioration in neurological status and for any indication of increasing intracranial pressure. Signs of increasing intracranial pressure signal impending cerebral disaster and potential death and require early and prompt intervention.

Equipment needed

Neurological observations chart
Penlight torch
Hand hygiene solution

PROCEDURES AND NORMAL FINDINGS	ABNORMAL FINDINGS AND CLINICAL ALERTS
Ongoing neurological observations and routine neurological screening assessment	
 A skills video (neurological assessment) is available to assist you in your skill development. Click on the QR code to access the video (instructions on the inside front cover of the book to access multimedia resources).	
General inspection	
When collecting subjective data, you will have noticed the condition of the person's skin, lips, hair and mucous membranes, as well as any breath odour, ease of breathing, body movements, height-to-weight ratio, body shape, posture, level of hygiene and grooming and general demeanour. All these factors provide clues to the person's neurological health. Neurological assessment begins as soon as you see the person. This enables the clinician to quickly determine the extent of the neurological assessment that is required.	

PROCEDURES AND NORMAL FINDINGS	ABNORMAL FINDINGS AND CLINICAL ALERTS
FAST	
FAST is an acronym devised to assist early recognition of signs of a stroke. • **F**ace—Check the person's face—has their mouth drooped? • **A**rm—Can they lift both arms? • **S**peech—Is their speech slurred? Do they understand you? • **T**ime is critical.	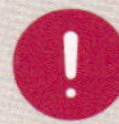 ***Clinical alert***: If these signs are positive, the person may be having a stroke, and they need urgent medical assessment.
Alertness	
• Do they appear to be aware of their surroundings? Are they conscious, unconscious or drowsy (in a stupor)?	This will enable the clinician to determine how to proceed with the neurological assessment.  ***Clinical alert:*** If any suspicion of change to conscious state the Glasgow Coma Scale should be conducted (Table 12.1).
Posture	
• Straight • Listing (leaning) to one side	Listing to one side may indicate a previous or current neurological condition (Table 12.9).
Dysmorphic features	
• Facial expressions (facies) • Skull shape and size • Skeleton, spine, hands and feet • Skin	Dysmorphic features may indicate underlying congenital neurological conditions and may require a complete neurological examination by a specialist practitioner (Table 12.10).
Hygiene and grooming	
• Cleanliness • Body odours • Appropriate dress for age and environment	The ability to care for oneself is often demonstrated in how we present ourselves. Although this may indicate underlying mental health concerns it may also indicate neurological disorder of the brain, in particular the frontal lobe.
Affect, attitude, mood	

• Behaviour: Are they acting appropriately to their current situation?
• Note speech
  • Volume (see Table 12.7 for common speech disorders)
  • Appropriateness
  • Incomprehensible
• Facial expressions
  • Grimacing
  • Contorting their face (Table 12.10)
  • Smiling
• Does what they convey relate to their facial expression?
• Do they appear relaxed?
• Can they make and maintain eye contact?
	The ability to interact with others may be inhibited by either neurological or mental health conditions.

PROCEDURES AND NORMAL FINDINGS	ABNORMAL FINDINGS AND CLINICAL ALERTS
Support aids	
• Glasses • Hearing aids • Walking stick • Communication board • Tracheostomy	Supports may determine to what extent the neurological examination can be performed.
General body movement (arms and legs)	
• Coordinated • Guarded • Uncoordinated	
Muscles	
• Bulk • Atrophy • Fasciculations	**Fasciculations:** Rapid, continuous twitching of resting muscle or part of muscle, without movement of limb, which can be seen or palpated may indicate underlying medical conditions which may affect the neurological assessment (Table 12.5).
Level of consciousness	
A *change* in the level of consciousness is the single most important factor in this assessment. A change can be subtle. Note the ease of arousal and state of awareness and orientation. A person is fully alert when: • their eyes are open or open spontaneously at your approach • they are oriented to person, place and time • they can follow verbal commands appropriately.	Note any decreasing level of consciousness, disorientation, memory loss, uncooperative behaviour or even complacency in a previously combative person. ! ***Clinical alert:*** If the person is not fully alert, increase the amount of stimulus used in this order: • light touch on person's arm • vigorous shake of shoulder • pain applied (pressure to nailbed, pinch trapezius muscle). Be careful not to inflict trauma/bruising on the person. ! ***Clinical alert:*** If the person is not responding, there is no point in repeatedly continuing to inflict pain. Note your findings and report any changes to a medical practitioner.
Assess orientation by asking questions about: • **person**—own name, occupation • **place**—where person is, nature of building, city, state • **time**—day of week, month, year.	! ***Clinical alert:*** If any sudden change in the person's orientation to person, place or time, complete a Glasgow Coma Scale score and then report the findings to a medical practitioner immediately.

PROCEDURES AND NORMAL FINDINGS	ABNORMAL FINDINGS AND CLINICAL ALERTS
Vary the questions during repeat assessments so the person is not merely memorising answers. Note the quality and the content of the verbal response—articulation, fluency, manner of thinking and any deficit in language comprehension or production (Chapter 7). If the person cannot speak, you will have to ask closed questions that require a nod or shake of the head: '*Are we in a hospital?*' '*Are you at home*?' '*Are we in (location/place)?*'	 ***Clinical alert:*** If the person cannot speak fluent English or if English is not their first language, you may need to get the assistance of a qualified interpreter to ensure accuracy in the assessment.
Using the Glasgow Coma Scale (ongoing neurological assessment)	
In addition to performing general inspection, level of consciousness, pupillary response, limb movement and strength and vital signs, you will also include use of the Glasgow Coma Scale as part of an ongoing neurological assessment (Table 12.1).	
The Glasgow Coma Scale[13] was developed as an accurate and reliable quantitative tool that assesses the functional state of the brain (Table 12.1). The Glasgow Coma Scale is a standardised, objective assessment that defines the level of consciousness by giving it a numeric value. This universal scale has good interrater reliability[14] and enhances interprofessional communication by providing a common language.[14] The scale is divided into three areas: • **eye opening** • **verbal response** • **motor response.** Each area is rated separately and a number is given for the person's best response. The three numbers are added: • The total score reflects the brain's functional level. • A fully alert, normal person has a score of 15, whereas **a score of 7 or less reflects coma.** • Serial assessments are plotted on a graph to illustrate visually whether the person is stable, improving or deteriorating.	Where possible, have one nurse conduct the assessments over a shift time frame. This will increase the reliability of the data over time. Before handing over to the next shift nurse, take the time to conduct the test together to increase the reliability of the data between the two nurses. • A score of 15 indicates normal consciousness. • A score of 7 indicates coma. • A score of 3 indicates a deep coma. 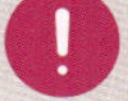 ***Clinical alert:*** Any downward trend (a change in score of 2 or more) in the Glasgow Coma Scale score should be **urgently** reported for medical review.

PROCEDURES AND NORMAL FINDINGS	ABNORMAL FINDINGS AND CLINICAL ALERTS

TABLE 12.1 Glasgow Coma Scale

GLASGOW COMA SCALE (GCS)			
(E) Eye opening – indicates the person's level of arousal	Open spontaneously	4	If the eyes are closed by swelling record as–C
	Open to sound or speech	3	
	Open to pressure or painful stimuli	2	
	None / no eye opening	1	
(V) Best verbal response – appropriateness of the person's speech	Orientated to time, place, person	5	If the person has a tracheostomy record as–T
	Confused	4	
	Inappropriate words	3	
	Incomprehensible sounds	2	
	Silent / no verbal response	1	
(M) Best motor response – awareness/ability to respond by movement	Obeys commands	6	Usually record the best arm response
	Localises to painful stimuli	5	
	Withdraws from painful stimuli	4	
	Abnormal flexion to painful stimuli (decorticate)	3	
	Abnormal extension to painful stimuli (decerebrate)	2	
	No motor response	1	
	Total GCS score/15 =		

Adapted from Mehta & Chinthapalli 2019[13] and Institute of Neurological Sciences 2015[15]

Eye opening

Best eye-opening response:

- Note the person's ability to open their eyes spontaneously.
- If the person does not open their eyes spontaneously, note whether they open their eyes to your request asking them to open their eyes (record if they open their eyes to speech).
- If they do not open their eyes to speech, apply painful stimuli as described above (start with light touch and increase as necessary).
- If they do not open their eyes to painful stimuli, record no response.

Verbal response

Best verbal response:

- Check the person's orientation to person, place, time (follow the instructions detailed above).
- Assess clarity and appropriateness of words/ speech or note if there is no verbal response.

If the person is unable to speak due to an endotracheal tube or tracheostomy tube, record this on the chart.

PROCEDURES AND NORMAL FINDINGS	ABNORMAL F NDINGS AND CLINICAL ALERTS
Motor response	
Best motor response: Ask the person, '*Can you wriggle your fingers (or toes)?*' • If the person can wriggle their fingers even faintly, they are scored as obeying commands. • This procedure also tests level of consciousness by noting the person's ability to follow commands. • If the person cannot obey your commands, you would then assess the person's best motor response to a painful stimulus. • For a person with decreased level of consciousness, movement may occur spontaneously and because of noxious stimuli such as airway suctioning.	Motor response is about the ability of the person to obey commands, not about muscular strength or coordination. In response to painful stimulus, if the person: • moves their hand above the nipple line, record '**localising to pain**' • moves their body away from the pain but does not localise, record '**withdraws from pain**' • bends their arm at the elbow, record '**flexion**' • extends their elbows and internally rotates their wrists, record '**extension to painful stimuli**'. If there is no physical response to painful stimulus, record '**no response**'.
Pupillary response	

• To test the **pupillary light reflex**, darken the room and ask the person to gaze into the distance. (This dilates the pupils.)
• Shine a fine light beam (from a penlight torch) in from the side and note the response. Normally you will observe:
  • constriction of the same-sided pupil (a direct light reflex)
  • simultaneous constriction of the other pupil (a consensual light reflex).
• Note the size, shape and symmetry of both pupils.
• Both pupils should constrict briskly. (Allow for the effects of any medication that could affect pupil size and reactivity.)
	Increasing intracranial pressure causes a sudden, unilateral, dilated and nonreactive pupil. **Cranial nerve III** runs parallel to the brainstem. When increasing intracranial pressure pushes the brainstem down (**brain herniation or 'coning'**), it puts pressure on cranial nerve III, causing pupil dilatation.
	Unequal, slowed response.
	
	! ***Clinical alert:*** Report changes in the pupil size immediately for urgent medical review. Continue to perform ongoing neurological observations.

In the acute care setting, gauge the pupil size in millimetres, both before and after the light reflex. Normally, the resting size is 3, 4 or 5 mm and decreases equally in response to light. This indicates that both pupils measure 3 mm in the resting state and that both constrict to 1 mm in response to light. A graduated scale printed on a handheld vision screener or taped onto a tongue blade facilitates your measurement.	! ***Clinical documentation***: Record the normal response to all these manoeuvres as PERRLA or **P**upils **E**qual, **R**ound, **R**eact to **L**ight and **A**ccommodation.

PROCEDURES AND NORMAL FINDINGS	ABNORMAL FINDINGS AND CLINICAL ALERTS

Pupil sizes in millimetres	
1 mm	
2 mm	
3 mm	
4 mm	
5 mm	
6 mm	
7 mm	
8 mm	

FIGURE 12.13 Pupil sizes

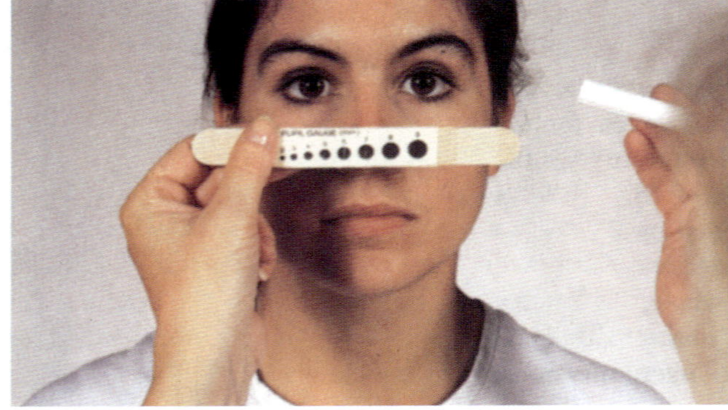

FIGURE 12.14 Measuring pupil sizes

Vital signs

Measure the temperature, pulse, respiration and blood pressure as often as the person's condition warrants. Vital signs should always be performed after a neurological assessment because the act of performing these activities may elicit a painful response to eye opening rather than to name.

Although they are vital to the overall assessment of a critically ill person, pulse and blood pressure are notoriously unreliable parameters of CNS deficit. Any changes are late consequences of rising intracranial pressure.

! ***Clinical alert:*** **The Cushing reflex** shows signs of increasing intracranial pressure: blood pressure—sudden elevation with widening pulse pressure; pulse—decreased rate, slow and bounding. **This is a medical emergency.**

Limb movement and strength

Upper extremities

- Check upper arm strength by checking hand grasps.
- Ask the person to squeeze your fingers. Offer your two fingers, one on top of the other, so that a strong hand grasp does not hurt your knuckles (Figure 12.15A, B and C).
- Begin by holding your fingers in a position that requires the person to raise their arms up and out to grasp your fingers.
- If they cannot reach their arms up and out, then move your fingers closer.
- Do not place fingers in the palm of the person's hand as some people with diffuse brain damage, especially frontal lobe injury, have a grasp that is a reflex only.

Unequal grasp.

! ***Clinical alert:*** Changes to limb movement, strength and/or balance can put the person at risk of falling and or being unable to perform activities of daily living. In such a situation a detailed assessment is required to be performed by a nurse or medical practitioner.

PROCEDURES AND NORMAL FINDINGS	ABNORMAL FINDINGS AND CLINICAL ALERTS

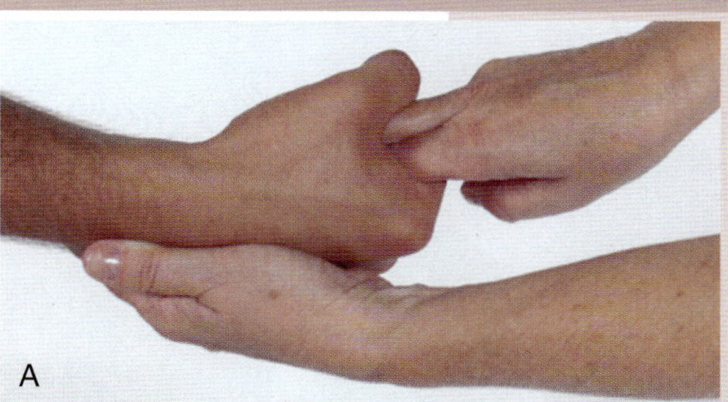

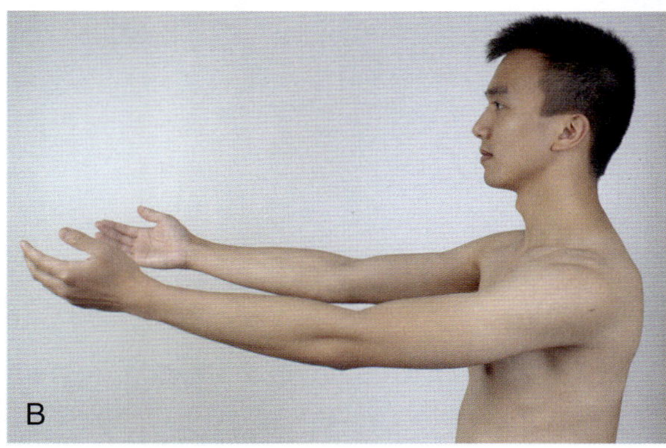

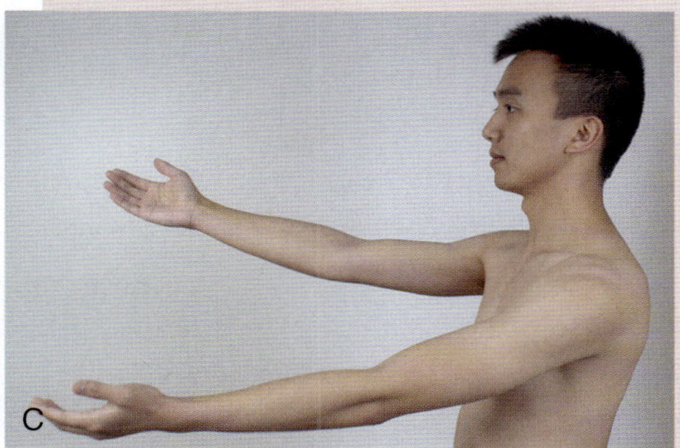

FIGURE 12.15 A, B and C Checking upper arm strength

- Alternatively, ask the person to lift each hand or to hold up one finger.
- You can also check upper extremity strength by palmar drift. Ask the person to extend both arms forwards or halfway up, palms up, eyes closed and hold for 10 to 20 seconds (Figures 12.15A, B and C).
- Normally, the arms stay steady with no downward drift.

Lower extremities

- Check lower extremities by asking the person to do straight leg raises.
- Ask the person to lift one leg at a time straight up off the bed (Figure 12.16A).
- Full strength allows the leg to be lifted 90 degrees. If multiple injuries, pain or equipment exclude this motion, ask the person to push one foot at a time against your hand's resistance, 'like putting your foot on the accelerator pedal of your car' (Figure 12.16B).

Unequal resistance.

Changes in motor function may indicate pathological conditions of the spinal cord or cerebral cortex.

Disorders of the neurological system may affect muscle tone and strength (Table 12.11).

PROCEDURES AND NORMAL FINDINGS	ABNORMAL FINDINGS AND CLINICAL ALERTS

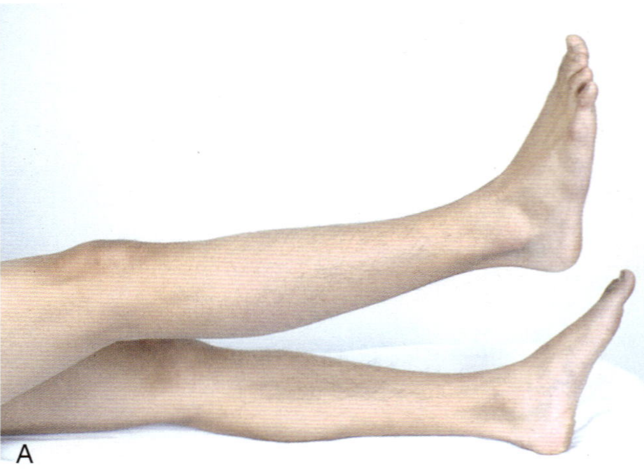

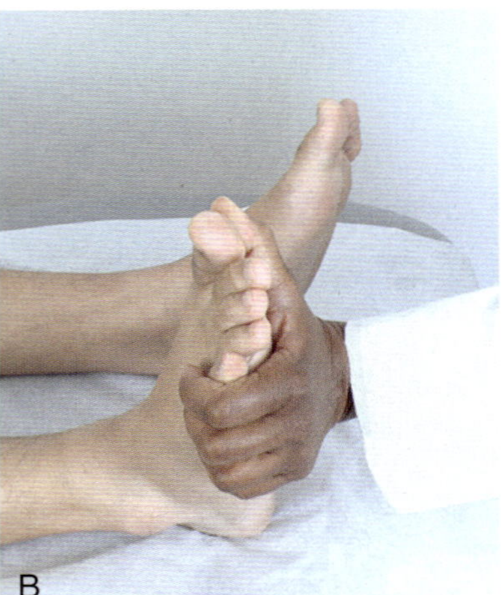

FIGURE 12.16 A and B Checking leg strength

Assessing delirium

For recognising delirium in hospitalised patients use one of the tools listed in the Clinical Care Standard.[3]

The Confusion Assessment Method tool requires the presence of features 1 and 2 and either 3 or 4 to diagnose delirium:[4]

1. Acute change in mental status with fluctuating course

   AND

2. Inattention

   AND EITHER

3. Disorganised thinking

   OR

4. Altered level of consciousness

A person suspected of being in delirium should be assessed (i.e. using a validated tool such as the Confusion Assessment Method) and closely monitored.

Measures should be taken to identify and, whenever possible, predict or eliminate potential contributing factors.

! ***Clinical alert:*** Escalating or fluctuating conscious state in delirium should be recognised as acute clinical deterioration and promptly reported to a treating medical practitioner.

See also Chapter 30.

Abnormal findings

TABLE 12.2 Warning signs of dementia

Sign	Explanation
Recent memory loss that affects job skills	• It is normal to forget meetings, colleagues' names or a business associate's telephone number occasionally but then remember them later. • A person with dementia may forget things more often and not remember them later.
Difficulty performing familiar tasks	• Busy people can be so distracted from time to time that they may leave the carrots on the stove and only remember to serve them when the meal has finished. • A person with dementia might prepare a meal and not only forget to serve it but also forget they made it.
Problems with language	• Everyone has trouble finding the right word sometimes. • A person with dementia may forget simple words or substitute inappropriate words.
Disorientation of time and place	• It is normal to forget the day of the week or your destination for a moment. • People with dementia can become lost on their own street, not know where they are, how they got there or how to get back home.
Poor or decreased judgement	• Dementia affects a person's memory and concentration and this in turn affects their judgement. Many activities, such as driving, require good judgement and when this ability is affected, the person will be a risk, not only to themselves but to others on the road.
Problems with abstract thinking	• Managing finances can be difficult for anyone. • Someone with dementia could forget completely what the numbers are and what needs to be done with them.
Misplacing things	• Anyone can temporarily misplace a wallet or keys. • A person with dementia may repeatedly put things in inappropriate places.
Changes in mood or behaviour	• Everyone becomes sad or moody from time to time. • Someone with dementia can have rapid mood swings from calm to tears to anger for no apparent reason.
Changes in personality	• People's personalities can change a little with age. • A person with dementia can become suspicious or fearful or just apathetic and uncommunicative. They may also become disinhibited, over-familiar or more outgoing than previously.
Loss of initiative	• It is normal to tire of housework, business activities or social obligations. • A person with dementia may become very passive and require cues prompting them to become involved.

Source: Dementia Australia 2023[2]

TABLE 12.3 Ischaemic and haemorrhagic stroke

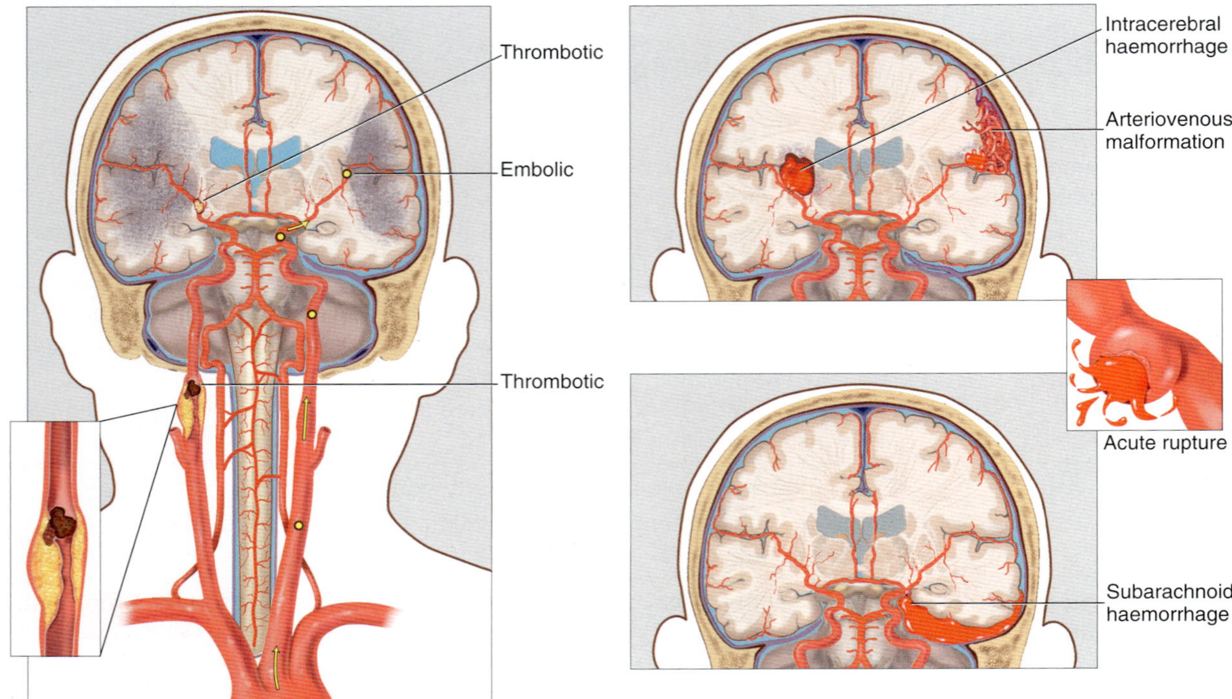

Ischaemic stroke is a sudden interruption of blood flow to the brain and accounts for 87% of all strokes. These are of two types. **Thrombotic** strokes result from atherosclerotic plaque formation. A vulnerable plaque ruptures and a local thrombus forms that deprives the brain tissue in the region of crucial oxygen and glucose. **Embolic** strokes result from a travelling clot caused by atrial fibrillation or flutter, recent heart attack, growth around prosthetic heart valves and endocarditis. Acute ischaemic stroke symptoms include unilateral facial droop, arm drift, weakness or paralysis on one half of the body, difficulty speaking or understanding speech, confusion, sudden onset of dizziness, loss of balance, clouding of vision.

Haemorrhagic stroke results from acute rupture and bleeding from a weakened artery in the brain and accounts for only 13% of all strokes. Most are intracerebral haemorrhages caused by ruptured aneurysm, arteriovenous malformation, disturbed coagulation cascade, tumour or cocaine abuse. Arteriovenous malformations are congenital networks of arteries and veins that do not have capillaries in between and are at risk for rupture. Think of a snarl of tendrils. A subarachnoid haemorrhage is less common and is due to an aneurysm between the base of the cerebral cortex and the arachnoid layer of the meninges. Symptoms include sudden severe headache, nausea and vomiting, sudden loss of consciousness and focal seizures.

TABLE 12.4 Primary headaches

	Tension	Migraine	Cluster
	Tension	Migraine*	Cluster
Definition	Headache (HA) of musculoskeletal origin; may be a mild-to-moderate, less disabling form of migraine	HA of genetically transmitted vascular and trigeminal nerve origin; HA plus prodrome, aura, other symptoms; 2–3 times as common in women as in men	Rare HA that is intermittent, excruciating, unilateral, with autonomic signs
Location	Usually both sides, across frontal, temporal and/or occipital region of head: forehead, sides and back of head	Commonly one-sided but may occur on both sides Pain is often behind the eyes, the temples or forehead	Always one-sided Often behind or around the eye, temple, forehead, cheek
Character	Bandlike tightness, vicelike Nonthrobbing, nonpulsatile	Throbbing, pulsating	Continuous, burning, piercing, excruciating
Duration	Gradual onset, lasts 30 minutes to days	Rapid onset, peaks 1–2 hours, lasts 4–72 hours, sometimes longer	Abrupt onset, peaks in minutes, lasts 45–90 minutes
Quantity and severity	Diffuse, dull aching pain Mild-to-moderate pain	Moderate-to-severe pain	Can occur multiple times a day, in 'clusters', lasting weeks Severe, stabbing pain
Timing	Situational, in response to overwork, posture	≈2 per month, last 1–3 days ≈1 in 10 patients have weekly headaches	1–2 per day, each lasting ½ to 2 hours for 1 to 2 months; then remission for months or years
Aggravating symptoms or triggers	Stress, anxiety, depression, poor posture Not worsened by physical activity	Hormonal fluctuations (premenstrual) Foods (e.g. alcohol, caffeine, MSG, nitrates, chocolate, cheese) Hunger Letdown after stress Sleep deprivation Sensory stimuli (e.g. flashing lights or perfumes) Changes in weather Physical activity	Exacerbated by alcohol, stress, daytime napping, wind or heat exposure

Continued

TABLE 12.4 Primary headaches cont'd

Associated symptoms	Fatigue, anxiety, stress Sensation of a band tightening around head, of being gripped like a vice Sometimes photophobia or phonophobia	Aura (visual changes such as blind spots or flashes of light, tingling in an arm or leg, vertigo) Prodrome (change in mood, behaviour, hunger, cravings, yawning) Nausea, vomiting, photophobia, phonophobia, abdominal pain Person looks sick Family history of migraine	Ipsilateral autonomic signs: Nasal congestion or runny nose, watery or reddened eye, eyelid drooping, miosis Feelings of agitation
Relieving factors, efforts to treat	Rest, massaging muscles in area, NSAID medication	Lie down, darken room, use eyeshade, sleep, take NSAID early, try to avoid opioid	Need to move, pace floor

TABLE 12.5 Abnormalities in muscle movement

	Condition	Description
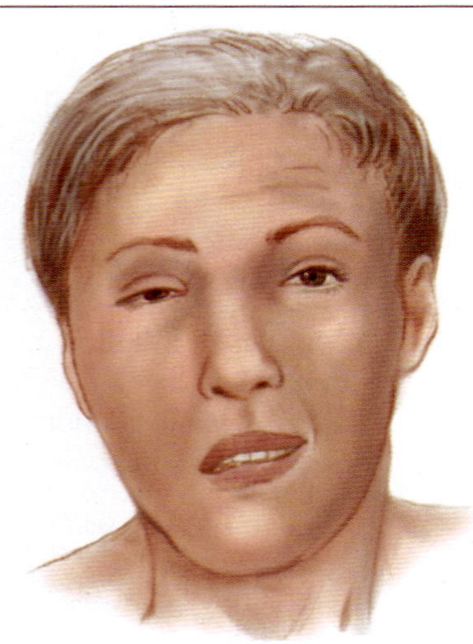	**Paralysis**	Decreased or loss of motor power due to problem with motor nerve or muscle fibres. Causes: acute—trauma, spinal cord injury, stroke, poliomyelitis, polyneuritis, Bell's palsy; chronic—muscular dystrophy, diabetic neuropathy, multiple sclerosis; episodic—myasthenia gravis. Patterns of paralysis: *hemiplegia*—spastic or flaccid paralysis of one side (right or left) of body and extremities; *paraplegia*—symmetrical paralysis of both lower extremities; *quadriplegia*—paralysis in all four extremities; *paresis*—weakness of muscles rather than paralysis.

TABLE 12.5 Abnormalities in muscle movement cont'd

	Condition	Description
	Fasciculation	Rapid, continuous twitching of resting muscle or part of muscle, without movement of limb, which can be seen or palpated. Types: fine—occurs with lower motor neuron disease, associated with atrophy and weakness; coarse—occurs with cold exposure or fatigue and is not significant.
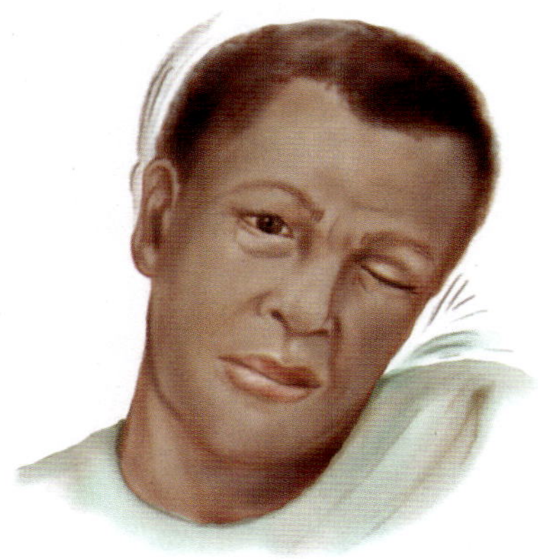	 **Tic**	Involuntary, compulsive, repetitive twitching of a muscle group, e.g. wink, grimace, head movement, shoulder shrug; due to a neurological cause, e.g. tardive dyskinesias, Tourette's syndrome or psychogenic cause (habit tic).
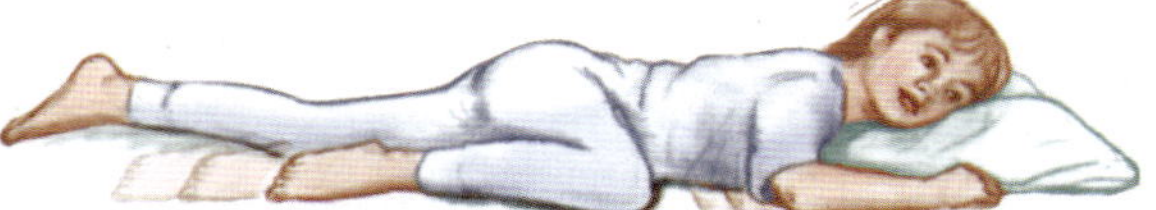	**Myoclonus**	Rapid, sudden jerk or a short series of jerks at fairly regular intervals. A hiccup is a myoclonus of diaphragm. Single myoclonic arm or leg jerk is normal when the person is falling asleep; myoclonic jerks are severe with tonic–clonic seizures.
	Tremor	Involuntary contraction of opposing muscle groups. Results in rhythmic, back-and-forth movement of one or more joints. May occur at rest or with voluntary movement. All tremors disappear while sleeping. Tremors may be slow (3–6 per second) or rapid (10–20 per second).

Continued

TABLE 12.5 Abnormalities in muscle movement cont'd

	Condition	Description
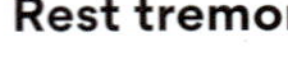 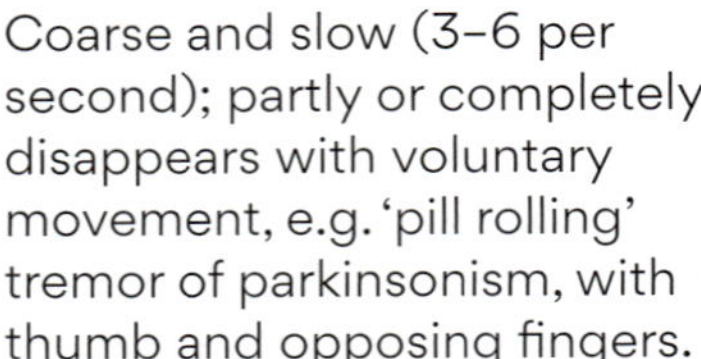	**Rest tremor**	Coarse and slow (3–6 per second); partly or completely disappears with voluntary movement, e.g. 'pill rolling' tremor of parkinsonism, with thumb and opposing fingers.
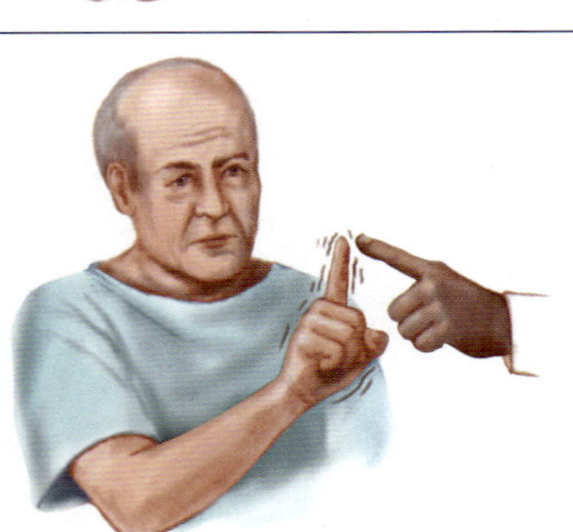	**Intention tremor**	Rate varies; worse with voluntary movement. Occurs with cerebellar disease and multiple sclerosis. Essential tremor (familial)—a type of intention tremor; most common tremor with older people. Benign (no associated disease) but causes emotional stress in business or social situations. Improves with the administration of sedatives, propranolol, alcohol, but use of alcohol is discouraged because of the risk of addiction.
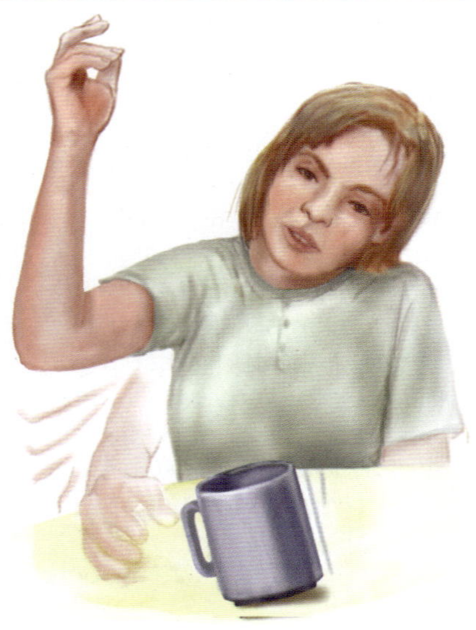	**Chorea**	Sudden, rapid, jerky, purposeless movement involving limbs, trunk or face. Occurs at irregular intervals, not rhythmic or repetitive, more convulsive than a tic. Some are spontaneous and some are initiated; all are accentuated by voluntary acts. Disappears with sleep. Common with Sydenham's chorea and Huntington's disease.

TABLE 12.5 Abnormalities in muscle movement cont'd

	Condition	Description
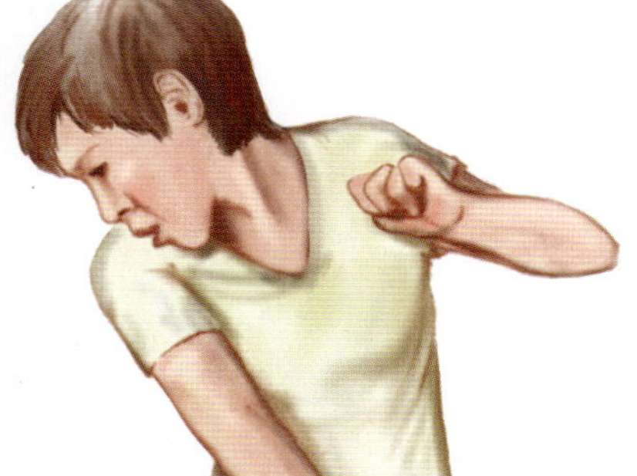	**Athetosis**	Slow, twisting, writhing, continuous movement, resembling a snake or worm. Involves distal part of limb more than the proximal part. Occurs with cerebral palsy. Disappears with sleep. 'Athetoid' hand—some fingers are flexed and some are extended.

TABLE 12.6 Abnormal gaits

Type	Characteristic Appearance	Possible causes
Hemiparesis with spasticity 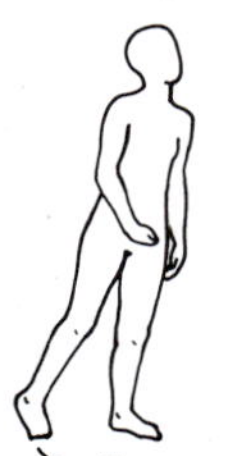	Arm is immobile against the body, with flexion of the shoulder, elbow, wrist, fingers and adduction of shoulder. The leg is stiff and extended and circumducts with each step (drags toe in a semicircle).	Upper motor neuron lesion of the corticospinal tract (e.g. stroke, trauma)
Cerebellar ataxia 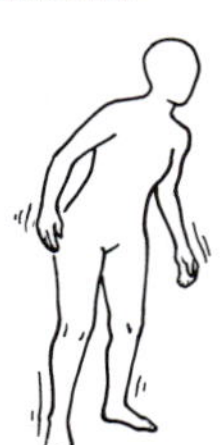	Staggering, wide-based gait; difficulty with turns; uncoordinated movement with positive Romberg sign.	Alcohol or barbiturate effect on cerebellum; cerebellar tumour; multiple sclerosis

Continued

TABLE 12.6 Abnormal gaits cont'd

Type	Characteristic Appearance	Possible causes
Parkinsonian (festinating)	Posture is stooped; trunk is pitched forwards; elbows, hips and knees are flexed. Steps are short and shuffling. Hesitation to begin walking and difficult to stop suddenly. The person holds the body rigid. Walks and turns body as one fixed unit. Difficulty with any change in direction.	Parkinsonism
Scissors	Knees cross or are in contact, like holding an orange between the thighs. The person uses short steps and walking requires effort.	Paraparesis of legs, multiple sclerosis
Steppage or footdrop	Slapping quality—looks as if walking up stairs and finds no stair there. Lifts knee and foot high and slaps it down hard and flat to compensate for footdrop.	Weakness of peroneal and anterior tibial muscles; due to lower motor neuron lesion at the spinal cord such as poliomyelitis and Charcot-Marie-Tooth disease (an inherited peripheral neuropathy)
Waddling	Weak hip muscles—when the person takes a step, the opposite hip drops, which allows compensatory lateral movement of pelvis. Often, the person also has marked lumbar lordosis and a protruding abdomen.	Hip girdle muscle weakness due to muscular dystrophy, dislocation of hips
Short leg	Leg length discrepancy greater than 2.5 cm. Vertical telescoping of affected side, which dips as the person walks. Appearance of gait varies depending on amount of accompanying muscle dysfunction.	Congenital dislocated hip; acquired shortening due to disease, trauma

TABLE 12.7 Speech disorders

Condition	Disorder of	Description
Dysphonia	Voice	Difficulty or discomfort in talking, with abnormal pitch or volume, due to laryngeal disease. Voice sounds hoarse or whispered, but articulation and language are intact.
Dysarthria	Articulation	Distorted speech sounds; speech may sound unintelligible; basic language (word choice, grammar, comprehension) intact.
Aphasia	Language comprehension and production secondary to brain damage	True language disturbance, defect in word choice and grammar or defect in comprehension; defect is in higher integrative language processing.

Types of aphasia

An earlier dichotomy classified aphasias as expressive (difficulty producing language) or receptive (difficulty understanding language). Since all people with aphasia have some difficulty with expression, beginning examiners tend to classify them all as expressive. The following system is more descriptive.

Condition	Description
Global aphasia	The most common and severe form. Spontaneous speech is absent or reduced to a few stereotyped words or sounds. Comprehension is absent or reduced to only the person's own name and a few select words. Repetition, reading and writing are severely impaired. Prognosis for language recovery is poor. Caused by a large lesion that damages most of the combined anterior and posterior language areas.
Broca's aphasia	Expressive aphasia. The person can understand language but cannot express themself using language. This is characterised by nonfluent, dysarthric and effortful speech. The speech is mostly nouns and verbs (high-content words) with few grammatic fillers, termed 'agrammatic' or 'telegraphic' speech. Repetition and reading aloud are severely impaired. Auditory and reading comprehensions are surprisingly intact. Lesion is in anterior language area called the motor speech cortex or Broca's area.
Wernicke's aphasia	Receptive aphasia. The linguistic opposite of Broca's aphasia. The person can hear sounds and words but cannot relate them to previous experiences. Speech is fluent, effortless and well-articulated but has many paraphasias (word substitutions that are malformed or wrong) and neologisms (made-up words) and often lacks substantive words. Speech can be totally incomprehensible. Often, there is a great urge to speak. Repetition, reading and writing also are impaired. Lesion is in posterior language area called the association auditory cortex or Wernicke's area.

TABLE 12.8 Common patterns of motor system dysfunction

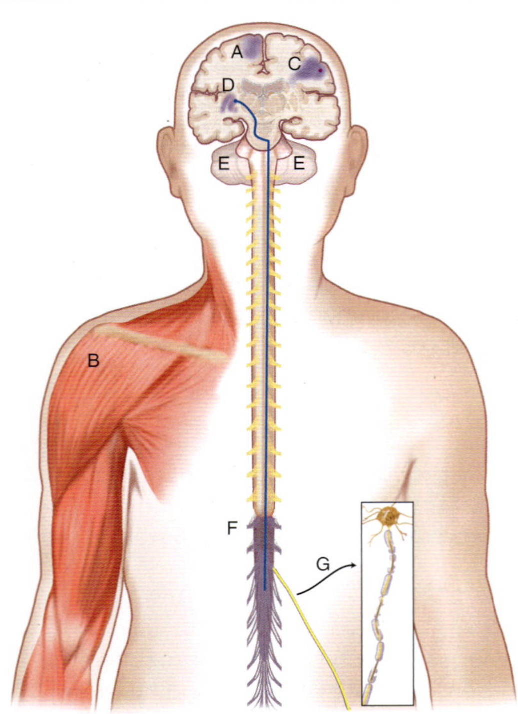

A—Cerebral palsy. Mixed group of paralytic neuromotor disorders of infancy and childhood; due to damage to cerebral cortex caused by a developmental defect, intrauterine meningitis or encephalitis, birth trauma, anoxia or kernicterus.

B—Muscular dystrophy. Chronic, progressive wasting of skeletal musculature, which produces weakness, contractures and, in severe cases, respiratory dysfunction and death. Onset of symptoms occurs in childhood. Many types exist; the most severe is Duchenne's dystrophy, characterised by the waddling gait described in Table 12.6.

C—Hemiplegia. Damage to corticospinal tract (e.g. stroke). Upper motor neuron damage occurs above the pyramidal decussation crossover, so motor impairment is on contralateral (opposite) side. Initially flaccid when the lesion is acute; later, the muscles become spastic and abnormal reflexes appear. Characteristic posture: arm—shoulder adducted, elbow flexed, wrist pronated, leg extended; face—weakness only in lower muscles. Hyperreflexia and possible clonus occur on the involved side; loss of corneal, abdominal and cremasteric reflexes; positive Babinski's and Hoffman's reflexes.

D—Parkinsonism. Defect of extrapyramidal tracts, in the region of the basal ganglia, with loss of the neurotransmitter dopamine. Classic triad of symptoms: tremor, rigidity, akinesia. Also, slower monotonous speech and diminutive writing. The body tends to stay immobile; facial expression is flat, staring, expressionless; excessive salivation occurs; reduced eye blinking. Posture is stooped; equilibrium is impaired; loses balance easily; gait is described in Table 12.6. Parkinsonian tremor; cogwheel rigidity on passive range of motion.

E—Cerebellar. A lesion in one hemisphere produces motor abnormalities on the ipsilateral side. Characterised by ataxia, lurching forward of affected side while walking, rapid alternating movements are slow and arrhythmic, finger-to-nose test reveals ataxia and tremor with overshoot or undershoot and eyes display coarse nystagmus.

F—Paraplegia. Lower motor neuron damage caused by spinal cord injury. A severe injury or complete transection initially produces 'spinal shock', which is defined as no movement or reflex activity below the level of the lesion. Gradually, deep tendon reflexes reappear and become increased, flexor spasms of legs occur; and finally, extensor spasms of legs occur; these spasms lead to prevailing extensor tone.

TABLE 12.9 Abnormal postures

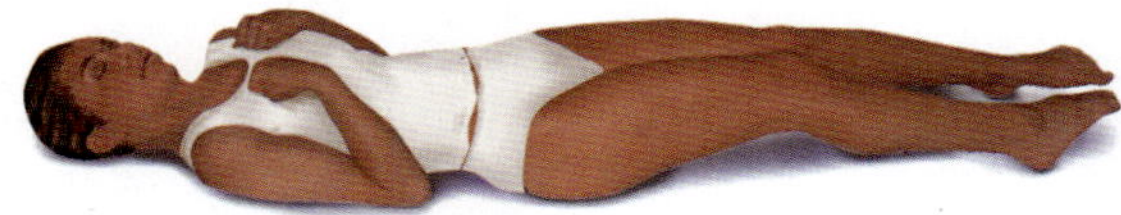

Decorticate rigidity

Upper extremities—flexion of arm, wrist and fingers; adduction of arm (tight against thorax). Lower extremities—extension, internal rotation, plantar flexion. This indicates hemispheric lesion of cerebral cortex.

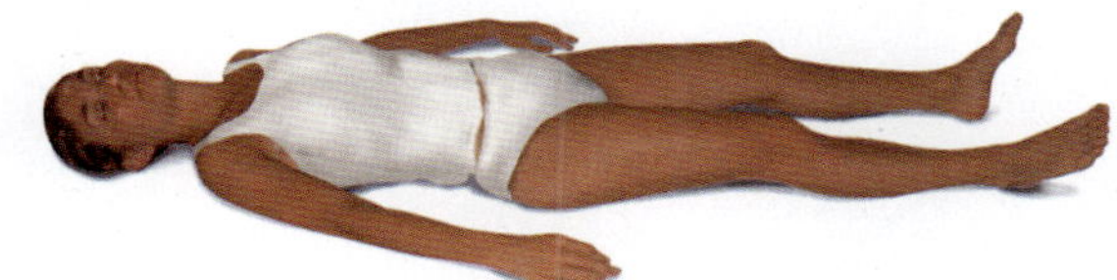

Flaccid quadriplegia

Complete loss of muscle tone and paralysis of all four extremities, indicating completely nonfunctional brainstem.

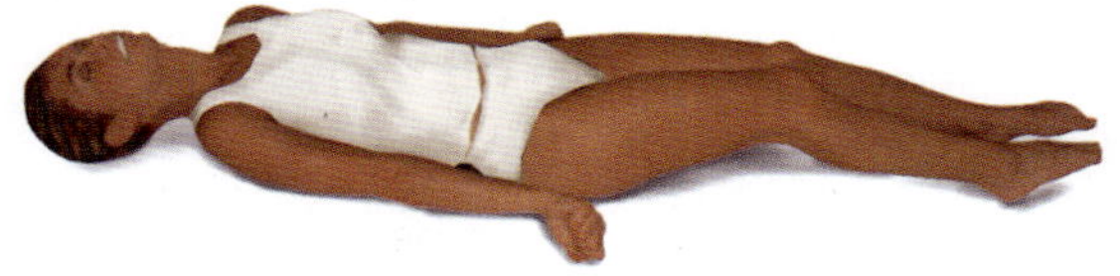

Decerebrate rigidity

Upper extremities stiffly extended, adducted, internal rotation, palms pronated. Lower extremities stiffly extended, plantar flexion; teeth clenched; hyperextended back. More ominous than decorticate rigidity; indicates lesion in brainstem at midbrain or upper pons.

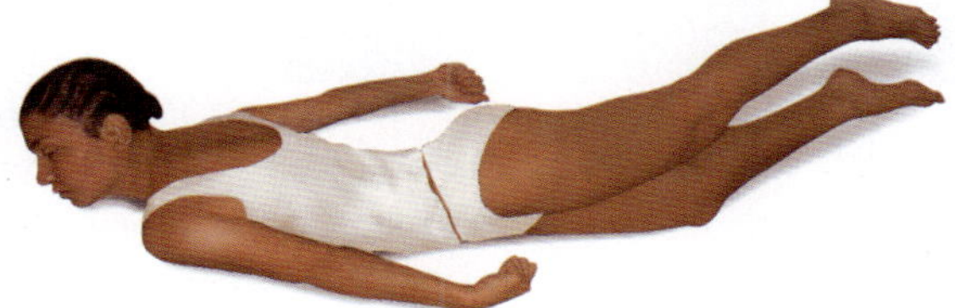

Opisthotonos

Prolonged arching of the back, with head and heels bent backwards. This indicates meningeal irritation.

TABLE 12.10 Abnormal facial appearances with neurological disorders

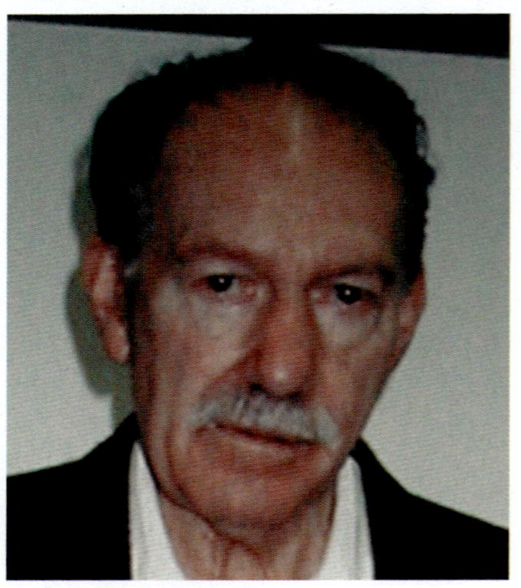

Parkinson's syndrome

A deficiency of the neurotransmitter dopamine and degeneration of the basal ganglia in the brain. The immobility of features produces a face that is flat and expressionless, 'mask-like', with elevated eyebrows, staring gaze, oily skin and drooling.

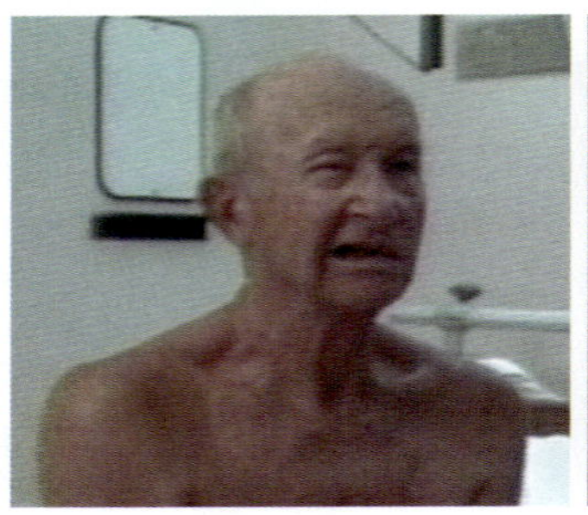

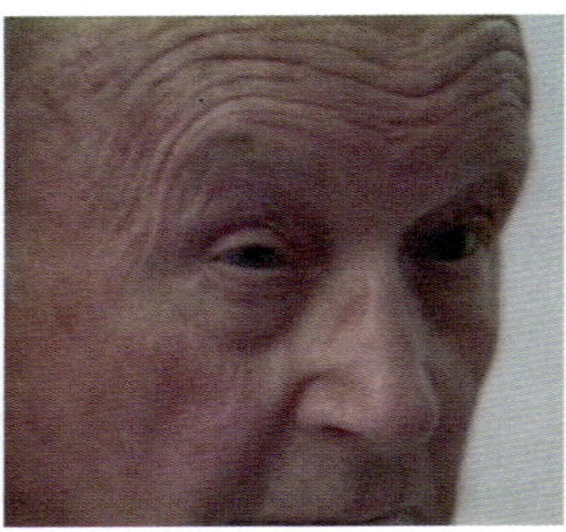

Stroke

An **upper motor neuron** lesion (**central**). A stroke is an acute neurological deficit caused by an obstruction of a cerebral vessel, as in atherosclerosis or a rupture in a cerebral vessel. Note paralysis of lower facial muscles, but also note that the upper half of the face is not affected because of the intact nerve from the unaffected hemisphere. The person can still wrinkle the forehead and close the eyes.

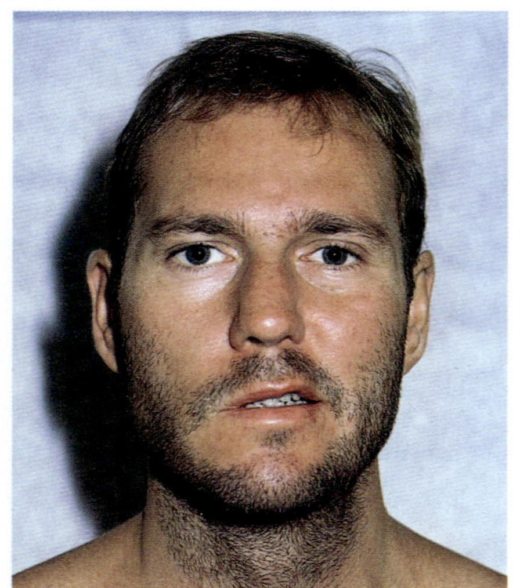

Bell's palsy (right side)

A **lower motor neuron** lesion **(peripheral)**, producing cranial nerve VII paralysis, which is almost always unilateral. It has a rapid onset and its cause is currently thought to be the herpes simplex virus. Note complete paralysis of half of the face; the person cannot wrinkle the forehead, raise the eyebrows, close the eyes, whistle or show teeth on the right side. Usually presents with smooth forehead, wide palpebral fissure, flat nasolabial fold, drooling and pain behind the ear.

TABLE 12.11 Abnormalities in muscle tone

Condition	Description	Associated with
Flaccidity	Decreased muscle tone or *hypotonia*; muscle feels limp, soft and flabby; muscle is weak and easily fatigued	Lower motor neuron injury anywhere from the anterior horn cell in the spinal cord to the peripheral nerve (peripheral neuritis, poliomyelitis, Guillain-Barré syndrome). Early stroke and spinal cord injury are flaccid at first.
Spasticity	Increased tone or *hypertonia*; increased resistance to passive lengthening; then may suddenly give way (clasp-knife phenomenon)	Upper motor neuron injury to corticospinal motor tract such as paralysis with stroke (chronic stage)
Rigidity	Constant state of resistance (lead-pipe rigidity); resists passive movement in any direction; dystonia	Injury to extrapyramidal motor tracts (e.g. basal ganglia with parkinsonism)
Cogwheel rigidity	Type of rigidity in which the increased tone is released by degrees during passive range of motion so it feels like small regular jerks	Parkinsonism

Advanced practice—additional data

The complete neurological assessment is described in this section of the chapter. Many parts of a neurological assessment require an appropriately orientated and cooperative person to collect reliable assessment data. The assessments described in the following sections require advanced skills and scope of practice. Nurses working in specialist settings need to develop these skills to assess specific aspects of neurological function or identify specific neurological problems.

Preparation

In addition to the assessment strategies described above, use the following sequence for a complete neurological examination:

1. mental health (Chapter 11)
2. head, face and neck
3. cranial nerves
4. motor system
5. sensory system
6. reflexes.

Equipment needed

Neurological observations chart
Hand hygiene solution
Penlight torch
Tongue blade
Cotton swab
Cotton ball
Tuning fork (128 Hz or 256 Hz)
Percussion hammer
(Possibly) familiar aromatic substances (peppermint, coffee, vanilla)
Stethoscope

PROCEDURES AND NORMAL FINDINGS	ABNORMAL FINDINGS AND CLINICAL ALERTS
Inspect head, face and neck	
Inspect and palpate the skull	
Note the general size and shape. **Normocephalic** is the term that denotes a round symmetrical skull that is appropriately related to body size. Be aware that 'normal' includes a wide range of sizes.	Abnormalities: **microcephaly** (abnormally small head); **macrocephaly** (abnormally large head)—as occurs in **hydrocephaly**, **acromegaly**, **Paget's disease**.
To assess shape, place your fingers in the person's hair and palpate the scalp. The skull normally feels symmetrical and smooth. The cranial bones that have normal protrusions are the forehead, the lateral edge of each parietal bone, the occipital bone and the mastoid process behind each ear. There is no tenderness to palpation.	Note lumps, depressions or abnormal protrusions.
Temporal area Palpate the temporal artery above the zygoma (cheek bone) between the eye and top of the ear.	The artery looks more tortuous and feels hardened and tender with **temporal arteritis** (inflammation of the temporal artery) causing headaches, scalp tenderness, jaw pain and vision problems.
The temporomandibular joint is just below the temporal artery and anterior to the tragus. Palpate the joint as the person opens the mouth and note normally smooth movement with no limitation or tenderness.	Crepitation, limited range of motion or tenderness.
Inspect the face	
Facial expression Appropriateness to behaviour or reported mood.	• Anxiety is common in a hospitalised or ill person. • Hostility or embarrassment. • Tense, rigid muscles may indicate anxiety or pain. • A flat affect may indicate depression. • Excessive smiling may be inappropriate.
Shape and symmetry of facial structures May vary somewhat among people; they should always be largely symmetrical. Note symmetry of eyebrows, palpebral fissures, nasolabial folds and sides of the mouth.	Marked asymmetry with central brain lesion (e.g. stroke) or with peripheral cranial nerve VII damage (Bell's palsy) (Table 12.10).
Note any abnormal facial structures (coarse facial features, exophthalmos, changes in skin colour or pigmentation) or any abnormal swelling. Also note any involuntary movements (tics) in the facial muscles. Normally none occur.	Oedema in the face occurs first around the eyes (periorbital) and the cheeks where the subcutaneous tissue is relatively loose. Note rhythmic movement of jaw, tics, fasciculations or excessive blinking (Table 12.10).

PROCEDURES AND NORMAL FINDINGS	ABNORMAL FINDINGS AND CLINICAL ALERTS
Inspect and palpate the neck	
Symmetry Head position is centred in the midline and the accessory neck muscles should be symmetrical. The head should be held erect and still.	Head tilt occurs with muscle spasm. Rigid head and neck occur with arthritis.
Range of motion (ROM) Note any limitation of movement during active motion. Ask the person to touch the chin to the chest, turn the head to the right and left, try to touch each ear to the shoulder (without elevating shoulders) and to extend the head backwards. When the neck is supple, motion is smooth and controlled.	Note pain at any movement. Note ratchety or limited movement from cervical arthritis or inflammation of neck muscles. The arthritic neck is rigid; the person turns at the shoulders rather than at the neck.
Muscle strength Test muscle strength and the status of cranial nerve XI by trying to resist the person's movements with your hands as the person shrugs the shoulders and turns the head to each side.	See Tables 12.12 and 12.13.
Palpate for swelling, masses, pulsations As the person moves their head, note enlargement of the salivary glands and lymph glands. Normally no enlargement is present. Note a swollen parotid gland when the head is extended; look for swelling below the angle of the jaw. Also, note thyroid gland enlargement. Normally none is present. Also note any obvious pulsations. The carotid artery runs medial to the sternocleidomastoid muscle, and it creates a brisk localised pulsation just below the angle of the jaw. Normally, there are no other pulsations while the person is in the sitting position (Chapter 17).	Thyroid enlargement may be a unilateral lump or it may be diffuse and look like a doughnut lying across the lower neck.

PROCEDURES AND NORMAL FINDINGS	ABNORMAL FINDINGS AND CLINICAL ALERTS

Test the cranial nerves

TABLE 12.12 Summary—testing cranial nerve function of adults

Cranial nerve	Response
I	Not tested routinely—should have sense of smell in both nostrils Sense of smell does decrease with age
II, III, IV, VI	Optical blink reflex—shine light in open eyes, note rapid closure Size, shape, equality of pupils Eyes follow movement
V	Chewing Sensation Ophthalmic Maxillary Mandibular
VII	Facial movements symmetrical when smiling
VIII	Facial muscles
IX, X	Swallowing, gag reflex Coordinated swallowing
XII	Movement of the tongue

Cranial nerve I—olfactory nerve

Do not test routinely. Test the sense of smell in those who report loss of smell, those with head trauma and those with altered mental status and when the presence of an intracranial lesion is suspected. First, assess patency by occluding one nostril at a time and asking the person to sniff. Then, with the person's eyes closed, occlude one nostril and present an aromatic substance. Use familiar, conveniently obtainable and non-noxious smells such as coffee, toothpaste, orange, vanilla, soap or peppermint.

You cannot test smell when air passages are occluded with upper respiratory infection or with sinusitis.

Anosmia—decrease or loss of smell occurs bilaterally with tobacco smoking, allergic rhinitis and cocaine use.

Normally, a person can identify an odour on each side of the nose. Smell is normally decreased bilaterally with ageing. Any asymmetry in the sense of smell is important.

Unilateral loss of smell in the absence of nasal disease is **neurogenic anosmia** (Table 12.13).

Cranial nerve II—optic nerve

Test visual acuity and test visual fields by confrontation (Chapter 14).

Visual field loss (Table 14.5).

Using the ophthalmoscope, examine the ocular fundus to determine the colour, size and shape of the optic disc (Chapter 14).

Papillo-oedema with increased intracranial pressure; optic atrophy (Table 14.9).

Cranial nerves III, IV and VI—oculomotor, trochlear and abducens nerves

Palpebral fissures are usually equal in width or nearly so (Figure 14.1).

Ptosis (drooping) occurs with myasthenia gravis, dysfunction of cranial nerve III or Horner's syndrome (Table 14.2).

PROCEDURES AND NORMAL FINDINGS	ABNORMAL FINDINGS AND CLINICAL ALERTS
Check pupils for size, regularity, equality, direct and consensual light reaction and accommodation (see above and Chapter 14).	Increasing intracranial pressure causes a sudden, unilateral, dilated and nonreactive pupil.  ***Clinical alert:*** Unilateral, dilated and nonreactive pupils are a medical emergency: report this finding immediately to a medical practitioner.
Assess extraocular movements by the cardinal positions of gaze (Chapter 14). Nystagmus is a back-and-forth oscillation of the eyes. End-point nystagmus, a few beats of horizontal nystagmus at extreme lateral gaze, occurs normally. Assess any other nystagmus carefully, noting the presence of abnormal movement in one or both eyes.	**Strabismus** (deviated gaze) or limited movement.
• Pendular movement (oscillations move equally left to right) or *jerk* (a quick phase in one direction, then a slow phase in the other). Classify the jerk nystagmus in the direction of the quick phase. • Amplitude. Judge whether the degree of movement is fine, medium or coarse. • Frequency. Is it constant, or does it fade after a few beats? • Plane of movement. Horizontal, vertical, rotary or a combination?	**Nystagmus** occurs with disease of the vestibular system, cerebellum or brainstem. Nystagmus leads to low vision: symptoms include: blurred vision and a reduction in depth perception which may put the person at risk of injury, falls or an inability to manage their activities of daily living.
Cranial nerve V—trigeminal nerve	
Motor function. Assess the muscles of mastication by palpating the temporal and masseter muscles as the person clenches the teeth (Figure 12.17). Muscles should feel equally strong on both sides. Next, try to separate the jaws by pushing down on the chin; normally you cannot.	Decreased strength on one or both sides. Asymmetry in jaw movement. Pain with clenching of teeth.  ***Clinical alert:*** Abnormalities in ability to chew may result in nutritional issues.

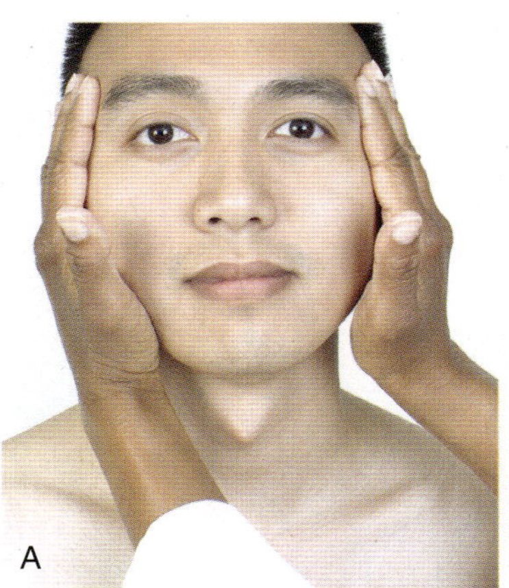

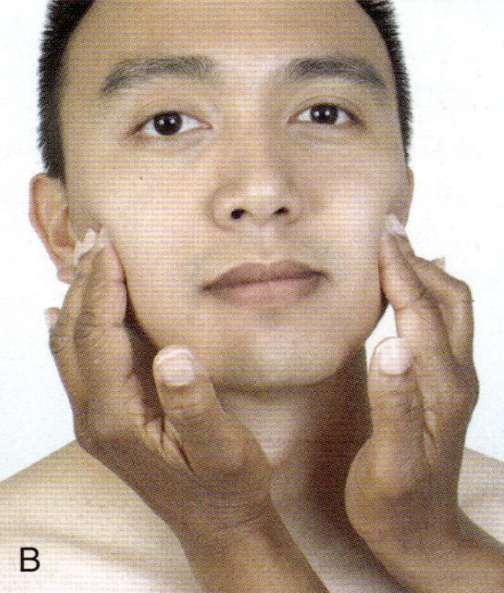

FIGURE 12.17 A & B Assess motor function—Cranial nerve V—trigeminal nerve

PROCEDURES AND NORMAL FINDINGS	ABNORMAL FINDINGS AND CLINICAL ALERTS

Sensory function. With the person's eyes closed, test light touch sensation by touching a cotton wisp to these designated areas on person's face: forehead, cheeks and chin (Figure 12.18). Ask the person to say 'Now', whenever the touch is felt. This tests all three divisions of the nerve: (1) ophthalmic, (2) maxillary and (3) mandibular.

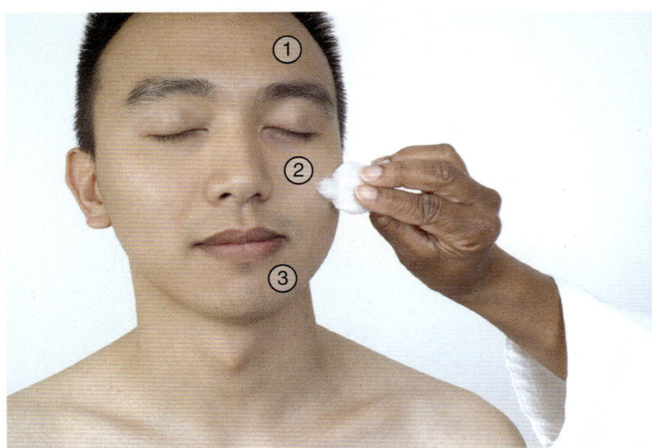

FIGURE 12.18 Assess sensory function—Cranial nerve V—trigeminal nerve

Abnormal findings: Decreased or unequal sensation.

Corneal reflex

This test is done if there is:

- a current or induced altered conscious state
- abnormal facial sensation
- abnormal facial movement such as Bell's palsy.

Normally, a person will blink bilaterally and frequently. If the person is not able to blink, then a wisp of clean cotton wool can be used to elicit the corneal reflex. This is done with the person looking forwards. Bring the wisp of cotton wool in laterally and lightly touch the cornea of the eye.

This procedure tests the sensory afferent pathway of cranial nerve V (sensation of cornea) and the motor efferent pathway of cranial nerve VII (muscles that close the eye). Check to see if the person is wearing contact lenses—assist to remove if necessary.

Abnormal findings: No blink occurs with a lesion of cranial nerve V or cranial nerve VII paralysis.

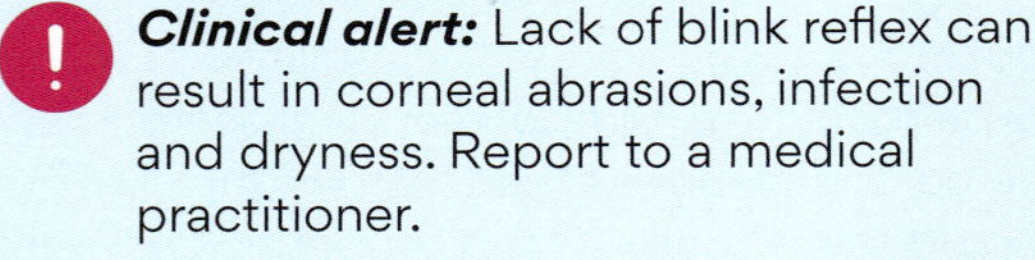

Clinical alert: Lack of blink reflex can result in corneal abrasions, infection and dryness. Report to a medical practitioner.

PROCEDURES AND NORMAL FINDINGS	ABNORMAL FINDINGS AND CLINICAL ALERTS

Cranial nerve VII—facial nerve

Motor function. Note mobility and facial symmetry as the person responds to these requests: smile (Figure 12.19A), frown, close eyes tightly (against your attempt to open them), lift eyebrows, show teeth and puff cheeks (Figure 12.19B). Then, press the person's puffed cheeks in and note that the air should escape equally from both sides.

Muscle weakness is shown by flattening of the nasolabial fold, drooping of one side of the face, lower eyelid sagging and escape of air from only one cheek that is pressed in.

Loss of movement and asymmetry of movement occur with both central nervous system lesions (e.g. stroke that affects the lower face on one side) and PNS lesions (e.g. Bell's palsy that affects the upper and lower face on one side).

Clinical alert: Facial nerve weakness can result in difficulty in chewing food and control of saliva in the mouth (Table 12.14).

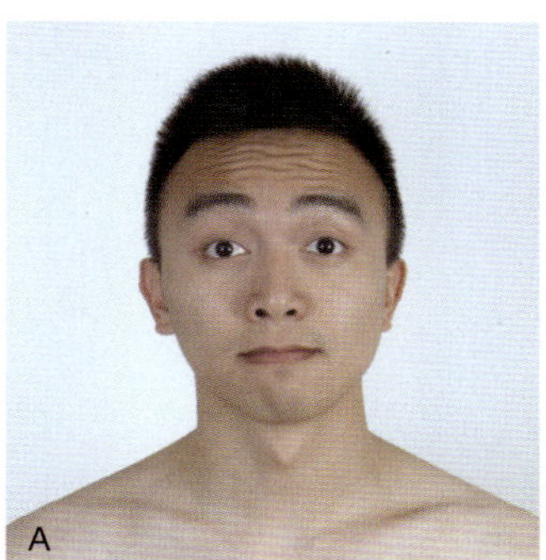

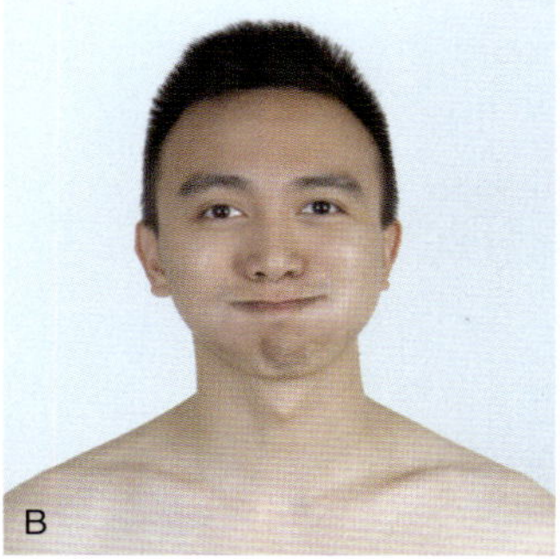

FIGURE 12.19 A & B Assess motor function—Cranial nerve VII—facial nerve

Sensory function. Test when you suspect facial nerve injury.
When indicated, test sense of taste by applying to the tongue a cotton applicator covered with a solution of sugar, salt or lemon juice (sour). Ask the person to identify the taste.

Cranial nerve VIII—acoustic (vestibulocochlear) nerve

Test hearing acuity by assessing the person's ability to hear normal conversation: by the whispered voice test (Chapter 15).

Cranial nerves IX and X—glossopharyngeal and vagus nerves

Motor function. Depress the tongue with a tongue blade and note pharyngeal movement as the person says 'ahhh' or yawns; the uvula and soft palate should rise in the midline and the tonsillar pillars should move medially.

Absence or asymmetry of soft palate movement.
Uvula deviates to side.
Asymmetry of tonsillar pillar movement.

If motor function abnormalities are detected or the person reports swallowing difficulties, touch the posterior pharyngeal wall with a tongue blade and note the gag reflex. Also note that the voice sounds smooth and not strained.

Hoarse or brassy voice occurs with vocal cord dysfunction; nasal twang occurs with weakness of soft palate.

PROCEDURES AND NORMAL FINDINGS	ABNORMAL FINDINGS AND CLINICAL ALERTS
Sensory function. Cranial nerve IX does mediate taste on the posterior one-third of the tongue, but technically this sensation is too difficult to test.	 ***Clinical alert:*** Abnormalities in the function of the glossopharyngeal and vagus nerves are likely to compromise the person's airway.

Cranial nerve XI—spinal accessory nerve

Examine the sternocleidomastoid and trapezius muscles for equal size. Check equal strength by asking the person to rotate the head forcibly against resistance applied to the side of the chin (Figure 12.20A). Then ask the person to shrug the shoulders against resistance (Figure 12.20B). These movements should feel equally strong on both sides.	Atrophy. Muscle weakness or paralysis.

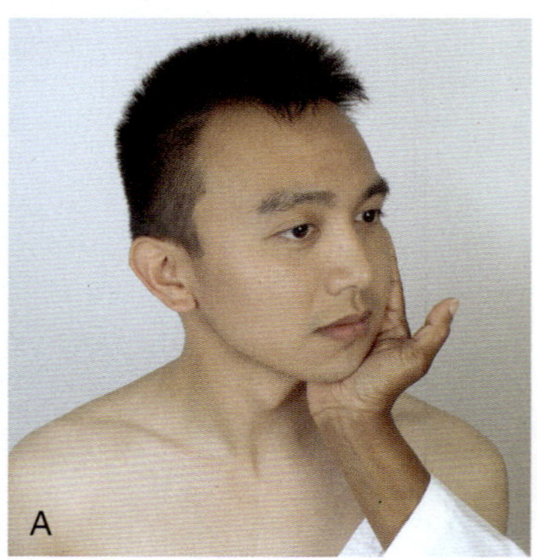
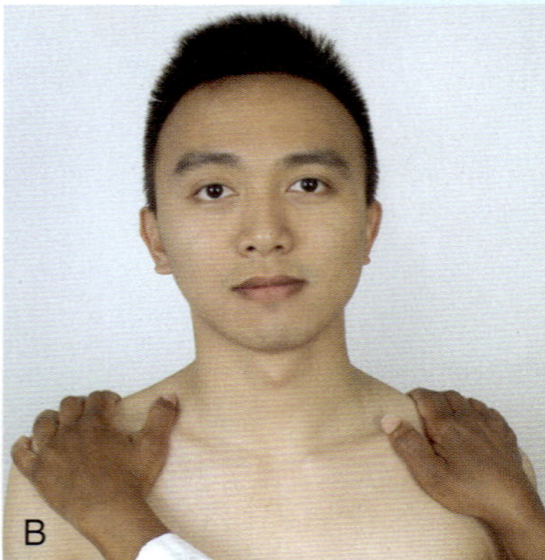

FIGURE 12.20 A & B Assess motor function—Cranial nerve XII—spinal accessory nerve

Inspect the tongue. No wasting or tremors should be present. Note the forward thrust in the midline as the person protrudes the tongue. Also ask the person to say 'light, tight, dynamite' and note that lingual speech (sounds of letters l, t, d, n) is clear and distinct.	Atrophy. Fasciculations. Tongue deviates to side with lesions of the hypoglossal nerve (when this occurs, deviation is towards the paralysed side).  ***Clinical alert:*** Abnormalities in the function of the hypoglossal nerve are likely to compromise the person's airway.

Inspect and palpate motor system

Muscles

Size. As you proceed through the examination, inspect all muscle groups for size. Compare the right side with the left. Muscle groups should be within the normal size limits for age and should be symmetrical bilaterally. When muscles in the extremities look asymmetrical, measure each in centimetres and record the difference. A difference of 1 cm or less is not significant. Note that it is difficult to assess muscle mass in very obese people.	**Atrophy**—abnormally small muscle with a wasted appearance; occurs with disuse, injury, lower motor neuron disease such as polio, diabetic neuropathy. **Hypertrophy**—increased size and strength; occurs with isometric exercise.

PROCEDURES AND NORMAL FINDINGS	ABNORMAL FINDINGS AND CLINICAL ALERTS
Strength. (See Chapter 20 Musculoskeletal assessment.) Test the power of muscle groups (extremities, neck and trunk) simultaneously.	**Paresis** or weakness is diminished strength; **paralysis** or plegia is absence of strength.
Tone. Tone is the normal degree of tension (contraction) in voluntarily relaxed muscles. It shows as a mild resistance to passive stretch. To test muscle tone, move the extremities through a passive range of motion. First, persuade the person to relax completely, to 'go loose like a rag doll'. Move each extremity smoothly through a full range of motion. Support the arm at the elbow and the leg at the knee (Figure 12.21). Normally, you will note a mild, even resistance to movement.	Limited range of motion. Pain with motion. **Flaccidity**—decreased resistance, hypotonic. **Spasticity and rigidity**—types of increased resistance (Tables 12.8 and 12.11).

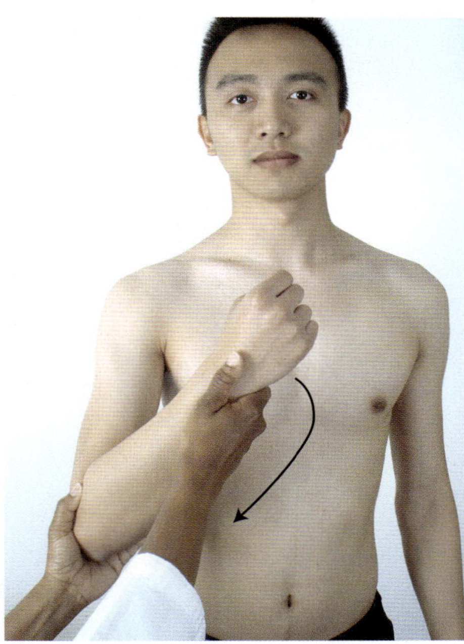

FIGURE 12.21 Assess muscle tone

Involuntary movements. Normally, no involuntary movements occur. If they are present, note their location, frequency, rate and amplitude. Note if the movements can be controlled at will.	Tic, tremor, fasciculation, myoclonus, chorea and athetosis (Table 12.5).

Cerebellar function

Balance tests

Gait. Observe as the person walks 5 to 10 metres, turns and returns to the starting point. Normally, the person moves with a sense of freedom. The gait is smooth, rhythmic and effortless; the opposing arm swing is coordinated; the turns are smooth. The step length is about 40 cm from heel to heel.	Stiff, immobile posture. Staggering or reeling. Wide base of support. Lack of arm swing or rigid arms. Unequal rhythm of steps. Slapping of foot. Scraping of toe of shoe. **Ataxia**—uncoordinated or unsteady gait (Table 12.6).

PROCEDURES AND NORMAL FINDINGS	ABNORMAL FINDINGS AND CLINICAL ALERTS
Tandem walking. Ask the person to walk a straight line in a heel-to-toe fashion (tandem walking) (Figure 12.22). This decreases the base of support and will accentuate any problem with coordination. Normally, the person can walk straight and stay balanced.	
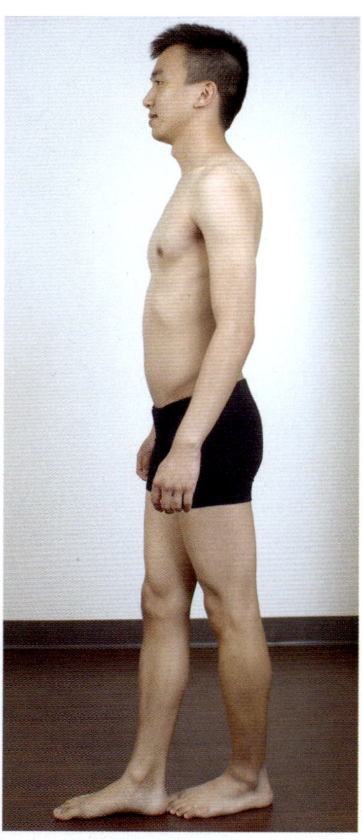 **FIGURE 12.22** Tandem walking	
You may also test for balance by asking the person to walk on their toes, then on their heels for a few steps.	Muscle weakness in the legs prevents this.
The Romberg test. Ask the person to stand up with feet together and arms at the sides. Once in a stable position, ask the person to close the eyes and to hold the position (Figure 12.23 A and B). Wait about 20 seconds. Normally, a person can maintain posture and balance even with the visual orienting information blocked, although slight swaying may occur. Stand close to catch the person in case they fall.	Sways, falls, widens base of feet to avoid falling. **A positive Romberg sign** is loss of balance that occurs when closing the eyes. You eliminate the advantage of orientation with the eyes, which had compensated for sensory loss. A positive Romberg sign occurs with cerebellar ataxia (multiple sclerosis, alcohol intoxication), loss of proprioception and loss of vestibular function.

PROCEDURES AND NORMAL FINDINGS	ABNORMAL FINDINGS AND CLINICAL ALERTS

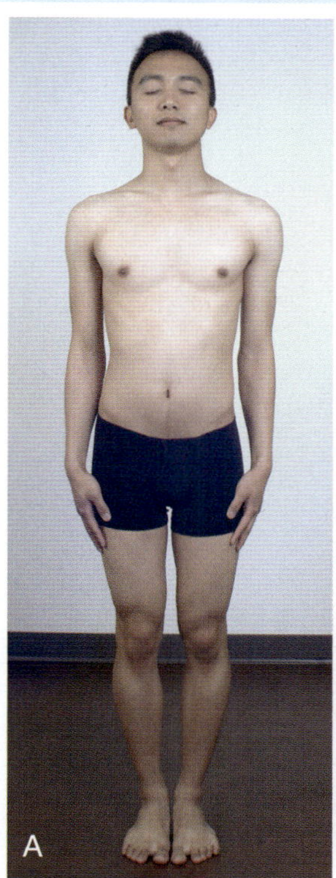

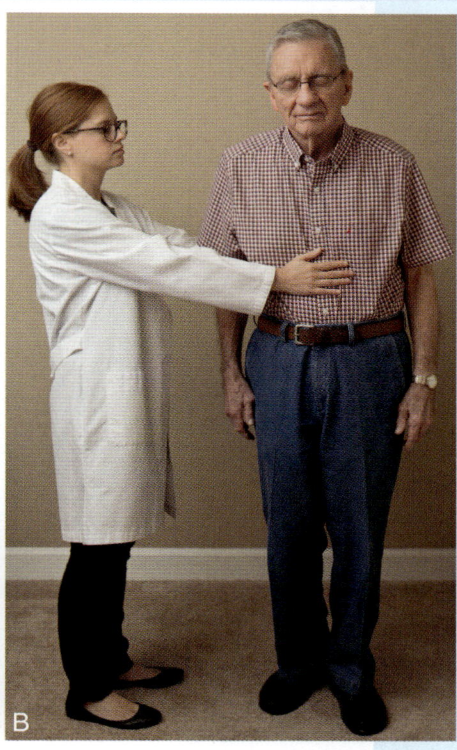

FIGURE 12.23 A & B Romberg test

Ask the person to perform a shallow knee bend first on one leg, then the other either standing alone or lightly supporting themselves by holding on to a bench or stable chair (Figure 12.24 A and B). Alternatively, the person can be asked to rise from a chair without using the arm rests for support. This demonstrates normal position sense, muscle strength and cerebellar function.

Unable to perform knee bend because of weakness in quadriceps muscle or hip extensors.

PROCEDURES AND NORMAL FINDINGS	ABNORMAL FINDINGS AND CLINICAL ALERTS

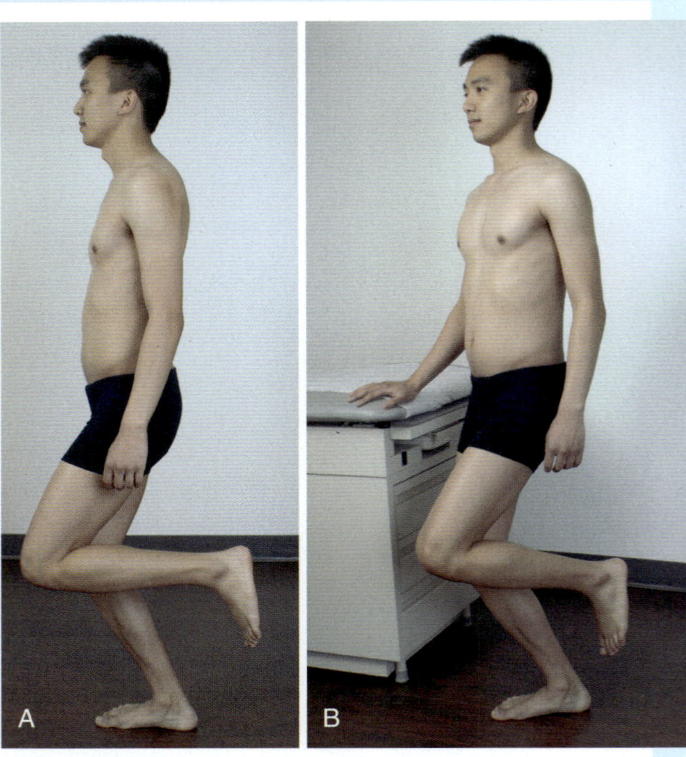

FIGURE 12.24 A & B Testing quadriceps muscle strength

Coordination and skilled movements

Rapid alternating movements (RAM). Ask the person to pat the knees with both hands, lift up, turn hands over and pat the knees with the backs of the hands (Figure 12.25 A and B). Then ask the person to do this faster. Normally, this is done with equal turning and a quick rhythmic pace.

Lack of coordination.

Slow, clumsy and sloppy response is termed **dysdiadochokinesia** and occurs with cerebellar disease.

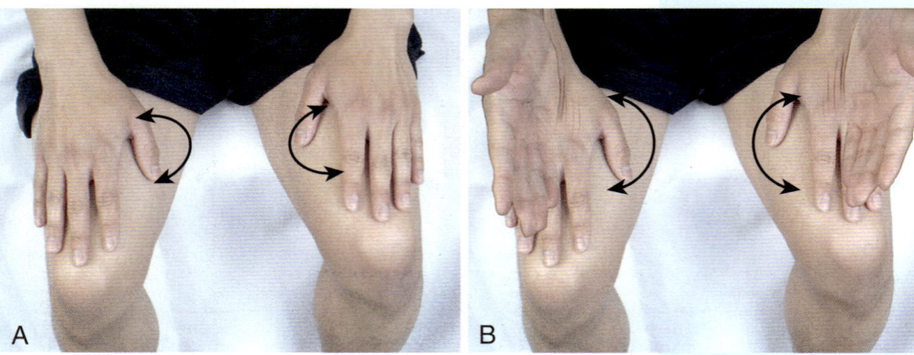

FIGURE 12.25 A & B Rapid alternating movements.

PROCEDURES AND NORMAL FINDINGS	ABNORMAL FINDINGS AND CLINICAL ALERTS
Alternatively, ask the person to touch the thumb to each finger on the same hand, starting with the index finger, then reverse direction (Figure 12.26). Normally, this can be done quickly and accurately.	Lack of coordination.

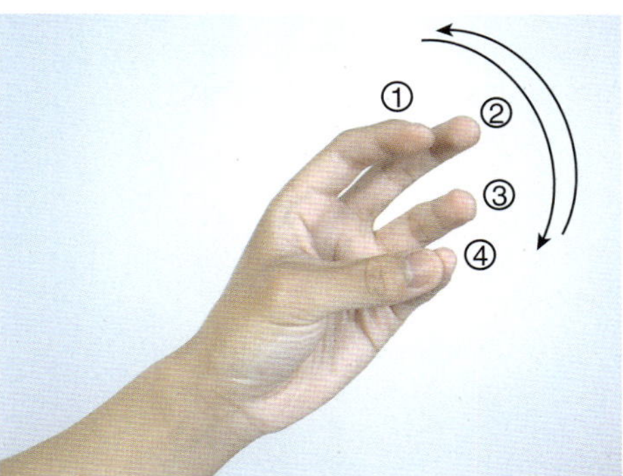

FIGURE 12.26 Assess coordination

Dysmetria is clumsy movement with overshooting the mark and occurs with cerebellar disorders or acute alcohol intoxication.

Past-pointing is a constant deviation to one side.

Finger-to-finger test. With the person's eyes open, ask them to use the index finger to touch your finger, then their own nose (Figure 12.27). After a few times move your finger to a different spot. The person's movement should be smooth and accurate.

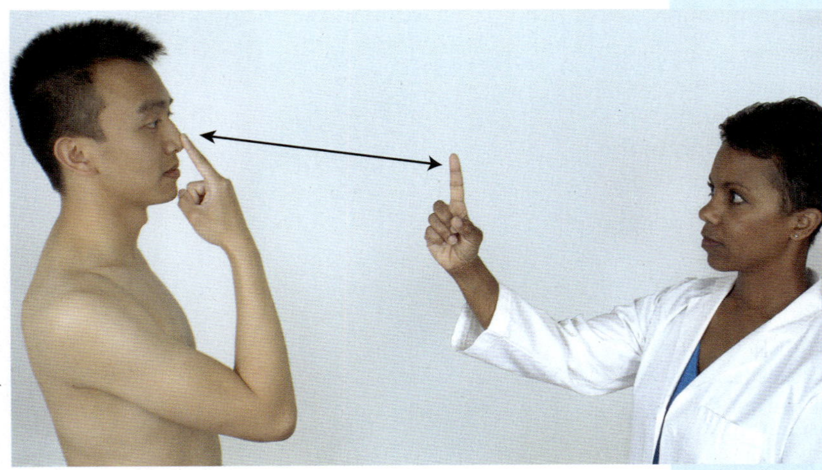

FIGURE 12.27 Finger-to-finger test

PROCEDURES AND NORMAL FINDINGS	ABNORMAL FINDINGS AND CLINICAL ALERTS
Finger-to-nose test. Ask the person to close their eyes and to stretch out their arms. Ask the person to touch the tip of their nose with each index finger, alternating hands and increasing speed. Normally this is done with accurate and smooth movement.	Misses nose. Worsening of coordination when the eyes are closed occurs with cerebellar disease or alcohol intoxication.
Heel-to-shin test. Test lower extremity coordination by asking the person, who is in a supine position, to place their heel on the opposite knee and run it down the shin from the knee to the ankle (Figure 12.28). Normally, the person moves the heel in a straight line down the shin.	Lack of coordination, heel falls off shin; occurs with cerebellar disease.

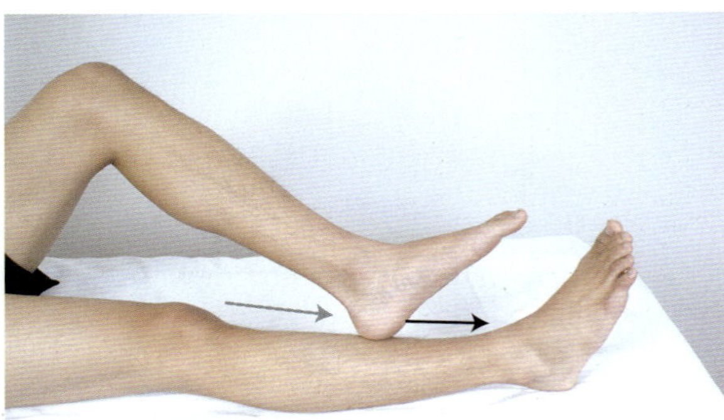

FIGURE 12.28 Heel-to-shin test

Assess the sensory system

Ask the person to identify various sensory stimuli to test the intactness of the peripheral nerve fibres, the sensory tracts and higher cortical discrimination.

Ensure validity of sensory system testing by making sure the person is alert, cooperative and comfortable and has an adequate attention span. Otherwise, you may get misleading and invalid results. Testing of the sensory system can be fatiguing. If the person is tired, you may need to repeat the examination later or to break it into parts.

You do not need to test the entire skin surface for every sensation. Routine screening procedures include testing superficial pain, light touch and vibration in a few distal locations and testing stereognosis (see below). This will suffice for all who have not demonstrated any neurological symptoms or signs. Complete testing of the sensory system is warranted in those with neurological symptoms (e.g. localised pain, numbness and tingling) or when you discover abnormalities (e.g. motor deficit). Then, test all sensory modalities and cover most dermatomes of the body (Figure 12.11).

Clinical alert: Abnormalities in sensory perception can pose an injury risk such as burns and pressure injury. See Table 12.15.

PROCEDURES AND NORMAL FINDINGS	ABNORMAL FINDINGS AND CLINICAL ALERTS
Compare sensations on symmetrical parts of the body. When you find a definite decrease in sensation, map it out by systematic testing in that area. Proceed from the point of decreased sensation towards the sensitive area. By asking the person to tell you where the sensation changes, you can map the exact borders of the deficient area. Draw your results on a diagram. Avoid asking leading questions, '*Can you feel this pinprick?*' This creates an expectation of how the person should feel the sensation, which is called *suggestion*. Instead, use unbiased directions such as, '*What can you feel?*' The person's eyes should be closed during each of the tests. Take time to explain what will be happening and exactly how you expect the person to respond.	Note if the topographic pattern of sensory loss is distal, i.e. over the hands and feet in a 'glove and stocking' distribution or if it is over a specific dermatome.
Spinothalamic tract	
Pain. Pain is tested by the person's ability to perceive a pinprick. Break a tongue blade lengthwise, forming a sharp point at the fractured end and a dull spot at the rounded end. Lightly apply the sharp point or the dull end to the person's body in a random, unpredictable order (Figure 12.29 A and B). Ask the person to say 'sharp' or 'dull', depending on the sensation felt. (Note that the sharp edge is used to test for pain; the dull edge is used as a general test of the person's responses.) Discard the tongue blade.	**Hypoalgesia**—decreased pain sensation. **Analgesia**—absent pain sensation. **Hyperalgesia**—increased pain sensation.

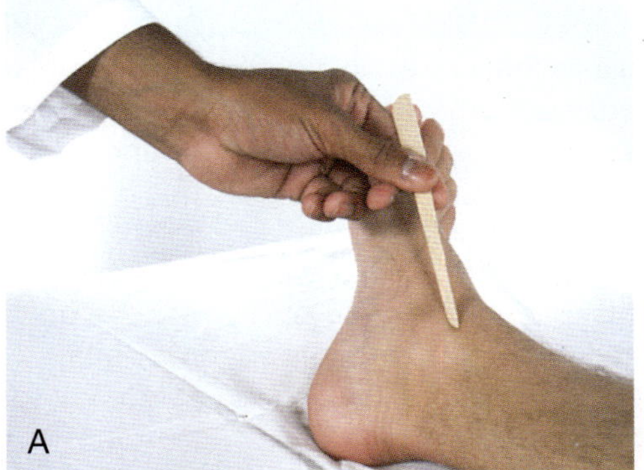

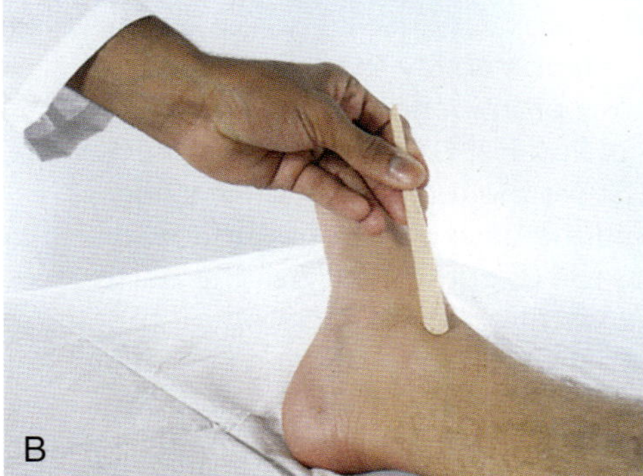

FIGURE 12.29 A & B Testing spinothalmic tract (pain perception)

PROCEDURES AND NORMAL FINDINGS	ABNORMAL FINDINGS AND CLINICAL ALERTS
Temperature. Test temperature sensation only when pain sensation is abnormal; otherwise, you may omit it because the fibres' tracts are much the same. Place a metal object (e.g. the flat side of a tuning fork) on the skin; the metal is almost always cold. Ask the person to describe the sensation.	
Light touch. Apply a wisp of cotton to the skin. Stretch a cotton ball to make a long end and brush it over the skin in a random order of sites and at irregular intervals (Figure 12.30). This prevents the person from responding just from repetition. Include the arms, forearms, hands, chest, thighs and legs. Ask the person to say 'now' or 'yes' when touch is felt. Compare symmetrical points. 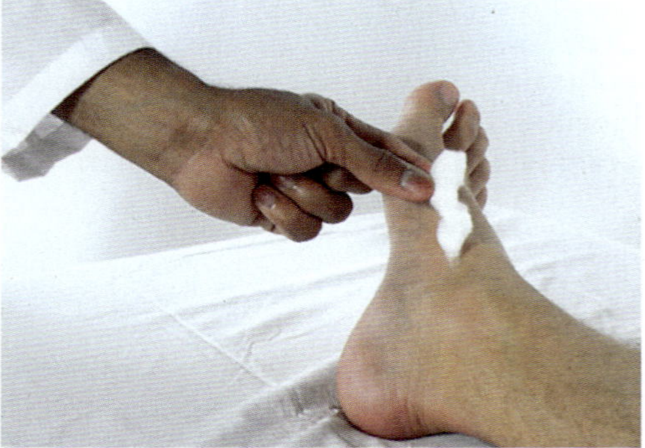 **FIGURE 12.30** Testing spinothalmic tract (light touch)	**Hypoaesthesia**—decreased touch sensation. **Anaesthesia**—absent touch sensation. **Hyperaesthesia**—increased touch sensation.
Posterior column tract	
Vibration. Test the person's ability to feel vibrations of a tuning fork over bony prominences. Use a low-pitch tuning fork (128 Hz or 256 Hz) because its vibration has a slower decay. Strike the tuning fork on the heel of your hand and hold the base on a bony surface of the fingers and great toe (Figure 12.31). Ask the person to indicate when the vibration starts and stops. If the person feels the normal vibration or buzzing sensation on these distal areas, you may assume proximal spots are normal and proceed no further. If no vibrations are felt, move proximally and test ulnar processes and ankles, patellae and iliac crests. Compare the right side with the left side. If you find a deficit, note whether it is gradual or abrupt.	Unable to feel vibration. Loss of vibration sense occurs with peripheral neuropathy (e.g. type 1 and type 2 diabetes and alcohol dependence). Often, this is the first sensation lost. Peripheral neuropathy is worse at the feet and gradually improves as you move up the leg, as opposed to a specific nerve lesion, which has a clear zone of deficit for its dermatome.

PROCEDURES AND NORMAL FINDINGS	ABNORMAL FINDINGS AND CLINICAL ALERTS

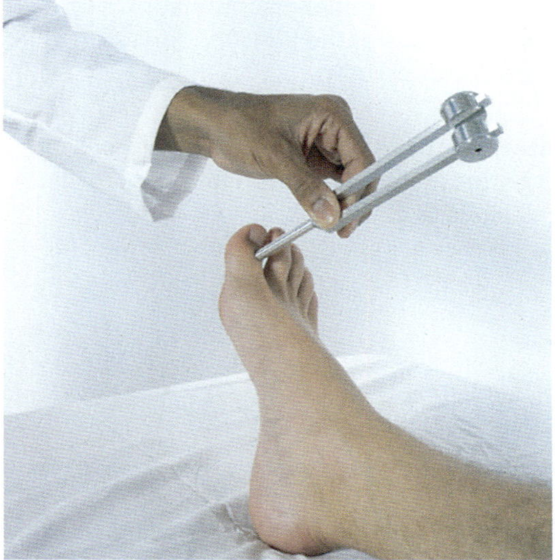

FIGURE 12.31 Testing posterior column tract (vibration)

Position (kinaesthesia). Test the person's ability to perceive passive movements of the extremities. Move a finger or the big toe up and down and ask the person to tell you which way it is moved (Figure 12.32). The test is done with the eyes closed, but to be sure it is understood, have the person watch a few trials first. Vary the order of movement up or down. Hold the digit by the sides, since upwards or downwards pressure on the skin may provide a clue as to how it has been moved. Normally, a person can detect movement of a few millimetres.

Loss of position sense.

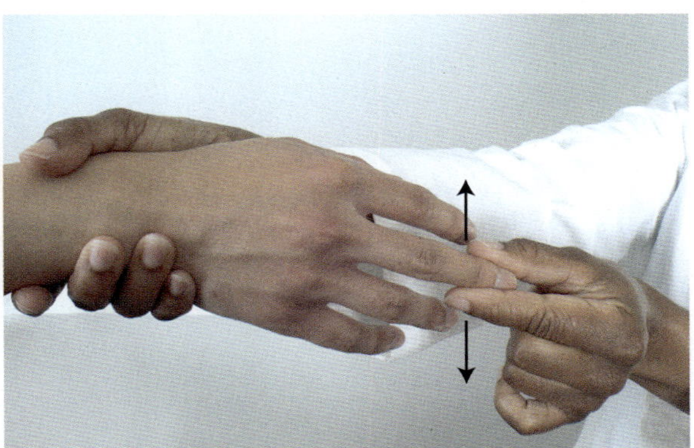

FIGURE 12.32 Testing posterior column tract (position)

PROCEDURES AND NORMAL FINDINGS	ABNORMAL FINDINGS AND CLINICAL ALERTS
Tactile discrimination (fine touch). The following tests also measure the discrimination ability of the sensory cortex. As a prerequisite, the person needs a normal or near-normal sense of touch and position sense.	Problems with tactile discrimination occur with lesions of the sensory cortex or posterior column.
Stereognosis. Test the person's ability to recognise objects by feeling their forms, sizes and weights. With the eyes closed, place a familiar object (paperclip, key, coin, cotton ball or pencil) in the person's hand and ask the person to identify it (Figure 12.33). Normally, a person will explore it with the fingers and correctly name it. Test a different object in each hand; testing the left hand assesses right parietal lobe functioning. 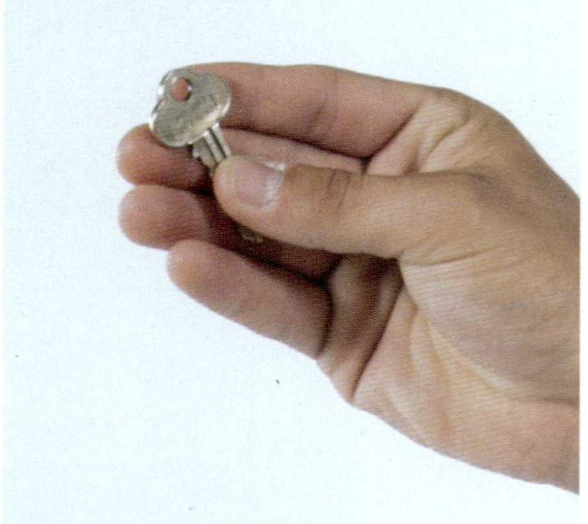 **FIGURE 12.33** Stereognosis	**Astereognosis**—inability to identify object correctly. Occurs in sensory cortex lesions (e.g. stroke).
Graphaesthesia. Graphaesthesia is the ability to 'read' a number by having it traced on the skin. With the person's eyes closed, use a blunt instrument to trace a single digit number or a letter on the palm (Figure 12.34). Ask the person to tell you what it is. Graphaesthesia is a good measure of sensory loss if the person cannot make the hand movements needed for stereognosis, as occurs in arthritis. 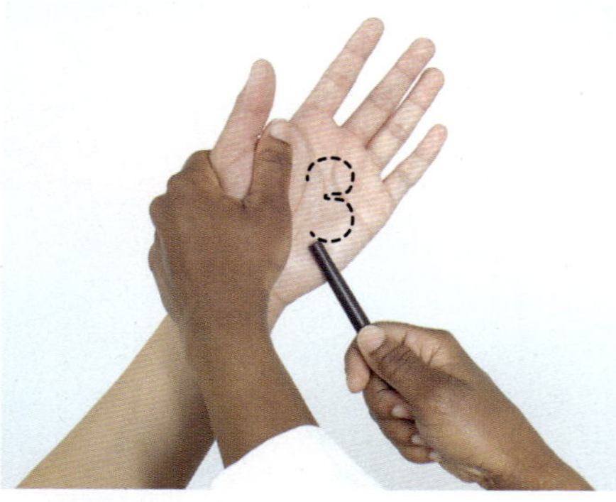 **FIGURE 12.34** Graphaesthesia	Inability to distinguish number occurs with lesions of the sensory cortex.

PROCEDURES AND NORMAL FINDINGS	ABNORMAL FINDINGS AND CLINICAL ALERTS
Two-point discrimination. Test the person's ability to distinguish the separation of two simultaneous pin-points on the skin. Apply the two points of an opened paper clip lightly to the skin in ever-closing distances. Note the distance at which the person no longer perceives two separate points. The level of perception varies considerably with the region tested; it is most sensitive in the fingertips (2–8 mm) and least sensitive on the upper arms, thighs and back (40–75 mm).	An increase in the distance it normally takes to identify two separate points occurs with sensory cortex lesions.
Extinction. Simultaneously touch both sides of the body at the same point. Ask the person to state how many sensations are felt and where they are. Normally, both sensations are felt.	The ability to recognise only one of the stimuli occurs with sensory cortex lesion; the stimulus is extinguished on the side *opposite* the cortex lesion.
Point location. Touch the skin and withdraw the stimulus promptly. Tell the person, '*Put your finger where I touched you*'. You can perform this test simultaneously with light touch sensation.	With a sensory cortex lesion, the person cannot localise the sensation accurately, even though light touch sensation may be retained.

Test the reflexes

Stretch or deep tendon reflexes

Measurement of the stretch reflexes reveals the intactness of the reflex arc at specific spinal levels as well as the normal override on the reflex of the higher cortical levels.

For an adequate response, the limb should be relaxed and the muscle partially stretched. Stimulate the reflex by directing a short, snappy blow of the reflex hammer onto the muscle's insertion tendon. Use a relaxed hold on the hammer.

As with the percussion technique, the action takes place at the wrist. Strike a brief, well-aimed blow and bounce up promptly; do not let the hammer rest on the tendon. Use the pointed end of the reflex hammer when aiming at a smaller target such as your thumb on the tendon site; use the flat end when the target is wider or to diffuse the impact and prevent pain.

Use just enough force to get a response. Compare right and left sides—the responses should be equal.

PROCEDURES AND NORMAL FINDINGS

The reflex response is graded on a four-point scale:
4+ Very brisk, hyperactive with clonus, indicative of disease
3+ Brisker than average, may indicate disease
2+ Average, normal
1+ Diminished, low normal
0 No response.
This is a subjective scale and requires some clinical practice. Even then, the scale is not completely reliable because no standard exists to say *how* brisk a reflex should be to warrant a grade of 3+. Also, a wide range of normal exists in reflex responses. Healthy people may have diminished reflexes or they may have brisk ones. Your best plan is to interpret the deep tendon reflexes *only* within the context of the rest of the neurological assessment and findings over time.

Sometimes the reflex response fails to appear. Try further encouragement of relaxation, varying the person's position or increasing the strength of the blow. **Reinforcement** is another technique to relax the muscles and enhance the response (Figure 12.35). Ask the person to perform an isometric exercise in a muscle group somewhat away from the one being tested. For example, to enhance a patellar reflex, ask the person to lock the fingers together and 'pull'. Then strike the tendon. To enhance a biceps response, ask the person to clench the teeth or to grasp the thigh with the opposite hand.

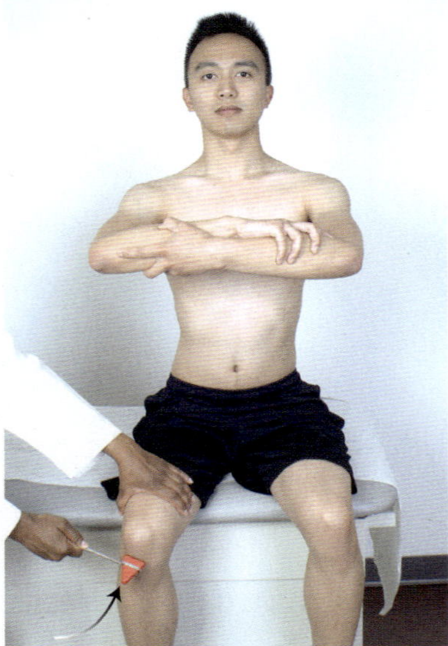

FIGURE 12.35 Reinforcement

ABNORMAL FINDINGS AND CLINICAL ALERTS

Clonus is a set of rapid, rhythmic contractions of the same muscle.

Hyperreflexia is the exaggerated reflex seen when the monosynaptic reflex arc is released from the usually inhibiting influence of higher cortical levels. This occurs with upper motor neuron lesions (e.g. a stroke).

Hyporeflexia, which is the absence of a reflex, is a lower motor neuron problem. It occurs with interruption of sensory afferents or destruction of motor efferents and anterior horn cells (e.g. spinal cord injury).

PROCEDURES AND NORMAL FINDINGS	ABNORMAL FINDINGS AND CLINICAL ALERTS

Biceps reflex (C5 to C6). Support the person's forearm on yours; this position relaxes, as well as partially flexes, the person's arm. Place your thumb on the biceps tendon and strike a blow on your thumb. You can feel as well as see the normal response, which is contraction of the biceps muscle and flexion of the forearm (Figure 12.36).

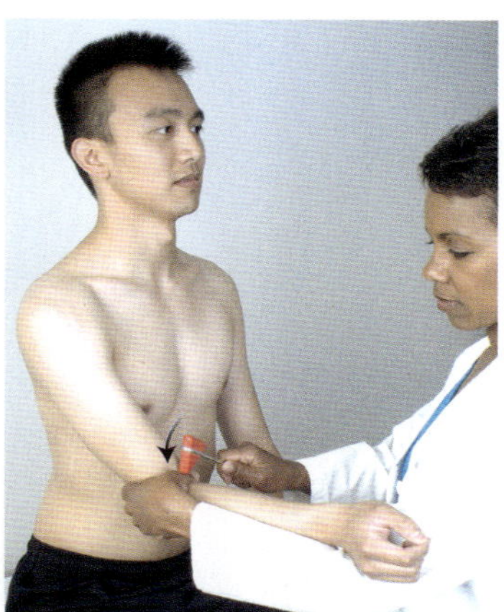

FIGURE 12.36 Biceps reflex

Triceps reflex (C7 to C8). Tell the person to let the arm 'just go dead' as you suspend it by holding the upper arm. Strike the triceps tendon directly just above the elbow (Figure 12.37). The normal response is extension of the forearm. Alternatively, hold the person's wrist across the chest to flex the arm at the elbow and tap the tendon.

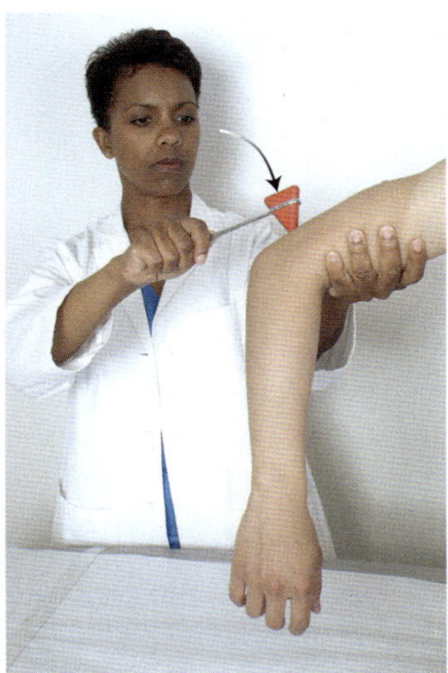

FIGURE 12.37 Triceps reflex

PROCEDURES AND NORMAL FINDINGS	ABNORMAL FINDINGS AND CLINICAL ALERTS

Brachioradialis reflex (C5 to C6). Hold the person's thumbs to suspend the forearms in relaxation. Strike the forearm directly, 2 to 3 cm above the radial styloid process (Figure 12.38). The normal response is flexion and supination of the forearm.

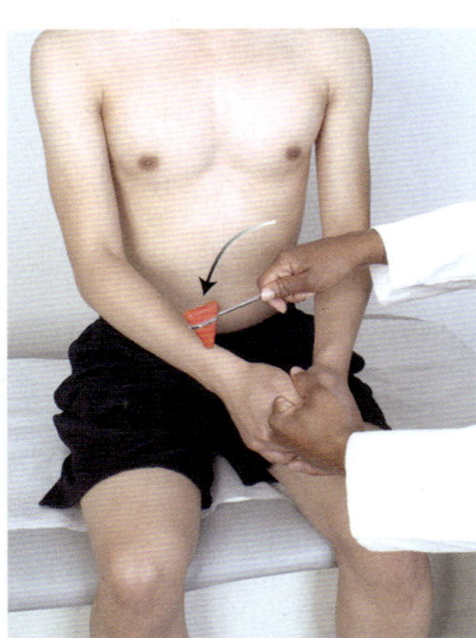

FIGURE 12.38 Brachioradialis reflex

Quadriceps reflex ('knee jerk') (L2 to L4). Let the lower legs dangle freely to flex the knee and stretch the tendons. Strike the tendon directly just below the patella (Figure 12.39). Extension of the lower leg is the expected response. You will also palpate contraction of the quadriceps.

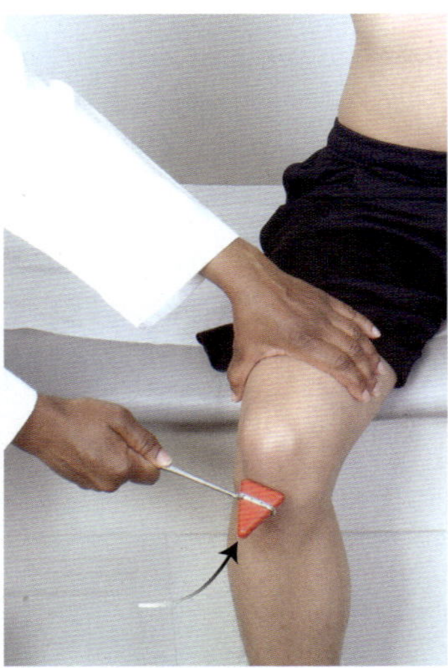

FIGURE 12.39 Quadriceps reflex

PROCEDURES AND NORMAL FINDINGS	ABNORMAL FINDINGS AND CLINICAL ALERTS

For the person in the supine position, use your own arm as a lever to support the weight of one leg against the other leg. This manoeuvre also flexes the knee (Figure 12.40).

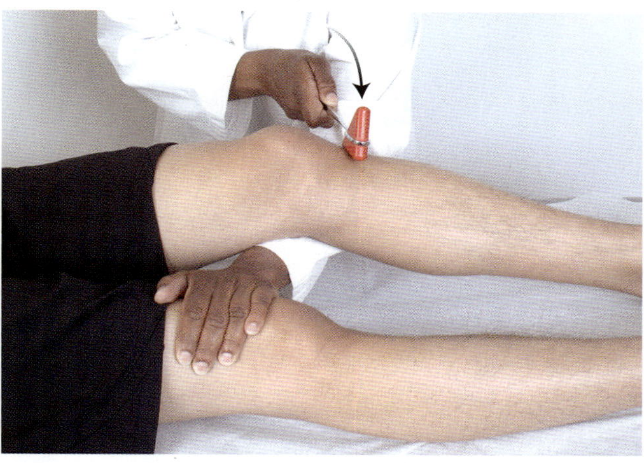

FIGURE 12.40 Supine quadriceps reflex

Achilles reflex ('ankle jerk') (L5 to S2). Position the person with the knee flexed and the hip externally rotated. Hold the foot in dorsiflexion and strike the Achilles tendon directly (Figure 12.41). Feel the normal response as the foot plantar flexes against your hand.

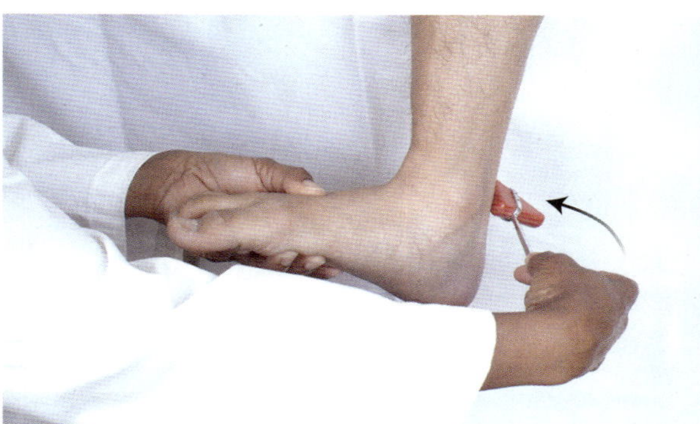

FIGURE 12.41 Achilles reflex

PROCEDURES AND NORMAL FINDINGS	ABNORMAL FINDINGS AND CLINICAL ALERTS

For the person in the supine position, flex one knee and support that lower leg against the other leg so that it falls 'open'. Dorsiflex the foot and tap the tendon (Figure 12.42).

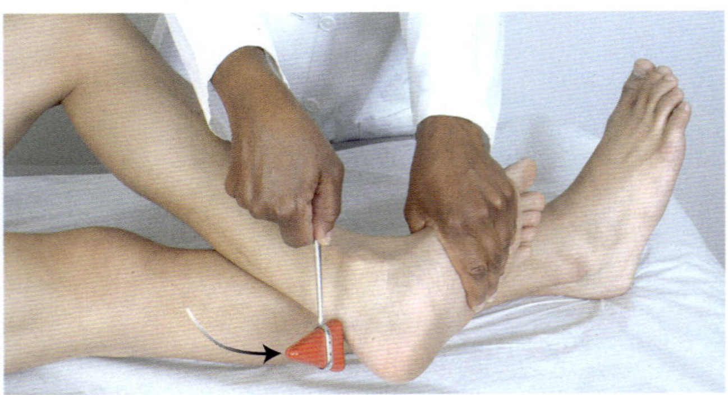

FIGURE 12.42 Supine Achilles reflex

Clonus. Test for clonus, particularly when the reflexes are hyperactive. Support the lower leg in one hand. With your other hand, move the foot up and down a few times to relax the muscle. Then stretch the muscle by briskly dorsiflexing the foot. Hold the stretch (Figure 12.43). With a normal response, you feel no further movement. When clonus is present, you will feel and see rapid rhythmic contractions of the calf muscle and movement of the foot.

Clonus is repeated reflex muscular movements. A hyperactive reflex with sustained clonus (lasting as long as the stretch is held) occurs with upper motor neuron disease.

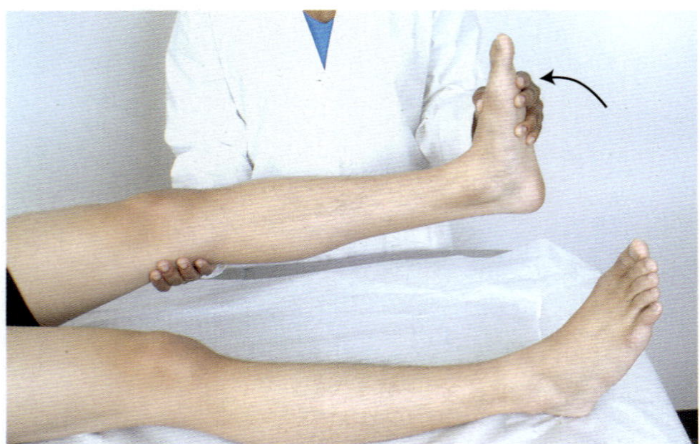

FIGURE 12.43 Test for clonus

PROCEDURES AND NORMAL FINDINGS	ABNORMAL FINDINGS AND CLINICAL ALERTS

Superficial (cutaneous) reflexes

Here, the sensory receptors are in the skin rather than in the muscles. The motor response is a localised muscle contraction.

Abdominal reflexes—upper (T8 to T10), lower (T10 to T12). Have the person assume a supine position, with the knees slightly bent. Use the handle end of the reflex hammer, a wood applicator tip or the end of a split tongue blade to stroke the skin. Move from the side of the abdomen towards the midline at both the upper and the lower abdominal levels (Figure 12.44). The normal response is ipsilateral contraction of the abdominal muscle with an observed deviation of the umbilicus towards the stroke. When the abdominal wall is very obese, pull the skin to the opposite side and feel it contract towards the stimulus.

Superficial reflexes are absent with diseases of the pyramidal tract—for example, they are absent on the contralateral side with stroke.

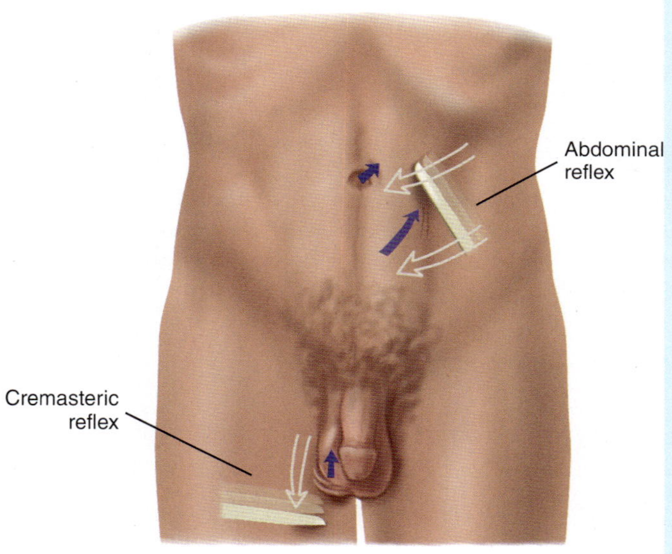

FIGURE 12.44 Abdominal reflexes

Cremasteric reflex (L1 to L2). This is not routinely done. On the male, lightly stroke the inner aspect of the thigh with the reflex hammer or tongue blade (Figure 12.44). Note elevation of the ipsilateral testicle.

Absent in both upper motor neuron and lower motor neuron lesions (Table 12.14).

Plantar reflex (L4 to S2). Position the thigh in slight external rotation. With the reflex hammer, draw a light stroke up the lateral side of the sole of the foot and inwards across the ball of the foot, like an upside-down J (Figure 12.45A). The normal response is plantar flexion of the toes and inversion and flexion of the forefoot.

Except in infancy, the abnormal response is dorsiflexion of the big toe and fanning of all toes, which is a positive **Babinski's sign**, also called 'upgoing toes' (Figure 12.45B). This occurs with upper motor neuron disease of the corticospinal (or pyramidal) tract (Table 12.17).

PROCEDURES AND NORMAL FINDINGS	ABNORMAL FINDINGS AND CLINICAL ALERTS

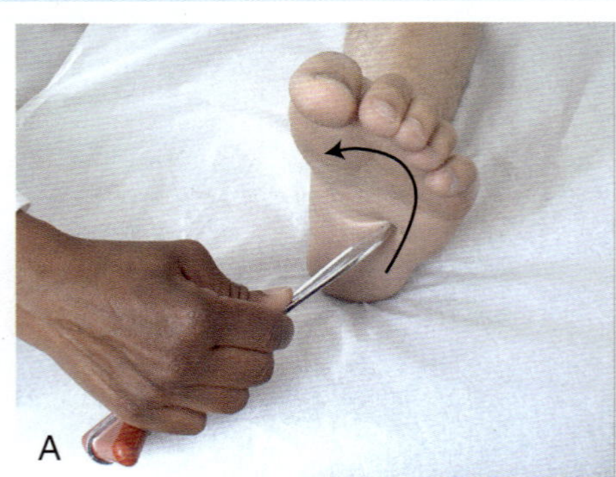

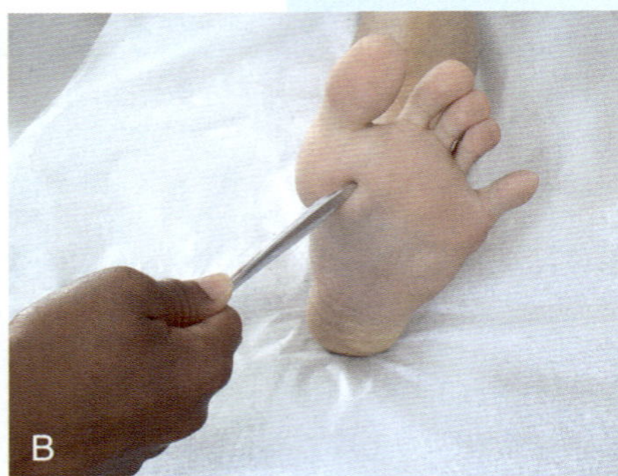

FIGURE 12.45 A & B Plantar reflex

Additional objective assessment for infants and toddlers

Skull

Measure an infant's **head size** with measuring tape at periodic health checks up to age 2 years, then yearly up to age 6 years. (Measurement of head circumference is presented in detail in Chapter 3.)

Note an abnormal increase in head size or failure to grow.

A newborn's head measures about 32 to 38 cm (average around 34 cm) and is 2 cm larger than chest circumference. At age 2 years, both measurements are the same. During childhood the chest circumference grows to exceed head circumference by 5 to 7 cm.

Microcephalic—head size below norms for age.

Macrocephalic—an enlarged head for age or rapidly increasing in size (e.g. hydrocephalus [increased cerebrospinal fluid]).

Observe the infant's head from all angles, not just the front. The contour should be symmetrical. Some variation occurs in normal head shapes.

Frontal bulges or 'bossing', occur with prematurity or rickets.

Two common variations in the newborn cause the shape of the skull to look markedly asymmetrical: a **caput succedaneum** is oedematous swelling and ecchymosis of the presenting part of the head caused by birth trauma (Figure 12.46). It feels soft and it may extend across suture lines. It gradually resolves during the first few days of life and needs no treatment.

PROCEDURES AND NORMAL FINDINGS	ABNORMAL FINDINGS AND CLINICAL ALERTS

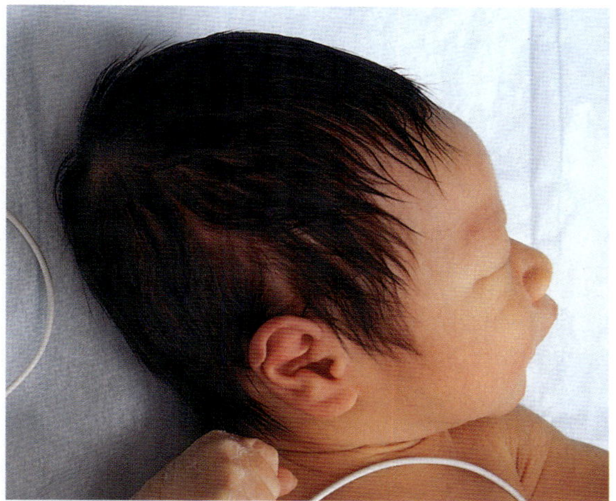

FIGURE 12.46 Caput succedaneum

A **cephalhaematoma** is a subperiosteal haemorrhage, which is also a result of birth trauma (Figure 12.47 A and B). It is soft, fluctuant and well defined over one cranial bone because the periosteum (i.e. the covering over each bone) holds the bleeding in place. It appears several hours after birth and gradually increases in size. No discolouration is present, but it looks bizarre, so parents need reassurance that it will be reabsorbed during the first few weeks of life without treatment. Rarely, a large haematoma may persist to 3 months.

An infant with cephalhaematoma is at greater risk for jaundice as the red blood cells within the haematoma are broken down and reabsorbed.

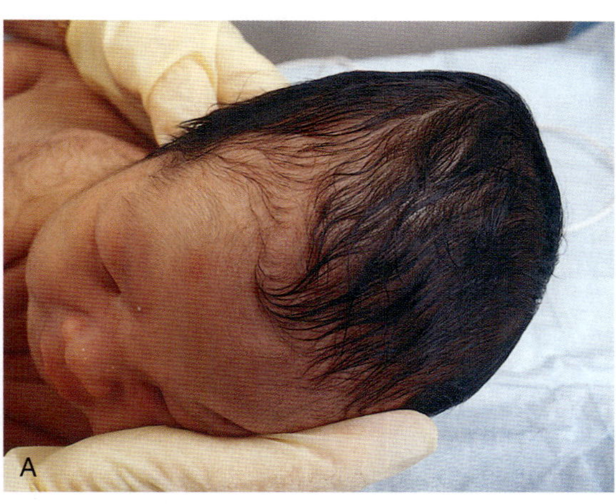

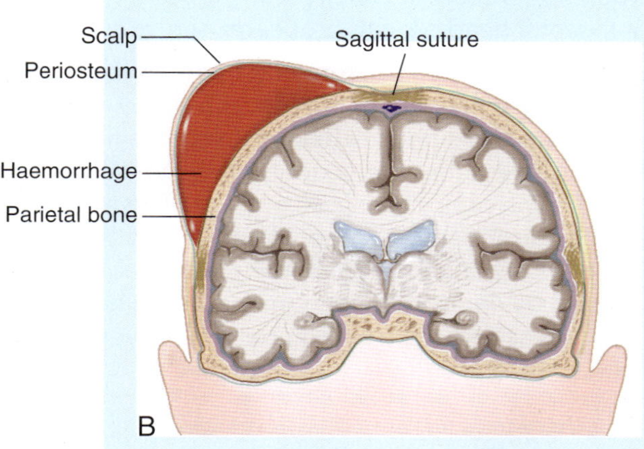

FIGURE 12.47 A & B Cephalhaematoma

PROCEDURES AND NORMAL FINDINGS	ABNORMAL FINDINGS AND CLINICAL ALERTS
As you palpate the newborn's head, the suture lines feel like ridges. By 5 to 6 months, they are smooth and not palpable.	Sutures palpable when the child is older than 6 months.
A newborn's head may feel asymmetrical and the involved ridges more prominent due to **moulding** of the cranial bones during engagement and passage through the birth canal. Moulding is overriding of the cranial bones; usually, the parietal bone overrides the frontal or occipital bone. Reassure parents that this lasts only a few days or a week. Babies delivered by caesarean section are noted for their evenly round heads. Also, some asymmetry may occur if an infant continually sleeps in one position; this is a flattening of the dependent cranial bone, usually the occiput.	Marked asymmetry, as in **craniosynostosis**, a severe deformity caused by premature closure of the sutures. Premature closing of the sutures results in a long, narrow head. Flattening also occurs with rickets or developmental delay.
Gently palpate the skull and **fontanels** while the infant is calm and somewhat in a sitting position (crying, lying down or vomiting may cause the anterior fontanel to look full and bulging). The skull should feel smooth and fused except at the fontanels. The fontanels feel firm, slightly concave and well-defined against the edges of the cranial bones. You may see slight arterial pulsations in the anterior fontanel.	A true tense or bulging fontanel occurs with acute increased intracranial pressure. Depressed and sunken fontanels occur with dehydration or malnutrition. Marked pulsations occur with increased intracranial pressure.
The posterior fontanel may not be palpable at birth. If it is, it measures 1 cm and closes by 1 to 2 months. The anterior fontanel may be small at birth and enlarge to 2.5 × 2.5 cm. A large diameter of 4 to 5 cm occasionally may be normal under 6 months. A small fontanel is usually normal. The anterior fontanel closes between 9 months and 2 years. Early closure may be insignificant if head growth proceeds normally.	Delayed closure or larger-than-normal fontanel size occurs with hydrocephalus, trisomy 21, hypothyroidism or rickets. A small fontanel is a sign of microcephaly, as is early closure.
Note the infant's **head posture** and **head control**. Infants can turn their heads side to side by 2 weeks and show the **tonic neck reflex** when supine and the head is turned to one side (extension of same arm and leg, flexion of opposite arm and leg). The tonic neck reflex disappears between 3 and 4 months, then the head is maintained in the midline. Head control is achieved by 4 months, when the baby can hold the head erect and steady when pulled to a vertical position.	Tonic neck reflex beyond 5 months may indicate brain damage. In children, head tilt occurs with habit spasm, poor vision and brain tumour. Head lag after 4 months may indicate developmental delay.
Face	
Check **facial features** for symmetry, appearance and presence of swelling. Note symmetry of wrinkling when the infant cries or smiles (e.g. both sides of the lips rise and both sides of forehead wrinkle). Parotid gland enlargement is seen best when the infant/toddler sits and looks up at the ceiling; the swelling appears below the angle of the jaw.	Unilateral immobility indicates nerve damage (central or peripheral) (e.g. note angle of mouth droop on paralysed side). Some facies are characteristic of congenital abnormalities or chronic allergy (Table 12.10).

PROCEDURES AND NORMAL FINDINGS	ABNORMAL FINDINGS AND CLINICAL ALERTS
Neck	
An infant's neck looks short; it lengthens during the first 3 to 4 years. You can see the neck better by supporting the infant's shoulders and tilting the head back a little. This positioning also enhances palpation of the trachea, which is buried deep in the neck. Feel for the row of cartilaginous rings in the midline or just slightly to the right of midline.	A short neck or webbing (loose fan-like folds) may indicate congenital abnormality (e.g. Trisomy 21 or Turner's syndrome) or it may occur alone.
Assess muscle development with gentle passive ROM. Cradle the infant's head with your hands and turn it side to side and test forward flexion, extension and rotation. Note any resistance to movement, especially flexion.	Head tilt and limited ROM occur with **torticollis** (wryneck) or from sternocleidomastoid muscle injury during birth or a congenital defect. Resistance to flexion (nuchal rigidity) and pain on flexion indicate meningeal irritation or meningitis.
The neurological system shows dramatic growth and development during the first year of life. Assessment includes noting that milestones you normally would expect for each month have indeed been achieved and that the early, more primitive reflexes cease at the appropriate developmental stage.	Failure to attain a skill by expected time. Persistence of reflex behaviour beyond the normal time.
At birth, newborns are very alert, with the eyes open and demonstrating strong, urgent sucking. The normal cry is loud, lusty and even angry. The next 2 or 3 days may be spent mostly sleeping as the baby recovers from the birth process. After that, the pattern of sleep and waking activity is highly variable; it depends on the baby's individual body rhythm as well as external stimuli.	A high-pitched, shrill cry or cat-sounding screech occurs with CNS damage. A weak, groaning cry or expiratory grunt occurs with respiratory distress.
The behavioural assessment should include your observations of the infant's spontaneous waking activity, responses to environmental stimuli and social interaction with the parents and others.	 ***Clinical alert:*** Lethargy, hyporeactivity, hyperirritability and parent's report of significant change in behaviour all warrant referral.
By 2 months of age, babies smile responsively and recognise the parents' faces. Babbling occurs at 4 months and one or two words (mama, dada) are used nonspecifically after 9 months.	
The motor system	
Observe spontaneous motor activity for smoothness and symmetry. Smoothness of movement suggests proper cerebellar function, as does the coordination involved in sucking and swallowing. To screen gross and fine motor coordination, use the Denver II test with its age-specific developmental milestones. You also can assess movement by testing the reflexes listed in the following section. Note their smoothness of response and symmetry. Also, note whether their presence or absence is appropriate for the infant's age.	Delay in motor activity occurs with brain damage, cognitive delay, peripheral neuromuscular damage, prolonged illness and parental neglect.

PROCEDURES AND NORMAL FINDINGS

Assess muscle tone by first observing resting posture. The newborn favours a flexed position; extremities are symmetrically folded inwards; the hips are slightly abducted and the fists are tightly flexed (Figure 12.48). Infants born by breech delivery, however, do not have flexion in the lower extremities.

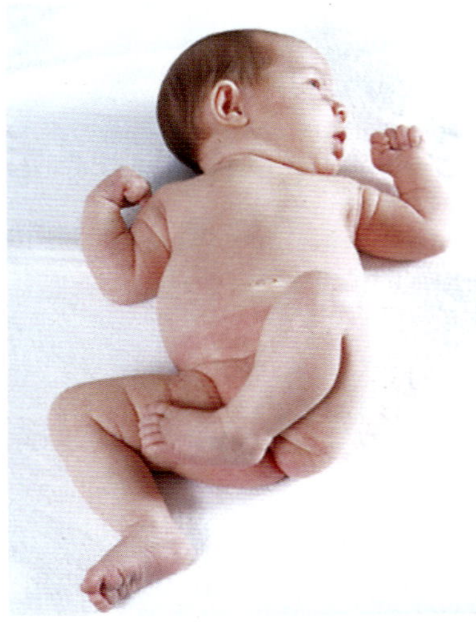

FIGURE 12.48 Assess muscle tone (newborn)

After 2 months of age, flexion gives way to gradual extension, beginning with the head and continuing in a cephalocaudal direction. Now is the time to check for spasticity; none should be present. Test for spasticity by flexing the infant's knees onto the abdomen and then quickly releasing them. They will unfold but not too quickly. Also, gently push the head forward—the baby should comply.

The fists are normally held in tight flexion for the first 3 months. Then the fists open for part of the time. A purposeful reach for an object with both hands occurs around 4 months of age, a transfer of an object from hand to hand at 7 months of age, a grasp using fingers and opposing thumb at 9 months of age and a purposeful release at 10 months of age. Babies are normally ambidextrous for the first 18 months.

Head control is an important milestone in motor development. You can incorporate the following two movements into every infant assessment to check the muscle tone necessary for head control.

ABNORMAL FINDINGS AND CLINICAL ALERTS

Abnormal postures:

Frog position—hips abducted and almost flat against the table, externally rotated (only normal after breech delivery).

Opisthotonos—head arched back, stiffness of neck and extension of arms and legs; occurs with meningeal or brainstem irritation and kernicterus (Table 12.9).

Extension of limbs may occur with intracranial haemorrhage.

Any type of continual asymmetry—for example, asymmetry of upper limbs occurs with **brachial plexus palsy.**

Spasticity is an early sign of cerebral palsy. After releasing flexed knees, legs will quickly extend and adduct, even to a 'scissoring' motion when spasticity is present. Also, the baby often resists head flexion and extends back against your hand when spasticity is present (Table 12.8).

Note a persistent one-hand preference in babies younger than 18 months of age, which may indicate a motor deficit on the opposite side.

PROCEDURES AND NORMAL FINDINGS

First, with the baby supine, pull to a sit holding the wrists and note head control (Figure 12.49A). The newborn will hold the head almost in the same plane as the body and it will balance briefly when the baby reaches a sitting position, then flop forward. (Even a premature infant shows some head flexion.) At 4 months of age, the head stays in line with the body and does not flop.

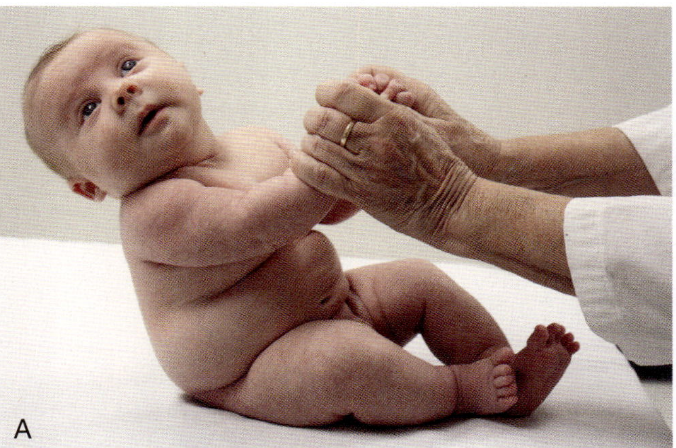

FIGURE 12.49A Assess head control

Second, lift up the baby in a prone position, with one hand supporting the chest (Figure 12.49B). The term newborn holds the head at an angle of 45 degrees or less from horizontal, the back is straight or slightly arched and the elbows and knees are partly flexed.

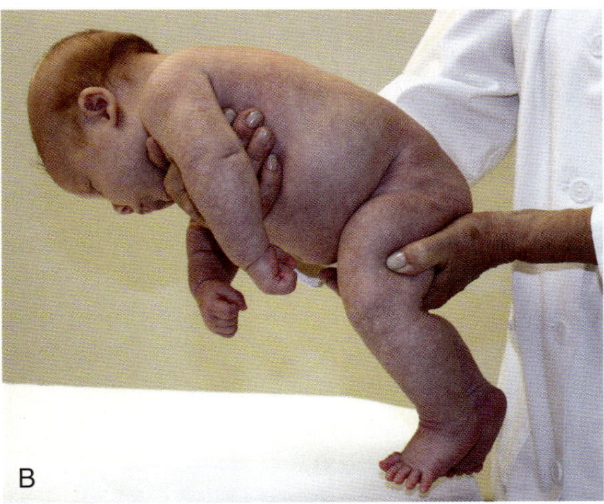

FIGURE 12.49B Assess head control

ABNORMAL FINDINGS AND CLINICAL ALERTS

Because development progresses in a cephalocaudal direction, head lag is an early sign of brain damage.

Clinical alert: After 6 months of age, refer any baby with failure to hold their head in midline when sitting.

PROCEDURES AND NORMAL FINDINGS	ABNORMAL FINDINGS AND CLINICAL ALERTS
At 3 months of age, the baby raises their head and arches the back, as in a swan dive. This is the **Landau reflex**, which persists until 18 months of age.	Head lag, a limp, floppy trunk and dangling arms and legs. Absence of the reflex indicates motor weakness, upper motor neuron disease or cognitive delay.
Assess muscle strength by noting the strength of sucking and of spontaneous motor activity. Normally, no tremors are present and no continual overshooting of the mark occurs when reaching (Figure 12.50).	

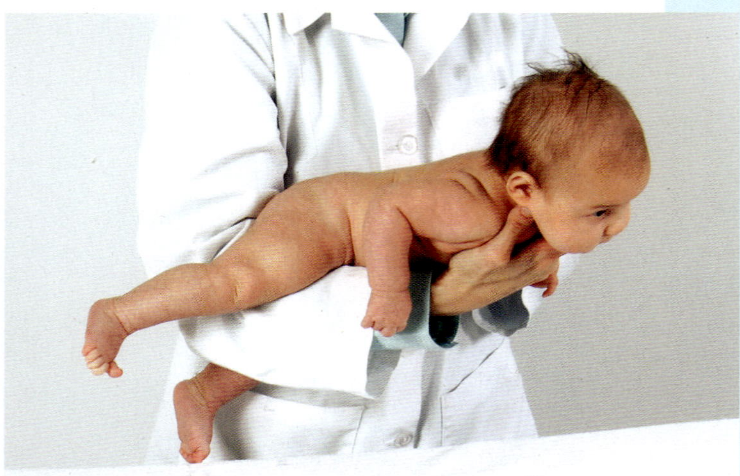

FIGURE 12.50 Assess muscle strength

The sensory system

You will perform very little sensory testing with infants and toddlers. The newborn normally has hypoaesthesia and requires a strong stimulus to elicit a response. The baby responds to pain by crying and a general reflex withdrawal of all limbs. By 7 to 9 months of age, the infant can localise the stimulus and shows more specific signs of withdrawal. Other sensory modalities are not tested.	Unusually rapid withdrawal is **hyperaesthesia**, which occurs with spinal cord lesions, CNS infections, increased intracranial pressure, peritonitis. No withdrawal is decreased sensation, which occurs with decreased consciousness, cognitive delay, spinal cord or peripheral nerve lesions.

The motor system—reflexes

Infantile automatisms are reflexes that have a predictable timetable of appearance and departure. The reflexes most tested are listed in the following section. For the screening examination, you can just check the rooting, grasp, tonic neck and Moro reflexes.

PROCEDURES AND NORMAL FINDINGS	ABNORMAL FINDINGS AND CLINICAL ALERTS
Rooting reflex. Brush the infant's cheek near the mouth. Note whether the infant turns the head towards that side and opens the mouth. Appears at birth and disappears at 3 to 4 months.	
Sucking reflex. Touch the lips and offer your gloved little finger to suck. Note strong sucking reflex. The reflex is present at birth and disappears at 10 to 12 months.	
Palmar grasp. Place the baby's head midline to ensure symmetrical response. Offer your finger from the baby's ulnar side, away from the thumb. Note the tight grasp of all the baby's fingers (Figure 12.51). Sucking enhances grasp. Often you can pull baby to a sit from grasp. The reflex is present at birth, is strongest at 1 to 2 months and disappears at 3 to 4 months.	The palmar grasp reflex is absent with brain damage and with local muscle or nerve injury. Persistence of palmar grasp reflex after 4 months of age occurs with frontal lobe lesion.

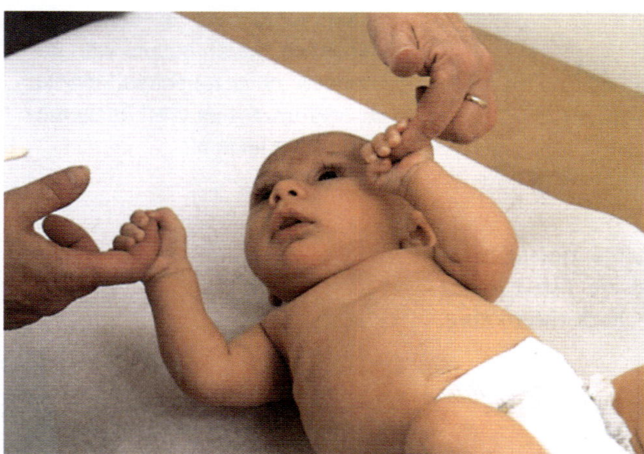

FIGURE 12.51 Assess palmar grasp

Plantar grasp. Touch your thumb at the ball of the baby's foot. Note that the toes curl down tightly (Figure 12.52). The reflex is present at birth and disappears at 8 to 10 months.

PROCEDURES AND NORMAL FINDINGS	ABNORMAL FINDINGS AND CLINICAL ALERTS
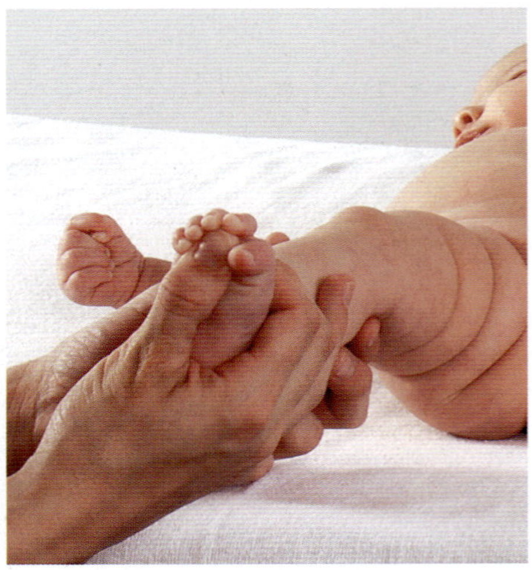 **FIGURE 12.52** Assess plantar grasp	
Babinski's reflex. Stroke your finger up the lateral edge and across the ball of the infant's foot. Note fanning of toes (positive Babinski's reflex) (Figure 12.53). The reflex is present at birth and disappears (changes to the adult response) by 24 months of age (variable).	Positive Babinski's reflex after 2 or 2½ years of age occurs with pyramidal tract disease. See Table 12.17.
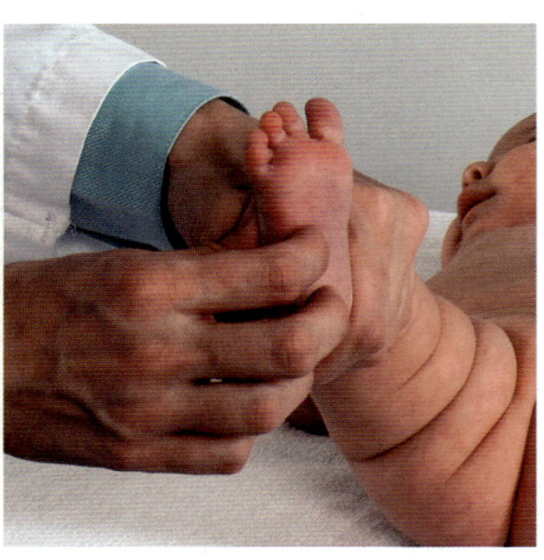 **FIGURE 12.53** Babinski's reflex	

PROCEDURES AND NORMAL FINDINGS	ABNORMAL FINDINGS AND CLINICAL ALERTS
Tonic neck reflex. With the baby supine, relaxed or sleeping, turn the head to one side with the chin over shoulder. Note ipsilateral extension of the arm and leg and flexion of the opposite arm and leg; this is the 'fencing' position. If you turn the infant's head to the opposite side, positions will reverse (Figure 12.54). The reflex appears by 2 to 3 months, decreases at 3 to 4 months and disappears by 4 to 6 months.	Persistence later in infancy occurs with brain damage.

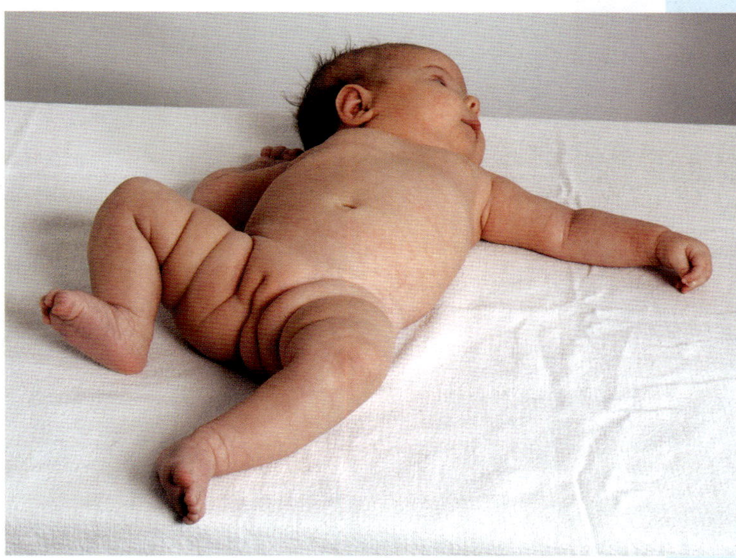

FIGURE 12.54 Tonic neck reflex

PROCEDURES AND NORMAL FINDINGS	ABNORMAL FINDINGS AND CLINICAL ALERTS
Moro reflex. Startle the infant by jarring the cot, making a loud noise or supporting the head and back in a semi-sitting position and quickly lowering the infant to 30 degrees. The baby looks as if they are hugging a tree. That is, symmetrical abduction and extension of the arms and legs, fanning fingers and curling of the index finger and thumb to C position occur. The infant then brings in both arms and legs (Figure 12.55). The reflex is present at birth and disappears at 1 to 4 months.	Absence of the Moro reflex in the newborn or persistence after 5 months of age indicates severe CNS injury. Absence of movement in just one arm occurs with fracture of the humerus or clavicle and with brachial nerve palsy. Absence in one leg occurs with a lower spinal cord problem or a dislocated hip. A hyperactive Moro reflex occurs with tetany or CNS infection.

PROCEDURES AND NORMAL FINDINGS	ABNORMAL FINDINGS AND CLINICAL ALERTS
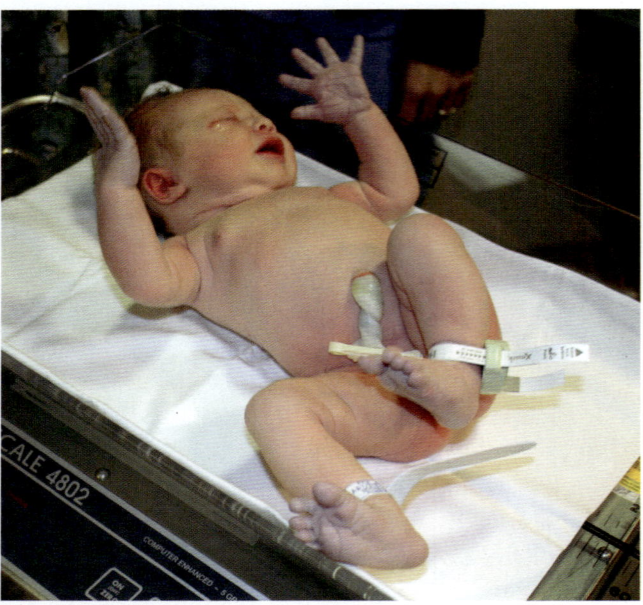 **FIGURE 12.55** Moro reflex	
Placing reflex. Hold the infant upright under the arms, close to a table. Let the dorsal 'top' of foot touch the underside of table. Note flexing of hip and knee, followed by extension at the hip, to place foot on table. Reflex appears at 4 days after birth.	
Stepping reflex. Hold the infant upright under the arms, with the feet on a flat surface. Note regular alternating steps. The reflex disappears before voluntary walking.	**Extensor thrust** or 'scissoring'; crossing of lower extremities.
Special procedures	
Palpation. Craniotabes is a softening of the skull's outer layer. With a newborn, pressure along the suture of the parietal and occipital bones above the ear produces a snapping sensation because of the pliable skull bone. It is like indenting a ping-pong ball and feeling it snap back. Do not attempt this unless craniotabes is suspected because of other abnormal findings and, even then, avoid excessive pressure. Craniotabes may be normal, especially with premature infants.	**Craniotabes** may occur with rickets, hydrocephaly or congenital syphilis.
Percussion. With an infant, you may directly percuss with your plexor finger against the head surface. This yields a resonant or 'cracked pot' sound, which is normal before closure of the fontanels.	The sound occurs with hydrocephalus from separation of cranial sutures (Macewen's sign).

PROCEDURES AND NORMAL FINDINGS	ABNORMAL FINDINGS AND CLINICAL ALERTS
Auscultation. Bruits are common in the skull in children under 4 or 5 years of age or in children with anaemia. They are systolic or continuous and are heard over the temporal area.	After 5 years of age, bruits indicate increased intracranial pressure, aneurysm or arteriovenous shunt. If you suspect an abnormal head size or an intracranial lesion refer to medical practitioner for further assessment.
Additional objective assessment for children	
Use the same sequence of neurological assessment as with the adult, with the omissions or modifications mentioned in the following section.	
Behaviour	
Assess the child's general behaviour during play activities, reaction to parent and cooperation with parent and with you. Complete details are described in Chapter 11.	
Cranial nerves	
Smell and taste are almost never tested, but if you need to test the child's sense of smell (cranial nerve I), use a scent familiar to the child such as peanut butter or orange peel. When testing visual fields (cranial nerve II) and cardinal positions of gaze (cranial nerves III, IV, VI), you often need to gently immobilise the head or the child will track with the whole head. Make a game out of asking the child to imitate your funny 'faces' (cranial nerve VII); thus, the child has fun and you win a friend.	See Table 12.18 Summary—testing cranial nerve function in infants

TABLE 12.18 Summary—testing cranial nerve function in infants

Cranial Nerve	Response
II, III, IV, VI	Optical blink reflex—shine light in open eyes, note rapid closure Size, shape, equality of pupils Regards face or close object Eyes follow movement
V	Rooting reflex, sucking reflex
VII	Facial movements (e.g. wrinkling forehead and nasolabial folds) symmetrical when crying or smiling
VIII	Loud noise yields Moro reflex (until 4 months)
	Acoustic blink reflex—infant blinks in response to a loud hand clap 30 cm from head (avoid making air current)
IX, X	Swallowing, gag reflex Coordinated sucking and swallowing
XII	Pinch nose, infant's mouth will open and tongue rise in midline

PROCEDURES AND NORMAL FINDINGS	ABNORMAL FINDINGS AND CLINICAL ALERTS

Motor system

Much of the motor assessment can be derived from watching the child undress and dress and manipulate buttons. This indicates muscle strength, symmetry, joint range of motion and fine motor skills. Use the Denver II test to screen gross and fine motor skills that are appropriate for the child's specific age. Be familiar with developmental milestones described in Chapter 3 for each age.

Note the child's gait during both walking and running. Allow for the normal wide-based gait of the toddler and the normal knock-kneed walk of the preschooler.

Normally, the child can balance on one foot for about 5 seconds by 4 years of age, can balance for 8 to 10 seconds at 5 years of age and can hop at 4 years. Children enjoy performing these tests (Figure 12.56).

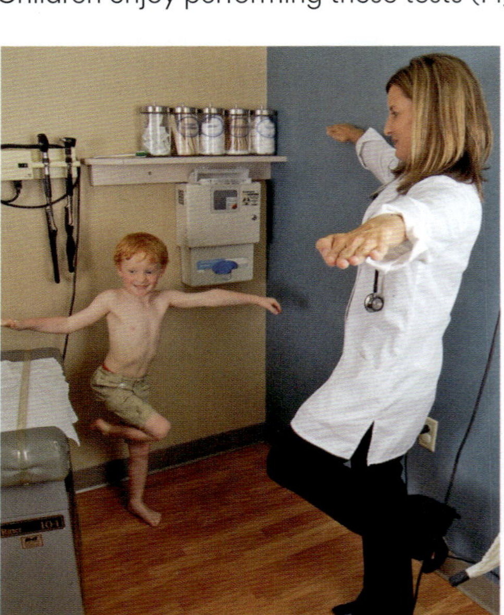

FIGURE 12.56 Assess motor system (Balance)

Observe the child as they rise from a supine position on the floor to a sitting position and then to a stand. Note the muscles of the neck, abdomen, arms and legs. Normally, the child curls up in the midline to sit up, then pushes off with both hands against the floor to stand (Figure 12.57).

Muscle hypertrophy or **atrophy** occurs with muscular dystrophy.

Muscle weakness.

Lack of coordination.

Causes of motor delay are listed earlier in the infant section.

Staggering, falling.

Weakness climbing up or down stairs occurs with muscular dystrophy.

Broad-based gait beyond toddlerhood, scissor gait (Tables 12.6, 12.8 and 12.11).

Failure to hop after 5 years of age indicates uncoordination of gross motor skill.

PROCEDURES AND NORMAL FINDINGS	ABNORMAL FINDINGS AND CLINICAL ALERTS
	Weak pelvic muscles are a sign of muscular dystrophy; from the supine position, the child will roll to one side, bend forward to all four extremities, plant hands on legs and literally 'climb' up themself. This is **Gower's sign** (Figure 12.57B). See also Tables 12.8 and 12.11.

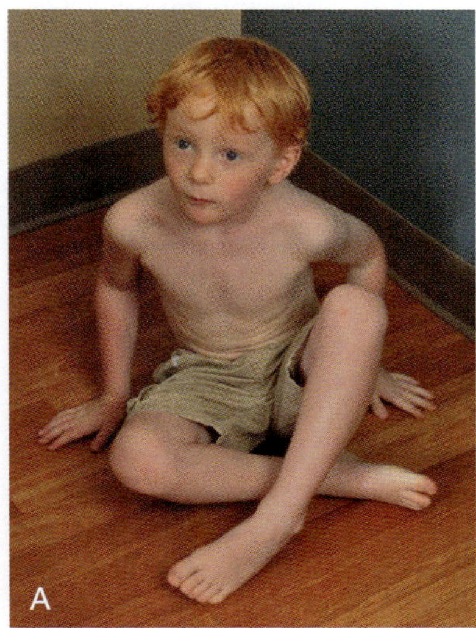

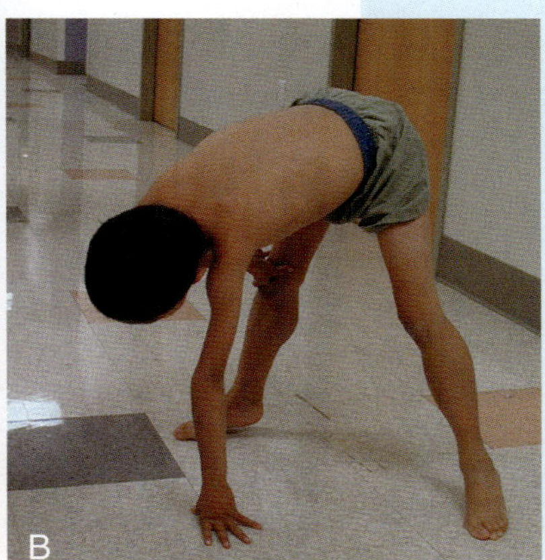

FIGURE 12.57 Gower's sign

Assess fine coordination by using the finger-to-nose test if you can be sure the young child understands your directions. Demonstrate the procedure first, then ask the child to do the test with the eyes open, then with the eyes closed. Fine coordination is not fully developed until the child has reached 4 to 6 years of age. Consider it normal if a younger child can bring the finger to within 2 to 5 cm of the nose.	Failure of the finger-to-nose test with the eyes open indicates gross uncoordination; failure of the test with the eyes closed indicates minor uncoordination or lack of position sense.
Sensation	
Testing sensation is very unreliable in toddlers and preschoolers. You may test light touch by asking the child to close the eyes and then to point to the spot where you touch or tickle. Testing of vibration, position, stereognosis, graphaesthesia or two-point discrimination usually is not done on a child younger than 6 years of age. Also, do not test for perception of superficial pain. In children older than 6 years of age, you may perform sensory testing as with adults. Use a fractured tongue blade if you need to test superficial pain.	Sensory loss occurs with decreased consciousness, mental deficiency or spinal cord or peripheral nerve dysfunction.

PROCEDURES AND NORMAL FINDINGS	ABNORMAL FINDINGS AND CLINICAL ALERTS
Reflexes	
The deep tendon reflexes are usually not tested in children younger than 5 years of age due to lack of cooperation in relaxation. When you need to test deep tendon reflexes in a young child, use your finger to percuss the tendon. Use a reflex hammer only with an older child. Coax the child to relax or distract and percuss discreetly when the child is not paying attention. The knee jerk is present at birth, then the ankle jerk and brachial reflex appear, and the triceps reflex is present at 6 months.	Hyperactivity of deep tendon reflexes occurs with upper motor neuron lesion, hypocalcaemia and hyperthyroidism and with muscle spasm associated with early poliomyelitis. Decreased or absent reflexes occur with a lower motor neuron lesion, muscular dystrophy and flaccidity or flaccid paralysis. Clonus may occur with fatigue, but it usually indicates hyperreflexia (Table 12.11).
Additional objective assessment for adults over 65 years	
Use the same examination as used with the younger adult. The findings discussed in the following sections are normal variants due to ageing.	
Motor system	
Any decrease in muscle bulk is most apparent in the hand, as seen by guttering between the metacarpals. These dorsal hand muscles often look wasted, even with no apparent arthropathy. The grip strength remains relatively good.	Hand muscle atrophy is worsened with disuse and degenerative arthropathy. See Table 12.14.
Tremors occasionally occur (Table 12.5). These benign tremors include an intention tremor of the hands, head nodding (as if saying yes or no) and tongue protrusion. **Dyskinesias** are the repetitive stereotyped movements in the jaw, lips or tongue that may accompany senile tremors. No associated rigidity is present.	Tremors associated with Parkinson's disease are accompanied by rigidity and slowness and weakness of voluntary movement.
The gait may be slower and more deliberate than that in the younger person, and it may deviate slightly from a midline path.	Absence of a rhythmic reciprocal gait pattern is seen in Parkinson's disease and hemiparesis (Table 12.6).
The rapid alternating movements (e.g. pronating and supinating the hands on the thigh) may be more difficult to perform by an older adult.	
Sensory	
After 65 years of age, loss of the sensation of vibration at the ankle malleolus is common and is usually accompanied by loss of the ankle jerk. Position sense in the big toe may be lost, although this is less common than vibration loss. Tactile sensation may be impaired. An older person may need stronger stimuli for light touch and especially for pain.	Note any difference in sensation between right and left sides, which may indicate a neurological deficit.

PROCEDURES AND NORMAL FINDINGS	ABNORMAL FINDINGS AND CLINICAL ALERTS
Reflexes The deep tendon reflexes are less brisk. Those in the upper extremities are usually present, but the ankle jerks are commonly lost. Knee jerks may be lost, but this occurs less often. The plantar reflex may be absent or difficult to interpret. Often, you will not see a definite normal flexor response. However, you still should consider a definite extensor response to be abnormal. The superficial abdominal reflexes may be absent, probably because of stretching of the musculature through pregnancy or obesity.	

Abnormal findings for advanced practice

TABLE 12.13 Abnormalities in cranial nerves

Nerve	Test	Abnormal findings	Possible causes
I: Olfactory	Identify familiar odours	Anosmia	Upper respiratory infection (temporary); tobacco or cocaine use; fracture of cribriform plate or ethmoid area; frontal lobe lesion; tumour in olfactory bulb or tract
II: Optic	Visual acuity	Defect or absent central vision	Congenital blindness, refractive error, acquired vision loss from numerous diseases (e.g. stroke, type 1 and type 2 diabetes), trauma to globe or orbit (see discussion of cranial nerve III)
	Visual fields	Defect in peripheral vision, hemianopsia	
	Shine light in eye	Absent light reflex	
	Direct inspection	Papillo-oedema Optic atrophy Retinal lesions	Increased intracranial pressure Glaucoma Type 1 and type 2 diabetes

Continued

TABLE 12.13 Abnormalities in cranial nerves cont'd

Nerve	Test	Abnormal findings	Possible causes
III: Oculomotor	Inspection	Dilated pupil, ptosis, eye turns out and slightly down	Paralysis in cranial nerve III from internal carotid aneurysm, tumour, inflammatory lesions, uncal herniation with increased intracranial pressure
	Extraocular muscle movement	Failure to move eye up, in, down	Ptosis from myasthenia gravis, oculomotor nerve palsy, Horner's syndrome
	Shine light in eye	Absent light reflex	Blindness, drug influence, increased intracranial pressure, CNS injury, circulatory arrest, CNS syphilis
IV: Trochlear	Extraocular muscle movement	Failure to turn eye down or out	Fracture of orbit, brainstem tumour
V: Trigeminal	Superficial touch—three divisions Corneal reflex	Absent touch and pain, paraesthesias No blink	Trauma, tumour, pressure from aneurysm, inflammation, sequelae of alcohol injection for trigeminal neuralgia
	Clench teeth	Weakness of masseter or temporalis muscles	Unilateral weakness with cranial nerve V lesion; bilateral weakness with upper or lower motor neuron disorder
VI: Abducens	Extraocular muscle movement to right and left sides	Failure to move laterally, diplopia on lateral gaze	Brainstem tumour or trauma, fracture of orbit
VII: Facial	Wrinkle forehead, close eyes tightly	Absent or asymmetric facial movement	Bell's palsy (lower motor neuron lesion) causes paralysis of entire half of face
	Smile, puff cheeks Identify tastes	Loss of taste	Upper motor neuron lesions (stroke, tumour, inflammatory) cause paralysis of lower half of face, leaving forehead intact Other lower motor neuron causes of paralysis: swelling from ear or meningeal infections
VIII: Acoustic	Hearing acuity	Decrease or loss of hearing	Inflammation, occluded ear canal, otosclerosis, presbycusis, drug toxicity, tumour
IX: Glossopharyngeal	Gag reflex	See cranial nerve X	

TABLE 12.13 Abnormalities in cranial nerves cont'd

Nerve	Test	Abnormal findings	Possible causes
X: Vagus	Phonates 'ahh'	Uvula deviates to side	Brainstem tumour, neck injury, cranial nerve X lesion
	Gag reflex	No gag reflex	Vocal cord weakness
	Note voice quality	Hoarse or brassy Nasal twang Husky	Soft palate weakness Unilateral cranial nerve X lesion
	Note swallowing	Dysphagia, fluids regurgitate through nose	Bilateral cranial nerve X lesion
XI: Spinal accessory	Turn head, shrug shoulders against resistance	Absent movement of sternocleidomastoid or trapezius muscles	Neck injury, torticollis
XII: Hypoglossal	Protrude tongue Wiggle tongue from side to side	Deviates to side Slowed rate of movement	Lower motor neuron lesion Bilateral upper motor neuron lesion

TABLE 12.14 Characteristics of upper and lower motor neuron lesions

	Upper motor neuron lesion	Lower motor neuron lesion
Weakness/ paralysis	In muscles corresponding to distribution of damage in pyramidal tract lesion; usually in hand grip, arm extensors, leg flexors	In specific muscles served by damaged spinal segment, ventral root or peripheral nerve
Location	Descending motor pathways that originate in the motor areas of cerebral cortex and carry impulses to the anterior horn cells of the spinal cord	Nerve cells that originate in the anterior horn of spinal cord or in brainstem and carry impulses by the spinal nerves or cranial nerves to the muscles, the 'final common pathway'
Example	Stroke	Poliomyelitis, herniated intervertebral disc
Muscle tone	Increased tone; spasticity	Loss of tone, flaccidity
Bulk	May have some atrophy from disuse; otherwise normal	Atrophy (wasting), may be marked
Abnormal movements	None	Fasciculations
Reflexes	Hyperreflexia, ankle clonus; diminished or absent superficial abdominal reflexes; positive Babinski's sign	Hyporeflexia or areflexia; no Babinski's sign, no pathological reflexes
Possible nursing diagnoses	Risk for contractures; impaired physical mobility	Impaired physical mobility

TABLE 12.15 Common patterns of sensory loss

Type	Characteristics	Possible causes
Peripheral neuropathy		
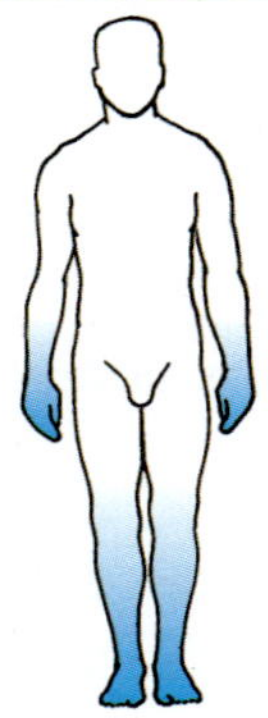	Loss of sensation involves all modalities. Loss is most severe distally (feet and hands); response improves as stimulus is moved proximally (glove-and-stocking anaesthesia). Anaesthesia zone gradually merges into a hypoaesthesia zone, then gradually becomes normal.	Type 1 and type 2 diabetes, chronic alcoholism, nutritional deficiency
Individual nerves or roots		
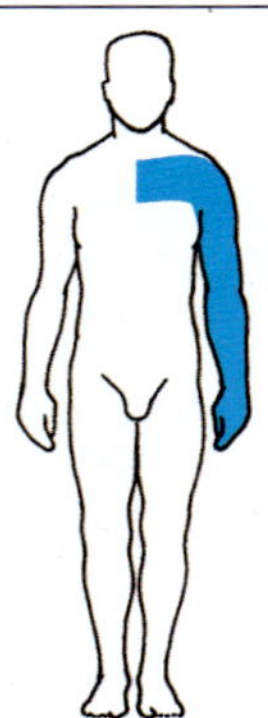	Decrease or loss of all sensory modalities. Area of sensory loss corresponds to distribution of the involved nerve.	Trauma, vascular occlusion
Spinal cord hemisection (Brown-Séquard syndrome)		
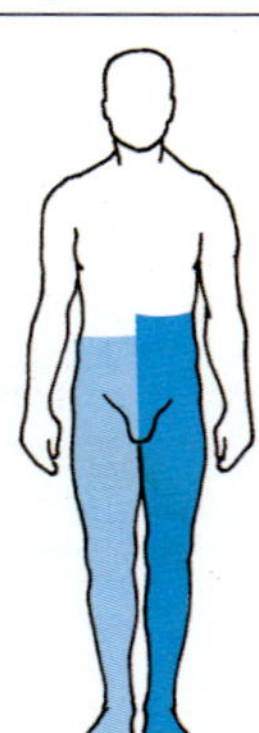	Loss of pain and temperature, contralateral side, starting one to two segments below the level of the lesion. Loss of vibration and position discrimination on the ipsilateral side, below the level of the lesion.	Meningioma, neurofibroma, cervical spondylosis, multiple sclerosis

TABLE 12.15 Common patterns of sensory loss cont'd

Type	Characteristics	Possible causes
Complete transection of the spinal cord		
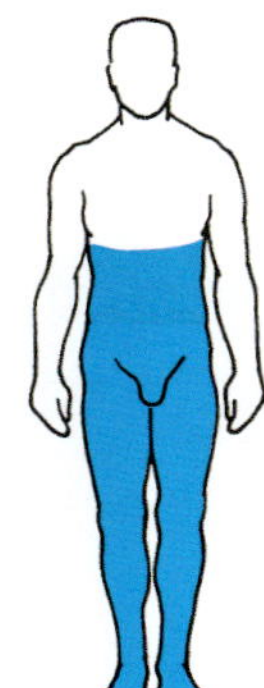	Complete loss of all sensory modalities below the level of the lesion. Condition is associated with motor paralysis and loss of sphincter control.	Spinal cord trauma, demyelinating disorders, tumour
Thalamus		
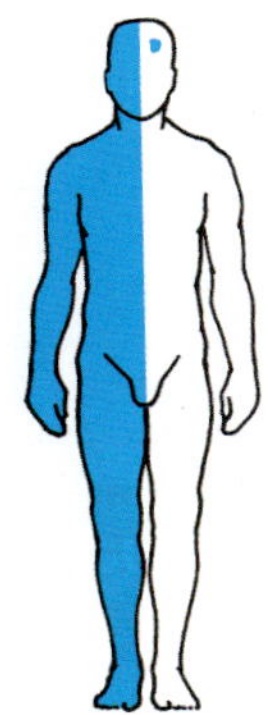	Loss of all sensory modalities on the face, arm and leg on the side contralateral to the lesion.	Vascular occlusion
Cortex		
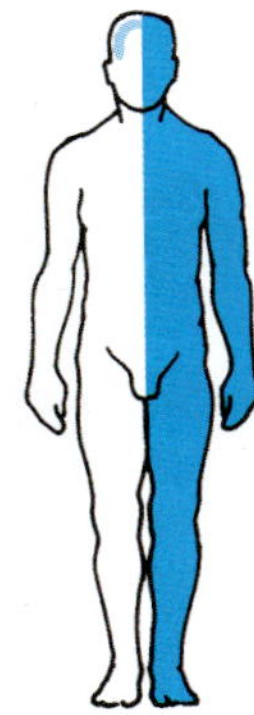	Since pain, vibration and crude touch are mediated by thalamus, little loss of these sensory functions occurs with a cortex lesion. Loss of discrimination occurs on the contralateral side. Loss of graphaesthesia, stereognosis, recognition of shapes and weights, finger finding.	Cerebral cortex, parietal lobe lesion (e.g. stroke)

TABLE 12.16 Frontal release signs

Reflex	
Snout	***Method of testing***
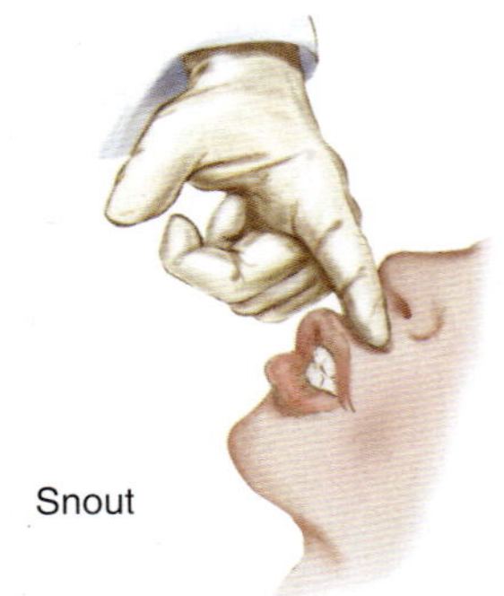 Snout	Gently percuss oral region
	Abnormal response (reflex is present)
	Puckers lips
	Indications
	Frontal lobe disease, cerebral degenerative disease (Alzheimer's), motor neuron disease, corticobulbar lesions
Sucking	***Method of testing***
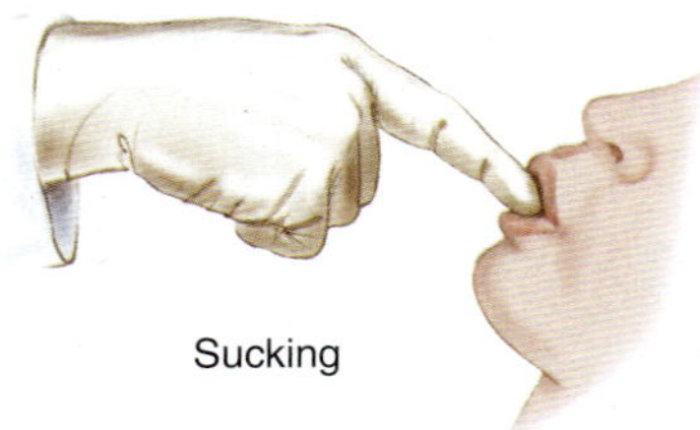 Sucking	Touch oral region
	Abnormal response (reflex is present)
	Sucking movement of lips, tongue, jaw, swallowing
	Indications
	Same as for snout reflex
Grasp	***Method of testing***
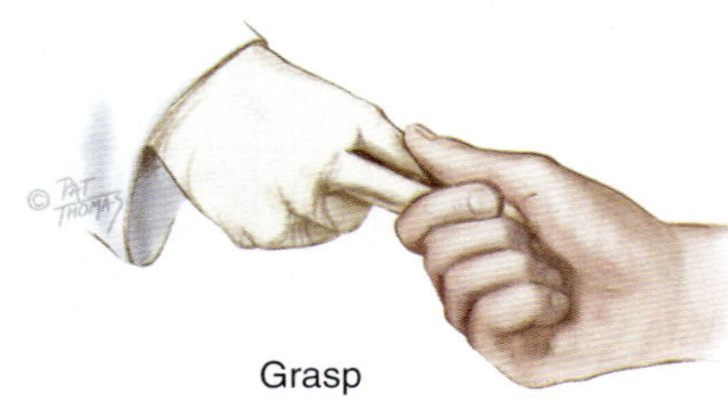 Grasp	Touch palm with your finger
	Abnormal response (reflex is present)
	Uncontrolled, forced grasping (grasp is usually last of these signs to appear, so its presence indicates severe disease)
	Indications
	When unilateral, frontal lobe lesion on contralateral side; when bilateral, diffuse bifrontal lobe disease

TABLE 12.17 Pathological reflexes

Reflex	Method of testing	Abnormal response (Reflex is present)	Indications
Babinski	Stroke the lateral aspect and across the ball of the foot	Extension of the great toe, fanning of toes	Corticospinal (pyramidal) tract disease (e.g. stroke, trauma)
Oppenheim	Using heavy pressure with your thumb and index finger, stroke the anterior medial tibial muscle	Same as above	Same
Gordon	Firmly squeeze the calf muscles	Same as above	Same
Hoffman	With the person's hand relaxed, wrist dorsified, fingers slightly flexed, sharply flick the nail of the distal phalanx of the middle or index finger	Clawing of the fingers and thumb	Same
Kernig	In a flat-lying supine position, raise the leg straight or flex the thigh on the abdomen, then extend the knee	Resistance to straightening (because of hamstring spasm), pain down the posterior thigh	Meningeal irritation (e.g. meningitis, infections)
Brudzinski	With one hand under the neck and the other hand on person's chest, sharply flex the chin on the chest, watch the hips and knees	Resistance and pain in the neck, with flexion of the hips and knees	Meningeal irritation (e.g. meningitis, infections)

Clinical reasoning and documentation

Case study 1 (continued)—Deterioration in cognitive function

The following is a continuation of the case study provided at the beginning of this chapter and the clinical reasoning process including problem/issue identification. Consult a fundamentals of nursing or medical-surgical Nursing text for information about goal setting, nursing interventions and evaluation.

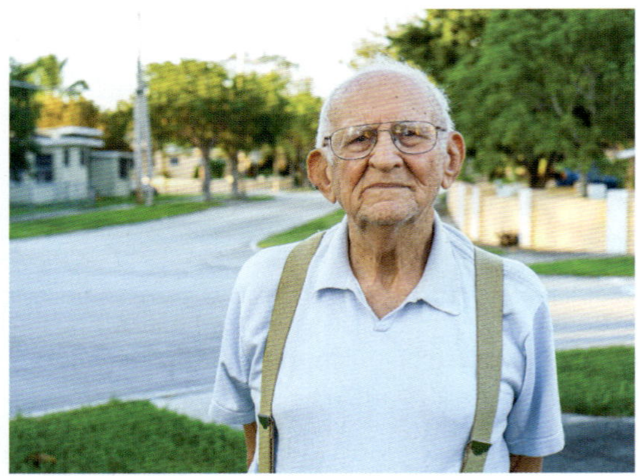

Context

You will recall from the case study described earlier in the chapter that you are a registered nurse working in an acute care ward where you are conducting a neurological assessment on Mr Adamik.

Consider the patient's situation

Mr Adamik, age 80 years, is a retired builder who lives with his son in a single-storey house. He was previously living independently performing his activities of daily living without assistance. He was initially referred to the neurosurgery department after a 2-month history of increasing confusion and generalised malaise. His GP ordered a CT scan, which showed a left-sided cerebral lesion.

Collect cues/information

Your further assessment reveals the following information.

Subjective data

Four hours ago, Mr Adamik returned to the ward from the operating room following a craniotomy and removal of a left temporal parietal lesion. Mr Adamik is currently stating that he is 'on the way to the bus stop'. This is despite being reoriented to time, place and person.

Objective data

Mental status: Dressed in hospital gown, lying in bed he appears alert with appropriate eye contact, listening intently to my questions. Speech is slow, requires great effort and voice tone is very soft. Verbal content confused to place and time.
Eye opening: In response to speech.
Motor: Obeying commands. Right-hand grip weak, right arm drifts, right leg weak. Spasticity in right arm and leg muscles, limited range of motion on passive movement.
Pupillary response: Size 3 mm, equal and responding briskly to light.
Vital signs: HR – 76 RR – 14 BP – 120/70
Glasgow Coma Scale score: 13/15 (E3V4M6). No change from previous assessment.

Process information and identify problems/issues

Collaborative problems

Deteriorating cognitive and neurological function related to craniotomy

Impaired physical mobility related to neuromuscular impairment

Problem statements/nursing diagnoses

Risk of altered conscious state related to recent brain surgery

Impaired verbal communication related to effects of neurological condition

Impaired physical mobility related to neuromuscular weakness

Self-care deficits: feeding, bathing, toileting, dressing/grooming related to muscular weakness

Risk for injury related to neuromuscular impairment

Clinical reasoning and documentation cont'd

Case study 2—Sudden onset of neurological symptoms

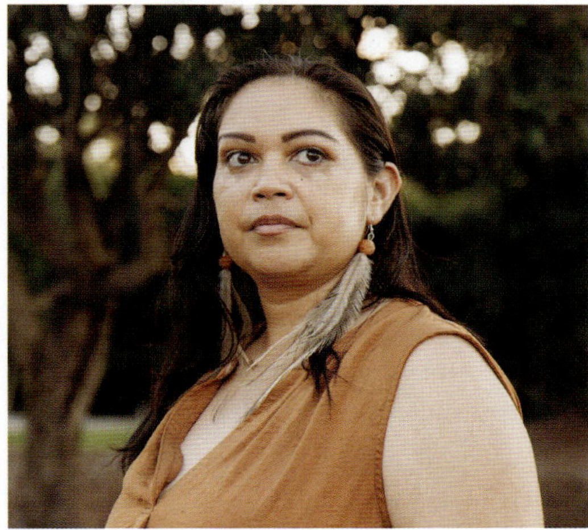

Context

You are a registered nurse working in the emergency department of a large tertiary hospital.

Consider the patient's situation

Sarah Mitchell (a Wurundjeri woman) has presented to the emergency department with sudden onset right-sided headache. She is 42 years old and is a primary school teacher who lives with her husband and three children, aged 10, 7 and 4.

Collect cues/information

Subjective data

Sarah has no significant past medical history. Her only hospital admissions have been for the births of her children. Sarah's mother and sister both experience migraines, though Sarah has never had one before. Her only regular medication is the oral contraceptive pill. Sarah became unwell at work today. She describes a sudden onset, severe, throbbing headache localised to the right side. She is experiencing nausea and vomited twice before a colleague became concerned about her and drove her to the hospital. A brain CT shows no signs of bleeding. Sarah describes increased sensitivity to light (photophobia), increased sensitivity to sound (phonophobia), blurred vision, difficulty concentrating and fatigue.

Objective data

Mental status: Dressed in hospital gown, lying in bed with eyes closed. Speech is slow, requires great effort and voice tone is very soft. Orientated to place and time.
Eye opening: In response to speech.
Motor: Obeying commands. Left- and right-hand grip slightly weak, no drift. Leg strength normal. Facial motor control symmetrical.
Pupillary response: Pupils equal. Size 5 mm and responding briskly to light.
Vital signs: HR – 87 RR – 17 BP – 135/68
Glasgow Coma Scale score: 14/15 (E3V5M6).

Process information and identify problems/issues

Collaborative problem

Headache, nausea and vomiting related to migraine

Problem statements/nursing diagnoses

Knowledge deficit related to first presentation of migraine
Pain related to migraine
Nausea related to migraine
Self-care deficit related to altered sensation and perception and fatigue
Altered sensation/perception related to photo- and phonophobia
Risk for falls related to altered sensation and perception
Risk for fluid and electrolyte imbalance related to nausea and vomiting

ADDITIONAL RESOURCES

You can further develop your knowledge and skills relevant to neurological assessment, related pathophysiology, common health issues and nursing interventions by:

- reading chapters of a fundamentals of nursing or medical-surgical nursing textbook
- answering chapter multiple choice questions online. Log onto ClinicalKey Student and search for the text 'Health Assessment, 4th edition'. Choose the section titled 'Teaching material'. In this section you will find question and answer documents for each chapter.
- visiting websites

  Dementia Australia: https://www.dementia.org.au/information/diagnosing-dementia

  Glasgow Coma Scale: https://www.glasgowcomascale.org

  Brain Injury Australia: https://www.braininjuryaustralia.org.au/

  Stroke Foundation Australia: https://strokefoundation.org.au

  Stroke Foundation of New Zealand: http://www.stroke.org.nz

REFERENCES

1. Castelli V, Benedetti E, Antonosante A, Catanesil M, Pitari G, Ippoliti R, et al. Neuronal cells rearrangement during aging and neurodegenerative disease: metabolism, oxidative stress and organelles dynamic. Frontiers in Molecular Neuroscience. 2019 May 28;12:132. doi: 10.3389/fnmol.2019.00132.
2. Dementia Australia. Warning signs of dementia. 2023. Available at: https://www.dementia.org.au/information/about-dementia/how-can-i-find-out-more/warning-signs-of-dementia
3. Australian Commission on Safety and Quality in Health Care (ACSQHC). Delirium Clinical Care Standard. Sydney: ACSQHC; 2021. Available at: https://www.safetyandquality.gov.au/sites/default/files/2021-09/delirium_clinical_care_standard_2021.pdf
4. Marcantonio ER. Delirium in hospitalized older adults. New England Journal of Medicine. 2017;377:1456–1466.
5. American Psychiatric Association. Diagnostic and statistical manual of mental disorders. 5th ed. Arlington, VA: American Psychiatric Association; 2013.
6. Stroke Foundation Australia. Top 10 facts about stroke. 2023a. Available at: https://strokefoundation.org.au/about-stroke/learn/facts-and-figures.
7. Stroke Foundation of New Zealand. Facts and FAQs. 2023. Available at: https://www.stroke.org.nz/facts-and-faqs
8. Australian Institute of Health and Welfare (AIHW). Heart, stroke and vascular disease: Australian facts. Canberra: AIHW; 2023. Available at: https://www.aihw.gov.au/reports/heart-stroke-vascular-diseases/hsvd-facts/contents/all-heart-stroke-and-vascular-disease/stroke
9. Talley NJ, O'Connor S. Clinical examination: a systematic guide to physical diagnosis. 8th ed. Chatswood: Elsevier; 2018.
10. Stroke Foundation Australia. Signs of Stroke. 2023b. Available at: https://strokefoundation.org.au/about-stroke/learn/signs-of-stroke
11. Stroke Foundation Australia. Understanding stroke. 2021. Available at: https://strokefoundation.org.au/news-and-events/latest-news/2021/07/understanding-stroke#:,:text=The%20truth%20is%2C%20

stroke%20can,modifiable%20risk%20factor%20for%20stroke.

12. Duncan PW, Bushnell C, Sissine M, Coleman S, Lutz BJ, Johnson AM, et al. Comprehensive stroke care and outcomes: time for a paradigm shift. Stroke. 2021 Jan;52(1):385–393.
13. Mehta R, Chinthapalli K. (2019). Glasgow coma scale explained. BMJ, 365, l1296.
14. Teasdale G, Maas A, Lecky F, et al. The Glasgow Coma Scale at 40 years: standing the test of time. Lancet Neurol. 2014;13(8): 844–854.
15. Institute of Neurological Sciences. (2015). Glasgow Coma Scale: Do it this way. NHS Greater Glasgow and Clyde. Available: https://www.glasgowcomascale.org/downloads/GCS-Assessment-Aid-English.pdf?v=3

CHAPTER 13

Pain assessment

Written by Carolyn Jarvis and Sarah Jarvis
Adapted by Helen Forbes and Elizabeth Watt

INTRODUCTION

Almost 50 years ago, McCaffery introduced the often-quoted definition of pain as 'what the person says it is and exists whenever he or she says it does'.[1] The recognition that pain is more than a physiological manifestation and that the person experiencing pain is the most reliable source (or 'gold-standard') for understanding their pain experience has shaped the way pain is assessed clinically. This definition has been a foundational principle of pain management in nursing practice ever since. More recently, the International Association for the Study of Pain updated the definition as 'an unpleasant sensory and emotional experience associated with or resembling that associated with actual or potential tissue damage'.[2]

The experience of pain is a complex biopsychosocial phenomenon. We are only now developing an understanding of pain at the cellular level, but more research is needed to fully understand the complexities of the pain experience. We still rely on the person's report as the best indicator of pain, but researchers continue to explore whether pain and certain objective measures (e.g. biomarkers) are associated with one another.

Case study

The following case study gives an example of a typical situation involving pain assessment and the initial clinical reasoning process. It will help you to identify your learning needs.

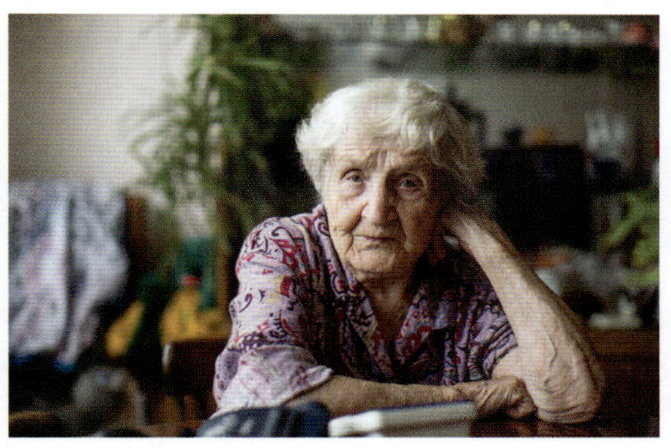

Context

You are nursing student on your third-year final clinical placement. Your clinical supervisor asks you to perform a pain assessment on Mrs Alberici.

Consider the patient's situation

Mrs Maria Alberici is an 85-year-old Italian-Australian female with a 20-year history of osteoarthritis.

Subjective

Mrs Alberici reports increased pain and stiffness in her hips and knees for the past year. However, she isn't experiencing any radiation of pain, tingling or numbness in the lower extremities.

Questions to further your learning

- What are the possible things that might be going on with Mrs Alberici?
- What knowledge do you need to be able to predict what might be going on?
- What approach to pain assessment will you take?
- What questions (subjective data) will you ask Mrs Alberici to extend the health history and why?
- What physical examination (objective data) will you conduct and why?
- What resources are available to assist in your assessment of Mrs Alberici?

Assessment plan

Pain is a distressing symptom; relief of which is a human right.[3] There are many known challenges to effective pain management including doctors and nurses lacking knowledge about pain mechanisms, personal biases, not working collaboratively and having concerns about addiction and overdosing. Also, people experiencing pain may also lack knowledge about pain mechanisms and may be reluctant to take analgesics because of fear of side effects and addiction.[4]

Pain is multidimensional in scope, encompassing physical, affective and functional domains. Assessment of pain is an important first step in effective pain management. Pain assessment is a complex process depending on the context of pain and the ability of the person to communicate their pain. The assessment of pain includes a thorough history, physical examination and an evaluation of associated functional impairment.[5]

The purpose of pain assessment is, where possible, to establish the person's perception of their experience of pain, identify how pain interferes with physical and psychosocial wellbeing and provide a baseline for decisions about pharmacological and non-pharmacological treatment. The main areas for subjective data collection are:

- initial pain assessment
- presenting concern
- other symptoms
- health and lifestyle management
- pain assessment tools.

Following subjective data collection, you will get a sense of the areas needed to be examined for objective data. Only the relevant areas should be examined. The main areas for physical examination and measurement are:

- general inspection (acute pain behaviours and chronic pain behaviours)
- limbs and joints
- muscles and skin
- abdomen
- other pain sites
- vital signs
- functional impact of pain.

Resources available

You will find additional resources and the reference list at the end of this chapter.

Structure and function

Pathological pain develops by two main processes: **nociceptive** (Figure 13.1) and/or **neuropathic** processing. It is important to understand how these two types of pain develop because people present with distinguishing sensations and respond differently to analgesics. An accurate pain assessment enables clinicians to more accurately select effective strategies to interrupt pain processing along multiple points within the pain messaging system and ultimately provide improved pain relief.

Neuroanatomical pathway

Pain is a highly complex and subjective experience that originates from the central nervous system, the peripheral nervous system or both. Specialised peripheral sensory nerve endings called nociceptors are designed to detect painful sensations from the periphery and transmit them to the central nervous system. Nociceptors are located within the skin, joints, connective tissue, muscle and the thoracic, abdominal and pelvic viscera. These nociceptors can be stimulated directly by trauma or injury or secondarily by chemical mediators that are released from the site of tissue damage.

Nociceptors carry the pain signal to the central nervous system by two primary sensory (or afferent) fibres: **A-delta fibres** and **C-fibres** (Figure 13.1). A-delta fibres are myelinated and large in diameter, thus

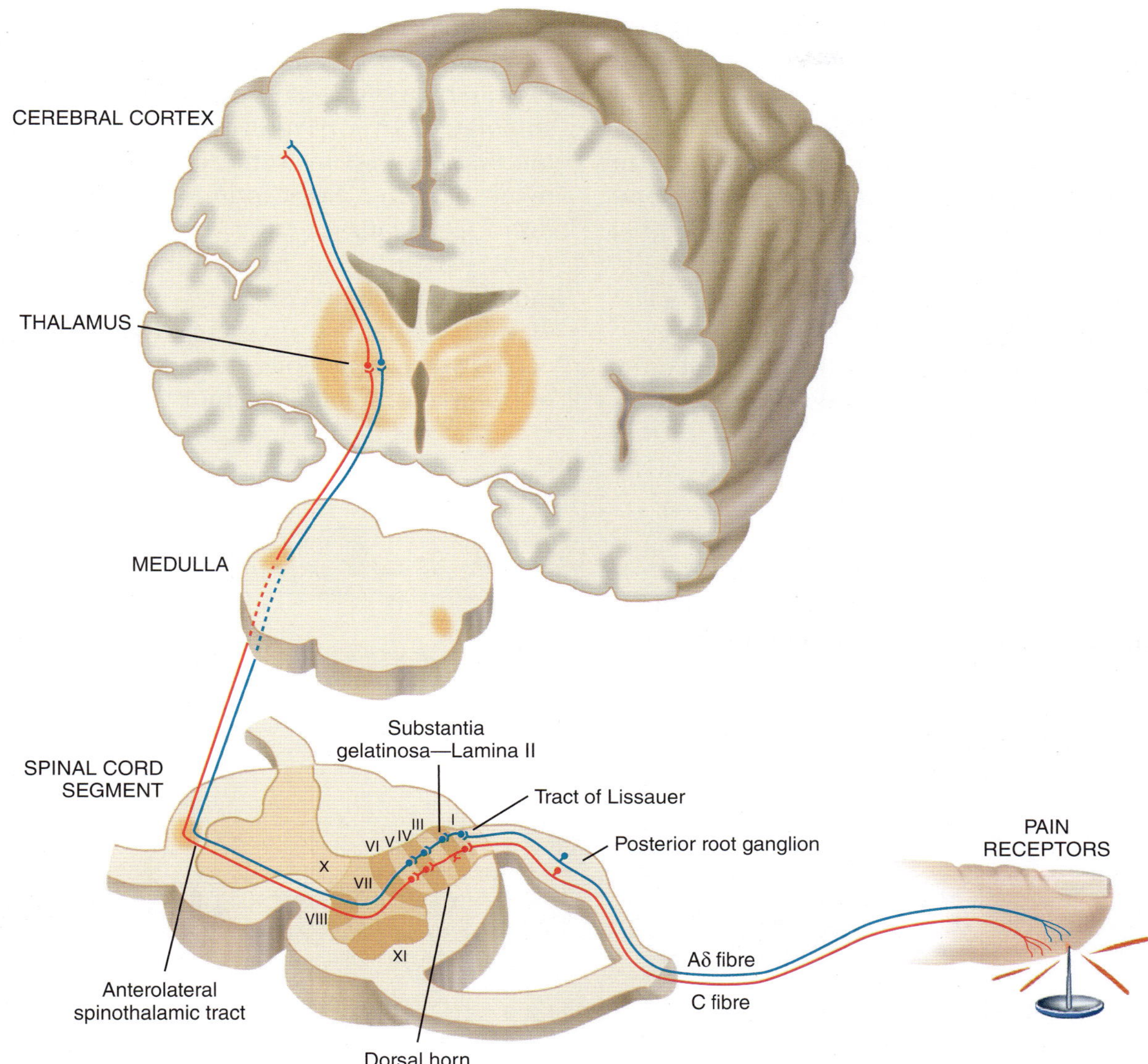

FIGURE 13.1 Neuroanatomical pathway

they transmit the pain signal rapidly to the central nervous system. Very localised, short-term and sharp sensations result from A-delta fibre stimulation. In contrast, C-fibres are unmyelinated and smaller, and they transmit the signal more *slowly*. These secondary sensations are diffuse and aching and they persist after the initial injury.

Peripheral sensory A-delta and C-fibres enter the spinal cord by posterior nerve roots within the dorsal horn by the tract of Lissauer. The fibres synapse with **interneurons** located within a specified area of the cord called the **substantia gelatinosa**. A cross-section shows that the grey matter of the spinal cord is divided into a series of consecutively numbered laminae (layers of nerve cells) (Figure 13.1). The substantia gelatinosa is lamina II, which receives sensory input from various areas of the body. The pain signals then cross over to the other side of the spinal cord and ascend to the brain via the **anterolateral spinothalamic tract**. When pain is poorly controlled over an extended period, structural plasticity and reorganisation of pain pathways occurs. Cells within the dorsal horn become altered in size and function, and this damage is associated with nociceptive hypersensitivity.

Nociceptive pain

Nociception is the term used to describe how noxious stimuli are typically perceived as pain. Nociceptive pain develops when *functioning and intact* nerve fibres in the periphery and the central nervous system are stimulated. It is triggered by events outside the nervous system from actual or potential tissue damage. Nociception can be divided into four phases: (1) transduction, (2) transmission, (3) perception and (4) modulation (Figure 13.2).

Initially, the first phase of **transduction** occurs when a noxious stimulus in the form of traumatic or chemical injury, burn, incision

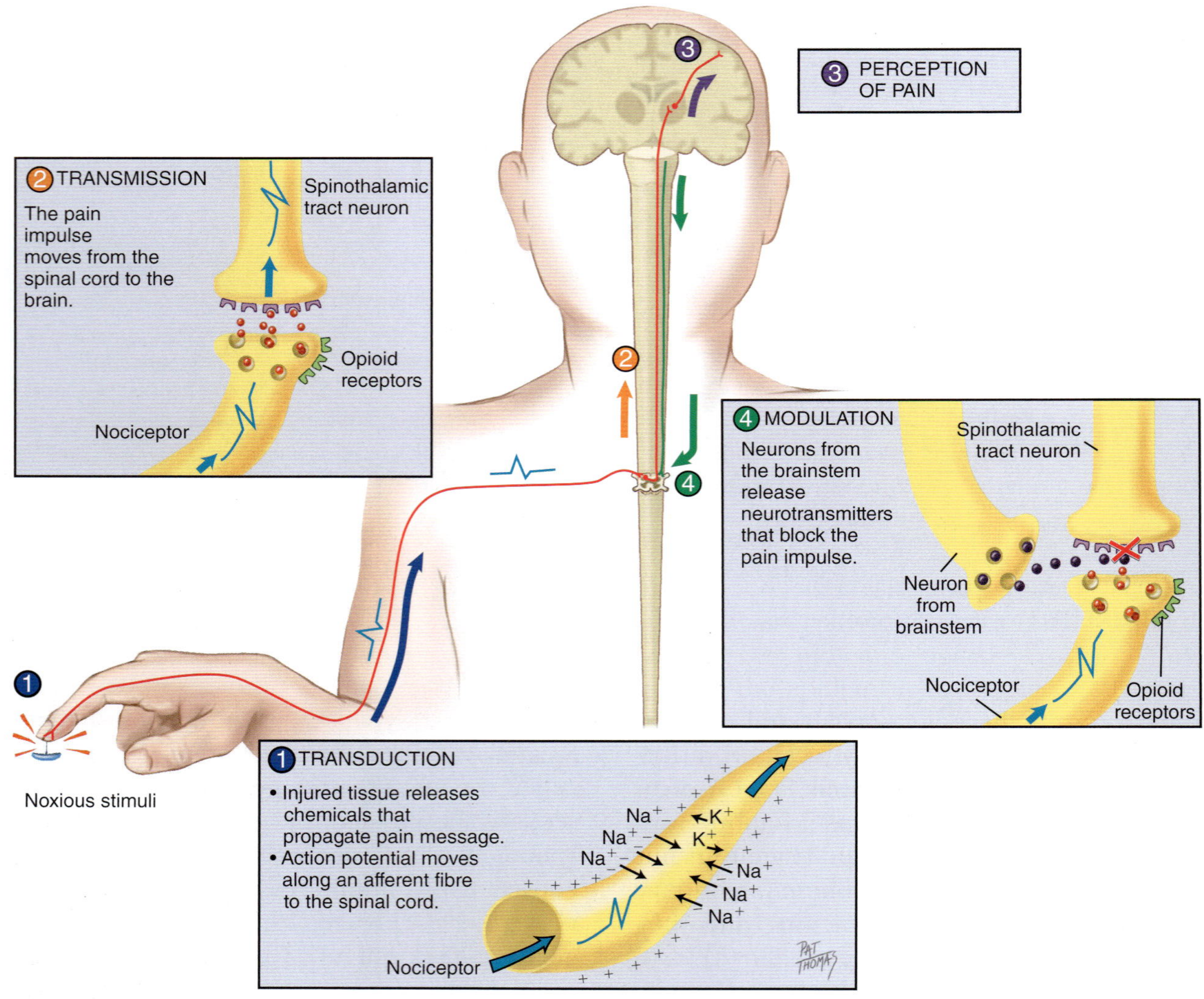

FIGURE 13.2 Nociceptive pain.

or tumour takes place in the periphery. The periphery includes the skin, as well as somatic and visceral structures. These injured tissues then release a variety of chemicals, including substance P, histamine, prostaglandins, serotonin and bradykinin. These chemicals are neurotransmitters that transmit a pain message or action potential, along sensory afferent nerve fibres to the spinal cord. These nerve fibres terminate in the dorsal horn of the spinal cord. Because the initial afferent fibres stop in the dorsal horn, a second set of neurotransmitters carry the pain impulse across the synaptic cleft to the dorsal horn neurons. These neurotransmitters include substance P, glutamate and adenosine triphosphate.

In the second phase, known as **transmission**, the pain impulse moves from the level of the spinal cord to the brain. Within the spinal cord, at the site of the synaptic cleft, are opioid receptors that can block this pain signalling with endogenous opioids or with exogenous opioids if they are administered. However, if left uninterrupted, the pain impulse moves to the brain via various ascending fibres within the spinothalamic tract to the thalamus. Once the pain impulse moves through the thalamus, the message is dispersed to higher cortical areas via mechanisms that are not clearly understood currently.

The third phase, **perception**, indicates the conscious awareness of a painful sensation. Cortical structures such as the limbic system account for the emotional response to pain, and somatosensory areas can characterise the sensation. Only when the noxious stimuli are interpreted in these higher cortical structures can this sensation be identified as 'pain'.

Last, the pain message is inhibited through the phase of **modulation**. Fortunately, our bodies have a built-in mechanism that will eventually slow down and stop the processing of a painful stimulus. If not for pain modulation, the experience of pain would continue from childhood injuries to adulthood. To inhibit and block the pain impulse, descending pathways from the brainstem to the spinal cord produce a third set of neurotransmitters that slow down or impede the pain impulse, producing an analgesic effect. These neurotransmitters include serotonin; noradrenaline; neurotensin; gamma-aminobutyric acid (GABA); and our own endogenous opioids, β-endorphins, enkephalins and dynorphins.

Normal nociceptive processing is protective and can be a warning signal that injury is about to take or has taken place.[6] We quickly learn to move our hand away from a hot stove. Other examples of nociceptive pain include a skinned knee, kidney stones, menstrual cramps, muscle strain, venipuncture or arthritic joint pain. Nociceptive pain is typically predictable and time-limited based on the extent of the injury.

Neuropathic pain

Neuropathic pain is pain that does not adhere to the typical and rather predictable phases in nociceptive pain. It is pain due to a lesion or disease in the somatosensory nervous system. Neuropathic pain implies abnormal processing of the pain message from an injury to the nerve fibres. This type of pain is the most difficult to assess and treat. Pain is often perceived long after the site of the injury heals, and it evolves into a chronic condition.[7]

Conditions and treatments that may cause neuropathic pain include diabetes mellitus, herpes zoster (shingles), HIV/AIDS, sciatica, trigeminal neuralgia, phantom limb pain and chemotherapy. Further examples include central nervous system lesions such as stroke, multiple sclerosis and tumour. Pain sustained on a neurochemical level cannot be identified by x-ray imaging, computed tomography (CT) scan or traditional magnetic resonance imaging (MRI). Recent advances in noninvasive neuroimaging techniques allow us to study the structural, functional and neurochemical changes in the brain caused by nociception.[8] Pain researchers are using functional MRI (fMRI) to visualise changes in brain activity while people experience pain. When these images are shown to a person in real time, they can learn to use neurofeedback to help control pain. Researchers can better understand how pain is processed and how cognitive influences (e.g. fear and anxiety) impact the experience of pain.

The abnormal processing of the neuropathic pain impulse can be continued by the peripheral or the central nervous system. An injury to peripheral neurons can result in spontaneous and repetitive firing of nerve fibres, almost seizure-like activity (Figure 13.3). Neuropathic pain may be sustained centrally in a phenomenon known as neuronal 'wind-up'. Central neuron hyper-excitability leads to maintenance of neuropathic pain. In neuropathic pain, even minor stimuli cause significant pain.[9]

Nociceptive pain can change into a neuropathic pain pattern over time when pain has been poorly controlled. This type of pain is known as nociplastic pain. **Nociplastic pain** occurs when there is increased sensitisation of the nervous system. There is no clear evidence of tissue damage. The constant irritation and inflammation caused by a pain stimulus alters nerve cells, making them more sensitive to any future stimulus.[10]

Sources of pain

Physical pain sources are based on their origin. **Visceral** pain originates from the larger interior organs (i.e. kidneys, stomach, intestines, gall bladder and pancreas). It is often described as dull, deep, squeezing or cramping. The pain can stem from direct injury to the organ or from stretching of the organ from tumour, ischaemia, distension or severe contraction. Examples of visceral pain include ureteric colic, acute appendicitis, ulcer pain and cholecystitis. The pain impulse

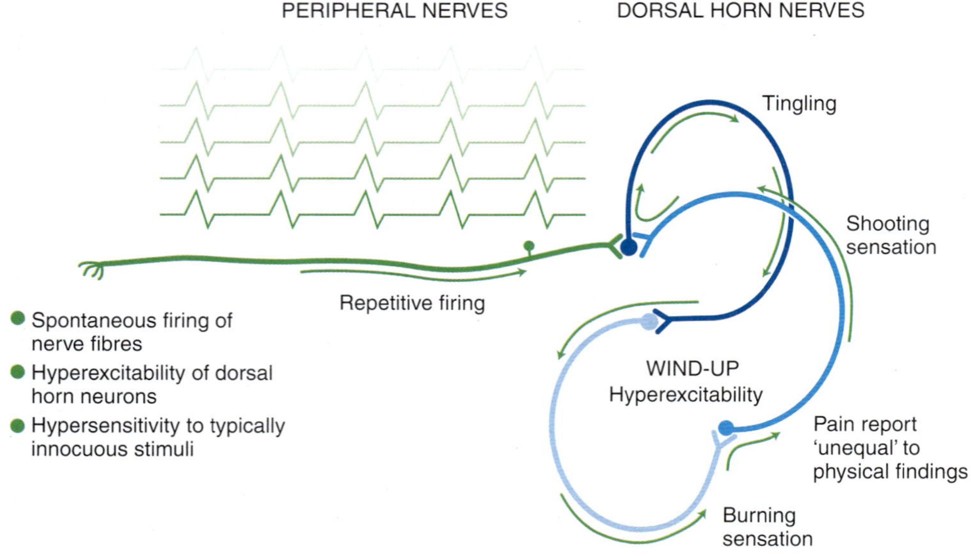

FIGURE 13.3 Neuropathic mechanisms

is transmitted by ascending nerve fibres and nerve fibres of the autonomic nervous system. That is why visceral pain often presents in association with autonomic responses such as vomiting, nausea, pallor and diaphoresis.

Somatic pain originates from musculoskeletal tissues or the body surface and can be classified as deep or superficial. **Deep somatic pain** comes from sources such as the blood vessels, joints, tendons, muscles and bone. Pain may result from pressure, trauma or ischaemia. Superficial or **cutaneous somatic pain** is derived from injury to the skin surface and subcutaneous tissues.

In general, somatic pain is well localised with surrounding tenderness and is characterised as sharp, stinging or burning, whereas visceral pain is poorly localised, dull, cramping or colicky in nature accompanied by local or referred tenderness.

Pain that is felt at a particular site but originates from another location is termed **referred pain**. Both sites are innervated by the same spinal nerve, and it is difficult for the brain to differentiate the point of origin. Referred pain may originate from visceral or somatic structures. Various structures maintain their same embryonic innervations. For example, an inflamed appendix in the right lower quadrant of the abdomen may have referred pain in the periumbilical area, or the pain from acute coronary syndrome may be felt in the left arm or neck. It is useful to have knowledge of areas of referred pain for diagnostic purposes (Table 23.3).

Types of pain

Pain can be classified by its duration into **acute or chronic** (also referred to as *persistent*) categories. The duration can provide information on possible underlying mechanisms and thus inform treatment decisions.

Acute pain is short term and self-limiting, often following a predictable trajectory and dissipates after an injury heals. Acute pain serves a self-protective purpose, warning the person of actual or potential tissue damage. Examples of acute pain include surgery, trauma and kidney stones. Incident pain is a type of pain that occurs predictably with certain movements. Examples include pain in the lower back on standing or turning from side to side. Acute pain may also present as recurrent pain, as occurs with migraines or the menstrual cycle, and, in these circumstances, these types of pain may be referred to as chronic pain conditions.[11] Acute pain may progress to chronic pain. The transition of acute pain to chronic pain is sometimes called the 'subacute phase' and refers to the pain that occurs after tissue healing and that persists up to the 3 months that is the defining duration for chronic pain.[12]

Chronic (or persistent) pain is diagnosed when there is constant daily pain for 3 months or more in the preceding 6 months. Chronic pain originates from abnormal processing of pain fibres in peripheral or central sites, and often the source of pain is unknown.[9]

Chronic pain can be further divided into:

- ***Chronic primary pain***. This is chronic pain in one or more anatomical regions characterised by significant emotional distress or functional disability.
- ***Chronic cancer-related pain***. This pain type often parallels the pathology created by the tumour cells. The pain is induced by tissue necrosis or stretching of an organ by the growing tumour. The pain fluctuates within the course of the disease.
- ***Chronic post-surgical or post-traumatic pain*** is pain developing or increasing in intensity after a surgical procedure or a tissue injury and persisting beyond the healing process (> 3 months).

- ***Chronic secondary musculoskeletal pain*** is associated with conditions such as arthritis, low back conditions or fibromyalgia.
- ***Chronic secondary visceral pain*** is persistent or recurrent pain originating from internal organs of the head/neck regions and of the thoracic, abdominal and pelvic cavities.
- ***Chronic neuropathic pain*** is pain caused by a lesion or disease of the somatosensory nervous system.
- ***Chronic secondary headache or orofacial pain*** comprises all headache and orofacial pain disorders that have an underlying cause and occur on at least 50% of the days in the preceding 3 months. The duration of the pain is at least 4 hours (untreated).[13]

Chronic pain does not stop when the injury heals. It persists after the predicted trajectory associated with injury. Chronic pain outlasts its protective purpose, and the level of pain intensity does not correspond with the physical findings. Chronic pain may not respond readily to therapy and, unfortunately, many people with chronic pain are not believed and are often labelled as malingerers, attention-seekers, drug-seekers and so forth.[5]

There may be misconceptions held by clinicians and carers about chronic pain that can influence how pain is assessed and treated.[14] These misconceptions include overemphasis on the contributing role of psychological factors on pain experience and misunderstandings about the meanings of pain tolerance.[15]

Breakthrough pain is a transient spike in pain level, moderate to severe in intensity, in an otherwise controlled pain syndrome. It can result from end-of-dose medication failure. This occurs when a person taking a long-acting opioid has a recurrence of pain before the next scheduled dose. Treating end-of-dose failure includes shortening the interval between doses or increasing the dose of medication. Breakthrough pain can also be the result of incident or episodic pain. This is a predictable breakthrough pain that may be triggered by a physical stimulus such as a return to activity after surgery or from a psychological event.[16]

Complex regional pain syndrome, also known as reflexive sympathetic dystrophy or Sudeck's atrophy, is a chronic progressive nerve condition characterised by burning pain, swelling, stiffness and discolouration of the affected extremity. It affects both men and women (although the prevalence is higher in women), usually around the age of 40 to 60 years and occurs weeks to months after a nerve injury (e.g. carpal tunnel syndrome, leg fracture, stroke or surgery). The prevalence of complex regional pain syndrome in Australia is not known but is estimated to account for 2 to 5% of adult and 20% of children seen in pain clinics.[17] The pathophysiology involves a complex interaction of sensory, motor and autonomic nerves and the immune system (Figure 13.4). The nerve injury may modify the usual pain pathway, causing a neuropathic 'wind-up' or 'short circuit' mechanism.

A key feature is that a typically innocuous stimulus (e.g. a light brush of a cotton ball or clothing) can create a severe, intense painful response. Subjective data include burning pain often disproportionate to the degree of injury and joint pain during movement. Objective data include swelling, disappearance of skin wrinkles, cool skin temperature, discolouration, brittle nails and atrophic changes (pale, dry, shiny skin and muscle atrophy). Treatment includes high doses of a combination of medications (e.g. prednisolone, amitriptyline, pregabalin and clonidine) to reduce symptoms and physical therapy to regain limb function. There is limited evidence for prevention strategies, but

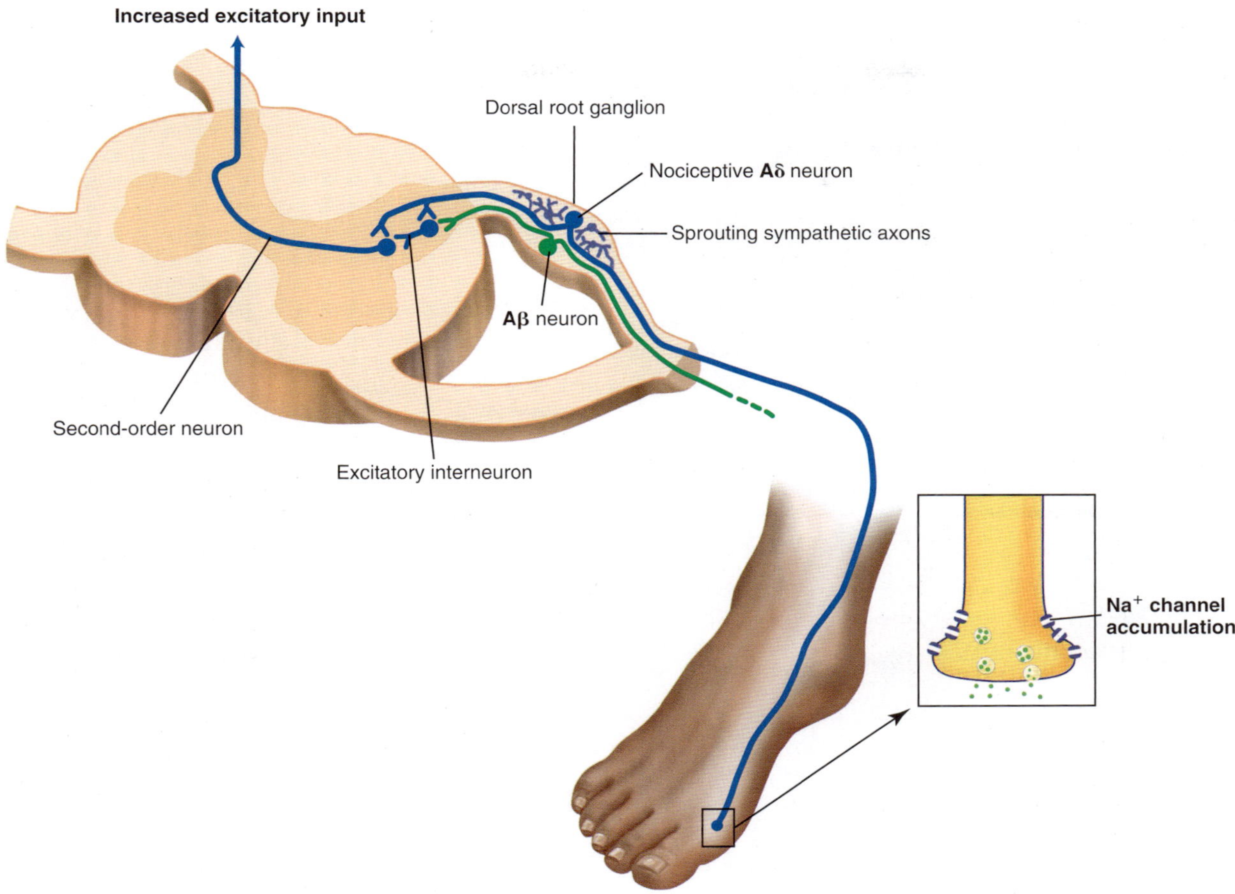

FIGURE 13.4 Complex regional pain syndrome

providing effective analgesia after surgery or trauma is recommended.[18]

Effects and use of opioids

Opioid medications must connect with **mu-opioid receptors** to achieve pain-relieving effects. Mu-opioid receptors are located throughout the body. There are high concentrations of mu-opioid receptors in the brain, including in the periaqueductal grey region, the thalamus, the cingulate cortex and the insula; these receptors regulate pain perception. Further, mu receptors in the amygdala mediate the emotional response to pain and mu receptors in the ventral tegmental area and nucleus accumbens mediate the perception of wellbeing and pleasure. Thus, opioid medications produce pain relief and euphoria. As to the side effects of opioid medications, mu receptors in the brainstem can lead to respiratory depression, and mu receptors in the small intestine produce troublesome constipation (Figure 13.5). Mu receptors in the dorsal horn of the spinal cord and peripheral nerves modulate the perception of pain.

Mu receptors are also responsible for the physical dependence associated with continued use of opioid pain medications.[19] Physical dependence means only that repeated dosing will lead to a predictable physical reaction when the drug is withdrawn

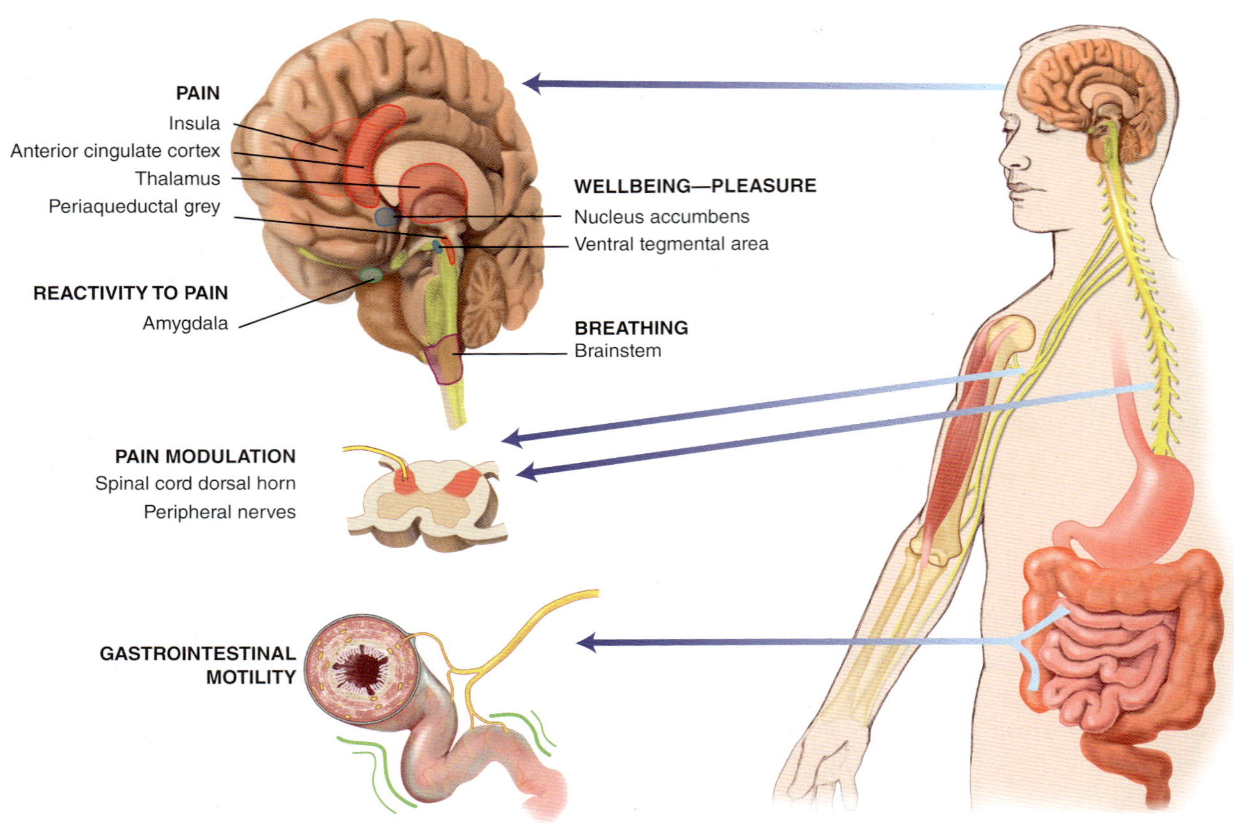

FIGURE 13.5 Response of mu receptor activation

abruptly after prolonged use; this is *not* the same as addiction. Certainly, the stimulation of mu receptors in the reward system of the brain can lead to addiction, especially when opioids are delivered rapidly, as happens when opioids are used for pleasure and reward or as can happen to persons in pain after months of opioid medication exposure. Refer to Chapters 6 and 11 for information relevant to substance misuse, withdrawal from opioids and mental health.

While opioid medications are effective in the management of severe pain, they also cause a variety of side effects based on the mechanism of action. Opioid medications are indispensable in treating certain types of pain (e.g. cancer pain, end-of-life pain, trauma and postoperative pain) and remain the mainstay of systemic analgesia for the treatment of moderate to severe acute pain but care should be taken in the long-term use of opioids.[20]

In 2017, in the United States, the Department of Health and Human Services declared the opioid crisis a public health emergency and announced a strategy to combat the epidemic. The 'opioid epidemic' has been linked to the increase in prescriptions and misuse of opioid medications. In the United States, although research indicates that the amount of pain experienced is stable, the prescription of opioids has quadrupled. It is estimated that more than 130 people die every day in the United States due to opioid overdose, and 115 million Americans misuse prescription opioids.[21] Deaths involving prescription opioids and heroin remained stable in 2018.[22]

There is little evidence that Australia has experienced the same trajectory of the problem as seen in the United States. However, there is evidence of an increase in harm associated with pharmaceutical opioids and heroin.[23] As such, there is a recognised need to introduce measures in Australia to reduce the harm associated with pharmaceutical opioids.[24] See Chapter 6 for further discussion of substance misuse.

While caution is needed in the use of opioids, we must also recognise that people in pain need adequate pain management. Addressing adequate pain management capability and appropriate education on opioid prescribing is necessary for all healthcare providers to ensure the safe use of pharmaceutical opioids while ensuring that people receive appropriate treatment.

Developmental considerations

Infants and children

Infants have the same capacity for pain as adults. During fetal development, ascending sensory fibres, neurotransmitters and connections to the thalamus are developed by 20 weeks' gestation. However, immaturity of the cortex and lack of conscious awareness may prevent the fetus from experiencing emotional 'pain' until 30 weeks' gestation. Conscious or not, pain-producing invasive fetal procedures elicit a stress response, and pain during gestation should be avoided until more is known about fetal pain. If invasive procedures must be performed on a developing fetus, adequate analgesia is necessary.[25] During the postnatal period, there is functional and structural immaturity in the nociceptive pathways that affects the pattern of activity in the infant's central nervous system This immaturity means that there is less discrimination between noxious and non-noxious stimuli. In addition, inhibitory networks and neurotransmitters are in insufficient supply in early development.[26] Therefore, neonates, contrary to popular belief, are rendered more sensitive to painful stimuli than older children.

Preverbal infants are at high risk for under-treatment of pain because of persistent myths and beliefs that infants have lower sensitivity to pain or do not remember pain.[27] Repetitive and poorly controlled pain in infants (daily heel sticks, venipunctures) can result in long-term adverse consequences such as neurodevelopmental problems, poor weight gain and learning disabilities.[28] Regardless of age, adequate use of analgesics during painful procedures is necessary.[9]

Late adulthood (65+ years)

The ageing population and advances in anaesthetic and surgical techniques have resulted in an increase in the age of people undergoing major surgery.[29] Also, older people are more likely to have chronic pain conditions. The most common pain-producing conditions for ageing adults include pathologies such as arthritis, osteoarthritis, osteoporosis, peripheral vascular disease, cancer, peripheral neuropathies, ischaemic heart disease and chronic constipation. There are many factors that combine to make effective pain management difficult in older adults. These include the higher incidence of comorbid conditions and concurrent medications, age-related changes in physiology, pharmacodynamics and pharmacokinetics and altered responses to pain.[30]

Although pain is a common experience among people 65 years of age or older, it is *not* a normal process of ageing. People over the age of 65 report more chronic pain and demonstrate a reduced tolerance to experimental pain than do people under the age of 65.[31] Pain indicates pathology or injury. Pain should never be considered something to tolerate or accept in one's later years. The experience of pain can be under-reported by older people for several reasons. Unfortunately, many clinicians and older adults wrongfully assume that pain should be expected in ageing, which leads to fewer investigations and less aggressive treatment. Older adults have additional fears about becoming dependent on others, undergoing invasive procedures, taking pain medications and having a financial burden.[32]

Altered cognitive function may present a challenge for pain assessment within this group, and the available evidence suggests that pain processing may be altered by different types and severity of dementia.[33] Further, autonomic reactions to pain such as diaphoresis and increased heart rate, blood pressure and respiratory rate can be blunted in people with dementia. Delirium during acute illnesses and in the postoperative period is more prevalent in older people and can also impact on pain assessment. The challenge for accurate pain assessment in older adults with altered cognitive function is the decreased reporting associated with diminished memory and communication difficulties requiring focused assessment strategies to detect and measure pain in this group of people.[14] In people with dementia or delirium, self-report of pain should be attempted, but this can be limited. In these circumstances, we can assess body language instead of verbal communications (e.g. a clenched fist or agitation may indicate pain). See further discussion on pain assessment with dementia later in this chapter.

Gender differences

Gender differences are influenced by societal expectations, hormones and genetic make-up. According to the Australian Health Survey, the prevalence of chronic pain is higher for women (16.0%) than it is for men (18.0%) in the years between 45 and 54 years.[34] Hormonal changes across the life span are found to have strong influences on pain sensitivity for women.[35] Women are two to three times more likely to experience migraines during childbearing years, are more sensitive to pain during the premenstrual period and are more likely to have fibromyalgia. Gender differences in reported pain intensity, frequency of pain conditions and reported pain coping strategies have been identified in children and adolescents from the age of 8 years onwards.

Findings from the Human Genome Project indicate that a pain gene exists, which helps to explain why some people feel more/less pain even with the same stimulus. Efforts are being made to tailor pharmacological agents to improve pain treatment based upon genetic sequencing.[36]

Cultural and social considerations

When clinicians speak a language or belong to a culture different from the person experiencing pain, the risk increases for misunderstanding, under-reporting and undertreating. Please review the methods for working with an interpreter in Chapter 7 and the discussion of cultural safety in Chapter 4.

The need to understand cultural differences when assessing and managing pain extends beyond just accounting for language. Culture influences the beliefs, attitudes, expectations and behaviours of people and health professionals. These factors affect how pain is interpreted, how pain is expressed and the person's pain relief–seeking behaviours. For example, people from cultures that value stoicism tend to avoid vocalising (moaning or screaming) when in pain, whereas other cultural groups may be more expressive.

In Australia, as in many other countries, there is significant cultural and ethnic diversity. The most recent national Census revealed that 27.6% of Australians were born overseas and 23% spoke a language other than English at home.[37] Disparities in the assessment and effectiveness of pain treatment exist across cultural groups, but pain assessment and treatment should be individualised to avoid cultural stereotyping that can lead to false assumptions about pain responses and its management.[20]

The pain experience of Aboriginal and Torres Strait Islander people has received very little research attention. Indigenous peoples are a heterogeneous group. This heterogeneity is evident in language, links to traditional cultural beliefs and links to the land and their understanding of western medicine.[20] Pain assessment and management of Indigenous people is often performed by non-Indigenous clinicians. Poor understanding of their cultures in relation to pain experiences can lead to inadequate pain management. Current pain assessment tools may have limited utility since they are set to standards based on data collected from non-Indigenous populations.[38] The use of a numerical rating scale of 0 to 10 is likely to produce inaccurate pain assessment as some Indigenous languages do not have a conceptual recognition of certain numbers.[39] Pain behaviours and language that may be unique to Indigenous people such as averting their eyes or turning their head away or feigning sleep can be misinterpreted and pain may be undertreated. The use of verbal description of pain and involving Aboriginal health workers to assist in communication should be encouraged. Clinical Yarning is recommended as a person-centred approach to improving communication between the person and the clinician because it has the potential to improve health outcomes.[40]

The experience of pain is more layered than just physical suffering. Pain and the expression of pain are influenced by social, cultural, emotional and spiritual concerns. It is imperative that pain assessment is thorough for all people, recognising that a lack of outward signs of pain does not indicate an absence of pain.

HEALTH EDUCATION

Chronic pain

Chronic pain is a common and complex condition characterised by persistent pain lasting generally 3 to 6 months longer than the expected healing time after an injury or illness. One in five Australians aged 45 years and over experience chronic pain that can be described as anything from mild to severe. Of those experiencing chronic pain they are more likely to be an older person, female, have limitations to their daily activities, have long-term medical conditions and longer hospital stays.[41] The problem is similar in Aotearoa New Zealand, where one in six people experience chronic pain that is persistent or episodic.

Pain seriously affects a person's physical state—for example, sleep, mobility and nutrition. The psychosocial aspects of the person are also affected—relationships, mental health, stress and coping. The person's ability to work and to participate in education or the community can be seriously affected. There is a significant economic impact of chronic pain. In 2020 the cost of chronic pain to the Australian Health Budget was $144.10 billion. There was $49.74 billion in lost productivity.[42] Conditions

Continued

HEALTH EDUCATION cont'd

associated with chronic pain include arthritis, trigeminal neuralgia, back pain, fibromyalgia, endometriosis, headaches, cancer and obesity.[41]

Nurse's role

Nurses have an important role in pain management, the beginning step of which is to perform a thorough pain assessment. Nurses should conduct pain assessment on a regular basis—for example, at least once per shift or more frequently depending on the person's situation and using a relevant assessment tool. Nurses must not let their personal beliefs guide their pain assessment practice but instead adhere to the principle that pain is what the person says it is. Familiarity with and use of relevant pain assessment tools is essential. There is a wide range of pain assessment tools available to take the guess work out of patient centred pain management. Nurses should also:

- consult with the person as to their knowledge and beliefs about pain
- find out the person's expectations about managing their pain
- use the most relevant pain assessment tool in relation to the person's need (verbal, nonverbal, older person, child, infant)
- reflect on own knowledge and beliefs about pain
- ensure pain management knowledge is up to date by engaging in continuing education programs
- access mentoring and guidance from senior health professionals in relation to pain assessment and management
- evaluate the effectiveness of pain strategies and, if the pain is unresolved, refer to a medical practitioner, nurse practitioner or pain service
- provide the person with readily available pain resources.

Websites

- Pain Australia—fact sheets: https://www.painaustralia.org.au/painaustralia-health-professionals/useful-resources-2021/painaustralia-fact-sheets
- Pain Australia—National Pain Services Directory: https://www.painaustralia.org.au/pain-services-directory/pain-directory
- Pain Australia—Clinical assessment of pain: http://painaustralia.staging3.webforcefive.com.au/static/uploads/files/painaust-factsheet3-jan-16-wfksvufhgrzc.pdf
- Pain Australia—Multidisciplinary pain management: http://painaustralia.staging3.webforcefive.com.au/static/uploads/files/painaust-factsheet4-aug-16-wfyaezqnplrj.pdf

Subjective data

Some people may be reluctant to discuss having pain for fear of dependency on others, the fear of further testing or invasive procedures, the cost of taking pain killers or the fear of becoming drug addicted. During subjective data collection establish an empathetic and caring rapport with the person or child to gain trust. As an alternative to the questions below you can collect a complete pain health history using the PQRST mnemonic described in Table 13.1 or the COLDSPA mnemonic described in Table 13.2.

Practice note

Before you start the assessment, introduce yourself to the person, confirm the person's identity, discuss the purpose and scope of the assessment, clarify any questions the person may have and obtain verbal consent from the person to perform the assessment.

ASSESSMENT GUIDELINES	CLINICAL SIGNIFICANCE AND CLINICAL ALERTS
Initial pain assessment	
Presenting concern	
• *Do you have pain? Discomfort or soreness? Tell me in your own words.*	Some people report pain only when it is severe. Try a variety of words.
• *Where is your pain? Tell me about all the places you have pain.*	Pain may be localised or occur in multiple sites.
• *When did your pain start? What were you doing when the pain started? Is it constant or does it come and go?*	Identifies onset and duration. **Chronic pain** persists after injury heals; it is pain that occurs for 3 months or longer.
• *What does your pain feel like?* – *Burning, stabbing, aching?* – *Throbbing, firelike, squeezing?* – *Cramping, sharp, itching, tingling?* – *Shooting, crushing, sharp, dull?*	Identifies the quality of pain and helps differentiate between nociceptive and neuropathic pain mechanisms. **Neuropathic pain** is described as burning, shooting and tingling. **Nociceptive pain** originating from visceral sites is described as aching if localised and cramping if poorly localised. **Nociplastic pain** is persistent pain arising from altered nociception. **Somatic site pain** is described as throbbing/aching.
• *How much pain do you have now?* Refer to various intensity scales—for example, the 0–10 numerical rating scale. Refer to 'Pain assessment tools' below.	Identifies current intensity and represents pain at rest.
• *How much pain do you have when you move?* Refer to various intensity scales—for example, the 0–10 numerical rating scale.	Identifies intensity of pain with activity. This pain is referred to as **dynamic pain**.
• *What makes your pain better or worse?* (e.g. behavioural, pharmacological and nonpharmacological interventions)	Identifies alleviating and aggravating factors.
• *Which medicines control your pain? Are doses adequate? How often do you take pain medicines?*	Evaluates effectiveness of current treatment. ! ***Clinical alert:*** If a person has unrelieved or increasing pain not relieved by their current treatment plan, report it to a medical practitioner.
• *How much does your pain interfere with your ability to:* – *do activities in bed such as turning, repositioning or sitting up?* – *do activities out of bed such as walking, sitting in a chair or standing?* • *What does the pain prevent you from doing?*	Identifies the dynamic nature of pain and the degree of impairment or effect on quality of life.

ASSESSMENT GUIDELINES	CLINICAL SIGNIFICANCE AND CLINICAL ALERTS
• *How does pain affect your sleep and mood?* • *Do you experience feelings of stress or anxiety when you have pain? How do you manage your stress or anxiety?*	Identifies degree of impairment and quality of life. Mood (feeling anxious or depressed) and sleep (falling asleep and staying asleep) may be particularly relevant for chronic pain.
• *Do you experience any other symptoms along with the pain* (nausea, vomiting, dizziness, heart racing, difficulty sleeping or fatigue)?	Will aid in detection, assessment and treatment. Unfortunately, clinical staff may inadvertently interpret an altered sleeping pattern, particularly day sleeping, as 'comfort' and fail to properly assess the person's pain and may fail to provide appropriate pharmacological intervention.
• *What does this pain mean to you? Why do you think you are having pain?*	Can identify myths, misconception and beliefs such as '*I'm getting old*'. Can reveal feelings of fear, depression or helplessness.
• *What are your expectations of and preferences for, pain treatment?*	Assists in planning pain relief interventions that reflect patient preferences and satisfaction with pain relief outcomes.
Other symptoms	
Nutrition and metabolic • *Has the pain affected your appetite?* • *Do you have any nausea or vomiting?* **Elimination** • *Have you experienced any changes in bowel habits?*	Nausea and vomiting are common side effects of pain medicines. Constipation is a side effect of some analgesics because of effects on smooth muscle.
Health and lifestyle management	
• *Tell me more about the medicines you are taking for pain.* • *How much? How often?* • *Do you experience any side effects?* Ask about smoking, alcohol and/or illicit drug use.	Analgesics include the following groups: • **non-opioids** such as acetaminophen (paracetamol) • **non-steroidal anti-inflammatory medications** such as ibuprofen, aspirin and diclofenac • **opioids** such as codeine, morphine, oxycodone, fentanyl and tramadol • **anticonvulsants** such as gabapentin and pregabalin • **corticosteroids** such as prednisolone and prednisone • **medicinal cannabis** • **antidepressants** such as amitriptyline.

ASSESSMENT GUIDELINES	CLINICAL SIGNIFICANCE AND CLINICAL ALERTS
Additional history for infants and children	
Include the parent or caregiver and use a relevant pain assessment tool depending on the age of the child/infant	
Additional history for adults over 65 years	
• *Do you have any chronic health conditions such as* osteoarthritis, peripheral vascular disease, cancer, osteoporosis, angina or chronic constipation? If there is cognitive impairment—use a relevant pain assessment tool (see information below).	

TABLE 13.1 PQRST mnemonic—pain assessment questions

P = Provocation/palliation
What were you doing when the pain started? What caused it? What makes it better? Worse? What seems to trigger it? Stress? Position? Certain activities? *What relieves it? Medications, massage, heat/cold, changing position, being active, resting?* *What aggravates it? Movement, bending, lying down, walking, standing?*
Q = Quality/quantity
What does it feel like? Use words to describe the pain, such as sharp, full, stabbing, burning, crushing, throbbing, nauseating, shooting, twisting or stretching.
R = Region/radiation
Where is the pain located? Does it radiate? Where? Does it feel as if it travels/moves around? Did it start elsewhere and is now localised to one spot?
S = Severity scale
How severe is the pain on a scale of 0 to 10, with zero being no pain and 10 being the worst pain ever? Does it interfere with activities? How bad is it at its worst? Does it force you to sit down, lie down or slow down? How long does an episode last?
T = Timing
When/at what time did the pain start? How long did it last? How often does it occur: Hourly? Daily? Weekly? Monthly? Is it sudden or gradual? What were you doing when you first experienced it? When do you usually experience it: Daytime? Night? Early morning? Are you ever awakened by it? Does it lead to anything else? Is it accompanied by other signs and symptoms? Does it ever occur before, during or after meals? Does it occur seasonally?

Table 13.2 COLDSPA mnemonic—pain assessment questions

First letter meaning	Questions
Character	*Can you describe the pain?* What does the pain feel like? Is it sharp, dull, crushing or burning?
Onset	When did the pain begin?
Location	*Where is the pain?* Does the pain go anywhere else?
Duration	Is the pain constant or does it come and go?
Severity	*How severe is the pain?* Can you rate the pain on a scale of 0 to 10, with 0 being 'no pain'?
Pattern	What makes it better or worse?
Associated factors	Do you have any other symptoms such as nausea or vomiting?
Affects	Does the pain stop you from doing things? Give examples please.

Pain assessment tools

Various tools have been developed to capture unidimensional aspects such as intensity or multidimensional components. The choice of tool depends on its purpose, time involved in its administration and the person's ability to comprehend and complete the tool.

Self-assessment pain scales can be used reliably for most people with mild-to-moderate cognitive impairment although dementia and delirium can limit a person's ability to report pain.[43]

In situations of acute pain and pain as a symptom of trauma or disease, assessment of the presence, intensity (at rest and with movement) and location of pain enables characterisation of pain and evaluation of the effectiveness of treatment. The following practice points will help you get the most useful information from the pain tool.

- The assessment tool should be used consistently before and after treatment to see whether the treatment has been effective.
- When first using a tool, familiarise the person with the format and purpose of the tool.
- It may be useful to enlarge the print for people with impaired vision.
- Where possible, involve an interpreter when the person's first language is other than English.
- For people with low literacy you will need to read out the statements/questions on the pain tool.
- Ask the person to rate and evaluate all their pain sites.
- Some pain tools allow for only one pain rating score, therefore if the person has pain at more than one site, you will need to document the pain score for each site.

Multidimensional pain assessment tools are more useful for chronic pain conditions or particularly problematic acute pain problems. These tools provide more information about the characteristics of pain and its impact on the person. A few examples include the Initial Pain Assessment, the Brief Pain Inventory and the McGill Pain Questionnaire.

In the **Initial Pain Assessment**[44] the clinician asks the person to answer eight questions concerning location, intensity, quality, duration and aggravating/relieving factors. Further, the clinician adds questions about manner of expressing pain and the effects of pain that impairs quality of life (Figure 13.6).

The **Brief Pain Inventory**[45] ask the person to rate the pain within the past 24 hours using graduated scales (0–10) with respect to its impact on areas such as mood, walking ability and sleep. It is available in multiple languages (Figure 13.7). The **Short-Form McGill Pain Questionnaire**[46] asks the person to rank a list of descriptors in terms

Initial pain assessment tool

Date ______

Patient's name ______ Age ______ Room ______

Diagnosis ______ Physician ______

Nurse ______

1. LOCATION: Patient or nurse mark drawing.

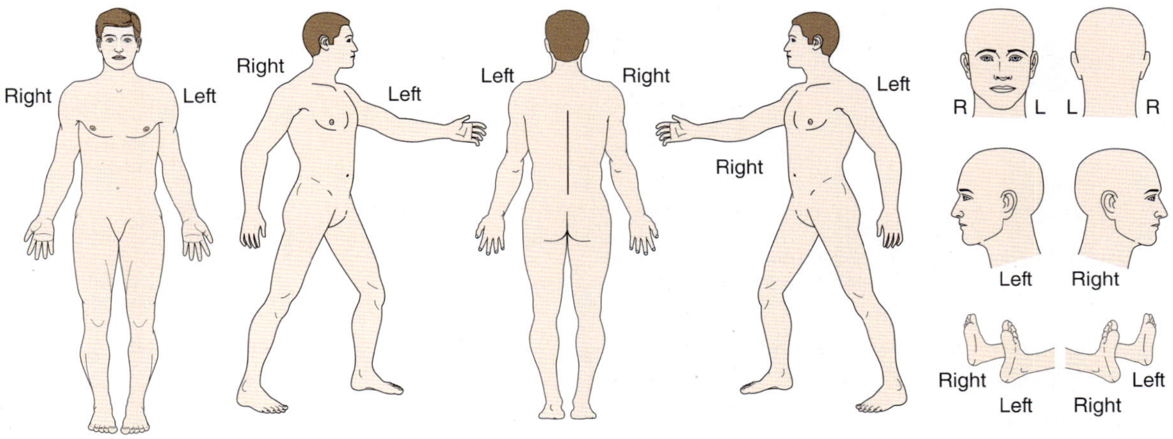

2. INTENSITY: Patient rates the pain. Scale used ______
   Present: ______
   Worst pain gets: ______
   Best pain gets: ______
   Acceptable level of pain: ______
3. QUALITY: (Use patient's own words, e.g. prick, ache, burn, throb, pull, sharp.) ______
4. ONSET, DURATION, VARIATION, RHYTHMS: ______
5. MANNER OF EXPRESSING PAIN: ______
6. WHAT RELIEVES THE PAIN? ______
7. WHAT CAUSES OR INCREASES THE PAIN? ______
8. EFFECTS OF PAIN: (Note decreased function, decreased quality of life.)
   Accompanying symptoms (e.g. nausea) ______
   Sleep ______
   Appetite ______
   Physical activity ______
   Relationship with others (e.g. irritability) ______
   Emotions (e.g. anger, suicidal, crying) ______
   Concentration ______
   Other ______
9. OTHER COMMENTS: ______
10. PLAN: ______

FIGURE 13.6 Initial pain assessment tool
Source: McCaffery & Pasero 1999[4]

Brief pain inventory

Date: ___/___/___ Time: ___________

Name: ______________________________

Last First Middle initial

1. Throughout our lives, most of us have had pain from time to time (such as minor headaches, sprains and toothaches). Have you had pain other than these everyday kinds of pain today?
   1. Yes 2. No

2. On the diagram, shade in the areas where you feel pain. Put an X on the area that hurts the most.

Right Left Left Right

3. Please rate your pain by circling the one number that best describes your pain at its **worst** in the past 24 hours.

0	1	2	3	4	5	6	7	8	9	10
No pain										Pain as bad as you can imagine

4. Please rate your pain by circling the one number that best describes your pain at its **least** in the past 24 hours.

0	1	2	3	4	5	6	7	8	9	10
No pain										Pain as bad as you can imagine

5. Please rate your pain by circling the one number that best describes your pain on the **average**.

0	1	2	3	4	5	6	7	8	9	10
No pain										Pain as bad as you can imagine

6. Please rate your pain by circling the one number that tells how much pain you have **right now**.

0	1	2	3	4	5	6	7	8	9	10
No pain										Pain as bad as you can imagine

7. What treatments or medications are you receiving for your pain?

____

____

8. In the past 24 hours, how much **relief** have pain treatments or medications provided? Please circle the one percentage that most shows how much relief you have received.

0%	10	20	30	40	50	60	70	80	90	100%
No relief										Complete relief

9. Circle the one number that describes how, during the past 24 hours, pain has **interfered** with your:

A: General activity

0	1	2	3	4	5	6	7	8	9	10
Does not interfere										Completely interferes

B: Mood

0	1	2	3	4	5	6	7	8	9	10
Does not interfere										Completely interferes

C: Walking ability

0	1	2	3	4	5	6	7	8	9	10
Does not interfere										Completely interferes

D: Normal work (includes both work outside the home and housework)

0	1	2	3	4	5	6	7	8	9	10
Does not interfere										Completely interferes

E: Relations with other people

0	1	2	3	4	5	6	7	8	9	10
Does not interfere										Completely interferes

F: Sleep

0	1	2	3	4	5	6	7	8	9	10
Does not interfere										Completely interferes

G: Enjoyment of life

0	1	2	3	4	5	6	7	8	9	10
Does not interfere										Completely interferes

FIGURE 13.7 Brief pain inventory.
Source: Cleeland & Ryan 1994[45]

Date: ____________

Subject ID: ____________

Short-form McGill Pain Questionnaire 2 (SF-MPQ-2)

For this questionnaire, I will provide you a list of words that describe some of the different qualities of pain and related symptoms. Please rate the intensity of each of the pain and related symptoms you felt during the past week on 0 to 10 scale, with 0 being no pain and 10 being the worst pain you can imagine. Use 0 if the word does not describe your pain or related symptoms. Limit yourself to a description of the pain related to your surgery or pelvic pain.

1. Throbbing pain	*none*	0	1	2	3	4	5	6	7	8	9	10	*worst possible*
2. Shooting pain	*none*	0	1	2	3	4	5	6	7	8	9	10	*worst possible*
3. Stabbing pain	*none*	0	1	2	3	4	5	6	7	8	9	10	*worst possible*
4. Sharp pain	*none*	0	1	2	3	4	5	6	7	8	9	10	*worst possible*
5. Cramping pain	*none*	0	1	2	3	4	5	6	7	8	9	10	*worst possible*
6. Gnawing pain	*none*	0	1	2	3	4	5	6	7	8	9	10	*worst possible*
7. Hot-burning pain	*none*	0	1	2	3	4	5	6	7	8	9	10	*worst possible*
8. Aching pain	*none*	0	1	2	3	4	5	6	7	8	9	10	*worst possible*
9. Heavy pain	*none*	0	1	2	3	4	5	6	7	8	9	10	*worst possible*
10. Tender	*none*	0	1	2	3	4	5	6	7	8	9	10	*worst possible*
11. Splitting pain	*none*	0	1	2	3	4	5	6	7	8	9	10	*worst possible*
12. Tiring-exhausting	*none*	0	1	2	3	4	5	6	7	8	9	10	*worst possible*
13. Sickening	*none*	0	1	2	3	4	5	6	7	8	9	10	*worst possible*
14. Fearful	*none*	0	1	2	3	4	5	6	7	8	9	10	*worst possible*
15. Punishing-cruel	*none*	0	1	2	3	4	5	6	7	8	9	10	*worst possible*
16. Electric-shock pain	*none*	0	1	2	3	4	5	6	7	8	9	10	*worst possible*

FIGURE 13.8 The short-form McGill Pain Questionnaire.
Source: Melzack 1987[46]

of their intensity and to give an overall intensity rating to their pain. The short form only takes 2 to 3 minutes to complete (Figure 13.8).

Pain rating scales are **unidimensional** and are intended to reflect pain intensity. They come in various forms. Pain rating scales can indicate baseline intensity, track changes due to changing disease state or recovery and give some degree of evaluation of treatment.

Numerical rating scales (NRS)[47] can be administered verbally or visually along a vertical or horizontal line (Figure 13.9). Typically, the person is asked to choose a number that rates the level of pain, with 0 being no pain and the highest anchor, 10, indicating the worst pain possible. The use of a numerical rating scale makes recording pain intensity among various clinicians easier and more consistent. The **Visual Analogue**

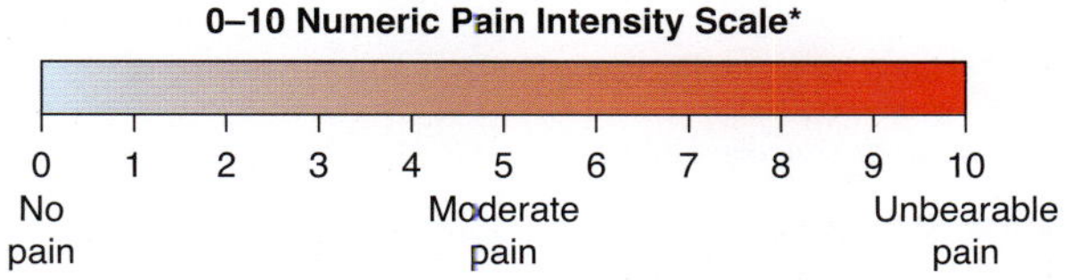

FIGURE 13.9 Numerical pain intensity scale.
Source: McCaffery & Beebe 1989[47]

Scale[20] is a numerical scale that allows patients to place a mark along a 10-centimetre line from no pain to the worst pain possible. There are minor variations in the anchors used for these scales (Figure 13.10).

An alternative to numerical scales is the use of **categorical scales** such as the simple **Verbal Descriptor Scale**[48] (Figure 13.11) where words are used to describe the magnitude of pain. The words describe different levels of pain intensity, such as *no pain*, *mild pain*, *moderate pain* and *severe pain*. The words can be converted to *numeric scores* (e.g. 0, 1, 2, 3, 4, 5).

Frail older adults may find the **numerical rating scales** too abstract and have difficulty responding, especially with a fluctuating chronic pain experience and will therefore often respond to scales such as the **Verbal Descriptor Scale**, in which words are selected rather than numbers. Again, it is essential to teach the person how to use the scale to enhance accuracy. There also needs to be awareness that personal, linguistic and cultural differences may affect interpretation of the descriptor words in situations where the person cannot communicate their pain because of altered conscious state, impaired cognition, language or developmental constraints; pain assessment needs to be modified to encompass behavioural and physiological manifestations of pain.

Visual Analogue Scale (VAS)†

No pain — Pain as bad as it could possibly be

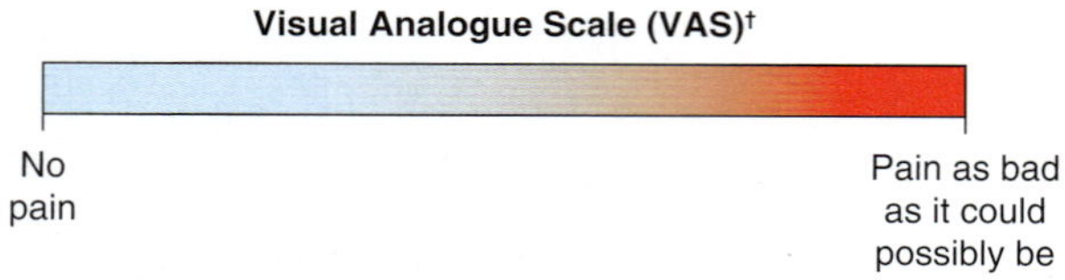

* If used as a graphic rating scale, a 10-cm baseline is recommended.

† A 10-cm baseline is recommended for VAS scales.

FIGURE 13.10 Visual analogue scale (VAS).
Source: Schug et al. 2020[20]

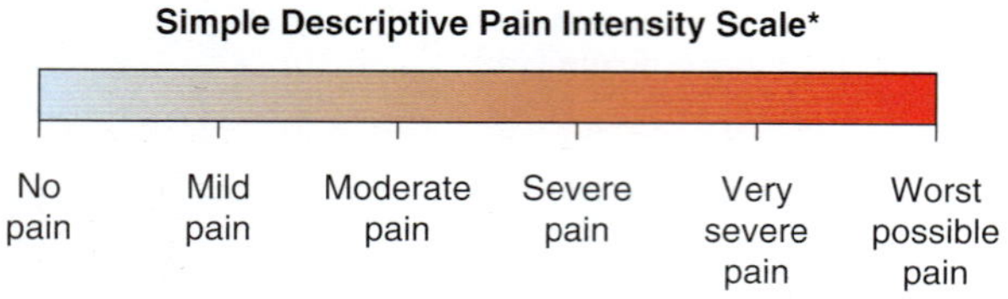

Simple Descriptive Pain Intensity Scale*

No pain — Mild pain — Moderate pain — Severe pain — Very severe pain — Worst possible pain

FIGURE 13.11 Simple descriptive pain intensity scale (categorical).
Source: Jensen et al. 1986[48]

TOOLS FOR ASSESSING PAIN IN PEOPLE WITH DEMENTIA

Several observational pain assessment scales have been developed and used in people with varying degrees of dementia. A commonly used scale in Australia is the Abbey Pain Scale[49] (Figure 13.12). This scale is a one-page assessment tool where the presence and severity of six observable cues (vocalisation, facial expression, change in body language, behavioural change, physiological change and physical changes) are scored to provide a total pain score.

The **PAINAD scale** is a simple, reliable and validated five-item observational tool that evaluates common behaviours: breathing; vocalisation; facial expression; body language and consolability[50] (Figure 13.13). Specific behaviours in these categories are quantified from 0 to 2, with a total score of 0 to 10. This is consistent with the commonly used 0 to 10 score on other pain assessment tools. For the PAINAD, a score of 4 or more indicates the need for pain management.

TOOLS FOR INFANTS AND CHILDREN

Most pain research on infants has focused on acute, procedural pain. We have a limited understanding of how to assess chronic pain in the infant. Currently, there is no one assessment tool that adequately identifies pain in the infant. Using a multidimensional approach for the whole infant is encouraged. Assessment of pain in infants and children requires the use of age- and context-appropriate assessment tools. It is recommended that behavioural and physiological signs are evaluated in conjunction with a child's self-report of pain.[20]

Place identification label here

Name: ....

DOB: ....

Room No: ....

ABBEY PAIN SCALE

For measurement of pain in people with dementia who cannot verbalise

How to use scale: While observing the resident, score questions 1 to 6.

Name of person completing the scale: ....

Date: .... Time: .... Designation: ....

Latest pain relief given was .... at .... hours.

Q1 Vocalisation **Q1** ☐
(e.g. whimpering, groaning, crying)

Absent 0 *Mild 1* *Moderate 2* *Severe 3*

Q2 Facial expression **Q2** ☐
(e.g. looking tense, frowning, grimacing, looking frightened)

Absent 0 *Mild 1* *Moderate 2* *Severe 3*

Q3 Change in body language **Q3** ☐
(e.g. fidgeting, rocking, guarding part of body, withdrawn)

Absent 0 *Mild 1* *Moderate 2* *Severe 3*

Q4 Behavioural change **Q4** ☐
(e.g. increased confusion, refusing to eat, alteration in usual patterns)

Absent 0 *Mild 1* *Moderate 2* *Severe 3*

Q5 Physiological change **Q5** ☐
(e.g. temperature, pulse or blood pressure outside normal limits, perspiring, flushing or pallor)

Absent 0 *Mild 1* *Moderate 2* *Severe 3*

Q6 Physical changes **Q6** ☐
(e.g. skin tears, pressure areas, arthritis, contractures, previous injuries)

Absent 0 *Mild 1* *Moderate 2* *Severe 3*

Add scores for 1–6 and record here **Total Pain Score** ☐

Now tick the box that matches the Total Pain Score

0–2 No pain	3–7 Mild	8–13 Moderate	14+ Severe

Finally, tick the box which matches the type of pain

Chronic	Acute	Acute on Chronic

FIGURE 13.12 The Abbey pain scale.
Source: Abbey et al. 2004[49]

Because infants are preverbal and incapable of self-report, pain assessment is dependent exclusively upon behavioural and physiological cues. Refer to the 'Objective data' section below. It is important to emphasise the understanding that infants *do* feel pain but are vulnerable to having their pain not recognised or underestimated.

By 2 years of age children can report pain and point to its location. They cannot rate pain intensity at this developmental level. It is helpful to ask the parent or caregiver what

Pain Assessment In Advanced Dementia (PAINAD) Scale

	0	1	2	Score
Breathing Independent of Vocalisation	Normal	Occasional laboured breathing, short period of hyperventilation	Noisy laboured breathing, long period of hyperventilation, Cheyne-Stokes respirations	
Negative Vocalisation	None	Occasional moan or groan, low level of speech with a negative or disapproving quality	Repeated troubled calling out, loud moaning or groaning, crying	
Facial Expression	Smiling or inexpressive	Sad, frightened, frown	Facial grimacing	
Body Language	Relaxed	Tense, distressed pacing, fidgeting	Rigid, fists clenched, knees pulled up, pulling or pushing away, striking out	
Consolability	No need to console	Distracted or reassured by voice or touch	Unable to console, distract or reassure	
			TOTAL	

FIGURE 13.13 Pain assessment in advanced dementia (PAINAD) scale.
Source: Warden et al. 2002[50]

Faces Pain Scale — Revised (FPS-R)

In the following instructions, say 'hurt' or 'pain', whichever seems right for a particular child.

'These faces show how much something can hurt. This face [point to left-most face] **shows no pain. The faces show more and more pain** [point to each from left to right] **up to this one** [point to right-most face] **— it shows very much pain. Point to the face that shows how much you hurt** [right now].'

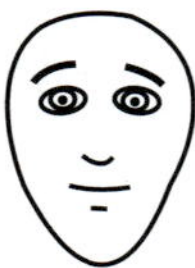
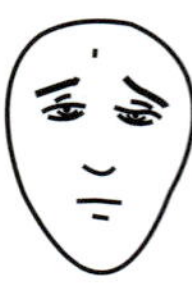
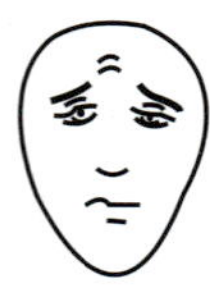
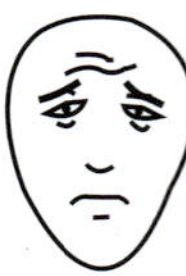
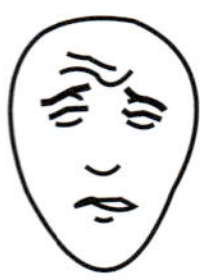
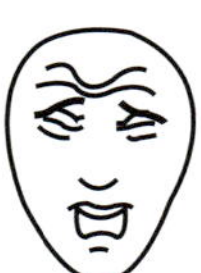

Score the chosen face 0, 2, 4, 6, 8 or 10, counting left to right, so '0' = 'no pain' and '10' = 'very much pain'. Do not use words like 'happy' and 'sad'. This scale is intended to measure how children feel inside, not how their face looks.

Sources. Hicks CL, von Baeyer CL, Spafford P, et al. The Faces Pain Scale—Revised: toward a common metric in pediatric pain measurement. *Pain*, *93*, 173–83. Bieri D, Reeve R, Champion GD, et al. The Faces Pain Scale for the self-assessment of the severity of pain experienced by children: development, initial validation and preliminary investigation for ratio scale properties. *Pain*, *41*, 139–50.

FIGURE 13.14 FACES pain scale—revised.
Source: International Association for the Study of Pain 2019[51]

words their child uses to report pain (e.g. ouch, sore). Be aware that some children will try to be 'grown up and brave' and often deny having pain in the presence of a stranger or if they are fearful of receiving a 'needle'.

Rating scales can be introduced at 3 or 4 years of age.[20] **The Faces Pain Scale—Revised (FPS-R)** has six drawings of faces that show pain intensity. The child is given an explanation that each face is a person with 'no pain' on the left (score of 0) to 'very much pain' on the right (score of 10) (Figure 13.14). The FPS-R has realistic facial expressions, with a furrowed brow and horizontal mouth. The advantage of the FPS-R is that it avoids smiles or tears so children will not confuse pain intensity with happiness or sadness.[51]

One tool that has been developed for postoperative pain in preterm and term neonates is the **CRIES tool**.[52] It measures physiological and behavioural indicators on a three-point scale (Figure 13.15).

The **FLACC scale** was developed to assess pain in young children and has been shown to have good interrater reliability and validity.[53] The FLACC scale is a simple framework that enables pain behaviours to be assessed objectively and quantified. The scale is composed of five categories of pain behaviours: F = face, L = legs, A = activity, C = cry, C = consolability. Each category receives a score of 0 to 2 to provide a total pain score range of 0 to 10 (Figure 13.16).

CRIES Neonatal Postoperative Pain Measurement Score

	0	1	2
Crying	No	High-pitched	Inconsolable
Requires O_2 for sat >95%	No	<30% from baseline	>30% from baseline
Increased vital signs	HR and BP = or < preop	HR or BP ↑ <20% of preop	HR or BP ↑ >20% of preop
Expression	None	Grimace	Grimace/grunt
Sleepless	No, continuously asleep	Wakes at frequent intervals	Constantly awake

FIGURE 13.15 CRIES Neonatal postoperative pain measurement score.
Source: Krechel & Bildner 1995[52]

FLACC Behavioral Pain Scale (Infants and Toddlers)

DATE/TIME						
Face 0–No particular expression or smile 1–Occasional grimace or frown, withdrawn, disinterested 2–Frequent to constant quivering chin, clenched jaw						
Legs 0–Normal position or relaxed 1–Uneasy, restless, tense 2–Kicking, or legs drawn up						
Activity 0–Lying quietly, normal position, moves easily 1–Squirming, shifting back and forth, tense 2–Arched, rigid or jerking						
Cry 0–No cry (awake or asleep) 1–Moans or whimpers; occasional complaint 2–Crying steadily, screams or sobs, frequent complaints						
Consolability 0–Content, relaxed 1–Reassured by occasional touching, hugging or being talked to, distractible 2–Difficult to console or comfort						
TOTAL SCORE						

FIGURE 13.16 FLACC Behavioral pain scale (infants and toddlers).
Source: Merkel et al. 1997[53]

The FLACC is recommended for use in emergency triage. Note that these tools assess acute pain. No biological markers have been identified for long-term chronic pain in infants or children. Therefore, evaluate the whole person.

Objective data

Preparation

Objective assessment of pain is sometimes necessary in circumstances when verbalisation of pain is not possible. The objective data collection process includes using pain assessment tools to help you further understand the person's experience and the nature of the pain. Consider whether this is an acute or chronic condition. Recall that physical findings may not always support the person's pain reports, particularly for chronic pain syndromes. Pain should not be discounted when objective physical evidence is not found. Based on the person's pain report, make every effort to reduce or eliminate the pain with appropriate analgesic and nonpharmacological intervention.

Equipment needed

Hand hygiene solution
Tape measure to measure circumference of swollen joints or extremities
Tongue depressor
Penlight

PROCEDURES AND NORMAL FINDINGS	ABNORMAL FINDINGS AND CLINICAL ALERTS
General inspection	
While collecting subjective data, you will have noticed the condition of the person's skin, lips, hair and mucous membranes, breath odour, ease of breathing, body movements, height-to-weight ratio, body shape, posture, level of hygiene and grooming and general demeanour. All these factors provide clues to the person's level of comfort. Identify pain-related features through observing alterations in mobility or guarding. Check for changes in the person's facial expression, posture, gait or mood.	For example, abdominal pain may result in a hunched posture; appearance of tiredness or grimacing; and uneven gait such as limping, which may indicate the site of injury.
When the person cannot verbally communicate their pain, you can (**to a limited extent**) identify pain using behavioural cues.	People react to painful stimuli with a wide variety of behaviours. Behaviours are influenced by many factors including the nature of the pain (acute versus chronic), age and cultural and gender expectations.

PROCEDURES AND NORMAL FINDINGS	ABNORMAL FINDINGS AND CLINICAL ALERTS
Acute pain behaviours	
Acute pain involves autonomic responses and has a protective purpose. Observe the person for pain behaviours.	People experiencing moderate to intense levels of pain *may* exhibit the following behaviours: **guarding, grimacing, vocalisations such as moaning, agitation, restlessness, stillness, diaphoresis** or change in vital signs. This list of behaviours is not exhaustive because they should not be used exclusively to deny or confirm the presence of pain. For example, in a postoperative patient, pulse and blood pressure can be altered by fluid volume, medications and blood loss.
Chronic (persistent) pain behaviours	
Observe for chronic pain behaviours.	People experiencing chronic pain may exhibit behaviours such as **bracing, rubbing, diminished activity, sighing and change in appetite**. Sleeping is one way people behave in response to chronic pain to self-distract.
Limbs and joints	
If the pain is in a limb or joint, note the size and contour of the joint/limb. Measure circumference of the involved joint/limb for comparison with baseline. Check active or passive range of motion (see complete technique, Chapter 20). Joint motion normally causes no tenderness, pain or crepitation.	Swelling, inflammation, injury, deformity, diminished range of motion, increased pain on palpation and crepitation (an audible and palpable crunching that accompanies movement).
Muscles and skin	
Inspect the skin and tissue for colour, swelling, temperature and any masses or deformity.	Bruising, lesions, open wounds, tissue damage, atrophy, bulging, change in hair distribution, heat or cold and pallor or redness.
To assess for changes in sensation, ask the person to close their eyes. Test the person's ability to perceive sensation by breaking a tongue depressor in two lengthwise. Lightly press the sharp and blunted ends on the skin in a random fashion and ask the person to identify it as sharp or dull (Figure 12.29A and 12.29B). This test will help you identify location and extent of altered sensation (Table 13.3).	Absent pain sensation (**analgesia**); increased pain sensation (**hyperalgesia**); or if a severe pain sensation is evoked with a stimulus that does not normally induce pain (e.g. the blunt end of the tongue blade, cotton ball, clothing) (**allodynia**).

PROCEDURES AND NORMAL FINDINGS	ABNORMAL FINDINGS AND CLINICAL ALERTS
Abdomen	
If the pain is in the abdomen, observe for contour and symmetry. Palpate superficially for muscle guarding. Note any areas of referred pain (Table 23.13). Observe person's face for nonverbal responses to palpation.	Swelling, bulging, herniation, inflammation and muscle guarding. Leave any reported area of tenderness until last so as not to cause guarding or unnecessary discomfort. Nonverbal responses to palpation may include, drawing up of legs, guarding, groaning.  ***Clinical alert:*** If the person experiences any significant abdominal tenderness on palpation stop the examination and refer the person to a medical practitioner for further assessment.
Other pain sites	
For example, the chest, mouth, face, nose, ear, lips, tongue, throat or symptoms such as dysuria, constipation, or pain on breathing. Refer to relevant chapters within the text for assessment guidelines.	
Vital signs	
A check of vital signs is recommended to determine any physiological changes (Table 13.4).	Vital sign changes may include tachycardia, high or low blood pressure, raised respiratory rate, pallor and perspiration. ***Clinical alert:*** A lack of change in vital signs is not a reliable indicator of the person's pain state. Be aware that tachycardia and tachypnoea also occur with anxiety and fear and are not specific to pain. However, poorly controlled pain can result in systemic physiological change (Table 13.4).
Functional impact of pain	
Measure pain intensity scores on movement and with deep breathing and coughing. Assess the person's ability to sit upright by themselves, to move and their ability to perform self-care. Use the **Functional Activity Scale** (FAS), the purpose of which is to assess whether a patient can undertake a certain activity.[20]	The FAS has a simple three-level ranked categorical score: • **A—No limitation** (the person can undertake the activity without limitation due to pain) (pain intensity score typically 0–3 on a 0–10 scale) • **B—Mild limitation** (the person can undertake the activity but experiences moderate to severe pain) (pain intensity score is typically 4–10) • **C—Significant limitation** (the person is unable to complete the activity due to pain or pain treatment-related side effects independent of pain intensity scores).

PROCEDURES AND NORMAL FINDINGS	ABNORMAL FINDINGS AND CLINICAL ALERTS
Additional objective data for adults over 65 years	
Pain should not be considered a 'normal' part of ageing. When an older adult reports a history of conditions such as osteoarthritis, peripheral vascular disease, cancer, osteoporosis, angina or chronic constipation, be alert and anticipate a pain problem. Use the FAS tool to assess functional ability such as dressing, walking, toileting, eating or involvement in daily activities.	Slowness and rigidity may be apparent.
Adults with cognitive impairment and/or aphasia	
A person with cognitive impairment and/or aphasia may experience pain but may not be able to alert others that they have pain, describe the pain, discern variations in pain or recall severity of pain. When this is the case, then observation of pain behaviours is an important component of pain assessment. The Abbey Pain Scale or similar will be useful for people with cognitive impairment or are aphasic. Look for a sudden onset of acute confusion, which may indicate poorly controlled pain (Figure 13.12).	Behaviours such as restlessness, frowning and grimacing and sounds such as grunting or groaning may be apparent; however, they may not always be valid indicators of pain in nonverbal adults. ! ***Clinical alert:*** Sudden onset of acute confusion may indicate poorly controlled pain. However, you will need to rule out other competing explanations such as infection, adverse reaction to medications or delirium.
Additional objective data for infants and children	
General inspection	
Look for changes in temperament, expression and activity. For example, observe facial activity and body movements. Crying can be described in terms of its presence or absence, duration and amplitude or pitch. Observe for facial expressions (e.g. taut tongue, bulging brow, eye squeeze, nasolabial furrow).	! ***Clinical alert:*** If a procedure or disease process is known to induce pain in adults (e.g. surgery, injury, cancer), it *will* induce pain in an infant or child. Because the sympathetic nervous system is engaged particularly in acute episodes of pain, physiological changes take place that may indicate the presence of pain. These include sweating, increases in blood pressure and heart rate, vomiting, nausea and changes in oxygen saturation. However, like in adults, these physiological changes cannot be used exclusively to confirm or deny pain because of other factors such as stress, medications and fluid changes.

Abnormal findings

TABLE 13.3 Peripheral neuropathy

Condition Description	Symptoms
Peripheral neuropathy is symmetrical damage to peripheral nerves (feet or hands), resulting in pain without stimulation of the nerves. This is a common neuropathic pain.	Numbness and tingling, with interspersed shooting or lancinating pain that is not attributed to a specific nociceptive source.
Diabetic neuropathy is a common complication of diabetes and may relate to demyelination of the larger peripheral nerves, with an increase in smaller myelinated nerves. Other aetiologies may include ischaemic damage to nerves or hyperglycaemia, causing changes in nerve microenvironment.	Burning pain in the feet bilaterally, which is often worse at night.
Chemotherapy-induced peripheral neuropathy occurs during or after chemotherapy treatment for cancer. The risk increases with the number or agents used during treatment, higher cumulative doses of neurotoxic agents, pre-existing neuropathy from diabetes or other causes and older age.	Depends on the nerves affected and include: tingling ('pins and needles'); burning pain that can be severe and constant or may come and go; decreased sensation; increased sensitivity to touch, temperature or pressure; and muscle weakness.[53]

Note: With any cancer survivor, you must address any new onset of pain promptly to rule out pathological recurrence of cancer.

TABLE 13.4 Physiological changes from poorly controlled pain

Pain is not a benign symptom. Poorly controlled acute pain and chronic pain have negative impacts on physiological systems.

Physiological System	Acute Pain Responses
Cardiac	Tachycardia Elevated blood pressure Increased myocardial oxygen demand Increased cardiac output
Pulmonary	Hypoventilation Hypoxia Decreased cough Atelectasis
Gastrointestinal	Nausea Vomiting Ileus
Renal	Oliguria Urinary retention

TABLE 13.4 Physiological changes from poorly controlled pain cont'd

Musculoskeletal	Spasm Joint stiffness
Endocrine	Increased adrenergic activity
Central nervous system	Fear Anxiety Fatigue
Immune	Impaired cellular immunity Impaired wound healing
Poorly controlled chronic pain	Depression Isolation Limited mobility and function Confusion Family distress Diminished quality of life

Clinical reasoning and documentation

Case study (continued)—Hip and knee pain

The following is a continuation of the case study provided at the beginning of this chapter and the clinical reasoning process including problem/issue identification and documentation. Consult a fundamentals of nursing or medical-surgical nursing text for information about goal setting, nursing interventions and evaluation.

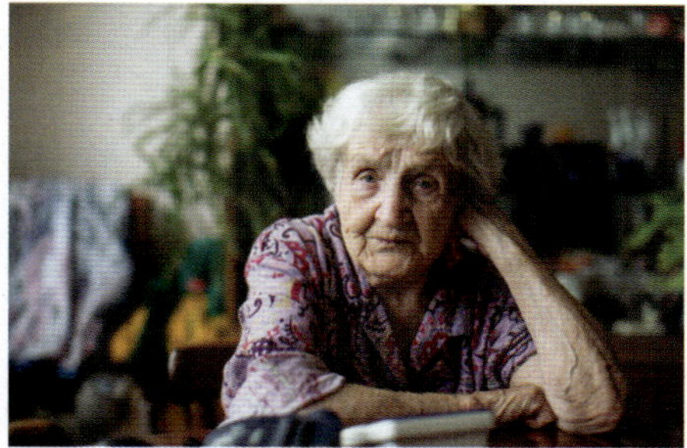

Context

You will recall from the case study described earlier in the chapter that you are on your final year clinical placement. Your clinical supervisor has asked you to undertake a pain assessment on Mrs Alberici.

Consider the patient's situation

Mrs Maria Alberici is an 85-year-old Italian-Australian female with a 20-year history of osteoarthritis.

Collect cues/information

Your further assessment reveals the following information.

Subjective data

Mrs Alberici reports increased pain and stiffness in her hips and knees for the past month. There is no radiation of pain, tingling or numbness in lower extremities. She tells you she has difficulty getting in and out of the bath and dressing herself. Describes pain as aching, with 'good and bad days'. Mrs Alberici becomes frustrated when asked to rate her pain intensity, replying: 'I don't know what number to give; it hurts a lot, on and off'. She takes Panadol Osteo, two tablets, when the pain 'really gets bad', with some degree of relief. She restricts her activities, such as walking to the local shops, because it 'hurts too much'.

Objective data

Localised tenderness noted upon palpation of knees; unable to fully flex knees. Crepitus

Continued

Clinical reasoning and documentation cont'd

noted in both knee joints. Swelling noted. Rubs lower knee area frequently. Gait slow and unsteady. Facial expression tense, clenching teeth.

Process information and identify problems/issues

Collaborative problems

Chronic pain related to osteoarthritis of hips and knees

Problem statements/nursing diagnoses

Chronic pain related to osteoarthritis of hips and knees
Partial self-care deficit: hygiene and dressing related to pain in knees
Impaired mobility related to painful knees

Case study 2: Postoperative abdominal pain

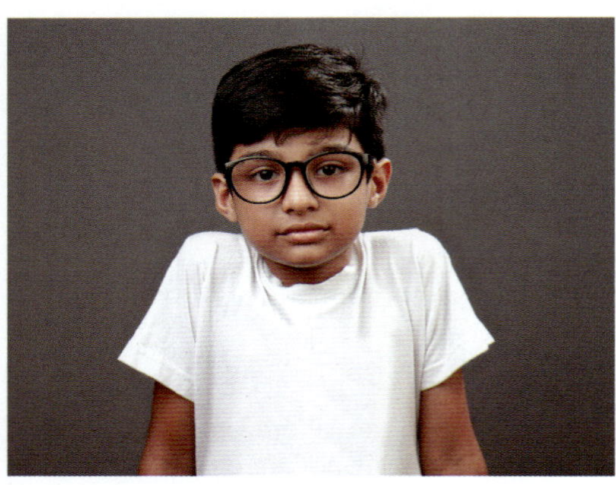

Context

You are a nursing student on a paediatric placement in the surgical ward.

Consider the patient's situation

Vivaan Patel is a 7-year-old boy who has just undergone a laparoscopic appendectomy earlier that day. He is awake, but his eyes are closed, and he is lying flat on the bed without movement.

Collect cues/information

Subjective data

When asked if he is in pain, Vivaan states 'a little', but he rates his pain as +8 using the Faces Pain Scale.

Objective data

Requiring assistance to move in the bed. Speaks only when spoken to. Diaphoretic, flushed, grimaces with slight touch.
Vital signs: Temp 37°C oral, BP 122/72 mmHg, HR 126 bpm, RR 22/min.
Lungs: Clear on auscultation. Pulse oximetry 98% on room air.
Abdomen: Hypoactive bowel sounds, tenderness on light palpation, dressings dry and intact at surgical sites.

Process information and identify problems/issues

Collaborative problem

Acute postoperative pain.

Problem statements/nursing diagnoses

Acute postoperative pain related to surgical wound.

ADDITIONAL RESOURCES

You can further develop your knowledge and skills relevant to pain assessment related pathophysiology, common health issues and nursing interventions by:

- reading chapters of a fundamentals of nursing or medical-surgical nursing textbook
- answering chapter multiple choice questions online. Log onto ClinicalKey Student and search for the text 'Health Assessment, 4th edition'. Choose the section titled 'Teaching material'. In this section you will find question and answer documents for each chapter.
- visiting websites

Commonwealth of Australia (Department of Health)—2021 National Strategic Action Plan for Pain Management: https://www.health.gov.au/sites/default/files/documents/2021/05/the-national-strategic-action-plan-for-pain-management-the-national-strategic-action-plan-for-pain-management.pdf

College of Emergency Nurses, New Zealand—Pain management nursing knowledge and skills framework for Registered Nurses: https://www.nzno.org.nz/groups/colleges_sections/colleges/college_of_emergency_nurses/resources/knowledge_skills_framework

Pain Australia: https://www.painaustralia.org.au

Aboriginal and Torres Strait Islander people: https://www.painaustralia.org.au/about-pain/who-it-affects-pages-2021/indigenous-australians-2021

REFERENCES

1. McCaffery M. Nursing practice theories related to cognition, bodily pain, and main-environment interactions. Los Angeles: University of Los Angeles; 1968.
2. Raja SN, Carr DB, Cohen M, Finnerup NB, Flor H, Gibson S, et al. The revised IASP definition of pain: Concepts, challenges, and compromises. Pain. 2020 Sep 9;161(9): 1976–1982.
3. Craig KD, Holmes C, Hudspith M, Moor G, Moosa-Mitha M, Varcoe C, Wallace B. Pain in persons who are marginalized by social conditions. Pain. 2020 Feb;161(2):261.
4. Aerts N, Van Bogaert P, Bastiaens H, Peremans L. Integration of nurses in general practice: a thematic synthesis of the perspectives of general practitioners, practice nurses and patients living with chronic illness. Journal of Clinical Nursing. 2020 Jan;29(1–2):251–264.
5. Cohen SP, Vase L, Hooten WM. Chronic pain: an update on burden, best practices, and new advances. The Lancet. 2021 May 29;397(10289): 2082–2097.
6. Coghill RC. The distributed nociceptive system: a framework for understanding pain. Trends in neurosciences. 2020 Oct 1;43(10):780–794.
7. Finnerup NB, Kuner R, Jensen TS. Neuropathic pain: from mechanisms to treatment. Physiological Reviews. 2021 Jan 1;101(1):259–301.
8. Xu A, Larsen B, Henn A, Baller EB, Scott C, Sharma V, et al. Brain responses to noxious stimuli in patients with chronic pain: a systematic review and meta-analysis. JAMA Network Open. 2021;4(1):e2032236. doi: 10.1001/jamanetworkopen.2020.32236

9. Banasik JL, Copstead LE. Pathophysiology. 7th ed. St Louis: Elsevier; 2022.
10. Fitzcharles MA, Cohen SP, Clauw DJ, Littlejohn G, Usui C, Häuser W. Nociplastic pain: towards an understanding of prevalent pain conditions. The Lancet. 2021 May 29;397(10289):2098–2110.
11. Commonwealth of Australia (Department of Health) 2021 National Strategic Action Plan for Pain Management. Available at: https://www.health.gov.au/sites/default/files/documents/2021/05/the-national-strategic-action-plan-for-pain-management-the-national-strategic-action-plan-for-pain-management.pdf
12. National Pain Summit Initiative. National pain strategy. Pain management for all Australians. 2010. Available at: www.painsummit.org.au
13. Benoliel R, Svensson P, Evers S, Wang SJ, Barke A, Korwisi B, et al. The IASP classification of chronic pain for ICD-11: chronic secondary headache or orofacial pain. Pain. 2019 Jan 1;160(1):60–68.
14. Jonsdottir T, Gunnarsson EC. Understanding nurses' knowledge and attitudes toward pain assessment in dementia: a literature review. Pain Management Nursing. 2021 Jun 1;22(3): 281–292.
15. Akca YA, Slootmaekers L, Boskovic I. Verifiability and symptom endorsement in genuine, exaggerated, and malingered pain. Psychological Injury and Law. 2020 Sep;13:235–245.
16. Hait B. Pain Management in Palliative Care: What Is Significant? 2023. Available at: https://www.intechopen.com/online-first/88692
17. Johnston-Devin C, Oprescu F, Gray M, Wallis M. Patients describe their lived experiences of battling to live with complex regional pain syndrome. The Journal of Pain. 2021 Sep 1;22(9):1111–1128.
18. Taylor SS, Noor N, Urits I, Paladini A, Sadhu MS, Gibb C, et al. Complex regional pain syndrome: a comprehensive review. Pain and Therapy. 2021 Dec;10(2):875–892.
19. Cuitavi J, Torres-Pérez JV, Lorente JD, Campos-Jurado Y, Andrés-Herrera P, Polache A, et al. Crosstalk between Mu-Opioid receptors and neuroinflammation: Consequences for drug addiction and pain. Neuroscience & Biobehavioral Reviews. 2023 Feb 1;145:1050211.
20. Schug SA, Palmer GM, Scott DA, Alcock MM, Halliwell R, Mott JF. Acute Pain Management Scientific Evidence 5th edition. Australian and New Zealand College of Anaesthetists and Faculty of Pain Medicine. 2020. Available at: https://airr.anzca.edu.au/anzcajspui/handle/11055/1071
21. Centers for Disease Control and Prevention. Understanding the opioid overdose epidemic. 2023. Available at: https://www.cdc.gov/opioids/basics/epidemic.html#:~:text=Combatting%20the%20Opioid%20Overdose%20Epidemic,-View%20Larger&text=CDC's%20work%20focuses%20on%3A,and%20to%20evaluate%20prevention%20efforts.
22. Wilson N, Kariisa M, Seth P, Smith H 4th, Davis NL. Drug and opioid-involved overdose deaths—United States, 2017–2018. Morbidity and Mortality Weekly Report. 2020 Mar 20;69(11):290–297. doi: 10.15585/mmwr.mm6911a4. PMID: 32191688; 'PMCID: PMC7739981.
23. Brown R, Morgan A. The opioid epidemic in North America: Implications for Australia. Trends & issues in crime and criminal justice no. 578. Canberra: Australian Institute of Criminology; 2019. Available at: https://www.aic.gov.au/sites/default/files/2020-05/ti578_the_opioid_epidemic_in_north_america-v2.pdf
24. Dunlop AJ, Lokuge B, Lintzeris N. Opioid prescribing in Australia: too much and not enough. The Medical Journal of Australia. 2021 Aug; 215(3):117.
25. Bellieni CV. Analgesia for fetal pain during prenatal surgery: 10 years of progress. Pediatric Research. 2021 May;89(7):1612–1618.
26. Meyers JM, Decker AS, Tryon C. Neonatal pain management. Perinatal Palliative Care: A Clinical Guide. 2020:155–178.
27. Bellieni CV. The communicative features of non-verbal patients. In: A New Holistic-Evolutive

Approach to Pediatric Palliative Care 2022 May 27 (pp. 63–76). Cham: Springer International Publishing.
28. Walker SM. Biological and neurodevelopmental implications of neonatal pain. Clinics in Perinatology 2013;40(3):471–491.
29. Australian Institute of Health and Wellbeing (IAHW). 2019. Hospitals at a glance. 2017-18. Available at: https://www.aihw.gov.au/reports/hospitals/hospitals-at-a-glance-2017-18/contents/surgery-in-australia-s-hospitals
30. Macintyre PE, Schug SA. Acute pain management: a practical guide. 5th ed. Florida: CRC Press; 2021.
31. Dagnino A, Campos MM. Chronic pain in the elderly: mechanisms and perspectives. Frontiers in Human Neuroscience. 2022 Mar 3;16:736688.
32. National Ageing and Research Institute (NARI). 2023. Improving pain detection and management. Available at: https://www.nari.net.au/improving-pain-detection-and-management
33. Bunk S, Zuidema S, Koch K, Lautenbacher S, De Deyn PP, Kunz M. Pain processing in older adults with dementia-related cognitive impairment is associated with frontal neurodegeneration. Neurobiology of Aging. 2021 Oct 1;106:139–152.
34. Australian Institute of Health and Wellbeing (IAHW). Chronic Pain in Australia. 2020. Available at: https://www.aihw.gov.au/getmedia/10434b6f-2147-46ab-b654-a90f05592d35/aihw-phe-267.pdf?v=20230605184320&inline=true
35. Osborne NR, Davis KD. Sex and gender differences in pain. International Review of Neurobiology 2022 Jan 1 (Vol. 164, pp. 277–307). Academic Press.
36. Packiasabapathy S, Sadhasivam S. Gender, genetics, and analgesia: understanding the differences in response to pain relief. Journal of Pain Research 2018;11:2729–2739.
37. Australian Bureau of Statistics. Cultural diversity: Census [Internet]. Canberra: ABS; 2021 [cited 2024 February 3]. Available from: https://www.abs.gov.au/statistics/people/people-and-communities/cultural-diversity-census/latest-release
38. Mittinty MM, McNeil DW, Jamieson LM. Limited evidence to measure the impact of chronic pain on health outcomes of Indigenous people. Journal of Psychosomatic Research. 2018 Apr; 107:53–54. doi: 10.1016/j.jpsychores.2018.02.001 Epub 2018 Feb 6. PMID: 29502764; PMCID: PMC5929123.
39. Fenwick C. Assessing pain across the cultural gap: central Australian Indigenous people's pain assessment. Contemporary Nurse 2006;22(2):218–227.
40. Lin I, Green C, Bessarab D. 'Yarn with me': applying clinical yarning to improve clinician–patient communication in Aboriginal health care. Australian Journal of Primary Health. 2016 Nov 8;22(5):377–382.
41. Australian Institute of Health and Wellbeing. 2020. Chronic pain. Available at: https://www.aihw.gov.au/reports/chronic-disease/chronic-pain-in-australia/summary
42. Pain Australia. Painful Facts. 2020. Available at: https://www.painaustralia.org.au/about-pain/painaustralia-painful-facts
43. Pautex S, Herrmann F, Le Louis P. Feasibility and reliability of four pain self-assessment scales and correlation with an observational rating scale in hospitalised elderly demented patients. The Journals of Gerontology. Series A, Biological Sciences and Medical Sciences, 2005;60(4):524–529.
44. McCaffery M, Pasero C. Pain: clinical manual. 2nd ed. St Louis: Mosby; 1999.
45. Cleeland CS, Ryan KM. Pain assessment: global use of the brief pain inventory. Annals of Academic Medicine Singapore 1994;23(2):129–138.
46. Melzack R. The short-form McGill Pain Questionnaire. Pain. 1987 Aug;30(2):191–197. doi: 10.1016/0304-3959(87)91074-8. PMID: 3670870.
47. McCaffery M, Beebe A (1989) Pain: Clinical Manual for Nursing Practice. Mosby, St. Louis.
48. Jensen MP, Karoly P, Braver S (1986) The measurement of clinical pain intensity: a comparison of six methods. Pain 27, 117–126.
49. Abbey J, Piller N, De Bellis A, Esterman A, Parker D, Giles L et al. The Abbey pain scale:

A 1-minute numerical indicator for people with end-stage dementia. International Journal of Palliative Nursing 2004;10(1):6–13.
50. Warden V, Hurley AC, Volicer L. Development and psychometric evaluation of the Pain Assessment in Advanced Dementia (PAINAD) scale. Journal of the American Medical Directors Association 2002;4(1):9–15.
51. International Association for the Study of Pain (IASP). Faces pain scale—revised. 2019. Available at: https://www.iasp-pain.org/resources/faces-pain-scale-revised/
52. Krechel SW, Bildner J. CRIES: a new neonatal postoperative pain measurement score. Initial testing of validity and reliability. Pediatric Anesthesia 1995;5(1):53–61.
53. Merkel SI, Voepel-Lewis T, Shayevitz JR, Malviya S. The FLACC: A behavioral scale for scoring postoperative pain in young children. Pediatric Nursing 1997;23(3):293–297.

CHAPTER 14

Eye assessment

Written by Carolyn Jarvis
Adapted by Amanda Wylie

INTRODUCTION

The eyes are the major source of sensory information, so the brain is heavily involved in the function of vision. Any alteration in vision has an impact on function and safety that needs to be considered in planning care. Processing visual information takes place in the cerebral cortex, and the visual association area occupies most of the occipital lobe. It is the largest of all the cortical sensory areas in the occipital lobe.[1] In this chapter we review the external and internal anatomy of the eye and accessory muscles, visual pathways, visual fields and visual light reflexes. This information is also relevant to neurological system assessment (Chapter 12).

Case study

The following case study gives an example of a typical situation involving assessing the eyes and the initial clinical reasoning process. It will help you to identify your learning needs.

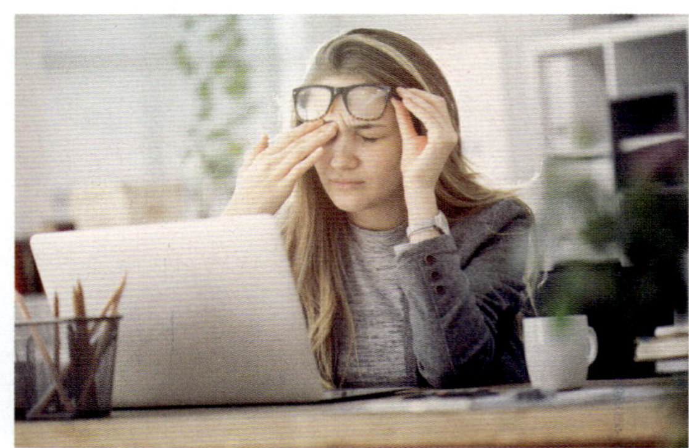

Context

You are on a clinical placement in a family medical clinic working alongside a nurse practitioner.

Consider the patient's situation

Ms Emma Jensen is an 18-year-old female who has attended the clinic complaining of red, gritty eyes.

Questions to further your learning

- What are the possible things that might be going on with Emma?
- What knowledge do you need to be able to predict what might be going on?
- What approach to Emma's health assessment will you undertake?
- What questions (subjective data) will you ask Emma to extend the health history and why?
- What physical examination (objective data) will you conduct and why?
- What resources are available to you to assist you in your assessment of Emma?

Assessment plan

Vision enables people to perform daily tasks and to learn about the world that surrounds them. Disorders of the eye can affect many parts of a person's functional life. Accurate, systematic assessment can identify issues and provide focus for early treatment that may lead to sight preservation.

Relevant areas that can affect the eye that you might consider when focusing your specific assessment questions include cardiac (Chapter 17), peripheral vascular (Chapter 16) and neurological function (Chapter 12). Impairment of eye function can also impact on other body systems such as the musculoskeletal system (Chapter 20)—for example, increasing the risk of falling or the inability to complete activities of daily living independently. Subjective data assessment focuses on the following:

- presenting concern
- vision difficulty (decreased acuity, blurring, blind spots)
- pain
- strabismus (turned eye), diplopia (double vision)
- redness, swelling
- watering, discharge
- history of ocular problems
- glaucoma
- use of glasses or contact lenses
- health and lifestyle management
- adjustment to vision loss (if relevant).

Following subjective data collection, you will get a sense of the areas needed to be examined for objective data collection. Only the relevant areas should be examined. The main areas for physical examination and measurement are:

- general inspection
- inspect external ocular structures—eyebrows, eyelids and eyelashes, eyeballs, conjunctiva and sclera
- inspect anterior eyeball structures—cornea and lens, iris and pupil
- visual acuity—test vision
- visual field—confrontation test.

Resources available

You will find additional resources and the reference list at the end of this chapter.

Structure and function

External anatomy

Because this sense is so important to humans, the eyes are well protected by the bony orbital cavity, which is surrounded with a cushion of orbital fat. The **eyelids** are like two movable shades that further protect the eyes from injury, strong light and dust. The upper eyelid is the larger and more mobile one. The eyelashes are short hairs in double or triple rows that curve outwards from the lid margins, filtering out dust and dirt.

When closed, the lid margins approximate completely. When open, the upper lid covers the upper part of the iris and the lower lid sits just at the **limbus**, the border between the cornea and sclera. The elliptical open space between the eyelids is called the **palpebral fissure** (Figure 14.1). The **canthus** is the corner of the eye, the angle where the lids meet. At the inner canthus, the **caruncle** is a small fleshy mass containing sebaceous glands.

Within the upper lid, **tarsal plates** are strips of connective tissue that give it shape (Figure 14.2). The tarsal plates contain the **meibomian glands**, modified sebaceous glands that secrete an oily lubricating material onto the inner lids. This stops the tears from overflowing and evaporating and helps to form an airtight seal when the lids are closed.

The exposed white part of the eyes (sclera) has a transparent protective covering, the **conjunctiva**. The conjunctiva is a thin mucous membrane folded like an envelope between the eyelids and the eyeball. The *palpebral* conjunctiva lines the lids and is clear, with many small blood vessels. It forms a deep recess or pocket and then folds back over the eye. The *bulbar* conjunctiva overlays the eyeball, with the white sclera showing through. At the limbus the conjunctiva merges with the cornea. The cornea covers and protects the iris and pupil.

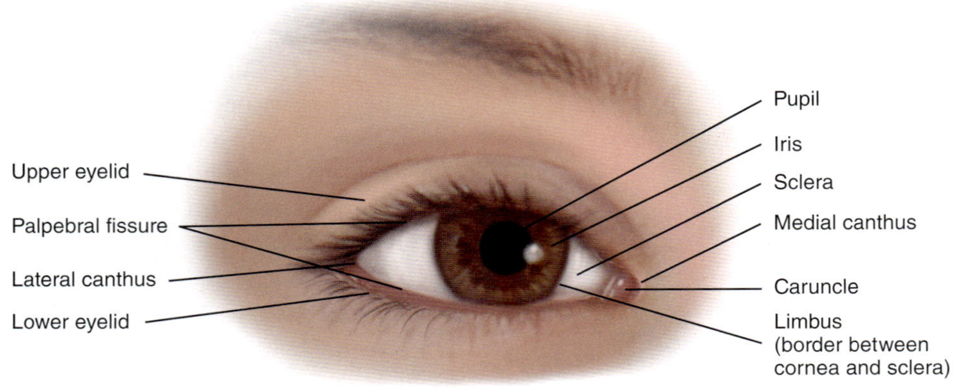

FIGURE 14.1 Structures of the external eye.

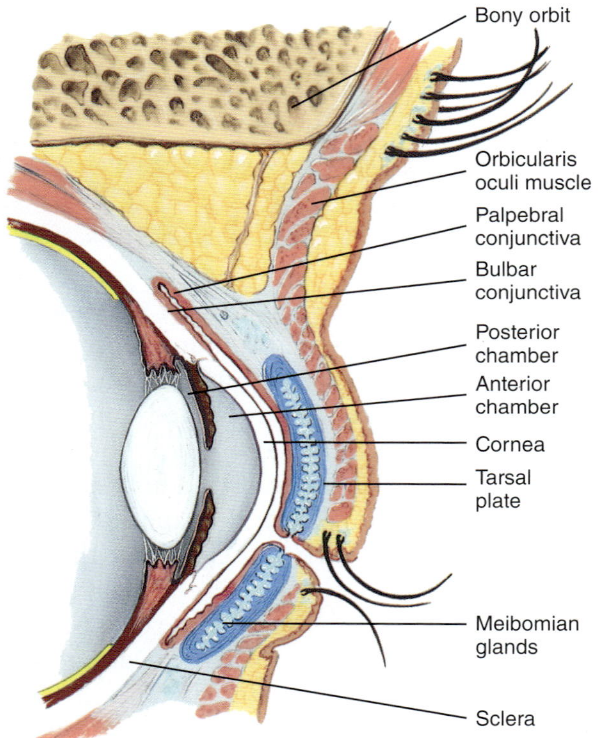

FIGURE 14.2 Cross-section of the eye and related structures

The **lacrimal apparatus** provides constant irrigation to keep the conjunctiva and cornea moist and lubricated (Figure 14.3). The **lacrimal gland**, in the upper outer corner over the eye, secretes aqueous tears. The tears wash across the eye and are drawn up evenly as the lid blinks. The tears drain into the **puncta**, visible on the upper and lower lid rims at the inner canthus. The tears then drain into the nasolacrimal sac, through the 7.5 cm **nasolacrimal duct** and empty into the inferior meatus inside the nose. A tiny fold of mucous membrane prevents air from being forced up the nasolacrimal duct when the nose is blown.

EXTRAOCULAR MUSCLES

Six muscles attach the eyeball to its orbit (Figure 14.4A and 14.4B) and serve to direct

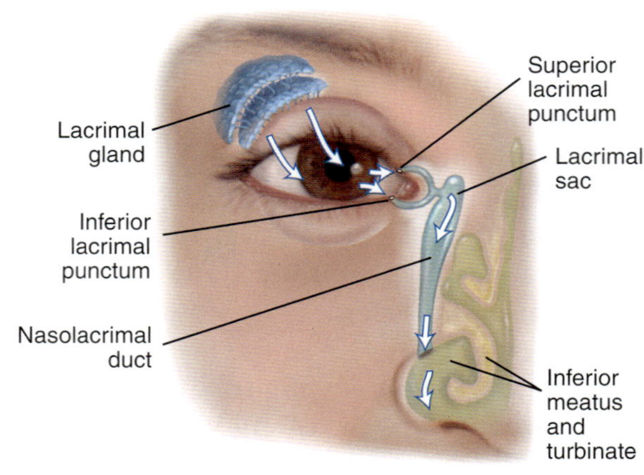

FIGURE 14.3 Lacrimal apparatus and related structures

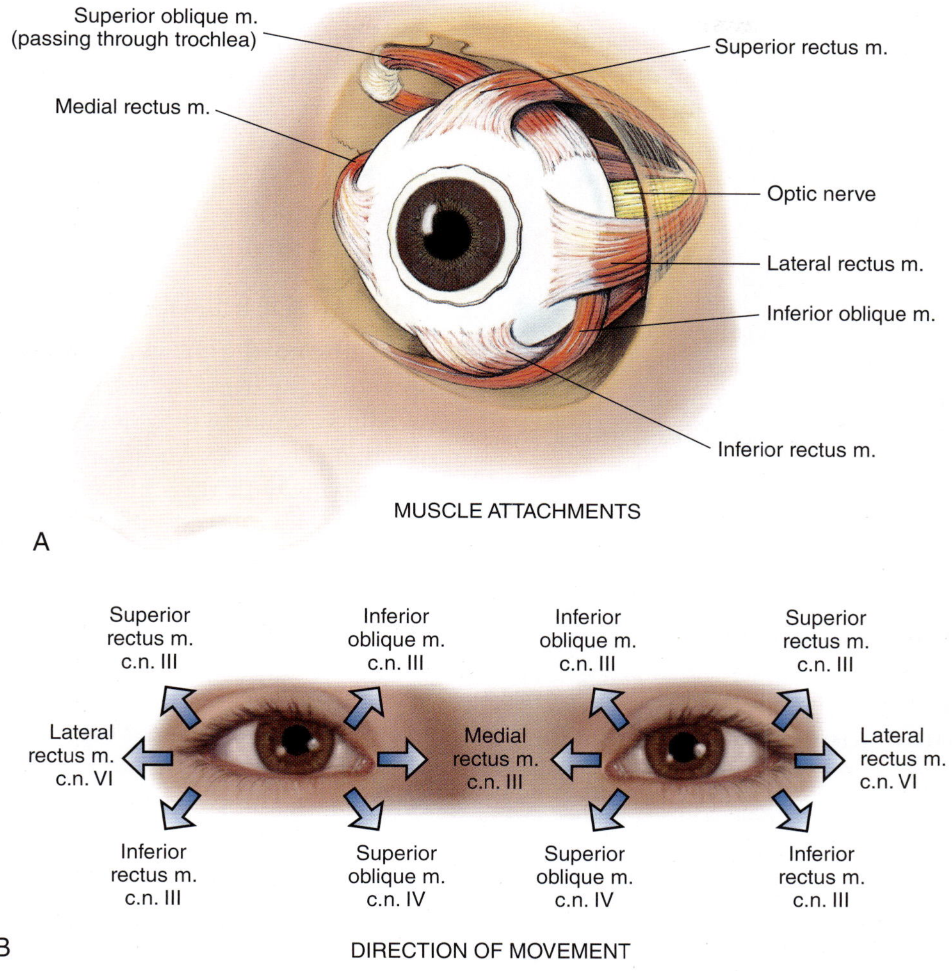

FIGURE 14.4 Extraocular muscles

the eye to points of the person's interest. These extraocular muscles give the eye both straight and rotary movement. The four straight, or *rectus*, muscles are the superior, inferior, lateral and medial rectus muscles. The two slanting, or *oblique*, muscles are the superior and inferior oblique muscles.

Each muscle is coordinated, or yoked, with one in the other eye. This ensures that when the two eyes move, their axes always remain parallel (called *conjugate movement*). Parallel axes are important because the human brain can tolerate seeing only one image. Although some animals can perceive two different pictures through each eye, human beings have a binocular, single-image visual system. This occurs because our eyes move as a pair. For example, the two yoked muscles that allow looking to the far right are the right lateral rectus and the left medial rectus.

Movement of the **extraocular muscles** (below) is stimulated by three **cranial nerves**. Cranial nerve VI, the abducens nerve, innervates the lateral rectus muscle (which abducts the eye); cranial nerve IV, the trochlear nerve, innervates the superior oblique muscle; and cranial nerve III, the oculomotor nerve, innervates all the rest—the superior, inferior and medial rectus and the inferior oblique muscles. Note that the superior oblique muscle is located on the superior aspect of the eyeball, but when it contracts, it enables the person to look downwards and inwards.

Internal anatomy

The eye is a sphere composed of three concentric coats: (1) the outer fibrous **sclera and cornea**, (2) the middle vascular **choroid, ciliary body and iris** and (3) the inner nervous **retina** (Figure 14.5).

THE OUTER LAYER

The sclera is a tough, protective, white covering. It is continuous anteriorly with the smooth, transparent cornea, which covers the iris and pupil.

The **cornea** is very sensitive to touch; contact with a wisp of cotton stimulates a blink in both eyes, called the *corneal reflex*. The trigeminal nerve (cranial nerve V) carries the afferent sensation into the brain, and the facial nerve (cranial nerve VII) carries the efferent message that stimulates the blink. The cornea is part of the refracting media of the eye, bending incoming light rays so they will be focused on the retina.

THE MIDDLE LAYER

The **choroid** has dark pigmentation to prevent light from reflecting internally and is heavily vascularised to deliver nutrients to the overlying retina. Anteriorly, the choroid is continuous with the ciliary body and the iris. The muscles of the ciliary body control the thickness of the lens and in turn its focusing power. The iris functions as a diaphragm, varying the opening at its centre, the pupil. This controls the amount of light admitted into the eye. The muscle fibres of the iris contract the pupil in bright light and to

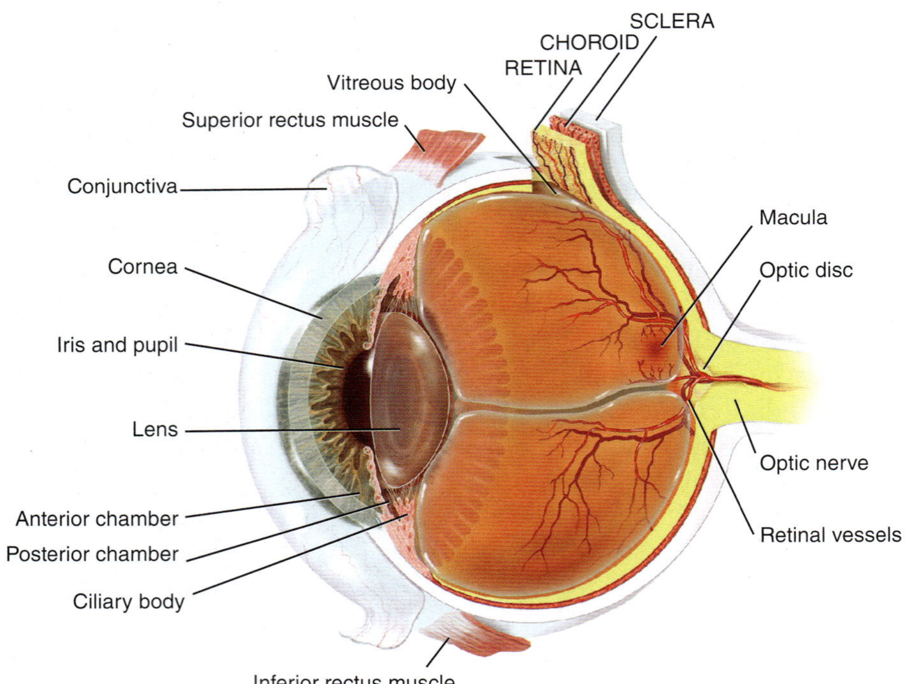

FIGURE 14.5 Internal anatomy of the eye.

accommodate for near vision and dilate the pupil when the light is dim and for far vision. The colour of the iris varies from person to person, depending on individual pigmentation.

The **pupil** is round and regular. Its size is determined by a balance between the parasympathetic and sympathetic chains of the autonomic nervous system. Stimulation of the parasympathetic branch, through cranial nerve III, causes constriction of the pupil. Stimulation of the sympathetic branch dilates the pupil and elevates the eyelid. As mentioned earlier, the pupil size also reacts to the amount of ambient light and to accommodation or focusing an object on the retina.

The **lens** is a biconvex disc located just posterior to the pupil. The transparent lens serves as a refracting medium, working with the clear cornea to focus a viewed object on the retina. Its thickness is controlled by the ciliary body; the lens bulges for focusing on near objects and flattens for far objects. The change in lens thickness in response to the distance at which an object is viewed is known as accommodation.

THE INNER LAYER

The **retina** is the visual receptive layer of the eye in which light waves are changed into nerve impulses. The retinal structures viewed through the ophthalmoscope are the optic disc, the retinal vessels, the general background and the macula (Figure 14.6).

The **optic disc** (or optic papilla) is the area in which fibres from the retina converge to form the optic nerve. Located towards the nasal side of the retina, it has these characteristics: a colour that varies from creamy yellow orange to pink; a round or oval shape; margins that are distinct and sharply demarcated, especially on the temporal side; and a physiological cup, the smaller circular area inside the disc where the blood vessels exit and enter.

The **retinal vessels** normally include a paired artery and vein extending to each quadrant, growing progressively smaller in

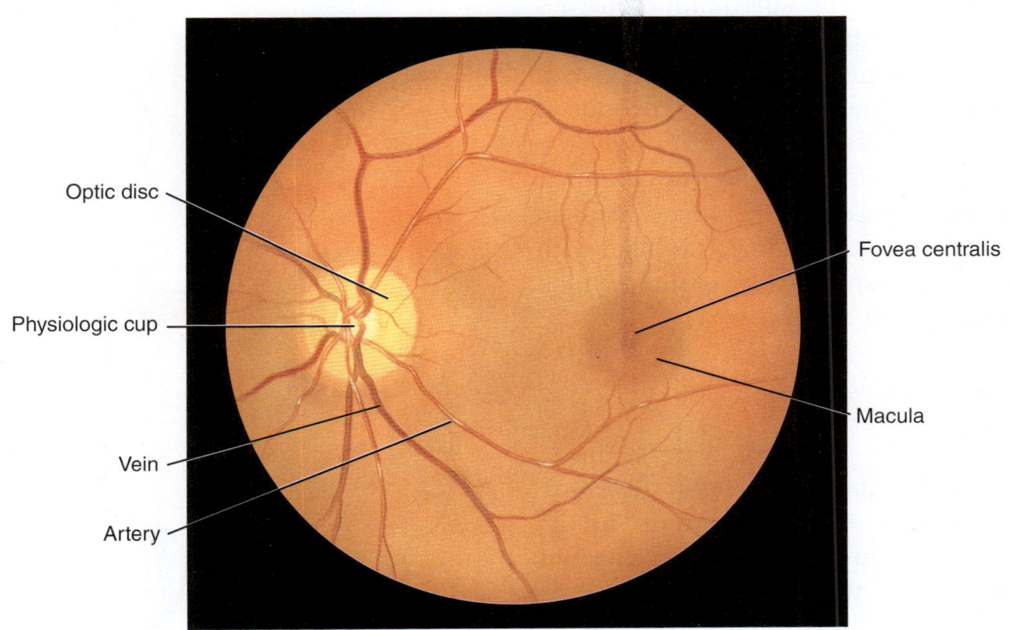

FIGURE 14.6 Ophthalmoscope image of the retina.

calibre as they reach the periphery. The arteries appear brighter red and narrower than the veins, and the arteries have a thin sliver of light on them (the arterial light reflex). The general background of the fundus varies in colour, depending on the person's skin colour. The **macula** is located on the temporal side of the fundus. It is a slightly darker pigmented region surrounding the **fovea centralis**; these areas are responsible for the most detailed and colour vision. The macula receives and transduces light from the centre of the visual field.

The eye is divided into **anterior** and **posterior segments**. The **anterior segment** is from the clear cornea to the posterior part of the lens. The anterior segment is divided into two chambers. The **anterior chamber** is from the clear cornea to the front of the iris. The **posterior chamber** lies behind the iris to the posterior lens. Both chambers of the anterior segment contain the clear, watery **aqueous humour** that is produced continually by the ciliary body. The continuous flow of fluid serves to deliver nutrients to the surrounding tissues and to drain metabolic waste. Intraocular pressure is determined by a balance between the amount of aqueous humour produced and resistance to its outflow through the trabecular meshwork in the anterior chamber. The **posterior segment** of the eye is from the posterior lens to the retina. It is filled with a gelatinous, transparent substance called **vitreous humour**.

Visual pathways and visual fields

Objects reflect light. The light rays are refracted through the transparent media (cornea, aqueous humour, lens and vitreous body) and strike the retina. The retina transforms the light stimulus into nerve impulses that are conducted through the optic nerve and the optic tract to the visual cortex of the occipital lobe (Figure 14.7).

The image formed on the retina is upside down and reversed from its actual appearance in the outside world. That is, an object in the upper temporal visual field of the right eye reflects its image onto the lower nasal area of the retina. All retinal fibres collect to form the optic nerve, but they maintain this same spatial arrangement, with nasal fibres running medially and temporal fibres running laterally.

At the **optic chiasm**, nasal fibres (from both temporal visual fields) cross over. The left optic tract now has fibres from the left half of each retina, and the right optic tract contains fibres only from the right. The right side of the brain therefore looks at the left side of the world.

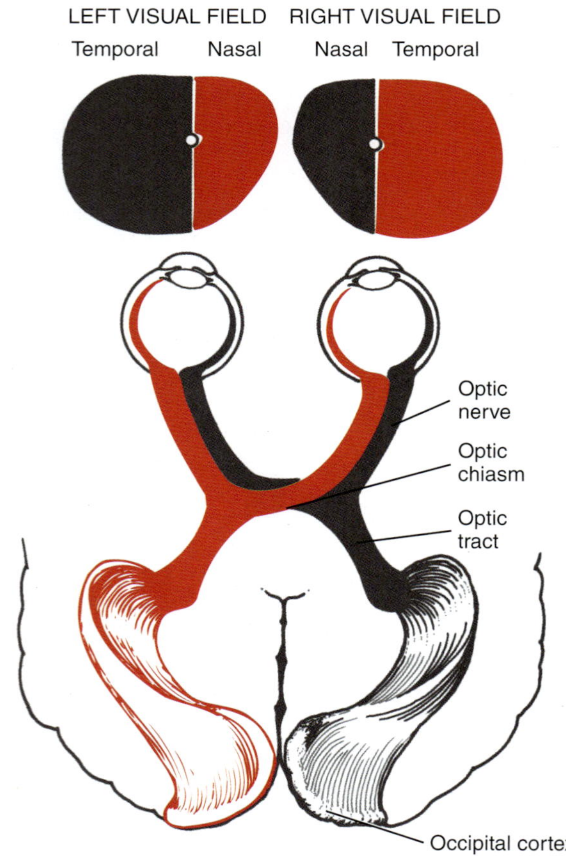

FIGURE 14.7 Visual pathways (viewed from above)

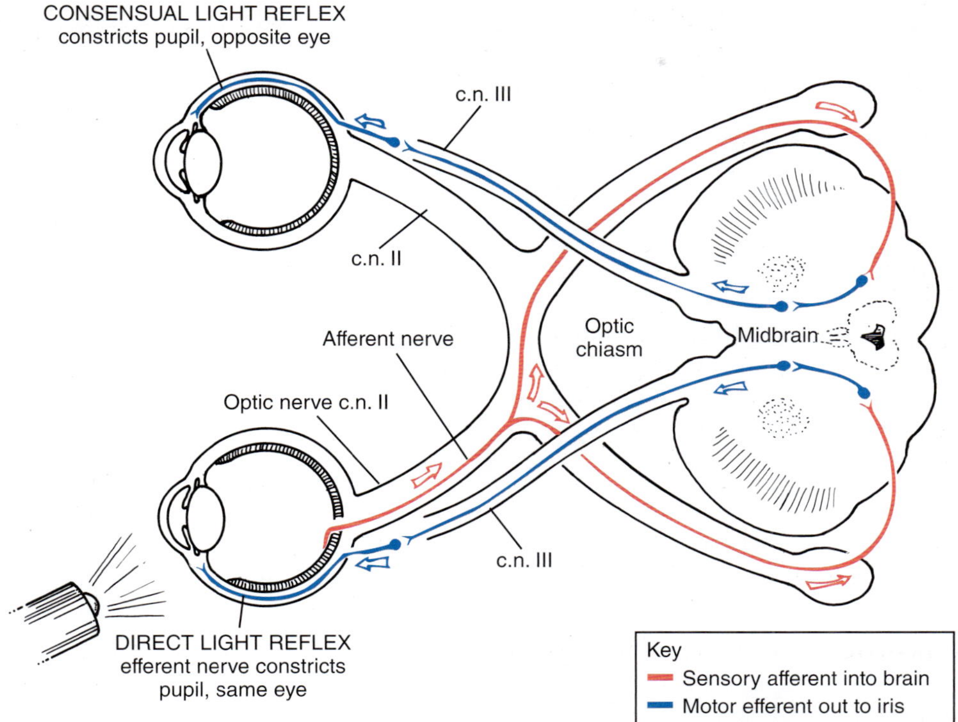

FIGURE 14.8 Diagram of the pupillary light reflex

Visual reflexes

PUPILLARY LIGHT REFLEX

The pupillary light reflex is the normal constriction of the pupils when bright light shines on the retina (Figure 14.8). It is a subcortical reflex arc (i.e. a person has no conscious control over it); the afferent link is cranial nerve II, the optic nerve, and the efferent path is cranial III, the oculomotor nerve. When one eye is exposed to bright light, a direct light reflex occurs (constriction of that pupil), as well as a consensual light reflex (simultaneous constriction of the other pupil). This happens because the optic nerve carries the sensory afferent message in and then synapses with both sides of the brain. For example, consider the light reflex in a person who is blind in one eye. Stimulation of the normal eye produces both a direct and a consensual light reflex. Stimulation of the blind eye causes no response because the sensory afferent in cranial nerve II is destroyed.

FIXATION

This is a reflex direction of the eye towards an object attracting a person's attention. The image is fixed in the centre of the visual field, the fovea centralis. This consists of very rapid ocular movements to put the target back on the fovea, and somewhat slower (smooth pursuit) movements to track the target and keep its image on the fovea. Drugs, alcohol, fatigue and inattention impair these ocular movements.

ACCOMMODATION

This is adaptation of the eye for near vision. It is accomplished by increasing the curvature of the lens through movement of the ciliary muscles. Although the lens cannot be observed directly, the components of accommodation that can be observed are convergence (motion towards) of the axes of the eyeballs and pupillary constriction.

Developmental considerations

Infants and children

Although prevalence data of common visual conditions in children in Australia and Aotearoa New Zealand is inconsistent, self-reported data suggests that 12% of the Australian population of children aged 0 to 14 are affected by chronic eye conditions.[2] An awareness of normal visual development in children is important when assessing an infant or child.

At birth, eye function is limited, but it matures fully during the early years. Peripheral vision is intact in newborns. The macula, the area of sharpest vision, is absent at birth but is developing by 4 months and is mature by 8 months. Eye movements may be poorly coordinated at birth. By 3 or 4 months of age, infants establish binocularity and can fixate on a single image with both eyes simultaneously. Most neonates (80%) are born farsighted; this gradually decreases after 7 or 8 years of age.

In structure, the eyeball reaches adult size by 8 years. At birth, the iris shows little pigment, and the pupils are small. The lens is nearly spherical at birth, growing flatter throughout life. Its consistency changes from that of soft plastic at birth to rigid glass in old age.

Late adulthood (65+ years)

In Australia, vision disorders are common and are often related to ageing. In 2017–18, long-term vision disorders affected 93% of people aged 65 or older.[3] Approximately 90% of vision impairment in both Indigenous and non-Indigenous Australians is preventable or treatable.[2] Similarly, in Aotearoa New Zealand, 11% of adults over 65 years old experience vision impairment, compared with 2% of adults aged 15 to 44.[4]

The leading causes of vision impairment for non-Indigenous Australians are refractive error (61%), cataract (13%) and age-related macular degeneration (10%). For Indigenous Australians they are refractive error (61%), cataract (20%) and diabetic retinopathy (5.2%).[5] Another notable cause of vision loss is glaucoma.[2] These are explained as the following:

1. **Uncorrected refractive error.** This is a condition where the light that passes through the front of the eye fails to focus precisely on the retina. This causes long or short sightedness and difficulties changing focus. Approximately 63.39% of Indigenous Australians and 61.69% of non-Indigenous Australians are affected by this condition.[2] Likewise in Aotearoa New Zealand 55% of the population aged over 40 is affected by uncorrected refractive error.[6]
2. **Cataract**, or lens opacity, results from a degeneration of proteins in the natural lens as the adult ages. Cataract formation varies globally and across age groups with a minimum prevalence of 1% reported in those aged 20 to 39, compared with a maximum prevalence of 88.17% in the over-60 age group.[7] In 2016, cataracts affected 20.22% of Australia's Indigenous population and 13.93% of non-Indigenous Australians.[2] In Aotearoa New Zealand, the prevalence of cataract varies from approximately 0.1% in 60- to 69-year-olds to 15% in the population aged over 90.[8]
3. **Age-related macular degeneration (AMD)** is the breakdown of cells in the macula of the retina. There are two types of AMD: *non-neovascular or atrophic* (dry), the most common form, and

neovascular (wet), the most severe form. It is a progressive, late-onset degenerative disease that affects central vision. Peripheral vision is not affected, so the person can usually manage self-care and will not become completely disabled. Over the past decade, understanding of the risk factors of the disease, along with advances in treatment options, have seen a reduction in the progression of the disease leading to a decrease in vision impairment and blindness due to AMD.[9] It is still the most common form of permanent visual impairment in non-Indigenous Australians over the age of 50 (71%). It has a lower prevalence in Indigenous Australians (1.09%).[2] In Aotearoa New Zealand AMD is the leading cause of visual loss in the non-Māori population.[10]

4. **Glaucoma**. The term glaucoma encompasses several diseases in which there is a progressive loss of retinal nerve fibres, with corresponding loss of visual field that results in a 'cupped' appearance in the optic nerve. Glaucoma results in irreversible loss of vision, usually starting in the periphery. The damage to the optic nerve is often but not always associated with elevation in intraocular pressure.[11] The prevalence of glaucoma is estimated to be 5.46% in Indigenous Australians and 0.55% in non-Indigenous Australians.[2] Chronic or primary open-angle glaucoma is the most common type and involves a gradual loss of peripheral vision that is usually unnoticed. As damage becomes extensive, symptoms such as reduced field of vision are noticeable. It is worth noting that high intraocular pressure is now considered a risk factor as opposed to a criterion for a diagnosis of glaucoma.[12]
5. **Retinopathy** refers to microvascular damage of the retina, which may develop slowly or rapidly, leading to blurred vision and progressive vision loss. Retinopathy is most often associated with chronic hypertension and type 1 or type 2 diabetes. Diabetic retinopathy is caused by complex neuronal, glial and microvascular abnormalities that disrupt retinal function. Diabetic macular oedema and proliferative diabetic retinopathy are the major sight-threatening end points of diabetes.[13] Occurrence of diabetic retinopathy is most often associated with duration of disease, poor glycaemic control, chronic hypertension, dyslipidaemia, pregnancy, smoking, obesity and diabetic nephropathy. Almost everyone with type 1 diabetes and more than 60% of those with type 2 diabetes will develop some form of diabetic eye disease.[14,15] There are two types of diabetic retinopathy: *non-proliferative retinopathy*, the most common form, and *proliferative retinopathy*, the most severe form, which leads to irreversible blindness. In its early forms, diabetic eye disease may be asymptomatic, which is why regular eye examinations for people with diabetes is vital. It is the leading cause of irreversible blindness in working-age Australian adults.[16] Both Indigenous Australians and Māori affected by diabetic retinopathy are over-represented in their respective populations.[2,6]

Aside from these leading causes of eye disease, other conditions are seen. Changes in eye structure contribute greatly to distinct facial changes in an ageing person. The skin loses its elasticity, causing wrinkling and drooping; fat tissues and muscles atrophy; and the external eye structures appear sunken. With ageing, **lacrimal glands** involute, causing decreased tear production and a feeling of dryness and burning (known as *dry eye disease*). This is more common in women and with age.[17] The **cornea** may show an infiltration of degenerative lipid material around the limbus. This is known as *arcus senilis*. As the person grows older, pupil size decreases and the lens progressively hardens and loses its ability to change shape (accommodate); this leads to a decreased ability to focus on close objects with no coinciding changes to distance vision. This is known as **presbyopia**. As these changes occur progressively with age, symptoms will usually manifest in the early to mid-40s and necessitate the use of reading glasses.[18] Visual acuity may diminish gradually after 50 years of age, and even more so after 70 years. Inside the posterior segment of the eye, **floaters** (vitreous opacities) may appear because of vitreous degeneration. People commonly describe these as blobs, spots or cobwebs in their vision.

Cultural and social considerations

Australia and Aotearoa New Zealand are culturally diverse societies, and health practitioners need to be familiar with specific variations and disease incidences that affect different cultural groups. Structural differences are evident in the palpebral fissures and epicanthic fold in peoples' eyes. Examples of this include narrowed palpebral fissures in people of Asian origin, which in non-Asian people may be diagnostic of a serious congenital anomaly like Trisomy 21 (Down syndrome).

There is variability in the colour of the iris and in retinal pigmentation, with darker irides having darker retinas behind them. People with light retinas generally have better night vision but can have pain in an environment that has too much light.

Specific populations within Australia and Aotearoa New Zealand are at higher risk for certain diseases that affect the eye. These groups include Aboriginal and Torres Strait Islander people, Māori, older adults, people with diabetes, those with a family history of eye disease and those who are considered marginalised and disadvantaged.[19]

Prevalence of eye disease is three times higher in the Aboriginal and Torres Strait Islander community compared with the non-Indigenous community, and 90% of vision loss in Aboriginal and Torres Strait Islanders is preventable or treatable.[3,20] Cataract, diabetic retinopathy, under-corrected refractive error and trachoma are the leading causes of blindness and vision impairment in Aboriginal and Torres Strait Islander communities.[20] Similarly, health inequities including disproportionate rates of almost all chronic and infectious diseases, including ocular conditions, are seen in Māori populations.[6]

Diabetic retinopathy is more prevalent in Aboriginal and Torres Strait Islander populations in Australia and the Māori and Pacific Islander population in Aotearoa New Zealand than in non-Indigenous populations.[6,20] This is due to higher rates of diabetes in these populations.[21]

With **cataract-related blindness** being higher in Aboriginal and Torres Strait Islander populations and the surgery rate less than other Australians, there appears to be a marked under-provision of resources to these populations.[22] Similarly, Māori and Pacific Islander populations have a 1.5 to 2 times higher prevalence of cataract than other New Zealanders.[23]

Trachoma is an infectious disease of the eye caused by *Chlamydia trachomatis* and is a significant factor in ocular morbidity in Aboriginal communities. Significant reductions in the incidence of trachoma in these populations have been made in recent years, with a rate of 4.5% of 5- to 9-year-old children affected in 2019; work continues in this area.[5] The higher rate of vision loss in these populations can be attributed to barriers to access and delays in diagnosis. Barriers to accessing eye health care include health service barriers (infrastructure and systems, cost, transport and distance, interpreters, escorts, consent, trust of specialists); community (family influence, community influence, culture and beliefs); and individual (ignorance, stoicism, fear, beliefs, demographics, other illnesses).[6,20]

HEALTH EDUCATION

Age-related macular degeneration

AMD is the most common cause of visual impairment in people over the age of 50 years in the developed world. The eye disease is the leading cause of vision loss in the non-Māori population of Aotearoa New Zealand and contributes 71% of blindness in non-Indigenous Australians over the age of 50.[10,20] AMD impairs central vision by progressive destruction of the macula and impacts significantly on a person's quality of life and independence. This includes affecting their ability to read, recognise faces, drive a car and watch TV. As this is often a bilateral condition, people with AMD often fear complete blindness. However, peripheral vision is unaffected, meaning that 'navigational' vision is preserved.

The disease can be classified into early (not visually impairing) and late (visually impairing) stages. Late AMD can be further divided into 'wet' (neovascular changes) and 'dry' (atrophic changes) forms. Non-modifiable risk factors that increase the speed of progression of the disease include age, genetic factors and ethnicity (e.g. Caucasian). Cigarette smoking is the major lifestyle risk factor predicting the presence and development of AMD. Dietary antioxidants also play a role in the occurrence, prevention and treatment of the disease.

Recent developments in treating wet AMD have resulted in some success in slowing the progression of vision loss and in some cases achieving an improvement in vision. There is currently no effective treatment for dry AMD.[9]

Prevention is the first approach to reducing vision loss in persons affected by AMD. These measures focus on modifiable risk factors. By controlling such risk factors as smoking, alcohol, high body mass index (BMI) and inadequate diet, the onset of AMD may be delayed.[9]

Nurses play an important role in assessing risk and screening for AMD. This forms part of any comprehensive eye evaluation. A person at risk of AMD or with signs of early AMD needs information and advice to slow or delay the onset or progression of the disease. This should include:

- information on how to quit smoking, including referral to support services if appropriate
- advice on controlling weight and exercising regularly
- advice on eating a well-balanced diet including:
  - eating fish two to three times a week, dark green leafy vegetables and fresh fruit daily, and a handful of nuts a week; limiting fats and oils
  - choosing low glycaemic index (GI) carbohydrates instead of high GI whenever possible
  - considering a suitable dietary supplement in consultation with an eye health professional (several supplements are currently available, formulated specifically for those at risk of AMD or who have been diagnosed with the disease)
- using the Amsler grid daily to check for symptoms of AMD—for example, distortion of lines or missing areas
- providing adequate protection for eyes from sunlight exposure, including for those who are very young
- encouragement to have regular eye examinations and referral to an eye health professional for further assessment and treatment as required.

Relevant websites

- Macular Disease Foundation Australia: https://www.mdfoundation.com.au
- Macular Degeneration New Zealand: http://mdnz.org.nz

Subjective data

Practice note

Before you start the assessment, introduce yourself to the person, confirm the person's identity, discuss the purpose and scope of the assessment, clarify any questions the person may have and get verbal consent from the person to perform the assessment.

ASSESSMENT GUIDELINES	CLINICAL SIGNIFICANCE AND CLINICAL ALERTS
Presenting concern	
• *Do you feel you have any problem with your vision or your eyes?* If a problem is perceived, ask: '*How does this impact on your quality of life?*' For example, have changes in vision affected their ability to participate in normal activities or social events?	It is important to ascertain the person's perception of their vision and eye health.
Vision difficulty (decreased acuity, blurring, blind spots)	
• *Do you have any difficulty seeing or any blurring?* • *When were symptoms first noticed? Did this begin suddenly or progress slowly?*	Any decrease in vision has an impact on function and safety, which needs to be considered in planning care. ***Clinical alert:*** Any sudden change or new change in vision requires immediate referral to a medical practitioner.
• *Is it in one eye or both eyes?*	Loss or change in vision or visual field in both eyes indicates the problem is after the *optic chiasm in the visual pathway*. The person may have suffered a stroke, brain injury or a tumour may be present.
• *Is it constant or does it come and go (intermittent)? How long does it last?*	Temporary blurring of vision in one or both eyes is most commonly due to migraine or transient lack of blood supply to the retina or the brain's visual cortex.[24]
• *What part of your vision is affected? (The central or peripheral vision?)* • *Is there a blind spot or part of the vision that is 'missing'? Does it move as you shift your gaze?*	If the central vision or colour vision is affected this suggests a problem with the **macula or optic nerve**. If the peripheral vision is affected, then **glaucoma** may be present. If only one part of the visual field is affected then this suggests a problem with the brain, visual pathway or retina—for example, **retinal detachment**.

ASSESSMENT GUIDELINES	CLINICAL SIGNIFICANCE AND CLINICAL ALERTS
	Scotoma, a partial loss of vision or blind spot in an otherwise normal visual field, occurs in several conditions including retinal, optic nerve, visual pathway and brain disease.
• *Is the vision distorted?*	When straight lines look wavy (**metamorphopsia**), this may indicate macular disease—for example, macular degeneration. See Table 14.1 for illustrations describing visual field loss.
• *Do spots move in front of your eyes (floaters)? Is there one or are there many? In one or both eyes? Are there also 'flashes' of light seen?*	Floaters are common with myopia or after middle age because of condensed vitreous fibres. ! ***Clinical alert:*** Usually not significant, but acute onset of floaters ('shade' or 'cobwebs'), especially with associated 'flashes', may indicate retinal detachment. People with these symptoms require immediate referral to a medical practitioner.
• *Are there any halos/rainbows around objects? Or rings around lights?*	Halos around lights occur with **acute angle-closure glaucoma**. ! ***Clinical alert:*** Halos with associated pain require immediate referral to a medical practitioner.
• *Do you have any trouble seeing in dim light (night blindness)?*	**Night blindness** occurs with optic atrophy, glaucoma or vitamin A deficiency.
Pain	
• *Do you have any eye pain? Please describe it.* • *Does it come on suddenly?*	! ***Clinical alert:*** *Sudden onset* of eye symptoms (pain, floaters, blind spot, loss of peripheral vision) may be an emergency (e.g. acute glaucoma or foreign body). Refer for medical assessment immediately.

ASSESSMENT GUIDELINES	CLINICAL SIGNIFICANCE AND CLINICAL ALERTS
Quality of pain	
• *Is it sharp, stabbing pain or pain with bright light (photophobia)?* • *Is burning or itching present?* • *Is there a foreign body sensation or grittiness?* • *Or deep aching? Or headache in the brow area or behind the eye?* • *Is there scalp tenderness, pain in jaw when chewing?*	**Photophobia** is inability to tolerate light. It is often associated with ocular inflammation. Itchy eyes are often due to **allergic conjunctivitis**. Grittiness is often due to dry eyes or **blepharitis** (inflammation of the eyelid), especially in older adults. **Temporal arteritis** is inflammation of blood vessels. Note: Some common eye problems cause no pain (e.g. refractive errors, cataract, open-angle glaucoma, detached retina).  ***Clinical alert:*** In older people, a headache with scalp tenderness and pain on chewing may indicate temporal arteritis, which is vision and life threatening. Refer to a medical practitioner for further assessment immediately.
Strabismus (turned eye), diplopia (double vision)	
• *Do you have any history of misaligned or crossed eyes? Now or in the past? Does this occur with eye fatigue?* • *Do you ever see double? Is this constant or does it come and go? Does your double vision go away if you cover one eye?*	**Strabismus** is a deviation in the anteroposterior axis of the eye**.** This is also sometimes referred to as a squint. **Diplopia** is the perception of two images of a single object. Diplopia (double vision) in one eye can be due to dry eye, uncorrected refractive error or cataract. Binocular diplopia only occurs when both eyes are open and is due to misalignment of the axes of the eyes. This type of visual change can significantly impact on a person's daily life.
Redness, swelling	
• *Have you noticed any redness or swelling in the eyes or eyelids?* • *Is one or both eyes affected?*	Redness occurs due to several causes. These include **conjunctivitis** and other 'red-eye conditions'. Many patients with red eye symptoms will have common, easily treated conditions, but others may have serious life-threatening diseases, therefore careful assessment is important.

ASSESSMENT GUIDELINES	CLINICAL SIGNIFICANCE AND CLINICAL ALERTS
• *Do you have a history of:* – *infections presently or in the past?* – *trauma or injury to the eye?* – *eye disease or operations?* – *recent viral upper respiratory tract infection?* – *contact lens wear?* • *When do/did these occur? Was this at a particular time of year?* Advise the person regarding infection control measures to protect the unaffected eye and other household members.	Eye infections may be a result of bacterial, viral or fungal sources. Foreign body–introduced infections are common from contact lens use, injuries, seasonal variations (pollens) and environmental factors (e.g. swimming in contaminated water). A recent viral upper respiratory tract infection can be associated with viral conjunctivitis.  ***Clinical alert:*** Eye infections can be very contagious and require immediate treatment by a medical practitioner.
Watering, discharge	
• *Have you noticed watering or excessive tearing?*	**Lacrimation** (tearing) and **epiphora** (excessive tearing) are due to increased reflex tearing (due to dry eye, soreness or irritants) or obstruction in drainage of tears.
• *Do you have any discharge from the eyes?* • *Does it feel like there is anything in the eye that should not be there?* • *Is it hard to open your eyes in the morning? What colour is the discharge?* • *How do you remove this from the eyes?*	Purulent discharge is thick and yellow. Crusts often form at night. This is commonly associated with bacterial conjunctivitis. Assess hygiene practices and knowledge of cross-contamination. More common in children. 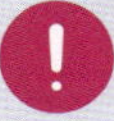 ***Clinical alert:*** A person with discharge and associated pain, photophobia and decreased vision requires urgent medical referral.
History of ocular problems	
• *Is there a history of eye disease, injury or surgery?* • *Any family history of ocular problems?* • *Is there any history of allergies?* • *Is there any history of diseases with eye symptoms/signs such as type 1 or type 2 diabetes, hypertension, thyroid disease, cardiac disease, high cholesterol, migraine?*	Some eye diseases have a genetic component; a family history of eye disease or blindness may be significant. Allergens may cause irritation of conjunctiva or cornea (e.g. make-up, contact lens solution, pollens).

ASSESSMENT GUIDELINES	CLINICAL SIGNIFICANCE AND CLINICAL ALERTS
Glaucoma	
• *Have you ever been tested for glaucoma? When and what were the results?* • *Is there any family history of glaucoma?*	**Glaucoma** represents a group of diseases where high intraocular pressure may or may not be present. Where there is a family history of glaucoma or if the person is more than 40 years of age, they should be advised to have regular eye examinations which should include dilation of the pupil and examination of the optic nerve.
If the person has glaucoma: • *How do you manage your eye drops?*	Adhering to the treatment regimen is often a problem because treatment manages the disease but does not cure it. Assess the person's ability to administer eye drops.
Use of glasses or contact lenses	
• *Do you wear **glasses** or **contact lenses**? How do they work for you? How long have you needed these? Do you wear them all the time or just for specific tasks? For example, reading or driving.*	
• *Has your prescription been stable? When was the last time your prescription was checked? Was it changed?*	Adults with glasses or contact lenses should have an annual eye examination to check their prescription and screen for age-related eye disease.
If the person wears contact lenses: • *Are there any problems such as pain, photophobia, watering or swelling?* • *What type of contact lens do you wear?* • *How do you care for contacts? How long do you wear them? How do you clean them?* • *Do you remove them/wear them for certain activities?*	Assess contact lens care routine and hygiene behaviours—for example, hand washing.
Health and lifestyle management	
• *When was your last vision test? Who tested it?* • *Have you ever had a colour vision test?*	The current recommendation is having the eyes tested every 2 years, or more often if recommended by a health professional or if there is a change in vision. In Australia, optometrists provide most eye examinations free under Medicare. In Aotearoa New Zealand, the Ministry of Health provides funding for children and low-income families.

ASSESSMENT GUIDELINES	CLINICAL SIGNIFICANCE AND CLINICAL ALERTS
• *Are there any environmental or occupational factors at home or at work that may affect your eyes? For example, flying sparks, metal shards, smoke, dust, chemical fumes. If so, do you wear goggles to protect your eyes?*	Provide education to prevent work-related eye injury (e.g. an auto mechanic with a foreign body from metal working or radiation damage from welding).
• *What medications are you taking? Are they systemic (like a tablet) or topical (applied to the skin)?* • *Do you take any medication specifically for the eyes?* • *Do you smoke?*	Some medications have ocular side effects; for example, prednisone may cause cataracts or increased intraocular pressure. Others can dilate or constrict the pupil, making it difficult to accommodate to changes in light. For example, narcotic medications and some antihypertensive medications can constrict the pupils; antidepressants, antinausea medications, atropine can dilate the pupils. Cigarette smoking is associated with age-related macular degeneration, cataract, diabetic retinopathy and eye inflammation. Advice or support on how to quit should be offered.
Adjustment to vision loss (if relevant)	
• *How has your life changed in terms of roles and relationships, employment, nutrition, activity and exercise, history of recent falls, for example?* • *What are some of the strategies you use to manage at home, like a change in layout within the home or reduced social activity?* • *Do you need extra lighting or magnification?* • *Have you been referred to/or are a current client of support services (Vision Australia, Blind Low Vision NZ)?* • *Do you use books with large print, audio books, Braille?*	Be alert to people in a hospital setting or new to residential care who are vision-impaired. They may need extra supports until they find their way around in new surroundings. They are at significant risk of injury. A constant spatial layout eases navigation through the home or new environment. If a person is an existing client of support services, collaboration with the service will assist in planning care.
Additional subjective data for infants and children (questions for parents or guardian)	
• *Did the mother have any vaginal infections at the time of delivery?*	Genital herpes and gonorrhoea vaginitis may have ocular sequelae for the newborn.

ASSESSMENT GUIDELINES	CLINICAL SIGNIFICANCE AND CLINICAL ALERTS

• *Have you noticed any visual difficulties in your child?*
  • *Have you noticed a 'turned' or 'crossed' eye?*
  • *Does the child have routine vision testing at school or elsewhere?*
  • *Does your child have reading problems or complain of difficulty seeing the screens, whiteboard or TV?*
  • *Have you noticed a white or pale pupil in a photograph?* (Usually, the pupil should appear black or red.)
  • *Which safety measures do you use to protect your child's eyes from trauma? Do you inspect toys?*
  • *Have you taught the child safe care with sharp objects and how to carry and how to use them?* (Can include specifics such as not looking directly at the sun.)
	The parent is most often the one to detect vision problems. While eye examinations are available under Medicare, vision testing in schools varies between states in Australia. Free testing for children is available in Aotearoa New Zealand through the Ministry of Health.
	An interruption in the pupillary red reflex indicates opacity in the cornea, lens or ocular media. This is often detected in family photographs.
	! ***Clinical alert:*** An absent red reflex occurs with congenital cataracts or retinal disorders. A white reflex or 'pupil' may indicate a serious intraocular tumour (retinoblastoma). The child should be referred urgently.

Additional subjective data for adults over 65 years	
• *Have you had to decrease any of your usual activities such as reading, driving or sewing?* • *Have you had any difficulty using equipment such as the telephone or computer? Or difficulty recognising people's faces?*	Age-related macular degeneration causes a loss in central vision acuity that can impact on activities of daily living.
• *Have you experienced a loss of independence such as problems climbing stairs, crossing the road or driving?*	! ***Clinical alert:*** Loss of depth perception, contrast sensitivity, peripheral or central vision may occur with age-related eye diseases such as cataract. If detected the person should be referred to a medical practitioner.
• *Do you have a history of cataracts? Any loss or progressive blurring of vision? Have you had cataract surgery?* • *Do you suffer from glare sensitivity such as from lights when driving at night?*	**Cataract** is opacity of the crystalline lens and commonly occurs in people over the age of 60. It is usually a bilateral condition, although degree of progression may vary between eyes. Cataract can cause glare sensitivity due to the opacities in the lens scattering light, rather than focusing it.
• *Do your eyes ever feel dry, burn or water excessively? What do you do for this?*	**Dry eye** is common in older people. Decreased tear production and quality may be due to medications, diseases, environmental triggers and changes in anatomy due to loss of elasticity in the tissues. Using artificial lubricants can improve comfort for these people.

Objective data

The insights you have gained from collecting subjective data will guide the objective data collection. Generalist nurses usually only perform a few of the techniques related to eye examination. Documentation of this data also takes a specific form and needs to follow a logical sequence.

Preparation

Have the person sitting comfortably in an upright position where possible. The examiner should sit or stand opposite the person so they can maintain a straight back. Ensure the examination takes place in a well-lit environment.

Equipment needed

Opaque card or occluder
Penlight
Hand hygiene solution

PROCEDURES AND NORMAL FINDINGS	ABNORMAL FINDINGS AND CLINICAL ALERTS
General inspection	
Already you will have noted the person's ability to move around the room, with vision functioning well enough to avoid obstacles and respond to your directions. Also note the facial expression, looking specifically for squinting, grimacing and so on. Also note the person's head posture and facial symmetry.	Note if the person is groping with their hands while walking and squinting or craning forwards. Abnormal head posture may indicate a problem with a particular area of the visual field. Asymmetrical facial appearance may indicate neurological involvement.
Inspect external ocular structures	
Begin with the most external points and logically work your way inwards.	
Eyebrows	
Normally the eyebrows are present bilaterally, move symmetrically as the facial expression changes and have no scaling or lesions.	Hypothyroidism often causes the lateral third of brow to be absent (can also be related to normal ageing). Unequal or absent movement of brows may be present with nerve damage. Scaling occurs with seborrhoea.

PROCEDURES AND NORMAL FINDINGS	ABNORMAL FINDINGS AND CLINICAL ALERTS
Eyelids and lashes	
The upper lids normally overlap the superior part of the iris and approximate completely with the lower lids when closed. The skin is intact without redness, swelling, discharge or lesions.	Hyperthyroidism causes lid lag. Incomplete closure of lids creates risk for corneal damage. **Ectropion** occurs when the lower lid turns outwards, **entropion** is when the lower lid turns inwards. Both findings are abnormal and can predispose the person to corneal damage and eye infection. **Ptosis** is drooping of the upper lid. See Tables 14.2 and 14.3 for examples of eyelid abnormalities and lesions. If detected, **eyelid lesions** require further investigation to rule out tumours, including **basal cell carcinoma** or **squamous cell carcinoma** (Table 14.3).
The **palpebral fissures** are horizontal in non-Asian people, whereas Asian people normally have an upward slant to the eye.	**Blepharospasm** is increased blink rate that occurs in spasms. It can be an inability to open eyelids. This is usually due to inflammation or malfunction of cranial nerves V (trigeminal) and VII (facial). It can occur in exposure to bright lights.
Note that the eyelashes are evenly distributed along the lid margins and curve outwards. Observe that the eyelid area is free of redness, swelling or rash.	**Periorbital oedema**, when the lids are swollen, may indicate local infection or systemic conditions (Table 14.2). ! ***Clinical alert:*** **Orbital cellulitis** is an acute purulent inflammation of the cellular tissue of the orbit. It is an ophthalmic emergency. The person should be referred urgently (Table 14.2).
Eyeballs	
The eyeballs are aligned normally in their sockets with no protrusion or sunken appearance.	**Exophthalmos** (protruding eyes) and **enophthalmos** (sunken eyes) (Table 14.2). Exophthalmos can be associated with thyroid eye disease and may result in exposure (drying) of the cornea.
Conjunctiva and sclera	
Ask the person to look up. Using your thumbs, slide the lower lids down along the bony orbital rim. Take care not to push against the eyeball. Inspect the exposed area (Figure 14.9). The eyeball looks moist and glossy. Numerous small blood vessels normally show through the transparent conjunctiva. Otherwise, the conjunctivae are clear and show the normal colour of the structure below, pink over the lower lids and white over the sclera. Note any colour change, swelling or lesions.	Note abnormal findings such as general reddening (Table 14.4). Pallor near the outer canthus of the lower lid may indicate anaemia (the inner canthus normally contains less pigment).

PROCEDURES AND NORMAL FINDINGS

FIGURE 14.9 Sclera

The sclera is china-white, although those with dark pigmented skin occasionally have a grey-blue or 'muddy' colour to the sclera. You may see small brown macules (like freckles) on the sclera, which are normal and should not be confused with foreign bodies or petechiae.

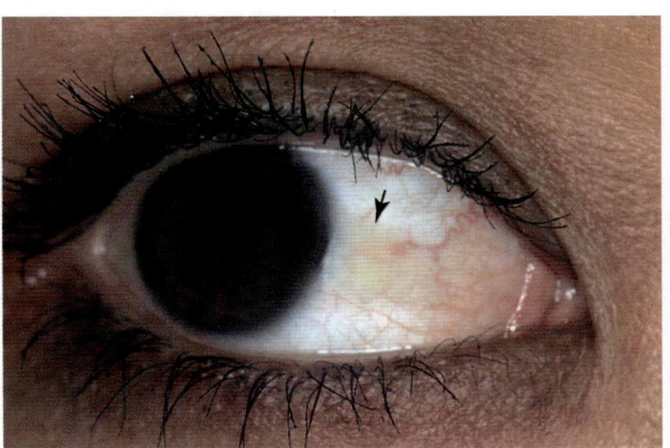

FIGURE 14.10 Pinguecula

ABNORMAL FINDINGS AND CLINICAL ALERTS

Scleral icterus is an even yellowing of the sclera extending up to the cornea, indicating jaundice.

Note any tenderness, foreign body, discharge or lesions.

Pinguecula is a growth on conjunctiva due to chronic ultraviolet light or other environmental exposure. (Figure 14.10).

PROCEDURES AND NORMAL FINDINGS	ABNORMAL FINDINGS AND CLINICAL ALERTS
Inspect anterior eyeball structures	
Cornea and lens	
Shine a light from the lateral side across the cornea and check for smoothness and clarity. This oblique view highlights any abnormal irregularities in the corneal surface. There should be no opacities (cloudiness) in or on the cornea, the anterior chamber or the lens behind the pupil. Do not confuse an **arcus senilis** with an opacity.	A **corneal abrasion** causes irregular ridges in reflected light, producing a shattered look to light rays (Table 14.5). The person may also report the sensation of a foreign body and/or pain. **Arcus senilis** is a grey-white arc or circle around the **limbus** (forms the border between the transparent cornea and the opaque sclera) due to deposition of lipid material. It is a normal finding in older people. **Pterygium** is an abnormal triangular growth over the cornea and sclera (Table 14.5).
Iris and pupil	
The iris normally appears flat, with a round regular shape and even colouration. Note the size, shape and equality of the pupils. Normally the pupils appear round, regular and of equal size in both eyes. In adults, resting size is from 3 to 5 mm. A small number of people (5%) normally have pupils of two different sizes, which is termed **anisocoria** (Table 14.6).	***Clinical alert***: Look for an irregular pupil shape. Ask if this is old or new. Irregularly shaped pupils may indicate intraocular inflammation or infection, previous eye surgery or injury. Although they may be normal, all unequally sized pupils should be investigated to rule out central nervous system injury, tumour or local trauma.
To test the **pupillary light reflex**, darken the room and ask the person to gaze into the distance (this dilates the pupils). Ensure you have a strong, bright light. Advance a light in from the lateral side and note the response. Normally you will see (1) constriction of the same-sided pupil (a *direct light reflex*) and (2) simultaneous constriction of the other pupil (a *consensual light reflex*) (Chapter 12). Always advance the light in from the side to test the light reflex. If you advance from the front, the pupils will constrict to accommodate for near vision and confuse the test results. In the acute-care setting record the pupil size in millimetres using a standardised gauge. Recording the pupil size in millimetres is more accurate when many health practitioners care for the same person or when small changes may be significant—for example, indicating increasing intracranial pressure. See Chapter 12 for a full description of pupil assessment as part of a neurological examination.	Abnormal findings include: • dilated pupils • dilated and fixed pupils • constricted pupils • unequal or no response to light (Table 14.6). Some systemic medications (e.g. opioids) or eye drops can affect the size of the pupil.

PROCEDURES AND NORMAL FINDINGS	ABNORMAL FINDINGS AND CLINICAL ALERTS
Visual acuity—test vision	
A simple but effective method to assess vision for most nurses includes asking the person to read a magazine or brochure (to test near vision) and a sign or clock on the wall (for distance vision), making the necessary adjustments for people who read a language other than English or who are unable to read. The information gained will assist you to adjust health information to meet the person's individual needs and to make referrals to other health professionals as necessary. Advanced practice nurses may use a range of techniques to test visual acuity (see 'Advanced practice—additional data').	Visual acuity only assesses the person's macular function. Even if a person has good visual acuity, they can be visually impaired due to other eye problems.
Visual field—confrontation test	
This is a gross measure of peripheral vision. It compares the person's peripheral vision with your own, assuming yours is normal (Figure 14.11). Position yourself at eye level with the person about 60 cm away. Direct the person to cover one eye with an opaque card, and with the other eye to look straight at you. Cover your own eye opposite to the person's covered one. You are testing the uncovered eye. Hold a pencil or your flicking finger as a target midline between you and the other person and slowly advance it in from the periphery in several directions. 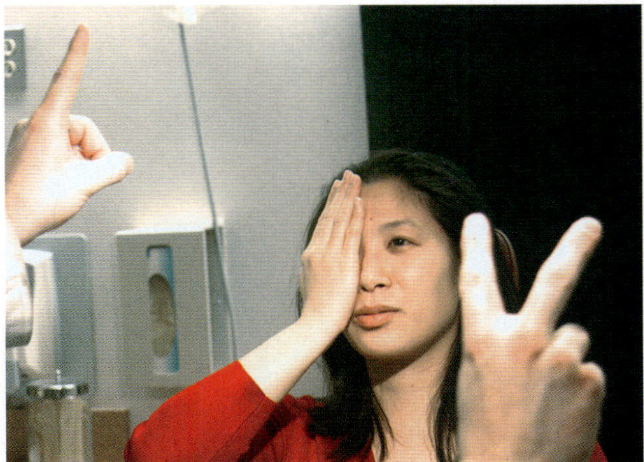 **FIGURE 14.11** Visual field—confrontation test	

PROCEDURES AND NORMAL FINDINGS	ABNORMAL FINDINGS AND CLINICAL ALERTS
Ask the person to say 'now' as the target is first seen; this should be just as you see the object also. (This works with all but the temporal visual field.) Estimate the angle between the anteroposterior axis of the eye and the peripheral axis where the object is first seen. Normal results are about 50 degrees upwards, 90 degrees temporal, 70 degrees down and 60 degrees nasal (Figure 14.12).	Abnormalities in peripheral vision can occur following stroke or head injury or with abnormalities of the eye or visual pathway Visual field loss can lead to risk of injury due to bumping into objects or falling and has implications for driving.

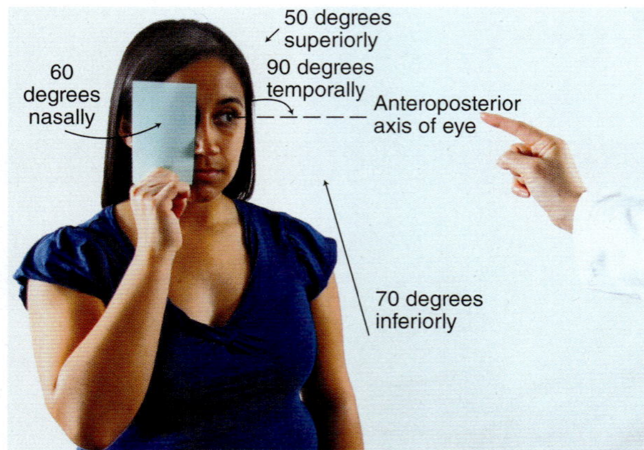

FIGURE 14.12 Range of peripheral vision

Additional objective data for infants and children (birth to 12 years)

The eye examination is often deferred at birth because of transient oedema of the lids from birth trauma. The eyes should be examined within a few days and at every child health visit thereafter.

Currently, in Australia, there is limited consistency in how and when visual screening is performed in children. This includes inconsistencies in the number of vision checks recommended, when age screening is undertaken, the tools and procedures used, the personnel conducting screening and referral and follow-up of the screening.[25]

The Centre for Community Child Health[26] advises that screening for vision should be undertaken from 18 months of age and no later than 5 years of age, in addition to the standard neonatal check. Exceptions are made for newborns with existing congenital vision conditions.

The child's age determines the screening measures used. Test **light perception** using the **blink reflex**; neonates blink in response to bright light (Figure 14.13). Also, the **pupillary light reflex** shows that the pupils constrict in response to light. These reflexes indicate that the lower portion of the visual apparatus is intact. But you cannot infer that the infant can *see*; that requires later observation to show that the brain has received images and can interpret them.

Clinical alert: Look for absence of blinking and pupillary light reflex, especially after 3 weeks, because this may indicate blindness.

Decreased vision may occur in premature infants or infants with neurological deficits.

PROCEDURES AND NORMAL FINDINGS	ABNORMAL FINDINGS AND CLINICAL ALERTS

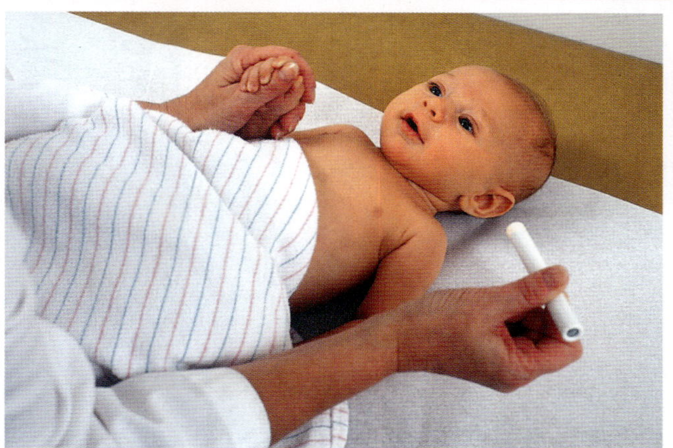

FIGURE 14.13 Testing light perception in an infant

Test visual reflexes and attending behaviours when you introduce an object into the infant's line of sight. Normal findings include:

Birth to 2 weeks—Infant refuses to reopen eyes after exposure to bright light; increasing alertness to object; infant may fixate on an object.

By 2 to 4 weeks—Infant can fixate on an object.

The Royal Australian and New Zealand College of Ophthalmologists Referral Guidelines for Eye and Vision Problems in Infants and Children[27] recommend referral in the case of:

- a baby with abnormal red reflex
- a child with ocular structural abnormalities or chronic watering eyes, not resolved in the first year of life
- a child for whom there is concern about poor vision with a family history of hereditary eye conditions
- a 4- or 5-year-old child with equally reduced distance vision in both eyes (< 6/19 or 6/12) or worse than 6/18 in either eye
- a 5-year-old (or older) with vision less than 6/6
- a child with vision that fails to improve following assessment and treatment by an optometrist
- various presentations of strabismus.

PROCEDURES AND NORMAL FINDINGS	ABNORMAL FINDINGS AND CLINICAL ALERTS

By 1 month—Infant can fixate and follow a light or bright toy.

By 6 weeks—Infant makes some visual response to your face.

By 3 to 4 months—Infant can fixate, follow and reach for the toy.

By 6 to 10 months—Infant can fixate and follow the toy in all directions.

External eye structures. Inspect the ocular structures as described in the earlier section. A neonate usually holds their eyes tightly shut. Do not attempt to pry them open; that just increases contraction of the orbicularis oculi muscle. Hold the newborn supine and gently lower the head; the eyes will open. Also, the eyes will open when you hold the infant at arm's length and slowly turn the infant in one direction. In addition to inspecting the ocular structures, this also tests the vestibular function reflex. That is, the baby's eyes will look in the same direction as the body is being turned. When the turning stops, the eyes will shift to the opposite direction after a few quick beats of nystagmus. Also termed 'doll's eyes', this reflex disappears by 2 months of age.

Eyelids and lashes. Normally, the upper lids overlie the superior part of the iris. In newborns the **setting-sun sign** is common. The eyes appear to deviate down, and you see a white rim of sclera over the iris. It may show as you rapidly change the neonate from a sitting to a supine position.

The setting-sun sign also occurs with hydrocephalus as the globes protrude.

Blank sunken eyes accompany malnutrition, dehydration and a severe illness.

Many infants have an epicanthal fold, an excess skinfold extending over the inner corner of the eye, partly or totally overlapping the inner canthus. It occurs frequently in children of Asian descent and in 20% of other children. In children of non-Asian descent, it disappears as the child grows, usually by 10 years of age. While they are present, epicanthal folds give a false appearance of malalignment, termed **pseudostrabismus** (Figure 14.14). In these cases, the ***corneal light reflex*** is normal.

The **corneal light reflex** is assessed by shining a bright torch towards both eyes from in front of the child. When the eyes are correctly aligned the light reflection from the torch will appear in the same location on each cornea.

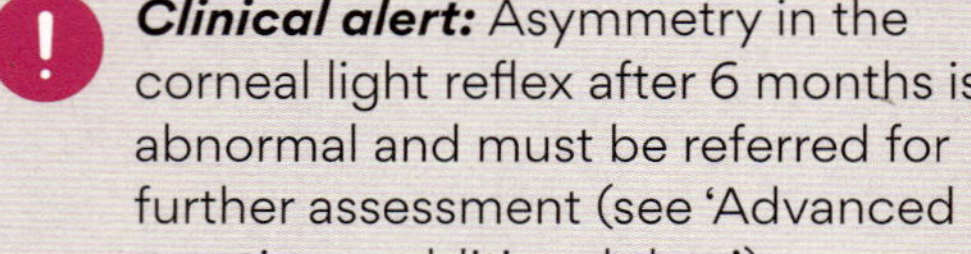
Clinical alert: Asymmetry in the corneal light reflex after 6 months is abnormal and must be referred for further assessment (see 'Advanced practice—additional data').

PROCEDURES AND NORMAL FINDINGS	ABNORMAL FINDINGS AND CLINICAL ALERTS
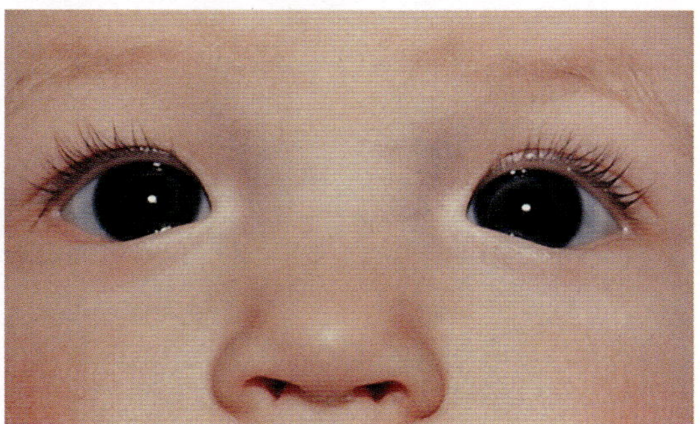 **FIGURE 14.14** Pseudostrabismus	
Infants of Asian descent normally have an upward slant of the palpebral fissures. Entropion, a turning inward of the eyelid, is found normally in some children of Asian descent. If the lashes do not abrade the corneas, it is not significant.	An upward lateral slope together with epicanthal folds and hypertelorism (large spacing between eyes) occurs with people with Trisomy 21 (Down syndrome) (Table 14.2).
Conjunctiva and sclera. The conjunctiva should be clear and show the normal colour of the structure below, pink over the lower lids and white over the sclera. Note any colour change or discharge. The sclera should be white and clear, although it may have a blue tint because of thinness at birth. The lacrimal glands are not functional at birth.	Conjunctivitis accounts for most general practice encounters involving children with eye conditions. ! ***Clinical alert:*** Ophthalmia neonatorum (conjunctivitis of the newborn) is a purulent discharge caused by a bacterial or viral agent from the birth canal. Refer to a medical practitioner.
Iris and pupils. The iris normally is blue or slate grey in light-skinned newborns and brown in dark-skinned infants. By 6 to 9 months, the permanent colour is differentiated. Brushfield's spots or white specks around the edge of the iris occasionally may be normal.	Absence of iris colour occurs with **albinism** (an inherited condition that leads to a person having very light coloured skin, hair and eyes). This results in poor vision due to excess light entering the eye resulting in glare symptoms. Brushfield's spots are frequently associated with Trisomy 21 (Down syndrome).
The **crystalline lens** of a newborn is colourless, clear and spherical.	**Cataract**, opacity of the crystalline lens, can occur congenitally. When a torch is shone in the eye, a white reflex in the pupil may be seen.
The ocular fundus. Examination of the ocular fundus in an infant is an advanced skill. However, it should be possible to check for a 'red reflex', indicating light returning from the healthy retina. The reflected light in the pupil should appear red, orange or yellow and be symmetrical across both eyes.	An abnormal or absent red reflex can indicate vision or life-threatening pathology including congenital cataract, retinal abnormalities, strabismus, refractive error or tumour. ! ***Clinical alert:*** Any child with an abnormal red reflex should be referred urgently to exclude retinoblastoma (ocular tumour).

PROCEDURES AND NORMAL FINDINGS	ABNORMAL FINDINGS AND CLINICAL ALERTS
A searching nystagmus is common just after birth. The pupils are small but constrict to light.	 ***Clinical alert:*** Constant nystagmus, prolonged setting-sun sign, marked strabismus and slow lateral movements suggest vision loss. Refer to a medical practitioner for further assessment.

Additional objective data for adults over 65 years

Ocular structures. The eyebrows may show a loss of the outer one-third to one-half of hair because of a decrease in hair follicles. The remaining brow hair is coarse (Figure 14.15). As a result of atrophy of elastic tissues, the skin around the eyes may show wrinkles or crow's feet. The upper lid may be so elongated as to rest on the lashes, resulting in a **pseudoptosis**.

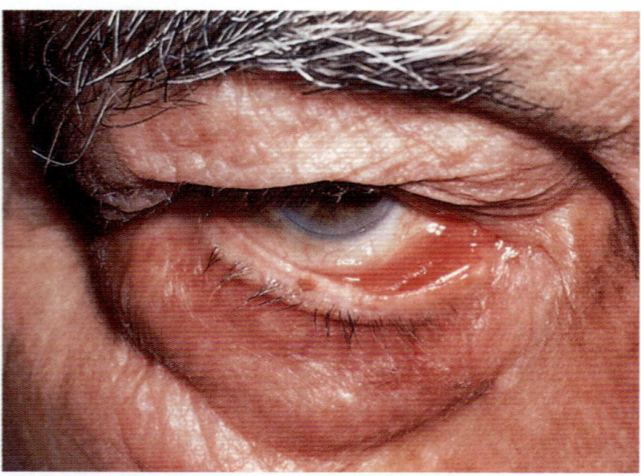

FIGURE 14.15 Pseudoptosis

The eyes may appear sunken from atrophy of the orbital fat. Also, the orbital fat may herniate, causing bulging at the lower lids and inner third of the upper lids.

Look for ectropion (lower lid dropping away) and entropion (lower lid turning in) (Table 14.2).

Xanthelasma are soft, raised, yellow plaques occurring on the lids at the inner canthus (Figure 14.16). They commonly occur around the fifth decade of life and more frequently in women. They occur with both high and normal blood levels of cholesterol and have no pathological significance.

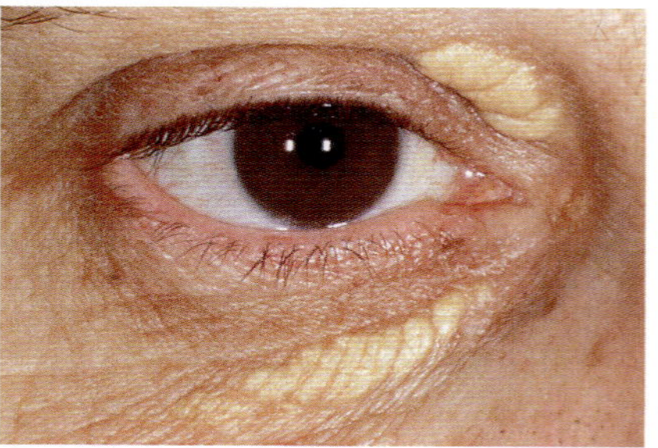

FIGURE 14.16 Xanthelasma

PROCEDURES AND NORMAL FINDINGS	ABNORMAL FINDINGS AND CLINICAL ALERTS
The **lacrimal apparatus** may decrease tear production, causing the eyes to look dry and lustreless. The person may report a burning sensation or grittiness associated with dry eye disease.	
Pingueculae commonly show on the sclera (Figure 14.10, earlier). These yellowish elevated nodules are due to a thickening of the bulbar conjunctiva from prolonged exposure to sun, wind and dust. Pingueculae appear at the 3 and 9 o'clock positions—first on the nasal side, then on the temporal side.	Distinguish **pinguecula** from the abnormal **pterygium**, also an opacity on the bulbar conjunctiva, but one that grows over the cornea (Figure 14.10 and Table 14.5). This subsequently disrupts the normal tear film, often causing a foreign body sensation.
The cornea may look cloudy with age. An **arcus senilis** is commonly seen around the cornea (Figure 14.17). This is a grey-white arc or circle around the limbus; it is due to deposition of lipid material. As more lipid accumulates, the cornea may look thickened and raised, but the arcus has no effect on vision.	
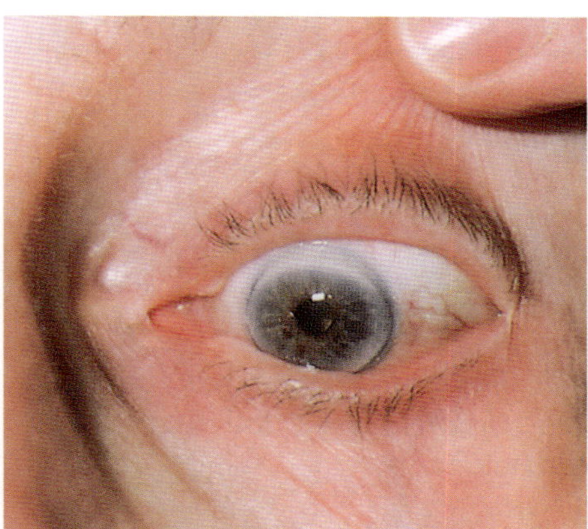 **FIGURE 14.17** Arcus senilis	
Pupils are small in old age, and the pupillary light reflex may be slowed. This can be marked when the person moves from a bright environment (e.g. outdoors) to a darker environment (inside the house) and is a potential risk factor for falls.	
The lens loses transparency and looks opaque. This has a subsequent effect on vision.	

Abnormal findings

TABLE 14.1 Visual field loss

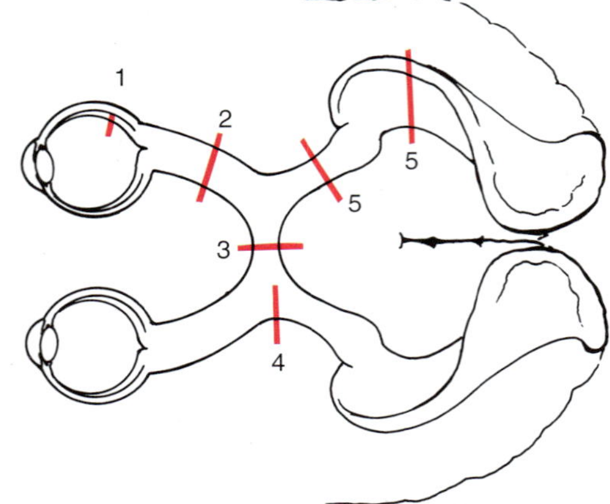

1. Retinal damage.

- **Macula**—central blind area (e.g. diabetes):

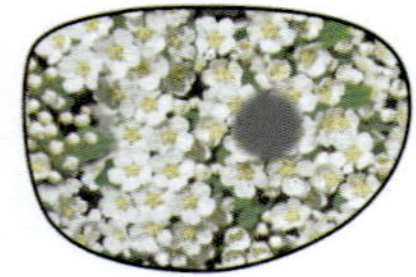
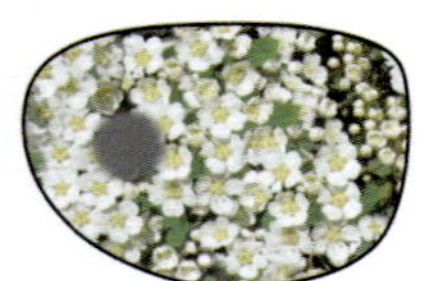

- **Increasing intraocular pressure**—decrease in peripheral vision (e.g. glaucoma). Starts with paracentral scotoma in the early stage:

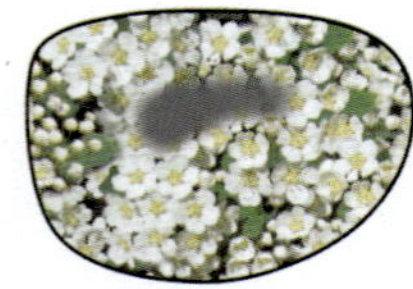
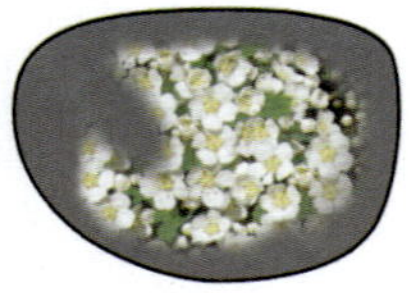

- **Localised damage**—blind spot (scotoma) corresponding to particular area:

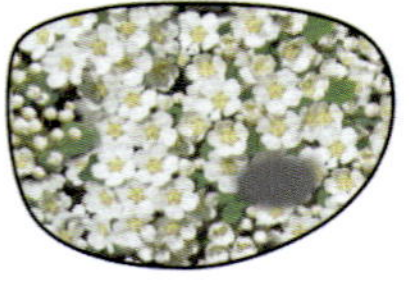
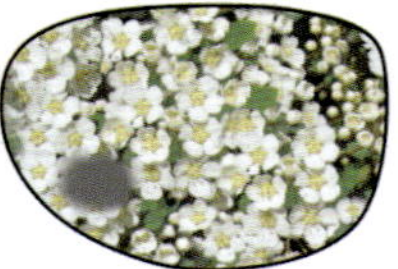

- **Retinal detachment.** Person has shadow or diminished vision in one quadrant or half of the visual field:

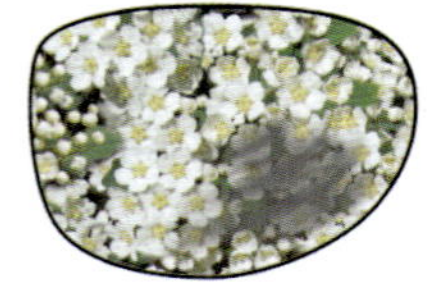
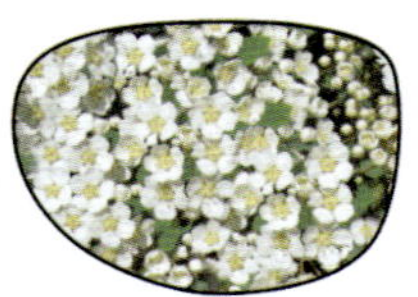

2. Lesion in globe or optic nerve.

Injury here yields one blind eye or unilateral blindness:

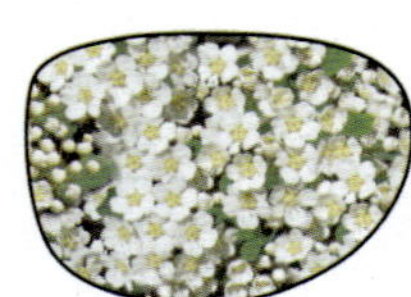

3. Lesion at optic chiasm (e.g. pituitary tumour)—injury to crossing fibres only yields a loss of nasal part of each retina and a loss of both temporal visual fields. Bitemporal (heteronymous) hemianopsia:

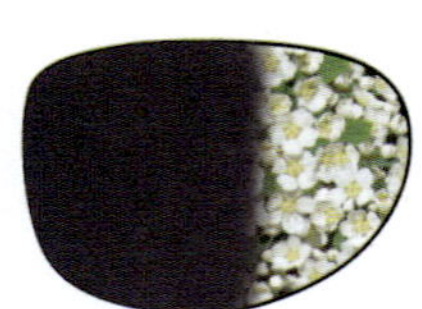
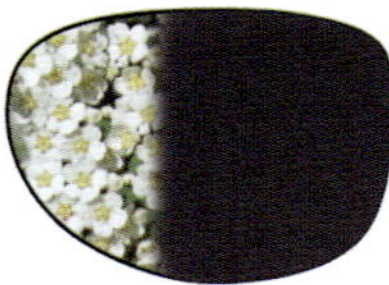

TABLE 14.1 Visual field loss cont'd

4. Lesion of outer uncrossed fibres at optic chiasm (e.g. aneurysm of the left internal carotid artery exerts pressure on uncrossed fibres). Injury yields left nasal hemianopsia:

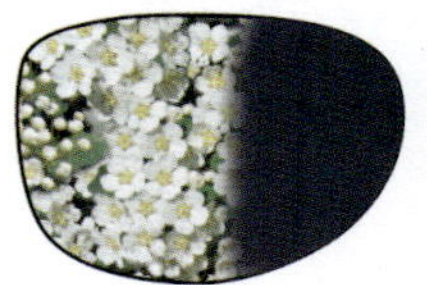
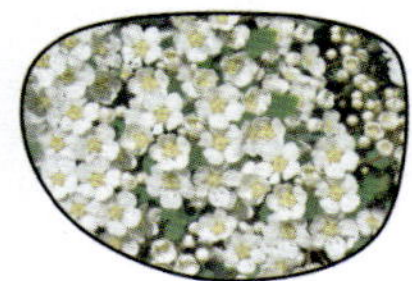

5. Lesion R optic tract or R optic radiation.

Visual field loss in R nasal and L temporal fields.

Loss of same half visual field in both eyes is homonymous hemianopsia:

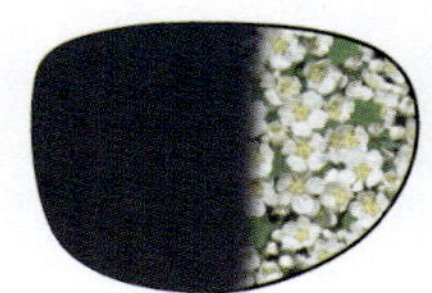
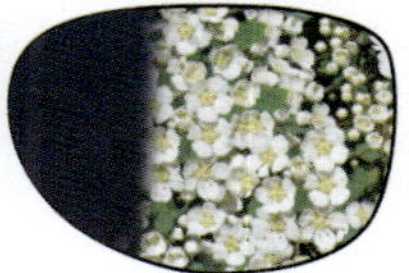

TABLE 14.2 Abnormalities of the eyelids

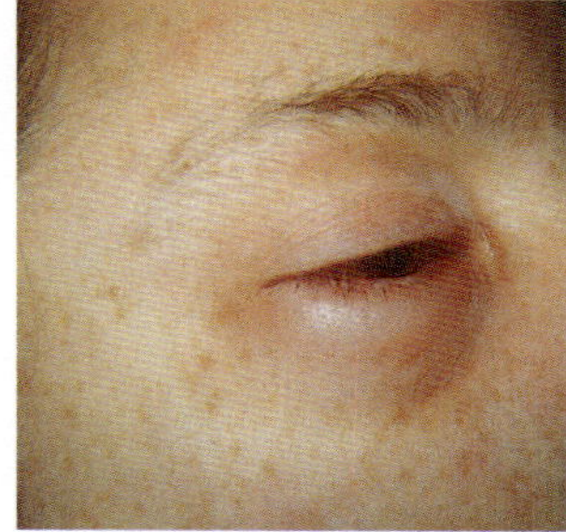

Periorbital oedema

Lids are swollen and puffy. Lid tissues are loosely connected so excess fluid is easily apparent. This occurs with local infections, crying and systemic conditions such as congestive heart failure, renal failure, allergy and hypothyroidism (myxoedema).

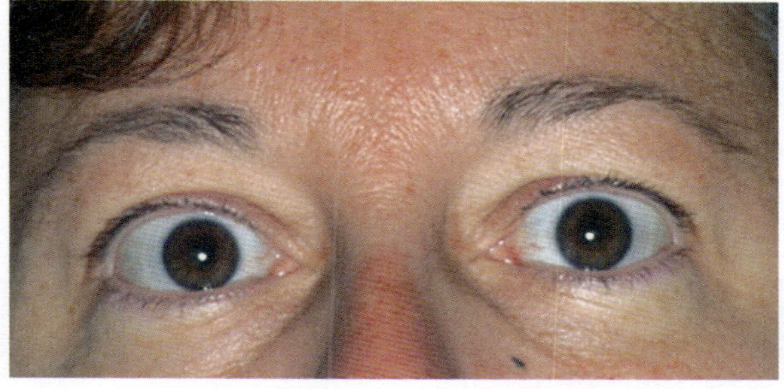

Exophthalmos (protruding eyes)

Exophthalmos is a forward displacement of the eyeballs and widened palpebral fissures. Note 'lid lag': the upper lid rests well above the limbus and white sclera is visible. Acquired bilateral exophthalmos is associated with thyrotoxicosis.

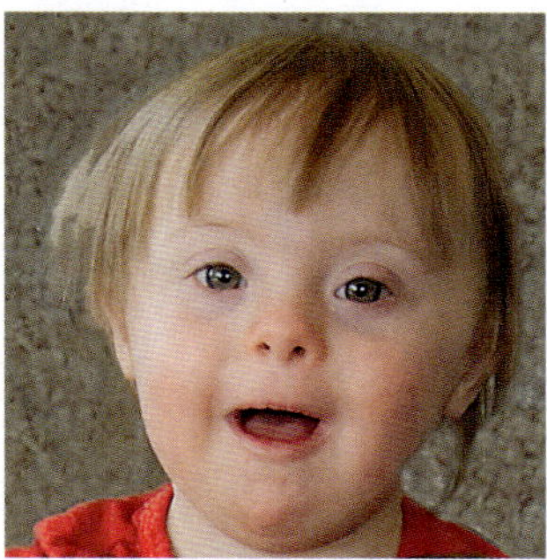

Upward palpebral slant

Although normal in many children, when combined with epicanthal folds, hypertelorism (large spacing between the eyes) and Brushfield spots (light-coloured areas in the outer iris) indicates Down syndrome.

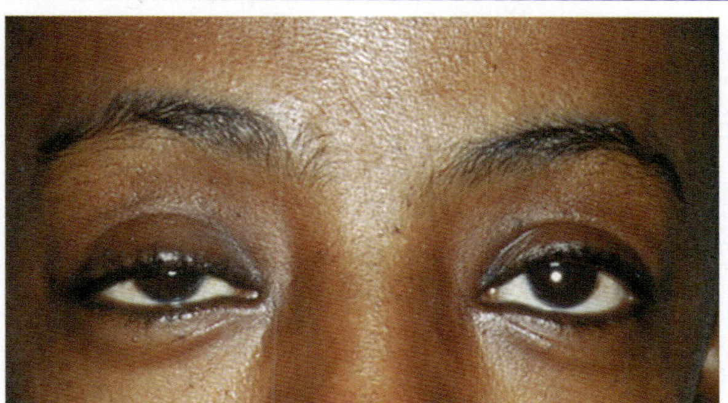

Ptosis (drooping upper lid)

Ptosis occurs from neuromuscular weakness (e.g. myasthenia gravis with bilateral fatigue as the day progresses), oculomotor cranial nerve III damage or sympathetic nerve damage (e.g. Horner's syndrome). It is a positional defect that gives the person a sleepy appearance and impairs vision.

Continued

TABLE 14.2 Abnormalities of the eyelids cont'd

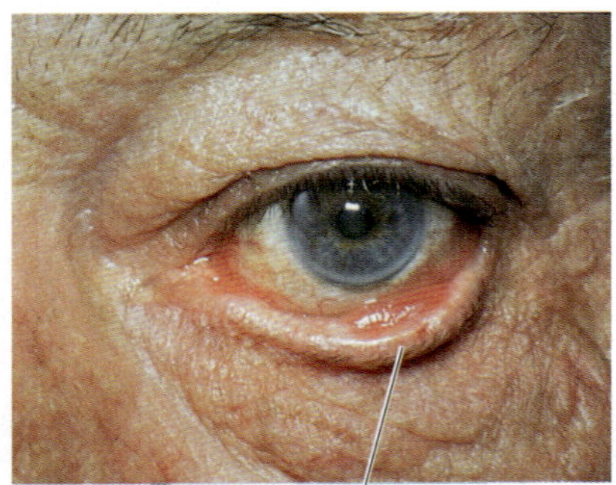

Ectropion

The lower lid is loose and rolling out and does not approximate to the eyeball. Puncta cannot siphon tears effectively, so excess tearing results. The eyes feel dry and itchy because the tears do not drain correctly over the corner and towards the medial canthus. Exposed palpebral conjunctiva increases the risk of inflammation. It occurs in ageing as a result of atrophy of elastic and fibrous tissues but may result from trauma.

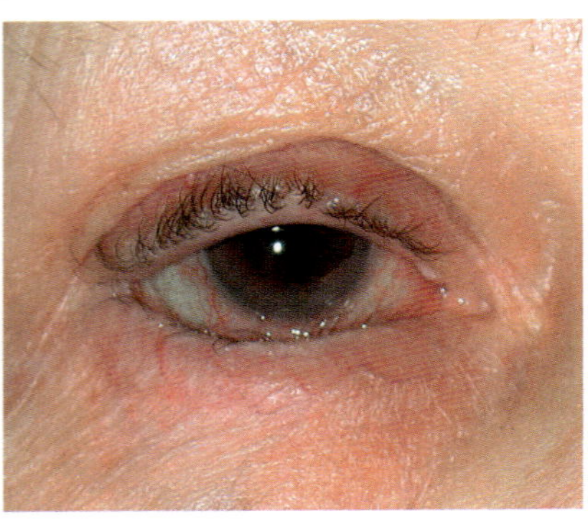

Entropion

The lower lid rolls in because of spasm of lids or scar tissue contracting. Constant rubbing of the lashes may irritate the cornea. The person feels a 'foreign body' sensation.

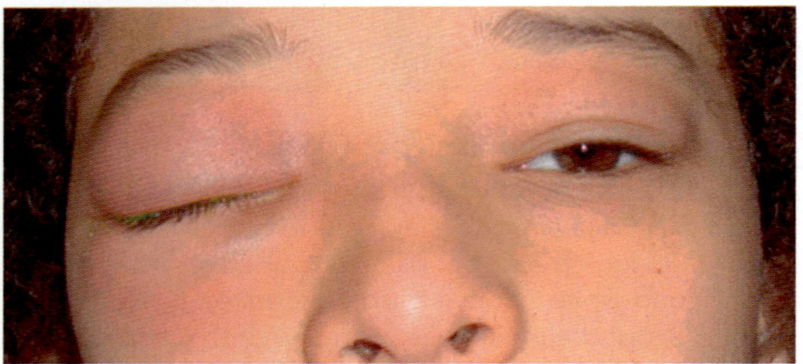

Orbital cellulitis

Orbital cellulitis is a severe and potentially life-threatening infection of the orbit soft tissues. Symptoms may include severe pain, blurred vision, diplopia (double vision), fever and malaise. Severe swelling and redness of the eyelid, with proptosis and decreased movement, is seen. The eyeball itself is also red. People with these symptoms require urgent referral.

TABLE 14.3 Lesions on the eyelids

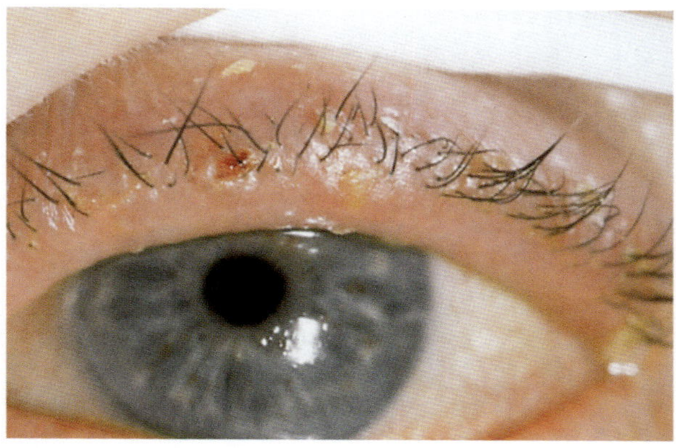

Blepharitis (inflammation of the eyelids)

Red, scaly, greasy flakes and thickened, crusted lid margins occur with staphylococcal infection or seborrhoeic dermatitis of the lid edge. Symptoms include burning, itching, tearing, foreign body sensation and some pain.

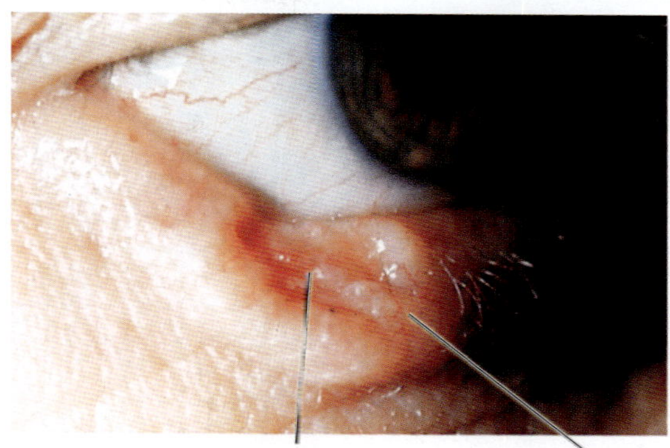

Basal cell carcinoma

Basal cell carcinoma occurs most often on the lower lid and presents as a small, painless nodule with central ulceration and sharp, rolled-out pearly edges. It occurs in older adults, associated with ultraviolet exposure and light skin tones. It is locally invasive, but metastases are rare.[28]

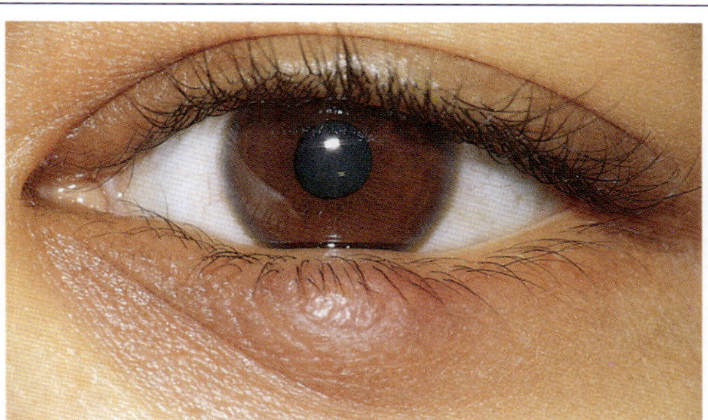

Chalazion

A beady nodule protruding on the lid, chalazion is an infection or retention cyst of a meibomian gland. It is a nontender, firm, discrete swelling with freely movable skin overlying the nodule. If it becomes inflamed, it points inside and not on lid margin (in contrast with stye).

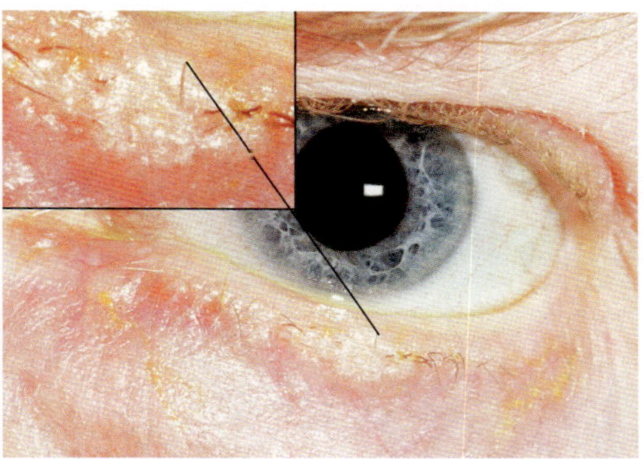

Squamous cell carcinoma

Squamous cell carcinoma is a rarer form of eyelid tumour but can be life threatening if it extends into the orbit. The lesion can be plaque-like, nodular or ulcerating. It is not usually vascularised.[29] Immediate referral is required.

Continued

TABLE 14.3 Lesions on the eyelids cont'd

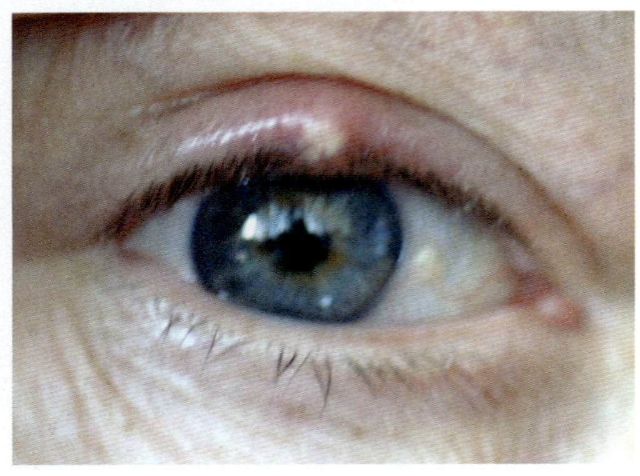

Hordeolum (stye)

Hordeolum is a localised staphylococcal infection of the hair follicles at the lid margin. It is painful, red and swollen—a pustule at the lid margin. Rubbing the eyes can cause cross-contamination and development of another stye.

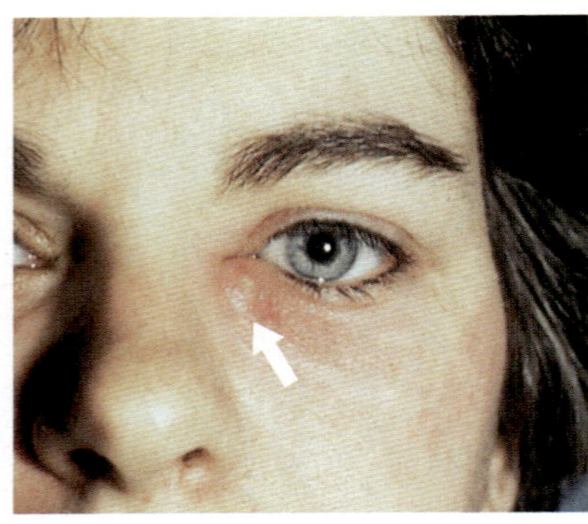

Dacryocystitis (Inflammation of the Lacrimal Sac)

Dacryocystitis is infection and blockage of sac and duct. Pain warmth, redness and swelling occur below the inner canthus towards the nose. Tearing is present. Pressure on sac yields purulent discharge from puncta.
Dacryoadenitis is an infection of the lacrimal gland (not illustrated). Pain, swelling and redness occur in the outer third of the upper lid. It occurs with mumps, measles and infectious mononucleosis or from trauma.

TABLE 14.4 Red eye

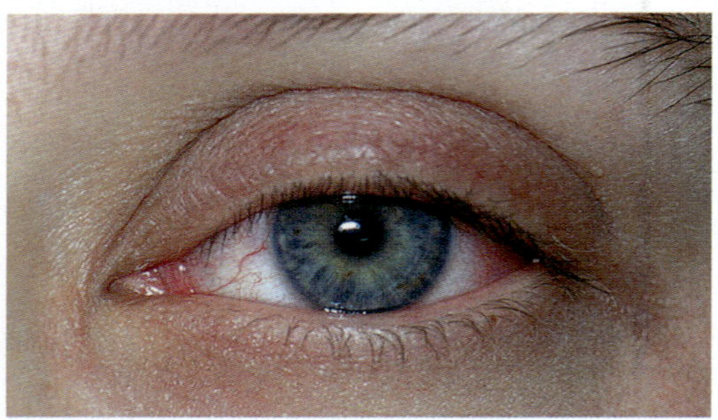

Conjunctivitis

Infection of the conjunctiva, 'red eye', has red beefy-looking vessels at periphery but usually clearer around iris (although here it is severe). This is common from bacterial or viral infection, allergy or chemical irritation. Purulent discharge accompanies bacterial infection. Preauricular lymph node is often swollen and painful, with a history of upper respiratory infection. Symptoms include itching, burning, foreign body sensation and eyelids stuck together on awakening.

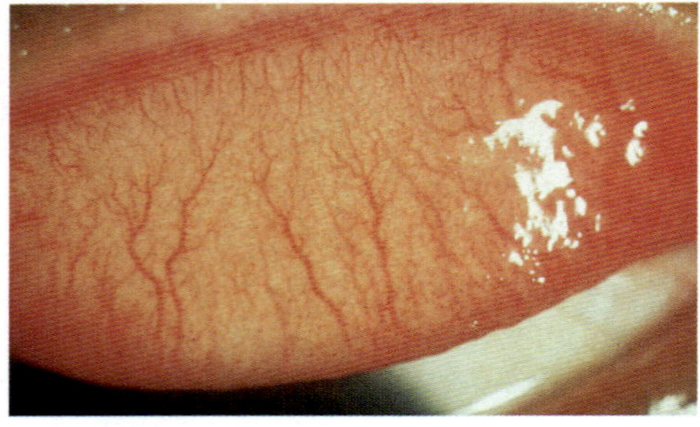

Allergic conjunctivitis

Note the upper lid, conjunctiva and cornea are inflamed from seasonal allergen (e.g. pollen, spores) or persistent allergen (e.g. house dust mite, animal dander). Symptoms include eye itching (not present in nonallergic conditions), redness, watering, discomfort. It does not obscure vision. Signs are diffuse redness of conjunctivae, lid swelling, upper tarsal surface that shows velvety thickening, redness, small papillae (shown above).

TABLE 14.4 Red eye cont'd

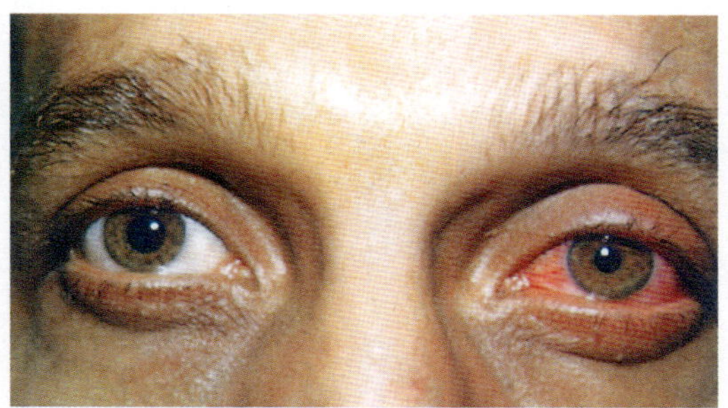

Iritis (circumcorneal redness)

Deep dull red halo around the iris and cornea. Note red is around iris, in contrast with conjunctivitis, in which redness is more prominent at the periphery. Pupil shape may be irregular from inflammation of iris. The person also has marked photophobia, a constricted pupil, blurred vision and throbbing pain. Requires immediate medical intervention.

Seropurulent vesicles due to HSV

Herpes simplex virus

Lid vesicles from primary HSV, associated with fever and preauricular lymphadenopathy. **Herpes zoster ophthalmicus** is a serious presentation of shingles involving the ophthalmic nerve. May have prodrome: numbness and tingling or burning along nerve route, fever, headache, malaise. Signs are acute, painful reddened conjunctivae; an unilateral maculopapular rash with vesicles and ulcers; and ocular signs that threaten vision. Severity increases with older age.

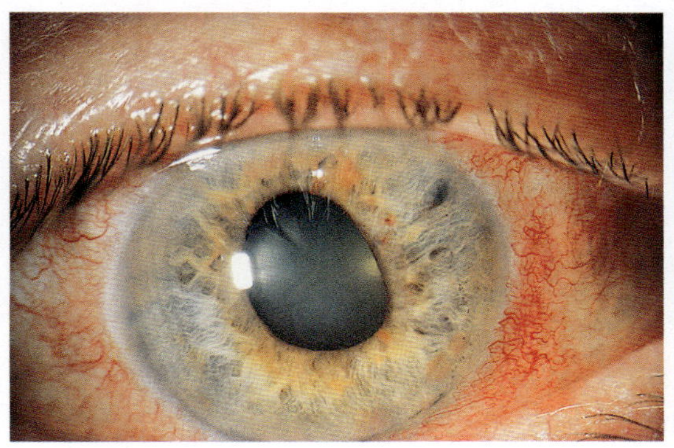

Primary angle-closure glaucoma

Angle-closure glaucoma shows a circumcorneal redness around the iris, with a dilated pupil. Pupil is irregular, dilated; cornea looks 'steamy' due to oedema; and anterior chamber is shallow. Primary angle-closure glaucoma occurs with sudden increase in intraocular pressure from blocked anterior chamber outflow. The person experiences a sudden decrease in vision, sudden eye pain and halos around lights. It is often accompanied by nausea and vomiting. This requires emergency treatment to avoid permanent vision loss.

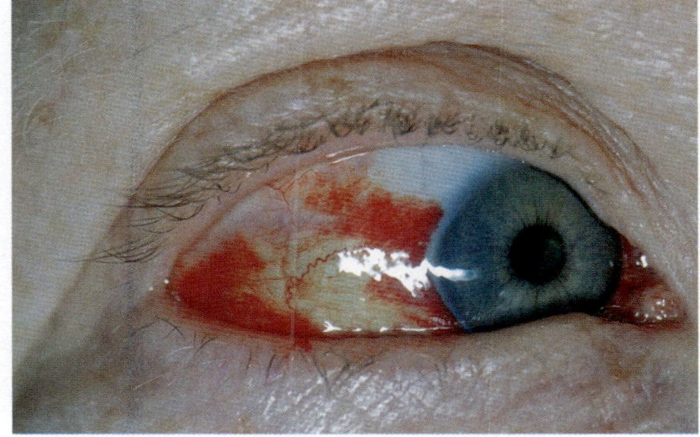

Subconjunctival haemorrhage

A red patch on the sclera, subconjunctival haemorrhage looks alarming but is usually not serious. The red patch has sharp edges like a spot of paint, although here it is extensive. It occurs from increased intraocular pressure from coughing, sneezing, weightlifting, labour during childbirth, straining at stool or trauma. Seen more commonly in people taking anticoagulation medications.

TABLE 14.5 Abnormalities on the cornea, iris and anterior chamber

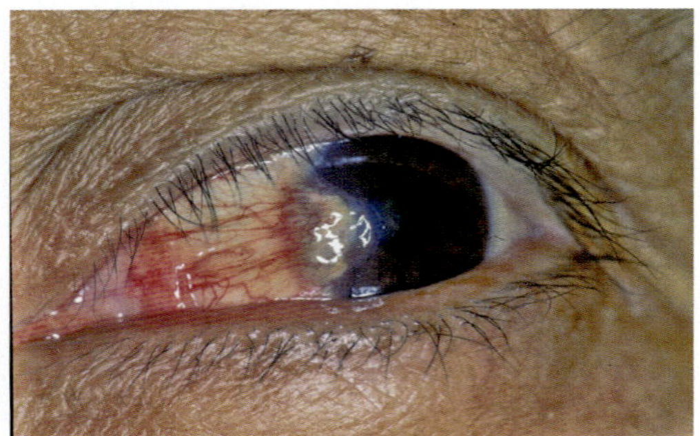

Pterygium

A triangular opaque wing of bulbar conjunctiva overgrows towards the centre of the cornea. It looks membranous, translucent and yellow to white, usually invades from nasal side and it may obstruct vision as it covers pupil. Occurs usually from chronic exposure to UV light. People who live in hot, dry, sunny regions are more likely to develop pterygia.

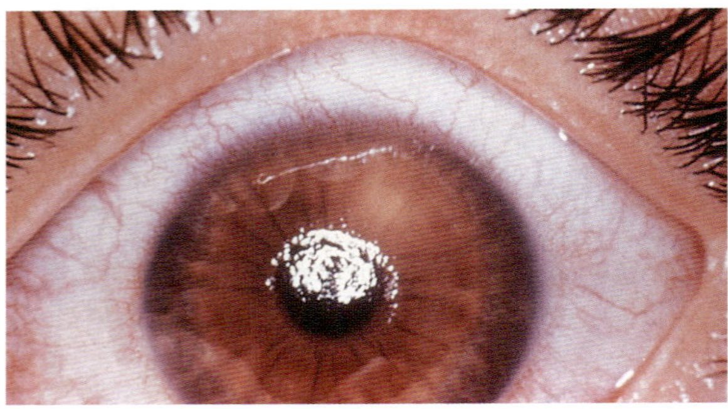

Corneal abrasion

This is the most common result of a blunt eye injury, but irregular ridges are usually visible only when a fluorescein stain reveals a yellow-green abraded area. The top layer of corneal epithelium is damaged from scratches or poorly fitting or overworn contact lenses. Because the area is rich in nerve endings, the person feels intense pain, a foreign body sensation and lacrimation, redness and photophobia.

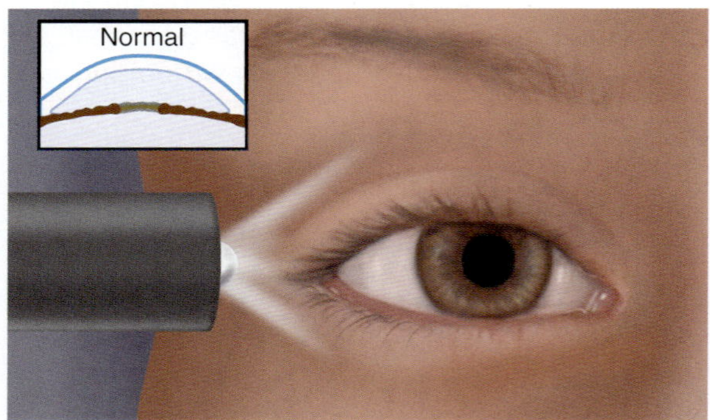

Normal anterior chamber (for contrast)

A light directed across the eye from the temporal side illuminates the entire iris evenly because the normal iris is flat and creates no shadow.

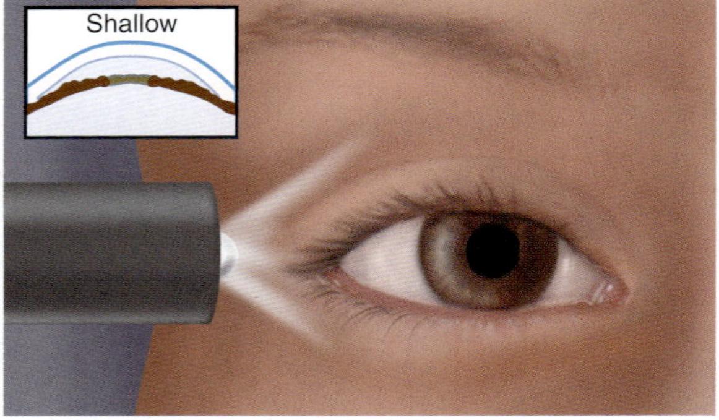

Shallow anterior chamber

The iris is pushed anteriorly because of increased intraocular pressure. Because direct light is received from the temporal side, only the temporal part of the iris is illuminated; the nasal side is shadowed, the 'shadow sign'. This may be a sign of acute angle-closure glaucoma; the iris looks bulging because aqueous humour cannot circulate.

TABLE 14.5 Abnormalities on the cornea, iris and anterior chamber cont'd

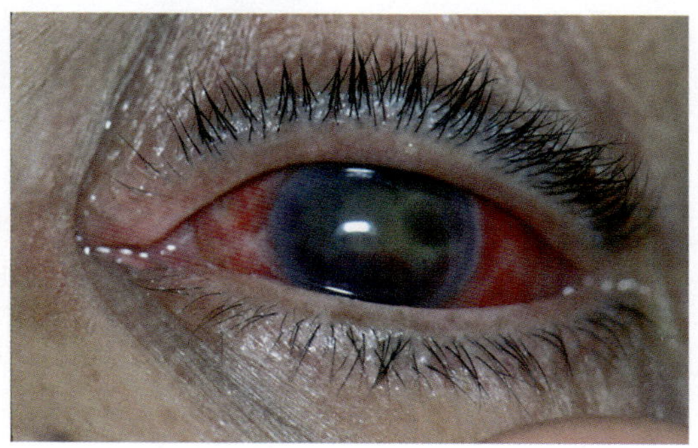

Hyphaema

Blood in anterior chamber is a serious result of blunt trauma (a fist or a tennis ball) or spontaneous haemorrhage. Suspect scleral rupture or major intraocular trauma. Note that gravity settles blood.

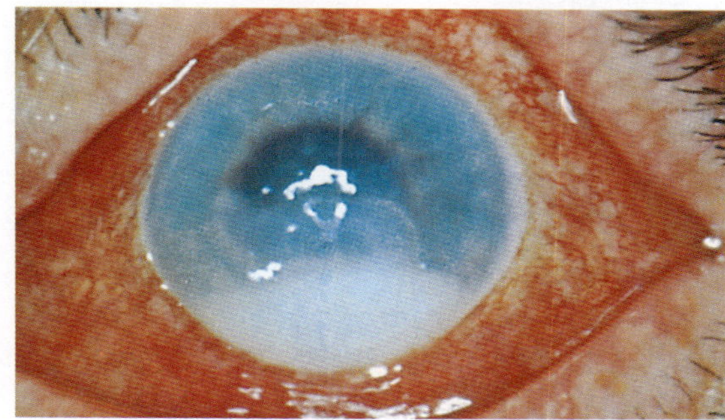

Hypopyon

Purulent matter (white blood cells) in the anterior chamber occurs with intraocular inflammation such as iritis or an intraocular infection.

TABLE 14.6 Abnormalities in the pupil

A Unequal pupil size—anisocoria

Although this exists normally in 5% of the population, it is considered a central nervous system disease.

C Constricted and fixed pupils—miosis

Miosis occurs with the use of pilocarpine drops for glaucoma treatment, the use of narcotics, with iritis and with brain damage of pons.

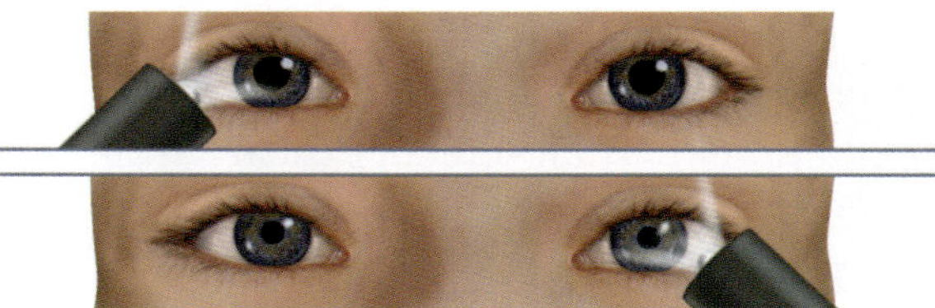

B Monocular blindness

When light is directed to the blind eye, no response occurs in either eye. When light is directed to the normal eye, both pupils constrict (direct and consensual response to light) as long as the oculomotor nerve is intact.

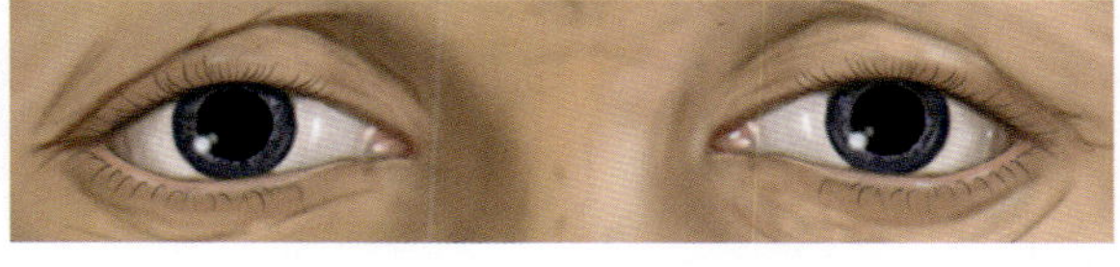

D Dilated and fixed pupils—mydriasis

Enlarged pupils occur with stimulation of the sympathetic nervous system, reaction to sympathomimetic drugs, use of dilating drops, acute glaucoma, past or recent trauma. Also, they herald central nervous system injury, cardiorespiratory arrest or deep anaesthesia.

Continued

TABLE 14.6 Abnormalities in the pupil cont'd

E Argyll Robertson pupil

No reaction to light, pupil does constrict with accommodation. Small and irregular bilaterally. Argyll Robertson pupil occurs with central nervous system syphilis, brain tumour, meningitis and chronic alcoholism.

G Cranial nerve III damage

Unilateral dilated pupil with no reaction to light or accommodation occurs with oculomotor nerve damage. It may also have ptosis with eye deviating down and laterally.

F Tonic pupil (Adie's pupil)

Sluggish reaction to light and accommodation. Tonic pupil is usually unilateral, a large regular pupil that does react but does so sluggishly after a long latent time. No pathological significance.

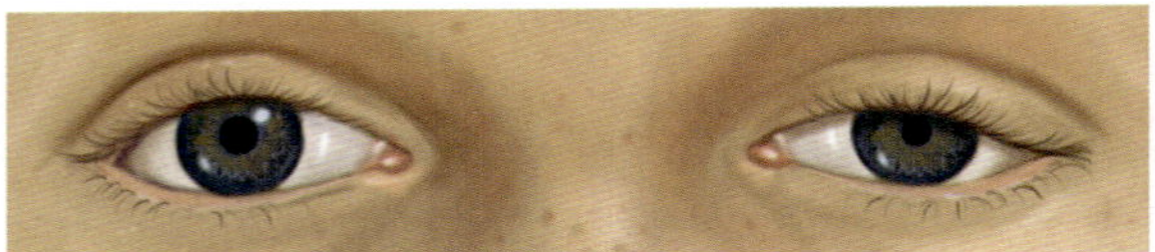

H Horner's syndrome

Unilateral, small, regular pupil does react to light and accommodation. It occurs with Horner's syndrome, a lesion of the sympathetic nerve. Also, note ptosis and the absence of sweat (anhidrosis) on the same side.

Adapted from Friedman et al. 2019[38]

Advanced practice—additional data

The assessments described in the following sections require advanced skill and scope of practice. Nurses working in specialist eye hospitals and clinics and in some community and emergency settings need to develop these skills.

Preparation

The person should be positioned at the distance specified on the eye chart (e.g. 3 m or 6 m). The examination environment should be well lit.

Equipment needed

In addition to the equipment listed previously you will require:

- Snellen eye chart (or other distance vision chart) and pinhole occluder
- handheld visual screener (near vision card)
- applicator stick
- ophthalmoscope
- Amsler grid.

PROCEDURES AND NORMAL FINDINGS	ABNORMAL FINDINGS AND CLINICAL ALERTS

Inspect the extraocular muscle function

Corneal light reflex (the Hirschberg test)

Assess the parallel alignment of the eye axes by shining a light towards the person's eyes. Direct the person to stare straight ahead as you hold the light about 30 cm away. Note the reflection of the light on the corneas; it should be in the same spot on each eye (symmetrical). See the bright white dots in an asymmetrical corneal light reflex in Figure 14.18. Some asymmetry (where one light falls off centre) under 6 months is normal.

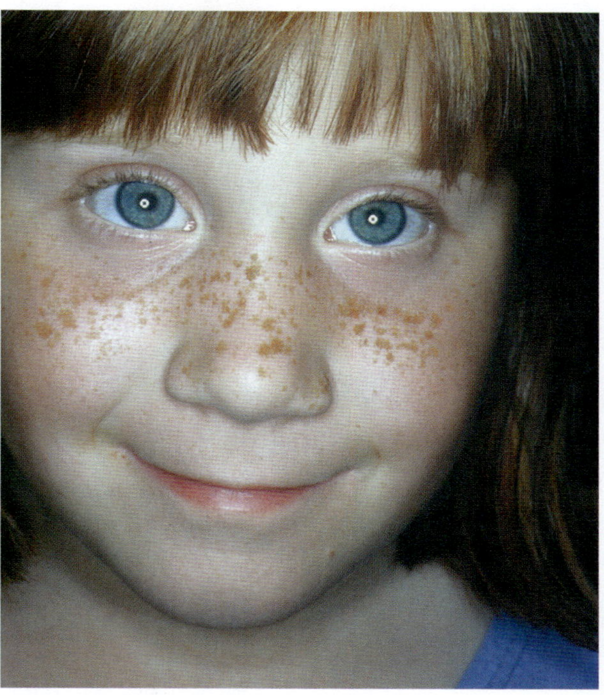

FIGURE 14.18 Corneal light reflex

Asymmetry of the light reflex indicates deviation in alignment from eye muscle weakness or paralysis. If you see this, perform the cover test.

Cover test

This test detects small degrees of deviated alignment by interrupting the **fusion reflex** (fusion refers to the brain's ability to gather information received from each eye and form a single unified image) that normally keeps the two eyes parallel. Ask the person to stare straight ahead at your nose even though the gaze may be interrupted. With an opaque card, cover one eye. As it is covered, note the uncovered eye. A normal response is a steady fixed gaze (Figure 14.19A).

If the eye 'jumps' to fixate on the designated point, it was out of alignment before.

Meanwhile, the macular image has been suppressed on the covered eye. If muscle weakness exists, the covered eye will drift into a relaxed position.

PROCEDURES AND NORMAL FINDINGS

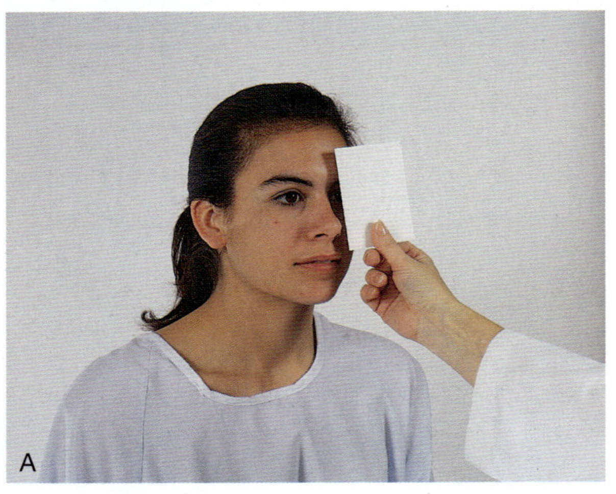

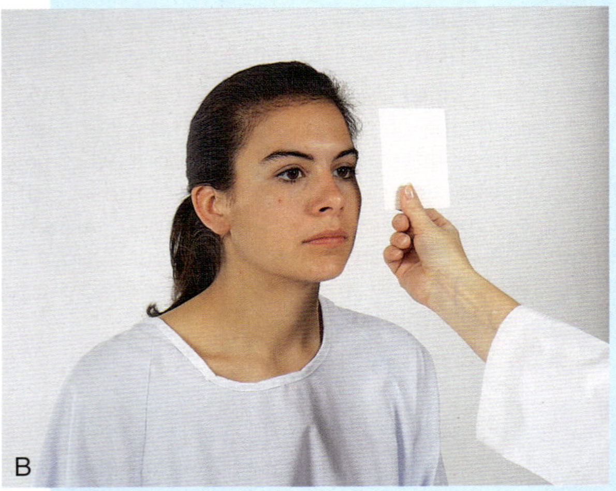

FIGURE 14.19 Cover test

Now uncover the eye and observe it for movement. It should stare straight ahead (Figure 14.19B). If it jumps to re-establish fixation, eye muscle weakness exists. Repeat with the other eye.

Diagnostic positions test

Leading the eyes through the six cardinal positions of gaze will elicit any muscle weakness during movement (Figure 14.20). Ask the person to hold the head steady and to follow the movement of your finger, pen or penlight torch only with the eyes. Hold the target back about 30 cm so the person can focus on it comfortably, and move it to each of the six positions, hold it momentarily, then back to centre. Progress clockwise. A normal response is parallel tracking of the object with both eyes.

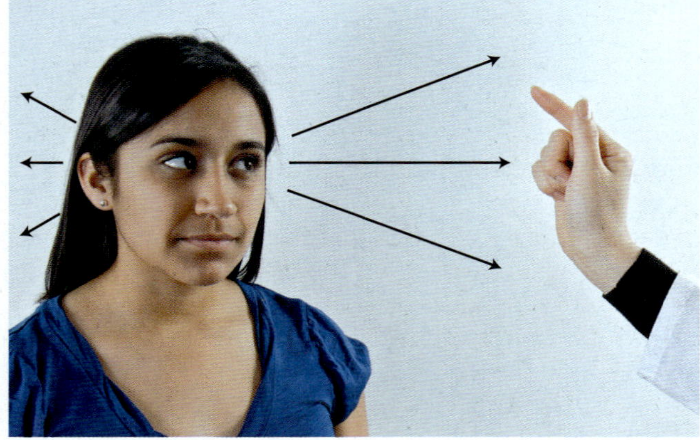

FIGURE 14.20 Diagnostic positions test

ABNORMAL FINDINGS AND CLINICAL ALERTS

A **phoria** is a mild weakness noted only during the cover test. A **tropia** is a constant malalignment of the eyes (Table 14.7C and D).

When eye movement is not parallel there is an abnormality. Failure to follow in a certain direction indicates weakness of an extraocular muscle (EOM) or dysfunction of the cranial nerve innervating it (see cranial nerves for each direction in Table 14.7).

PROCEDURES AND NORMAL FINDINGS	ABNORMAL FINDINGS AND CLINICAL ALERTS
In addition to parallel movement, note any **nystagmus**, a fine oscillating movement best seen around the iris. Mild nystagmus at extreme lateral gaze is normal; nystagmus at any other position is not. Finally, note that the upper eyelid continues to overlap the superior part of the iris, even during downward movement. You should not see a white rim of sclera between the lid and the iris. If noted, this is termed 'lid lag'.	**Nystagmus** is caused by disease of the semicircular canals in the ears, a paralysed eye muscle, multiple sclerosis or brain lesions. **Lid lag** occurs with hyperthyroidism.

Test central—visual acuity

Snellen eye chart

PROCEDURES AND NORMAL FINDINGS	ABNORMAL FINDINGS AND CLINICAL ALERTS
The Snellen alphabet chart is the most used measure of distance visual acuity. It has lines of letters arranged in decreasing size. Place the Snellen alphabet chart in a well-lit spot at eye level. Position the person on a mark exactly 6 m from the chart (or 3 m if you are using a 3 m chart). Hand the person an opaque card with which to shield one eye at a time during the test; inadvertent peeking may result when shielding the eye with the person's own fingers (Figure 14.21). If the person wears glasses or contact lenses, leave them on. Remove glasses worn only for reading because they will blur distance vision. Ask the person to read through the chart to the smallest line of letters possible. Encourage the person to try the next smallest line also. (Note: Use a Snellen picture chart or tumbling 'E' chart for people who cannot read letters.)	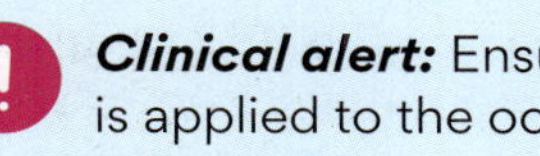 ***Clinical alert:*** Ensure that no pressure is applied to the ocular surface during testing. In a typical acute care ward environment it is unlikely that a Snellen chart would be available to test visual acuity. For advanced practice nurses, use the Snellen chart and note hesitancy, squinting, leaning forwards, misreading letters.

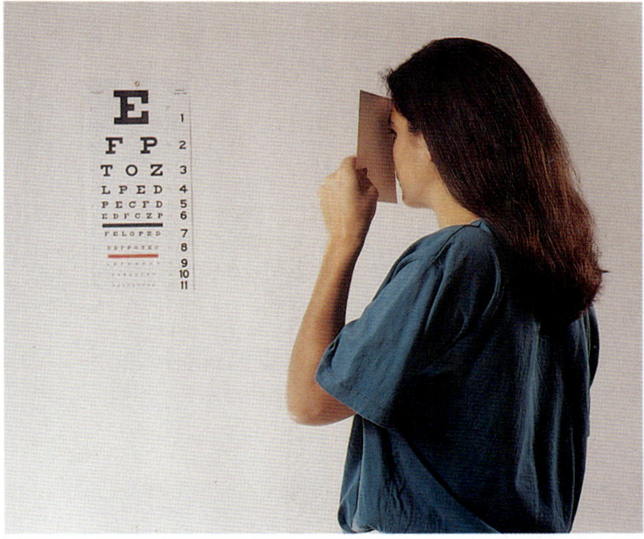

FIGURE 14.21 Distance vision test

PROCEDURES AND NORMAL FINDINGS	ABNORMAL FINDINGS AND CLINICAL ALERTS
Record the result using the numeric fraction at the end of the last successful line read. Indicate whether the person missed any letters or if corrective lenses were worn—for example, 'right 6/12, with glasses' (with the right eye, at the test distance of 6 m the person read to line 12 with their glasses on). If the person is unable to see even the largest letters, shorten the distance to the chart until the top letter is seen and record that distance (e.g. '4/60' at 4 m, line 60 (the top letter) was read). If visual acuity is even lower, assess whether the person can count your fingers (CF), see hand movement (HM) or distinguish light perception (PL) from your penlight. The standard distance for these tests is 30 cm. If the person is unable to perceive light, vision is recorded as 'no perception of light' (NPL).	Visual acuity is a ratio recorded as a fraction. This is not a percentage of vision, but a measurement that is affected by the eye chart that is used (e.g. 6 m or 3 m Snellen chart). The ratio equals test distance/ smallest line that the person can read the majority of the letters.[30]
Normal visual acuity is 6/6 using a 6 m chart and means, 'You can read at 6 m what the normal eye could have read at 6 m'.	Impaired vision may be due to refractive error, opacity in the media (cornea, lens, vitreous) or disorder in the retina or optic pathway. In Australia, a visual acuity of 6/12 or better with both eyes is the legal driving limit. Visual acuity of 6/18 or worse is termed moderate vision impairment.[31]
Pinhole test	
A pinhole test is used when visual acuity is diminished. A pinhole occluder (solid occluder with multiple 19-gauge needle holes) is held over the eye being tested and the solid occluder over the other eye. The test is performed as described above. Results are recorded noting that the pinholes were used to look through, e.g. right eye 6/6 with pinhole.	A test using the pinhole occluder can identify those people with poor vision due to refractive error and in some cases of cataract or corneal scarring. The occluder has very small holes in the area in front of the pupil. People who have visual acuity improved with the pinhole should be referred for examination and treatment by an eye care practitioner as their reduced vision is likely to be due to refractive error and thus could be improved with glasses or contact lenses.
Near vision	
For people over 40 years of age or for those who report increasing difficulty reading, a test of near vision is performed. A handheld vision screener with various sizes of print, with each size attributed a number (e.g. a Jaeger card) is used (Figure 14.22). Hold the card in good light at a comfortable reading distance (about 35 cm from the eye). Test each eye separately, with glasses on. Near visual acuity is recorded in point notation (the same as for computer font), which relates to the smallest line of print the person reads comfortably. A person with normal near vision can read four-point type at 35 cm. The person should be able to read without hesitancy and without moving the card closer or further away.	**Presbyopia**, the decrease in the lens' ability to accommodate with ageing, is suspected when the person moves the card further away to achieve focus. In case you do not have a Jaeger card, normal newspaper print is 8-point type (N8).

PROCEDURES AND NORMAL FINDINGS	ABNORMAL FINDINGS AND CLINICAL ALERTS

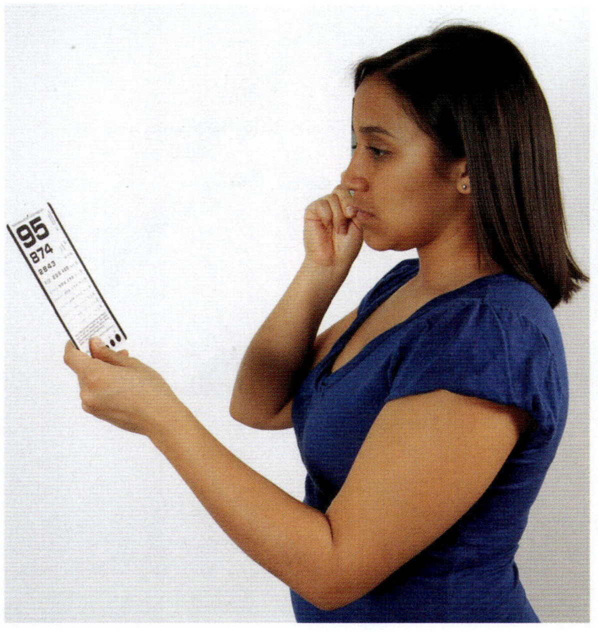

FIGURE 14.22 Near vision test

Inspect the external ocular structures

Eversion of the upper lid

This manoeuvre is not part of the normal examination, but it is useful when you need to inspect the conjunctiva of the upper lid, as with eye pain or suspicion of a foreign body. Most people are apprehensive of any eye manipulation. Enhance their cooperation by using a calm and gentle, yet deliberate, approach.

1. Ask the person to keep both eyes open and look down. This relaxes the eyelid, whereas closing it would tense the orbicularis muscle.
2. Slide the upper lid up along the bony orbit to lift up the eyelashes.
3. Grasp the lashes between your thumb and forefinger and gently pull down and outwards.
4. With your other hand, place the tip of an applicator stick on the upper lid above the level of the internal tarsal plates (Figure 14.23A).

Clinical alert: Eyelid eversion should not be attempted if a penetrating eye injury is suspected.

PROCEDURES AND NORMAL FINDINGS

ABNORMAL FINDINGS AND CLINICAL ALERTS

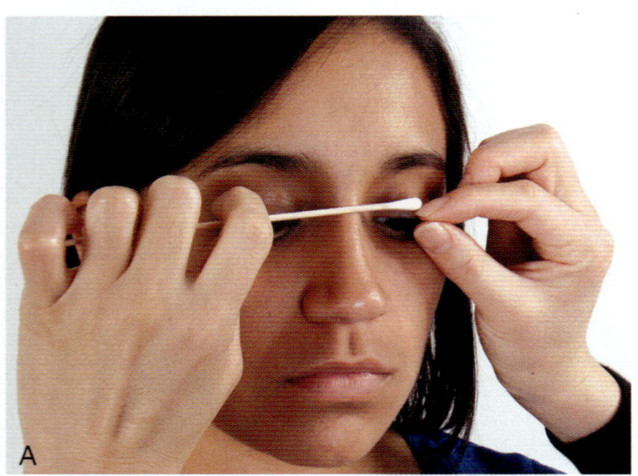

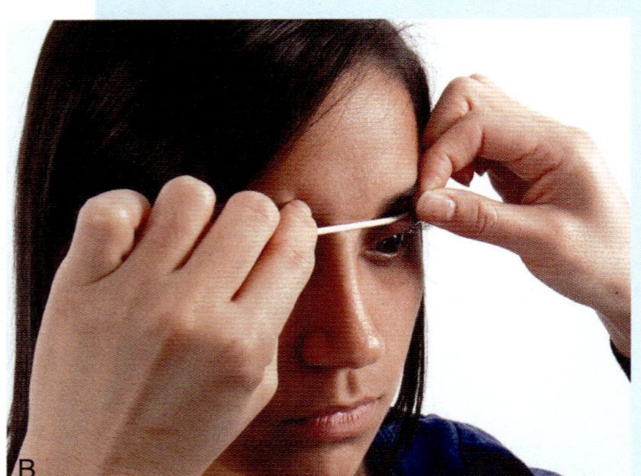

FIGURE 14.23 Eyelid eversion

5. Gently push down with the stick as you lift the lashes up. This uses the edge of the tarsal plate as a fulcrum and flips the lid inside out. Take special care not to push in on the eyeball.
6. Secure the everted position by holding the lashes against the bony orbital rim (Figure 14.23B).
7. Inspect for any colour change, swelling, lesion or foreign body.
8. To return to normal position, gently pull the lashes outwards as the person looks up.

Lacrimal apparatus

Ask the person to look down. With your thumbs, slide the outer part of the upper lid up along the bony orbit to expose under the lid. Inspect for any redness or swelling.

Swelling of the lacrimal gland may show as a visible bulge in the outer part of the upper lid.

Normally, the puncta drain the tears into the lacrimal sac. Presence of excessive tearing may indicate blockage of the nasolacrimal duct. Check this by pressing the index finger against the sac, just inside the lower orbital rim, not against the side of the nose (Figure 14.24). Pressure will slightly evert the lower lid, but there should be no other response to pressure.

Note if puncta are red, swollen or tender to pressure. This may be associated with **dacryocystitis** (infection of the lacrimal sac) (Table 14.3).

Watch for any regurgitation of fluid out of the puncta, which confirms duct blockage.

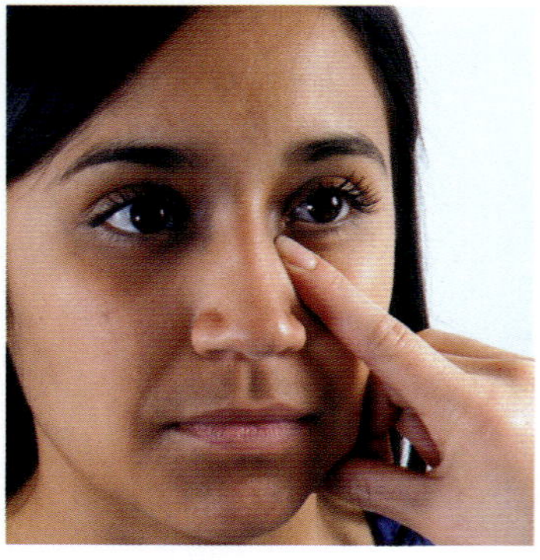

FIGURE 14.24 Punctal inspection

PROCEDURES AND NORMAL FINDINGS	ABNORMAL FINDINGS AND CLINICAL ALERTS
Inspect the anterior eyeball structures	
Test pupillary response to **accommodation** by asking the person to focus on a distant object (Figure 14.25). This process dilates the pupils. Then have the person shift the gaze to a near object, such as your finger held about 7 to 8 cm from the nose. A normal response includes (1) pupillary constriction and (2) convergence of the axes of the eyes.	Note any absence of constriction or convergence or an asymmetric response.

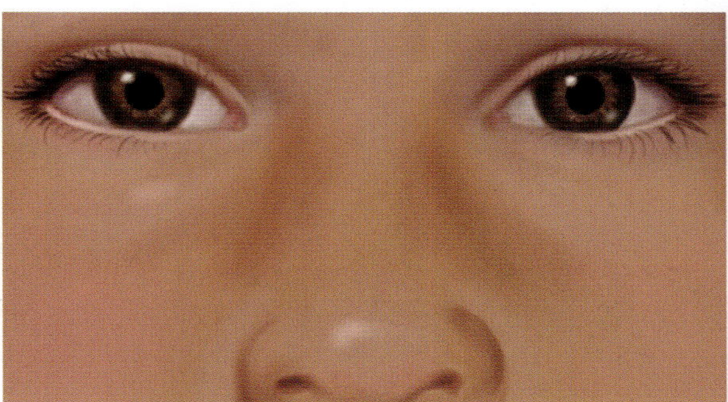

Far vision—pupils dilate

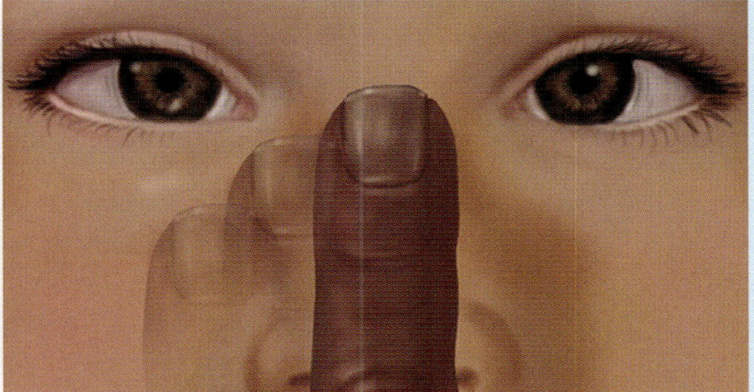

Near vision—pupils constrict

FIGURE 14.25 Pupillary response to accommodation

PROCEDURES AND NORMAL FINDINGS	ABNORMAL FINDINGS AND CLINICAL ALERTS
Test for relative afferent papillary defect (RAPD) by performing the 'swinging torch test'. Dim or turn off room lights and use the brightest light available. Ask the person to focus in the distance. First observe the **pupillary light reflex** (as described earlier), noting *direct* and *consensual* constriction of the pupil in response to the light. Next, move the light briskly from one eye to the other. A normal response is for each pupil to **constrict** when the torch is shone on it. A relative pupillary defect (abnormal response) is when the torch is swung from one eye to the other and the pupil of the illuminated eye **dilates** (becomes larger) instead of constricting as is normal.[32]	 ***Clinical alert:*** The presence of a relative afferent pupil defect alerts you that the person has seriously reduced visual acuity.[32]
Inspect the ocular fundus	
The ophthalmoscope enlarges your view of the eye so you can inspect the **media** (anterior chamber, lens, vitreous) and the **ocular fundus** (the internal surface of the retina). It accomplishes this by directing a beam of light through the pupil to illuminate the inner structures.	

PROCEDURES AND NORMAL FINDINGS

The ophthalmoscope should function as an appendage of your own eye. This takes some practice. Practice holding the instrument and focusing on objects around the room before you approach the person.

Hold the ophthalmoscope right up to your eye, braced firmly against the cheek and brow. Extend your index finger onto the lens selector dial so you can refocus as needed during the procedure without taking your head away from the ophthalmoscope to look. Now look about the room, moving your head and the instrument together as one unit. Keep both your eyes open; just view the field through the ophthalmoscope.

The ophthalmoscope contains a set of lenses that control the focus (Figure 14.26). The unit of strength of each lens is the **diopter**. The black numbers indicate a positive diopter; they focus on objects nearer in space to the ophthalmoscope. The red numbers show a negative diopter and are for focusing on objects further away.

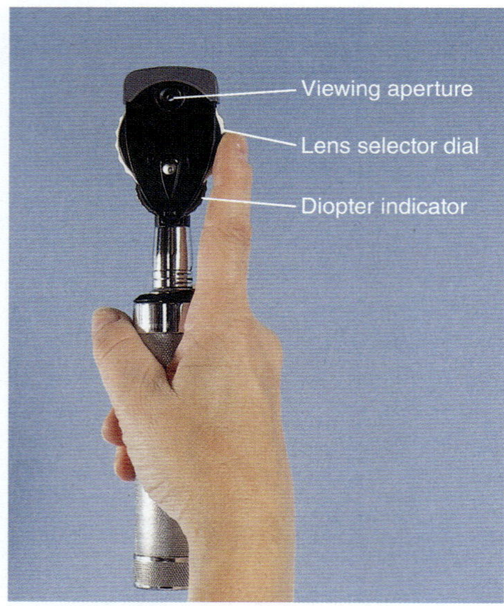

FIGURE 14.26 Ophthalmoscope

To examine a person, darken the room to help dilate the pupils. Remove eyeglasses from yourself or the other person; they obstruct close movement, and you can compensate for their correction by using the diopter setting. Contact lenses may be left in; they pose no problem if they are clean.

ABNORMAL FINDINGS AND CLINICAL ALERTS

PROCEDURES AND NORMAL FINDINGS	ABNORMAL FINDINGS AND CLINICAL ALERTS
Dilating eye drops are not needed during a screening examination. When indicated, they dilate the pupils for a wider look at the fundus background and macular area. Eye drops are used only when history of angle closure glaucoma can be completely ruled out, because dilating the pupils in the presence of glaucoma can precipitate an acute episode. Care should also be taken when dilating the pupils of persons with high degrees of long-sightedness, as they are also predisposed to angle closure.	
Select the large round aperture with the white light for the routine examination. If the pupils are small, use the smaller white light. The light must have maximum brightness; replace old or dim batteries.	Although the instrument has other shaped and coloured apertures, these are rarely used in a screening examination.
Tell the person: '*Please keep looking at that light switch (or mark) on the wall across the room, even though my head will get in the way.*'	Staring at a distant fixed object helps to dilate the pupils and to hold the retinal structures still.
Match sides with the person. That is, hold the ophthalmoscope in your *right* hand up to your *right* eye to view the person's *right* eye. You must do this to avoid bumping noses during the procedure. Place your free hand on the person's shoulder or forehead (Figure 14.27A). This helps orient you in space, because once you have the ophthalmoscope in position, you have only a very narrow range of vision. Also, your thumb can anchor the upper lid and help prevent blinking.	

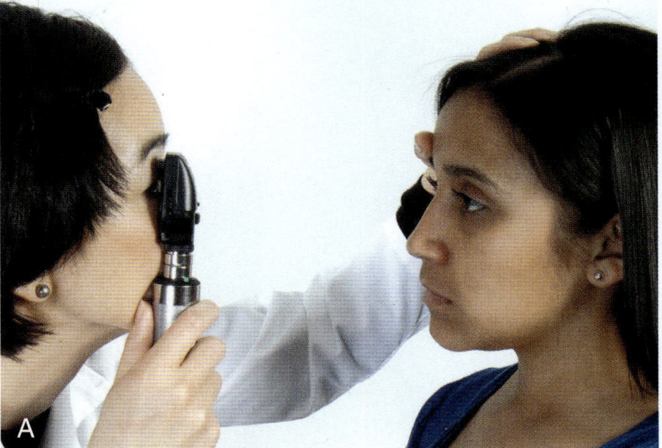

FIGURE 14.27A Examination using an ophthalmoscope

PROCEDURES AND NORMAL FINDINGS	ABNORMAL FINDINGS AND CLINICAL ALERTS
Begin about 25 cm away from the person at an angle about 15 degrees lateral to the person's line of vision. Note the red glow filling the person's pupil. This is the red reflex, caused by the reflection of your ophthalmoscope light off the inner retina. Keep sight of the red reflex and steadily move closer to the eye. If you lose the red reflex, the light has wandered off the pupil and onto the iris or sclera. Adjust your angle to find it again.	
As you advance, adjust the lens to +6 and note any opacity in the media. These appear as dark shadows or black dots interrupting the red reflex. Normally, none are present.	Cataracts appear as opaque black areas against the red reflex (Table 14.8).
Progress towards the person until your foreheads almost touch (Figure 14.27B). Adjust the diopter setting to bring the ocular fundus into sharp focus. If you and the person have normal vision, this should be at 0. Moving the diopters compensates for nearsightedness or farsightedness. Use the red lenses for nearsighted eyes and the black for farsighted eyes (Figure 14.28).	

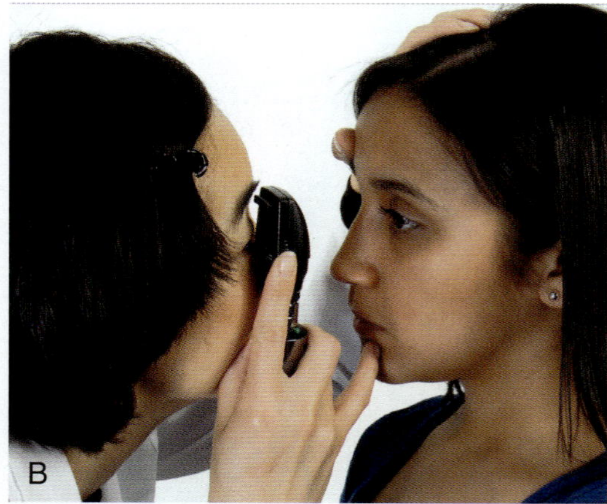

FIGURE 14.27B Examination using an ophthalmoscope

PROCEDURES AND NORMAL FINDINGS	ABNORMAL FINDINGS AND CLINICAL ALERTS

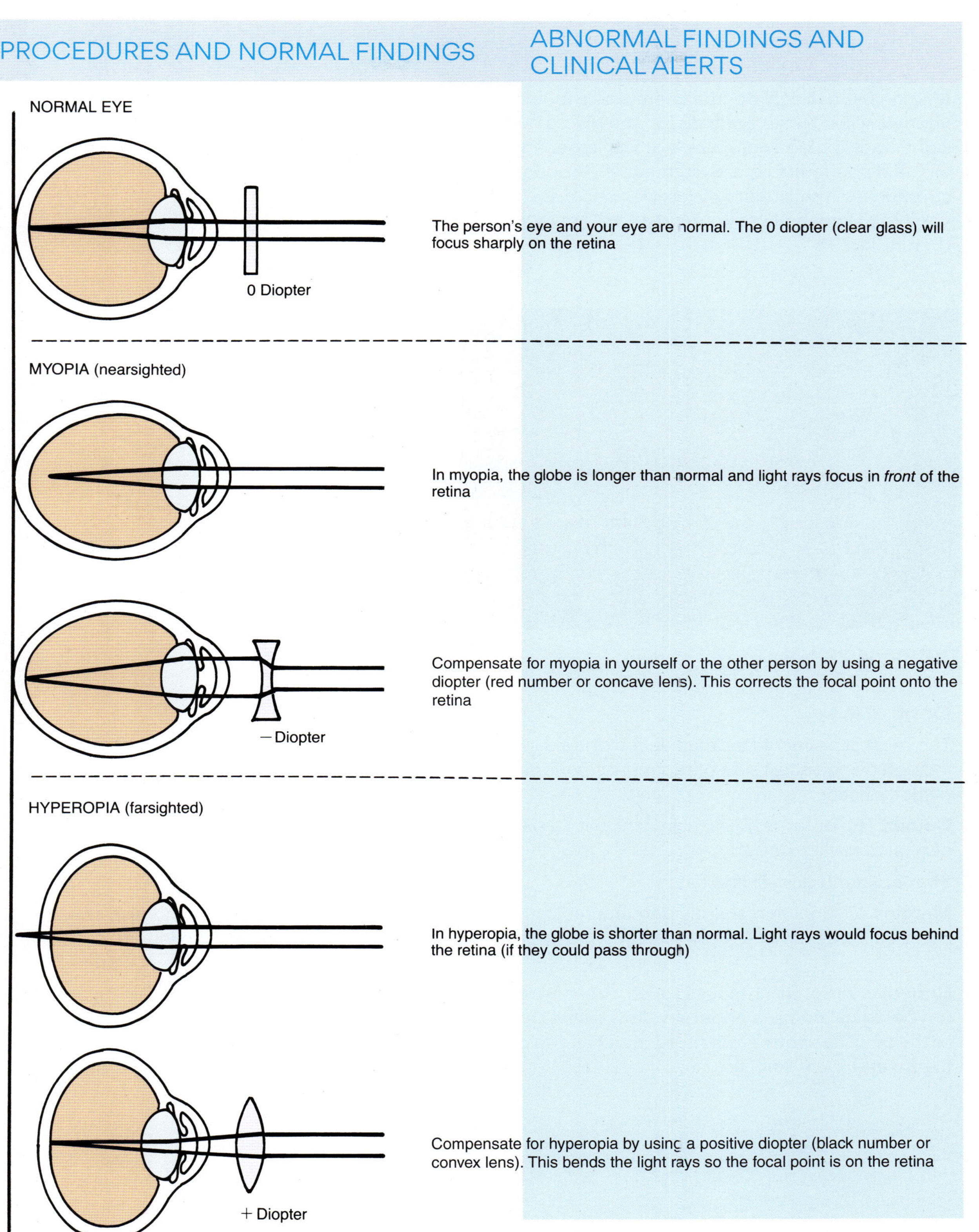

FIGURE 14.28 Using lenses in the ophthalmoscope

PROCEDURES AND NORMAL FINDINGS

Moving in on the 15-degree lateral line should bring your view just to the optic disc. If the disc is not in sight, track a blood vessel as it grows larger and it will lead you to the disc. Systematically inspect the structures in the ocular fundus: (1) optic disc, (2) retinal vessels, (3) general background and (4) macula (Figure 14.29).

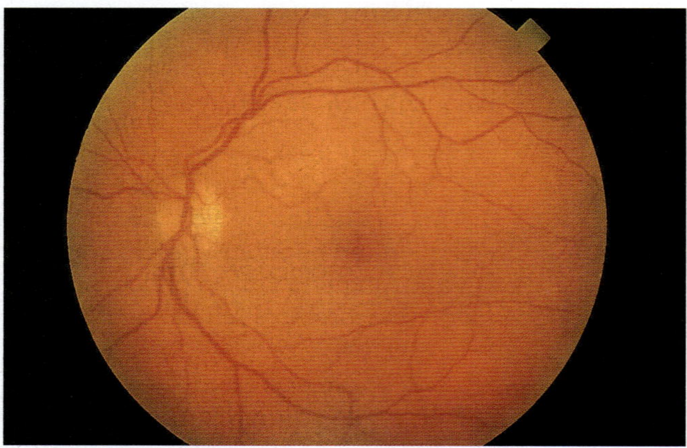

FIGURE 14.29 Normal ocular fundus

Optic disc

The most prominent landmark is the optic disc, located on the nasal side of the retina. Explore these characteristics:

Colour. The outer 'rim' is usually pink with a paler central excavated 'cup'.

Shape. Round or oval and flat.

Margins. Distinct and sharply demarcated, although the nasal edge may be slightly fuzzy.

Cup–disc ratio. Distinctness varies. When visible, physiological cup is a brighter yellow-white than rest of the disc. Its width is not more than half the disc diameter (Figure 14.30).

ABNORMAL FINDINGS AND CLINICAL ALERTS

Note the illustration here shows a large area of the fundus. Your actual view through the ophthalmoscope is much smaller—slightly larger than 1 disc diameter.

Note pallor or **hyperaemia** (excess of blood flow to the area).

Note irregular shape.

Look for blurred margins and disc swelling (**papillo-oedema**). Swollen optic discs may indicate high intracranial pressure.

Discs are abnormally 'cupped' in glaucoma (have an enlarged and deepened central cup or high cup–disc ratio). In such cases the cup can extend to the disc border (Table 14.9).

PROCEDURES AND NORMAL FINDINGS

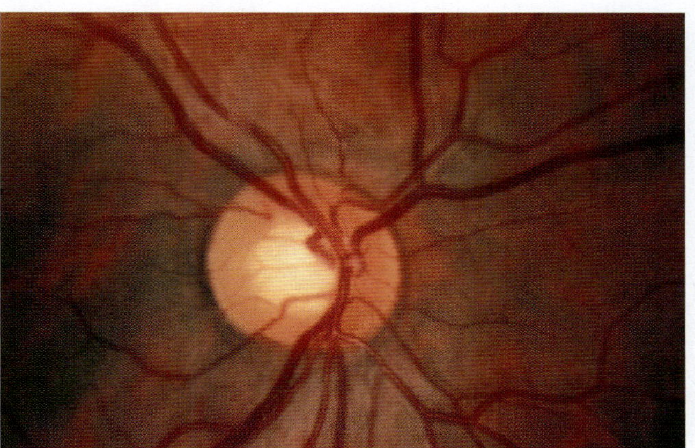

FIGURE 14.30 Normal optic disc

Two normal variations may occur around the disc margins. A **scleral crescent** is a grey-white new moon shape (Figure 14.31). It occurs when pigment is absent in the choroid layer and you are looking directly at the sclera. A **pigment crescent** is black; it is due to accumulation of pigment in the choroid.

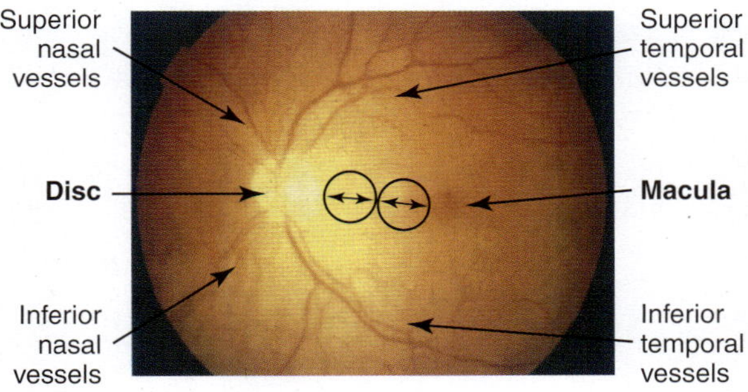

FIGURE 14.31 Scleral crescent

The diameter of the disc, or DD, is a standard of measure for other fundus structures. To describe a finding, note its clock-face position as well as its relationship to the disc in size and distance (e.g. the macula is at 3:00, 2 DD from the disc).

ABNORMAL FINDINGS AND CLINICAL ALERTS

PROCEDURES AND NORMAL FINDINGS	ABNORMAL FINDINGS AND CLINICAL ALERTS
Retinal vessels	
This is the only place in the body where you can view blood vessels directly. Many systemic diseases that affect the vascular system show signs in the retinal vessels. Follow a paired artery and vein out to the periphery in the four quadrants (Figure 14.31). 1. Number: a paired artery and vein pass to each quadrant 2. Colour: arteries are brighter red than veins. They also have the arterial light reflex (a thin stripe of light down the middle) 3. A:V ratio: the ratio of artery and vein width (should be 2:3 or 4:5) 4. Calibre: vessels show a regular decrease in calibre as they extend to the periphery 5. Tortuosity: mild tortuosity in both eyes is normal 6. Pulsations: mild vein pulsation adjacent to the disc is normal (can be difficult to see)	Abnormal findings include: • absence of major vessels • arteries constricted or veins dilated • proliferation of new vessels termed neovascularisation • extreme tortuosity or marked asymmetry between eyes • absent pulsations.
General background of the fundus	
The colour normally varies from light red to dark brown-red, generally corresponding with the person's skin colour. Your view of the fundus should be clear; no lesions should obstruct the retinal structures.	Abnormal lesions: haemorrhages, exudates, microaneurysms. These are often associated with diabetic retinopathy (Table 14.10).
Macula	
The macula is 1 DD in size and located 2 DD temporal to the disc. Inspect this area last in the fundoscopic examination. A bright light on this area of central vision causes some watering and discomfort and pupillary constriction. Note that the normal colour of the area is somewhat darker than the rest of the fundus but is even and homogeneous. Clumped pigment may occur with ageing.	Clumped pigment occurs with trauma or retinal detachment.
Within the macula, you may note the foveal light reflex. This is a tiny white glistening dot reflecting your ophthalmoscope light.	Haemorrhage or exudate in the macula occurs with age-related macular degeneration (Tables 14.9 and 14.10).
Additional objective data for infants and children (birth to 12 years)	
Visual field	
Assess peripheral vision with the confrontation test in children older than 3 years when the child can stay in position. As with the adult, the child should see the moving target at the same time as your normal eyes do. It's useful to use a small toy as the target to make the test a game. Often a young child forgets to say 'now' or 'stop' as the moving object is seen. Rather, note the instant the child's eyes deviate or head shifts position to gaze at the moving object. Match this nearly automatic response with your own sighting.	Visual field testing in children is usually only performed by advanced practice nurses.

PROCEDURES AND NORMAL FINDINGS

External muscle function

Testing for **strabismus** (squint or turned eye) is an important screening measure during early childhood. Strabismus causes disconjugate vision because one eye deviates off the fixation point. To avoid diplopia (double vision) or unclear images, the brain begins to suppress data from the weak eye (a suppression scotoma). Then visual acuity in this otherwise normal eye begins to deteriorate from disuse. Early recognition and treatment are essential to restore binocular vision. Diagnosis after 6 years of age has a poor prognosis. Test malalignment by the corneal light reflex and the cover test.

Corneal light reflex (Hirschberg test)

Check the **corneal light reflex** by shining a light towards the child's eyes. The light should be reflected at the same spot in the two corneas (Figure 14.18). Some asymmetry (where one light falls off centre) under 6 months of age is normal.

Cover test

Perform the **cover test** on all children as described for adults. Some examiners omit the opaque card and place a hand on the child's head. The examiner's thumb extends down and blocks vision over the eye without touching the eye. You can use a familiar character puppet to attract the child's attention. The normal results are the same as those listed in the adult section.

Diagnostic positions test

A brightly coloured toy can be used as a target to assess function of the extraocular muscles during the early weeks. An older infant can sit on the parent's lap as you move the toy in all directions. After 2 years of age, direct the child's attention through the six cardinal positions of gaze as described for adults earlier (Figure 14.20). You may stabilise the child's chin with your hand to prevent them from moving the entire head.

ABNORMAL FINDINGS AND CLINICAL ALERTS

Untreated strabismus can lead to permanent visual damage and can impact on a child's general development and learning. The resulting loss of vision from disuse is termed **amblyopia** and is commonly referred to as 'lazy eye'.

Strabismus (turned eye) affects 0.14–5.65% of children.[33]

Amblyopia (poor or indistinct vision in an eye that is otherwise physically normal) affects approximately 1.9% of children.[34]

Clinical alert: Asymmetry in the corneal light reflex after 6 months is abnormal and must be referred.

If asymmetry is seen perform the cover test.

PROCEDURES AND NORMAL FINDINGS	ABNORMAL FINDINGS AND CLINICAL ALERTS
Visual acuity	
The child's age determines the method used to assess visual acuity. Until children reach school age, naming letters on visual acuity charts such as the Snellen chart is usually not possible (Figure 14.21). By the age of 4, most children can complete a recognition acuity task, which involves either naming or matching letters or pictures of standard sizes. Testing may include: • picture charts • letter charts • nonsense symbol recognitions. In Australia and Aotearoa New Zealand, the Sheridan-Gardiner test is widely used for testing visual acuity in children who cannot yet read or those who are illiterate.[35] This test is conducted by providing the child with a seven-letter card and the examiner with a set of single-letter cards corresponding in size to Snellen letters. The child is then asked to point on their card to the letter shown to them by the examiner. For children above 3 years of age, the examiner may use cards containing lines of letters.	At-risk groups for further eye problems include those born prematurely, those with multiple disabilities and children in remote Aboriginal and Torres Strait Islander communities. For children in remote communities, education and health assessment needs to be tailored towards detection of uncorrected refractive error and prevention of trachoma.[26]
Colour vision	
Colour blindness (red, green) is an inherited recessive X-linked trait affecting about 8% of males and 0.4% of females. Only 5% of people who are colour blind have blue colour blindness—for these people this is not inherited but a change in the chromosome during development. In assessment, this may be identified when children are not able to recognise different colours and separate items by colour.	'Colour deficient' is a more accurate term because the condition is relative and not disabling. Often, it is just a social inconvenience, although it may affect the person's ability to discern traffic lights, or it may affect school performance when colour is a learning tool. Abnormal colour vision may also affect employment later in life.
The ocular fundus	
The amount of data gathered during the fundoscopic examination depends on the child's ability to hold the eyes still and on your ability to glean as much data as possible in a brief period.	

PROCEDURES AND NORMAL FINDINGS

A complete fundoscopic examination is difficult to perform on an infant. Position the infant (up to 18 months) lying on the table. The fundus appears pale, and the vessels are not fully developed. There may be no foveal light reflection because the macula area will not be mature until 1 year.

Inspect the fundus of the young child and school age child as described in the preceding section on the adult. Allow the child to handle the equipment. Explain why you are darkening the room and that you will leave a small light on. Assure the child that the procedure will not hurt. Direct the young child to look at an appealing picture, perhaps a toy or an animal, during the examination.

ABNORMAL FINDINGS AND CLINICAL ALERTS

An interruption in or abnormal red reflex indicates opacity in the cornea, lens or ocular media. This may be due to congenital cataract, retinal disorder or a serious intraocular tumour (retinoblastoma).

! ***Clinical alert:*** Any child with an abnormal red reflex should be referred urgently.

Papillo-oedema (swollen optic discs) is rare in the infant because the fontanels and open sutures will absorb any increased intracranial pressure if it occurs.

Additional objective data for adults over 65 years

Visual acuity

Perform the same examination as described in the adult section. Central acuity may decrease, particularly after 70 years of age. Peripheral vision may be diminished.

Central visual field

To assess the central visual field an **Amsler grid** test is used. This is a small sheet of paper with a grid of black lines on it (Figure 14.32). To use the grid, ask the person to cover one eye at a time, with glasses on if usually worn. Holding the grid about 30 cm away, ask them to focus on the central dot and ask if the lines look clear and straight.[36]

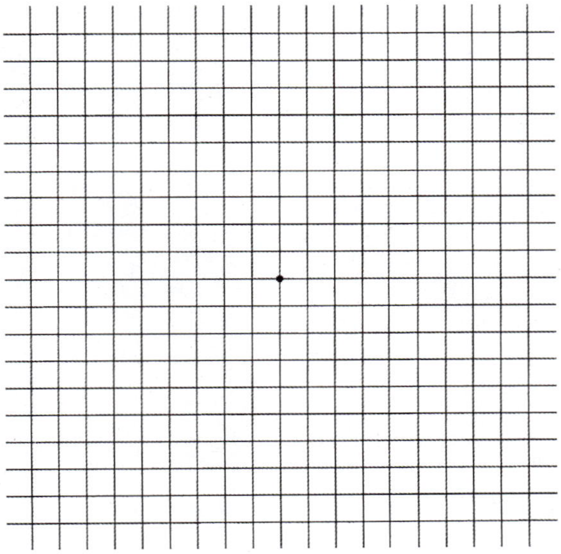

Amsler grid testing is used to assess the central visual field. People with macular disease, for example age-related macular degeneration, will often report the lines on the grid look distorted, curved or missing. These people may also report that straight lines, such as the edges of doors or windows, look wavy (metamorphopsia).

FIGURE 14.32 Amsler grid

PROCEDURES AND NORMAL FINDINGS	ABNORMAL FINDINGS AND CLINICAL ALERTS
The ocular fundus	
Retinal structures generally have less shine. The blood vessels look paler, narrower and attenuated. Arterioles appear paler and straighter, with a narrower light reflex.	
A normal development on the retinal surface is **drusen** or benign degenerative hyaline deposits (Figure 14.33). They are small, round, yellow dots that are scattered haphazardly on the retina. Although they do not occur in a pattern, they are usually symmetrically placed in the two eyes. They have no effect on vision.	**Drusen** are easily confused with the abnormal finding *hard exudates*, which occur with a more circular or linear pattern. The presence of hard exudates indicates chronic vascular leakage, such as in diabetic retinopathy or hypertensive retinopathy, Drusen are usually seen in the macular area and are commonly seen with age-related macular degeneration.
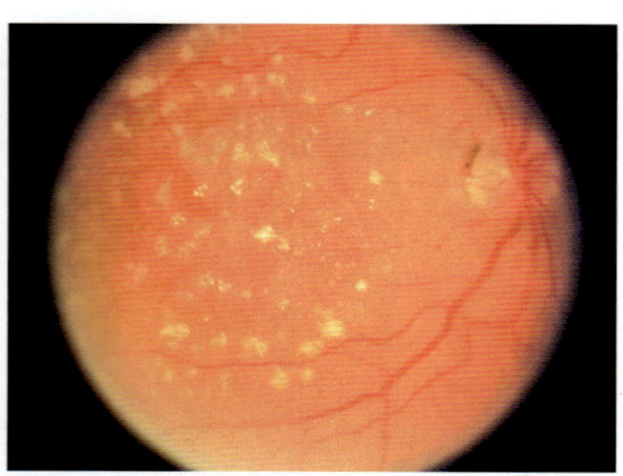 **FIGURE 14.33** Drusen	

Abnormal findings for advanced practice

TABLE 14.7 Extraocular muscle dysfunction

Asymmetrical corneal light reflex

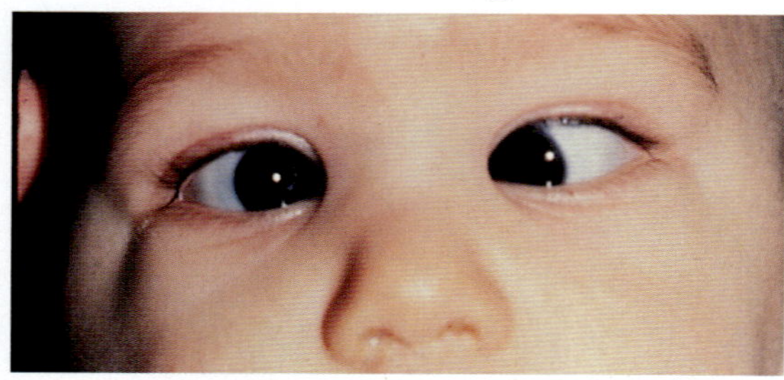

A Esotropia—inward turn of the eye. **Strabismus** is a true disparity of the eye axes. This constant malalignment is also termed *tropia* and is likely to cause amblyopia.

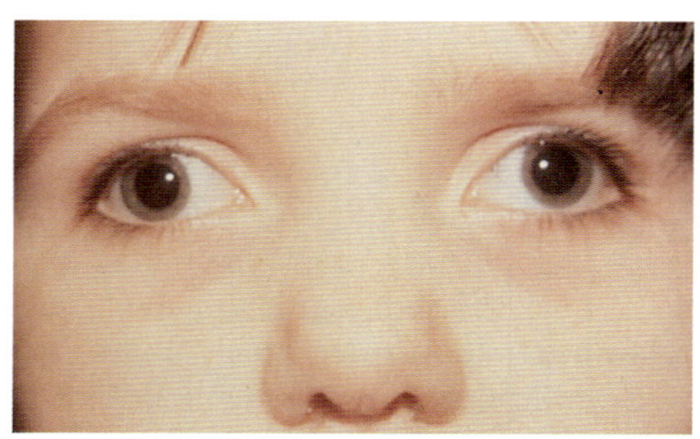

B Exotropia—outward turning of the eyes.

TABLE 14.7 Extraocular muscle dysfunction cont'd

Cover test

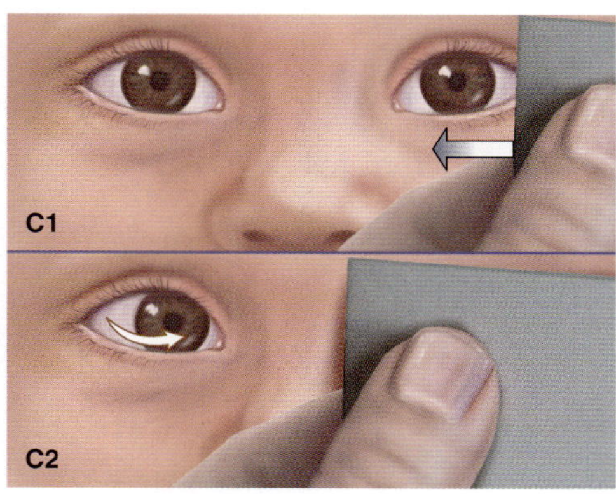

C Right, or uncovered eye, is weaker
Uncovered eye—if it jumps to fixate on designated point, it was out of alignment before (i.e. when you cover the stronger eye (C1), the weaker eye now tries to fixate (C2)).

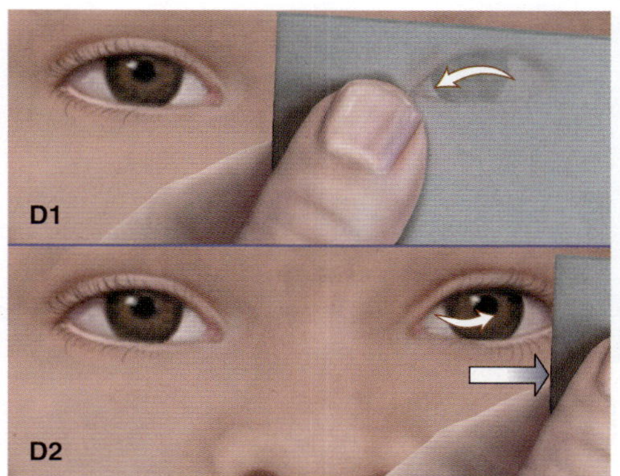

D Left, or uncovered eye, is weaker
Covered eye—if this is the weaker eye, once macular image is suppressed it will drift to relaxed position (D1).
As eye is uncovered—if it jumps to reestablish fixation (D2), weakness exists.
Phoria—mild weakness, apparent only with the cover test and less likely to cause amblyopia than a tropia but still possible.
Esophoria—nasal (inward) drift.
Exophoria—temporal (outward) drift.

Diagnostic positions test

Paralysis apparent during movement through six cardinal positions of gaze.

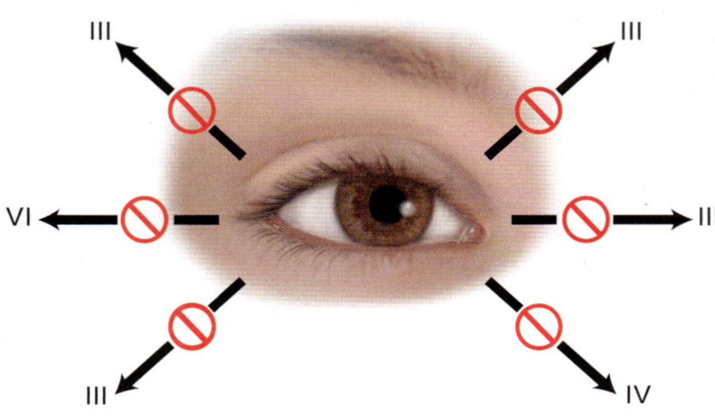

If eye will not turn:	Indicates paralysis in:	or cranial nerve:
Straight nasal	Medial rectus	III
Up and nasal	Inferior oblique	III
Up and temporal	Superior rectus	III
Straight temporal	Lateral rectus	VI
Down and temporal	Inferior rectus	III
Down and nasal	Superior oblique	IV

Source: McIntire et al. 2021[37]

TABLE 14.8 Lens opacities

Acquired cataract

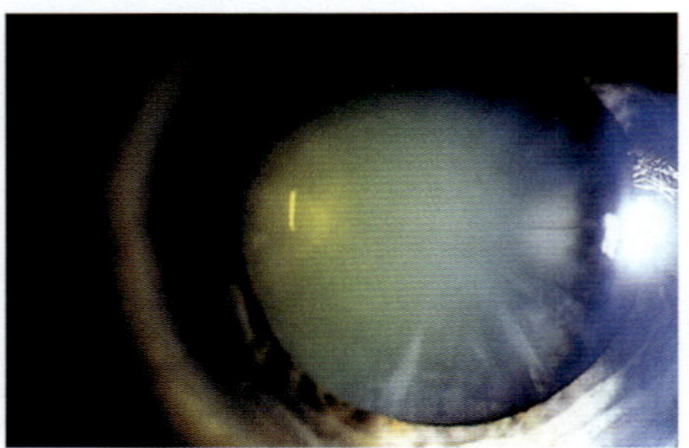

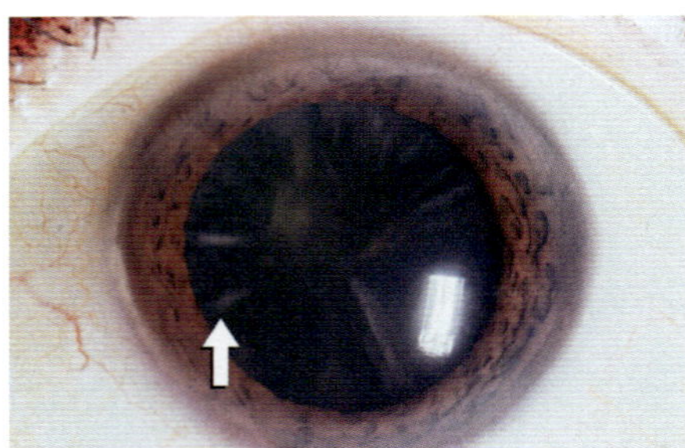

Central grey opacity—nuclear cataract

Nuclear cataract shows as an opaque grey surrounded by black background as it forms in the centre of lens nucleus. Through the ophthalmoscope, it looks like a black centre against the red reflex. It begins after age 40 years and develops slowly, gradually obstructing vision.

Star-shaped opacity—cortical cataract

Cortical cataract shows as asymmetrical, radial, white spokes with black centre. Through the ophthalmoscope, black spokes are evident against the red reflex. This forms in outer cortex of lens, progressing faster than nuclear cataract.

TABLE 14.9 Optic disc abnormalities

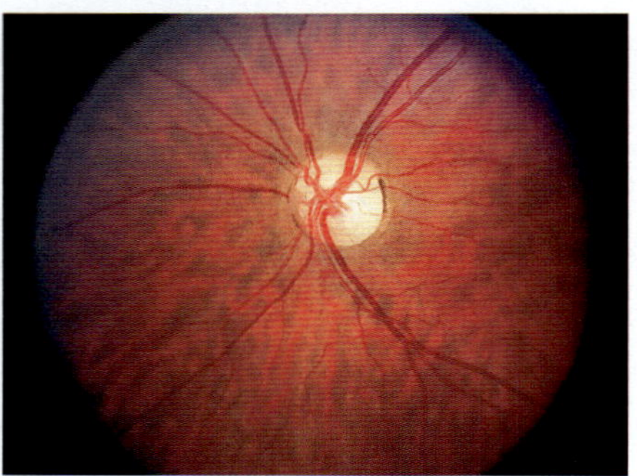

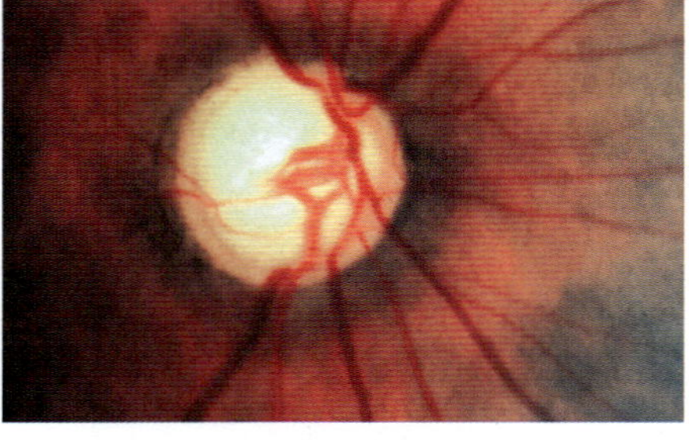

Optic atrophy (disc pallor)

Optic atrophy is a white or grey colour of the disc because of partial or complete death of the optic nerve. This results in decreased visual acuity, decreased colour vision and decreased contrast sensitivity.

Excessive cup–disc ratio

With primary, open-angle glaucoma, the increased intraocular pressure decreases blood supply to retinal structures. The physiological cup enlarges to more than half of the disc diameter, vessels appear to plunge over the edge of the cup and the vessels are displaced nasally. This is asymptomatic, although the person may have decreased vision or visual field defects in the late stages of glaucoma.

TABLE 14.9 Optic disc abnormalities cont'd

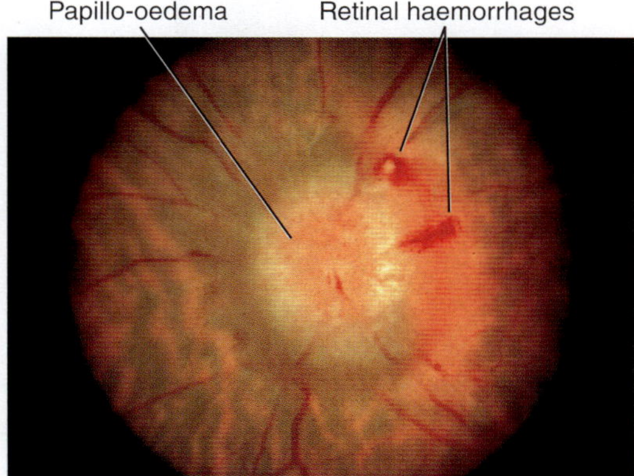

Papillo-oedema

Increased intracranial pressure causes venous stasis in the globe, showing redness, congestion and elevation of the disc; blurred margins; haemorrhages; and absent venous pulsations. This is a serious sign of intracranial pressure, usually caused by a space-occupying mass (e.g. a brain tumour or haematoma). Visual acuity is not affected.

TABLE 14.10 Retinal vessel and background abnormalities

Diabetic retinopathy (DR)
Findings are nonproliferative changes that occur *within* the retina (microaneurysms, dot haemorrhages, blot haemorrhages, lipid exudates) and proliferative changes that occur on the inner surface of the retina or vitreous. Proliferative changes are new vessel formations or neovascularisation, which increase the risk of retinal detachment or vitreous haemorrhage.

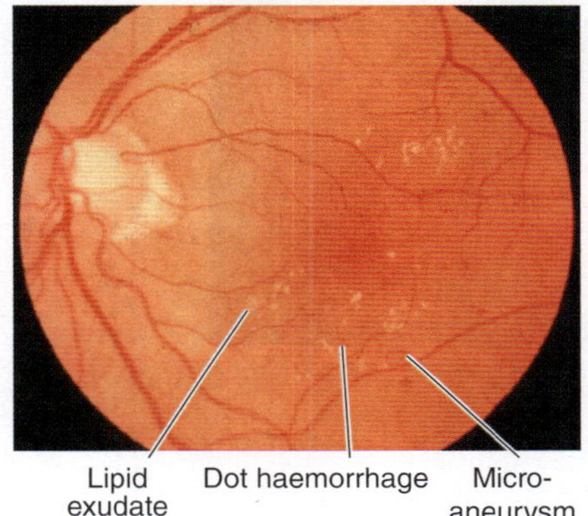

Continued

TABLE 14.10 Retinal vessel and background abnormalities cont'd

Moderate nonproliferative diabetic retinopathy. *Microaneurysms* are round, punctate red dots that are localised dilations of a small vessel. Their edges are smooth and discrete. The vessel itself is too small to view with the ophthalmoscope; only the isolated red dots are seen. *Dot haemorrhages* are deep intraretinal haemorrhages that look splattered on. They are distinguished from microaneurysms by the blurred irregular edges. *Lipid (hard) exudates* are small yellow-white spots with distinct edges and a smooth, solid-looking surface. They often form a circular or linear pattern (this is in contrast with drusen when have a scattered haphazard location).

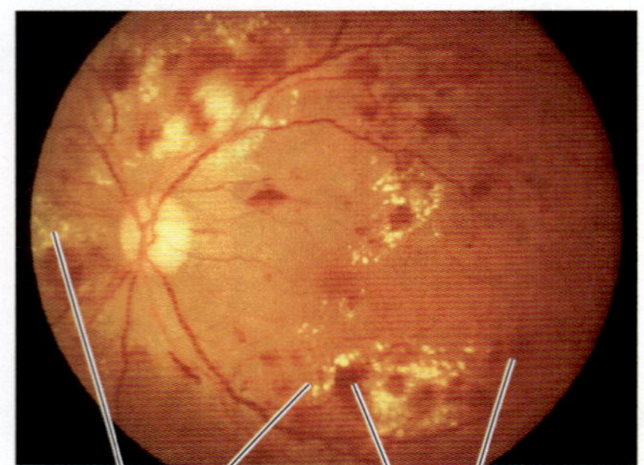

Severe nonproliferative diabetic retinopathy. Note *lipid (hard) exudates* as described and larger *flame-shaped haemorrhages* that look linear or spindle-shaped. These also occur with hypertension.

Proliferative diabetic retinopathy (not shown). *Neovasculariston* is new vessel formation that looks like radiating spokes.

Soft exudates or 'cotton wool-like' areas (both images). They are arteriolar microinfarctions that envelop and obscure the vessels. They occur with diabetes, hypertension, subacute bacterial endocarditis, lupus and papillo-oedema of any cause.

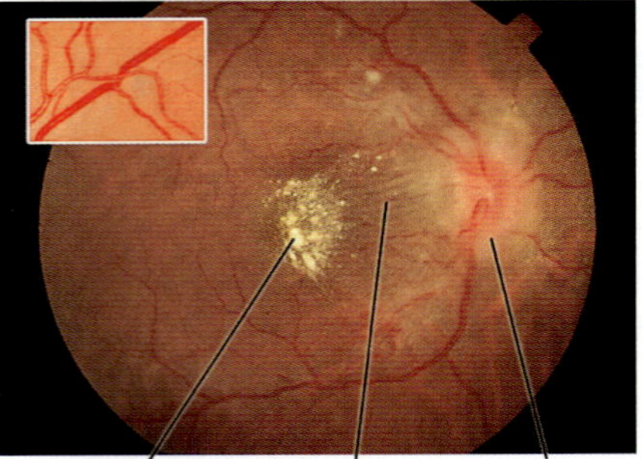

Arteriovenous crossing (nicking)

The inset shows arteriovenous crossing with interruption of blood flow. When a vein is occluded, it dilates distal to crossing. This person also has disc oedema and *hard exudates* in a macular star pattern that occur with acutely elevated (malignant) hypertension. With hypertension, the arteriole wall thickens and becomes opaque, so no blood is seen inside it (silver-wire arteries).

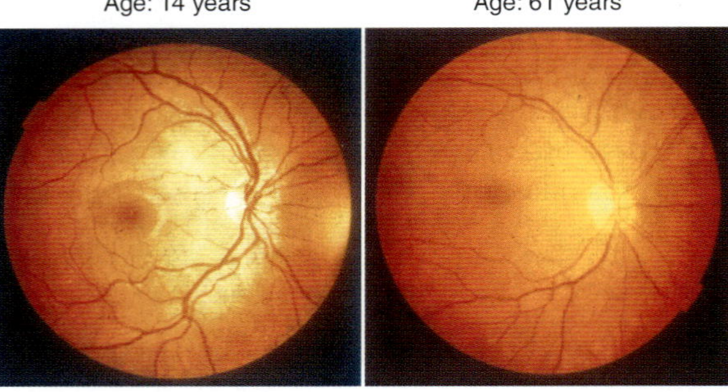

Narrow (attenuated) arteries

Narrow arteries indicate a generalised decrease in arteriole diameter. The light reflex also narrows. It occurs with severe hypertension (shown above on right) and with occlusion of the central retinal artery and retinitis pigmentosa.

Clinical reasoning and documentation

The following is a continuation of the case study provided at the beginning of this chapter and the clinical reasoning process including problem/issue identification. Consult a fundamentals of nursing or medical-surgical nursing text for information about goal setting, nursing interventions and evaluation.

Case study (continued)—Eye symptoms

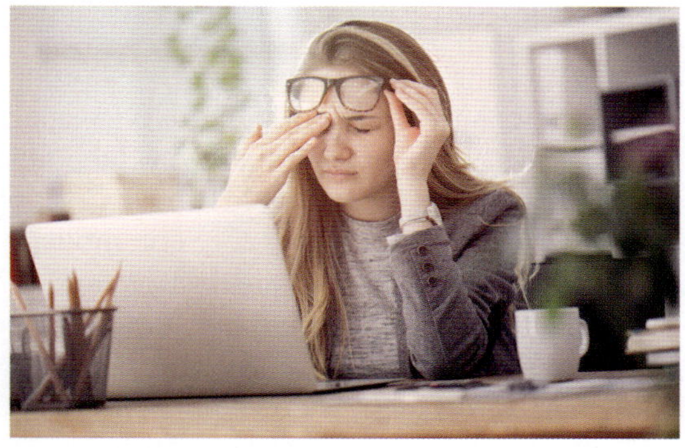

Context

You will recall from the case study described earlier in the chapter that you are on a clinical placement in a family medical clinic working alongside a nurse practitioner.

Consider the patient's situation

Ms Emma Jensen (an 18-year-old female) has attended complaining of red, gritty eyes.

Collect cues/information

Your further assessment reveals the following information.

Subjective data

Emma states her right eyelid was 'stuck together', red and gritty when she woke up that morning. The left eye has become progressively red and gritty during the day, with both eyes now affected equally. She says her vision is 'the same as it usually is'. She doesn't have any pain but finds very bright lights uncomfortable (mild photophobia).

She describes a gritty, foreign body sensation in both eyes. She states there has been some thick, yellow discharge from her eyes during the day. There is no history of trauma or eye injury. Emma does not wear contact lenses. Apart from the problem with her eyes, Emma has been otherwise well.

Objective data

The eyelids are slightly red and oedematous, and the conjunctivae are quite red. When the lower lid is pulled away from the eyeball, the forniceal conjunctiva are noted to be very red and mucopurulent discharge is seen in the lower fornix.

On inspection with a pen torch, there is no obvious injury to the conjunctiva, although Emma finds the bright light uncomfortable. The pupils are equal, round and briskly reactive to light.

Process information and identify problems/issues

Collaborative problem

Probable eye infection—refer to a medical practitioner for further assessment and swabs for micro and culture

Problem statements/nursing diagnoses

Discomfort related to photophobia, mucopurulent discharge and foreign body sensation

Potential for spread of infection related to knowledge deficit of hygiene and infection control practices

ADDITIONAL RESOURCES

You can further develop your knowledge and skills relevant to assessing the eyes, related pathophysiology, common health issues and nursing interventions by:

- reading chapters of a fundamentals of nursing or medical-surgical nursing textbook
- answering chapter multiple choice questions online. Log onto ClinicalKey Student and search for the text 'Health Assessment, 4th edition'. Choose the section titled 'Teaching material'. In this section you will find question and answer documents for each chapter. Please check instructions on the inside front cover of the book to access online resources.
- visiting websites

refer to Health Education section

REFERENCES

1. Marieb EM, Keller SM. Essentials of human anatomy & physiology. 13th Global ed.UK: Pearson; 2022.
2. Foreman J, Keel S, Xie J, et al. The national eye health survey. Melbourne: Vision 2020 Australia; 2016.
3. Australian Institute of Health and Welfare (AIHW). Eye health, Cat no PHE 206. Canberra: AIHW; 2023.
4. Statistics New Zealand. Disability survey: 2014. Tatauranga: Statistics New Zealand; 2014. Available at: https://www.stats.govt.nz/information-releases/disability-survey-2013
5. Australian Institute of Health and Welfare (AIHW). Eye health measures for Aboriginal and Torres Strait Islander people. Canberra: AIHW; 2022.
6. Rapata M, Cunningham W, Harwood M, Niederer R. Te hauora karu o te iwi Māori: a comprehensive review of Māori eye health in Aotearoa/New Zealand. Clinical & Experimental Ophthalmology. 2023; 1–14. doi: 10.1111/ceo.14279.
7. Hashemi, H, Pakzad, R, Abbasali, Y, Mohamadreza, Pakbin M, Ramin S, et al. Global and regional prevalence of age-related cataract: a comprehensive systemic review and meta-analysis. Eye (Lond). 2020 Aug; 34(8): 1357–1370. doi: 10.1038/s41433-020-0806-3
8. Taylor P, Mapp K. Clear focus: the economic impact of vision loss in New Zealand in 2009. Canberra: Access Economics; 2010. Available at: https://bf-website-uploads-production.s3.amazonaws.com/uploads/2016/04/Cost_of_vision_loss_in_NZ_report_27_September.pdf
9. Mitchell P, Liew G, Gopinath B, Wong TY. Age-related macular degeneration. Lancet 2018; 392:1147–1159.
10. Worsley D, Worsley A. Prevalence predictions of age-related macular degeneration in New Zealand have implications for provision of healthcare services. New Zealand Medical Journal. 2015; 128:44–45.
11. Barton K, Hitchings, R. Medical Management of Glaucoma. London: Springer Healthcare; 2013.
12. Jonas JB, Aung T, Bourne RR, Bron AM, Ritch R, Panda-Jonas S. Glaucoma. Lancet 2017;390:2083–2093.
13. Liew G., Tsang T, Marshall B, Saw M, Khachigian LM, Ong S, et al. Proportion of people with diabetic retinopathy and macular oedema varies by ethnicity in a tertiary retinal clinic in Australia: findings from the Liverpool Eye and Diabetes Study (LEADS). BMJ Open; 2023:13(2). https://doi.org/10.1136/bmjopen-2021-055404
14. Lee R, Wong TY, Sabanayagam C. Epidemiology of diabetic retinopathy, diabetic macular edema and related vision loss. Eye and Vision. 2015; 2:17. doi: 10.1186/s40662-015-0026-2
15. Lechner J, O'Leary O, Stitt A. The pathology associated with diabetic retinopathy. Vision

Res 2017; 139:7–14. doi: 10.1016/j.visres. 2017.04.003

16. Lake AJ, Hateley-Browne J, Rees G, Speight J. Effect of a tailored leaflet to promote diabetic retinopathy screening among young adults with type 2 diabetes: a randomised controlled trial. BMC Ophthalmology 2020; 20:1–12. doi: https://doi.org/10.1186/s12886-020-1311-y
17. Findlay Q, Reid K. Dry eye disease: when to treat and when to refer. Australian Prescriber 2018;41(5):160–163.
18. Katz JA, Karpecki PM, Dorca A, Chiva-Razavi S, Floyd H, Barnes E, et al. Presbyopia: a review of current treatment options and emerging therapies. Clinical Ophthalmology (Auckland, N.Z.) 2021;15:2167–2178.
19. Department of Health and Ageing (DOHA). Third progress report on the implementation of the national framework for action to promote eye health and prevent avoidable blindness and vision loss. Canberra: DOHA, Commonwealth of Australia; 2015. Available at: https://health.gov.au/internet/main/publishing.nsf/Content/8F3A179870AE7DC2CA258035007E09C1/$File/3rd%20Progress%20report%20under%20National%20Framework%20for%20Eye%20Health.pdf
20. Foreman J, Xie J, Keel S, van Wijngaarden P, Sandhu SS, Ang GS, et al. The prevalence and causes of vision loss in Indigenous and non-Indigenous Australians. Ophthalmology 2017;124(12):1743–1752.
21. New Zealand Ministry of Health. Diabetes, 2018. Available at: www.health.govt.nz/your-health/conditions-and-treatments/diseases-and-illnesses/diabetes
22. Razavi H, Burrow S, Trzesinki A. Review of eye health among Aboriginal and Torres Strait Islander people. Australian Indigenous Health Bulletin 2018; 18(4): 1–39. https://healthbulletin.org.au/articles/review-of-eye-health-among-aboriginal-and-torres-strait-islander-people
23. Royal Australian and New Zealand College of Ophthalmologists. Maori and Pasifika eye health. Community Engagement. 2021. Available at: https://test-ranzco-website.eluminaelearning.com.au/home/community-engagement/maori-and-pasifika-eye-health/
24. Pane A, Simcock P. Practical Ophthalmology. A survival guide for doctors and optometrists. Edinburgh: Elsevier Churchill Livingstone. 2005.
25. White SLJ, Wood JM, Black AA, Hopkins S. Vision screening outcomes of Grade 3 children in Australia: differences in academic achievement. International Journal of Educational Research 2017;83:154–159.
26. Centre for Community Child Health. National children's vision screening project. Final report. Melbourne: Centre for Community Child Health; 2009. Available at: https://www.iapb.org/wp-content/uploads/Final-Report-Vision-Screening-May-2009.pdf
27. Royal Australian and New Zealand College of Ophthalmologists. Referral Guidelines for Eye and Vision Problems in Infants and Children. 2018. Available at: https://ranzco.edu/wp-content/uploads/2018/11/GUIDELINES-Paediatric-Referral-Guidelines.pdf
28. Salmon JF. Kanski's Clinical Ophthalmology E-Book: A Systematic Approach. Elsevier Health Sciences; 2019 Oct 31.
29. Friedman NJ, Kaiser PK, Pineda II R. The Massachusetts Eye and Ear Infirmary Illustrated Manual of Ophthalmology E-Book. Elsevier Health Sciences; 2019.
30. Marsden J. Ophthalmic care. 2nd ed. London: M&K Publishing; 2017.
31. World Health Organization. Blindness and vision impairment. 2023. Available at: https://www.who.int/news-room/fact-sheets/detail/blindness-and-visual-impairment
32. Talley NJ, O'Connor S. Clinical examination: a systematic guide to physical diagnosis. 9th ed. Chatswood: Elsevier; 2021.
33. Agaje BG, Delelegne D, Abera E, Destak K, Girum M, Mossie M, et al. Strabismus prevalence and associated factors among pediatric patients in southern Ethiopia: a cross-sectional study. Journal of International Medical Research. 2020;48(10): 0300060520964339. doi: 10.1177/0300060520964339

34. Pai AS, Rose KA, Leone JF, Sharbini S, Burlutsky G, Varma R, et al. Amblyopia prevalence and risk factors in Australian preschool children. Ophthalmology 2012;119(1):138–144. doi: 10.1016/j.ophtha.2011.06.024.
35. Anstice NS, Thomson B. The measurement of visual acuity in children: an evidence-based update. Clinical and Experimental Optometry. 2014;29:3–11.
36. Macular Disease Foundation of Australia, Amsler grid. 2020. Available at: https://www.mdfoundation.com.au/content/testing-amsler-grid
37. McIntire SC, Nowalk AJ, Garrison J, Zitelli BJ, editors. Zitelli and Davis' atlas of pediatric physical diagnosis. Elsevier Health Sciences; 2021.

CHAPTER 15

Ear assessment

Written by Carolyn Jarvis
Adapted by Suzanne Sharrad

INTRODUCTION

The ear is the sensory organ for hearing and maintaining equilibrium. In this chapter the structure and function of the external and internal ear are reviewed. The chapter also provides guidance for conducting a comprehensive ear assessment for adults, infants and children and adults older than 65 years. However, as changes in neurological function can affect hearing, it is advisable to also review the relevant sections in Chapter 12.

Case study

The following case study provides you with an example of a typical situation involving assessment of the ears and the initial clinical reasoning process. It will help you to identify your learning needs.

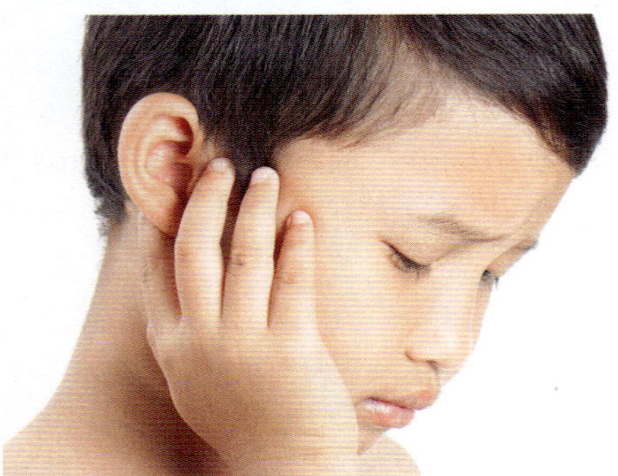

Context

You are working as a practice nurse in a busy local multidisciplinary health clinic. This role includes screening assessments for clients who attend.

Consider the patient's situation

Matthew Williams is a 4-year-old child who was brought into the clinic by his mother after he had been crying for most of the night and was difficult to settle. The only sleep the child had was when he was held upright against his mother's chest, but he slept for short periods only. The child feels warm to touch.

Questions to further your learning

- What are the possible things that might be going on with Matthew?
- What knowledge do you need to be able to predict what might be going on?
- What approach to Matthew's health assessment will you take?
- What questions (subjective data) will you ask Matthew's mother to extend the health history and why?
- What physical examination (objective data) will you conduct and why?
- What resources are available to assist in your assessment of Matthew?

Assessment plan

Determination of what a person feels or experiences in recent and past times contributes subjective data to the assessment of ear health. Questions focus on the presence of pain and associated symptoms, changes in hearing, discharge, infection, tinnitus, vertigo, the environmental circumstances, the impact of hearing loss on daily living, and how the person cares for their ears.

The main areas for subjective assessment are:

- presenting concern
- pain
- associated symptoms
- changes in hearing
- discharge
- infections
- past history
- tinnitus
- vertigo

- environmental noise
- health and lifestyle management.

Following subjective data collection, you will get a sense of the areas needed to be examined for objective data. Only the relevant areas should be examined. The main areas for physical examination are:

- general inspection
- inspect and palpate the external ear
- inspect and palpate the external auditory meatus
- test hearing acuity—whispered voice test.

Resources available

You will find additional resources and the reference list at the end of this chapter.

Structure and function

The ear has three parts: the external, the middle and the inner ear. The external ear is called the **auricle** or **pinna** and consists of movable cartilage and skin (Figure 15.1). Note the landmarks of the auricle and use these terms to describe any assessment findings. Although the mastoid process, which is the bony prominence behind the lobule, is not part of the ear, it remains an important landmark during assessment.

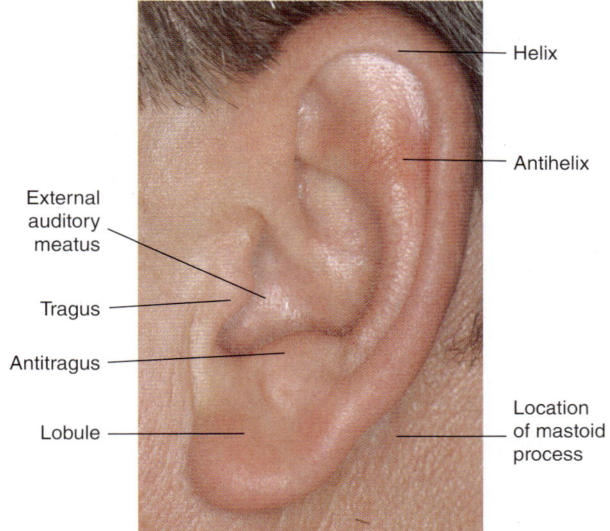

FIGURE 15.1 The external ear

External ear

The external ear has a characteristic shape and serves to funnel sound waves into its opening, the **external auditory canal** (Figure 15.2). The canal is a cul-de-sac 2.5 to 3 cm long in adults and terminates at the eardrum, or tympanic membrane. It is lined with glands that secrete cerumen (commonly referred to as earwax), a yellow waxy material that lubricates and protects the ear. Cerumen in the ear canal repels water and traps dust and stops small particles from entering and damaging the ear. Ordinarily it migrates out to the meatus by the movements of chewing and talking. However, its presence in the ear can press against the eardrum and occlude the auditory canal and impair hearing. Cerumen can be either grey and flaky or described as 'wet', in which case, it is honey brown to dark brown in colour and moist in consistency. The presence and composition of cerumen are not related to poor hygiene.

The outer one-third of the canal is made up of cartilage that is covered by skin. The inner two-thirds consists of bone that is also covered by thin sensitive skin. The canal has a slight S-curve in adults. The outer third curves up and towards the back of the head,

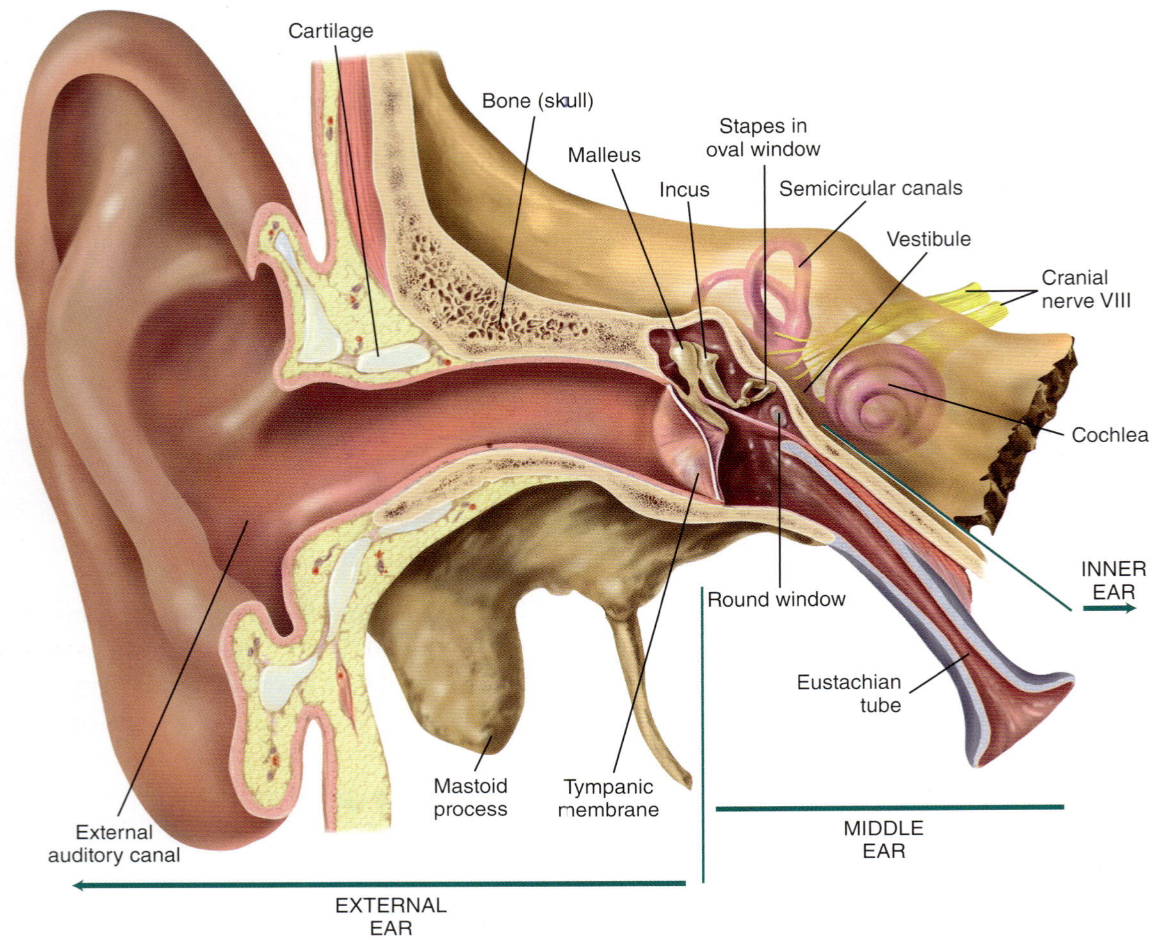

FIGURE 15.2 Structures of the external and middle ear

whereas the inner two-thirds angles down and forwards towards the nose.

The **tympanic membrane**, or **eardrum**, separates the external and middle ear and is tilted obliquely to the ear canal, facing downwards and somewhat forwards. It is a translucent membrane, pearly grey in colour, with a prominent cone of light in the anteroinferior quadrant, which is the reflection of the otoscope light (Figure 15.3). The drum is oval and slightly concave, pulled in at its centre by one of the middle ear ossicles, the **malleus**. The parts of the malleus show through the translucent drum; these include the **umbo**, the **manubrium** (handle) and the **short process**. The small, slack, superior section of the tympanic membrane is called the **pars flaccida**. The remainder of the drum, which is thicker and tauter, is the **pars tensa**. Last, the **annulus** is the outer fibrous rim of the drum.

Lymphatic drainage of the external ear flows to the parotid, mastoid and superficial cervical nodes.

Middle ear

The middle ear is a tiny air-filled cavity inside the temporal bone (Figure 15.2). It contains

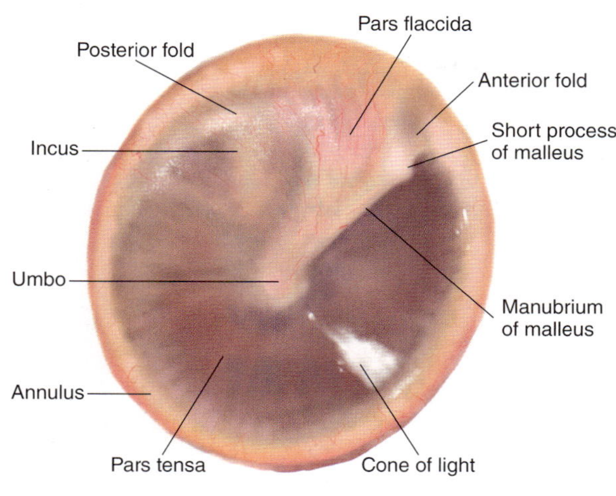

FIGURE 15.3 The eardrum

tiny ear bones, or auditory ossicles, known as the **malleus**, the **incus** and the **stapes**. In the middle ear, several openings are present. One of the openings is between the middle ear and the outer ear and is covered by the tympanic membrane. Other openings are to the inner ear and are known as the oval window at the end of the stapes and the round window. The final opening is the **Eustachian tube**, which connects the middle ear with the nasopharynx and allows the passage of air. Ordinarily the Eustachian tube is closed but can open with swallowing or yawning.

The middle ear has three functions: (1) it conducts sound vibrations from the outer ear to the central hearing apparatus in the inner ear, (2) it protects the inner ear by reducing the amplitude of loud sounds and (3) its Eustachian tube allows equalisation of air pressure on each side of the tympanic membrane so the membrane does not rupture (e.g. during altitude changes in an aeroplane).

Inner ear

The inner ear contains the **bony labyrinth**, which holds the sensory organs for equilibrium and hearing. Within the bony labyrinth, the **vestibule** and the **semicircular canals** compose the vestibular apparatus, and the **cochlea** (Latin for 'snail shell') contains the central hearing apparatus. Although the inner ear is not accessible to direct examination, its functions can be assessed.

Hearing

In relation to the function of hearing, the auditory system can be divided into three levels including the peripheral, brainstem and cerebral cortex (Figure 15.4). At the peripheral level, the ear transmits sound by converting longitudinal sound wave vibrations into electrical impulses that are subsequently analysed by the brain. For example, when an alarm bell ringing in the hall is heard, its sound waves travel instantly to the ears. The *amplitude* of the sound wave reflects the loudness of the alarm; its *frequency* is the pitch of the wave (in this case, high) or the number of cycles per second. The sound waves produce vibrations of the tympanic membrane that are carried by the middle ear ossicles to the oval window. Then the sound waves travel through the cochlea (which is coiled like a snail's shell) and are dissipated against the round window. Along the way, the **basilar membrane** vibrates at a point specific to the frequency of the sound. In this case, the alarm's high frequency stimulates the basilar membrane at its base near the stapes. The numerous fibres along the basilar membrane are the receptor hair cells of the **organ of Corti**, which is the sensory organ of hearing. As the hair cells bend, they mediate the vibrations into electrical impulses which are subsequently conducted by the auditory portion of cranial nerve VIII to the brainstem.

The function at the brainstem level is *binaural interaction*, where the sound is identified and its direction is determined. How does this occur? Each ear is one half of

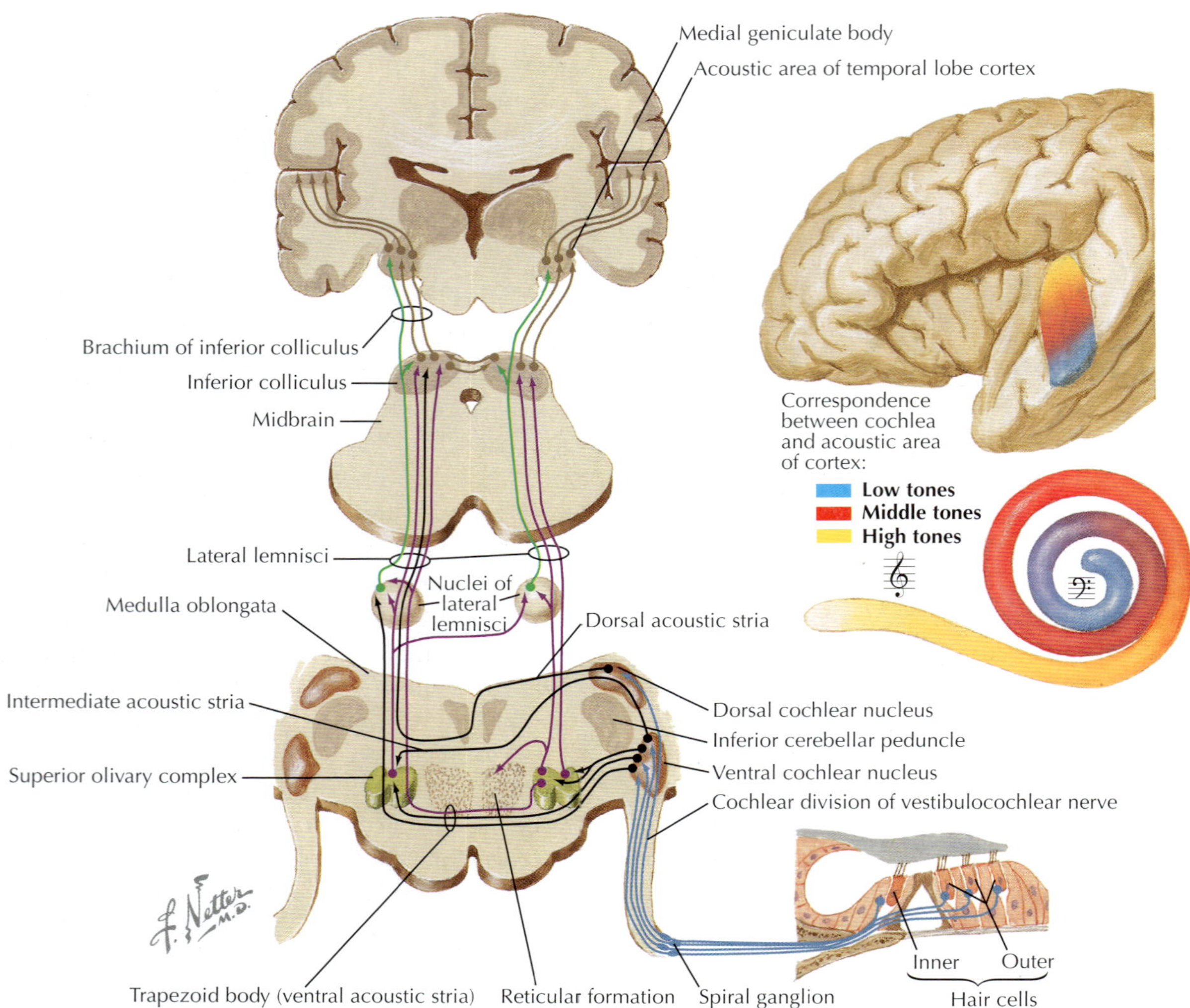

FIGURE 15.4 The auditory system

the total sensory organ. Because the ears are located on each side of a movable head, the cranial nerve VIII from each ear sends signals to both sides of the brainstem. Areas in the brainstem are sensitive to differences in intensity and timing of the messages from the two ears, depending on the way the head is turned.

Finally, the function of the cortex is to interpret the meaning of the sound and begin the appropriate response. Incredibly, all this happens in the split second it takes for a person to react to the alarm.

PATHWAYS OF HEARING

The normal pathway of hearing is air conduction as described above. This pathway is the most efficient pathway. However, an alternative pathway is available, and it is hearing by bone conduction. In the alternative pathway, it is the bones of the skull that vibrate. Bony vibrations are transmitted directly to the inner ear and to cranial nerve VIII.

HEARING LOSS

Obstruction to the transmission of sound caused by a problem in the outer, the middle or the inner hearing pathway or the auditory nerve pathway can cause hearing loss. Hearing loss may be mild, moderate, severe or profound. It is classified as conductive or sensorineural, or congenital or acquired.[1] Conductive hearing loss involves a mechanical dysfunction of the external or middle ear (Figure 15.5). It is a partial loss because an individual will be able to hear if the sound amplitude is increased enough to reach normal nerve elements in the inner ear. Conductive hearing loss may be caused by impacted cerumen, foreign bodies, a perforated tympanic membrane, pus or serum in the middle ear and otosclerosis (a decrease in mobility of the ossicles).

Sensorineural (or perceptive) **loss** signifies pathology of the inner ear, cranial nerve VIII or the auditory areas of the cerebral cortex. A simple increase in amplitude may not enable an individual to understand words. This classification of hearing loss may be caused by *presbycusis*, a gradual nerve degeneration that occurs with advancing years of age and by ototoxic drugs that affect the hair cells in the cochlea.

A third type of hearing loss can be caused by a combination of conductive and sensorineural hearing loss in the same ear. This is known as **mixed hearing loss**. It is caused by problems in the conductive pathways of the ear, that is, in the outer or middle ear and in the nerve pathways of the inner ear. An example of mixed hearing loss is a conductive loss resulting from a middle ear infection combined with a sensorineural loss caused by ageing.

EQUILIBRIUM

The labyrinth in the inner ear constantly feeds information to your brain about your

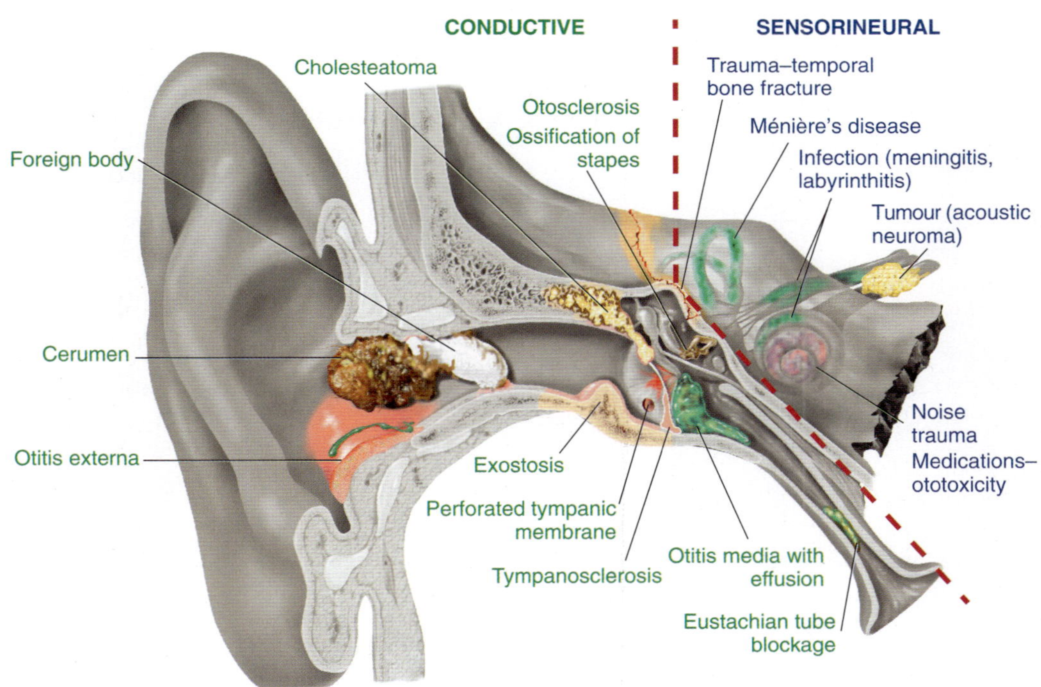

FIGURE 15.5 Conductive and sesorineural hearing loss

body's position in space. It works like a plumb line to determine verticality or depth. The ear's plumb lines register the angle of your head in relation to gravity. If the labyrinth ever becomes inflamed, it feeds the wrong information to the brain, creating a staggering gait and a strong, spinning, whirling sensation called *vertigo*.

Developmental considerations

Infants and children

The inner ear starts to develop early in the fifth week of gestation. In early development, the ear is posteriorly rotated and lowset; it ascends later to its normal placement around eye level. A child may be born with hearing loss (pre-lingual), putting them at risk for delayed speech, social development and learning deficit(s). Hearing loss in an infant may present if maternal rubella infection occurs during the first trimester, which leads to organ of Corti damage and impaired hearing. Post-lingual hearing loss develops **after** the acquisition of speech and language and usually **after** the age of 6 years.

An infant's Eustachian tube is relatively shorter and wider and its position is more horizontal than an adult's. At this stage, it is easier for pathogens from the nasopharynx to migrate through to the middle ear (Figure 15.6). The lumen of the Eustachian tube is surrounded by lymphoid tissue, which increases during childhood. Thus,

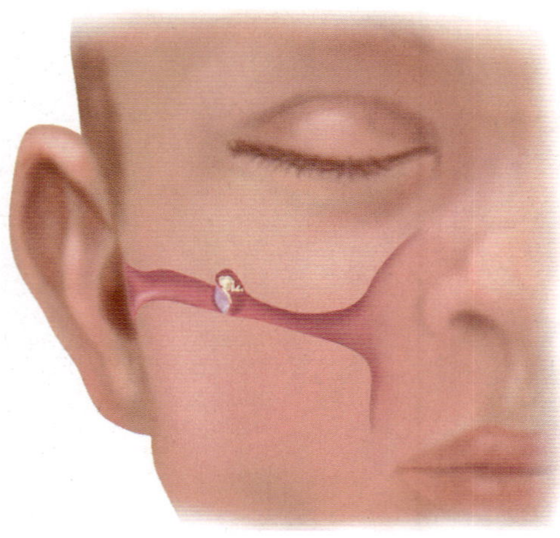

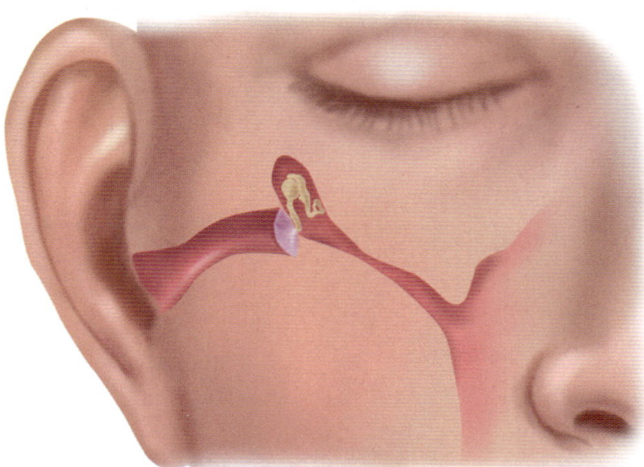

FIGURE 15.6 A child's Eustachian tube compared with an adult's

during this time, it can be easily occluded. Such factors place an infant at greater risk of middle ear infections than an adult.

The external auditory canal of an infant and toddler is shorter and has a slope opposite to that of an adult's (Figure 15.6).

Otitis media is an infection or inflammation of the middle ear and can affect all ages. Infection ascends into the middle ear cavity via the throat and causes swelling of the lining and blockage of the Eustachian tube and reduction of airflow.[2] A lack of ventilation, resulting from obstruction of the Eustachian tube or passage of nasopharyngeal secretions into the middle ear, leads to an accumulation of fluid. This fluid may be serous, as in acute otitis media, or purulent, as occurs in suppurative otitis media and causes the tympanic membrane to bulge. Persistent otitis media and fluid in the middle ear may lead to effusion and hearing loss, placing the child at risk of delayed cognitive development.[3]

The incidence of otitis media is also increased in premature infants, in those with trisomy 21 (Down syndrome) and in babies fed by bottle in a supine position. In the supine position, the effects of gravity and sucking tend to draw the nasopharyngeal contents directly into the middle ear.[4]

Adults

Otosclerosis is a common cause of conductive hearing loss in the early adult years between the ages of 20 and 40 years. It is a gradual hardening that causes the foot plate of the stapes to become fixed in the oval window, impeding the transmission of sound and causing progressive deafness.

Late adulthood (65+ years)

In a person aged over 65 years, cilia lining the ear canal can become coarse and stiff. This change may cause decreased hearing because it impedes sound waves travelling towards the tympanic membrane. It also causes cerumen to accumulate and oxidise, which greatly reduces hearing. The cerumen itself is drier because of atrophy of the apocrine glands. Also, a life history of frequent ear infections may result in scarring of the tympanic membrane.

Impacted cerumen is a common but reversible cause of hearing loss in people over 65 years. After removal of cerumen, most people have significantly improved hearing ability. Improvement of the hearing health of people over 65 years can be achieved by the routine performance of otoscopic examinations and irrigation of the ear canal when impacted cerumen occurs.

A person living in a noise-polluted area (e.g. near an airport or a busy highway) has a greater risk of hearing loss due to damage to the inner ear cells located in the cochlea. But **presbycusis** is a type of hearing loss that occurs with ageing, even in people living in a quiet environment. It is a gradual sensorineural loss caused by nerve degeneration in the inner ear or auditory nerve. Its onset usually occurs in the fifth decade, after which it slowly progresses. The person first notices a high-frequency tone loss; hearing consonants (high-pitched components of speech) becomes more difficult than vowels making words sound garbled. The ability to localise sound is also impaired. This communication dysfunction is accentuated when unfavourable background noise is present (e.g. with music, with dishes clattering or at a large noisy party).

Also, the auditory reaction time increases after age 70 years, meaning there is a delay in receiving and sending nerve impulses associated with hearing in an ageing adult.[5]

Cultural and social considerations

Today, the most significant cause of hearing loss is noise-induced hearing loss. Other causes include accidents, the effects of ototoxic drugs or chemicals and normal ageing.

Noise-induced hearing loss results from damage to the hearing cells of the cochlea of the inner ear. The damage, which results from either exposure to very loud noise or long-term exposure to 'reasonably loud noise', can often be attributed to prolonged employment in high-noise industries. Any noise louder than 85 decibels (dB) has the potential to cause hearing loss. Hearing loss in children is associated with lifelong negative consequences of language development, socialisation, education (including numeracy and literacy), social and emotional wellbeing and self-esteem, training and employment opportunities, mental health[6] and self-harm and domestic violence.[7] People of all ages with hearing loss are at risk of feeling isolated and frustrated.[6] A recently published study found that in Australia, across middle age, there is high and rising prevalence of slight and mild hearing loss, which implies Australia has an opportunity to prevent progression of hearing loss in significant numbers of its population to reduce the profound later burden of age-related hearing loss.[8] For younger age groups, the great concern about the use of digital devices remains.[9]

In Aotearoa New Zealand, the prevalence of hearing loss was estimated to be from 7.5 to 20.8% across the population.[10] Prevalence is higher among males, and it increases with age such that it is believed that most people will have mild hearing loss in their old age (90+ years old). Hearing loss is a major cause of disability.

Over many years, extraordinarily high and disproportionate levels of ear disease and hearing loss have been reported in the First Nations peoples of Australia and Aotearoa New Zealand when compared with non-Indigenous populations.[11] In 2018–19, 43% of Indigenous Australians aged 7 or older had hearing loss in one or both ears.[12] Notably, 29% of children aged 7 to 14 years had hearing loss in one or both ears, and this number increased to 40% in remote or very remote areas. After adjusting for differences in the age structure of the two populations, otitis media among Indigenous Australians was 3.6 times as high as the non-Indigenous rate.[12]

Aboriginal and Torres Strait Islander children experience one of the highest rates of middle ear disease in the world.[13] A recent inquiry into otitis media and hearing loss among Aboriginal and Torres Strait Islander children revealed that while only 7% of 1-year-old children had bilaterally normal ears, half (51%) of the children investigated had 'glue ear', and 41% had bulging or perforated ear drums.[14] It was noted that parents reported that the children were not experiencing pain. Perhaps even more alarming are the results of the birth cohort study of almost 400 Aboriginal and Torres Strait Islander infants recruited at 1 month of age and reviewed again at 2, 4, 6, 12, 18 and 36 months of age. In this study it was reported that only one baby had normal ears at every visit to age 7 months, whereas 40% of 1-month-old infants had otitis media in one ear, and 95% had bilateral otitis media. Chronic suppurative otitis media was seen in 5% of infants at 4 months of age and 27% at 36 months of age. By the time the infants in this study were 1 month of age, 50% had multiple bacteria colonisations of the nasopharynx.[14]

Hearing loss is a critical public health concern for Māori and Pacific Islander people in Aotearoa New Zealand. Recent reports indicate that 7.5% of New Zealanders aged over 15 years experience hearing impairment,[15] and the prevalence increases with age. It has been reported that 32% of Māori aged 65 years or older experience hearing loss compared with 28% of the total 65+ Aotearoa New Zealand population.[16] Not only are the Indigenous people of Aotearoa New Zealand disadvantaged by the higher prevalence of hearing loss, but they also experience more unmet needs for special equipment (30.4%) in comparison with older non-Māori (17.4%).[16] One of the reasons this is concerning relates to the known increased risk of accelerated cognitive decline in older adults with untreated hearing loss.[17]

The significant risk of severe otitis media in Indigenous Australians and New Zealanders is compounded by poverty, overcrowded living conditions and frequent exposure to nonpathogenic bacteria, inadequate access to clean water and functional sewerage systems, nutritional problems and lack of access to health care.[12] Otitis media may not only impair hearing but is also associated with problems in language development, educational outcomes and reduced employment opportunities.[14]

In Australia, funding has been provided for ear health initiatives aiming to give Aboriginal and Torres Strait Islander children a better start to education and to reduce the number of people experiencing avoidable hearing loss.[18] In Aotearoa New Zealand, the Universal Newborn Hearing Programme is administered via the National Screening Unit.[19] Strategies implemented by the Australian and Aotearoa New Zealand governments include creating agencies such as Hearing Australia[20] and the National Foundation for the Deaf and Hard of Hearing[21] to provide quality hearing resources to all people with hearing loss; conducting inquiries into hearing health; conducting research; providing national codes of practice; and initiating screening programs for all children.

HEALTH EDUCATION

The modern world: earbuds/headphones, loud music, industrial noise and hearing loss

More than 1 billion young people globally (aged 12–35 years) are at risk of hearing loss due to unsafe recreational hearing practices.[9,22] Of those in middle and high-income countries, nearly 40% are exposed to potentially damaging sound levels in recreational venues such as nightclubs and pubs. Nearly 50% face the risk of hearing loss due to listening at loud volumes or for prolonged periods on their personal audio listening devices such as smartphones, headphones and earbuds.[9] When wearing headphones or earbuds regularly for listening to music or podcasts, the devices are placed either over the ear or directly in the ear canal. Either way, the sound transmitted by the devices is placed closer to the eardrum. Listening with earbuds boosts sound signals. For example, an increase of 10 dB increases the impact of the sound tenfold. That is, sound conducted at 70 dB transmits 1,000 times as much energy as sound at 40 dB. Normal conversation takes place at about 60 dB, whereas a chainsaw typically records at 100 dB and a rock concert at 110 dB.[23] Because sound is digital, there is virtually no distortion, no matter how loud the volume, so most earbud wearers are not necessarily aware of its significance. Digital music devices can hold thousands of songs and play for hours without the need for recharging, which means users can listen continuously for hours at a time. In this example, hearing loss occurs slowly and often goes unnoticed until it is quite extensive. It is feared that exposure to

Continued

HEALTH EDUCATION cont'd

audio played directly into our ears will lead to a prematurely deaf generation of Australians.[24]

How much noise is too much?

'Noise dose' refers to the relationship between the level of noise and the time of exposure. Many experts suggest that digital music players should be designed either to prevent playing of music above 85 dB or to be limited to a maximum volume of 100 dB.

Exposure to excessive noise on worksites is also considered dangerous to employees' hearing.[25] Noise induced hearing loss, whether caused by use of digital music devices or exposure to continuous loud sounds in a social or work environment, cannot be reversed.[8] Early prevention is the key.

To maintain a safe level of hearing (no more 85 dB over an 8-hour period) it is recommended that the noise level should be lower than:

- 50 decibels, if work involves high concentration or lots of conversation
- 70 decibels, if work is routine, fast-paced and demands attentiveness and conversations are needed.[25]

Halving the time of exposure for every increase of 3 dB of noise level above 85 dB (music devices) and using larger headphones that rest over the ear opening or noise-cancelling headphones that eliminate background noise means listeners do not have to increase the volume.

Nurse's role

- assess noise levels in a work environment
- conduct hearing assessments
- refer employees of concern to a medical practitioner or an audiologist for further assessment
- act as advocate for employers in relation to noise abatement
- arrange for workers to have individually customised hearing protection devices
- ensure each worker understands how to use and maintain hearing protection
- educate on the importance of consistent usage.[25]

Subjective data

Practice note

Before you start the assessment, introduce yourself to the person, confirm the person's identity, discuss the purpose and scope of the assessment, clarify any questions the person may have and obtain verbal consent from the person to perform the assessment. It is important that you adjust your assessment techniques if the person is hearing impaired.

ASSESSMENT GUIDELINES	CLINICAL SIGNIFICANCE AND CLINICAL ALERTS
Presenting concern	
• *Do you have any problems concerning your hearing or your ears?* It is important to ascertain the person's perception of their presenting health concern. If the person does perceive a problem, ask: *How does this impact on your quality of life?*	During history taking, the following clues from normal conversation indicate possible hearing loss: • the person lip reading or watching your face and lips closely rather than your eyes • the person frowning or straining forwards to hear you

ASSESSMENT GUIDELINES	CLINICAL SIGNIFICANCE AND CLINICAL ALERTS
	• posturing of the head to catch sounds with their better ear • misunderstanding your questions or frequently asking you to repeat what you have said • irritability or showing startle reflex when you raise your voice (recruitment) • speech sounding garbled, possibly with vowel sounds distorted • an inappropriately loud voice • flat, monotonous tone of voice.
Pain	
• *Are you experiencing any earache or other pain in your ears?* **Location** • *Does the pain feel close to the surface or deep in the head?* • *Does it hurt when you push on the ear or pull on the earlobe?* Assess the **character** of the earache or pain by asking the person: • *Can you describe the pain?* • *Is it dull, aching, sharp or stabbing?* • *Is it constant or does it come and go?* • *Is it affected by changing the position of your head?* • *Have you ever experienced this kind of pain before?*	**Otalgia** (ear pain) may be directly due to ear disease or it may be referred pain from a problem in the person's teeth or oropharynx. Pain that occurs when the person puts pressure on the ear or pulls the earlobe may indicate the presence of an inner ear infection. The character of the pain may indicate the severity of the ear problem.  ***Clinical alert:*** People with severe or persistent earache should be referred to a medical practitioner.
Associated symptoms	
• *Do you have any cold symptoms or a sore throat?* • *Have there been any problems with sinuses or teeth?* • *Do you have any allergies?*	Virus/bacteria from upper respiratory tract infections may migrate up the Eustachian tube to involve middle ear. **Allergic rhinitis** can commonly occur alongside otitis media. The inflammation and oedema of the nasopharynx can lead to Eustachian tube obstruction. If the obstruction persists for long enough, pressure in the middle ear results in the development of middle ear fluid by transudation.

ASSESSMENT GUIDELINES	CLINICAL SIGNIFICANCE AND CLINICAL ALERTS
Changes in hearing	
Hearing loss • *Are you having trouble hearing?* **Onset** • *Did the loss come on slowly or all at once?*	Sensorineural, conductive and mixed losses are the causes of hearing loss. **Presbycusis** is gradual onset over years. Sounds cannot get through from the outside to the inner ear. Hearing loss resulting from trauma is often sudden.  ***Clinical alert:*** Refer any sudden loss of hearing in one or both ears *not* associated with upper respiratory tract infection for further investigation.
Character • *Has your hearing decreased in both ears or one ear?* • *Are there certain sounds you can't hear?*	
• *In what situations do you notice hearing loss—conversations, using the telephone, listening to TV or at a party?*	Loss is apparent when competition from background noise is present, as at a party.
• *Do people seem to shout at you?*	**Recruitment** is a marked loss when sound is at low intensity, but sound becomes painful when repeated in a loud voice.
• *Do ordinary sounds seem hollow, as if you are hearing in a barrel or under water?* • *Have you recently travelled by aeroplane?* • *Is there any family history of hearing loss?* • *Have you tried to treat the hearing loss with a hearing aid or other device?* • *Have you tried anything to help with your hearing?*	Characteristic of hearing loss when cerumen expands and becomes impacted—for example, after swimming or showering.
Discharge	
• *Has there been ever any discharge from your ears?*	Discharge (**otorrhoea**) suggests an infected canal or a perforated eardrum. Consider the following characteristics:
Colour of discharge • *Does it look like pus or is the discharge bloody?*	**External otitis media**—purulent, sanguineous or watery discharge. **Acute otitis media with perforation**—purulent discharge.
Odour • *Is there any odour/smell associated with the discharge?*	**Cholesteatoma**—dirty yellow/grey discharge, which is malodorous.
• *Is there any relationship between the discharge and the ear pain?*	Typically, with perforation of the ear drum, ear pain occurs first, then stops with a popping sensation when drainage occurs.

ASSESSMENT GUIDELINES	CLINICAL SIGNIFICANCE AND CLINICAL ALERTS
Infections	
• *Have you experienced any ear infections either as an adult or in childhood?* • *How frequent were they? How were they managed?*	A history of chronic ear problems suggests possible sequelae.
• *Has there been any past or recent trauma of the ear area such as a sports injury or trauma from a foreign body?*	Trauma may rupture the tympanic membrane.
• *What have you done to try to relieve the earache/ pain?*	Assess self-initiated interventions and the person's coping strategies.
Past history	
Hearing loss • *Do you or anyone in your family have a history of hearing loss?* **Onset** • *Did the loss come on slowly or all at once?* **Ear infections** • *Have you experienced any ear infections either as an adult or in childhood?* • *How frequent were they? How were they managed?* **Trauma** • *Has there been any past or recent trauma to the ear area?* • *Have you ever been hit on the ear or on the side of the head?* • *Have you experienced any sports injury that has involved the head or ears?* • *Have you ever experienced any trauma from a foreign body?* **Ear wax** • *Have you had any problems with a build-up of ear wax (cerumen)?*	***Clinical alert:*** Refer any sudden loss in one or both ears *not* associated with upper respiratory tract infection for further investigation. Trauma may rupture the tympanic membrane.
Tinnitus	
• *Have you ever felt ringing, crackling or buzzing in your ears?* • *When did this occur?* • *Does this seem louder at night?*	Tinnitus originates within the person. It accompanies some hearing or ear disorders.

ASSESSMENT GUIDELINES	CLINICAL SIGNIFICANCE AND CLINICAL ALERTS
Vertigo	
• *Have you ever felt dizzy—that is, the room spinning around or yourself spinning?*	(Vertigo is a true twirling motion.) True rotational spinning occurs with dysfunction of labyrinth. **Objective vertigo** feels like room spins. **Subjective vertigo** is where the person feels as if they are spinning. Dizziness and lightheadedness are likely to be due to changes in blood pressure (Chapter 12).
• *Have you ever felt not quite steady or like you are falling or losing your balance? Have you ever felt giddy or lightheaded?*	Distinguish true vertigo from dizziness or lightheadedness. People who experience vertigo are at risk of falling or another form of traumatic injury.
Environmental noise	
• *Have you experienced any loud noises at home or at work?* For example: • *Do you currently or have you ever lived in a noise-polluted area, near an airport or busy traffic area?* • *Are you exposed to other noises such as heavy machinery or a loud persistent noise or loud music?*	Old trauma to hearing initially goes unnoticed but results in further decibel loss in later years.
Health and lifestyle management	
• *How do you clean your ears?*	Assess potential trauma from invasive instruments. Cotton-tipped applicators can impact cerumen, causing hearing loss.
• *When was the last time you had your hearing checked?* • *If a hearing loss was noted, did you get a hearing aid?* • *How long have you had it? Do you wear it? How does it work? Any trouble with upkeep, cleaning, changing batteries?* • *Are you taking any medications?*	Recommend frequent hearing assessments according to the person's age or risk factors. **Ototoxic medications** that may cause temporary or permanent hearing loss include gentamycin, cancer chemotherapy drugs, aspirin, quinine, ACE inhibitors, beta-blockers, calcium blockers and illicit drugs (e.g. oxycontin, fentanyl, heroin, morphine and methadone).
Assess the person's coping strategies • *How does hearing loss affect your daily life?* • *Does it interfere with your occupation?* • *Does it cause you to feel embarrassed or frustrated?* • *How do your family and friends react?*	Hearing loss can cause social isolation, can interfere with professional roles and can lessen pleasure of leisure activities.

ASSESSMENT GUIDELINES	CLINICAL SIGNIFICANCE AND CLINICAL ALERTS
Additional history for infants and children (questions for parents or guardians)	
Ear infections	
• *How many ear infections in the last 6 months?* • *How many in total?* • *At what age was the child's first episode?* • *How were these managed?*	A first episode occurring within 3 months of life increases the risk of recurrent otitis media. Recurrent otitis media is defined as 'the occurrence of at least three episodes of acute otitis media within 6 months or four episodes within 12 months, with at least one of those episodes occurring in the immediately preceding 6 months'.[26]
• *Are the infections increasing in frequency or severity or is it staying the same?*	
Assess the infant's feeding type	
• *Is the child bottle or breastfed?* • *What is the child's usual position during feeding?* • *Has the child had any surgery such as insertion of tympanoplasty tubes/ventilation tubes (commonly called grommets) or removal of tonsils?*	Bottle feeding, particularly in the supine position, is a risk factor for developing ear infections in infants and younger children.
Environment	
• *Does anyone in the home smoke cigarettes or a pipe?*	Passive and gestational smoke is a risk factor for otitis media.[27]
• *Does your child receive childcare outside your home? In a daycare centre or someone else's home?* • *How many children in the group being cared for?*	Attendance at daycare and bottle feeding (as opposed to breastfeeding) are also risk factors for otitis media.[28]
Hearing	
• *Have you noticed that the infant startles with loud noise?* • *Did the infant babble around 6 months?* • *Do they talk?* • *At what age did your child start talking?* • *Was the speech intelligible?* • *Has the child's hearing ever been tested?*	Children at risk for hearing deficit include those who were: • exposed to maternal rubella, syphilis, cytomegalovirus or toxoplasmosis or to maternal ototoxic drugs in utero • premature infants • low-birthweight infants • trauma or hypoxia at birth • infants with congenital liver or kidney disease. Diseases such as meningitis, measles, mumps, otitis media and any illness with persistent high fever may increase risk of hearing deficit in children.[29]
If hearing loss was detected: • *Was it a consequence of another condition in the child or in the mother during pregnancy?* • *Is the older child or adolescent active in contact sports?* • *Has the child ever put objects in their ears?*	 ***Clinical alert:*** Early identification of hearing loss is essential to avoid delayed speech and problems with social development and learning. These children are at increased risk of ear-related trauma.

ASSESSMENT GUIDELINES	CLINICAL SIGNIFICANCE AND CLINICAL ALERTS
Additional subjective data for adults over 65 years	
• *Have you ever been treated for an ear problem such as surgery, medications, hearing aids or ear syringing?* • *When did this occur?* • *Was it successful?*	Hearing loss may occur because of: • **presbycusis** (gradual loss over years) • **sensorineural degeneration** which results from a problem within the cochlea or the neural pathway to the auditory cortex • **otosclerosis** (abnormal bone remodelling in the middle ear), which disrupts the transmission of sound to travel from the middle ear to the inner ear (it tends to run in families) • previous measles infection • stress fractures to the bony tissue surrounding the inner ear or immune disorders • excessive or impacted cerumen.

Objective data

Collecting objective data is an important part of any ear assessment. The focus of ear examination includes screening for hearing loss and assessing for other ear problems such as ear pain, discharge or lumps or lesions in the outer ear and surrounds.

The objective ear assessment is used for screening infants, children or adults for hearing loss, investigating symptoms such as ear pain and monitoring the effectiveness of a treatment plan for an ear problem. Social isolation is also a common consequence of hearing loss for adolescents, adults and older adults.[30] As a person ages, changes in ear function can result in risk of injury due to dizziness or hearing loss.

Preparation

Arrange the adult in a position of comfort.

Equipment needed

Hand hygiene solution
Additional personal protective equipment as appropriate

PROCEDURES AND NORMAL FINDINGS	ABNORMAL FINDINGS AND CLINICAL ALERTS
General inspection	
You will have already noted the ability of the person to hear your instructions and questions during subjective data collection. During subjective data collection you will also have noticed the colour of the person's skin and mucous membranes, ease of breathing, tone of voice, height-to-weight ratio, level of hygiene and grooming and general demeanour. Make note of your findings.	
Inspect and palpate the external ear	
Size and shape The ears are of equal size bilaterally with no swelling or thickening. Ears of unusual size and shape may be a normal familial trait with no clinical significance.	**Microtia**—ears smaller than 4 cm vertically. **Macrotia**—ears larger than 10 cm vertically. Oedema.
Skin condition The skin is intact, with no lumps or lesions. On some people you may note **Darwin's tubercle**, a small painless nodule at the helix. This is a congenital variation and is not significant (Table 15.1).	Reddened, excessively warm skin indicates inflammation (Table 15.2). Crusts and scaling occur with otitis externa, eczema, contact dermatitis, seborrhoea. Enlarged tender lymph nodes in the region indicate inflammation of the pinna or mastoid process. Red-blue discolouration indicates frostbite. Tophi, sebaceous cyst, chondrodermatitis, keloid, carcinoma (Table 15.1).
Palpate for tenderness Move the pinna and push on the tragus. They should feel firm, and movement should produce no pain. Palpating the mastoid process should not be painful.	Pain with movement occurs with otitis externa and furuncle (infection of a hair follicle). Pain at the mastoid process may indicate mastoiditis or lymphadenitis of the posterior auricular node.
Inspect and palpate the external auditory meatus	
No swelling, redness or discharge should be present.	**Atresia**—absence or closure of the ear canal. A sticky yellow discharge accompanies otitis externa or may indicate otitis media if the tympanic membrane has ruptured. ! ***Clinical alert:*** Frank blood or clear, watery drainage may be cerebrospinal fluid after trauma, which could suggest a basal skull fracture. A person presenting with this sign should be referred for urgent medical review.

PROCEDURES AND NORMAL FINDINGS	ABNORMAL FINDINGS AND CLINICAL ALERTS
Some cerumen is usually present. The colour varies from grey-yellow to light brown and black, and the texture varies from moist and waxy to dry and desiccated. A large amount of cerumen obscures visualisation of the canal and drum.	Impacted cerumen is a common cause of conductive hearing loss.
Test hearing acuity—whispered voice test	
Test one ear at a time while masking hearing in the other ear to prevent sound transmission around the head. This is done by placing one finger on the tragus and rapidly pushing it in and out of the auditory meatus. Shield your lips so the person cannot compensate for a hearing loss (consciously or unconsciously) by lip reading or using the 'good' ear. With your head 30 to 60 cm from the person's ear, exhale and whisper slowly some two-syllable words, such as Tuesday, armchair, football and fourteen. Normally, the person repeats each word correctly after you say it.	The person is unable to hear whispered words. A whisper is a high-frequency sound and is used to detect high-tone loss. If the **whisper test** is positive (hearing loss indicated) or the person reports deafness or significant recent or sudden change in hearing they should be referred for formal hearing testing (audiometry).[31]

Abnormal findings

TABLE 15.1 Lumps and lesions on the external ear

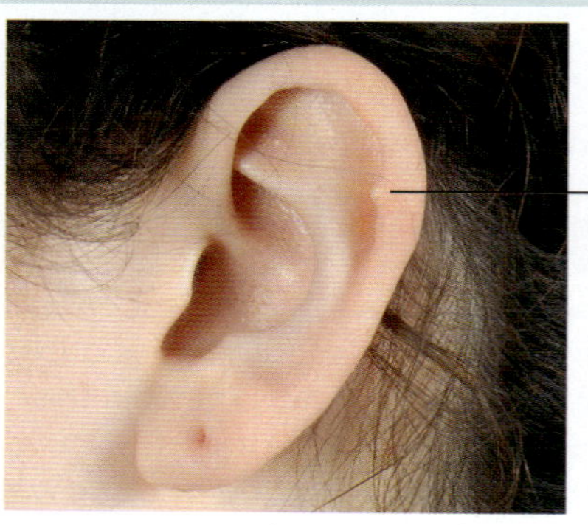

Darwin's tubercle

Small painless nodule at the helix. It is a congenital variation and is not significant. Distinguish this condition from tophus.

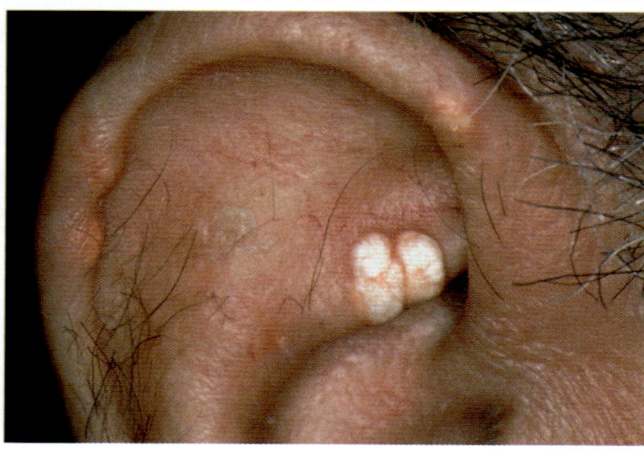

Tophi

Small, whitish-yellow, hard, nontender nodules in or near the helix or antihelix; contain greasy, chalky material of uric acid crystals and are a sign of gout.

TABLE 15.1 Lumps and lesions on the external ear cont'd

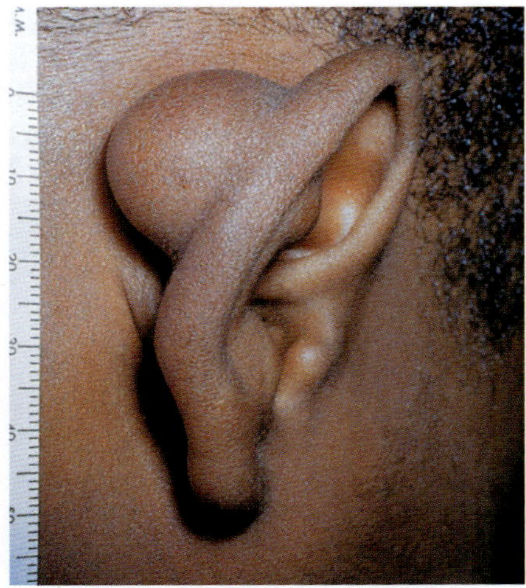

Sebaceous cyst

Location is commonly behind the lobule, in the postauricular fold. A nodule with central black punctum indicates a blocked sebaceous gland. It is filled with waxy sebaceous material and is painful if it becomes infected. Often occur in multiples.

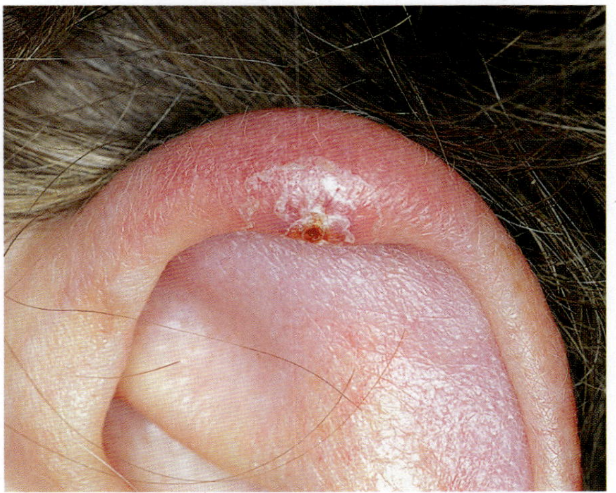

Chondrodermatitis nodularis helices

Painful nodules develop on the rim of the helix (where there is no cushioning subcutaneous tissue) as a result of repetitive mechanical pressure or environmental trauma (sunlight). They are small, indurated, dull red, poorly defined and very painful.

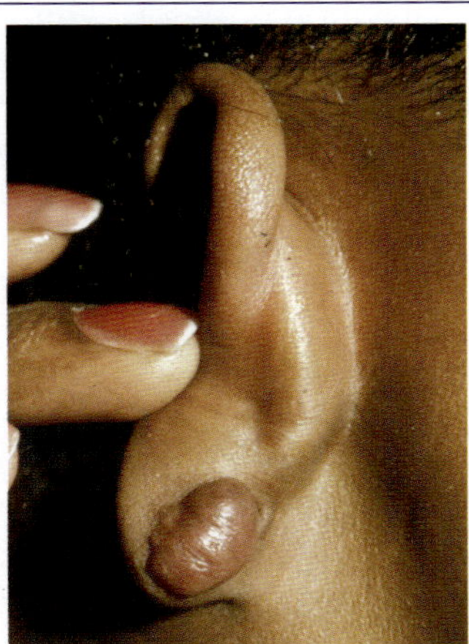

Keloid

Overgrowth of scar tissue, which invades original site of trauma. It is more common in dark-skinned people. In the ear it is most common at the lobule at the site of a pierced ear. Overgrowth shown here is unusually large.

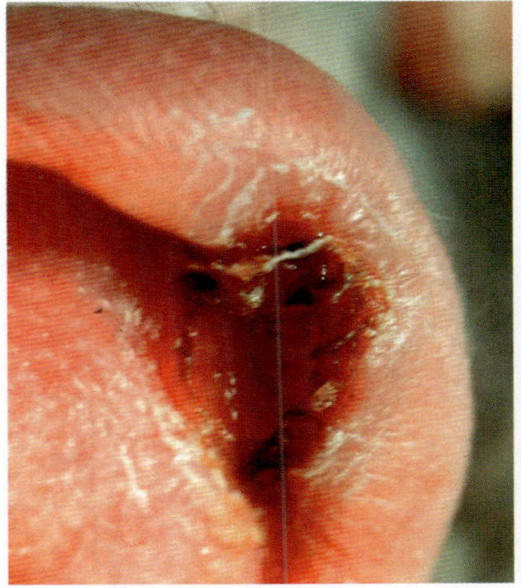

Carcinoma

Ulcerated crusted nodule with indurated base that fails to heal. Bleeds intermittently. This must be referred for biopsy. Usually occurs on the superior rim of the pinna, which has the most sun exposure. May occur also in the ear canal and show chronic discharge that is either serosanguineous or sanguineous.

TABLE 15.2 Abnormalities of the external ear

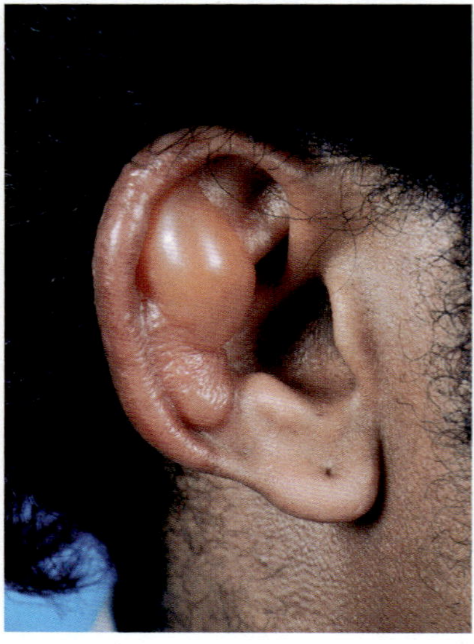

Frostbite

Reddish blue discolouration and swelling of auricle after exposure to extreme cold. Vesicles or bullae may develop, the person feels pain and tenderness and ear necrosis may ensue.

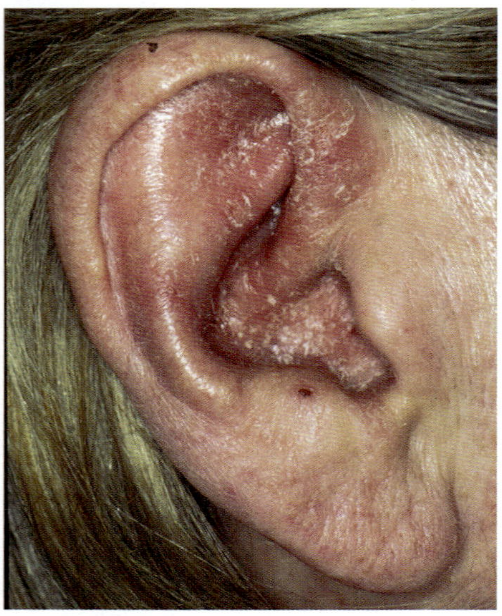

Otitis externa (swimmer's ear)

An infection of the outer ear, with severe painful movement of the pinna and tragus, redness and swelling of pinna and canal, scanty purulent discharge, scaling, itching, fever and enlarged tender regional lymph nodes. Hearing is normal or slightly diminished. More common in hot humid weather. Swimming causes the canal to become waterlogged and swell; skinfolds are set up for infection. Prevent by using rubbing alcohol or 2% acetic acid ear drops after every swim.

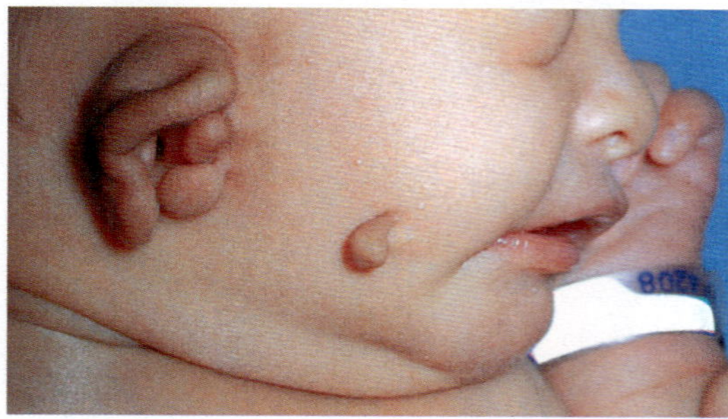

Branchial remnant and ear deformity

A facial remnant or leftover of the embryological branchial arch usually appears as a skin tag, in this case one containing cartilage. They occur most often in the preauricular area, in front of the tragus. When bilateral, there is increased risk of renal anomalies.

Advanced practice—additional data

As well as the objective data described previously, nurses working in advanced practice roles will need additional physical examination skills. The objective ear assessment is used for screening infants and children for hearing loss, investigating symptoms such as ear pain, pressure and fullness, checking for excessive cerumen or other objects in the ear canal and locating the site of an ear infection. A nurse will be able to detect problems in the ear canal or tympanic membrane. Signs of infection, excessive cerumen or foreign objects will clearly be seen. Middle ear infections are often associated with upper respiratory tract infections (Chapter 18). Changes in the objective data have significant implications. Infants and children with ear problems might be irritable, display signs of stress and anxiety and be socially isolated.

The table below includes views seen on otoscopy (Table 15.3) and images of tuning fork tests (Table 15.4).

Preparation

Position the adult sitting up straight with their head at your eye level. Occasionally, the ear canal is partially filled with cerumen, which obstructs your view of the tympanic membrane. In this case, the person should be referred to a medical practitioner for further assessment.

Equipment needed

Hand hygiene solution
Additional personal protective equipment as appropriate
Otoscope with bright light (fresh batteries give off white—not yellow—light)
256 or 512 Hz tuning fork

PROCEDURES AND NORMAL FINDINGS	ABNORMAL FINDINGS AND CLINICAL ALERTS
Inspect the external ear canal	
Note any redness and swelling, lesions, foreign bodies or discharge. If any discharge is present, note the colour and odour. For a person with a hearing aid, note any irritation on the canal wall from poorly fitting hearing aid ear moulds.	Redness and swelling occur with otitis externa; or the ear canal may be completely closed with swelling. This condition clearly will induce temporary unilateral hearing loss and has implications for communication. **Purulent otorrhoea** suggests otitis externa or otitis media if the drum has ruptured. Presence of foreign body, polyp, furuncle, exostosis (Table 15.5).
Inspection with the otoscope	
As you inspect the external ear, note the size of the auditory meatus. Then choose the largest speculum that will fit comfortably in the ear canal and attach it to the otoscope. Tilt the person's head slightly away from you towards the opposite shoulder. This method brings the obliquely sloping eardrum into better view.	

PROCEDURES AND NORMAL FINDINGS	ABNORMAL FINDINGS AND CLINICAL ALERTS
Pull the pinna up and back on a pre-adolescent child or adult; this helps straighten the S-shape of the canal (Figure 15.7). Hold the pinna gently but firmly. Do not release traction on the ear until you have finished the examination, and the otoscope is removed.	Pulling on the pinna may cause and increase pain if the person has otitis media.
Hold the otoscope 'upside down' along your fingers and have the dorsa (back) of your hand along the person's cheek braced to steady the otoscope (Figure 15.8). This position feels awkward to you only at first. It soon will feel natural, and you will find it useful to prevent forceful insertion. Also, your stabilising hand acts as a protecting lever if the person suddenly moves their head.	
Insert the speculum slowly and carefully along the axis of the canal. Watch the insertion; then put your eye up to the otoscope. Avoid touching the inner 'bony' section of the canal wall, which is covered by a thin epithelial layer and is sensitive to pain. Sometimes you cannot see anything but canal wall. If so, try to reposition the person's head, apply more traction on the pinna and re-angle the otoscope to look forwards and towards the person's nose.	

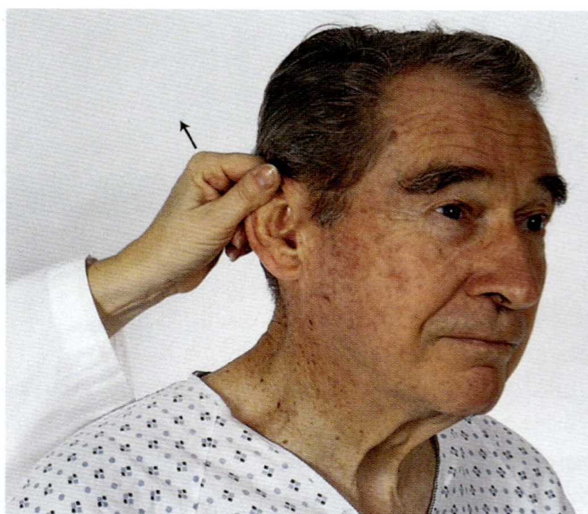

FIGURE 15.7 Pulling on an adult pinna

PROCEDURES AND NORMAL FINDINGS	ABNORMAL FINDINGS AND CLINICAL ALERTS
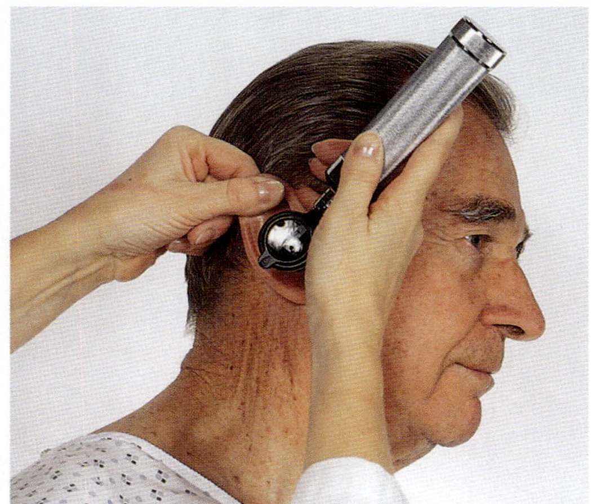 **FIGURE 15.8** Holding the otoscope	Once it is in place, you may need to rotate the otoscope slightly to visualise the entire eardrum; do this gently. Last, perform the otoscopic examination. Once the otoscope is in place, you may need to rotate it slightly to visualise the entire eardrum; do this gently. Last, perform the otoscopic examination before you test hearing; ear canals with impacted cerumen give the erroneous impression of pathological hearing loss (Table 15.5).
Tympanic membrane	
Colour and characteristics. Systematically explore its landmarks (Figure 15.9). The normal eardrum is shiny and translucent, with a pearl-grey colour. The cone-shaped light reflex is prominent in the anteroinferior quadrant (at 5 o'clock in the right drum and 7 o'clock in the left drum). This is the reflection of your otoscope light. Sections of the malleus are visible through the translucent drum: the umbo, manubrium and short process. (Infrequently, you also may see the incus behind the drum; it shows as a whitish haze in the upper posterior area.) At the periphery the annulus looks whiter and denser.	Yellow–amber drum colour occurs with otitis media with effusion (serous). Red colour occurs with acute otitis media. Absent or distorted landmarks. Air/fluid level or air bubbles behind drum indicate otitis media with effusion (Table 15.6).
Position. The eardrum is flat, slightly pulled in at the centre and flutters when the person performs the Valsalva manoeuvre or holds the nose and swallows (insufflation). You may elicit these manoeuvres to assess drum mobility. Avoid them with an ageing person because they may disrupt equilibrium. Also, avoid middle ear insufflation in a person with upper respiratory infection because it could propel infectious matter into the middle ear.	Retracted drum resulting from vacuum in middle ear with obstructed Eustachian tube. Bulging drum from increased pressure in otitis media. Drum hypomobility is an early sign of otitis media (Table 15.6).

PROCEDURES AND NORMAL FINDINGS	ABNORMAL FINDINGS AND CLINICAL ALERTS
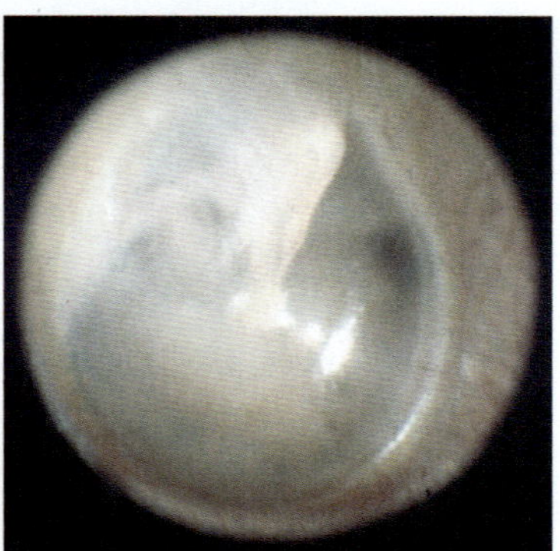 **FIGURE 15.9** Normal tympanic membrane	
Integrity of membrane. Inspect the eardrum and the entire circumference of the annulus for perforations. The normal tympanic membrane is intact. Some adults may show scarring, which is a dense white patch on the drum. This is a sequela of repeated ear infections (Table 15.3). Clean any discharge from the speculum before examining the other ear to avoid contamination with possibly infectious material.	Perforation shows as a dark oval area or as a larger opening on the drum. Vesicles on drum (Table 15.6).
Test hearing acuity as per previous section	
Weber test	
The tuning fork test measures hearing by air conduction or bone conduction, in which the sound vibrates through the cranial bones to the inner ear. This test may help differentiate the type of hearing loss such as conductive or sensorineural. Using a 256 or 512 Hz tuning fork, the tines are activated by striking them on the ulnar border of the palm. The stem of the fork is placed firmly in the middle of the person's forehead or midline on the top of the head. Ask the person where the sound is heard (centrally or towards one side). Sound should be heard equally in both ears (Table 15.5).	**Air conduction**—transmission of sound through the ear canal to inner ear to the auditory nerve. **Bone conduction**—transmission of sound through skull bones to the cochlea to the auditory nerve. If the sound is heard in one ear this might indicate unilateral conductive hearing loss. However, up to 40% of normal hearing people lateralise the Weber test—that is, they hear the tone louder in one ear. Because the Weber test is not a reliable indicator, audiometry is highly recommended.

PROCEDURES AND NORMAL FINDINGS	ABNORMAL FINDINGS AND CLINICAL ALERTS
Rinne test	
The Rinne test is where a vibrating tuning fork is placed on the mastoid process behind the ear. When the sound disappears, the tuning fork is placed in line with the external meatus (Table 15.5). Normally the sound is heard at the external meatus.	If the sound is not audible at the external meatus, this may indicate middle ear (conduction) deafness. Both the Weber and the Rinne tests should be followed up with audiometry where tests of mechanical sound transmission (middle ear function), neural sound transmission (cochlear function) and speech discrimination ability are conducted by an audiologist.
Test the vestibular apparatus	
The **Romberg test** assesses the ability of the vestibular apparatus in the inner ear to help maintain standing balance. The Romberg test also assesses intactness of the cerebellum and proprioception and therefore it is also discussed in Chapter 12 (Figure 12.28).	
Additional objective data for infants and children	
Inspect external ear structure	
Examination of the external ear is like that described for an adult, with the addition of examination of position and alignment on head. Note the ear position. The top of the pinna should match an imaginary line extending from the corner of the eye to the occiput. Also, the ear should be positioned within 10 degrees of vertical (Figure 15.10). Low-set ears or deviation in alignment may be associated with some congenital syndromes.	

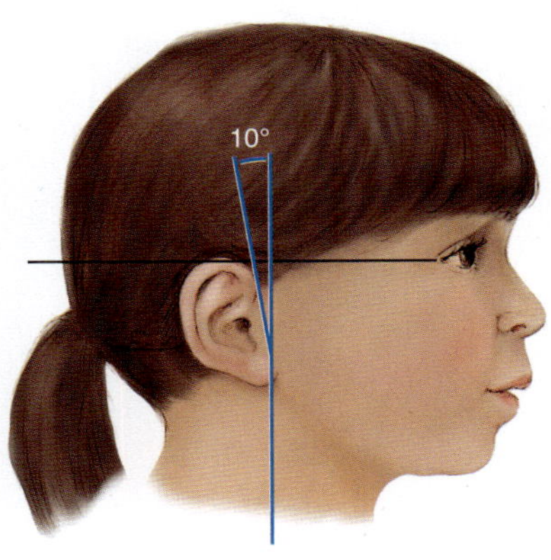

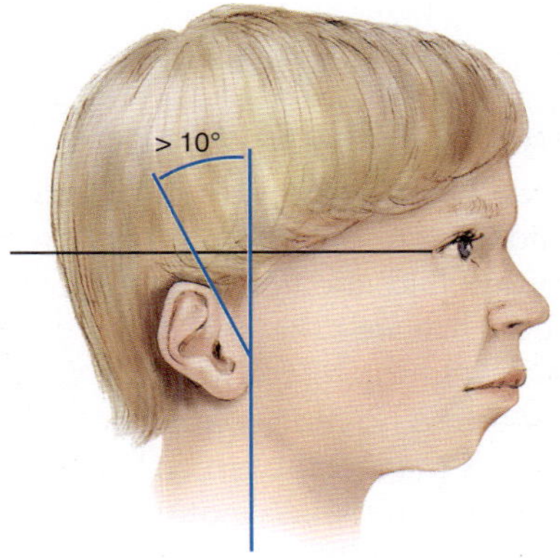

FIGURE 15.10 Ear alignment (child)

PROCEDURES AND NORMAL FINDINGS	ABNORMAL FINDINGS AND CLINICAL ALERTS

Test hearing acuity

Newborn—startle (Moro) reflex, acoustic blink reflex
3–4 months—acoustic blink reflex, infant stops movement and appears to 'listen', halts sucking, quiets if crying, cries if quiet

Absence of alerting behaviour may indicate congenital deafness.

6–8 months—infant turns head to localise sound, responds to own name

Failure to localise sound.

Preschool and school-age child—child must be screened with audiometry.
Note that a young child may be unaware of a hearing loss because the child does not know how one 'ought' to hear.

No intelligible speech by 2 years of age.
Note these behavioural manifestations of hearing loss:

- The child is inattentive in casual conversation.
- The child reacts more to movement and facial expression than to sound.
- The child's facial expression is strained or puzzled.
- The child frequently asks to have statements repeated.
- The child confuses words that sound alike.
- The child has an accompanying speech problem: speech is monotonous or garbled; the child mispronounces or omits sounds.
- The child appears shy and withdrawn and 'lives in a world of their own'.
- The child frequently complains of earaches.
- The child hears better at times when the environment is more conducive to hearing.

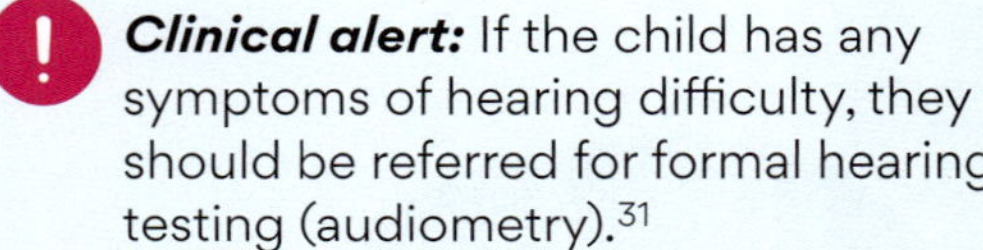

Clinical alert: If the child has any symptoms of hearing difficulty, they should be referred for formal hearing testing (audiometry).[31]

Inspection with otoscope

Eardrum assessment is mandatory for any infant or child requiring care for illness or fever. For an infant or young child, the timing of the otoscopic examination is best towards the end of the complete examination. Many young children protest vigorously during this procedure no matter how well you prepare, and it is difficult to re-establish cooperation afterwards. Save the otoscopic examination until last. Then the parent/caregiver can hold and comfort the child.

To help prepare the child, let the child hold your funny-looking 'torch' that is the otoscope. You may wish to have the child look in the parent's/caregiver's ear as you hold the otoscope (Figure 15.11).

PROCEDURES AND NORMAL FINDINGS

ABNORMAL FINDINGS AND CLINICAL ALERTS

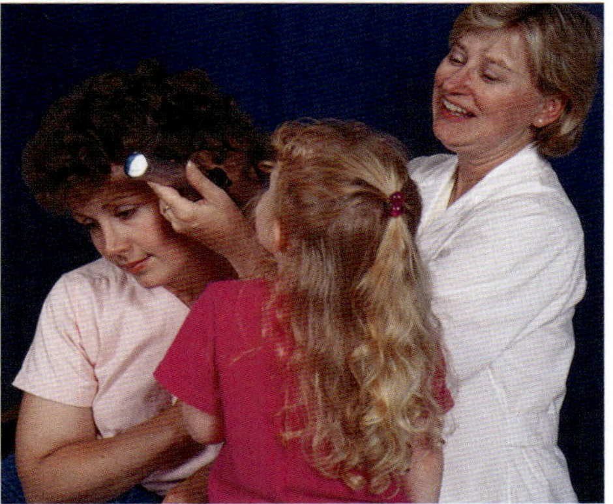

FIGURE 15.11 Preparing a child for an otoscopic examination

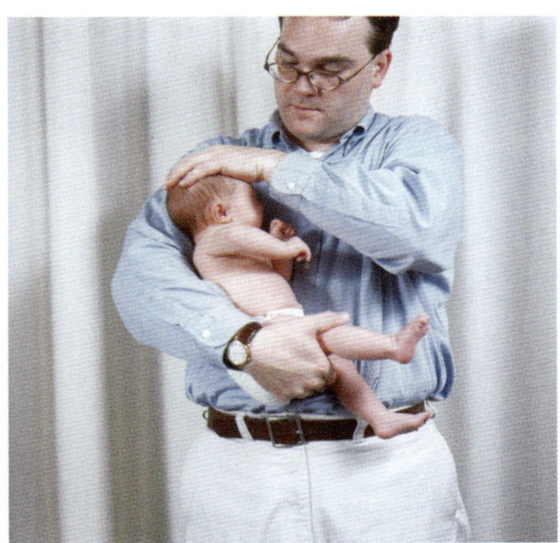

FIGURE 15.12 Holding an infant for an otoscopic examination

Positioning of the child is important. You need a clear view of the canal. Avoid harsh restraint, but you must protect the eardrum from injury in case of sudden head movement. Enlist the aid of a cooperative parent/caregiver. Prop an infant upright against the adult's chest or shoulder, with the adult's arm around the upper part of the head (Figure 15.12). A toddler can be held in the parent's/caregiver's lap or may lie on the examining table with their arms secured (Figure 15.13). In each case, the child's head is stabilised to avoid movement against the otoscope.

PROCEDURES AND NORMAL FINDINGS

ABNORMAL FINDINGS AND CLINICAL ALERTS

FIGURE 15.13 Positioning a child for an otoscopic examination

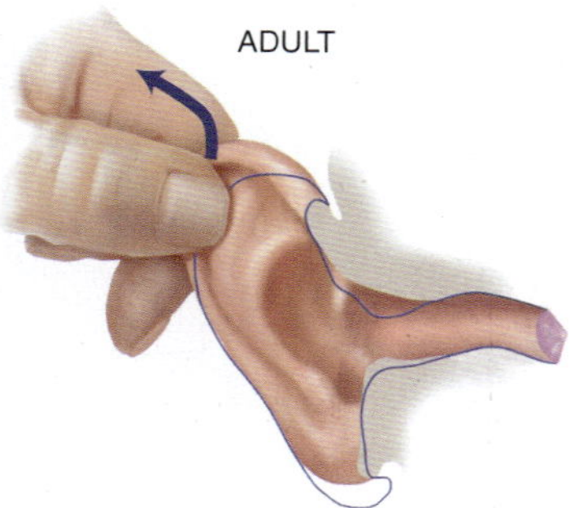

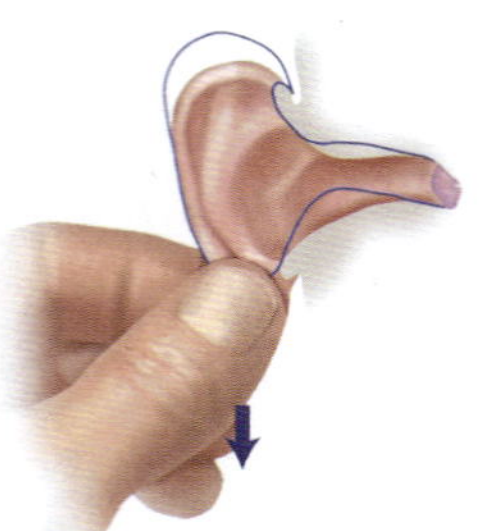

FIGURE 15.14 Pulling a child's pinna in an otoscopic examination

Remember to pull the pinna straight down on an infant or a child under 3 years old. This method will match the slope of the ear canal (Figure 15.14).

At birth the patency of the ear canal is determined, but the otoscopic examination is not performed because the canal is filled with amniotic fluid and vernix caseosa. After a few days the tympanic membrane is examined. During the first few days, the tympanic membrane often looks thickened and opaque. It may look 'injected' and have a mild redness from increased vascularity. The eardrum may look red, with prominent blood vessels in infants after crying.

PROCEDURES AND NORMAL FINDINGS	ABNORMAL FINDINGS AND CLINICAL ALERTS
The position of the eardrum is more horizontal in the neonate, making it more difficult to see completely and harder to differentiate from the canal wall. By 1 month of age, the drum is in the oblique (more vertical) position as in the older child and examination is a bit easier.	
Normally the tympanic membrane is intact. In a child being treated for chronic otitis media, you may note the presence of a tympanostomy tube (grommet) in the central part of the eardrum. This is inserted surgically to equalise pressure and drain secretions. Finally, although the condition is not normal, it is not uncommon to note a foreign body in a child's canal, such as a small stone or a bead.	**Chronic otitis media** relieved by tympanostomy tubes (Table 15.6). Foreign body (Table 15.5).
Additional objective data for adults over 65 years	
Inspect external ear structure	
An older person may have pendulous earlobes with linear wrinkling because of loss of elasticity of the pinna. Coarse, wiry hairs may be present at the opening of the ear canal.	
Test hearing acuity	
A high-tone frequency hearing loss is apparent for those affected with presbycusis, the hearing loss that occurs with ageing. This condition is revealed in difficulty hearing whispered words in the voice test and in difficulty hearing consonants during conversational speech. Older adults may think 'people are mumbling' and feel isolated in family or friendship groups.	If an older adult has any symptoms of hearing difficulty or a sudden hearing loss they should be urgently referred for formal hearing testing (audiometry).[32] Some people have had poor results from hearing aids and refuse to wear them. Hearing aids may be rejected because of negative self-image. Hearing loss can have a negative impact on a person's quality of life. Loss of hearing is associated with anxiety and depression and is a predictor of poor cognitive function in older adults.[34]
Inspection with otoscope	
During otoscopy the eardrum may be whiter in colour and more opaque, duller than in the early or middle adult. It may also look thickened.	If an older adult has any symptoms of hearing difficulty or a sudden hearing loss they should be urgently referred for formal hearing testing (audiometry).[35]

Abnormal findings for advanced practice

TABLE 15.3 Abnormal views seen on otoscopy

Appearance of Eardrum	Indicates	Suggested Condition
Yellow–amber colour	Serum or pus	Otitis media with effusion or chronic otitis media
Prominent landmarks	Retraction of drum	Vacuum in middle ear from obstructed Eustachian tube
Air–fluid level or air bubbles	Serous fluid	Otitis media with effusion
Absent or distorted light reflex	Bulging of eardrum	Acute otitis media
Bright red colour	Infection in middle ear	Acute otitis media
Blue or dark red colour	Blood behind drum	Trauma, skull fracture
Dark, round or oval areas	Perforation	Drum rupture
White dense areas	Scarring	Sequelae of infections
Diminished or absent landmarks	Thickened drum	Chronic otitis media
Black or white dots on drum or canal	Colony of growth	Fungal infection

TABLE 15.4 Tuning fork tests

Weber Test

Normal

Normal—Sound is equally loud in both ears; sound does not lateralise.

Rinne Test

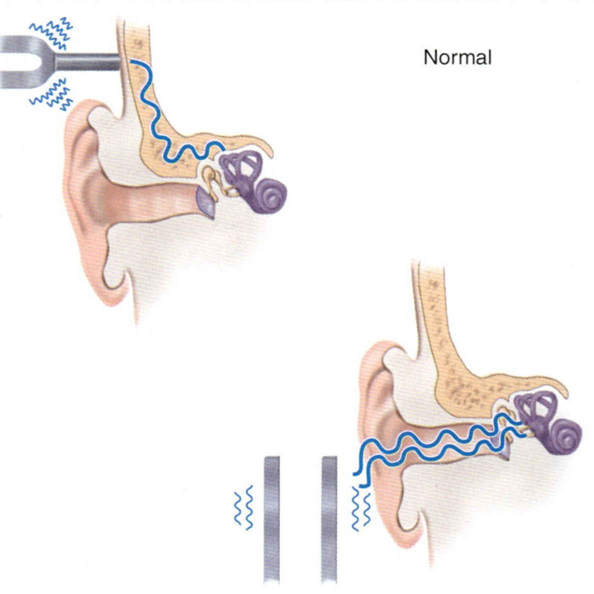

Normal—Sound is heard twice as long by air conduction (AC) as by bone conduction (BC); a 'positive' Rinne, or AC > BC.

TABLE 15.4 Tuning fork tests cont'd

Weber Test	Rinne Test
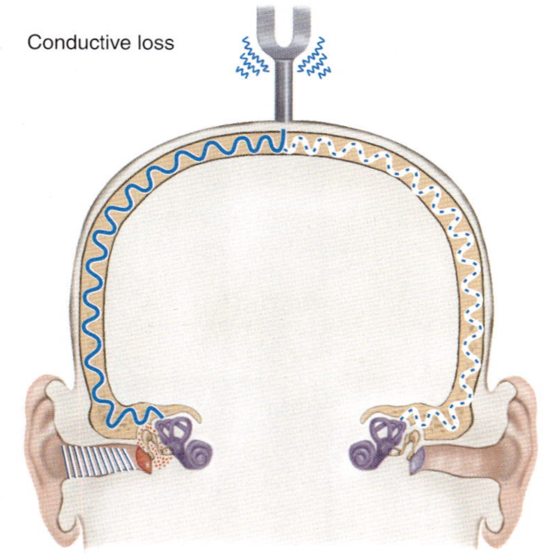	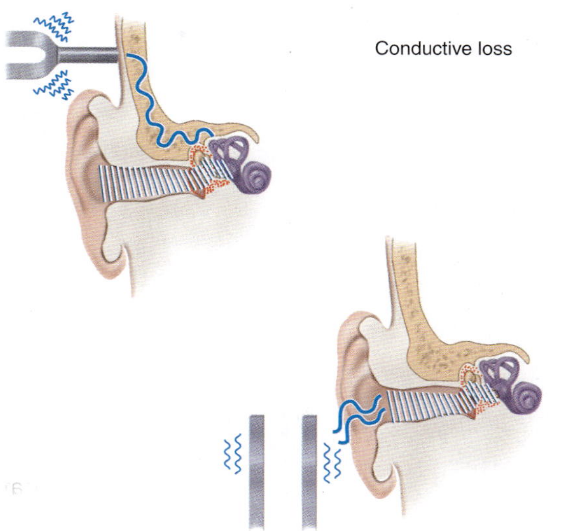
Conductive loss—Sound lateralises to 'poorer' ear from background room noise, which masks hearing in normal ear. 'Poorer' ear (the one with conductive loss) is not distracted by background noise and so has a better chance to hear bone-conducted sound. Examples: transient conductive loss with serous or purulent otitis media.	**Conductive loss**—Person hears equally long by bone conduction as by air conduction (AC = BC) or even longer (AC < BC). The Rinne test may be accurate to detect conductive loss, and loss can be confirmed by audiometry.[33]

Continued

TABLE 15.4 Tuning fork tests cont'd

Weber Test

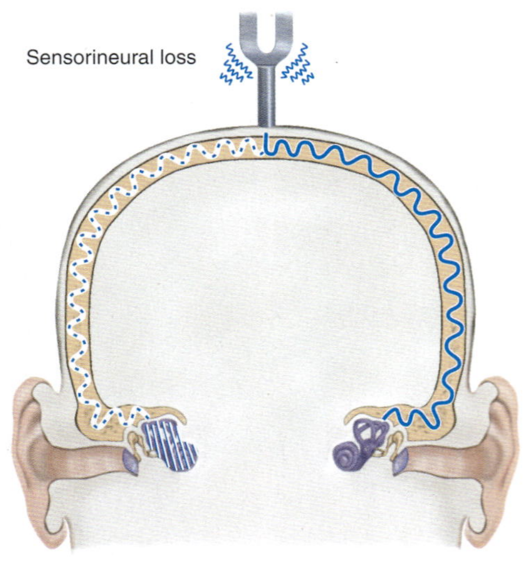

Sensorineural loss—Sound lateralises to 'better' ear or unaffected ear. Poorer ear (the one with nerve loss) is unable to perceive the sound. However, many people with unilateral loss (conductive or sensorineural) still localise the sound in the midline. Confirm with audiometry.

Rinne Test

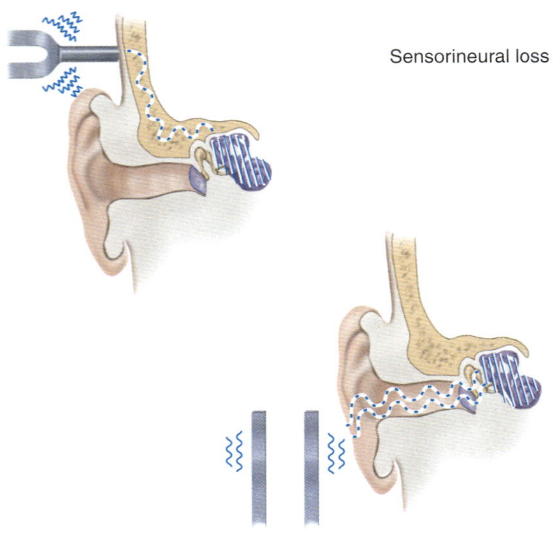

Sensorineural loss—Normal ratio of AC > BC is intact but is reduced overall. That is, the person hears poorly both ways. Confirm with audiometry.

TABLE 15.5 Abnormalities in the ear canal

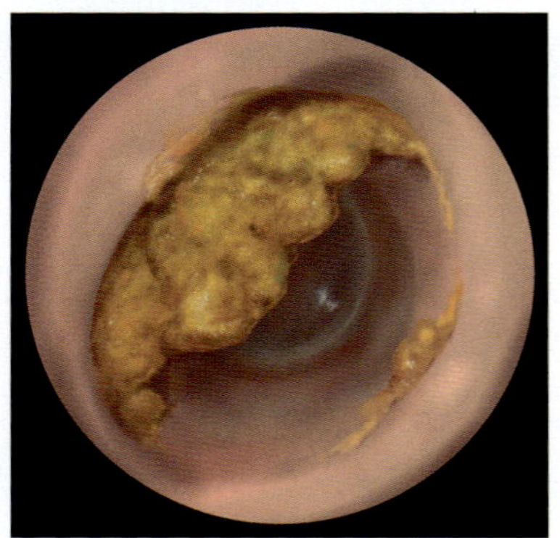

Excessive cerumen

Excessive cerumen is produced or is impacted because of narrow tortuous canal or poor cleaning method. May show as round ball partially obscuring drum or totally occluding canal. Even when canal is 90 to 95% blocked, hearing stays normal. But when the last 5 to 10% is totally occluded (when cerumen expands after swimming or showering), the person has ear fullness and sudden hearing loss.

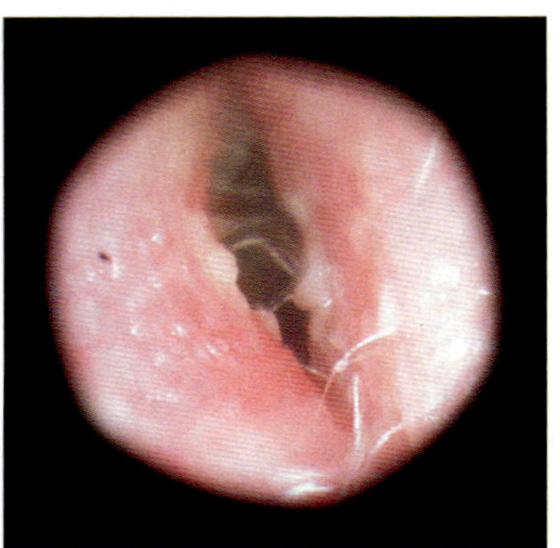

Otitis externa

Severe swelling of the canal, inflammation, tenderness. Here canal lumen is narrowed to one-quarter of its normal size. (See complete description in Table 15.2.)

TABLE 15.5 Abnormalities in the ear canal cont'd

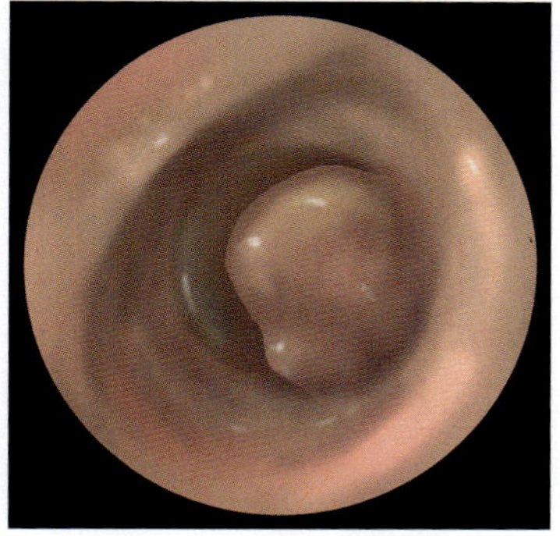

Osteoma

Single, stony hard, rounded nodule that obscures the drum; nontender; overlying skin appears normal. Attached to inner third, the bony part, of the canal. Benign, but refer for removal.

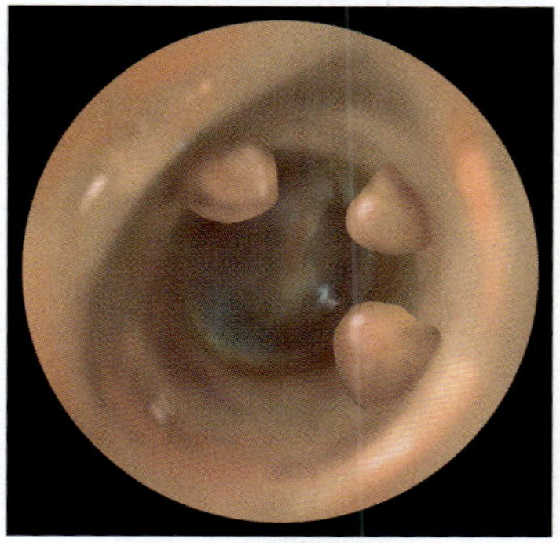

Exostosis

More common than osteoma. Small, hard, rounded nodules of hypertrophic bone covered with normal epithelium. They arise near the drum but usually do not obstruct the view of the drum. They are usually multiple and bilateral. They may occur more frequently in cold-water swimmers. The condition needs no treatment, although it may cause accumulation of cerumen, which blocks the canal.

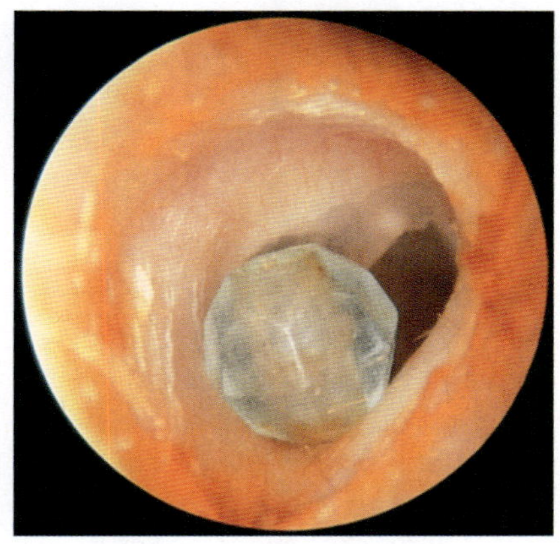

Foreign body

Usually it is children who place a foreign body in the ear (here, a stone completely occludes the canal), which is later noted on routine examination. Common objects are beans, corn, breakfast cereals, jewellery beads, small stones, sponge and rubber. Cotton is most common in adults and becomes impacted from cotton-tipped applicators. A trapped live insect is uncommon but makes the person especially frantic.

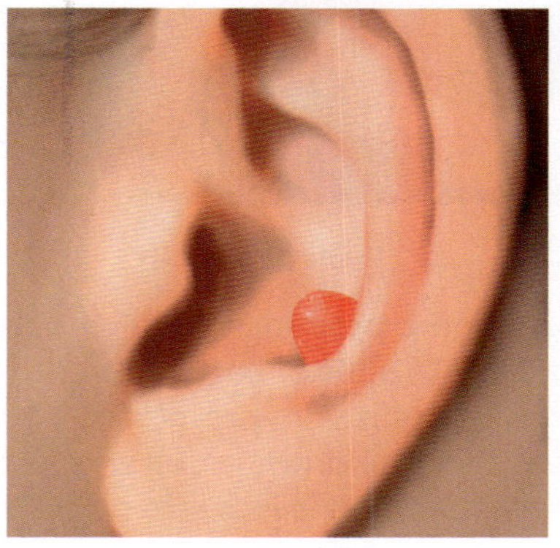

Furuncle

Exquisitely painful, reddened, infected hair follicle. Here, it occurs on the tragus but also may be on cartilaginous part of ear canal. Regional lymphadenopathy often accompanies a furuncle.

Continued

TABLE 15.5 Abnormalities in the ear canal cont'd

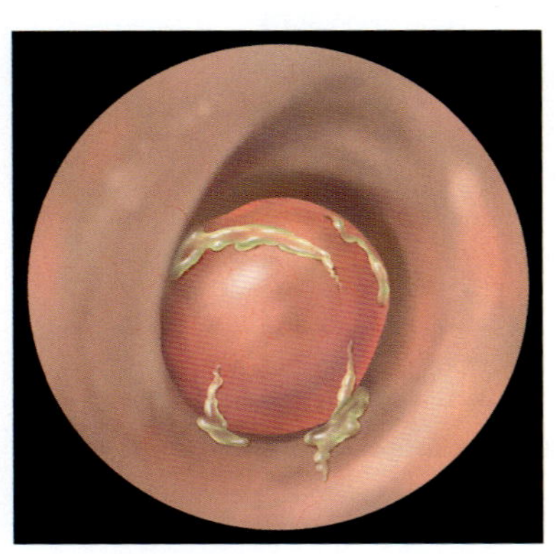

Polyp

Arises in canal from granulomatous or mucosal tissue; redder than surrounding skin and bleeds easily; bathed in foul purulent discharge; indicates chronic ear disease. Benign, but refer for excision.

TABLE 15.6 Abnormalities of the tympanic membrane

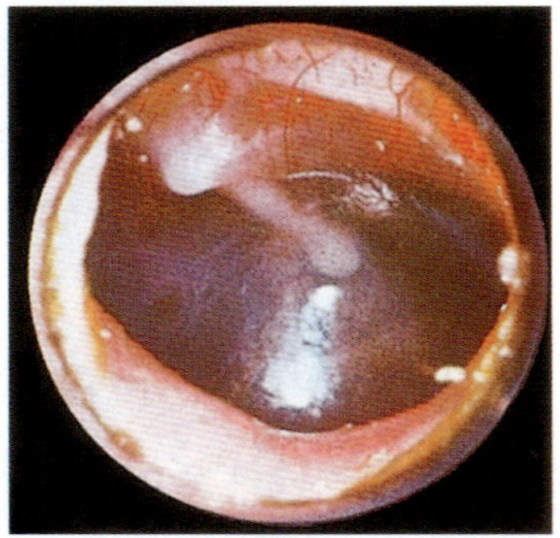

Retracted drum

Landmarks look more prominent and well defined. Malleus handle looks shorter and more horizontal than normal. Short process is very prominent. Light reflex is absent or distorted. The drum is dull and lustreless and does not move. These signs indicate negative pressure and middle ear vacuum from obstructed Eustachian tube and serous otitis media.

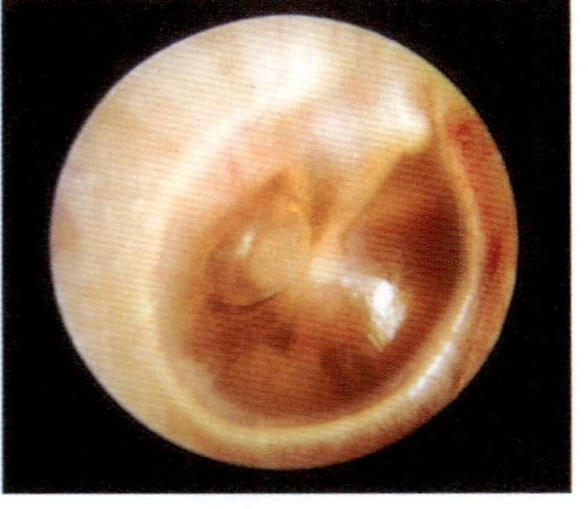

Otitis media with effusion

An amber–yellow drum suggests serum in middle ear that transudates to relieve negative pressure from the blocked Eustachian tube. You may note an air–fluid level with fine black dividing line or air bubbles visible behind drum. Symptoms are feeling of fullness, transient hearing loss, popping sound with swallowing. Also called serous otitis media or glue ear.

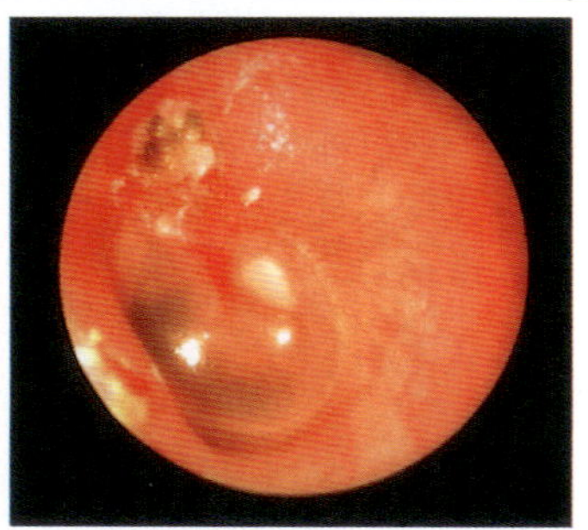

Cholesteatoma

An overgrowth of epidermal tissue in the middle ear or temporal bone may result over the years after a marginal tympanic membrane perforation. It has a pearly white, cheesy appearance. Growth of cholesteatoma can erode bone and produce hearing loss. Early signs include otorrhoea, unilateral conductive hearing loss and tinnitus.

TABLE 15.6 Abnormalities of the tympanic membrane cont'd

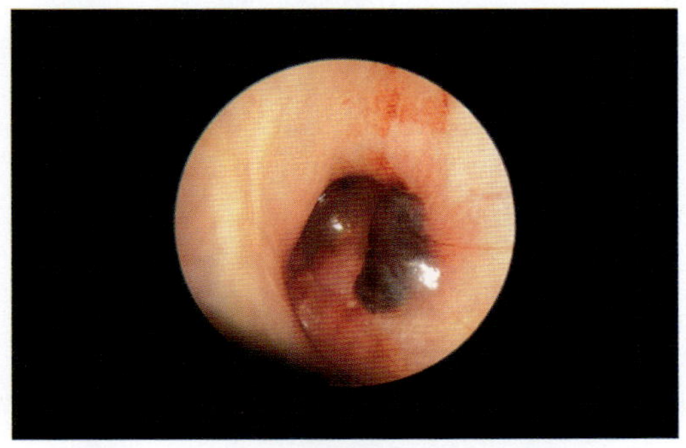

Bullous myringitis

Small vesicles containing blood on the drum; accompany mycoplasma pneumonia and virus infections. May have blood-tinged discharge and severe otalgia.

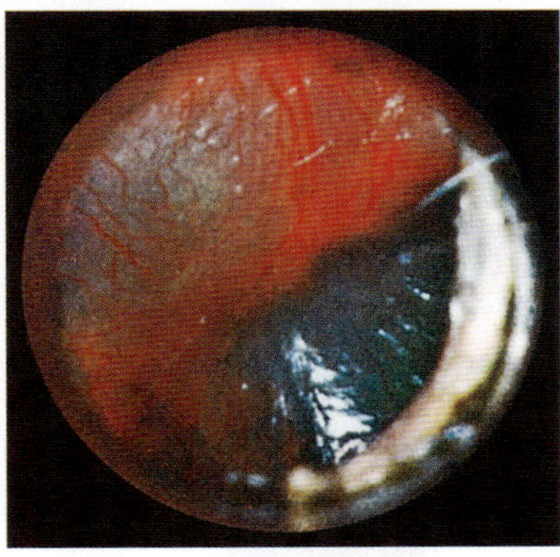

Early stage

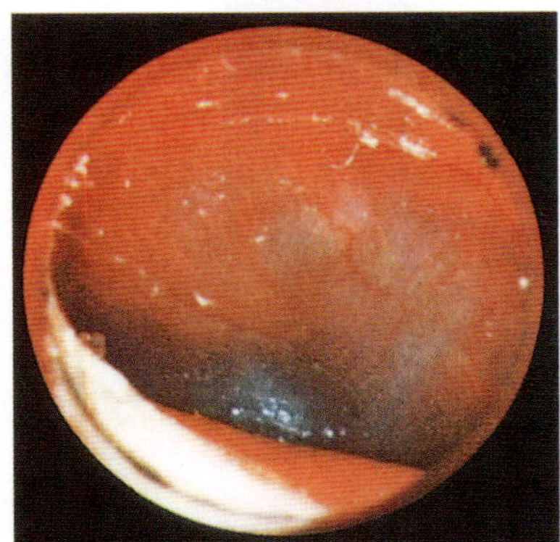

Later stage

Acute (purulent) otitis media

This results when the middle-ear fluid is infected. An absent light reflex from increasing middle ear pressure is an early sign. Redness and bulging are first noted in the superior part of the drum (pars flaccida), along with earache and fever. Then fiery red bulging of entire drum occurs; deep throbbing pain; fever and transient hearing loss. Pneumatic otoscopy reveals drum hypomobility.

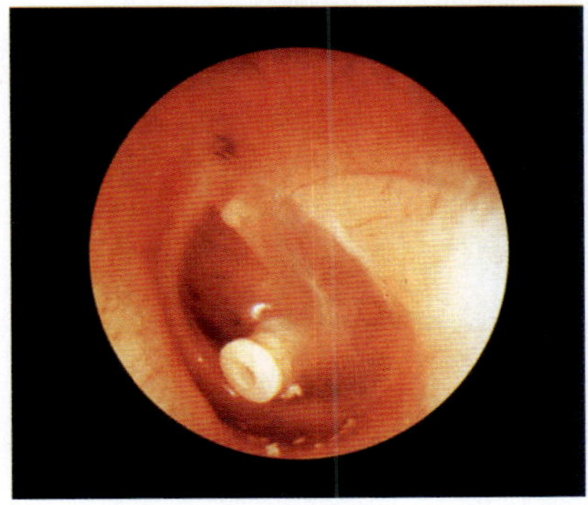

Insertion of tubes (grommets)

Polyethylene tubes are inserted surgically into the eardrum to relieve middle-ear pressure and promote drainage of chronic or recurrent middle-ear infections. The number of acute infections tends to decrease because of improved aeration. Tubes extrude spontaneously in 12 to 18 months. In Australia and Aotearoa New Zealand these tubes are called ventilation tubes or grommets.

Continued

TABLE 15.6 Abnormalities of the tympanic membrane cont'd

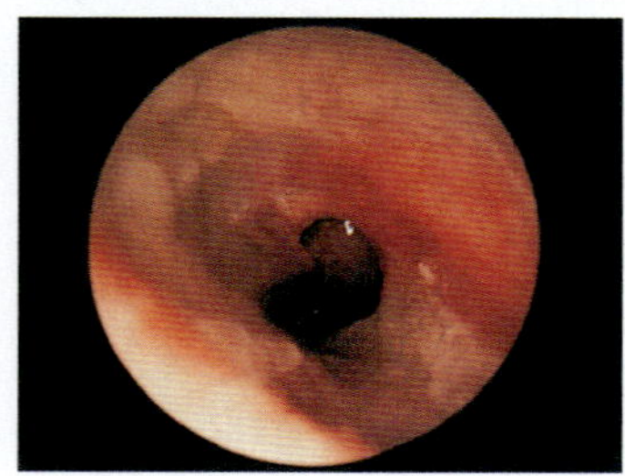

Perforation

If the acute otitis media is not treated, the drum may rupture from increased pressure. Perforations also occur from trauma (e.g. a slap on the ear). Usually the perforation appears as a round or oval darkened area on the drum, but in this photo the perforation is very large. *Central* perforations occur in the pars tensa. *Marginal* perforations occur at the annulus. Marginal perforations are called *attic perforations* when they occur in the superior part of the drum, the pars flaccida.

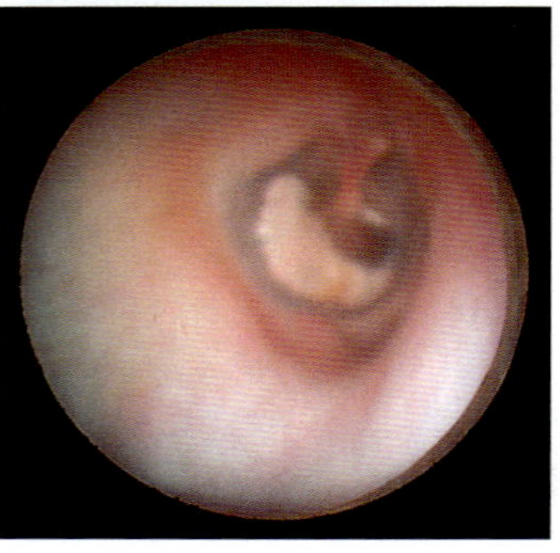

Scarred drum

Dense white patches on the eardrum are sequelae of repeated ear infections. They do not necessarily affect hearing.

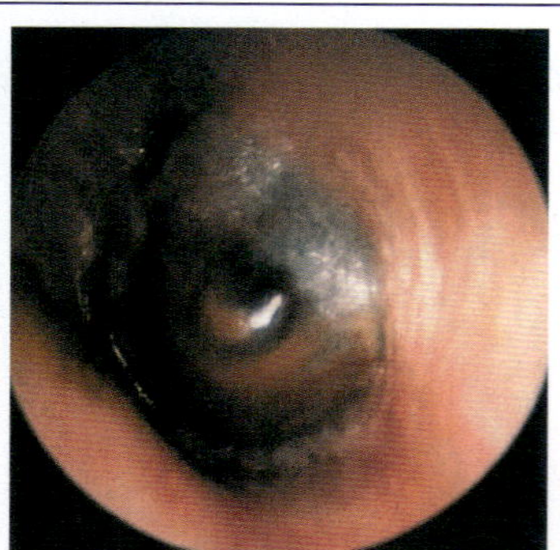

Blue drum (haemotympanum)

This indicates blood in the middle ear, as in trauma resulting in skull fracture.

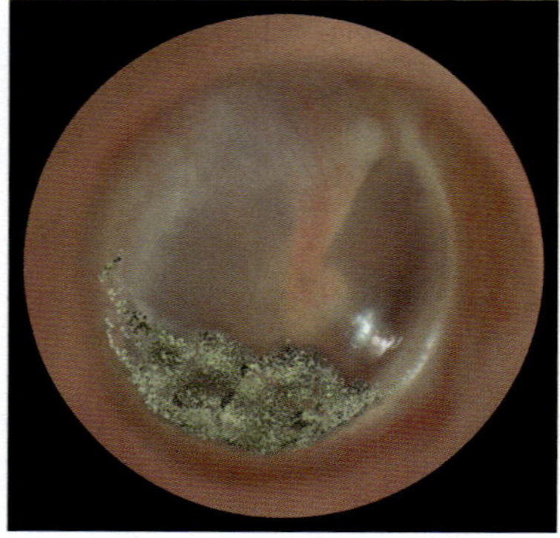

Fungal infection (otomycosis)

Colony of black or white dots on drum or canal wall suggests a yeast or fungal infection.

Clinical reasoning and documentation

The following case studies give examples of typical situations involving ear assessment and the clinical reasoning process including problem/issue identification. Consult a fundamentals of nursing or medical-surgical nursing text for information about goal setting, nursing interventions and evaluation.

Case study 1 (continued)—Middle ear infection

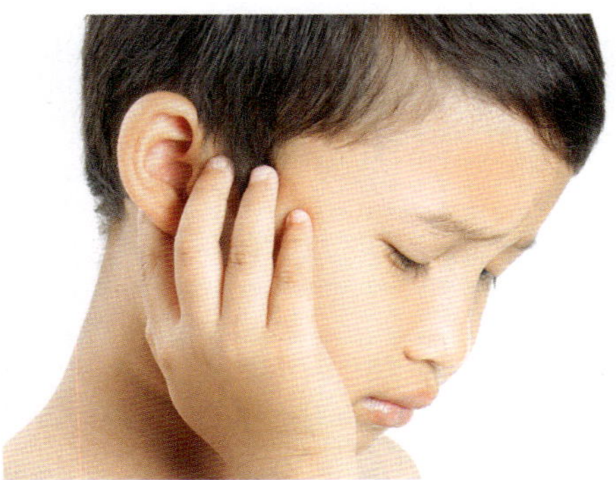

Context

You will recall from the case study described earlier in the chapter that you are working as a practice nurse in a busy local multidisciplinary health clinic. Your role includes screening assessments for clients who attend.

Consider the patient's situation

Matthew Williams is a 4-year-old child who was brought into the clinic by his mother after he had been crying for most of the night and was difficult to settle. The only sleep the child had was when he was held upright against his mother's chest, but he slept for short periods only. The child feels warm to touch.

Collect cues/information

Your further assessment reveals the following information.

Subjective data

Matthew is the second child born to Mr and Mrs Williams. He was born at term. The pregnancy, labour and delivery were uncomplicated. Matthew is up to date with all childhood immunisations and has no significant previous medical history. His mother reports that Matthew has recently had a mild cold.

Matthew and his parents live in a small two-bedroom house approximately 40 km north of the central business district. He shares a bedroom with his older sister who is aged 6 years. Matthew's father works at the local council undertaking park and garden maintenance, and Matthew's mother works as a receptionist in a community centre. While the parents are working, the children are cared for by their maternal grandmother. The grandmother also cares for two other grandchildren every day. Both parents and Matthew's grandmother smoke up to 10 cigarettes each per day.

Yesterday, Matthew's grandmother put him to bed for his afternoon sleep. He did not sleep very long before he awoke crying and tugging at his right ear. Although he would drink only small amounts of cordial, he refused to eat solid food. When his mother collected him at the end of the day after work, she found his temperature was 38°C (tympanic). Matthew has been fussing and crying most of the night. His mother has not tried to give him any medication.

Objective data

Temp 38.4°C (tympanic), HR 100, RR 20.

Alert, developmentally appropriate for age.

Skin: Warm and dry, no rashes or lesions.

Eyes: No exudate, conjunctivae clear, sclerae white.

Ears: Left tympanic membrane is intact and pearly grey in appearance. Right tympanic membrane dull red and bulging, no light reflex.

Nose: Sniffly breathing with small amount of clear nasal discharge

Mouth/throat: Oral mucosa pink, no lesions or exudate, tonsils 1+

Lungs: Breath sounds clear and equal bilaterally, no laboured breathing

Process information and identify problems/issues

Collaborative problem

Probable acute otitis media—needs referral to a GP for review and treatment.

Continued

Clinical reasoning and documentation cont'd

Problem statements/nursing diagnoses

Pain related to inflammation in right ear
Risk for chronic ear infection injury related to risk factors
Discomfort related to high temperature
Knowledge deficit for parents and guardians about risk factors and aspects of care

Case study 2: Ringing sound in ears

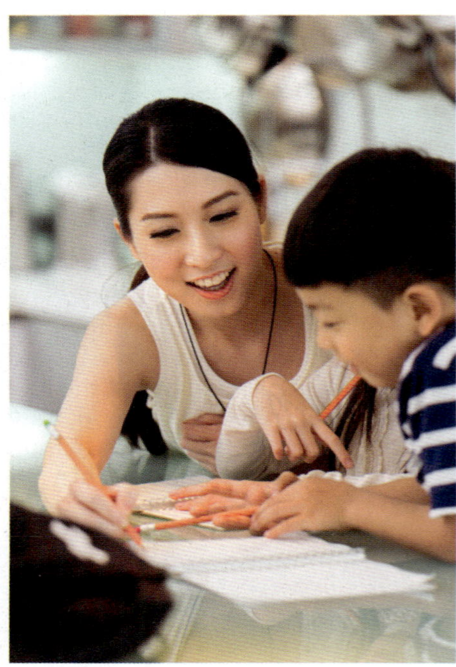

Context

You are on a clinical placement at a health clinic. You are working alongside a practice nurse.

Consider the patient's situation

Julia Chong is a 35-year-old single woman. She is employed as a teacher in a local primary school, teaching children who are in year 2.

Collect cues/information

Subjective data

Julia has presented to the health clinic reporting (1) 'ringing in her ears' that she has experienced consistently since attending a concert on Saturday night and (2) being unable to hear the students clearly when they spoke to her over the last couple of days at school.
She reports that in her early 20s she went out to see local bands or visit nightclubs almost every weekend. Over the past year or so, she has found it hard to hear when she is in the company of a group of people or if there is background noise. She has been frustrated when she can't take part in conversations with others and is left feeling isolated.
She also says she has had intermittent periods of tinnitus that did not bother her and for which she has never sought medical attention.

Objective data

Temp 37°C oral, HR 72, BP 120/70.
Ears: Right and left tympanic membranes are intact and pearly grey in appearance. Small amount of yellow cerumen in left ear canal.
Nose: Able to breath effectively through both nostrils.
Throat: Moist and pink. Tonsils present.
Hearing: Whisper test—reduced hearing in right and left ears.

Process information and identify problems/issues

Collaborative problem

Probable noise-induced hearing loss—requires referral for testing of auditory function and to GP for examination and management.

Problem statements/nursing diagnoses

Disturbed sensory perception related to ringing in ears and hearing impairment
Risk of impaired verbal communication related to hearing loss and its implications on personal and professional life.
Lack of knowledge related to preventative measures and management strategies.

ADDITIONAL RESOURCES

You can further develop your knowledge and skills relevant to ear assessment, related pathophysiology, common health issues and nursing interventions by:

- reading chapters of a fundamentals of nursing or medical-surgical nursing textbook
- answering chapter multiple choice questions online. Log onto ClinicalKey Student and search for the text 'Health Assessment, 4th edition'. Choose the section titled 'Teaching material'. In this section you will find question and answer documents for each chapter. Please check instructions on the inside front cover of the book to access online resources
- visiting websites

Australian Government (Department of Human Services)—Hearing Services Program: https://www.health.gov.au/our-work/hearing-services-program

Australian Indigenous Health InfoNet—Ear Health: https://healthinfonet.ecu.edu.au/learn/health-topics/ear-health/

'Be Healthy, Be Mobile'—World Health Organization: https://www.who.int/initiatives/behealthy

Ministry of Disabled People—Hearing and vision services: https://www.whaikaha.govt.nz/support-and-services/specific-disability-services/hearing-and-vision-services/

The Deaf Society: https://deafsociety.org.au/

The National Foundation for the Deaf Inc.: https://www.nfdhh.org.nz/

World Health Organization—Deafness and Hearing Loss: https://www.who.int/news-room/fact-sheets/detail/deafness-and-hearing-loss.

REFERENCES

1. Eggermont JJ. Acquired hearing loss and brain plasticity. Hearing Research. 2017 Jan 1;343: 176–190.
2. Clay-Williams R, Stephens JH, Williams H, Hallahan A, Dalton C, Hibbert P, et al. (2020). Assessing the appropriateness of the management of otitis media in Australia: A population-based sample survey. Journal of Paediatrics and Child Health, 56(2), 215–223. https://doi.org/10.1111/jpc.14560
3. Coleman A, Cervin A. Probiotics in the treatment of otitis media: the past, the present and the future. International Journal of Pediatric Otorhinolaryngology. 2019 Jan 1;116:135–140.
4. Hardani AK Sr, Moghimi Esfandabadi F, Delphi M, Ali Samir M, Zamiri Abdollahi F (2020). Risk factors for otitis media in children referred to Abuzar Hospital in Ahvaz: a case-control study. Cureus, 12(8), e9766. https://doi.org/10.7759/cureus.9766
5. Doiphode RS, Vinchurkar AS (2020). A comparative study of auditory and visual reaction time in young and elderly males. International Journal of Health Sciences and Research, 10(12), 333–337. https://www.ijhsr.org/IJHSR_Vol.10_Issue.12_Dec2020/48.pdf
6. Bennett RJ, Saulsman L, Eikelboom RH, Olaithe M (2022). Coping with the social challenges and emotional distress associated with hearing loss: a qualitative investigation using Leventhal's self-regulation theory. Internatinal Journal of Audiology, 61(5), 353–364. https://doi.org/10.1080/14992027.2021.1933620

7. Jervis-Bardy J, Carney AS, Duguid R, Leach AJ. Microbiology of otitis media in Indigenous Australian children. The Journal of Laryngology & Otology. 2017 Jul;131(S2):S2–11.
8. Wang T-C, Chang T-Y, Tyler R, Lin Y-J, Liang W-M, Shau Y-W, et al. (2020). Noise induced hearing loss and tinnitus—new research developments and remaining gaps in disease assessment, treatment, and prevention. Brain Sciences, 10(10), 1. https://doi.org/10.3390/brainsci10100732
9. World Health Organization. World report on hearing. 2021. Available at: https://www.who.int/publications/i/item/9789240020481
10. Bealing M (2023). Economic effects of hearing loss. NZIER, Wellington.
11. Coleman A, Wood A, Bialasiewicz S, Ware RS, Marsh RL, Cervin A. The unsolved problem of otitis media in indigenous populations: a systematic review of upper respiratory and middle ear microbiology in indigenous children with otitis media. Microbiome. 2018 Dec;6(1):1–5.
12. Institute of Health & Welfare. (2022). Ear and hearing health of Aboriginal and Torres Strait Islander people 2021. https://www.aihw.gov.au/reports/indigenous-australians/ear-and-hearing-health-of-aboriginal-torres-strait
13. Delacy J, Dune T, MacDonald JJ (2020). The social determinants of otitis media in aboriginal children in Australia: Are we addressing the primary causes? A systematic content review. BMC Public Health, 20(1), 492. https://doi.org/10.1186/s12889-020-08570-3
14. Leach AJ, Morris PS, Coates, Nelson S, O'Leary SJ, Richmond PC, et al. (2021). Otitis media guidelines for Australian Aboriginal and Torres Strait Islander children: summary of recommendations. Medical Journal of Australia, 214(5), 228–233. https://doi.org/https://doi.org/10.5694/mja2.50953
15. Reddy R, Welch D, Lima I, Thorne P, Nosa V (2019). Identifying hearing care access barriers among older Pacific Island people in New Zealand: a qualitative study. BMJ Open, 9(8), e029007. https://doi.org/10.1136/bmjopen-2019-029007
16. Manuel AR, Searchfield G, Curtis E (2021). Hearing loss and hearing service experiences among older Māori and whānau: a scoping review. New Zealand Medical Journal, 134 (1535), 55–70.
17. Azeem A, Julleekeea A, Knight B, Sohail I, Bruyns-Haylett M, Sastre M. (2023). Hearing loss and its link to cognitive impairment and dementia [Review]. Frontiers in Dementia, 2. https://www.frontiersin.org/articles/10.3389/frdem.2023.1199319
18. Department of Health and Aged Care. (2023, 2 June 2023). Indigenous Australians' Health Programme. Commonwealth of Australia Department of Health and Aged Care. Available at: https://www.health.gov.au/our-work/indigenous-australians-health-programme?language=en
19. Ministry of Health. (2023, 2 December 2014). Universal Newborn Hearing Screening Programme. New Zealand Government Ministry of Health – Manatū Hauora. Available at: https://www.nsu.govt.nz/health-professionals/universal-newborn-hearing-screening-programme
20. Hearing Australia. (2023). Hearing Australia. Available at: https://www.hearing.com.au/
21. National Foundation of the Deaf and Hard of Hearing Inc. (2023). Hearing Matters. Available at: https://www.nfdhh.org.nz/
22. Dillard LK, Arunda MO, Lopez-Perez L, Martinez RX, Jiménez L, Chadha S (2022). Prevalence and global estimates of unsafe listening practices in adolescents and young adults: a systematic review and meta-analysis. BMJ Global Health, 7(11), e010501. https://doi.org/10.1136/bmjgh-2022-010501
23. World Health Organization. (2019). Safe listening devices and systems: a WHO-ITU standard. Geneva: Available at: https://www.who.int/publications/i/item/9789241515276
24. Gopal KV, Mills LE, Phillips BS, Nandy R. Risk assessment of recreational noise–induced hearing loss from exposure through a personal audio system—ipod touch. Journal of the American Academy of Audiology. 2019 Jul;30(07):619–633.

25. WorkSafe Australia. Noise. Available at: https://www.safeworkaustralia.gov.au/safety-topic/hazards/noise/overview
26. Wald ER (2021). Management of recurrent acute otitis media. New England Journal of Medicine, 384(19), 1859–1860. https://doi.org/10.1056/NEJMe2104952
27. Vanker A, Gie RP, Zar HJ. The association between environmental tobacco smoke exposure and childhood respiratory disease: a review. Expert Review of Respiratory Medicine. 2017 Aug 3;11(8):661–673.
28. Megged O, Abdulgany S, Bar-Meir M. Does acute otitis media in the first month of life increase the risk for recurrent otitis?. Clinical Pediatrics. 2018 Jan;57(1):89–92.
29. Dimitrov L, Gossman W (2023). Pediatric Hearing Loss. National Library of Medicine. Available at: https://www.ncbi.nlm.nih.gov/books/NBK538285/
30. Speedie L, Middleton A, Hockenberry MJ, Wilson D, Rodgers CC (Eds.). (2021). Wong's nursing care of infants and children (1st Australian and New Zealand ed.). Elsevier.
31. Salmon MK, Brant J, Hohman MH, Leibowitz D (2023). Audiogram Interpretation. National Library of Medicine. Available at: https://www.ncbi.nlm.nih.gov/books/NBK578179/
32. Talley N, O'Connor S. Talley and O'Connor's Clinical Examination. 2023. 9th Ed. Elsevier. Sydney.
33. McGee S (2022). Evidence-based physical diagnosis (5th ed). Philadelphia: Elsevier.
34. Cosh S, Helmer C, Delcourt C, Robins TG, Tully PJ. Depression in elderly patients with hearing loss: current perspectives. Clinical Interventions in Aging. 2019 Aug 14:1471–1480.
35. Caplan RM (2023). The care of the older person/edited by Ronald Caplan (Fifth edition. ed.). Boca Raton, Florida : CRC Press.

CHAPTER 16

UNIT 4

Assessing cardiovascular function

Peripheral vascular assessment

Written by Carolyn Jarvis

Adapted by Niki Lillibridge

INTRODUCTION

The vascular system consists of the blood vessels of the body. Arteries carry oxygenated blood from the heart to the peripheries. Arterial walls stretch during systole and recoil during diastole, resulting in a palpable pulse. Veins carry deoxygenated blood to the heart. Because veins are low pressure vessels they do not usually produce pulsations. The exceptions are large veins such as the right internal carotid vein. Veins distend when there is an increase in intravascular volume. Any disruption or disease in the vascular system creates problems with delivering oxygen and nutrients to the tissues or elimination of waste products from cellular metabolism.

The lymphatic system consists of lymph nodes that filter lymphatic fluid. Body tissue fluids are drained first to lymphatic vessels then to lymphatic channels that empty into the bloodstream through lymphatic ducts in the thorax. Any disease in the lymphatic system results in tissue swelling from obstructions to lymph flow. Infection may cause enlarged, painful lymph nodes. Neoplasms (abnormal growth of cells in the body) may result in enlarged lymph nodes.

Diseases that affect the peripheral vascular or lymphatic systems can have a significant impact on a person's quality of life and their ability to carry out activities of daily living. To appreciate the impact of disease and trauma to these complex and dynamic systems you are advised to also review the structure and function of the heart and major blood vessels (Chapter 17).

Case study

The following case study gives an example of a typical situation involving peripheral vascular assessment and the initial clinical reasoning process. It will help you identify your learning needs.

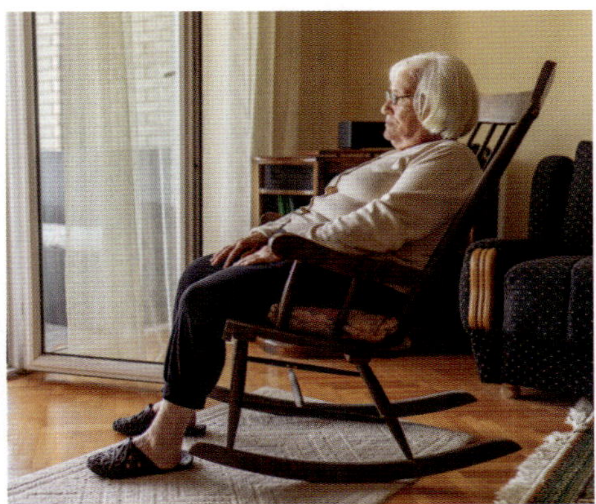

Context

You are on a clinical placement working alongside a community nurse specialist who works with people needing care in their home.

Consider the patient's situation

Mrs Margaret Sheffield, a 79-year-old woman, has been referred to the community nursing service for ongoing assessment and treatment of a venous leg ulcer (right lower leg).

Questions to further your learning

- What are the possible things that might be going on with Mrs Sheffield?
- What knowledge do you need to be able to predict what might be going on?
- What approach to peripheral vascular assessment will you take?
- What questions (subjective data) will you ask Mrs Sheffield to extend the health history and why?
- What physical examination (objective data) will you conduct and why?
- What resources are available to assist in your assessment of Mrs Sheffield?

Assessment plan

As you work through the assessment of peripheral vascular function you need to keep in mind that this area is usually assessed in connection with assessing cardiac function. An accurate assessment requires the nurse to obtain a careful history of the symptoms experienced, which will guide physical examination. This subjective data has been grouped under the following headings:

- presenting concern
- leg pain or cramps
- skin changes on arms or legs
- swelling of hands or feet
- past and family history
- health and lifestyle management.

The focus of the objective data collection is to examine the person for clinical signs that support or are in addition to their report of symptoms. Assessing the peripheral vascular system focuses on identifying risk factors for skin breakdown, pain, immobility and changes to the person's everyday activities. Objective data collection includes:

- inspecting and palpating the arms
- inspecting and palpating the legs
- assessing peripheral pulses using the Doppler.

Resources available

You will find additional resources and the reference list at the end of this chapter.

Structure and function

Arteries

The heart pumps newly oxygenated blood through the arteries to all body tissues. The pumping heart makes this a high-pressure system. The artery walls are strong, tough and tense to withstand the pressure exerted on the vessels by circulating blood. Arteries contain elastic fibres, which allow their walls to stretch with systole and recoil with diastole. Arteries also contain muscle fibres (vascular smooth muscle), which control the amount of blood delivered to the tissues. The vascular smooth muscle contracts or dilates, which changes the diameter of the arteries to control the rate of blood flow.

Each heartbeat creates a pressure wave, which makes the arteries expand then recoil. It is the recoil that propels blood through like a wave. All arteries have this pressure wave, or **pulse**, throughout their length, but you can feel it only at body sites where the artery lies close to the skin and over a bone. The arteries described in the following sections are accessible for examination.

TEMPORAL ARTERY

The temporal artery is palpated in front of the ear.

CAROTID ARTERY

The carotid artery is palpated in the groove between the sternocleidomastoid muscle and the trachea and is covered in Chapter 17 with the great vessels.

ARTERIES IN THE ARM

The major artery supplying the arm is the brachial artery, which runs in the biceps–triceps furrow of the upper arm and surfaces at the antecubital fossa in the elbow medial to the biceps tendon (Figure 16.1). Immediately below the elbow, the brachial artery bifurcates into the ulnar and radial arteries. These run distally and form two arches supplying the hand; these are called

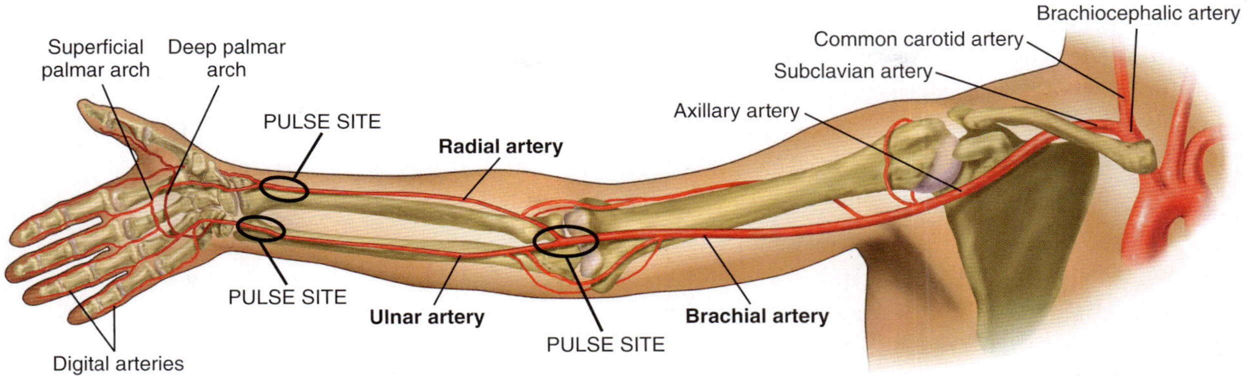

FIGURE 16.1 Arteries in the arm and shoulder and pulse sites

the *superficial* and *deep palmar arches*. The radial pulse lies just medial to the radius at the wrist; the ulnar artery runs parallel to the ulna, but it is deeper and often difficult to feel.

ARTERIES IN THE LEG

The major artery to the leg is the femoral artery, which passes under the inguinal ligament (Figure 16.2). The femoral artery travels down the thigh. At the lower thigh, it courses posteriorly; then it is termed the popliteal artery. Below the knee, the popliteal artery divides. The anterior tibial artery travels down the front of the leg on to the dorsum of the foot, where it becomes the dorsalis pedis. In the back of the leg, the posterior tibial artery travels down behind the medial malleolus and in the foot forms the plantar arteries.

The function of the arteries is to supply oxygen and essential nutrients to the tissues. **Ischaemia** is a deficient supply of oxygenated arterial blood to a tissue caused by obstruction of a blood vessel. A complete blockage leads to death of the distal tissue. A partial blockage creates an insufficient blood supply and the ischaemia may be apparent only at exercise when oxygen demand increases. Peripheral arterial disease affects non-coronary arteries and usually refers to

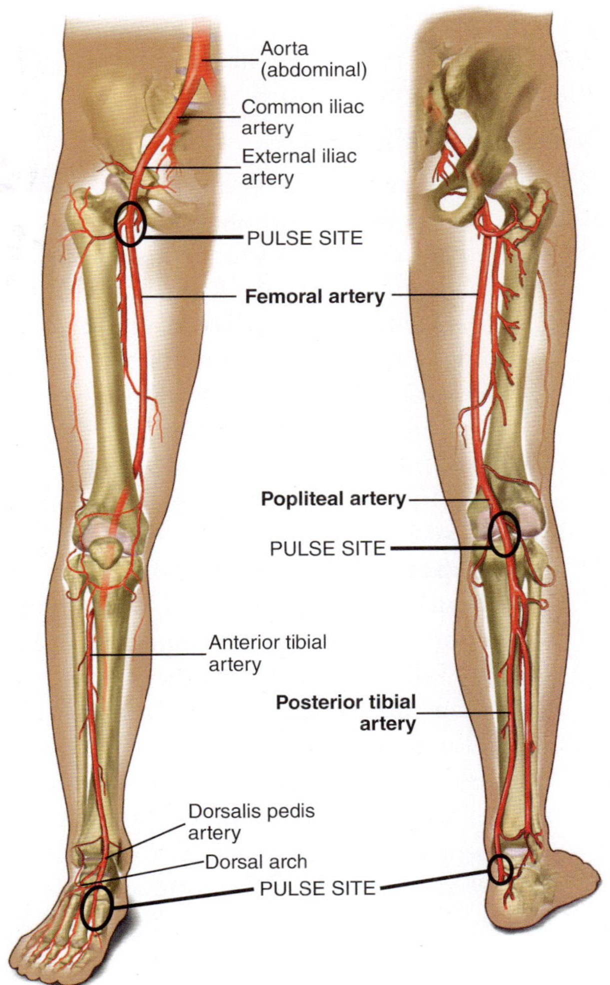

FIGURE 16.2 Arteries in the legs and pulse sites

arteries in the limbs. It is usually caused by atherosclerosis and less commonly by embolism, arterial dissection or other injury to the major arteries.

Veins

The course of veins parallels that of arteries, but the body has more veins, and they lie closer to the skin surface. The following veins are accessible to examination.

JUGULAR VEINS

Assessment of the jugular veins is presented in Chapter 17.

VEINS IN THE ARM

Each arm has two sets of veins: superficial and deep. The superficial veins are in the subcutaneous tissue and are responsible for most of the venous return.

VEINS IN THE LEG

The legs have three types of veins (Figure 16.3):

1. The **deep veins** run alongside the deep arteries and conduct most of the venous return from the legs. These are the **femoral** and **popliteal** veins. As long as these veins remain intact, the superficial veins can be excised without harming the circulation—for example, excising the saphenous vein to then use in coronary artery bypass surgery.
2. The **superficial veins** are the **great** and **small saphenous** veins. The great saphenous vein, inside the leg, starts at the medial side of the dorsum of the foot. You can see it ascend in front of the medial malleolus; then it crosses the tibia obliquely and ascends along the medial side of the thigh. The small saphenous vein, outside the leg, starts on the lateral side of the dorsum of the foot, ascends behind the lateral malleolus, up the back of the leg, where it joins the popliteal vein.

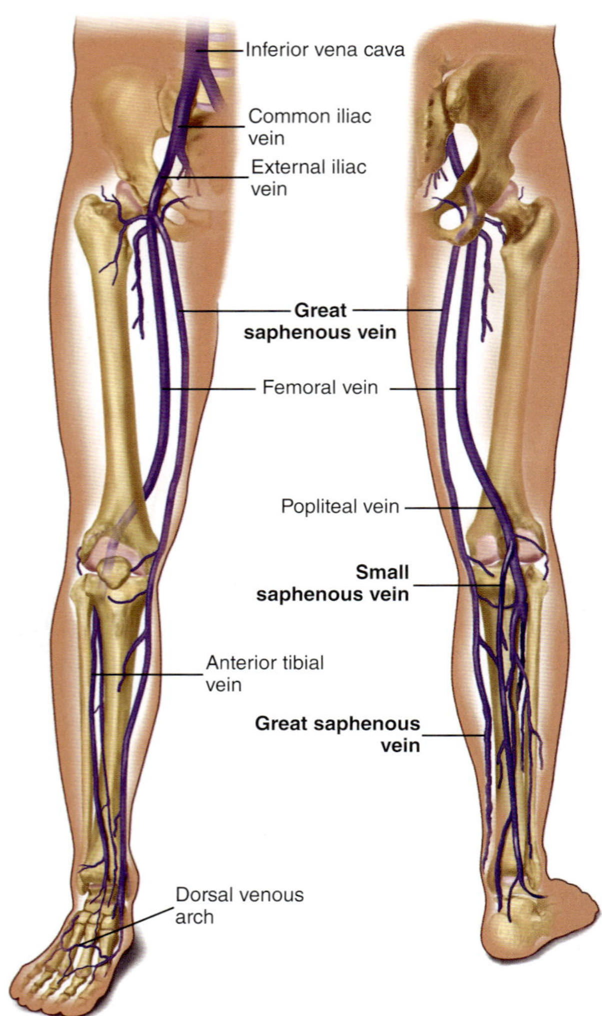

FIGURE 16.3 Veins in the legs

3. **Perforators** (not illustrated) are connecting veins that join the two sets. They also have one-way valves that direct blood from the superficial into the deep veins.

Venous flow

Veins drain the deoxygenated blood and its waste products from the tissues and return it to the heart. Unlike the arteries, veins are a low-pressure system. Because veins do not have a pump to generate their blood flow, the veins need a mechanism to keep blood

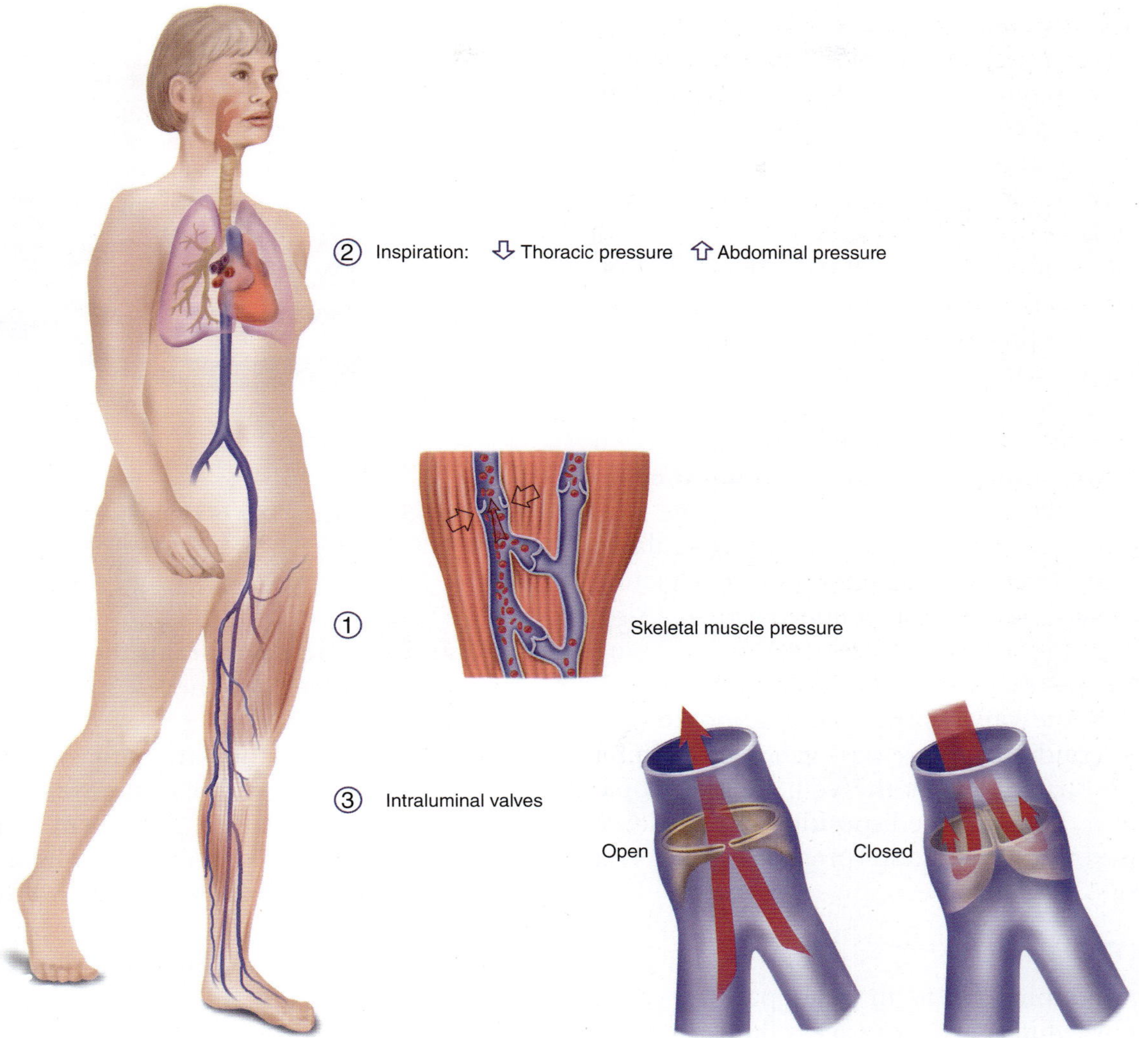

FIGURE 16.4 Mechanisms of venous flow

moving (Figure 16.4). This is accomplished by (1) the contracting skeletal muscles that milk the blood proximally, back towards the heart; (2) the pressure gradient caused by breathing, in which inspiration makes the thoracic pressure decrease and the abdominal pressure increase; and (3) the one-way valves, called the intraluminal valves, which ensure unidirectional flow. Each valve is a paired semilunar pocket that opens towards the heart and closes tightly when filled to prevent backflow of blood.

In the legs, this mechanism is called the *calf pump*. While walking, the calf muscles alternately contract (systole) and relax (diastole). In the contraction phase, the gastrocnemius and soleus muscles squeeze the veins and direct the blood flow proximally. Because of the valves, venous blood flows just one way—towards the heart.

Besides the presence of intraluminal valves, venous structure differs from arterial structure. Because venous pressure is lower, the walls of the veins are thinner than those of the arteries. Veins have a larger diameter and are more distensible; they can expand and hold more blood when blood volume increases. This is a compensatory mechanism to reduce stress on the heart. Because of this ability to stretch, veins are called **capacitance vessels**.

Efficient venous return depends on contracting skeletal muscles, competent valves in the veins and a patent lumen. Problems with any of these three elements lead to venous stasis. At risk for venous disease are people who undergo prolonged standing, sitting or bed rest because they do not benefit from the milking action that walking accomplishes. Hypercoagulable states and vein wall trauma are other factors that increase risk for venous disease. Also, dilated and tortuous (varicose) veins create **incompetent valves**, wherein the lumen is so wide the valve cusps cannot approximate. This condition increases venous pressure, which further dilates the vein. Some people have a genetic predisposition to varicose veins, but obesity and pregnancy are risk factors.

Lymphatics

The lymphatics form a separate vessel system, which retrieves excess fluid from the tissue spaces and returns it to the bloodstream (Figure 16.5). During circulation of the blood, somewhat more fluid leaves the capillaries than the veins can absorb. Without lymphatic drainage, fluid would build up in the interstitial spaces and produce oedema.

The vessels drain into two main trunks, which empty into the venous system at the subclavian veins (Figure 16.6):

1. The **right lymphatic duct** empties into the right subclavian vein. It drains the right side of the head and neck, right arm, right side of the thorax, right lung and pleura, right side of the heart and right upper section of the liver.

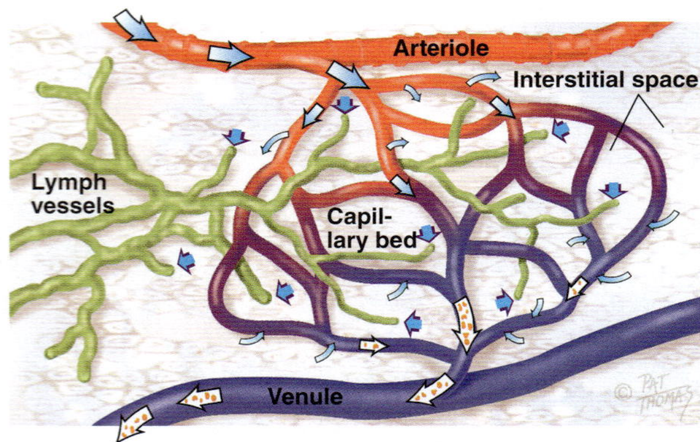

FIGURE 16.5 Mechanisms of blood flow from arterioles to venules in the microcirculation

2. The **thoracic duct** drains the rest of the body. It empties into the left subclavian vein.

The functions of the lymphatic system are (1) to conserve fluid and plasma proteins that leak out of the capillaries; (2) to form a major part of the immune system that defends the body against disease; and (3) to absorb lipids from the intestinal tract.

The processes of the immune system are complicated and not fully understood. The immune system detects and eliminates microorganisms that could be harmful to the body (pathogens), both those that come in from the environment and those arising from inside (abnormal or mutant cells). It accomplishes this by phagocytosis (ingestion and elimination) of the substances by neutrophils and monocytes/macrophages and by production of specific antibodies or specific immune responses by the lymphocytes.

The lymphatic vessels have a unique structure. Lymphatic capillaries start as microscopic open-ended tubes, which siphon interstitial fluid. The capillaries converge to form vessels. The vessels, like veins, drain into larger ones. The vessels have valves, so

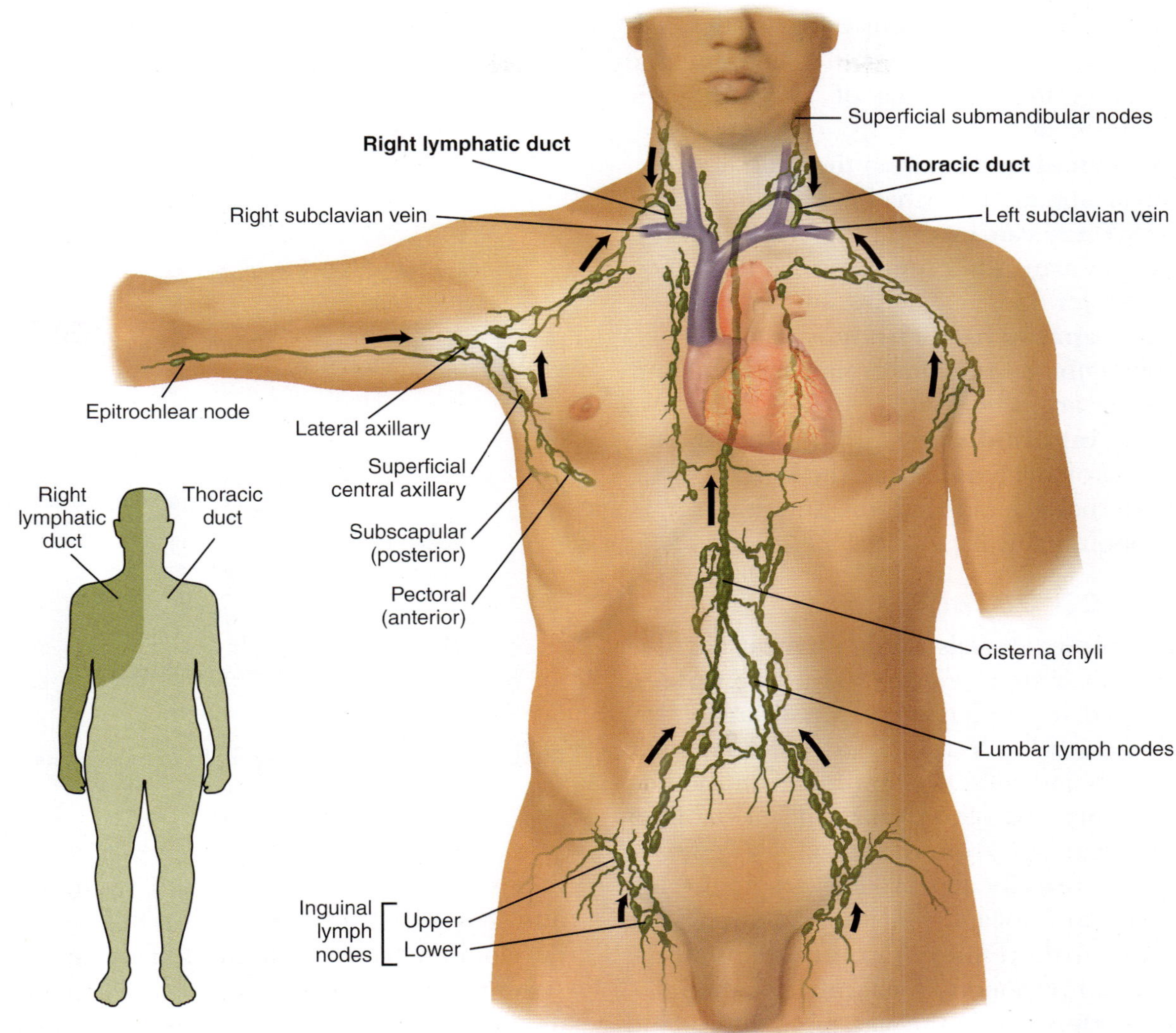

FIGURE 16.6 Lymphatic nodes, ducts and drainage patterns

flow is one way from the tissue spaces into the bloodstream. The many valves make the vessels look beaded. The flow of lymph is slow compared with that of the blood. Lymph flow is propelled by contracting skeletal muscles, by pressure changes secondary to breathing and by contraction of the vessel walls themselves.

Lymph nodes are small oval-shaped clumps of lymphatic tissue located at intervals along the vessels. Most nodes are arranged in groups, both deep and superficial, in the body. Nodes filter the fluid before it is returned to the bloodstream and filter out pathogens. The pathogens are exposed to lymphocytes in the lymph nodes. The lymphocytes mount an antigen-specific response to eliminate the pathogens. With local inflammation, the nodes in that area become swollen and tender.

The superficial groups of nodes are accessible to inspection and palpation and give clues to the status of the lymphatic system:

- **Cervical nodes** drain the head and neck and are described in Chapter 18.
- **Axillary nodes** drain the breast and upper arm. They are described in Chapter 28.
- The **epitrochlear node** is in the antecubital fossa and drains the hand and lower arm.
- The **inguinal nodes** in the groin drain most of the lymph from the legs, the external genitalia and the anterior abdominal wall.

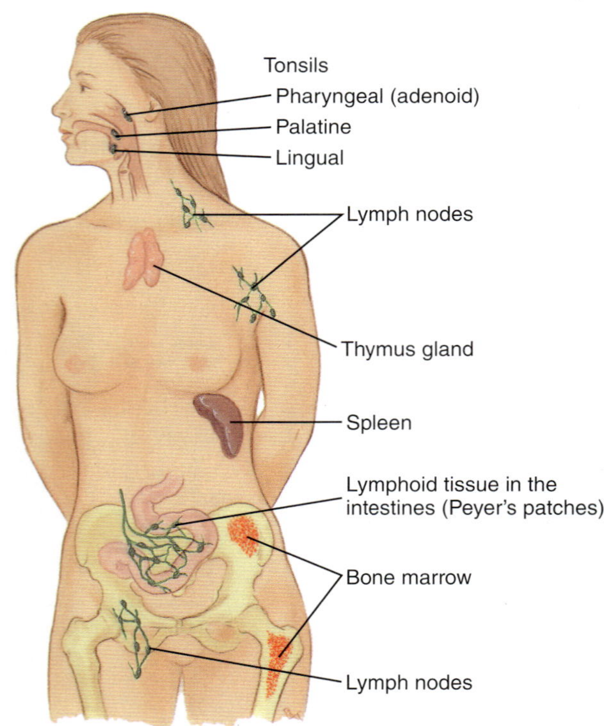

FIGURE 16.7 Related organs in the immune system

Related organs

The spleen, tonsils and thymus aid the lymphatic system (Figure 16.7). The **spleen** is located in the left upper quadrant of the abdomen. It has four functions: (1) to destroy old red blood cells; (2) to produce antibodies; (3) to store red blood cells; and (4) to filter microorganisms from the blood.

The **tonsils** (palatine, adenoid and lingual) are located in the throat at the entrance to the respiratory and gastrointestinal tracts and respond to local inflammation.

The **thymus** is the flat, pink-grey gland located in the superior mediastinum behind the sternum and in front of the aorta. It is relatively large in the fetus and young child and atrophies after puberty. It is important in developing the T lymphocytes of the immune system in children, but it serves no function in adults. The T and B lymphocytes originate in the bone marrow and mature in the lymphoid tissue.

Developmental considerations

Infants and children

The lymphatic system has the same function in children as in adults. It is well developed at birth and grows rapidly until age 10 or 11 years. By age 6 years, the lymphoid tissue reaches adult size; it surpasses adult size by puberty, then it slowly atrophies. It is possible that the excessive antigen stimulation in children causes the early rapid growth.

Lymph nodes are relatively large in children, and the superficial ones are often palpable even when the child is healthy. With infection, excessive swelling and hyperplasia occur. Enlarged tonsils are familiar signs in respiratory infections. The excessive lymphoid response may also account for the common childhood symptom of abdominal pain with seemingly unrelated problems such as upper respiratory infections. It is possible that the inflammation of mesenteric lymph nodes produces the abdominal pain.

Pregnant women

Hormonal changes cause vasodilation and the resulting drop in blood pressure described in Chapter 27. The growing uterus obstructs drainage of the iliac veins and the inferior vena cava. This condition causes low blood flow and increases venous pressure. This, in turn, causes dependent oedema, varicosities in the legs and vulva and haemorrhoids.

Late adulthood (65+ years)

Peripheral blood vessels grow more rigid with age, resulting in a condition called **arteriosclerosis**. This condition produces the rise in systolic blood pressure. Do not confuse this process with another one—**atherosclerosis**—or the deposition of fatty plaques on the intima of the arteries. Both processes are present with peripheral arterial disease (PAD) in ageing adults. The risk factors and impact of peripheral vascular disease (PVD) is further discussed in the section on cultural and social considerations below.

Ageing produces a progressive enlargement of the intramuscular calf veins. Prolonged bed rest, prolonged sitting and heart failure increase the risk of deep venous thrombosis and subsequent pulmonary embolism. These conditions are common in ageing and can occur after myocardial infarction. The care for a person after myocardial infarction includes early mobilisation and low-dose anticoagulant medication, which reduce the risk of pulmonary embolism.

Loss of lymphatic tissue leads to fewer numbers of lymph nodes and a decrease in the size of remaining nodes in people over 65.

Cultural and social considerations

Peripheral vascular health issues can have profound impact on the person and their family. PVD/PAD indicate systemic atherosclerosis, yet are underdiagnosed and undertreated and a significant cause of morbidity (painful walking, poor wound healing) and mortality in Australia.[1]

There is no definitive national data on Australians living with PAD,[2] but it is estimated to affect 10 to 20% of the Australian population, with approximately 50% having no symptoms.[3] Some estimates suggest more than 230 million people worldwide are afflicted with PAD.[4] PAD is a common reason for hospitalisation in people over 70 years of age.[2] Because there is a relationship between PAD and generalised cardiovascular health, it is important for people with PAD to have frequent heart health screening.

Advancing age, male sex, cigarette smoking, hypertension, diabetes, dyslipidaemia, hypertension, obesity and the presence of other cardiovascular diseases account for most of the risk factors for PAD.[5,6] Like coronary artery disease, PVD progression can be modified by pharmacological and lifestyle interventions that address the person's risk factors. A retrospective cohort study in Australia reported a comparison of the presenting characteristics and clinical outcomes of Indigenous Australians and non-Indigenous Australians with PAD.[1] Current smoking status and diabetes were recorded as more prevalent in the Indigenous study participants. The conclusion by Alahakoon and colleagues[1] suggests Indigenous study participants present at a younger age with PAD vascular risk factors and have poorer clinical outcomes compared with non-Indigenous Australians.

There are currently no Australian or Aotearoa New Zealand guidelines recommending routine screening for PVD, although screening should be considered in people over 50 years of age with a history of smoking, hypertension or diabetes.[7] There is further discussion of the major modifiable cardiovascular risk factors in Chapter 17.

HEALTH EDUCATION

Foot care

Foot problems often herald more serious health conditions such as arthritis, diabetes and nerve or circulatory disorders. Healthcare providers should not only remember to examine the feet for common foot problems but also be prepared to explain what 'good' foot care really means. Too often healthcare providers will advise good foot care but do not take the time to explain what it entails. You can advise the person with any health problem that affects the circulation or lymphatic drainage to their legs to do the following:

Monitor foot health

- Check the feet every day. If the person cannot see the bottoms of their feet, advise them to use a mirror or to ask someone to help.
- Examine each foot daily for red spots or sensitive areas, discolouration of skin or nails, ingrown nails, pain, cuts, swelling or blisters. A good time to examine feet is after a shower or bath.

Pay attention to foot hygiene

- Use mild soap when washing the feet and dry feet carefully, especially between the toes.
- Keep toenails trimmed, straight across and filed at the edges with a nail file. If circulation is severely impaired or feet lack sensation, suggest a referral to a podiatrist for further foot care.
- Apply a thin coat of a non-scented moisturising skin lotion over the tops and bottoms of the feet—this helps to keep skin soft and smooth. However, the lotion should not go between toes because it may make the area moist and increase the risk of skin breakdown.

Take action to prevent further damage to feet

- Keep blood circulating to the feet by increasing activity such as walking, which is one of the best exercises for overall circulation.
- Put the feet up when sitting or lying down, stretching, wiggling toes, having a gentle foot massage or warm foot bath are great alternatives if the person cannot walk.
- Avoid crossing the legs for long periods.
- Avoid smoking and vaping—give advice for quitting.
- Wear shoes that fit well and are comfortable.

For more information on foot care or to find a podiatrist:

- Health Care Direct—foot care: www.healthdirect.gov.au/foot-care
- Better Health Channel—Diabetes foot care: www.betterhealth.vic.gov.au/health/conditionsandtreatments/diabetes-foot-care
- Australian Podiatry Association: www.podiatry.org.au
- New Zealand Society of Podiatrists: www.podnz.org

Subjective data

Practice note

Before you start the assessment, introduce yourself to the person, confirm the person's identity, discuss the purpose and scope of the assessment, clarify any questions the person may have and obtain verbal consent from the person to perform the assessment.

ASSESSMENT GUIDELINES	CLINICAL SIGNIFICANCE AND CLINICAL ALERTS
Presenting concern	
• *Do you have any problem with the circulation in your legs, feet, arms or hands?* It is important to ascertain the person's perception of their circulation. If they do perceive a problem, ask: *How does this impact on their quality of life?*	Questionnaires are additional measures to record the impact of the vascular condition on the person's overall health.
Leg pain or cramps	
• *Do you have any leg pain (cramps)? Where exactly is the pain?*	
• *Can you describe the type of pain? Is it burning, aching, cramping or stabbing?* • *Did this come on gradually or suddenly?* • *Is it aggravated by activity such as walking?*	**Peripheral vascular disease** (Table 16.1)
• *How far can you walk? Blocks? Stairs? To your letterbox?* • *What stops you?*	**Claudication distance** is the number of blocks walked or stairs climbed to produce pain in the calf. Confirm that claudication distance is the primary symptom affecting mobility.
• *Has this amount changed recently?* • *Is the pain worse with elevation?* • *Is it worse with cool temperatures?*	Note sudden decrease in claudication distance or pain not relieved by rest.
• *Does the pain wake you up at night?*	Night leg pain is not uncommon in ageing adults. It may indicate the ischaemic rest pain of PVD, severe night muscle cramping (usually the calf) or **restless leg syndrome**.
• *Have you experienced any recent change in exercise, a new exercise or increasing exercise?*	Pain of musculoskeletal origin rather than vascular. Musculoskeletal pain can be made worse with walking and relieved by rest.

ASSESSMENT GUIDELINES	CLINICAL SIGNIFICANCE AND CLINICAL ALERTS
• *What relieves this pain: dangling your legs, walking, rubbing?* • *Is the leg pain associated with any skin changes?*	Location and interventions that relieve the pain help identify the cause. Foot pain relieved by dangling, walking or rubbing the foot relieves an ischaemic pain. Insufficient blood flow to the foot is assisted by gravity. Leg cramps reported up and down the lower limb and relieved by rest can occur with diabetes.
• *Is the pain associated with any change in sexual function?* (males)	**Aortoiliac occlusion** is associated with impotence (Leriche's syndrome). This is an important sign that the man should be referred for further medical assessment because erectile dysfunction has a strong association with cardiovascular disease.
Skin changes on arms or legs	
• *Have you noticed any skin changes in arms or legs? What colour? Redness, pallor, blueness, brown discolourations? Hyperpigmentation?*	Hyperpigmentation, pallor/cyanosis and oedema are associated with venous stasis.
• *Have you noticed any change in temperature—excess warmth or coolness?* • *Have you noticed a reduction or absence of hair on your lower legs?* • *Have you noticed any numbness or tingling in your feet or hands?*	Coolness, pallor and hair loss are associated with arterial disease.
• *Do your leg veins look bulging and crooked?* • *How have these been treated?* • *Do you use support stockings?*	**Varicose veins.** A common condition of the lower and/or upper legs caused by weak or damaged vein walls and valves. Blood pools in these vessels and the veins appear overfilled and twisted on the skin surface. Support stockings provide graduated compression to the lower legs that help to reduce swelling. They are designed to increase blood flow return by compression of the deep venous system.
• *Do you have any leg sores or ulcers? Where on the leg?* • *How long have they been there?* • *Is there any pain with the leg ulcer?* • *Can you describe the pain? Is it dull, sharp, burning?* • *Can you rate the pain on a scale of 0 to 10 (10 being the worst pain you have experienced)?* • *What makes the pain worse? Does anything improve it?*	**Leg ulcers** occur with chronic arterial and chronic venous disease (Table 16.2).

ASSESSMENT GUIDELINES	CLINICAL SIGNIFICANCE AND CLINICAL ALERTS
Swelling of hands or feet	
• *Have you noticed any swelling in your hands or legs?* • *When did this swelling start?* • *What time of day is the swelling at its worst: morning or after you have been up most of the day?* • *Does the swelling come and go, or is it constant?* • *What seems to bring it on: trauma, standing all day, sitting?* • *What relieves swelling: elevation, support hose?* • *Is swelling associated with pain, heat, redness, ulceration or hardened skin?*	**Oedema** is bilateral when caused by a systemic problem such as heart failure or unilateral when the result of a local obstruction or inflammation.
Past and family history	
• *Do you have any past history of vascular problems such as varicose veins or heart problems?* • *Do you have a history of diabetes, smoking, physical trauma to the pelvis and lower limbs?* • *Have you ever been pregnant?* (if relevant) • *Is there anyone in your family that has had any problems with their veins or arteries?*	Risk factors for PAD include diabetes and cigarette smoking. A family history of vascular problems such as varicose veins is a risk factor in other family members.
Health and lifestyle management	
• **Medications.** *What medications are you taking? Oral contraceptives, hormone replacement, antihypertensives, cardiac drugs?* • **Nutrition.** *Please describe your usual daily diet.* (Note if this diet is representative of the basic food groups, the number of kilojoules, cholesterol and any additives such as salt.) • **Weight.** *What is your usual weight? Has there been any recent change?* • **Travel.** *Have you been on a long-haul flight recently?*	**Thrombophlebitis** is an inflammatory process that causes a blood clot to form and block one or more veins, usually in the lower legs/calves. Can be precipitated by prolonged bed rest or lack of movement on a long-haul flight. Inflammation may also occur as an adverse reaction when taking oral contraceptives.
• **Smoking.** *Do you smoke cigarettes or vape? At what age did you start? How many packs per day? For how many years have you smoked this amount? Have you ever tried to quit? If so, how did this go?* • **Alcohol.** *How much alcohol do you usually drink each week or each day? Beer/wine/spirits? When was your last drink? What was the number of drinks that episode? Have you ever been told you had a drinking problem?* • **Exercise.** *What is your usual amount of exercise each day or week? What stops you?* (e.g. fatigue, leg pains, other, specify). *What type of exercise* (state type or sport)? If a sport, *what is your usual amount* (light, moderate, heavy)?	Tobacco constricts arteries, increases coagulability, injures endothelium and promotes inflammation. Smoking is the strongest risk factor for PAD. Drinking alcohol increases both blood pressure and heart rate. Moderate to heavy alcohol consumption is associated with an increased risk for PAD.

Objective data

Preparation

During the physical examination, assess the arms at the very beginning when you are checking the vital signs, when the person is sitting. Examine the legs directly after the abdominal examination while the person is still supine. Then have the person stand up to evaluate the leg veins.

Examination of the arms and legs includes peripheral vascular characteristics (described below), the skin (Chapter 22), musculoskeletal findings (Chapter 20) and neurological findings (Chapter 12).

Use inspection and palpation. Compare your findings with the opposite extremity.

Equipment needed

Hand hygiene solution
Occasionally needed:

- tape measure
- tourniquet or blood pressure cuff
- stethoscope
- Doppler

PROCEDURES AND NORMAL FINDINGS	ABNORMAL FINDINGS AND CLINICAL ALERTS
Inspecting and palpating the arms	
Lift both of the person's hands in your hands. Inspect, then turn the person's hands over, noting colour of skin and nailbeds; temperature, texture and turgor of skin; and the presence of any lesions, oedema or clubbing. Use the **profile sign** (viewing the finger from the side) to detect early clubbing. The normal nail bed angle is 160 degrees. (See Chapter 22 for a full discussion of skin colour, lesions and clubbing.)	Flattening of angle and **clubbing** (diffuse enlargement of terminal phalanges) occur with congenital cyanotic heart disease and cardiopulmonary disease.
With the person's hands near the level of their heart, check **capillary refill**. This is an index of peripheral perfusion and cardiac output. Depress and blanch the nail beds; release and note the time for colour return. Usually, the vessels refill within a fraction of a second. Consider it normal if the colour returns in less than 1 or 2 seconds. Note conditions that can skew your findings: a cool room, decreased body temperature, cigarette smoking, peripheral oedema and anaemia.	Refill lasting more than 1 or 2 seconds signifies vasoconstriction or decreased cardiac output (hypovolaemia, heart failure, shock). The hands are cold, clammy and pale.
The two arms should be symmetrical in size.	**Oedema** of upper extremities occurs when lymphatic drainage is obstructed, which may occur after breast surgery (Table 16.4).

PROCEDURES AND NORMAL FINDINGS	ABNORMAL FINDINGS AND CLINICAL ALERTS
Note the presence of any scars on hands and arms. Many occur normally with usual childhood abrasions or with occupations involving hand tools.	Needle tracks (small marks along a vein from repeated punctures) occur with prolonged intravenous drug use. Some may show signs of inflammation or infection; linear scars on wrists may signify past self-inflicted injury.
Palpate upper limb pulses	
Palpate both **radial pulses**, noting rate, rhythm, elasticity of vessel wall and equal force (Figure 16.8). Grade the strength on a three-point scale.	Pulses may be more difficult to palpate in an obese person.
3+, increased, full, bounding 2+, normal 1+, weak 0, absent	**Full, bounding pulse** (3+) occurs with hyperkinetic states (exercise, anxiety, fever), anaemia and hyperthyroidism. **Weak, 'thready' pulse** (1+) occurs with shock and PAD. See Table 16.3 for illustrations of these and irregular pulse rhythms.
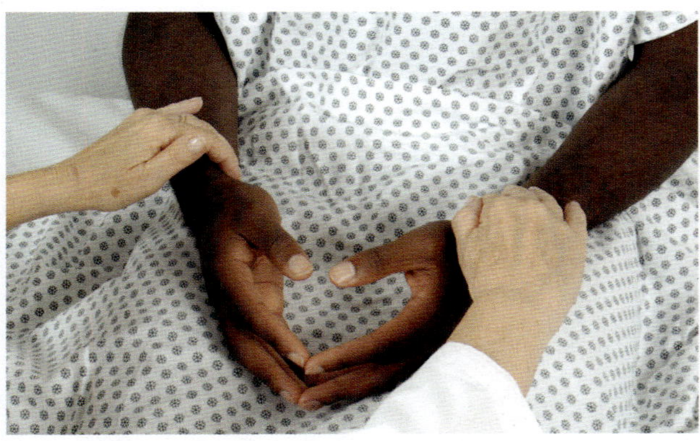 **FIGURE 16.8** Palpation of radial pulses	
It is not usually necessary to palpate the **ulnar pulses**. If indicated, palpate along the medial side of the inner forearm (Figure 16.9), although the ulnar pulses are often not palpable in the normal person.	The ulnar arterial pulses are palpated when a radial artery has been harvested for coronary artery bypass graft surgery.

PROCEDURES AND NORMAL FINDINGS	ABNORMAL FINDINGS AND CLINICAL ALERTS

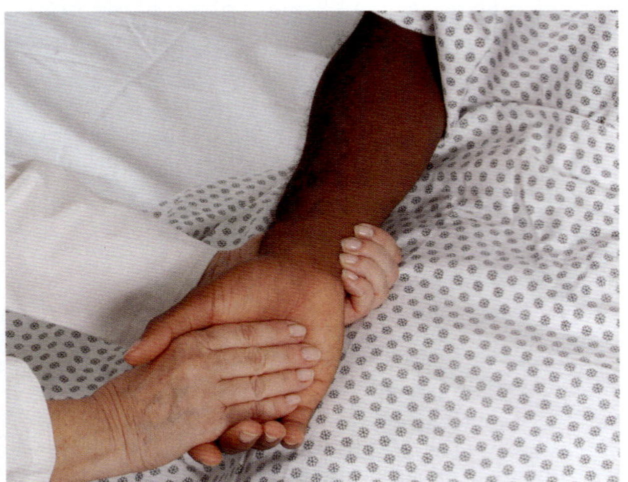

FIGURE 16.9 Palpation of ulnar pulses

Palpate the **brachial pulses**—their strength should be equal bilaterally (Figure 16.10).

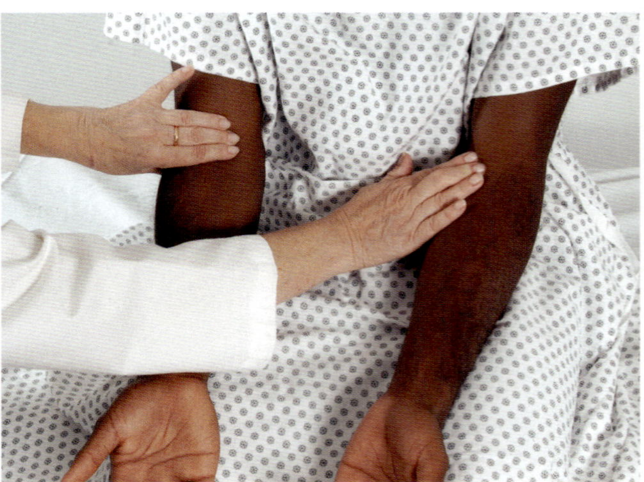

FIGURE 16.10 Palpation of brachial pulses

Inspecting and palpating the legs

PROCEDURES AND NORMAL FINDINGS	ABNORMAL FINDINGS AND CLINICAL ALERTS
Uncover the legs while keeping the genitalia draped. Inspect both legs together, noting skin colour, hair distribution, venous pattern, size (swelling or atrophy) and any skin lesions or ulcers.	**Pallor** with vasoconstriction; **erythema** with vasodilatation; **cyanosis**.
Normally hair covers the legs. Even if leg hair is shaved, you may still note hair on the dorsa of the toes. Hair distribution decreases with age.	**Malnutrition**—thin, shiny atrophic skin, thick-ridged nails, loss of hair, ulcers, gangrene. Malnutrition, pallor and coolness occur with arterial insufficiency.

PROCEDURES AND NORMAL FINDINGS

The venous pattern is normally flat and barely visible. Note obvious varicosities, although these are best assessed while standing.

Both legs should be symmetrical in size without any swelling or atrophy. If the lower legs look asymmetrical or if deep venous thrombosis is suspected, measure the calf circumference with a tape measure (Figure 16.11). Measure at the widest point, taking care to measure the other leg in the same place (i.e. the same number of centimetres down from the patella or other landmark). If lymphoedema is suspected, measure also at the ankle, knee and thigh. Record your findings in centimetres.

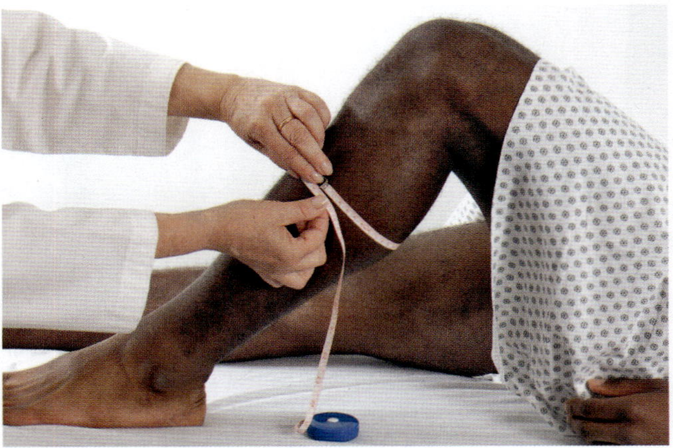

FIGURE 16.11 Measuring calf circumference for symmetry

In the presence of skin discolouration, skin ulcers or gangrene, note the size and the exact location.

ABNORMAL FINDINGS AND CLINICAL ALERTS

The one-way valves in the venous system return blood to the heart. When standing, there is also the additional effect of gravity. Valves that close properly prevent this backflow from occurring.

Diffuse bilateral oedema occurs with systemic illnesses.

Clinical alert: Acute, unilateral, painful swelling and asymmetry of calves of 1 cm or more is abnormal; refer the person to a medical practitioner to determine whether deep venous thrombosis is present.

Asymmetry of 1 to 3 cm occurs with mild lymphoedema; 3 to 5 cm with moderate lymphoedema; and more than 5 cm with severe lymphoedema (Table 16.4).

Brown discolouration occurs with chronic venous stasis due to **haemosiderin** deposits from red blood cell degradation and leakage from fragile capillaries.

Venous ulcers are caused by chronic venous insufficiency from damaged veins (Table 16.2).

Arterial ulcers occur with chronic lack of blood flow to the tissues of the legs and feet. Arterial ulcers usually occur on tips of toes, metatarsal heads and lateral malleoli.

PROCEDURES AND NORMAL FINDINGS	ABNORMAL FINDINGS AND CLINICAL ALERTS
Palpate for temperature along the legs down to the feet, comparing symmetrical spots (Figure 16.12). The skin should be warm and equal bilaterally. Bilateral cool feet may be due to environmental factors such as cool room temperature. If any increase in temperature is present higher up the leg, note if it is gradual or abrupt.	A unilateral cool foot or leg or a sudden temperature drop as you move down the leg occurs with arterial deficit.

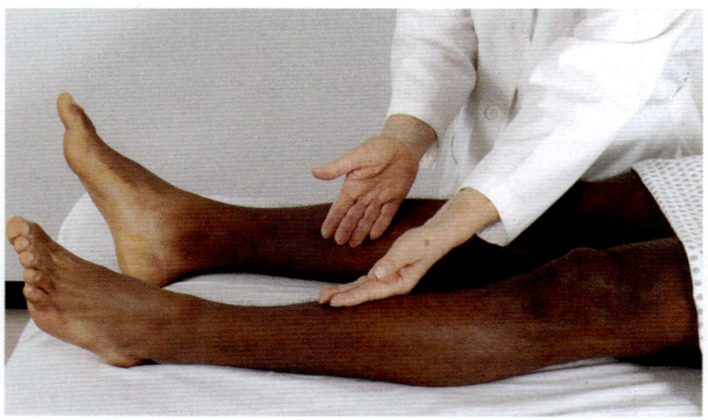

FIGURE 16.12 Light palpation for temperature of the skin

Flex the person's knee, then gently compress the gastrocnemius (calf) muscle anteriorly against the tibia; no tenderness should be present.	***Clinical alert:*** If tenderness on flexion of calf causes pain, do not continue with palpation. Pain can be a sign of deep vein thrombosis, superficial phlebitis, Achilles tendinitis, gastrocnemius and plantar muscle injury and lumbosacral disorders. Where there is any concern that the person could have a deep vein thrombosis, they should be referred to a medical practitioner for further assessment.

Palpate peripheral pulses

Palpate the peripheral arteries in both legs: femoral, popliteal, dorsalis pedis and posterior tibial. Grade the strength on the four-point scale. Locate the **femoral arteries** just below the inguinal ligament halfway between the pubis and the anterior superior iliac spines (Figure 16.13). The simplest method of locating the femoral artery is to recall that the femoral artery is always located at a 45-degree angle to the person's umbilicus. Press firmly and then slowly release, noting the pulse tap under your fingertips.	The femoral artery in a healthy person is easily palpable. Atherosclerosis may be evident if this pulse is not palpable or difficult to palpate.

PROCEDURES AND NORMAL FINDINGS

FIGURE 16.13 Palpation of the femoral artery and pulse

The **popliteal pulse** is a more diffuse pulse and can be difficult to localise.

With the leg extended but relaxed, anchor your thumbs on the knee and curl your fingers around into the popliteal fossa (Figure 16.14). Press your fingers forwards to compress the artery against the bone (the lower edge of the femur or the upper edge of the tibia). Often it is just lateral to the medial tendon.

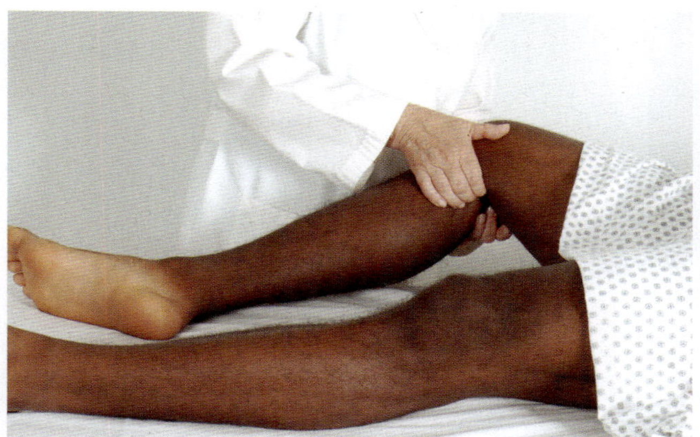

FIGURE 16.14 Palpation of the popliteal pulse (knee raised)

If you have difficulty, turn the person prone and lift the lower leg (Figure 16.15). Let the leg relax against your arm and press in deeply with your two thumbs. Often a normal popliteal pulse is impossible to palpate.

ABNORMAL FINDINGS AND CLINICAL ALERTS

PROCEDURES AND NORMAL FINDINGS	ABNORMAL FINDINGS AND CLINICAL ALERTS

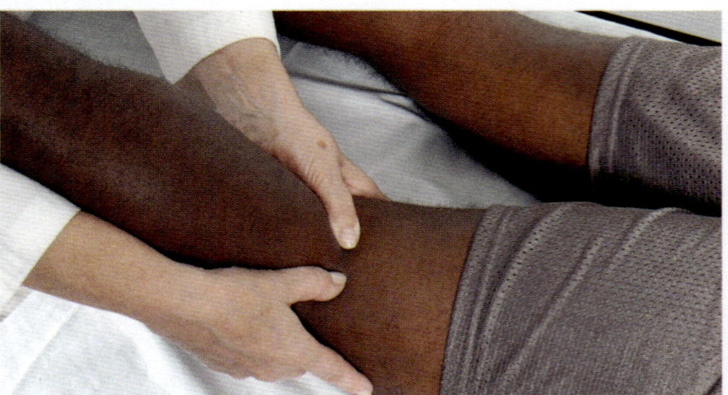

FIGURE 16.15 Palpation of the popliteal pulse (knee relaxed)

For the **posterior tibial** pulse, curve your fingers around the medial malleolus (Figure 16.16). You will feel the tapping right behind it in the groove between the malleolus and the Achilles tendon. If you cannot, try passive dorsiflexion of the foot to make the pulse more accessible.

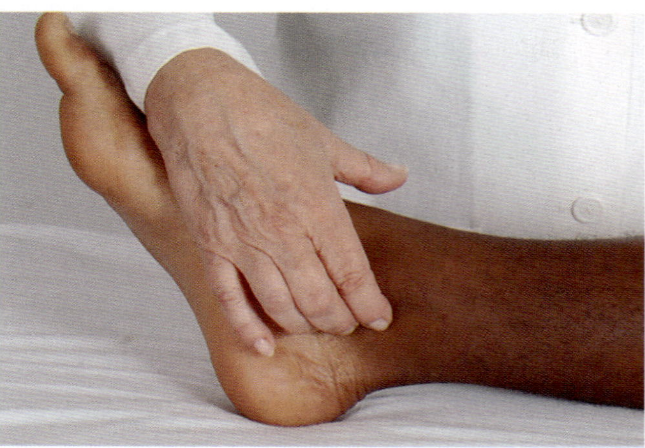

FIGURE 16.16 Palpation of the posterior tibial pulse

The **dorsalis pedis** pulse requires a very light touch. Normally it is just lateral to and parallel with the extensor tendon of the big toe (Figure 16.17). Do not mistake the pulse in your own fingertips for that of the person.

PROCEDURES AND NORMAL FINDINGS

ABNORMAL FINDINGS AND CLINICAL ALERTS

In adults over 45 years, occasionally either the dorsalis pedis or the posterior tibial pulse may be hard to find but not both on the same foot.

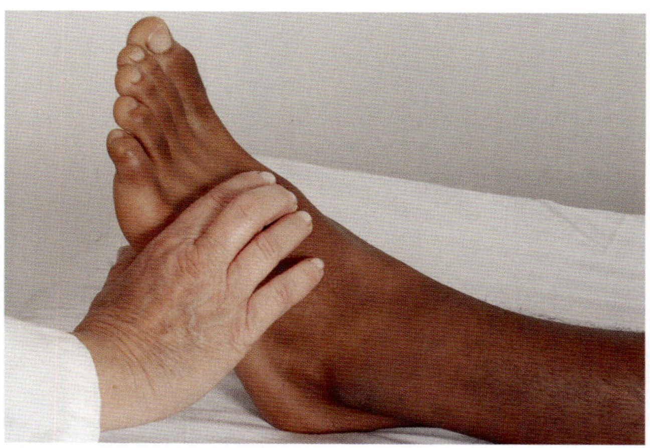

FIGURE 16.17 Palpation of the dorsalis pedis pulse

Pretibial oedema

Check for pretibial oedema. Firmly depress the skin over the tibia or the medial malleolus for 5 seconds and release (Figure 16.18A).
Normally, your finger should leave no indentation, although a pit is commonly seen if the person has been standing all day or during pregnancy.

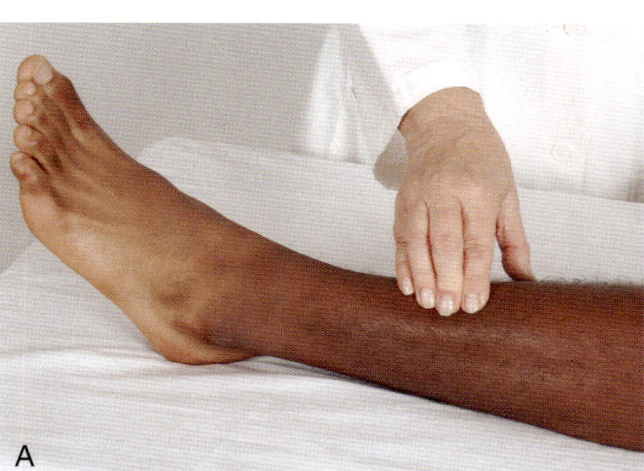

FIGURE 16.18A Palpation for pretibial oedema

Bilateral, dependent, pitting oedema occurs with heart failure, diabetic neuropathy and hepatic cirrhosis (Figure 16.18B).

PROCEDURES AND NORMAL FINDINGS	ABNORMAL FINDINGS AND CLINICAL ALERTS

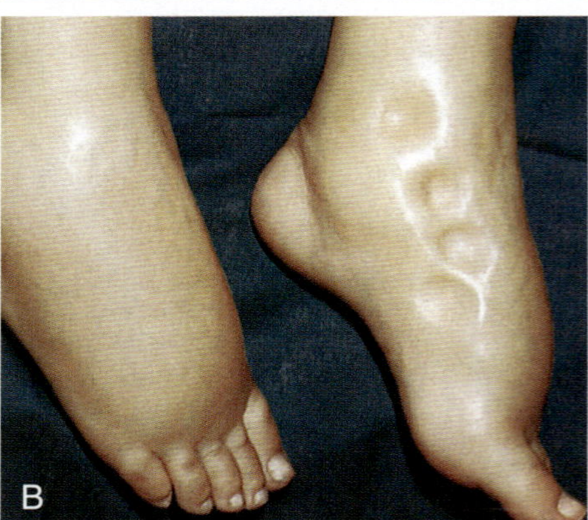

FIGURE 16.18B Pitting oedema of the feet and ankles

If pitting oedema is present, grade it on the following scale:

1+ Mild pitting, slight indentation, no perceptible swelling of the leg
2+ Moderate pitting, indentation subsides rapidly
3+ Deep pitting, indentation remains for a short time, leg looks swollen
4+ Very deep pitting, indentation lasts a long time, leg is very swollen.

However, this scale has not been established to be reliable although it is commonly used clinically. The amount of pressure used is arbitrary, as is the judgement of the depth and rate of pitting. Clinicians need a standard quantified scale to ensure consistent clinical measurements and management. Many classify the oedema by measuring the depth of the pitting in centimetres (1+ = 1 cm, 2+ = 2 cm, etc.)

Ankle circumference is more reliable using a non-stretchable tape at a point 7 cm proximal to the midpoint of the medial malleolus. Because peripheral oedema is a common clinical sign, it is important to detect true changes in the most accurate way available. Check with your own institution to conform to a consistently used scale.

Unilateral oedema occurs with occlusion of a deep vein (Table 16.5). Unilateral or bilateral oedema occurs with lymphatic obstruction. With these factors, it is 'brawny' or nonpitting and feels hard to the touch.

Leg veins

Ask the person to stand so that you can assess the venous system. Note any visible, dilated and tortuous veins.

Varicosities occur in the saphenous veins (Table 16.2).

PROCEDURES AND NORMAL FINDINGS

Skin colour changes

If you suspect an arterial deficit, raise the legs about 30 cm off the bed and ask the person to wag the feet for about 30 seconds to drain off venous blood (Figure 16.19). The skin colour now reflects only the contribution of arterial blood. A light-skinned person's feet normally will look a little pale but still should be pink. A dark-skinned person's feet are more difficult to evaluate, but the soles should reveal extreme colour change.

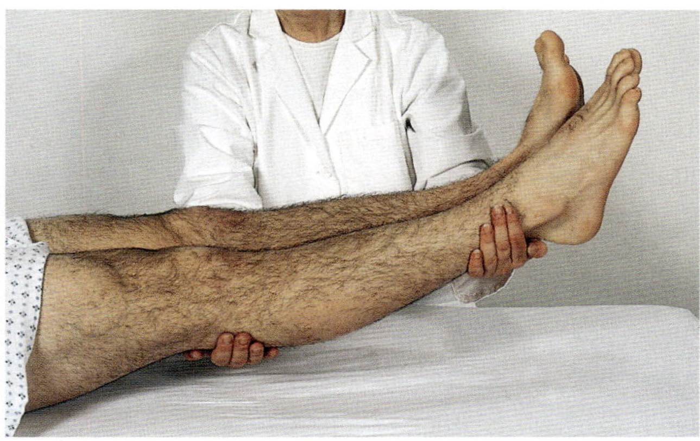

FIGURE 16.19 Inspection for skin colour change on leg raise

Now have the person sit up with the legs over the side of the bed (Figure 16.20A). Compare the colour of both feet. Note the time it takes for colour to return to the feet. Normally, this is 10 seconds or less. Also note the time it takes for the superficial veins around the feet to fill—the normal time is about 15 seconds. This test is unreliable if the person has concomitant venous disease with incompetent valves.

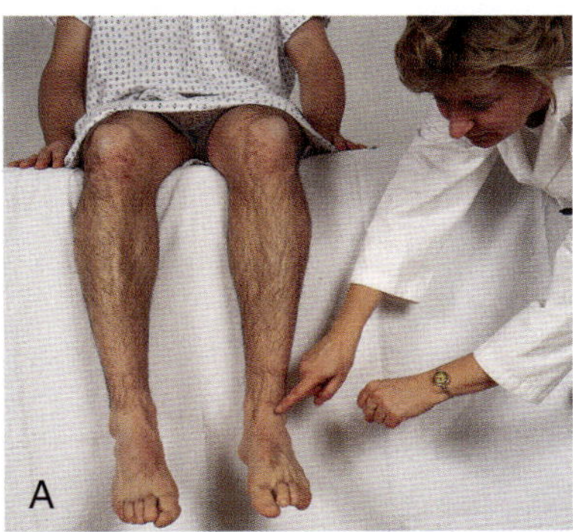

FIGURE 16.20A Inspection for skin colour change when feet dangling

ABNORMAL FINDINGS AND CLINICAL ALERTS

Elevational pallor (marked) indicates arterial insufficiency.

Dependent rubor (deep blue-red colour) occurs with severe arterial insufficiency (Figure 16.20B). Chronic hypoxia produces a loss of vasomotor tone and a pooling of blood in the veins.

Delayed venous filling occurs with arterial insufficiency.

PROCEDURES AND NORMAL FINDINGS	ABNORMAL FINDINGS AND CLINICAL ALERTS

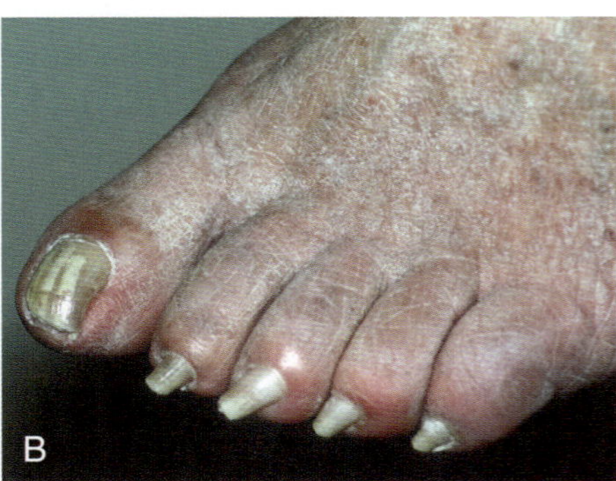

FIGURE 16.20B Severe arterial insufficiency of the feet

Lower leg strength and sensation

Test the lower legs for strength (Chapter 12). Test the lower legs for sensation (Chapter 12).

Motor loss occurs with severe arterial deficit.

Sensory loss occurs with arterial deficit, especially diabetes.

Assessing peripheral pulses using a Doppler

Use this device to detect a weak peripheral pulse, to monitor blood pressure in infants or children or to measure a low blood pressure or blood pressure in a lower extremity (Figure 16.21). The Doppler magnifies pulsatile sounds from the heart and blood vessels. Place the person in a supine position, with the legs externally rotated so you can reach the medial ankles easily. Place a drop of coupling gel on the end of the handheld transducer. Place the transducer over a pulse site, swivelled at a 45-degree angle. Apply very light pressure; locate the pulse site by the swishing, whooshing sound. See also Chapter 10.

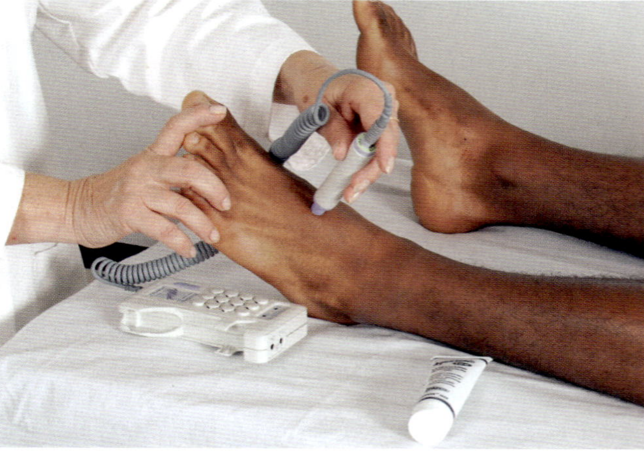

FIGURE 16.21 Using a Doppler to assess peripheral pulses

PROCEDURES AND NORMAL FINDINGS	ABNORMAL FINDINGS AND CLINICAL ALERTS
Additional objective data for infants and children	
Transient acrocyanosis and skin mottling at birth are discussed in Chapter 22. The pulse strength should be strong and symmetrical. The pulse strength should also be the same in the upper and lower extremities.	**Acrocyanosis** is a vasomotor condition characterised by persistent, painless, usually symmetrical cyanosis of the distal parts of the body (the hands, feet or, rarely, the face) caused by vasospasm of the small vessels of the skin in response to cold.[8] Weak pulses occur with vasoconstriction of diminished cardiac output. Full, bounding pulses occur with patent ductus arteriosus because of the large left-to-right shunt. Diminished or absent femoral pulses while upper extremity pulses are normal suggest **coarctation of aorta** (congenital narrowing of the aorta).
Additional objective assessment data for pregnant women	
Expect diffuse bilateral pitting oedema in the lower extremities, especially at the end of the day and into the third trimester. Varicose veins in the legs are also common in the third trimester.	 ***Clinical alert:*** Generalised oedema with hypertension is a sign of preeclampsia, a serious obstetric health issue. The woman should be referred to her midwife, nurse practitioner or medical practitioner for further assessment.
Additional objective assessment data for adults over 65 years	
The dorsalis pedis and posterior tibial pulse may become more difficult to find. Trophic changes associated with arterial insufficiency (thin, shiny skin, thick-ridged nails, loss of hair on lower legs) also occur normally with ageing.	

Abnormal findings

TABLE 16.1 History profiles of pain of peripheral vascular disease

Symptom Analysis	Chronic Arterial Symptoms	Acute Arterial Symptoms
Location	Deep muscle pain, usually in calf, but may be lower on leg or dorsum of foot	Varies, distal to occlusion, may involve entire leg
Character	Intermittent claudication, feels like 'cramp', 'numbness and tingling', 'feeling of cold'	Throbbing
Onset and duration	Chronic pain, onset gradual after exertion	Sudden onset (within 1 hour)

Continued

TABLE 16.1 History profiles of pain of peripheral vascular disease cont'd

Symptom Analysis	Chronic Arterial Symptoms	Acute Arterial Symptoms
Aggravating factors	Activity (walking, stairs) 'Claudication distance' is specific number of blocks, stairs it takes to produce pain Elevation (rest pain indicates severe involvement)	
Relieving factors	Rest—usually within 2 minutes (e.g. lying) Dangling (severe involvement)	
Associated symptoms	Cool, pale skin	Six Ps: pain, pallor, pulselessness, paraesthesia, poikilothermia (coldness), paralysis (indicates severe)
Those at risk	Adults over 65 years, more males than females, inherited predisposition, history of hypertension, smoking, diabetes, hypercholesterolaemia, obesity, vascular disease	History of vascular surgery; arterial invasive procedure; abdominal aneurysm (emboli) (Table 16.5); trauma, including injured arteries, chronic atrial fibrillation
Symptom Analysis	***Chronic Venous Symptoms***	***Acute Venous Symptoms***
Location	Calf, lower leg	Calf
Character	Aching, tiredness, feeling of fullness	Intense, sharp; deep muscle tender to touch
Onset and duration	Chronic pain, increases at end of day	Sudden onset (within 1 hour)
Aggravating factors	Prolonged standing, sitting	Pain may increase with sharp dorsiflexion of foot
Relieving factors	Elevation, lying, walking	
Associated symptoms	Oedema, varicosities, weeping ulcers at ankles	Red, warm, swollen leg
Those at risk	Job with prolonged standing or sitting; obesity; pregnancy; prolonged bed rest; history of heart failure, varicosities or thrombophlebitis; veins crushed by trauma or surgery	

TABLE 16.2 Peripheral vascular disease in the legs

Chronic Arterial Insufficiency

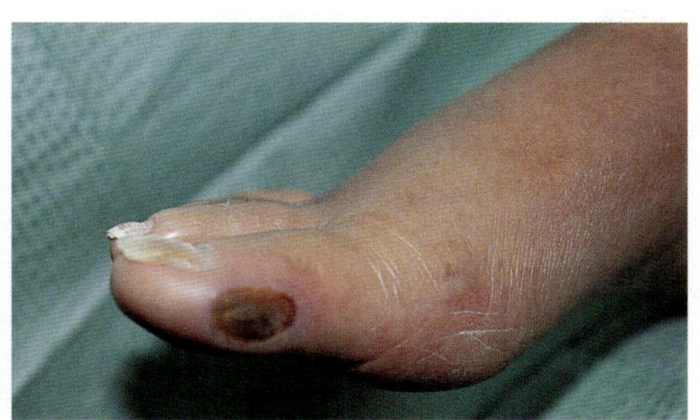

Arterial foot ulcer

Cause: Build-up of fatty plaques on inner layer (intima) (atherosclerosis) plus hardening and calcification of arterial wall (arteriosclerosis).
Symptoms: Deep muscle pain in calf or foot, claudication (pain with walking), pain at rest indicates worsening of condition.
Signs: Coolness, pallor, elevational pallor and dependent rubor; diminished pulses; systolic bruits; trophic skin; signs of malnutrition (thin, shiny skin, thick-ridged nails, absence of hair, atrophy of muscles); xanthoma formation; distal gangrene.
Ulcers: Occur at toes, metatarsal heads, heels, lateral ankle and are characterised by pale ischaemic base, well-defined edges and no bleeding.

Chronic Venous Insufficiency

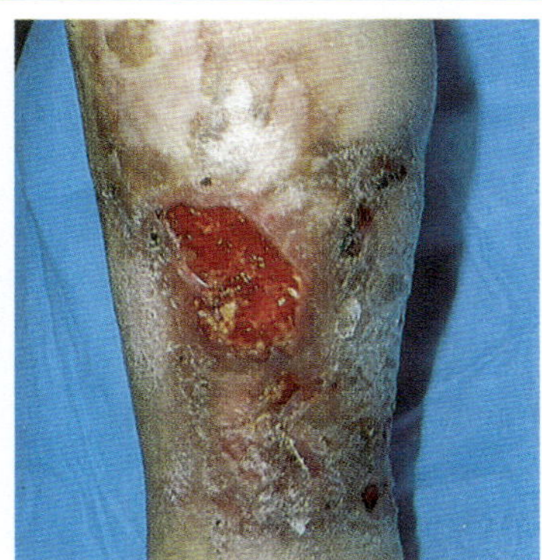

Venous ulcer

Venous ulcers account for 80% of lower leg ulcers.
Symptoms: Aching pain in calf or lower leg, which is worse at end of the day and worse with prolonged standing or sitting. Itching with stasis ulcers.
Signs: Lower leg oedema; coarse, thickened skin; pulses normal; brown pigment discolouration; petechiae; dermatitis.
Ulcers: Occur at medial malleolus and are characterised by bleeding, uneven edges.

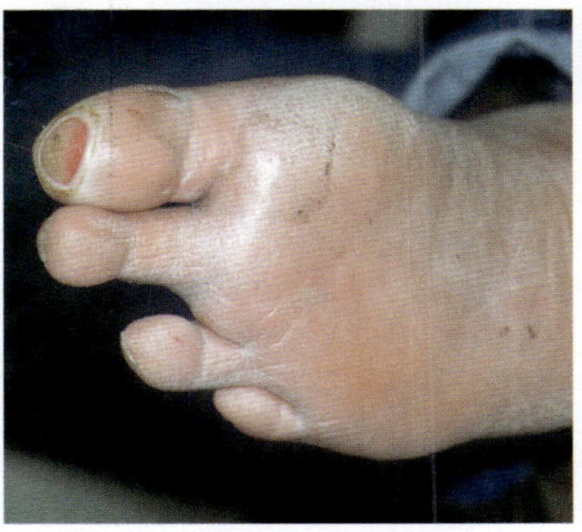

Diabetic (neuropathic) related foot ulcer

Diabetes hastens changes described with arterial ischaemic ulcer, with generalised dysfunction in all arterial areas (peripheral, coronary, cerebral, retinal and renal). A peripheral diabetic ulcer has its pathogenesis in sensory neuropathy with loss of protective sensation, autonomic neuropathy with decreased sweating and dry skin and motor neuropathy with foot deformity.
Ulcers: Occur with repetitive stress over these at-risk areas.

Continued

TABLE 16.2 Peripheral vascular disease in the legs cont'd

Chronic Venous Disease	Acute Venous Disease
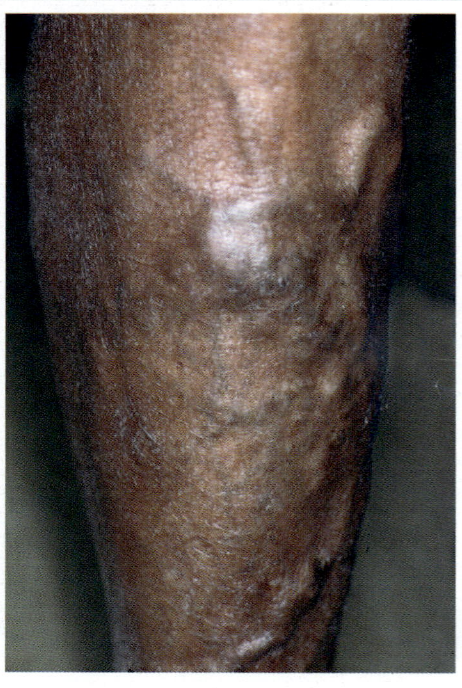	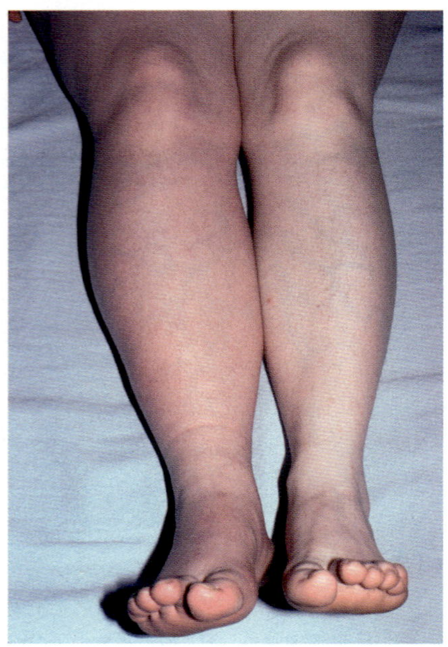
Superficial varicose veins Incompetent valves permit reflux of blood, producing dilated, tortuous veins. Unremitting hydrostatic pressure causes distal valves to be incompetent and causes worsening of the varicosity. Over age 45 years, occurrence is three times more common in women than in men. **Symptoms:** Aching, heaviness in calf, easy fatiguability, night leg or foot cramps. **Signs:** Dilated, tortuous veins, foot oedema.	***Deep vein thrombophlebitis*** A deep vein is occluded by a thrombus, causing inflammation, blocked venous return, cyanosis and oedema. **Symptoms:** Sudden onset of intense, sharp, deep muscle pain; may increase with sharp dorsiflexion of foot. **Signs:** Increased warmth; swelling (compare both legs); redness; dependent cyanosis is mild or may be absent; tender to palpation.

TABLE 16.3 Variations in arterial pulse

Description	Associated With
Weak, 'thready' pulse—1+ Hard to palpate, need to search for it, may fade in and out, easily obliterated by pressure.	Decreased cardiac output; PAD; aortic valve stenosis

TABLE 16.3 Variations in arterial pulse cont'd

Description	Associated With
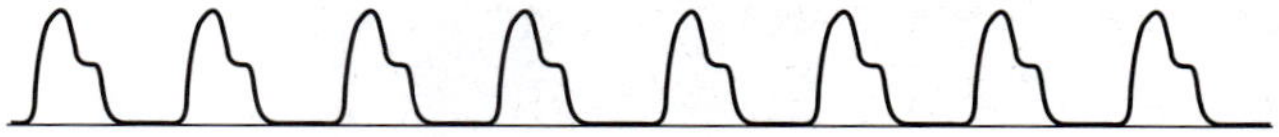 **Full, bounding pulse—3+** Easily palpable, pounds under your fingertips.	Hyperkinetic states (exercise, anxiety, fever), anaemia, hyperthyroidism
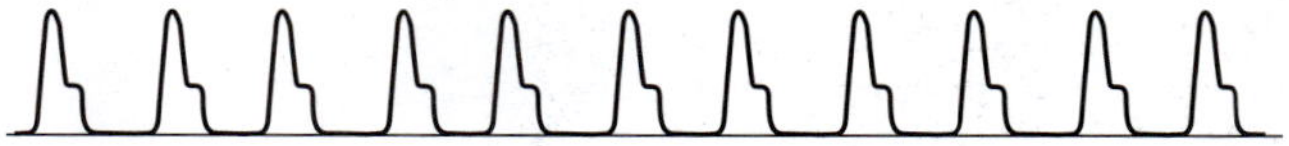 **Water-hammer (Corrigan's) pulse—3+** Greater than normal strength, then collapses suddenly.	Aortic valve regurgitation; patent ductus arteriosus
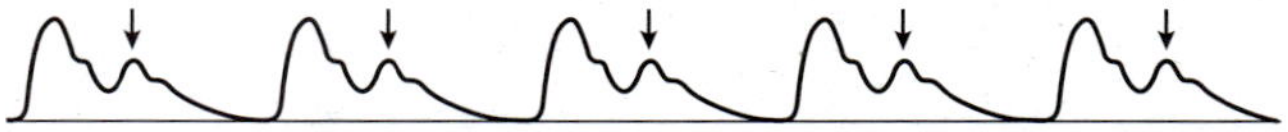 **Pulsus bigeminus** Rhythm is coupled, every other beat comes early or normal beat followed by premature beat. The strength of the premature beat is decreased because of shortened cardiac filling time.	Conduction disturbance (e.g. premature ventricular contraction, premature atrial contraction)
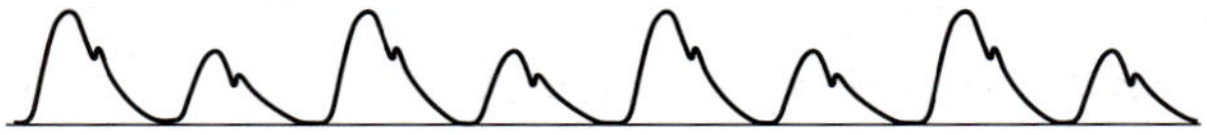 **Pulsus alternans** Rhythm is regular, but the strength varies with alternating beats of large and small amplitude.	Heart failure
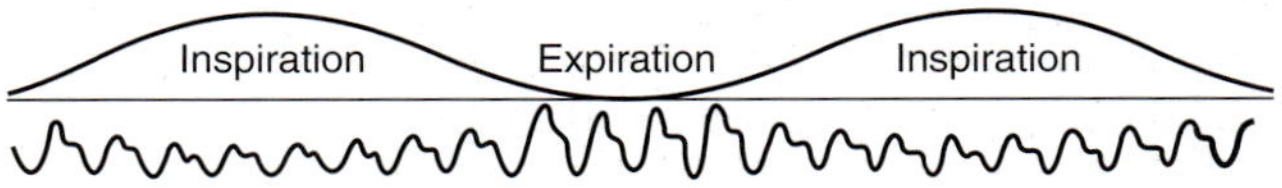 Inspiration Expiration Inspiration **Pulsus paradoxus** Beats have weaker amplitude with inspiration, stronger with expiration. Best determined during blood pressure measurement; reading decreases (> 10 mmHg) during inspiration and increases with expiration.	Any condition that blocks venous return to the right side of the heart or blocks left ventricular filling (e.g. cardiac tamponade; constrictive pericarditis, pulmonary embolism)
Pulsus bisferiens Each pulse has two strong systolic peaks, with a dip in between. Best assessed at the carotid artery.	Aortic valve stenosis plus regurgitation

TABLE 16.4 Peripheral vascular disease in the arms

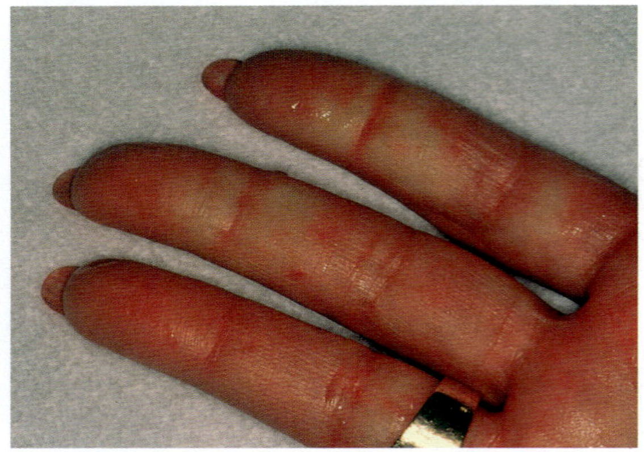

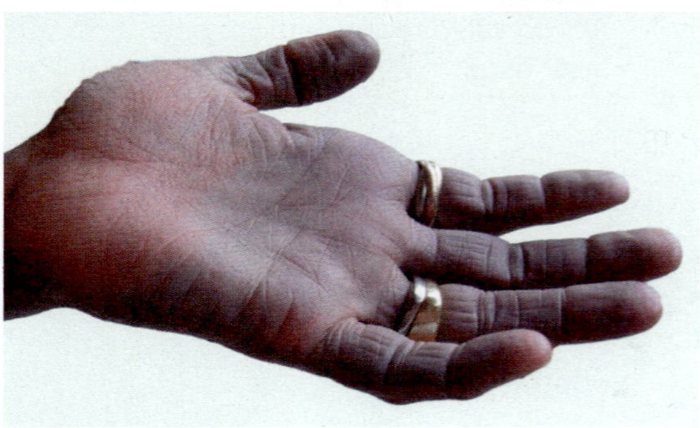

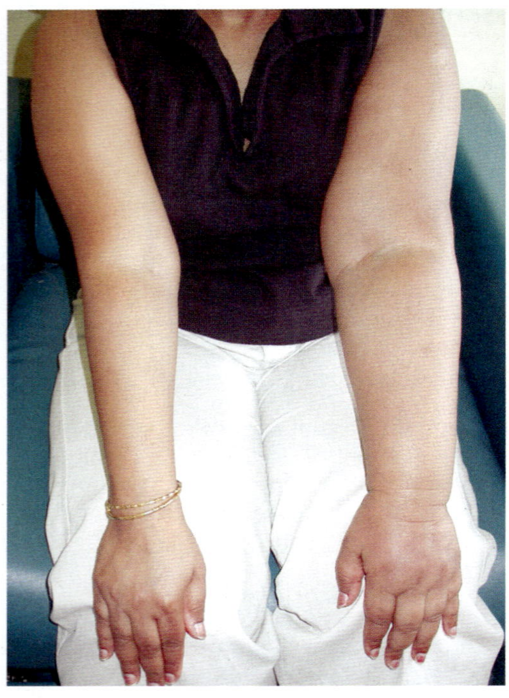

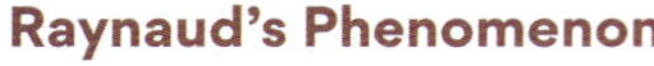

Raynaud's Phenomenon

Symptoms: May have cold, numbness or pain along with pallor or cyanosis stage; then burning, throbbing pain, swelling along with rubor. Lasts minutes to hours; occurs bilaterally.
Signs: Episodes of abrupt progressive tricolour change of the fingers in response to cold, vibration or stress: first white (pallor) from arteriospasm and resulting deficit in supply; then blue (cyanosis) from slight relaxation of the spasm that allows a slow trickle of blood through the capillaries and increased oxygen extraction of haemoglobin; finally red (rubor) due to return of blood into the dilated capillary bed or reactive hyperaemia.

Lymphoedema

Removal of axillary lymph nodes with breast surgery or damage to lymph nodes and channels with radiation therapy for breast cancer; can impede drainage of lymph. Protein-rich lymph builds up in the interstitial spaces, which further raises local colloid oncotic pressure and promotes more fluid leakage. Stagnant lymphatic fluid can lead to infection, delayed wound healing, chronic inflammation and fibrosis of surrounding tissue.
Signs: Chronic lymphoedema is unilateral, non-pitting 'brawny' oedema, with overlying skin indurated.

Advanced practice—additional data

The assessments that are described in the following sections require advanced skill and scope of practice. Nurses working in specialist cardiac units and nurses working in community centres may need to develop these skills. See Chapter 15 for reference.

PROCEDURES AND NORMAL FINDINGS	ABNORMAL FINDINGS AND CLINICAL ALERTS
Inspect and palpate the arms	
Lymph nodes	
Check the epitrochlear lymph node in the depression above and behind the medial condyle of the humerus. Do this by 'shaking hands' with the person and reaching your other hand under the person's elbow to the groove between the biceps and triceps muscles, above the medial epicondyle (Figure 16.22). This node is not normally palpable.	An enlarged epitrochlear node occurs with infection of the hand or forearm.
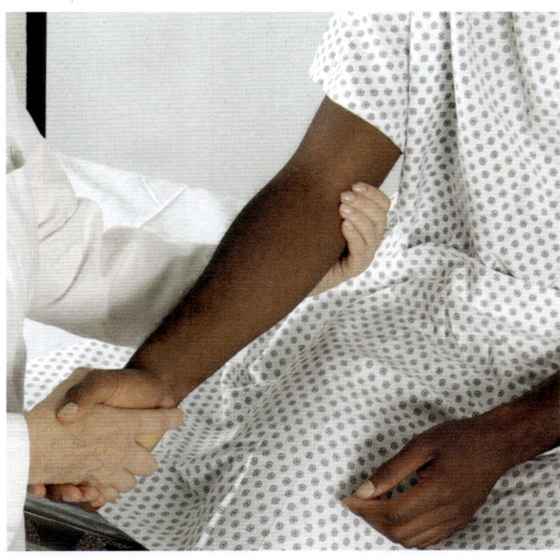 **FIGURE 16.22** Palpation of the epitrochlear lymph node	
In addition to the techniques related to inspection and palpation of the arms described previously, the modified Allen test will give you additional data on peripheral circulation of the arms.	

PROCEDURES AND NORMAL FINDINGS	ABNORMAL FINDINGS AND CLINICAL ALERTS

The Allen test—radial artery patency

The **modified Allen test** is used to evaluate the adequacy of collateral circulation before cannulating the radial artery (Figure 16.23).
A Firmly occlude both the ulnar and the radial arteries of one hand while the person makes a fist several times. This causes the hand to blanch.
B Ask the person to open the hand without hyperextending it; then release pressure on the ulnar artery while maintaining pressure on the radial artery. Adequate circulation is suggested by a return to the hand's normal colour in approximately 2 to 5 seconds.
The modified Allen test is a valid tool in primary screening.[9]

Pallor persists or a sluggish return to colour suggests occlusion of the collateral arterial flow. Avoid radial artery cannulation until adequate circulation is shown.

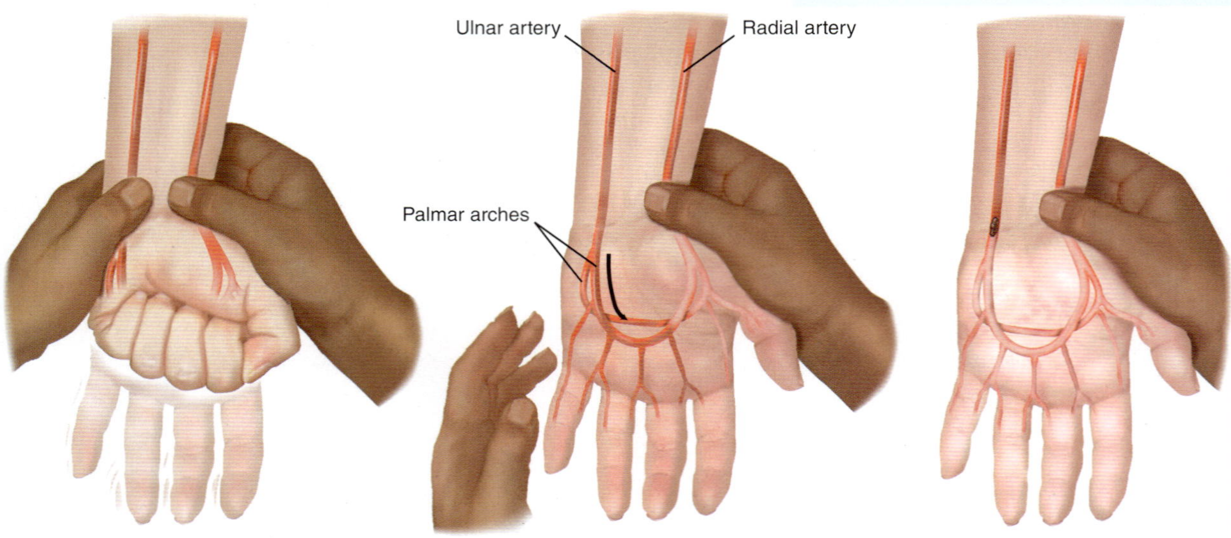

FIGURE 16.23 Modified Allen test

Inspect and palpate the legs

In addition to the techniques related to inspection and palpation of the legs described previously, palpation of inguinal lymph nodes will extend assessment data for the advanced practice nurse.
The manual compression test and the ankle brachial index will give you additional data on peripheral circulation of the legs.

Palpate the inguinal lymph nodes. It is not unusual to find palpable nodes that are small (1 cm or less), movable and nontender.

Enlarged nodes, tender or fixed in area.

The ankle-brachial index (ABI)

Use of the Doppler stethoscope is a highly specific, noninvasive and readily available way to determine the extent of PAD.

PROCEDURES AND NORMAL FINDINGS	ABNORMAL FINDINGS AND CLINICAL ALERTS
The person is lying flat with the head and heels fully supported. Confirm no smoking within 2 hours of the measurement and allow a 5- to 10-minute rest period supine before measurement. Choose the correct cuff width for the arm and the ankle; width should be 40% of limb circumference. Position the ankle cuff just above the malleoli with straight wrapping. Use the Doppler probe for both brachial and ankle measurements. In all sites, locate the pulse by Doppler and inflate the cuff 20 mmHg above disappearance of flow signal; then deflate slowly to detect reappearance of flow signal.[10] Measure each site twice and use the average as the recorded pressure. Moving counterclockwise, measure: right arm, right posterior tibial (PT), right dorsalis pedis (DP), left PT, left DP, left arm. Calculate both ABI using this formula:	
$\text{Right ABI} = \dfrac{\text{highest right average ankle pressure (DP or PT)}}{\text{Highest average arm pressure (right or left)}}$	An ABI of 0.91 to 1.0 is borderline for cardiovascular risk.[11] An ABI of 0.91 or less indicates the presence of PAD: • 0.90 to 0.70—mild PAD • 0.71 to 0.40—moderate to severe PAD • 0.41 to 0.30—severe PAD, usually with rest pain except in the presence of diabetic neuropathy • $<$ 0.30—ischaemia, with impending loss of tissue.
For example: $\dfrac{\text{132 ankle systolic}}{\text{124 arm systolic}} = \text{1.06 or 106, indicating no flow reduction}$	
$\text{Left ABI} = \dfrac{\text{highest left ankle pressure (DP or PT)}}{\text{highest average arm pressure (right or left)}}$ The normal ankle pressure is slightly greater than or equal to the brachial pressure; thus, a normal ABI is usually 1.0 to 1.2. In people with diabetes, the ABI may be less reliable because of calcification (which makes their arteries noncompressible and may give a falsely high measurement).[4]	
Additional objective data for infants and children	
Palpable lymph nodes often occur in healthy infants and children. They are small, firm, mobile and nontender. They may be the sequelae of past infection, such as inguinal nodes from a nappy rash or cervical nodes from a respiratory infection. Vaccinations can also produce local lymphadenopathy. Note characteristics of any palpable nodes and whether they are local or generalised.	Enlarged, warm, tender nodes indicate current infection. Look for the source of infection.

Abnormal findings for advanced practice

TABLE 16.5 Other vascular abnormalities

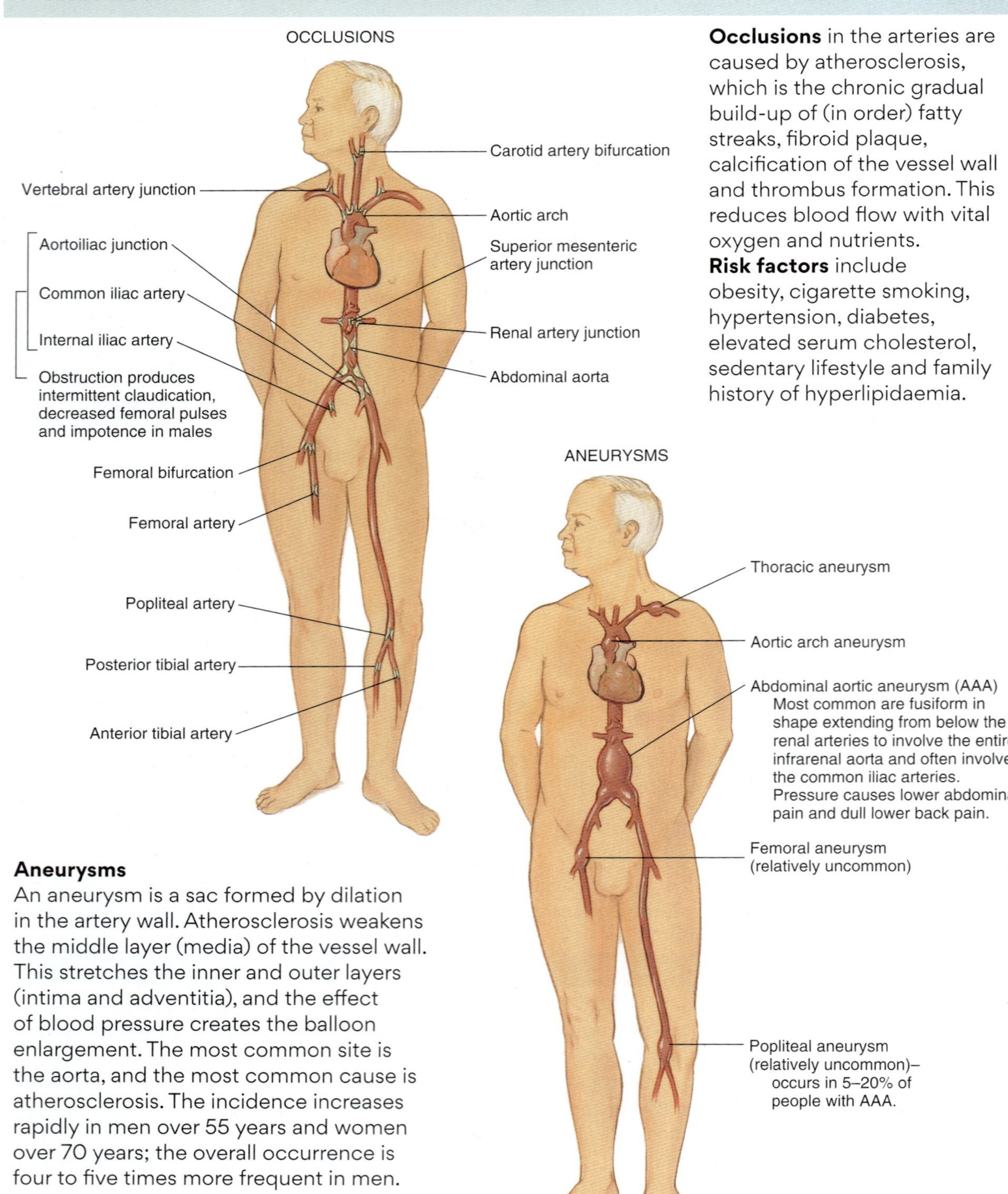

Occlusions in the arteries are caused by atherosclerosis, which is the chronic gradual build-up of (in order) fatty streaks, fibroid plaque, calcification of the vessel wall and thrombus formation. This reduces blood flow with vital oxygen and nutrients. **Risk factors** include obesity, cigarette smoking, hypertension, diabetes, elevated serum cholesterol, sedentary lifestyle and family history of hyperlipidaemia.

Aneurysms
An aneurysm is a sac formed by dilation in the artery wall. Atherosclerosis weakens the middle layer (media) of the vessel wall. This stretches the inner and outer layers (intima and adventitia), and the effect of blood pressure creates the balloon enlargement. The most common site is the aorta, and the most common cause is atherosclerosis. The incidence increases rapidly in men over 55 years and women over 70 years; the overall occurrence is four to five times more frequent in men.

Documentation and clinical reasoning

The following are case studies that illustrate the documentation of clinical data related to peripheral vascular assessment and the clinical reasoning process including problem/issue identification. Consult a fundamentals of nursing or medical-surgical nursing text for information about goal setting, nursing interventions and evaluation.

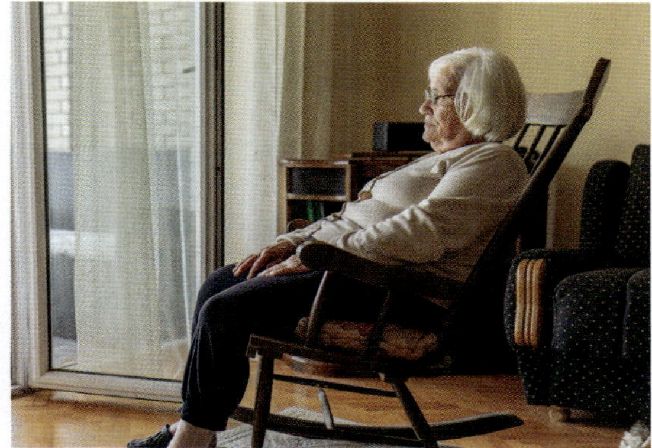

Case study 1 (continued)—Chronic venous leg ulcer

Context

You will recall that you are on a clinical placement working alongside a community nurse specialist who works with people requiring care in their home.

Consider the patient's situation

Mrs Margaret Sheffield, a 79-year-old woman, has been referred to the community nursing service for ongoing assessment and treatment of a venous leg ulcer (right lower leg).

Collect cues/information

Your further assessment reveals the following information.

Subjective data

Mrs Sheffield has been living in a retirement village for 5 years. She enjoys the social life in the village and has many friends. Her husband died 6 years ago. She has three adult children who all visit her regularly. She worked in a fabric shop until she was 60 years of age.

Her relevant past medical history includes varicose veins that developed during pregnancy and have been treated by a vascular surgeon 'many years ago'. She is receiving treatment for high blood pressure—*Perindopril* (4 mg bd), which is monitored by her GP. She says her blood pressure has been stable for a few years. She smoked cigarettes (a few a day) until she was in her mid-20s when she first became pregnant. Her husband smoked cigarettes (a pack per day) until he was in his early 40s. He did not smoke in the house.

She has noticed that the skin on her shins and ankles has been itchy and scaly for about 6 months. She has not noticed any changes to sensation or temperature of her feet. She has no pain on walking. Three weeks ago she knocked the outer aspect of her lower leg on a shelf in the local supermarket. She didn't pay much attention to it at the time, but a few days later she noticed that the wound was not healing and leaking clear fluid. She tried to manage it herself with bandaids and Dettol washes. She found that the wound continued to leak, and the bandaids seemed to be pulling her 'good' skin off. She was worried about it and mentioned it to her daughter who said she should go to see her GP, who diagnosed a chronic venous leg ulcer.

She says the wound is not painful, but she is finding it difficult to keep it dry and it sticks to her clothes. She says that she is otherwise well and able to manage her own personal care, shopping and social activities. She says she gets help with the weekly vacuuming, changing her bed sheets and quilt cover and cleaning of the toilet and bathroom. She does her own shopping using the retirement village bus service and does most of her own meal preparation and cooking, which she enjoys. She loves reading and sewing.

Her diet includes a variety of meats and vegetables and she has breakfast and an early dinner every day. She says she doesn't need lunch but likes a biscuit or two with her cup of tea in the morning and in the afternoon. She doesn't eat much fruit unless it is cooked. She says she sometimes snacks on potato chips or nuts. She attends a village group meal and movie night twice a week. She says she has no problem eating or chewing.

Documentation and clinical reasoning cont'd

Objective data

Mrs Sheffield looks well, can move about her home unit independently without any mobility aids and is well groomed. Her home is clean and tidy. She appears slightly over a healthy weight; her BMI is 31.

Vital signs: Temp 36.8°C, BP 130/85, RR 12, HR 84

Left leg: Skin on lower leg dry and scaly. Left femoral, popliteal pulse strong and regular. Dorsalis pedis pulse palpable. Capillary return moderate to brisk. Toes pink and warm. Sensation normal to touch. Slight (+) pitting oedema in the feet and ankles.

Right leg: Skin on lower leg very dry and scaly. Right femoral and popliteal pulse strong and regular. Dorsalis pedis pulse palpable. Capillary return moderate. Toes pink and warm. Sensation normal to touch. Slight (+) pitting oedema in the feet, ankles and lower leg.

She had a bandage, combine pad and Jelonet type dressing in situ (applied by the GP 3 days ago). Combine is moist with a yellow tinge but no foul odour.

An ulcerated area is located on the lower outer aspect of her leg above the lateral malleolus. It is 50 mm × 30 mm and about 2 mm deep. It has a well demarcated edge with some granulation tissue. The wound is pink, with a small amount of yellow sloughy tissue in the centre. The surrounding tissue is pink and slightly moist. There is obvious serous exudate coming from the wound surface.

Process information and identify problems/issues

Collaborative problem

Chronic venous ulcer related to recent injury and moderate PVD. Refer to medical or nurse practitioner.

Problem statement/nursing diagnoses

Risk for further skin injury due to impaired skin integrity on the lower legs and impaired venous return.

Knowledge deficit about how to reduce the risk of further skin injury.

Knowledge deficit about signs of infection and when to get further assistance.

Knowledge deficit about the process of wound healing and the need for regular wound assessment and wound dressings.

Knowledge deficit about how to optimise her health status to promote wound healing.

Case study 2—Aortic stenosis causing poor peripheral arterial circulation

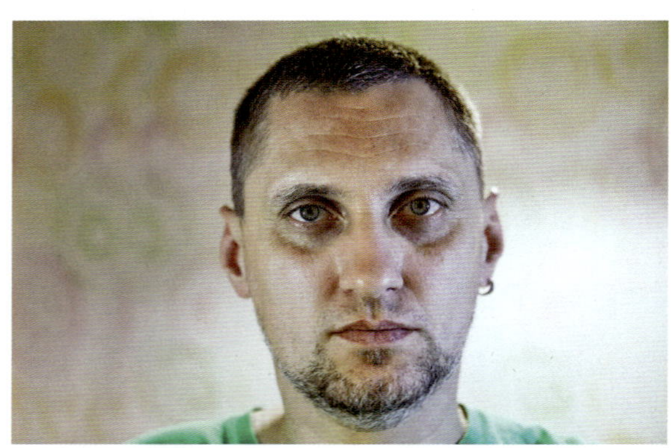

Context

Mr James Kerrigan is a 43-year-old council employee, admitted to hospital today for 'bypass surgery tomorrow to fix my aorta and these dark-coloured toes'.

Collect clues/information

Subjective data

6 years ago: Motorcycle accident with handlebars jammed into groin and lower abdominal area. Treated and discharged from local hospital. There was a lot of abdominal bruising but no apparent significant abdominal or other injury, although the cardiovascular surgeon now thinks accident may have precipitated present stenosis of aorta.

1 year ago: Radiating pain in right calf on walking 0.5 km. Pain relieved with rest.

3 months ago: Began experiencing erectile dysfunction, unable to maintain erection during intercourse.

1 month ago: Leg pain present after walking two blocks. Numbness and tingling in right foot and calf. Tips of three toes on right foot look dusky in colour. Referred to a surgeon.

Documentation and clinical reasoning cont'd

Present: Leg pain at rest, constant and severe, worse at night, partially relieved by dangling legs over side of bed.
History: No history of heart or vessel disease, hypertension, diabetes or obesity.
Current smoker: 1 packet per day. History of 25 pack years.
Walking is part of occupation, although has been driving a council truck past 3 months due to leg pain. Not currently on medication.
Social: Is married with two young children. Supportive family. Wife will be taking leave from work to care for him when he is discharged home.

Objective data

Inspection: Lower extremity size equal bilaterally with no swelling or atrophy. No varicosities. Colour L leg pink, R leg pink when supine, but marked pallor to R foot on elevation. Gangrene at tips of R 2nd, 3rd, 4th toes. Leg hair present but absent on involved toes.
Palpation: R foot cool and temperature progressively warms on palpation up R leg.
Pulses: Femorals, both 1+; popliteals, both 0; posterior tibial, both 0 but present with Doppler; dorsalis pedis both 0, but left dorsalis pedis is present with Doppler, and right is not present with Doppler.
Diagnostic studies: Showed stenosis of abdominal aorta below kidneys.

Process information and identify problems/issues

Collaborative problem

Ineffective tissue perfusion related to interruption of blood flow resulting from past injury.

Problem statements/nursing diagnoses

Ischaemic rest pain in right leg related to poor blood flow.
Impaired tissue integrity in the right toes related to altered circulation.
Risk of skin breakdown related to altered circulation.
Activity intolerance related to leg pain.
Potential for anxiety related to uncertain outcome of surgery and possible need for amputation of toes.

ADDITIONAL RESOURCES

You can further develop your knowledge and skills relevant to peripheral vascular assessment, related pathophysiology, common health issues and nursing interventions by:

- reading chapters of a fundamentals of nursing or medical-surgical nursing textbook
- answering chapter multiple choice questions online. Log onto ClinicalKey Student and search for the text 'Health Assessment, 4th edition'. Choose the section titled 'Teaching material'. In this section you will find question and answer documents for each chapter. Please check instructions on the inside cover of the book to access online resources
- visiting websites

The Australian and New Zealand Society for Vascular Nursing: www.anzsvn.org

The Australian and New Zealand Society for Vascular Surgery: www.anzsvs.org.au

The Australian Lymphology Association: www.lymphoedema.org.au

REFERENCES

1. Alahakoon C, Singh TP, Morris, D, Charles J, Fernando M, Lazzarini P, et al. Cohort study examining the presentation, distribution, and outcomes of peripheral artery disease in Aboriginal, Torres Strait Islander, and Non-Indigenous Australians. European Journal of Vascular and Endovascular Surgery, 2023;66(2): 237–244.
2. Australian Institute of Health and Welfare. Heart, stroke and vascular disease: Australian facts [Internet]. Canberra: Australian Institute of Health and Welfare, 2023. Available from: https://www.aihw.gov.au/reports/heart-stroke-vascular-diseases/hsvd-facts
3. Aitken SJ. Peripheral artery disease in the lower limbs. Australian Journal of General Practice, 2020: 49: 239–244.
4. Polonsky TS, McDermott MM. Lower extremity peripheral artery disease without chronic limb-threatening ischemia: a review. JAMA: The Journal of the American Medical Association, 2021; 325(21): 2188–2198.
5. GBD 2019 Peripheral Artery Disease Collaborators. Global burden of peripheral artery disease and its risk factors, 1990–2019: a systematic analysis for the Global Burden of Disease Study 2019. The Lancet Global Health, 2023; 11(10): e1553–e1565.
6. Mena C. and Jayasuriya S. Peripheral vascular disease: a clinical approach. Philadelphia, Pennsylvania: Wolters Kluwer. 2020
7. Rosenberg H, Rosenberg E, Kubelik D. Acute limb ischemia, Canadian Medical Association Journal, 2023;195(40):E1383.
8. Takeuchi Y, Tsukagoshi J. Primary acrocyanosis. Journal of General and Family Medicine; 2021:22(3):156–157.
9. Sivaharini S, Babu KY, Mohanraj KG. Comparative analysis of Allen's test with modified Allen's test and its clinical importance. Drug Invention Today 2018;(10):1936–1938.
10. Chan KA, Junia A. Lower extremity peripheral artery disease: a basic approach, British Journal of Hospital Medicine, 2020;81(3):1–9.
11. Aboyans V, Criqui MH, Abraham P, Allison MA, Creager MA, Diehm C, et al. Measurement and interpretation of the ankle-brachial index: a scientific statement from the American Heart Association. Circulation 2012;126(24): 2890–2909.

CHAPTER 17

Cardiac assessment

Written by Carolyn Jarvis
Adapted by Elizabeth Watt and Helen Forbes

INTRODUCTION

The cardiovascular system consists of the **heart**, a muscular pump, and the **blood vessels**. The blood vessels are arranged in two continuous loops, the pulmonary circulation and the systemic circulation. When the heart contracts, it pumps blood simultaneously into both loops. Heart disease, stroke (Chapter 12) and vascular diseases (Chapter 16), collectively known as cardiovascular disease, are common health issues that can have a significant impact on the person's activities of daily living and quality of life.

The focus of this chapter is on assessing cardiac function. You are advised to read this chapter in conjunction with Chapter 16 because cardiac assessment is commonly performed with peripheral vascular assessment. Changes in cardiac function have the potential to affect all body systems including cognitive function and mental health. To appreciate the impact of disease and trauma to this complex and dynamic system you are advised to first review the structure and function of the cardiovascular system.

Case study

The following case study gives an example of a typical situation involving cardiac assessment and the initial clinical reasoning process. It will help you to identify your learning needs.

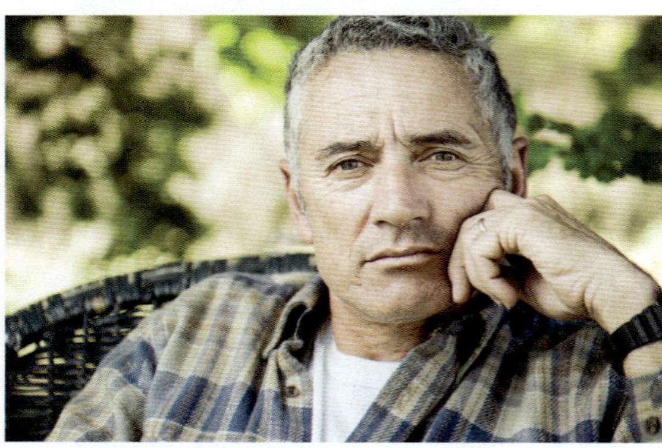

Context

You are on a clinical placement in a cardiac ward and are assisting the registered nurse to complete the admission assessment.

Consider the patient's situation

Mr Neil Andrews is a 53-year-old male who runs his own building company and was admitted to the cardiac ward via the emergency department with chest pain.

Questions to further your learning

- What are the possible things that might be going on with Mr Andrews?
- What knowledge do you need to be able to predict what might be going on?
- What approach to cardiac assessment will you take?
- What questions (subjective data) will you ask Mr Andrews to extend the health history and why?
- What physical examination (objective data) will you conduct and why?
- What resources are available to assist in your assessment of Mr Andrews?

Assessment plan

As you work through the assessment of cardiac function, keep in mind that this area is usually conducted with assessment of peripheral vascular and respiratory function. It is important to investigate the symptoms the person is presenting with because these will give clues to the underlying pathophysiology of the symptoms and will guide physical examination. The main areas for subjective data collection are:

- presenting concern
- chest pain

- dyspnoea
- orthopnoea
- cough
- fatigue
- cyanosis or pallor
- oedema
- nocturia
- cardiac history
- family cardiac history
- health and lifestyle management.

Following subjective data collection, you will get a sense of the areas needed to be examined for objective data. The focus of the physical examination is to check over the person for clinical signs that support or are in addition to their reported symptoms. Assessment of cardiac function is aimed at assessing risk factors, pain, fatigue, dyspnoea, risk of falling and the impact of symptoms on the person's usual activities of daily living. Only the relevant areas should be examined. The main areas for physical examination and measurement are:

- general inspection
- detailed inspection and vital signs
- identify relevant surface landmarks
- inspect and palpate neck vessels
- inspect and palpate the praecordium
- auscultation of apical (mitral) area
- laboratory studies.

Resources available

You will find additional resources and the reference list at the end of this chapter. This chapter also has a video available demonstrating objective data collection related to cardiac assessment. You will find a QR code in the objective data section that will allow you to access the video easily on your device.

Structure and function

Heart position and surface landmarks

The **praecordium** is the area on the anterior chest overlying the heart and great vessels (Figure 17.1). The great vessels are the major arteries and veins connected to the heart. The heart and the great vessels are located between the lungs in the middle third of the thoracic cage, called the **mediastinum**. The heart extends from the second to the fifth intercostal space and from the right border of the sternum to the left midclavicular line.

Think of the heart as an upside-down triangle in the chest. The 'top' of the heart is the broader base and the 'bottom' is the apex, which points down and to the left (Figure 17.2). During contraction, the apex beats against the chest wall, producing an apical impulse. This is palpable in most people, normally at the fifth intercostal space, 7 to 9 cm from the midsternal line on the left side.

Inside the body, the heart is rotated so that its right side is anterior, and its left side is mostly posterior. Of the heart's four chambers, the right ventricle forms the greatest area of anterior cardiac surface. The left ventricle lies behind the right ventricle and forms the apex and slender area of the left border. The right atrium lies to the right and above the right ventricle and forms the right border. The left atrium is located posteriorly, with only a small portion, the left atrial appendage, showing anteriorly.

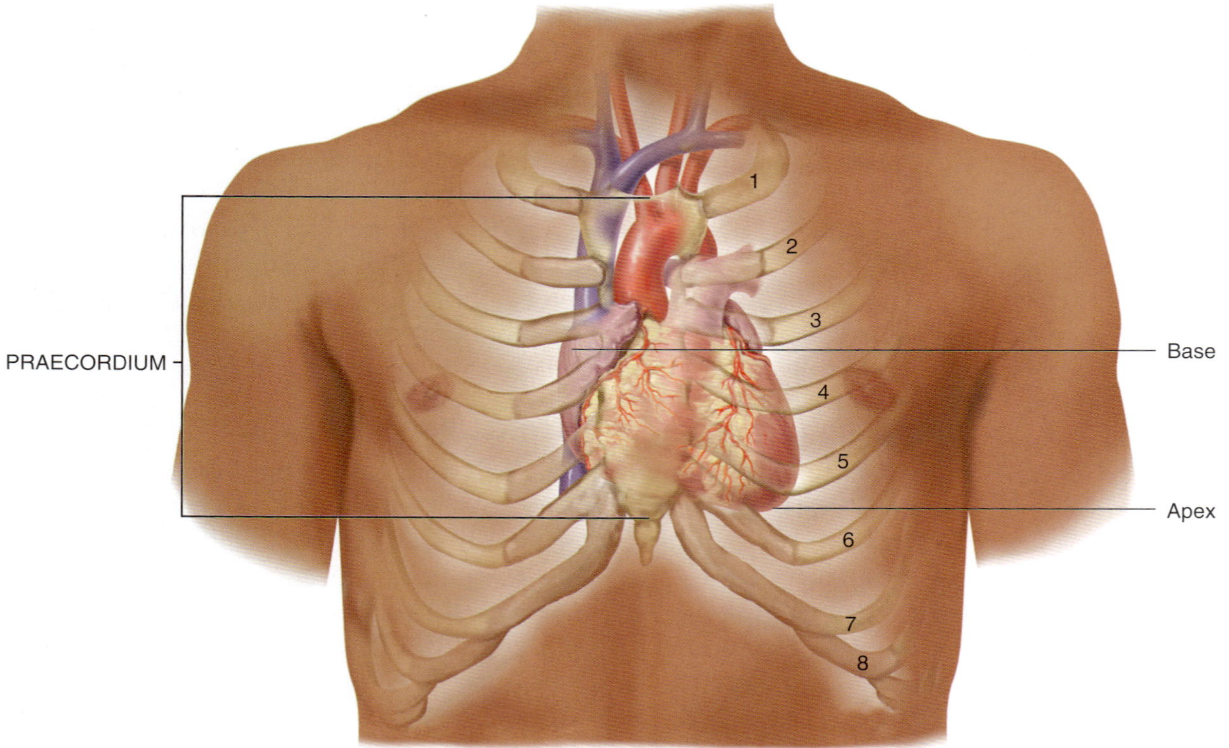

FIGURE 17.1 Anterior chest—position of the heart and major blood vessels

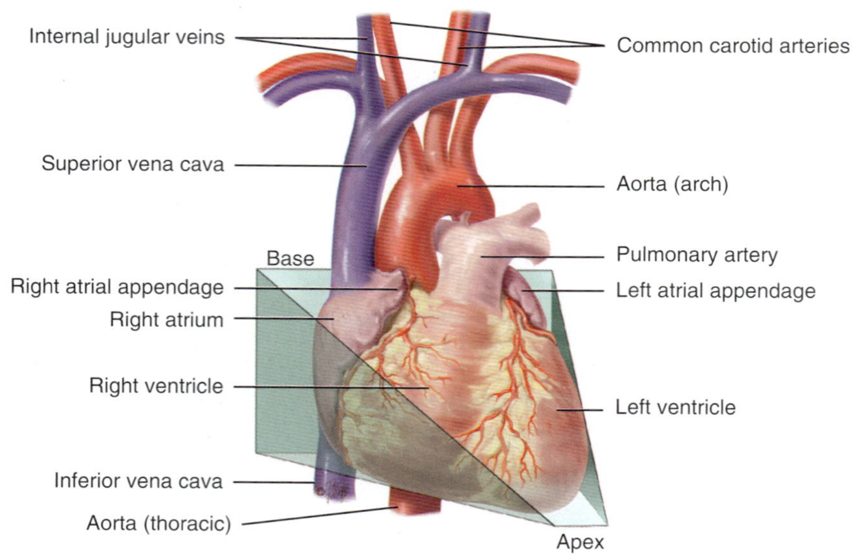

FIGURE 17.2 Anatomical features of the external heart and major blood vessels

The **great vessels** lie above the base of the heart. The **superior** and **inferior vena cava** return deoxygenated venous blood to the right side of the heart. The **pulmonary artery** leaves the right ventricle, bifurcates and carries the venous blood to the lungs. The **pulmonary veins** return the freshly oxygenated blood to the left side of the heart, and the aorta carries it out to the body. The aorta ascends from the left ventricle, arches back at the level of the sternal angle and descends behind the heart.

Heart wall, chambers and valves

The **heart wall** has three layers. The **pericardium** is a tough, fibrous, double-walled sac that surrounds and protects the heart (see its cut edge in Figure 17.3). It has two layers that contain 10 to 30 mL of serous pericardial fluid. This ensures smooth, friction-free movement of the heart muscle. The pericardium is adherent to the great vessels, oesophagus, sternum and pleurae and is anchored to the diaphragm. The **myocardium** is the muscular wall of the heart; it does the pumping. The **endocardium** is the thin layer of endothelial tissue that lines the inner surface of the heart chambers and valves.

The common metaphor is to think of the heart as a pump. But consider that the heart is actually two pumps; the right side of the heart pumps blood into the lungs, and the left side of the heart simultaneously pumps blood

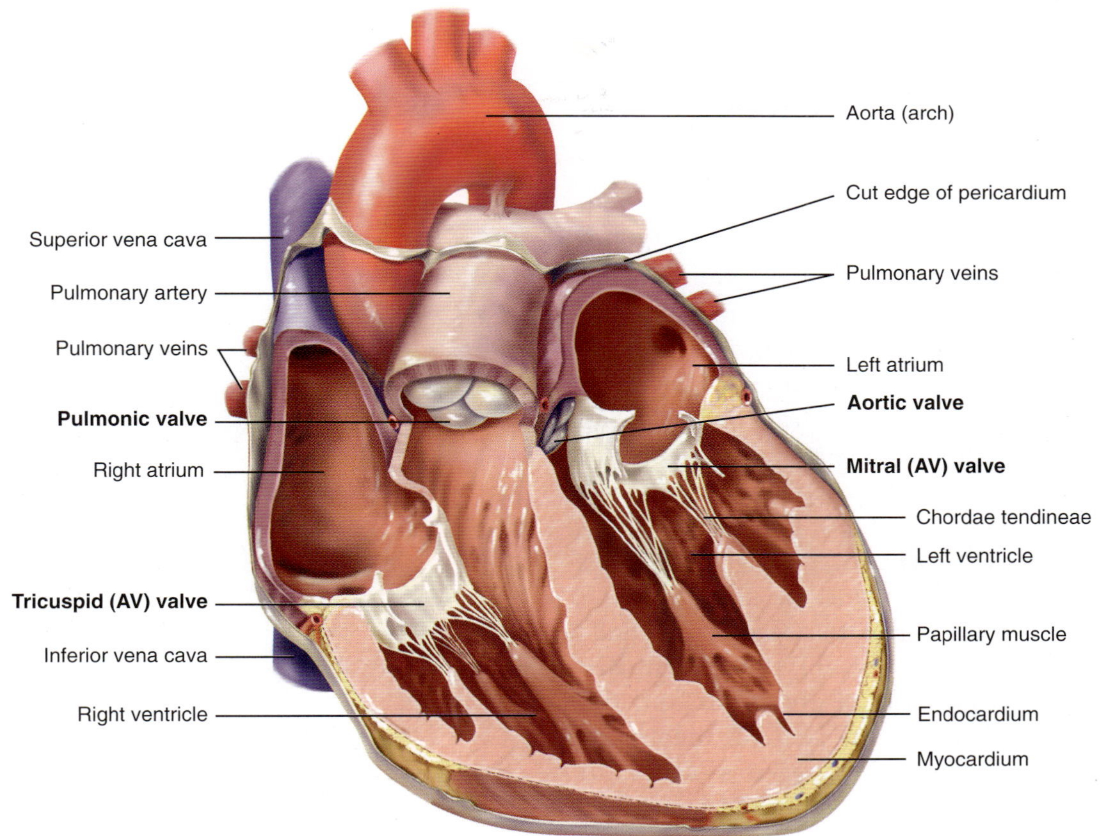

FIGURE 17.3 Anatomical features of the internal heart and major blood vessels

into the body. The two pumps are separated by an impermeable wall, the septum. Each side has an **atrium** and a **ventricle**. The atrium is a thin-walled reservoir for holding blood, and the thick-walled ventricle is the muscular pumping chamber. It is common to use the following abbreviations to refer to the chambers: RA, right atrium; RV, right ventricle; LA, left atrium; and LV, left ventricle.

The four **chambers** are separated by swinging door–like structures, called valves, whose main purpose is to prevent backflow of blood. The valves are unidirectional; they can only open one way. The valves open and close passively in response to pressure gradients in the moving blood.

There are four **valves** in the heart (Figure 17.3). The two **atrioventricula**r (AV) valves separate the atria and the ventricles. The right AV valve is the **tricuspid**, and the left AV valve is the bicuspid or **mitral** valve. The valves are thin leaflets that are anchored by collagenous fibres (**chordae tendineae**) to papillary muscles embedded in the ventricle floor. The AV valves open during the heart's filling phase, or **diastole**, to allow the ventricles to fill with blood. During the pumping phase, or **systole**, the AV valves close to prevent regurgitation of blood back up into the atria. The papillary muscles contract at the same time so the valve leaflets meet and unite to form a perfect seal without turning themselves inside out.

The **semilunar** (SL) valves are set between the ventricles and the arteries. Each valve has three cusps that look like half-moons. The SL valves are the **pulmonic** valve in the right side of the heart and the **aortic** valve in the left side of the heart. They open during pumping, or **systole**, to allow blood to be ejected from the heart.

Note: There are no valves present between the vena cava and the RA, nor between the pulmonary veins and the LA. For this reason, abnormally high pressure in the left side of the heart results in symptoms of pulmonary congestion, and abnormally high pressure in the right side of the heart shows in the neck veins and abdomen.

Direction of blood flow

Think of a deoxygenated red blood cell being drained downstream into the vena cava. It is swept along with the flow of venous blood and follows the route illustrated in Figure 17.4.

1. From the liver to the RA through the inferior vena cava.
   The superior vena cava drains venous blood from the head and upper extremities
   From the RA, venous blood travels through the tricuspid valve to the RV.

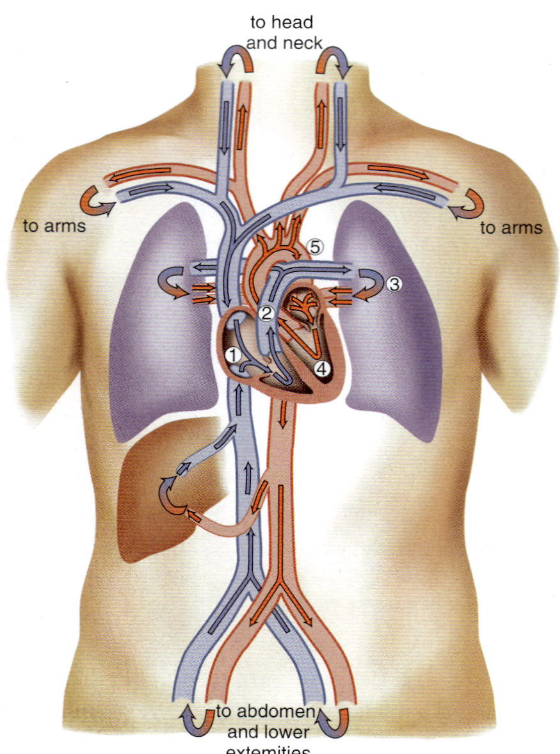

FIGURE 17.4 Direction of blood flow through the heart and circulatory system

2. From the RV, venous blood flows through the pulmonic valve to the pulmonary artery The pulmonary artery delivers deoxygenated blood to the lungs.
3. The lungs oxygenate blood. Pulmonary veins return oxygenated blood to the LA.
4. From the LA, arterial blood travels through the mitral valve to the LV.
5. The LV ejects blood through the aortic valve into the aorta.
6. The aorta delivers oxygenated blood to the body.

Remember that the circulation is a continuous loop. The blood is kept moving along by continually shifting pressure gradients. The blood flows from an area of higher pressure to one of lower pressure.

Cardiac cycle

The rhythmic movement of blood through the heart is the **cardiac cycle**. It has two phases, **diastole** and **systole**. In diastole, the ventricles relax and fill with blood. This takes up two-thirds of the cardiac cycle. The heart's contraction is systole. During systole, blood is pumped from the ventricles and fills the pulmonary and systemic arteries. This is one-third of the cardiac cycle.

DIASTOLE

In diastole, the ventricles are relaxed and the AV valves (i.e. the tricuspid and the mitral) are open (Figure 17.5). (Opening of the normal valve is acoustically silent.) The pressure in the atria is higher than that in the ventricles, so blood pours rapidly into the ventricles. This first passive filling phase is called early or protodiastolic filling.

Towards the end of diastole, the atria contract and push the last amount of blood (about 25% of the stroke volume) into the ventricles. This active filling phase is called **presystole**, or **atrial systole**. It causes a small rise in the LV pressure. Note that atrial systole occurs during ventricular diastole, a confusing but important point.

SYSTOLE

Now so much blood has been pumped into the ventricles that the ventricular pressure is finally higher than that in the atria, so the mitral and tricuspid valves swing shut. The closure of the AV valves contributes to the first heart sound (**S_1**) and signals the beginning of systole. The AV valves close to prevent any regurgitation of blood back up into the atria during contraction.

For a moment, all four valves are closed. The ventricular walls contract. This contraction against a closed system works to build pressure inside the ventricles to a high level (isometric contraction). Consider first the left side of the heart. When the pressure in the ventricle finally exceeds pressure in the aorta, the aortic valve opens, and blood is ejected rapidly.

After the ventricle's contents are ejected, its pressure falls. When its pressure falls below the pressure in the aorta, some blood flows backwards towards the ventricle, causing the aortic valve to swing shut. This closure of the semilunar valves causes the **second heart sound (S_2)** and signals the end of systole.

Diastole again. Now all four valves are closed and the ventricles relax (called isometric or isovolumic relaxation). Meanwhile, the atria have been filling with oxygenated blood delivered from the lungs. The atrial pressure is now higher than the relaxed ventricular pressure. The mitral valve drifts open and diastolic filling begins again.

Events in the right and left sides. The same events are happening in the right side of the heart, but pressures in the right side of the heart are much lower than those of the left side because less energy is needed to pump blood to its destination, the pulmonary circulation. Also, events occur just slightly later in the right side of the heart because of

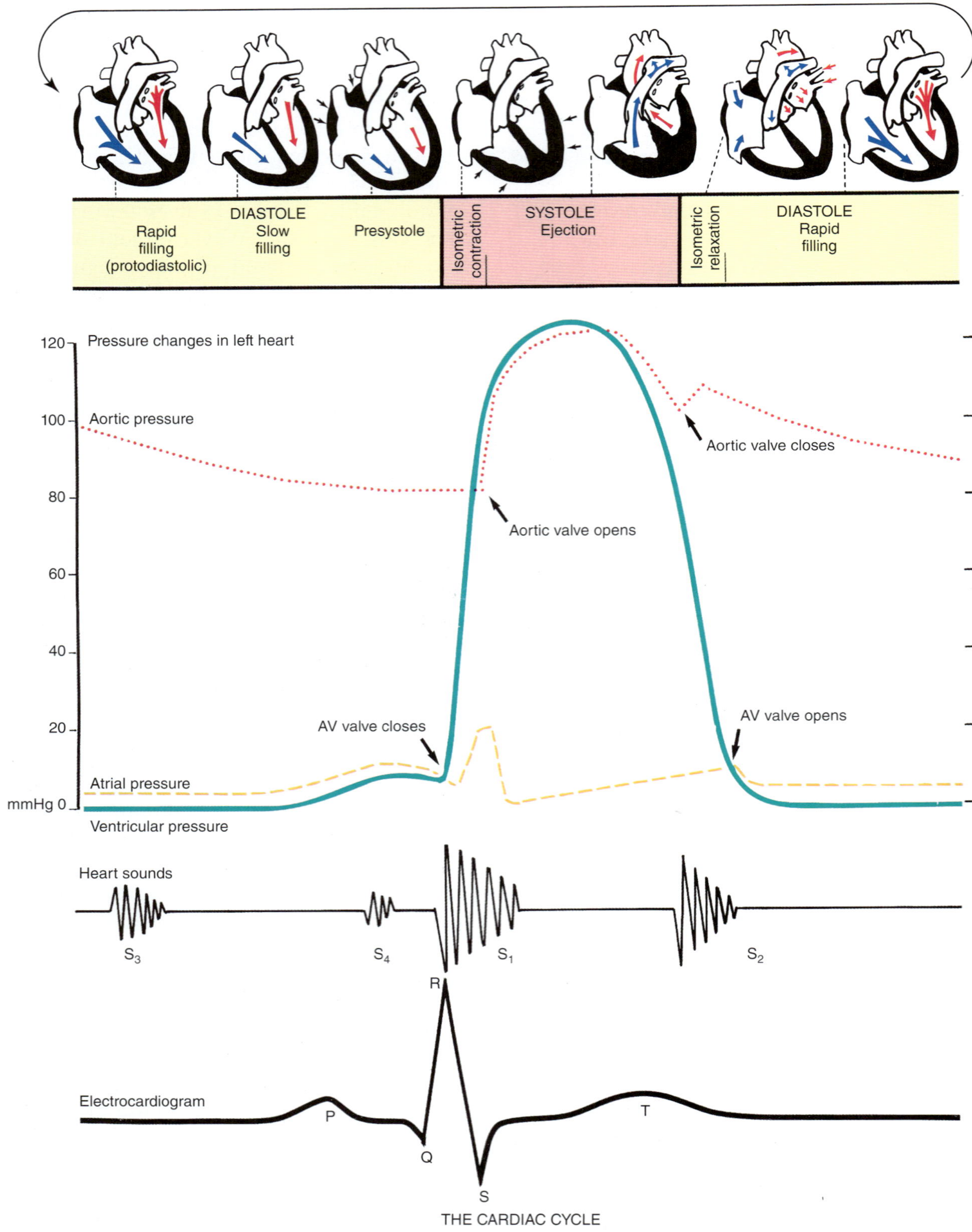

FIGURE 17.5 The cardiac cycle—blood flow, ventricular pressure changes, heart sounds and electrocardiogram

the route of myocardial depolarisation. As a result, two distinct components to each of the heart sounds exist and sometimes you can hear them separately. In **S_1**, the mitral component closes just before the tricuspid component. And with **S_2**, aortic closure occurs slightly before pulmonic closure.

Heart sounds

Events in the cardiac cycle generate sounds that can be heard through a stethoscope over the chest wall. These include normal heart sounds and, occasionally, extra heart sounds and murmurs (Figure 17.6).

Normal heart sounds

S_1 occurs with closure of the AV valves and thus signals the beginning of systole. The mitral component of the first sound slightly precedes the tricuspid component, but you usually hear these two components fused as one sound. You can hear **S_1** over all the praecordium, but usually it is loudest at the apex.

S_2 occurs with closure of the semilunar valves and signals the end of systole. The aortic component of the second sound slightly precedes the pulmonic component. Although it is heard over all the praecordium, **S_2** is loudest at the base.

EFFECT OF RESPIRATION

The volume of RV and LV systole is just about equal, but this can be affected by respiration. During inspiration, intrathoracic pressure is decreased. This pushes more blood into the vena cava, increasing venous return to the right side of the heart, which increases RV stroke volume. The increased volume prolongs RV systole and delays pulmonic valve closure.

Meanwhile, on the left side, a greater amount of blood is sequestered in the lungs during inspiration. This momentarily decreases the amount returned to the left side of the heart, decreasing LV stroke volume. The decreased volume shortens LV systole and allows the aortic valve to close a bit earlier. When the aortic valve closes significantly earlier than the pulmonic valve, you can hear the two components separately. This is a **split** S_2.

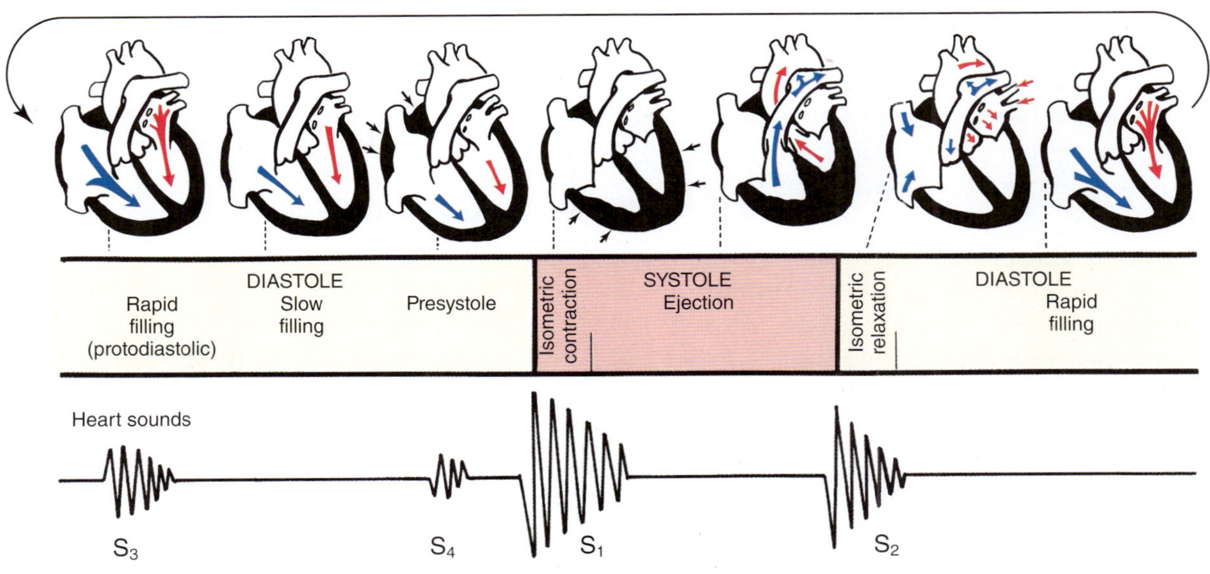

FIGURE 17.6 The cardiac cycle—blood flow, heart sounds and electrocardiogram

Extra heart sounds

THIRD HEART SOUND (S_3)

Normally diastole is a silent event. However, in some conditions, ventricular filling creates vibrations that can be heard over the chest. These vibrations are S_3. The S_3 occurs when the ventricles are resistant to filling during the early rapid filling phase. This occurs immediately after S_2, when the AV valves open and atrial blood first pours into the ventricles. See a complete discussion of S_3 in Table 17.9, later in the chapter.

FOURTH HEART SOUND (S_4)

The S_4 occurs at the end of diastole, at presystole, when the ventricle is resistant to filling. The atria contract and push blood into a noncompliant ventricle. This creates vibrations that are heard as S_4. The S_4 occurs just before S_1.

MURMURS

Blood circulating through normal cardiac chambers and valves usually makes no noise. However, some conditions create turbulent blood flow and collision currents. These result in a murmur, much like a pile of stones or a sharp turn in a creek creates a noisy water flow. A murmur is a gentle, blowing, swooshing sound that can be heard on the chest wall. Conditions resulting in a murmur are that the:

- velocity of blood increases (flow murmur) (e.g. in exercise, thyrotoxicosis)
- viscosity of blood decreases (e.g. in anaemia)
- structural defects in the valves (narrowed valve, incompetent valve) or unusual openings occur in the chambers (dilated chamber, wall defect).

Characteristics of sound

All heart sounds are described by:

- **frequency** (pitch)—heart sounds are described as high pitched or low pitched, although these terms are relative because all are low-frequency sounds and you need a good stethoscope to hear them
- **intensity (loudness)**—loud or soft
- **duration**—very short for heart sounds; silent periods are longer
- **timing**—systole or diastole.

Conduction

Of all organs, the heart has a unique ability; the heart can contract by itself, independent of any signals or stimulation from the body. The heart contracts in response to an electrical current conveyed by a conduction system (Figure 17.7). Specialised cells in the sinoatrial node near the superior vena cava initiate an electrical impulse. Because the sinoatrial node has an intrinsic rhythm, it is the 'pacemaker'. The current flows in an orderly sequence, first across the atria to the AV node low in the atrial septum. There, it is delayed slightly so that the atria have time to contract before the ventricles are stimulated. Then, the impulse travels to the **Bundle of His**, the right and left bundle branches, then through the ventricles.

The electrical impulse stimulates the heart to do its work, which is to contract. A small amount of electricity spreads to the body surface, where it can be measured and recorded on the electrocardiograph (ECG). The ECG waves are arbitrarily labelled PQRST, which stand for the following elements:

- **P wave**—depolarisation of the atria
- **PR interval**—from the beginning of the P wave to the beginning of the QRS complex (the time necessary for atrial depolarisation plus time for the impulse to travel through the AV node to the ventricles)
- **QRS complex**—depolarisation of the ventricles
- **T wave**—repolarisation of the ventricles.

Electrical events slightly precede the mechanical events in the heart. The ECG

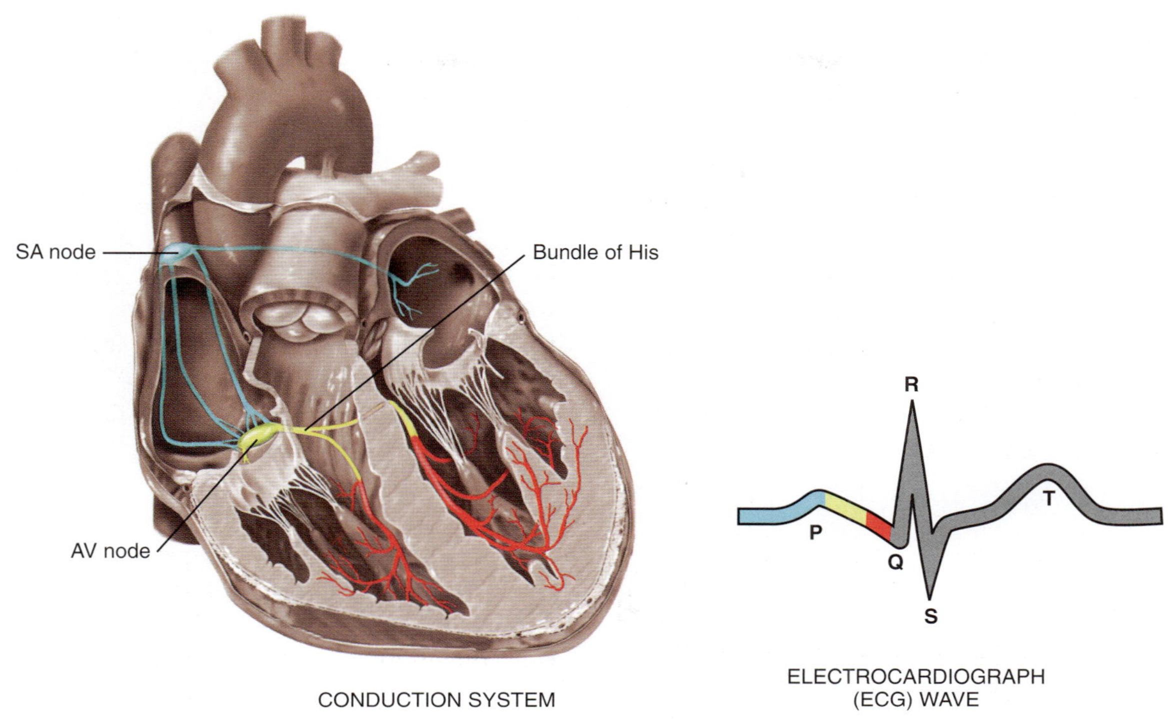

FIGURE 17.7 Conduction system of the heart and ECG representing the various phases

juxtaposed on the cardiac cycle is illustrated in Figure 17.5.

Pumping ability

In the resting adult, the heart normally pumps between 4 and 6 L of blood per minute throughout the body. This **cardiac output** equals the volume of blood in each systole (called the stroke volume) times the number of beats per minute (heart rate). This is described as:

$$CO = SV \times HR$$

The heart can alter its cardiac output to adapt to the metabolic needs of the body. Preload and afterload affect the heart's ability to increase cardiac output.

Preload is the venous return that builds during diastole. It is the length to which the ventricular muscle is stretched at the end of diastole just before contraction (Figure 17.8).

When the volume of blood returned to the ventricles is increased (as when exercise stimulates skeletal muscles to contract and force more blood back to the heart), the muscle bundles are stretched beyond their normal resting state to accommodate. The force of this switch is the preload. According to the Frank-Starling law, the greater the stretch, the stronger is the heart's contraction. This increased contractility results in an increased volume of blood ejected (increased stroke volume).

Afterload is the opposing pressure the ventricle must generate to open the aortic valve against the higher aortic pressure. It is the resistance against which the ventricle must pump its blood. Once the ventricle is filled with blood, the ventricular end diastolic pressure is 5 to 10 mmHg, whereas that in the aorta is 70 to 80 mmHg. To overcome this difference, the ventricular muscle tenses

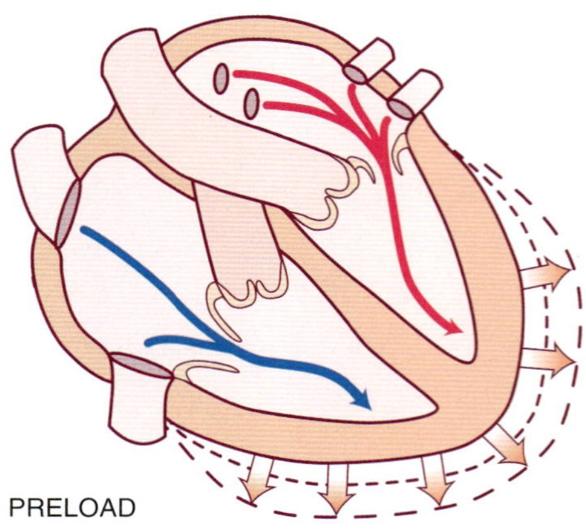

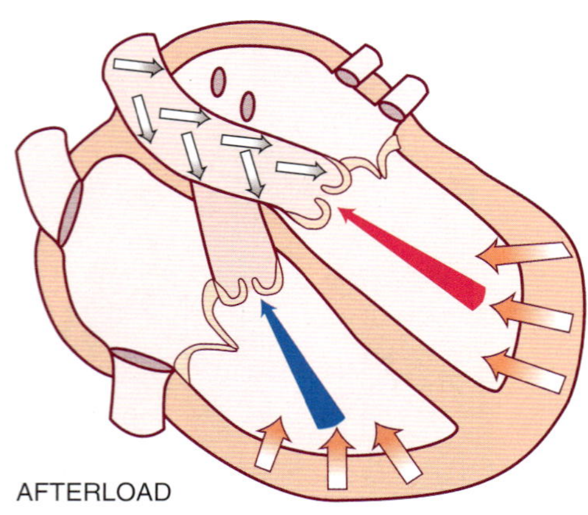

FIGURE 17.8 The heart's pumping ability

(isovolumic contraction). After the aortic valve opens, rapid ejection occurs.

The neck vessels

Cardiac assessment includes the survey of vascular structures in the neck—the carotid artery and the jugular veins (Figure 17.9). These vessels reflect the efficiency of cardiac function.

The carotid artery pulse

The pulse can be described as a pressure wave generated by each systole pumping blood into the aorta. The carotid artery is a central artery—that is, it is close to the heart. Its timing closely coincides with ventricular systole. Assessment of the peripheral pulses is found in Chapter 16 and blood pressure assessment is found in Chapter 10.

The **carotid artery** is located in the groove between the trachea and the sternocleidomastoid muscle, medial to and alongside that muscle. Note the characteristics of its waveform (Figure 17.10): a smooth rapid upstroke, a summit that is rounded and smooth and a downstroke that is more gradual and that has a dicrotic notch caused by closure of the aortic valve (marked D in the figure).

Jugular venous pulse and pressure

The **jugular veins** empty deoxygenated blood directly into the superior vena cava. Because no cardiac valve exists to separate the superior vena cava from the RA, the jugular veins give information about activity on the right side of the heart. Specifically, they reflect filling pressure and volume changes. Because volume and pressure increase when the right side of the heart fails to pump efficiently, the jugular veins expose this.

Two jugular veins are present in each side of the neck (Figure 17.9). The larger **internal jugular** lies deep and medial to the sternocleidomastoid muscle. It is usually not visible, although its diffuse pulsations may be seen in the sternal notch when the person is supine. The external jugular vein is more superficial; it lies laterally to the sternocleidomastoid muscle, above the clavicle.

Although an arterial pulse is caused by forward propulsion of blood, the jugular pulse is different. The jugular pulse results from a backwash, a waveform moving backwards caused by events upstream. The jugular pulse has five components, as shown in Figure 17.11.

The five components of the jugular venous pulse occur because of events in the right side

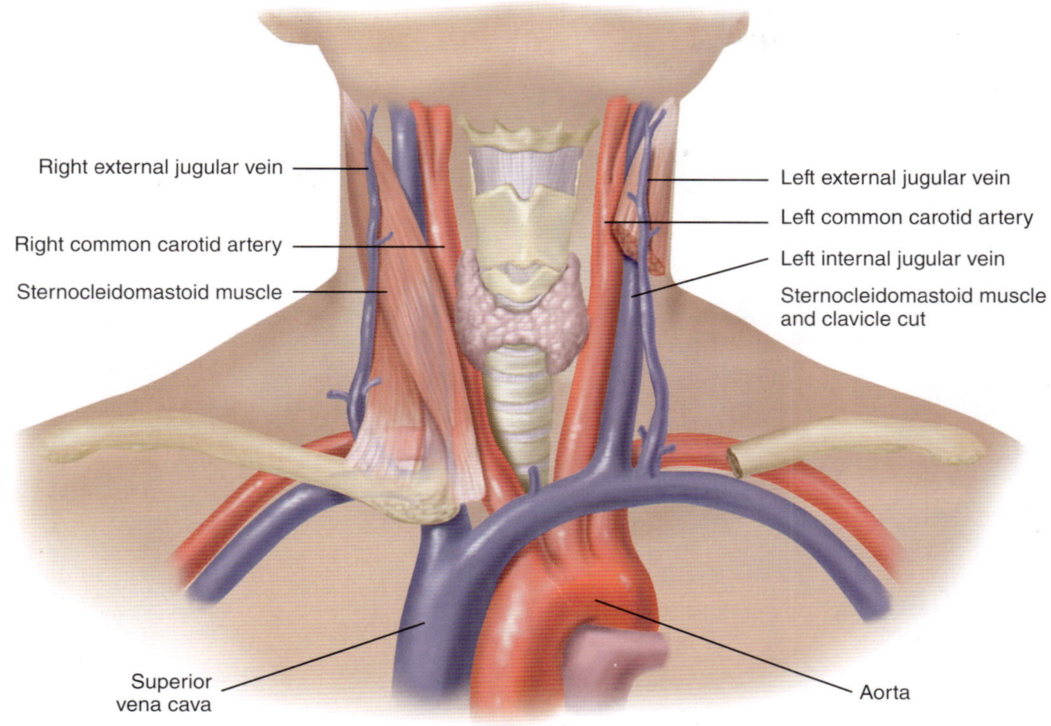

FIGURE 17.9 Major blood vessels in the neck

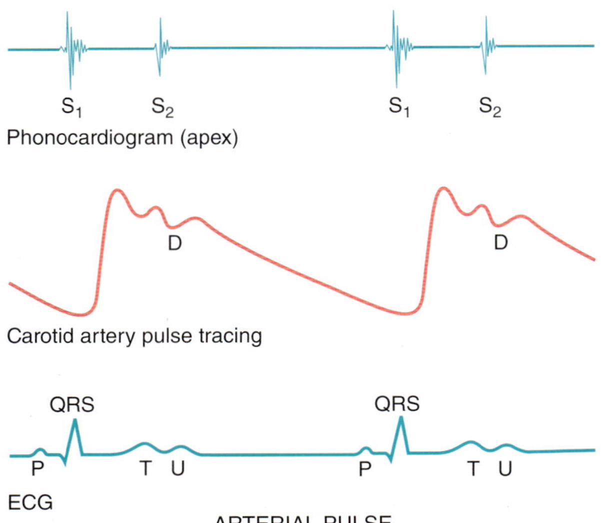

FIGURE 17.10 The carotid artery pulse waveform

of the heart. The A wave reflects atrial contraction because some blood flows backwards to the vena cava during right atrial contraction. The C wave, or ventricular contraction, is backflow from the bulging upwards of the tricuspid valve when it closes at the beginning of ventricular systole (not from the neighbouring carotid artery pulsation). Next, the X descent shows atrial relaxation when the RV contracts during systole and pulls the bottom of the atria downwards. The V wave occurs with passive atrial filling because of the increasing volume in the right atria and increased pressure. Finally, the Y descent reflects passive ventricular filling when the tricuspid valve opens and blood flows from the RA to the RV.

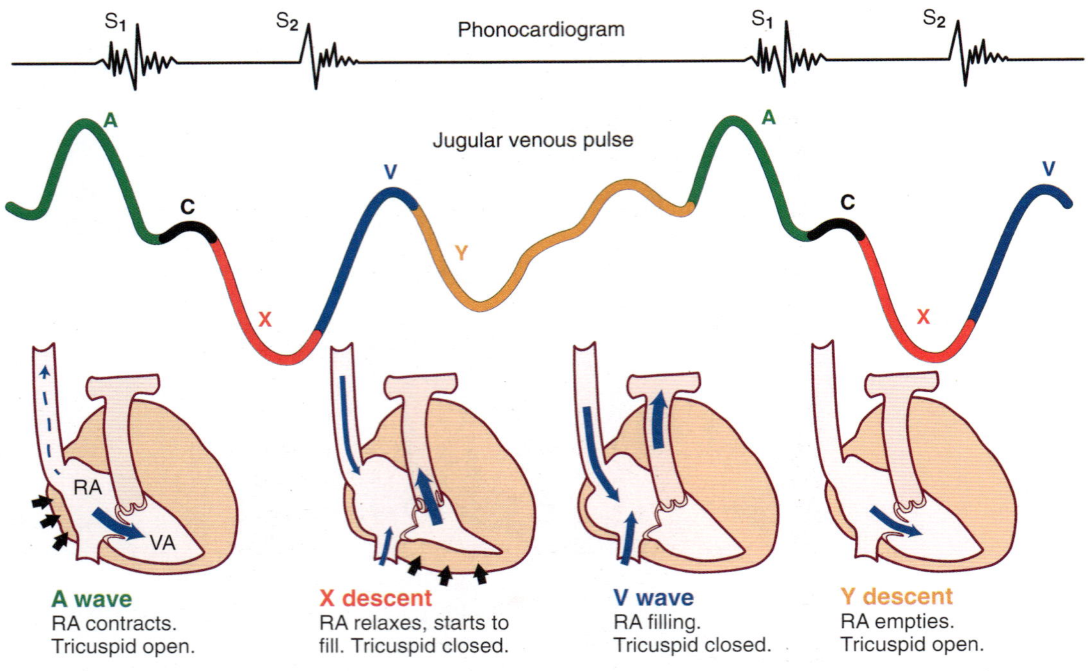

FIGURE 17.11 The jugular venous pulse waveform
Note: Match colour on waveform with its description.

Developmental considerations

Infants and children

The fetal heart functions early; it begins to beat at the end of 3 weeks' gestation. The lungs are nonfunctional, but the fetal circulation compensates for this (Figure 17.12). Oxygenation takes place at the placenta and the arterial blood is returned to the right side of the heart. There is no point in pumping all this freshly oxygenated blood through the lungs, so it is rerouted in two ways. First, about two-thirds of it is shunted through an opening in the atrial septum, the **foramen ovale**, into the left side of the heart, where it is pumped out through the aorta. Second, the rest of the oxygenated blood is pumped by the right side of the heart out through the pulmonary artery, but it is detoured through the **ductus arteriosus** to the aorta. Because they are both pumping into the systemic circulation, the RV and LV are equal in weight and muscle wall thickness.

Inflation and aeration of the lungs at birth produces circulatory changes. Now the blood is oxygenated through the lungs rather than through the placenta. The foramen ovale closes within the first hour because of the new lower pressure in the right side of the heart than in the left side. The ductus arteriosus closes later, usually within 10 to 15 hours of birth. Now, the LV has the greater workload of pumping into the systemic circulation so when the baby has reached 1 year of age, the LV's mass increases to reach the adult ratio of 2:1 LV to RV.

The heart's position in the chest is more horizontal in infants than in adults, so the

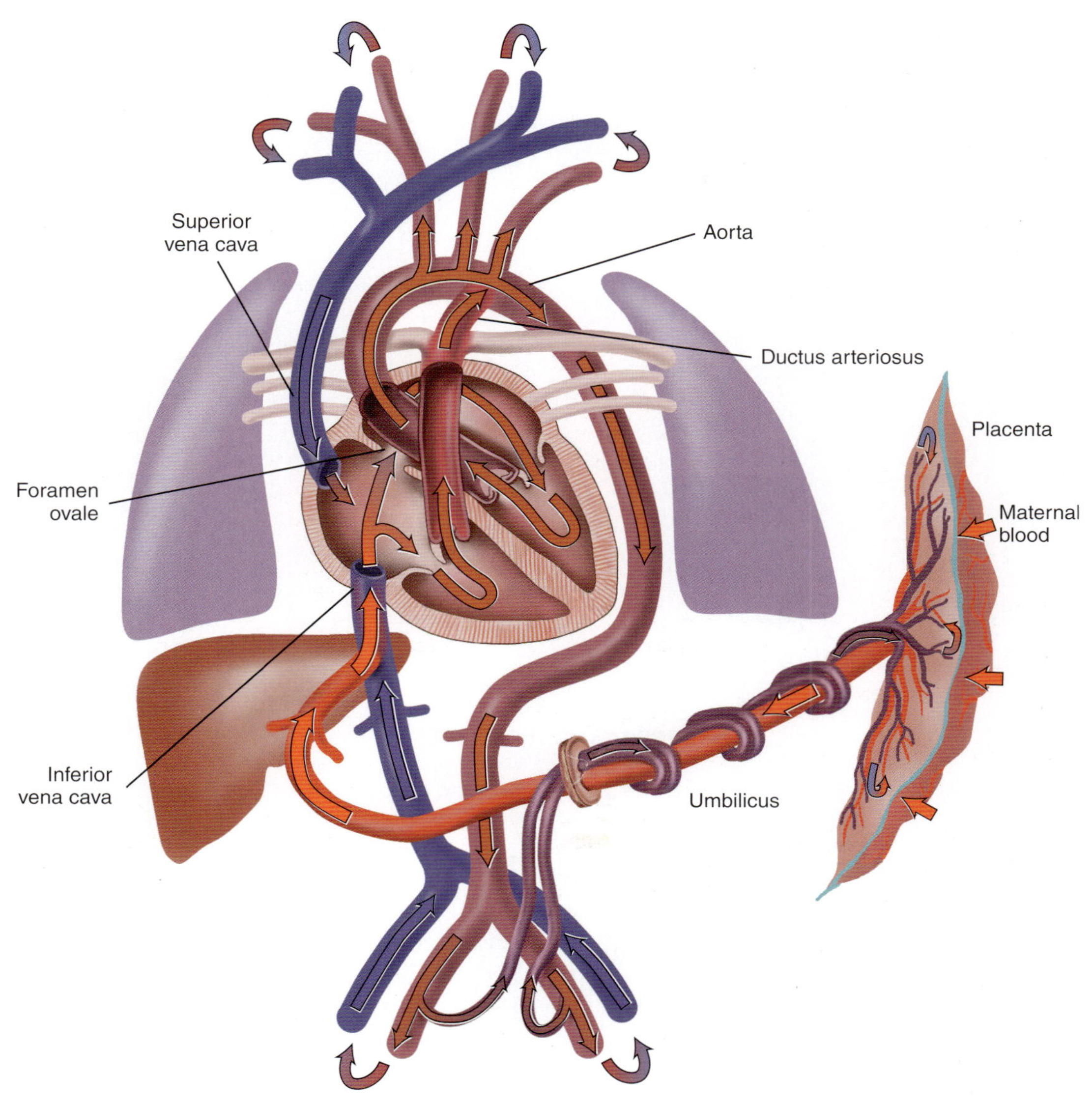

FIGURE 17.12 Fetal circulation

apex is higher, located at the fourth left intercostal space (Figure 17.13). It reaches the adult position when the child reaches age 7 years.

Pregnancy

The cardiovascular system adapts to ensure adequate blood supply to the uterus and placenta, to deliver oxygen and nutrients to the fetus and to allow the mother to function normally during the pregnancy. Blood volume increases by 30 to 40% during pregnancy, with the most rapid expansion occurring during the second trimester. This creates an increase in stroke volume and cardiac output and an increased pulse rate of 10 to 15 beats

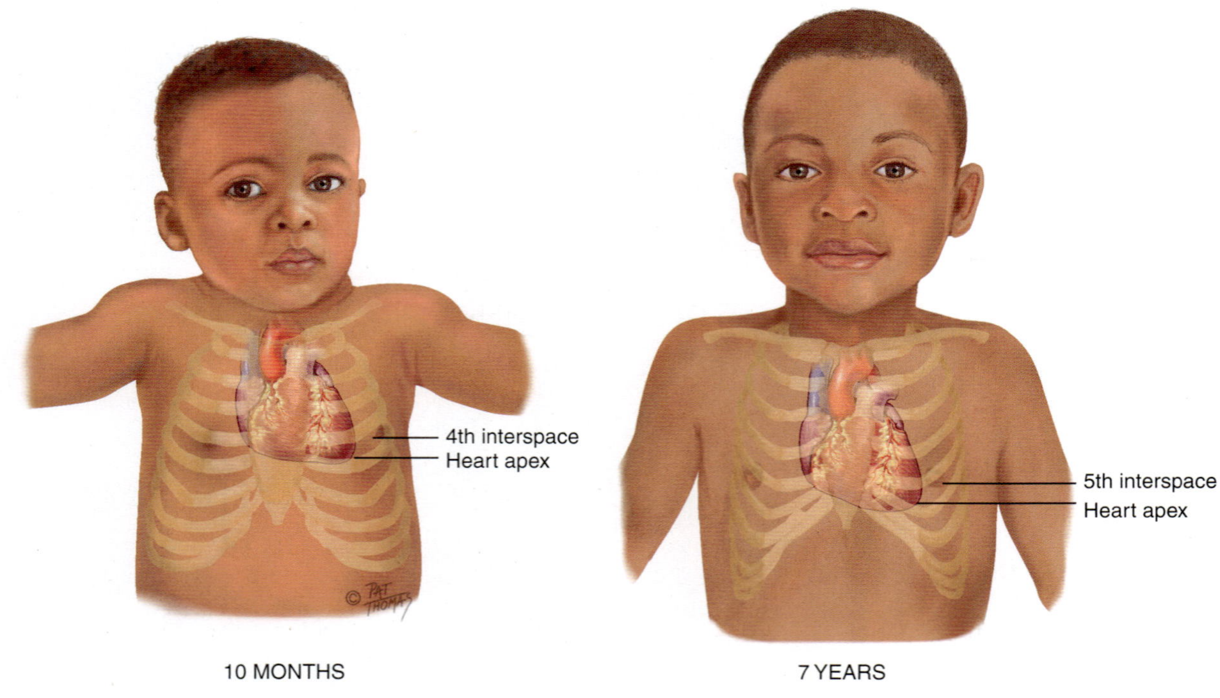

FIGURE 17.13 The position of the heart in the chest of an infant and child

per minute. The heart rate rises in the first trimester, peaks in the third trimester and returns to baseline within the first 10 postpartum days. Despite the increased cardiac output, arterial blood pressure decreases in pregnancy because of peripheral vasodilation. The blood pressure drops to its lowest point during the second trimester and then rises after that.

Late adulthood (65+ years)

It is difficult to isolate the 'ageing process' of the cardiovascular system per se because it is so closely interrelated with lifestyle, habits and diseases. We now know that lifestyle is a significant modifying factor in the development of cardiovascular disease; smoking, diet, alcohol use, exercise patterns and stress have an influence on coronary artery disease. Lifestyle also affects the ageing process; cardiac changes once thought to be part of the process of ageing are partially due to the sedentary lifestyle. However, a decrease in the rate of cardiovascular disease and overall mortality can be achieved by increasing the physical activity of older adults, even at a moderate level.[1]

There is no change in resting heart rate or cardiac output at rest with ageing. However, there are several changes to structure and function of the cardiac system that can occur with ageing.

CHANGE IN SYSTOLIC BLOOD PRESSURE

With ageing, there is a rise in the systolic blood pressure. This is caused by thickening and stiffening of the large arteries which, in turn, is caused by collagen and calcium deposits in the vessel walls and loss of elastic fibres. This stiffening (arteriosclerosis) creates an increase in pulse wave velocity because the less compliant arteries cannot store the volume ejected.

HEART WALL THICKNESS

The overall size of the heart does not increase with age, but the LV wall thickness increases. This is an adaptive mechanism to accommodate the vascular stiffening mentioned earlier that creates an increased workload on the heart.

CHANGE IN DIASTOLIC BLOOD PRESSURE

Diastolic blood pressure may decrease after the sixth decade of life. A rising systolic pressure with a relatively constant diastolic pressure increases the pulse pressure (the difference between the two).

DECREASE CARDIAC RESPONSE TO EXERCISE

There is a decreased ability of the heart to augment cardiac output with exercise. This is shown by a decreased maximum heart rate with exercise and diminished sympathetic response. Non-cardiac factors also cause a decrease in maximum work performance with ageing: decrease in skeletal muscle performance, increase in muscle fatigue and increased sense of dyspnoea.

DYSRHYTHMIAS

The presence of supraventricular and ventricular dysrhythmias increases with age. Ectopic beats are common in ageing people; although these are usually asymptomatic in healthy older people, they may compromise cardiac output and blood pressure when disease is present.

Tachyarrhythmias may not be tolerated as well in older people. The myocardium is thicker and less compliant and early diastolic filling is impaired at rest due to the structural changes that occur in ageing.[2] Thus, a tachycardia may not be well tolerated because of shortened diastole. There are several types of tachyarrhythmias, however **atrial fibrillation** is the most common type of arrhythmia in older people. Episodes can be short or persistent. The person may notice, for example, breathlessness, feeling lightheaded, a racing heart, chest pain or discomfort. The heart rate will be fast and sometimes irregular. Atrial fibrillation poses a significant long-term risk of stroke, heart failure and death. Apart from screening and early intervention, treatment involves medications to regulate the heart rhythm, anticoagulants to reduce the risk of stroke and sometimes synchronised electrical cardioversion.[2]

ELECTROCARDIOGRAPH

Age-related changes in the ECG occur because of histological changes in the conduction system. These changes include:

- prolonged P-R interval (first-degree AV block) and prolonged Q-T interval, but the QRS interval is unchanged
- left axis deviation from age-related mild LV hypertrophy and fibrosis in left bundle branch
- increased incidence of bundle branch block.

Although the haemodynamic changes associated with ageing alone do not seem severe, the fact remains that the incidence of cardiovascular disease, hypertension and heart failure increases with advancing age.

Cultural and social considerations

As stated previously, heart disease, stroke and vascular disease are collectively known as cardiovascular diseases. The most common cardiac health issue is coronary heart disease (CHD). CHD, also known as ischaemic heart disease, occurs when there is a narrowing or blockage in the vessels that supply blood to the heart muscle.[3] Ischaemic heart disease includes acute myocardial infarction (heart attack, or AMI) and angina.

An AMI occurs when there is acute ischaemia from partial or complete blockage of one or more coronary blood vessels causing necrosis of the heart muscle from lack of oxygenated blood.[4] It can be life threatening. Angina (angina pectoris) is chest pain that results from myocardial ischaemia when the blood flow to the heart is insufficient to support demand. It is usually due to the presence of atherosclerotic plaque in the coronary vessel lumen.[5] There are several types including stable angina and unstable angina. People with angina are at increased risk for AMI. For typical symptoms of AMI and angina please read the section titled 'Health education' below and see Table 17.1.

CHD is the leading single cause of disease burden and death in Australia representing 10% of all deaths.[3] It is estimated that 2.9% of the adult population is living with CHD. Prevalence increases with age with one in nine adults aged 75 years and over affected.[3] The rate of acute coronary events (AMI) has dropped significantly over the past 20 years due to a reduction in risk factors (smoking rates), better assessment of risk and treatment options. The most recent Australian data estimates that, over a 1-year period, there were 391 acute coronary events per 100,000 males and 172 acute coronary events per 100,000 females over 25 years of age. Of these 12% were fatal.[3]

The impact of CHD varies between population groups. For example, Indigenous Australians are 2.8 times more likely to develop CHD than non-Indigenous Australians. People living in remote areas are 0.9 times more likely to develop CHD, and those from lower socioeconomic groups are 1.6 times more likely to develop CHD than those living in regional towns or cities or those with a higher socioeconomic status. In Aotearoa New Zealand there are similar prevalence trends. More than one in 23 Aotearoa New Zealand adults are living with heart disease.[6] Of these, male New Zealanders from a European background and Māori males have the highest prevalence. The incidence rises with age, with approximately 28% of males and 15% of females over 75 years of age having CHD.[7]

Given the varying prevalence of CHD in socioeconomic groups, ethnic groups, people with other health conditions such as diabetes, chronic kidney disease and severe mental illness, there are guidelines in Australia and Aotearoa New Zealand that recommend that cardiovascular risk screening should start earlier than populations without known risk factors. Recommendations are, for example, 30 years of age for Indigenous Australians, 30 to 40 years of age for Māori, Pacific and South-Asian populations and earlier for those with known risk factors.[8,9]

The major modifiable risk factors for heart disease and stroke are high blood pressure, smoking, high cholesterol levels, obesity, physical inactivity and diabetes. However, other known risk factors—for example, family stress, depression, anxiety, social isolation and lack of social support—also need to be addressed.[10]

Hypertension

Hypertension causes heart disease by decreasing vascular compliance which results in stiff, inelastic blood vessels and initiates endothelial injury. This process causes a cascade of events accelerating the development of atherosclerosis (thickening or hardening of the arteries).[11] Untreated hypertension risks damage to heart, main blood vessels, heart valves, brain and kidneys and can cause cardiac arrhythmias including atrial fibrillation.[12]

The most current National Health Survey found that 11.6% of Australians reported having hypertension, with similar rates in males and females. However, three in four people who did not report having high blood pressure had high blood pressure when measured by a health professional. Most people are unaware they have high blood pressure. Prevalence increases with age, with approximately 45% of people over 75 years of age reporting hypertension.[13] Indigenous Australians have higher rates of hypertension than non-Indigenous Australians, but the highest disparity is in the 25–34-year-old age group, who had nearly twice the rate of non-Indigenous Australians.[14] In Aotearoa New Zealand, it is estimated that approximately 16.8% of adults are receiving medication for hypertension. Māori and Pacific Islander adults are 1.4 times more likely to have measured high blood pressure than other New Zealanders.[15]

Because hypertension and the organ damage it causes can be asymptomatic, identifying people most at risk, making blood pressure screening important. Blood pressure can easily be measured in a clinic situation by a health professional although many people will have a raised blood pressure simply due to their anxiety of being examined. Intermittent blood pressure measurements by the person in their home can be performed twice per day for 7 days and an average reading can be calculated.[16] For those who cannot manage measuring their own blood pressure or where more detailed records are needed, continuous ambulatory blood pressure measurement over a 24- to 48-hour period has been found to be accurate and cost-effective. It also gives the clinician insight into changes in blood pressure over time including when the person is sleeping.[16]

Smoking

Tobacco smoking and exposure to environmental tobacco smoke (sometimes referred to as passive smoking) causes atherosclerosis by impairing endothelial function in blood vessels, increasing arterial stiffness, promoting an inflammatory response, insulin resistance and increasing low-density lipoprotein deposition and reducing high-density lipoprotein levels.[17]

Tobacco smoking is a major cause of preventable death and disease in Australia and Aotearoa New Zealand and there is a strong inverse relationship between tobacco use and socioeconomic indicators. Australian Indigenous people and Aotearoa New Zealand Māori and Pacific Islander peoples are more likely to smoke than non-Indigenous people and are therefore most at risk of smoking-related cardiovascular and other health-related adverse effects. For a more detailed discussion of smoking related statistics and health implications see Chapter 19.

While tobacco smoking significantly increases the incidence of acute and chronic cardiovascular disease, the harmful effects are substantially reversible after quitting.[17] All smokers need to be encouraged to quit smoking for the sake of their health on each presentation to a health service. 'Quit' services are government-funded, and printed information is available in many languages. See Chapter 19 for more information about quitting smoking.

Abnormal blood lipids

The blood lipids comprise several components including total cholesterol, high-density lipoproteins, low-density lipoproteins ('bad' cholesterol) and triglycerides. While essential for many bodily functions, abnormal levels of blood lipids (**dyslipidaemia**) can contribute to cardiovascular disease. The most recent published survey found that approximately 63% of adults had abnormal blood lipid levels and 33% had a total cholesterol level that was high.[3] There are no significant differences in the proportion of Australian adults who have abnormal blood lipid levels across socioeconomic groups or whether living in cities, regionally or remotely.[3] In Aotearoa New Zealand, 11.4% of adults are taking lipid-lowering medication. Of these, about 1.4 times more Māori and 1.53 times more Pacific Islander people are currently taking lipid-lowering medication than other New Zealanders.[15]

Obesity

The World Health Organization[18] has reported that obesity has grown to epidemic proportions in most Western countries. Obesity compounds any health problem and increases the incidence of many diseases including cardiovascular disease, diabetes, musculoskeletal disorders and some cancers. For a detailed discussion of the health implications of overweight and obesity and the social and cultural considerations, see Chapter 21.

Diabetes

Diabetes increases the risk of microvascular and macrovascular dysfunction and increases the risk of coronary artery disease, chronic renal disease and blindness.[19] The incidence of type 2 diabetes has been rising dramatically internationally.[20] This is attributed to increasing rates of obesity, insufficient physical activity, unhealthy diet, tobacco smoking and an ageing population. For a detailed discussion of the health implications of diabetes and the social and cultural considerations see Chapter 21.

Rheumatic heart disease

Rheumatic heart disease (RHD) usually begins in childhood after an episode of acute rheumatic fever which is an abnormal immune response to Group A streptococcal throat infection.[21] RHD is caused by one or several untreated episodes of acute rheumatic fever causing a systemic inflammatory response affecting the heart, joints, subcutaneous tissue and central nervous system. For many people, acute rheumatic fever resolves without permanent damage, but in approximately 33% of children, the cardiac inflammatory response leads to RHD.[21] RHD causes heart failure from scarring and fibrosis of the mitral and aortic valves.[21] People with heart valve damage because of RHD may require heart valve replacement surgery and often have a significant reduction in their quality of life and life expectancy.

Acute rheumatic fever and RHD are treatable and preventable diseases.[22] However, RHD is described as a disease of poverty, overcrowding, poor access to health services and social disadvantage.[21] It is not surprising therefore that 92% of Australians with acute rheumatic fever are Indigenous, with the highest rate in the 5- to 14-year-old age group.[22] Of those with RHD, 78% are Indigenous Australians and most (66%) are females with a median age of 33 years.[22] In Aotearoa New Zealand, acute rheumatic fever and RHD almost exclusively affects Pacific Islander and Māori peoples under 30 years of age living in socioeconomically deprived areas.[23]

In addition to addressing the social and economic factors that contribute to developing acute rheumatic fever and/or RHD, preventing recurrences of acute rheumatic fever by using prophylactic antibiotics for episodes of streptococcal throat infection is critical to controlling the incidence. Currently Australia is leading the world in the development of a strep A vaccine.[24] See the list of websites in the 'Additional resources' section of this chapter for information on preventing RHD in Australia and Aotearoa New Zealand.

HEALTH EDUCATION

Women and heart disease

CHD remains the leading cause of death in Australia and the second most frequent cause of death in Aotearoa New Zealand.[25,26] Myocardial infarction (heart attack, or MI) causes almost one in 20 deaths, with one person being hospitalised in Australia for a heart attack every 9 minutes.[27] Traditionally, the assessment and care of people who have an MI has been based on male-focused typical symptoms, risk factors and treatments. It is now known that women have several different risk factors and symptoms. While there are well-established guidelines for caring for people who have an MI, there is evidence that women are less likely to receive guideline-directed care than men and are therefore likely to have delayed care and suboptimal outcomes.[28] In part this is because of lack of awareness of the sex-specific differences in clinical signs and symptoms and risk factors for MI for both health professionals and the general public. In recent years there has been public awareness campaigns to increase understanding of the risk factors and warning signs in women.

The key factor in surviving an acute MI is the time it takes to get professional help via an ambulance or emergency department. Therefore, it is important for all people to know the warning signs and know how to get help quickly. Typically, people recognise chest pain as the most common heart attack symptom, but women are more likely than men to have non-chest pain symptoms[29] such as:

- indigestion
- shortness of breath or difficulty breathing
- jaw, shoulder and back pain
- nausea and vomiting
- fatigue and tiredness
- dizziness.

All these symptoms are easy to attribute to something else other than the heart and are often ignored.

In addition to the cardiovascular disease risk factors described previously, women who have polycystic ovarian syndrome, premature menopause, an autoimmune disorder (and their treatments), undergone cancer treatments (for breast cancer), depression or a history of pregnancy complications such as gestational diabetes and pre-eclampsia are at higher risk of cardiovascular disease.[29]

Nurse's role:

- provide information about cardiac symptoms and risk factors for women
- inform the woman to seek immediate emergency care should symptoms arise
- provide information about resources.

The following resources have up-to-date information for women about heart disease:

- Heart Foundation (Australia): https://www.heartfoundation.org.au/Bundles/Your-heart/heart-conditions-in-women
- Heart Foundation (New Zealand): https://www.heartfoundation.org.nz/your-heart/women-and-heart-disease

Subjective data

Practice note

Before you start the assessment, introduce yourself to the person, confirm the person's identity, discuss the purpose and scope of the assessment, clarify any questions the person may have and get verbal consent from the person to perform the assessment.

ASSESSMENT GUIDELINES	CLINICAL SIGNIFICANCE AND CLINICAL ALERTS
Presenting concern	
• *Do you have any problems with your heart and your ability to exercise and go about your daily activities?* It is important to ascertain the person's perception of their cardiac function. If they do perceive a problem, ask: *How does this affect your quality of life?*	The person's response to this question will guide areas to focus on in further subjective and objective data collection.
Chest pain	
• *Have you experienced any chest pain, tightness or heaviness?* **Onset** • *When did it start? How long have you had it this time? Have you had this type of pain before? How often have you experienced it?* **Location** • *Where did the pain start? Does the pain radiate to any other spot?* **Character** • *How would you describe it? Crushing, stabbing, burning, vice-like?* (Allow the person to offer adjectives before you suggest them.) Note if the person uses a clenched fist to describe the pain. **Precipitating factors** • *Do you experience chest pain after activity—what type; during rest; emotional upset; after eating; during sexual intercourse; with cold weather?*	**Angina**, an important cardiac symptom, occurs when the heart's vascular supply cannot keep up with metabolic demand. Chest pain also may also be of pulmonary, musculoskeletal or gastrointestinal origin; it is important to differentiate. See Table 17.1 for a description of varying conditions that can present with chest pain. **Character** Typical descriptors of cardiac chest pain are central location, tight heavy sensation, a crushing sensation, may radiate to the jaw or left arm. Some people may describe a dull, aching sensation or discomfort, particularly with angina on exertion.[30] ! ***Clinical alert:*** Be aware that many women may not have 'typical' chest pain but may still be experiencing MI or angina. Pay close attention to associated symptoms.

ASSESSMENT GUIDELINES	CLINICAL SIGNIFICANCE AND CLINICAL ALERTS
Associated symptoms • *Have you experienced any sweating, ashen grey or pale skin, heart skips beat, shortness of breath, nausea or vomiting, indigestion, racing of heart, jaw/shoulder pain, extreme fatigue or tiredness that can't be explained?*	Note that the presence of chest pain and/or a squeezing sensation in the chest and the associated symptoms described here are typical of serious cardiac circulatory insufficiency. However, women may only experience non-chest pain symptoms such as indigestion, shortness of breath/difficulty breathing, jaw, shoulder and back pain, nausea and vomiting, fatigue and tiredness, dizziness. See also the section titled 'Health education' for more information on women and heart disease.
• *Is the pain made worse by moving the arms or neck, breathing, lying flat?* • *Is the pain relieved by rest or glyceryl trinitrate? How many tablets/sprays?*	This question is trying to focus on the origin of the chest pain—cardiac or non-cardiac. ***Clinical alert:*** In the presence of ongoing chest pain, if the person has taken more than three glyceryl-trinitrate tablets (0.3–0.6 mg) or sprays (0.4–0.8 mg) every 5 minutes without relief[31] they must be urgently referred for further assessment and treatment by a medical practitioner or ambulance service.
Dyspnoea	
• *Have you experienced any shortness of breath?* • *What type of activity and how much brings on shortness of breath? Is this different to what you were experiencing 6 months ago?* **Onset** • *Does the shortness of breath come on unexpectedly?* **Duration** • *Is it constant or does it come and go?* **Associated factors** • *Does it seem to be affected by position such as lying down?* • *Does this awaken you from sleep at night?* • *Does your heart feel like it is racing when you feel breathless?* • *Does the shortness of breath interfere with activities of daily living? If so, what does your shortness of breath prevent you from doing?*	**Dyspnoea**—the subjective feeling of shortness of breath. Dyspnoea can be caused by several health issues including asthma, chronic lung diseases, as well as heart disease, cardiomyopathy (disease of the heart muscle), atrial fibrillation and heart failure. **Dyspnoea on exertion**—shortness of breath on exertion (SOBOE)—quantify exactly (e.g. after walking two level blocks). **Paroxysmal nocturnal dyspnoea** (PND) occurs with heart failure. Lying down increases volume of intrathoracic blood and the weakened heart cannot accommodate the increased load. Classically, the person awakens after 2 hours of sleep with the perception of needing fresh air.
Orthopnoea	
• *How many pillows do you use when sleeping or lying down?*	**Orthopnoea** is the need to assume a more upright position to breathe. Note the exact number of pillows used.

ASSESSMENT GUIDELINES	CLINICAL SIGNIFICANCE AND CLINICAL ALERTS
Cough	
• *Do you have a cough?* **Duration** • *How long have you had a cough?* **Frequency** • *Is it worse at a particular time of day?* **Type** • *Can you describe it?* (For example, dry, hacking, barking, hoarse or congested.)	
Productive • *Do you cough up mucus? What colour is the mucus? Is it watery or thick? Does it have any odour? Is it blood-tinged?*	By asking for specific information about the nature of the cough, you are trying to differentiate between possible pulmonary or heart related causes of the symptoms. **Haemoptysis** (blood in sputum) is often a pulmonary disorder but also occurs with mitral stenosis.
• *Is it associated with a particular activity, position (lying down), anxiety, talking?* **Shortness of breath on exertion** • *What activities make it better or worse* (sit, walk, exercise)*?* • *Is the cough relieved by rest or medication?*	
Fatigue	
• *Do you seem to tire easily?* • *Are you able to keep up with your family and co-workers?* • *Do you feel like your heart is racing or irregular when you feel fatigued?* **Onset** • *When did fatigue start? Was this sudden or gradual? Has any recent change occurred in energy level?*	**Fatigue** can be from several cardiac related causes including the presence of an arrhythmia such as atrial fibrillation.
• *Is the fatigue occurring all day, morning, evening?*	Fatigue from decreased cardiac output is worse in the evening, whereas fatigue from anxiety or depression occurs all day or is worse in the morning.
• *How have these symptoms (chest pain, fatigue, breathlessness) affected your life?*	
Cyanosis or pallor	
• *Have you ever noted that your facial skin turns blue or ashen?*	**Cyanosis or pallor** occurs with MI or low cardiac output states because of decreased tissue perfusion.

ASSESSMENT GUIDELINES	CLINICAL SIGNIFICANCE AND CLINICAL ALERTS
Oedema	
• *Have you ever noticed any swelling of your feet and legs?*	**Oedema** is dependent when caused by heart failure.
Onset • *When did you first notice this? Has there been any recent change?*	
Timing • *What time of day does the swelling occur? Do your shoes feel tight at the end of the day?*	**Cardiac related peripheral oedema** is worse in the evening and less so in the morning after elevating the legs all night.
Amount • *How much swelling would you say there is? Are both legs equally swollen?*	
Alleviating factors • *Does the swelling go away with rest, elevation or after a night's sleep?* • *Are there any associated symptoms such as shortness of breath? If so, does the shortness of breath occur before leg swelling or after?*	
Nocturia	
• *Do you awaken at night needing to urinate? If so, how many times do you get up to urinate? How long has this been occurring? Has there been any recent change?*	**Nocturia**—recumbency at night promotes fluid reabsorption and excretion; this occurs with heart failure in people who are ambulatory during the day. See also Chapter 24 for assessment related to urinary function.
Cardiac history	
• *Do you have any history of hypertension, elevated cholesterol, heart murmur, changes to the rhythm of your heart, congenital heart disease, rheumatic fever or unexplained joint pains as a child or youth, recurrent tonsillitis, anaemia or iron deficiency?* • *Have you ever been told that you have heart disease? When was this? Have you been treated by medication, percutaneous intervention (e.g. insertion of a stent) or heart surgery?* • *Have you ever had any investigations for heart disease?* • *If so, when did you have your last ECG, cardiac stress test, blood cholesterol (blood lipids) test or other heart tests?*	

ASSESSMENT GUIDELINES	CLINICAL SIGNIFICANCE AND CLINICAL ALERTS
Family cardiac history	
• *Do you have any family history of hypertension, obesity, diabetes, cardiovascular disease, sudden death at younger age (under 50 years)?*	A family history of heart disease is a significant alert that the person may be at higher risk of cardiovascular disease.
Health and lifestyle management	
Nutrition • *Please describe your usual daily diet.* (Note if the person's diet is representative of the basic food groups, the amount and type of highly processed foods consumed, the number of kilojoules and any additives such as salt.) **Weight** • *What is your usual weight? Has there been any recent change?* **Exercise** • *What is your usual amount of exercise each day or week? What stops you?* (e.g. fatigue, leg pains, other—specify). *What type of exercise?* (state type or sport). If a sport, ask: *What is your usual amount?* (light, moderate, heavy)	To identify risk factors for cardiovascular disease.
Medications • *Do you take any prescribed medications? Are you aware of side effects? Have you recently stopped taking any medication? If so, why?* • *Are you using any complementary therapies? If so, what are you taking and for how long?* **Smoking** • *Do you smoke cigarettes or use vapes? At what age did you start? How many packs per day? For how many years have you smoked this amount? Have you ever tried to quit? If so, how did this go?* **Alcohol** • *How much alcohol do you usually drink each week or each day? What type—beer/wine/spirits? When was your last drink? What was the number of drinks that episode? Have you ever been told you had a drinking problem?*	Common cardiovascular-related medications include diuretics, antihypertensives, antiarrhythmics, cardiac glycosides (digoxin), vasodilators (e.g. glyceryl trinitrate) and lipid-modifying drugs.
Health screening For adults over 45 years or Indigenous . *Have you had a heart health check with your GP or practice nurse? When?*	Heart health checks include blood pressure, smoking status, blood lipids, diabetes status, chronic kidney disease, family history of cardiovascular disease, weight, etc.

ASSESSMENT GUIDELINES	CLINICAL SIGNIFICANCE AND CLINICAL ALERTS
Additional subjective data for infants (questions for parents or guardians)	
Ask about the mother's health during pregnancy: • *Did you experience any unexplained fever, rubella in the first trimester or another infection? Did you have hypertension or take medications?* • *Have you noted any change in the infant's skin colour while feeding or crying? Is the baby able to eat, suckle or complete feed without tiring?*	To screen for heart disease in infants, note fatigue during feeding. An infant with heart failure takes small amounts at each feed; becomes dyspnoeic with sucking; may be diaphoretic, then falls into exhausted sleep; awakens after a short time hungry again.
Growth • *Has the baby grown as expected by growth charts and about the same as their siblings or peers?*	Poor weight gain is an indicator of heart abnormalities.
Activity • *Were developmental milestones achieved as expected? Is the baby able to play without tiring? How many sleeps does the baby take each day? How long does a sleep last?*	
Additional subjective data for children (questions for parents or guardians)	
Growth • *Has the child grown as expected by growth charts?*	Fatigue. Record specific limitations. Cyanosis is a serious indication of heart or lung dysfunction.
Activity • *Is the child able to keep up with siblings or friends? Is the child willing or reluctant to go out to play? Is the child able to climb stairs, ride a bike? Does the child squat to rest during play or to watch television or assume a knee–chest position while sleeping? Have you noted any change in skin colour during daily activities?* • *Has the child had any unexplained joint pains or unexplained fever?* • *Does the child have frequent headaches or nosebleeds?* • *Does the child have more than an average number of respiratory infections? How many per year? How are they treated? Have any of these proved to be streptococcal infections?*	
Family history • *Does the child have a sibling with a heart defect? Is anyone in the child's family known to have chromosomal abnormalities, such as Trisomy 21 (Down syndrome)?*	

ASSESSMENT GUIDELINES	CLINICAL SIGNIFICANCE AND CLINICAL ALERTS
Additional subjective data for pregnant women	
Blood pressure	
• *Have you had high blood pressure during this or earlier pregnancies? What was your usual blood pressure level before pregnancy? How has your blood pressure been monitored during pregnancy?*	
• *If you have high blood pressure, what treatment has been started?*	
• *Have you experienced any associated symptoms such as weight gain, protein in the urine or swelling in the feet, legs or face?*	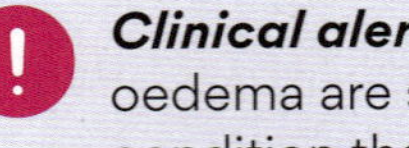 ***Clinical alert:*** Hypertension, proteinuria and oedema are signs of pre-eclampsia, a serious condition that can occur during pregnancy, placing the mother and fetus at risk. Pregnant women with these symptoms should be referred to their medical practitioner or midwife.
• *Have you had any faintness or dizziness with this pregnancy?*	
Additional subjective data for adults over 65 years	
History of heart or lung disease	
• *Do you have any of the following conditions: hypertension, coronary artery disease, issues with your heart rate or rhythm or chronic obstructive pulmonary disease?*	
• *What treatments have been started?*	
• *Have the usual symptoms changed recently? Does your illness interfere with activities of daily living?*	
Medications	
• If relevant—*Do you take any medications for your heart condition such as digoxin or beta-blockers? Are you aware of side effects? Have you recently stopped taking your medication? Why?*	Not taking medication may be related to side effects or lack of understanding of the chronic nature of heart disease.
Environment	
• *Do you have any difficulty moving around your house and completing your daily activities? If so, does your home have any stairs? How often do you need to climb them? Does this have any effect on activities of daily living?*	

Objective data

Preparation

Ideally the room should be warm; chilling can make a person uncomfortable, and shivering interferes with heart sounds. Where possible, try to conduct the assessment in a quiet room; heart sounds are very soft, and any ambient room noise masks them.

When performing a cardiac assessment, the person can be sitting up in a chair or a bed. If you are right-handed, stand on the person's right side; this will facilitate your hand placement and auscultation of the praecordium.

Ensure a female's privacy by keeping her breasts draped. The female's left breast overrides part of the area you will need to examine. Gently displace the breast upwards or ask the woman to hold it out of the way.

Equipment needed

Stethoscope with diaphragm and bell endpieces
Alcohol wipe (to clean endpiece)
Hand hygiene solution

PROCEDURES AND NORMAL FINDINGS	ABNORMAL FINDINGS AND CLINICAL ALERTS
A skills video (Cardiac assessment) is available to assist you in your skill development. Scan the QR code to access the video (instructions on the inside front cover of the book to access multimedia resources).	
General inspection	
While collecting subjective data, you will have noticed the colour of the person's skin and mucous membranes, ease of breathing, height-to-weight ratio, level of hygiene and grooming and general demeanour. All these factors provide clues to the functioning of the cardiovascular system. Refer to Chapter 8.	
Detailed inspection and vital signs	
Physical appearance, level of consciousness, skin colour, body structure, mobility, behaviour, measurement of height, weight, waist circumference and vital signs. Refer to Chapter 10.	
Identify relevant surface landmarks	
Identify position of clavicles, sternum, ribs and apex of heart (fifth intercostal space, midclavicular line) (Figure 17.1).	
Inspect and palpate the neck vessels	
Palpate the carotid artery	
Located central to the heart, the carotid artery yields important information on cardiac function.	

PROCEDURES AND NORMAL FINDINGS	ABNORMAL FINDINGS AND CLINICAL ALERTS
Palpate each carotid artery medial to the sternocleidomastoid muscle in the neck (Figure 17.14). Avoid excessive pressure on the carotid sinus area higher in the neck; excessive vagal stimulation here could slow down the heart rate, especially in adults over 65. Take care to palpate gently. Palpate only one carotid artery at a time to avoid compromising arterial blood to the brain. 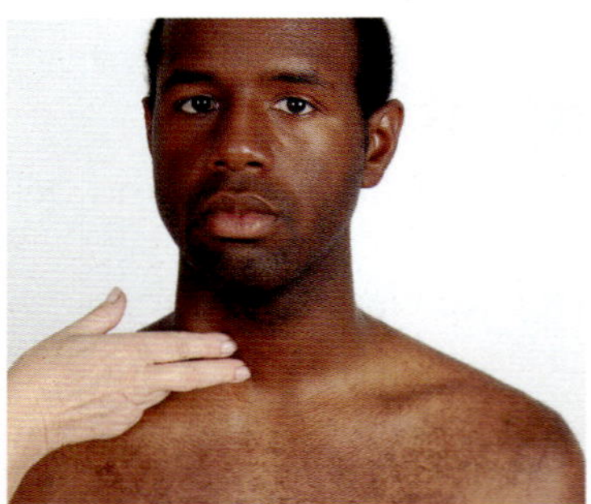 **FIGURE 17.14** Palpation of the carotid artery	**Carotid sinus hypersensitivity** is the condition in which pressure over the carotid sinus leads to a decreased heart rate, decreased blood pressure and cerebral ischaemia with syncope. This may occur in older adults with hypertension or occlusion of the carotid artery.
Feel the rate, rhythm and strength of the pulse. Normally the pulse is easy to palpate, and the normal strength is 2+ or moderate (Chapter 16). Your findings should be the same bilaterally.	Diminished pulse feels small and weak **(decreased stroke volume)**. Increased pulse feels full and strong **(hyperkinetic states)** (Table 16.1).

Inspect the jugular venous pulse

Jugular venous pressure reflects filling volume and pressure on the right side of the heart. The level of the jugular venous pulse gives an indirect estimation of jugular venous pressure.

Observe the right side of the neck because the right internal jugular vein most accurately reflects the right heart haemodynamics.

You won't see the internal jugular vein itself, but you can see its pulsation.

- The person should be placed in the supine position anywhere from a 30- to a 45-degree angle, wherever you can best see the pulsations. In general, the higher the venous pressure is, the higher the position you need.
- Remove the pillow to avoid flexing the neck; the head should be in the same plane as the trunk.
- Turn the person's head slightly away from the examined side and direct a strong light tangentially onto the neck to highlight pulsations and shadows.

PROCEDURES AND NORMAL FINDINGS	ABNORMAL FINDINGS AND CLINICAL ALERTS
• Note the external jugular veins overlying the sternocleidomastoid muscle. In some people, the veins are not visible at all, whereas in others they are full in the supine position. As the person is raised to a sitting position, these external jugulars flatten and disappear, usually at 45 degrees.	Unilateral distension of external jugular veins is due to local cause (kinking or aneurysm). Full distended external jugular veins above 45 degrees reflects increased central venous pressure and RV failure (and is a late finding in LV failure).[32]
Now observe for pulsations of the internal jugular veins in the area of the suprasternal notch or around the origin of the sternocleidomastoid muscle around the clavicle. You must be able to distinguish internal jugular vein pulsation from that of the carotid artery. It is easy to confuse them because they lie close together. Use the guidelines shown in Table 17.2.	
Inspect and palpate the praecordium	
Inspect the anterior chest	
Arrange tangential lighting to accentuate any flicker of movement. **Pulsations** You may or may not see the **apical impulse**, the pulsation created as the LV rotates against the chest wall during systole. When visible, it occupies the fourth or fifth intercostal space, at or inside the midclavicular line. It is easier to see in children and in those with thinner chest walls.	A **lift (heave) and thrill** are abnormal pulsations that may be observed on the praecordium. See Table 17.3 for a full description of abnormal pulsations on the praecordium.
Palpate the apical impulse	
• Localise the apical impulse precisely by using one finger pad (Figure 17.15A). • Asking the person to 'exhale and then hold it' aids the examiner in locating the pulsation. You may need to roll the person midway to the left to find it; note that this also displaces the apical impulse further to the left (Figure 17.15B).	The point at which you can palpate the apical impulse is the point at which you place your stethoscope to auscultate the apical heart sounds.

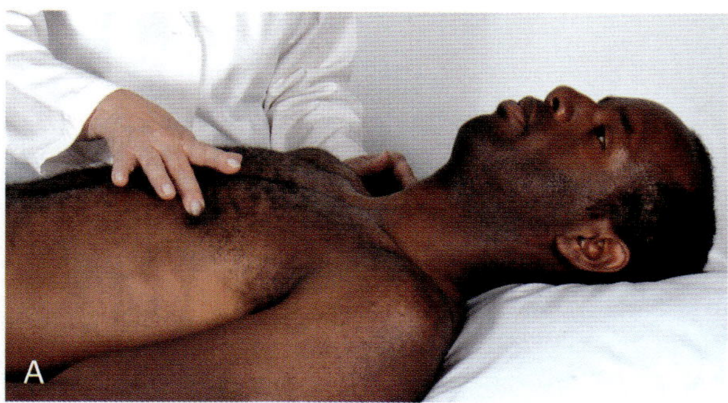

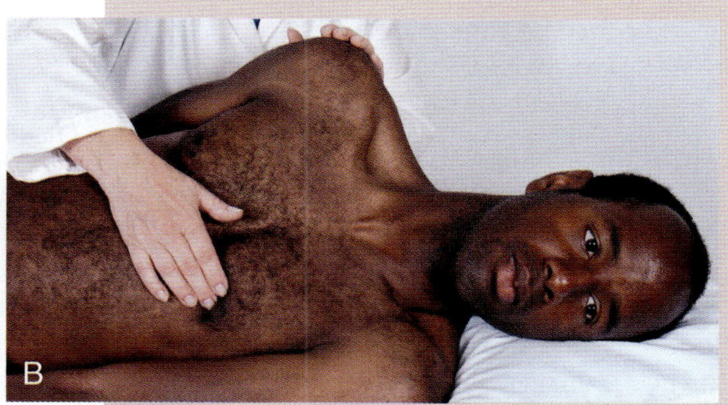

FIGURE 17.15 A, B Palpation of the apical impulse.

PROCEDURES AND NORMAL FINDINGS	ABNORMAL FINDINGS AND CLINICAL ALERTS
Note: **Location:** The apical impulse should occupy only one interspace, the fourth or fifth and be at or medial to the midclavicular line **Size:** Normally 1 cm × 2 cm **Amplitude:** Normally a short, gentle tap **Duration:** Short, normally occupies only first half of systole The apical impulse is easily palpated in most adults. It is not palpable in obese people or in people with thick chest walls. With high cardiac output states (anxiety, fever, hyperthyroidism, anaemia), the apical impulse increases in amplitude and duration.	Cardiac enlargement: **LV dilatation** (volume overload) displaces impulse down and to left and increases size more than one space. Increased force and duration but no change in location occurs with LV hypertrophy and no dilatation (pressure overload) (Table 17.3). Not palpable with chronic obstructive pulmonary disease due to hyperinflated lungs.
Auscultation of the apical (mitral) area	
In most situations, a generalist registered nurse will only need to perform the skill of auscultation of the two heart sounds at the apex of the heart. To do this, you will use both endpieces of your stethoscope when auscultating heart sounds. Although all heart sounds are low frequency, the diaphragm is for relatively higher pitched sounds and the bell is for relatively lower pitched ones. Before you begin, alert the person: '*I always listen to the heart in several places on the chest. Just because I am listening for a long time does not necessarily mean that something is wrong*'. • Locate the fifth intercostal space at the left midclavicular line—mitral valve area. • After you place the stethoscope, try closing your eyes briefly to tune out any distractions. Concentrate and listen selectively to *one sound at a time*. Consider that at least two, and perhaps three or four, sounds may be happening in less than 1 second. You cannot process everything at once. • Begin with the diaphragm endpiece and use the following routine: 1. note the rate and rhythm 2. identify S_1 and S_2 3. assess S_1 and S_2 separately.	
Note the rate and rhythm. The rate ranges normally from 60 to 100 beats per minute. (Review the full discussion of the pulse in Chapter 10 and the normal rates across age groups.) The rhythm should be regular, although **sinus arrhythmia** occurs normally in young adults and children. With sinus arrhythmia, the rhythm varies with the person's breathing, increasing at the peak of inspiration and slowing with expiration. Note any other irregular rhythm. If one occurs, check if it has any pattern or if it is totally irregular.	**Premature beat**—an isolated beat is early or a pattern occurs in which every third or fourth beat sounds early. **Irregularly irregular**—no pattern to the sounds; beats come rapidly and at random intervals. In a person with **rapid atrial fibrillation**, auscultation of the heart rate may be easier than palpating a peripheral pulse.

PROCEDURES AND NORMAL FINDINGS	ABNORMAL FINDINGS AND CLINICAL ALERTS
When you notice any irregularity, check for a **pulse deficit** by auscultating the apical beat while simultaneously palpating the radial pulse. • Count a serial measurement (one after the other) of apical beat and radial pulse. Normally, every beat you hear at the apex should perfuse to the periphery and be palpable. • The two counts should be identical. When different, subtract the radial rate from the apical and record the remainder as the pulse deficit. • **S_1** is louder than **S_2** at the apex; **S_2** is louder than **S_1** at the base. • **S_1** coincides with the carotid artery pulse. Feel the carotid gently as you auscultate at the apex; the sound you hear as you feel each pulse is **S_1** (Figure 17.16). • **S_1** coincides with the R wave (the upstroke of the QRS complex) if the person is on an ECG monitor. • **Listen to S_1 and S_2 separately.** Note whether each heart sound is normal, accentuated, diminished or split. Inch your diaphragm across the chest as you do this. **First heart sound (S_1).** Caused by closure of the AV valves, **S_1** signals the beginning of systole. You can hear it over the entire praecordium, although it is loudest at the apex (Figure 17.17). (Sometimes the two sounds are equally loud at the apex, because **S_1** is lower pitched than **S_2**.) You can hear **S_1** with the diaphragm with the person in any position and equally well in inspiration and expiration. **Second heart sound (S_2).** The **S_2** is associated with closure of the semilunar valves. You can hear it with the diaphragm, over the entire praecordium, although **S_2** is loudest at the base (Figure 17.18).	A **pulse deficit**—a difference in the apical heart rate and radial pulse—signals a weak contraction of the ventricles; it occurs with atrial fibrillation, premature beats and heart failure (Table 17.4).

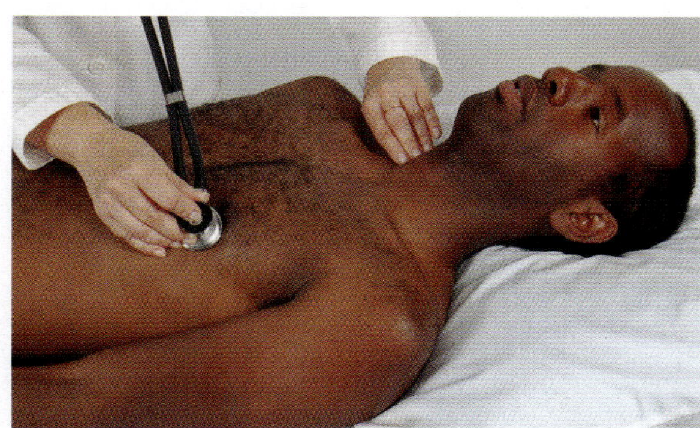

FIGURE 17.16 Auscultation of the apical (mitral) area

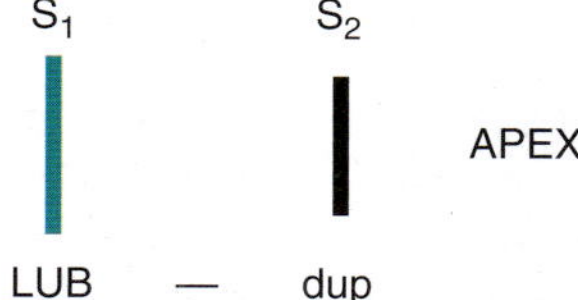

FIGURE 17.17 Diagrammatic representation of the first heart sound (S_1)

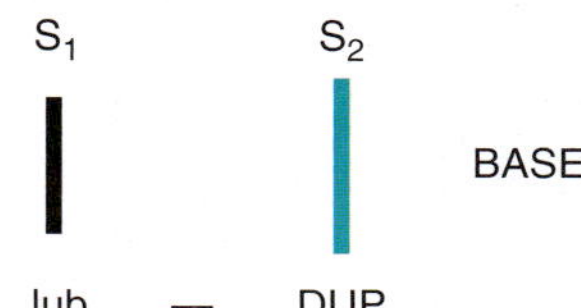

FIGURE 17.18 Diagrammatic representation of the second heart sound (S_2)

PROCEDURES AND NORMAL FINDINGS	ABNORMAL FINDINGS AND CLINICAL ALERTS

Additional objective data for adults over 65 years

- A gradual rise in systolic blood pressure is common with ageing; the diastolic blood pressure stays constant with a resulting widening of pulse pressure.
- Use caution in palpating and auscultating the carotid artery. Avoid pressure in the carotid sinus area, which could cause a reflex slowing of the heart rate. Also, pressure on the carotid artery could compromise circulation if the artery is already narrowed by atherosclerosis.
- When measuring jugular venous pressure, view the right internal jugular vein. The aorta stiffens, dilates and elongates with ageing, which may compress the left neck veins and obscure pulsations on the left side.
- The chest often increases in anteroposterior diameter with ageing. This makes it more difficult to palpate the apical impulse and to hear the splitting of $\mathbf{S_2}$. The $\mathbf{S_4}$ often occurs in people over 65 with no known cardiac disease. Systolic murmurs are common, occurring in over 50% of such people.
- Occasional premature ectopic beats are common and do not necessarily indicate underlying heart disease. When in doubt, obtain an ECG. However, consider that the ECG only records for one isolated minute in time and may need to be supplemented by a test of 24-hour ambulatory heart monitoring.

Some adults over 65 experience **orthostatic hypotension**, a sudden drop in blood pressure when rising to sit or stand.

The $\mathbf{S_3}$ is associated with heart failure and is always abnormal over age 35 years (Table 17.4).

Laboratory studies

There are many relevant specialist laboratory tests done to assess heart function. We have listed the most common tests that are undertaken as part of clinical assessment.

Reference values may vary by healthcare service depending on the laboratory testing procedures.

Clinical alert: Notify a medical practitioner or nurse practitioner of any abnormal results.

Troponin I or T: Troponin levels are very sensitive and specific for myocardial damage. Increased amounts of troponin are released into the circulating blood with myocardial damage. This blood test helps confirm a clinical diagnosis. The normal levels rise within a few hours of onset of pain and remain elevated for at least a week.

Elevated troponin levels confirm the diagnosis of MI.

Levels vary according to a specific laboratory, but an example of a cut-off for elevation (> 99th percentile of a reference population) is:[33]

- cTnI males 26 nanogram/L, females 16 nanogram/L
- cTnT males 15.5 nanogram/L, females 9 nanogram/L.

PROCEDURES AND NORMAL FINDINGS	ABNORMAL FINDINGS AND CLINICAL ALERTS
• **Potassium:** K^+ is an intracellular ion and is an essential ion for cardiac function. The test becomes abnormal within 12 hours of commencement of chest pain and remains abnormal for about 7 days. Normal levels vary by age. Normal reference interval:[34] • 3.5–5.2 mmol/L (adults—18 years or older).	**Hypokalaemia** (< 3.5 mm/L in adults) is commonly associated with excessive heat, dehydration, chronic kidney disease, excessive vomiting and diarrhoea, endocrine disorders and some drugs (e.g. diuretics). It can cause weakness, fatigue, muscle cramps and cardiac arrhythmias. **Hyperkalaemia** (> 5.5 mmol/L in adults) is associated with chronic kidney disease, diabetes, heart failure, trauma and medications that disrupt potassium balance (e.g. some drugs for hypertension). At moderately raised levels, there may be no symptoms, but higher levels can lead to potentially fatal cardiac arrhythmias. Variation in potassium levels may be evident on the 12-lead ECG.
Haemoglobin (Hb): This test is part of a full blood count and is used to exclude anaemia. Haemoglobin levels vary by gender, with adults, in pregnancy and in a child or a newborn. Values will also increase in high altitudes. Levels vary according to a specific laboratory, but an example reference interval is:[35] • non-pregnant women (15+ years of age)—115–165 g/L • men—125–185 g/L.	**Anaemia** (Hb < 115 g/L in non-pregnant adult women and < 125 g/L in adult men) can result from many causes including blood loss and iron deficiency. Symptoms include tiredness, lethargy and breathlessness. Anaemia is associated with heart failure in people with comorbidities and advancing age and can exacerbate heart failure symptoms. Insufficient haemoglobin may be a trigger for activating angina symptoms.
Brain-type natriuretic peptide (BNP): BNP levels rise with the severity of heart failure. When pressure in the ventricles rises, BNP levels become elevated. The serum levels can rise before the person becomes symptomatic with heart failure. This test can be done when the person reports fatigue or dyspnoea and it assists in generating a clinical diagnosis. BNP levels are higher in women than men, increase with age and have an inverse relationship with BMI (lower in obesity). Reference interval:[34] • BNP < 100 ng/L—heart failure unlikely.	BNP levels are elevated in the presence of heart failure. BNP levels may be elevated by factors other than heart failure such as acute coronary syndrome, pulmonary embolism, shock, atrial arrhythmia, severe pneumonia and renal disease. BNP 100–500 ng/L: equivocal range (unable to make a definitive diagnosis) BNP > 500 ng/L: consistent with the diagnosis of heart failure.

Abnormal findings

TABLE 17.1 Differential diagnosis of chest pain

	Common Pain Description	Location/Radiation	Possible Associated Symptoms
Cardiovascular (ischaemic)			
Angina pectoris: stable (no change in pain pattern within last 60 days)	Pressure-like discomfort (e.g. tightness, squeezing, burning, heaviness that lasts 3 to 5 minutes precipitated by activity and often resolves with rest)	Generalised substernal or retrosternal: can radiate to teeth, jaw, neck, one or both arms or shoulders; or there may be no pain and only associated symptoms	Diaphoresis, nausea, vomiting, dyspnoea
Prinzmetal or variant angina	Pressure-like discomfort often occurring at rest and early morning hours	Retrosternal: can radiate to jaw, neck, left arm or shoulder	Palpitations, syncope or feelings of syncope
Acute coronary syndrome (unstable angina, MI)	Heaviness; vice-like, squeezing, crushing, tightness; vague, burning, constricting or pressure; poorly localised pain lasting 20 to 30 minutes to hours and does not resolve with rest	Generalised substernal or retrosternal: can radiate to teeth, jaw, neck, one or both arms or shoulders; or there may be no pain and only associated symptoms	Indigestion-like feeling, nausea, vomiting, dizziness, flushing, perspiration, palpitations, dyspnoea **Note:** These are common symptoms in women and may be present without the typical description of chest pain
Cardiovascular (non-ischaemic)			
Pericarditis	Sudden sharp and stabbing pain relieved often by sitting or leaning forwards and worsens by lying down or with inspiration	Substernal, which can radiate to trapezius muscle region	Dry cough, muscle and joint aches, fever
Mitral valve prolapse	Sharp pain not associated with activity	Chest pain without radiation	Fatigue, light-headedness, dyspnoea, irregular heartbeat, palpitations, exercise intolerance

TABLE 17.1 Differential diagnosis of chest pain cont'd

	Common Pain Description	Location/Radiation	Possible Associated Symptoms
Aortic dissection	Sudden severe pain with change in location and/or tearing sensation lasting for hours	Anterior chest pain with radiation to the neck, jaw or intrascapular region of the back	Mental status changes, limb pain and weakness, dyspnoea
Pulmonary hypertension (secondary)	Cardiac-like chest pain with exertion	Chest region	Dyspnoea, lower-extremity oedema, fatigue
Pulmonary			
Pulmonary embolism	Sharp, stabbing pain worsening with deep breaths	Pain can be experienced in chest, back, shoulder or upper abdomen	Dyspnoea, haemoptysis, cough
Pneumonia	Sharp or stabbing pain associated with cough	Mostly generalised to one side of chest but can have upper abdominal pain	Cough, fever, dyspnoea, chills, sputum, myalgia, malaise
Pneumothorax	Acute/sudden and sharp	Lateral region of the chest but can have referred pain to shoulder	Acute dyspnoea, cough
Gastrointestinal			
Gastro-oesophageal reflux	May be angina-like; however, usually burning sensation with eating large meals reproduced by lying down and relieved by sitting up	Retrosternal region	Cough, regurgitation of food, abdominal pain
Oesophageal spasm	Crushing chest pain	Substernal	Dysphagia, sensation of object in throat or oesophagus
Cholecystitis	Sudden onset of pain that crescendos and can last for up to 20 minutes, usually after eating a fatty meal	Epigastrium or right upper abdomen that can radiate to right intrascapular region, shoulder or back	Nausea, vomiting, anorexia, fever
Pancreatitis	Sudden dull, boring, steady pain unrelieved by lying supine; leaning forwards or the fetal position may ease pain	Epigastrium or periumbilical pain radiating to the back	Nausea, vomiting, anorexia and sometimes diarrhoea

Continued

TABLE 17.1 Differential diagnosis of chest pain cont'd

	Common Pain Description	Location/Radiation	Possible Associated Symptoms
Dermatological			
Herpes zoster	Unilateral, burning, bore-like pain	Chest region in dermatome distribution	Tingling, itching, burning
Musculoskeletal/neurological			
Costochondritis	Sharp, pleuritic-type pain worsens with deep breathing, palpation or movement	Area from 2nd through to 5th intercostal spaces; can radiate to arm, depending on where initial inflammation occurs	Chest tightness, warmth at area of pain
Chest wall muscle strain	Sharp pain with moving, stretching or pushing movements of the arms; palpation of area reproduces the pain	Area around the strained muscle, sternum or ribs	Muscle spasm, crepitation, swelling, loss of strength
Psychogenic			
Depression	Heaviness	Chest region	Fatigue, restlessness, withdrawal, weight gain or loss, depressed mood
Anxiety	Sharp pain	Chest region	Palpitations, dizziness, sweating, shaking, restlessness, fatigue, irritability

Adapted from Zitkus 2010[38]

TABLE 17.2 Characteristics of jugular versus carotid pulsations

	Internal Jugular Pulse	Carotid Pulse
Location	Lower, more lateral, under or behind the sternocleidomastoid muscle	Higher and medial to this muscle
Quality	Undulant and diffuse, two visible waves per cycle	Brisk and localised, one wave per cycle
Respiration	Varies with respiration; its level descends during inspiration when intrathoracic pressure is decreased	Does not vary
Palpable	No	Yes
Pressure	Light pressure at the base of the neck easily obliterates	No change
Position of person	Level of pulse drops and disappears as the person is brought to a sitting position	Unaffected

TABLE 17.3 Abnormal pulsations on the praecordium

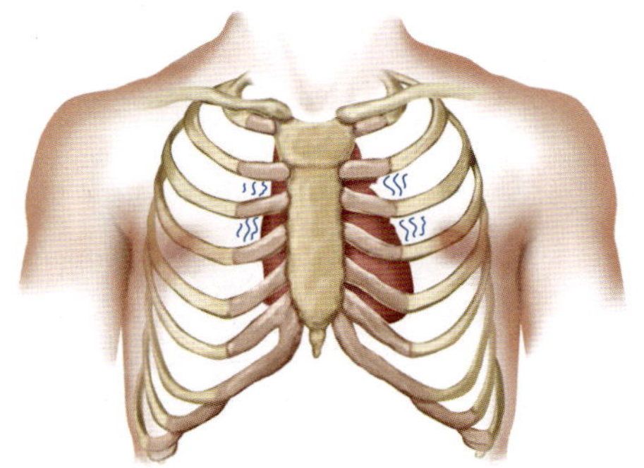

Base

A **thrill** in the second and third right interspaces occurs with severe aortic stenosis and systemic hypertension.

A thrill in the second and third left interspaces occurs with pulmonary valve stenosis and pulmonary hypertension.

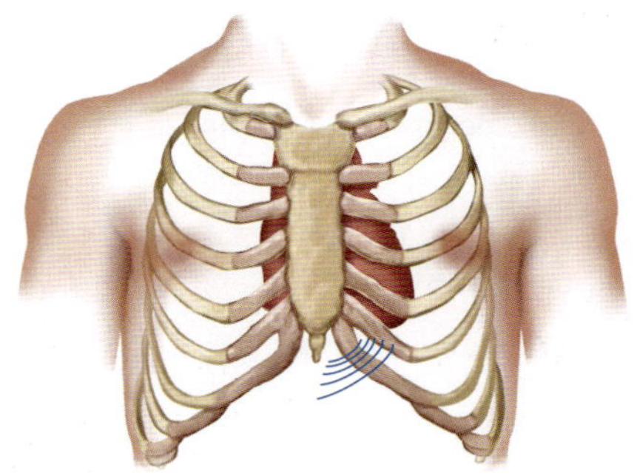

Left sternal border

A **lift (heave)** occurs with RV hypertrophy, as found in pulmonic valve disease, pulmonary hypertension and chronic lung disease. You will feel a diffuse lifting impulse during systole at the left lower sternal border. It may be associated with retraction at the apex because the LV is rotated posteriorly by the enlarged RV.

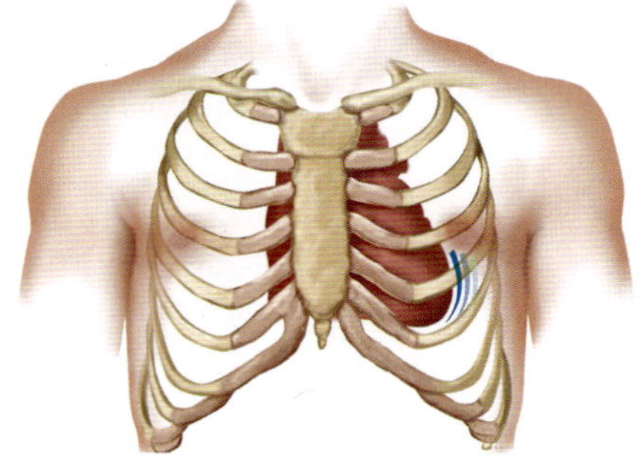

Apex

Cardiac enlargement displaces the apical impulse laterally and over a wider area when LV hypertrophy and dilatation are present. This is **volume overload**, as in mitral regurgitation, aortic regurgitation and left-to-right shunts.

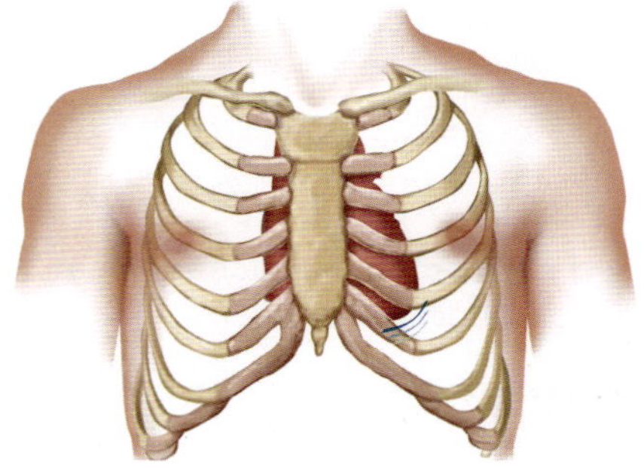

Apex

The apical impulse is increased in force and duration but is not necessarily displaced to the left when LV hypertrophy occurs alone without dilatation. This is **pressure overload**, as found in aortic stenosis or systemic hypertension.

TABLE 17.4 Clinical portrait of heart failure

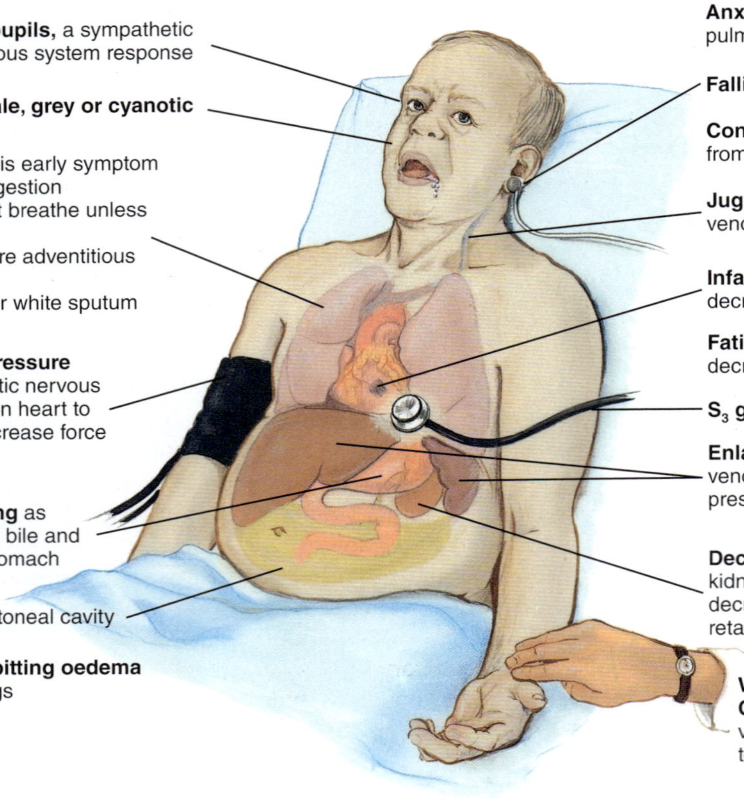

Dilated pupils, a sympathetic nervous system response

Skin pale, grey or cyanotic

Dyspnoea, SOBOE is early symptom from pulmonary congestion
Orthopnoea, cannot breathe unless sitting up
Crackles, wheeze are adventitious breath sounds
Cough, frothy pink or white sputum

Decreased blood pressure stimulates sympathetic nervous system, which acts on heart to increase rate and increase force of contraction

Nausea and vomiting as peristalsis slows and bile and fluids back up into stomach

Ascites, fluid in peritoneal cavity

Dependent, pitting oedema in sacrum, legs

Anxiety, gasping from pulmonary congestion

Falling O_2 saturation

Confusion, unconsciousness from decreased O_2 to brain

Jugular vein distension from venous congestion

Infarct, may be cause of decreased cardiac output

Fatigue, weakness from decreased cardiac output

S_3 gallop, tachycardia

Enlarged spleen and liver from venous congestion, which causes pressure on breathing

Decreased urine output as kidneys compensate for decreased cardiac output by retaining sodium and H_2O

Weak pulse
Cool, moist skin as peripheral vasoconstriction shunts blood to vital organs

Decreased cardiac output occurs when the heart fails as a pump, and the circulation becomes backed up and congested.

Signs and symptoms of heart failure come from two basic mechanisms: (1) the heart's inability to pump enough blood to meet the metabolic demands of the body; and (2) the kidney's compensatory mechanisms of abnormal retention of sodium and water to compensate for the decreased cardiac output. This increases blood volume and venous return, which causes further congestion.

Onset of heart failure may be: (1) acute, as following an MI when direct damage to the heart's contracting ability has occurred; or (2) chronic, as with hypertension, when the ventricles must pump against chronically increased pressure.

Advanced practice—additional data

The assessments that are described in the following section require advanced skill and scope of practice. Nurses working in specialist cardiac care units, intensive care units as well as community health centres may need to develop these skills. Advanced assessment for infants and children is performed by specialist neonatal and paediatric nurses, some midwives and maternal and child health nurses.

Equipment

Ruler

PROCEDURES AND NORMAL FINDINGS	ABNORMAL FINDINGS AND CLINICAL ALERTS
Estimate the jugular venous pressure	
As a follow-on from inspecting the jugular venous pulse, think of the jugular veins as a central venous pressure manometer attached directly to the RA. You can measure the jugular venous pressure at the highest level of pulsations (Figure 17.19 A, B). • Use the angle of Louis (sternal angle) as an arbitrary reference point and compare it with the highest level of venous pulsation. Hold a vertical ruler on the sternal angle. • Align a straight edge on the ruler like a T-square and adjust the level of the horizontal straight edge to the level of pulsation. • Read the level of intersection on the vertical ruler. • Normal jugular venous pulsation is 2 cm or less above the sternal angle. • When documenting the result, state the person's position—for example, 'internal jugular vein pulsations 3 cm above sternal angle when elevated 30 degrees'. If you cannot find the internal jugular veins, use the external jugular veins, and note the point where they look collapsed. Be aware that the technique of estimating venous pressure is difficult and is not always a reliable predictor of central venous pressure. Consistency in grading among examiners is difficult to achieve.	**Central venous pressure** is a measure of pressure in the vena cava. Central venous pressure is often used as an assessment of hemodynamic status, particularly in critically ill people.[36] Elevated pressure is a level of pulsation that is more than 3 cm above the sternal angle while at 45 degrees. There are several causes of raised jugular venous pressure including right heart failure and hypervolaemia.[32]
Auscultate the carotid artery	
For people middle-aged or older or who show symptoms or signs of cardiovascular disease, follow on from inspecting the neck vessels and auscultate each carotid artery for the presence of a **bruit** (pronounced bru-ee) (Figure 17.20). This is a blowing, swishing sound indicating blood flow turbulence; normally none is present.	A **bruit** indicates turbulence due to a local vascular cause, such as atherosclerotic narrowing.

PROCEDURES AND NORMAL FINDINGS	ABNORMAL FINDINGS AND CLINICAL ALERTS

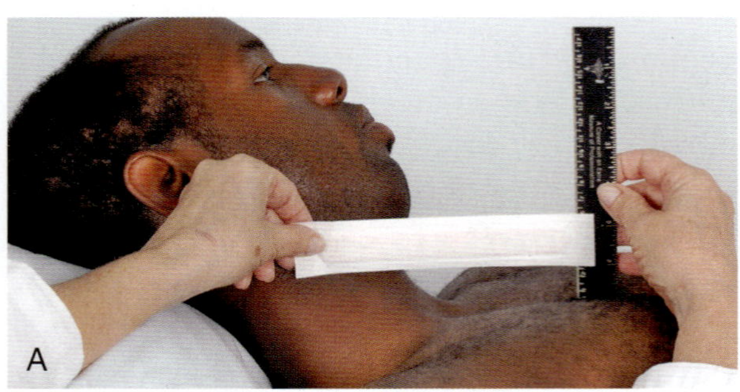

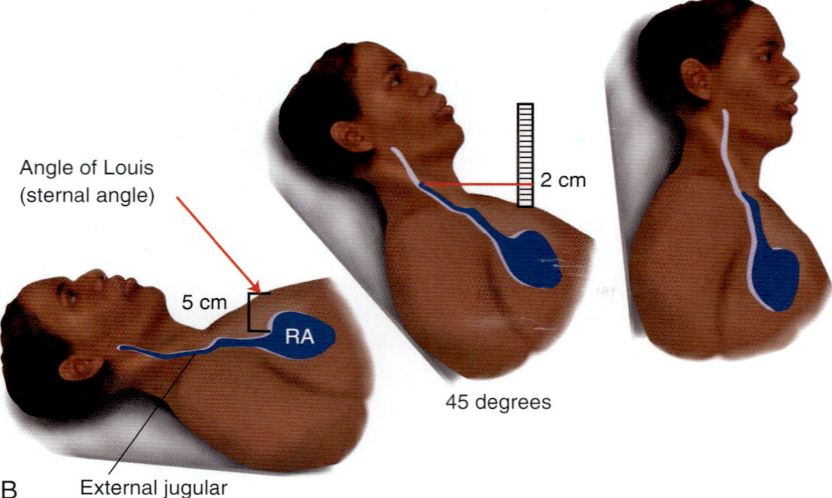

FIGURE 17.19 A, B Estimation of jugular venous pressure

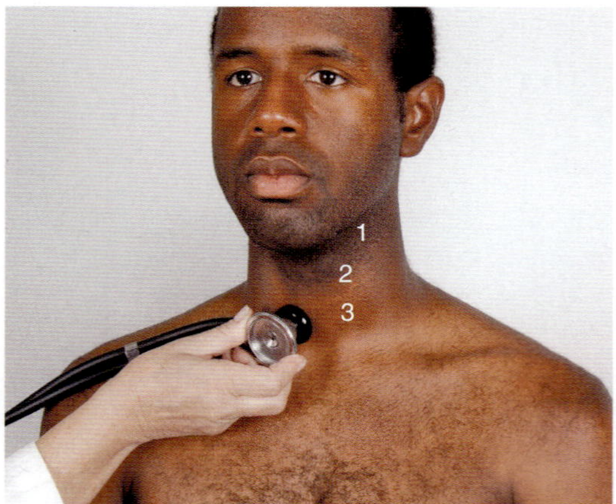

FIGURE 17.20 Auscultation of the carotid artery

PROCEDURES AND NORMAL FINDINGS	ABNORMAL FINDINGS AND CLINICAL ALERTS
• Keep the neck in a neutral position. • Lightly apply the bell of the stethoscope over the carotid artery at three levels: (1) the angle of the jaw, (2) the midcervical area and (3) the base of the neck (Figure 17.20). • Avoid compressing the artery because this could create an artificial bruit, and it could compromise circulation if the carotid artery is already narrowed by atherosclerosis. • Ask the person to take a breath, exhale and hold it briefly while you listen so tracheal breath sounds do not mask or mimic a carotid artery bruit. (Holding the breath on inhalation will also tense the levator scapulae muscles, which makes it hard to hear the carotids.) Sometimes you can hear normal heart sounds transmitted to the neck; do not confuse these with a bruit.	A **carotid bruit** is audible when the lumen is occluded by half to two-thirds. Bruit loudness increases as the atherosclerosis worsens until the lumen is occluded by two-thirds. After that, bruit loudness decreases. When the lumen is completely occluded, the bruit disappears. Thus, absence of a bruit does not ensure absence of a carotid lesion. A **murmur** sounds much the same but is caused by a cardiac disorder. Some aortic valve murmurs (aortic stenosis) radiate to the neck and must be distinguished from a local bruit.
Auscultate the praecordium	
In addition to auscultation at the apical area, some advanced practice nurses need to develop skills in auscultation across the praecordium. First you need to identify the auscultatory areas where you will listen. These include the four traditional valve 'areas' (Figure 17.21). The valve areas are not over the actual anatomical locations of the valves but are the sites on the chest wall where sounds produced by the valves are best heard. The sound radiates with the direction of blood flow. The valve areas are: • second right interspace—aortic valve area • second left interspace—pulmonic valve area • left lower sternal border—tricuspid valve area • fifth interspace at around left midclavicular line—mitral valve area. Do not limit your auscultation to only four locations. Sounds produced by the valves may be heard all over the praecordium. (For this reason, many experts even discourage the naming of the valve areas.) Learn to inch your stethoscope in a rough **Z pattern**, from the base of the heart across and down, then over to the apex. Or start at the apex and work your way up. Include the sites shown in Figure 17.21. After you place the stethoscope, try closing your eyes briefly to tune out any distractions. Concentrate and listen selectively to ***one sound at a time***. Consider that at least two, and perhaps three or four, sounds may be happening in less than 1 second. You cannot process everything at once. Begin with the diaphragm endpiece and use the following routine: (1) note the rate and rhythm, (2) identify $\mathbf{S_1}$ and $\mathbf{S_2}$, (3) assess $\mathbf{S_1}$ and $\mathbf{S_2}$ separately, (4) listen for extra heart sounds and (5) listen for murmurs.	

PROCEDURES AND NORMAL FINDINGS	ABNORMAL FINDINGS AND CLINICAL ALERTS

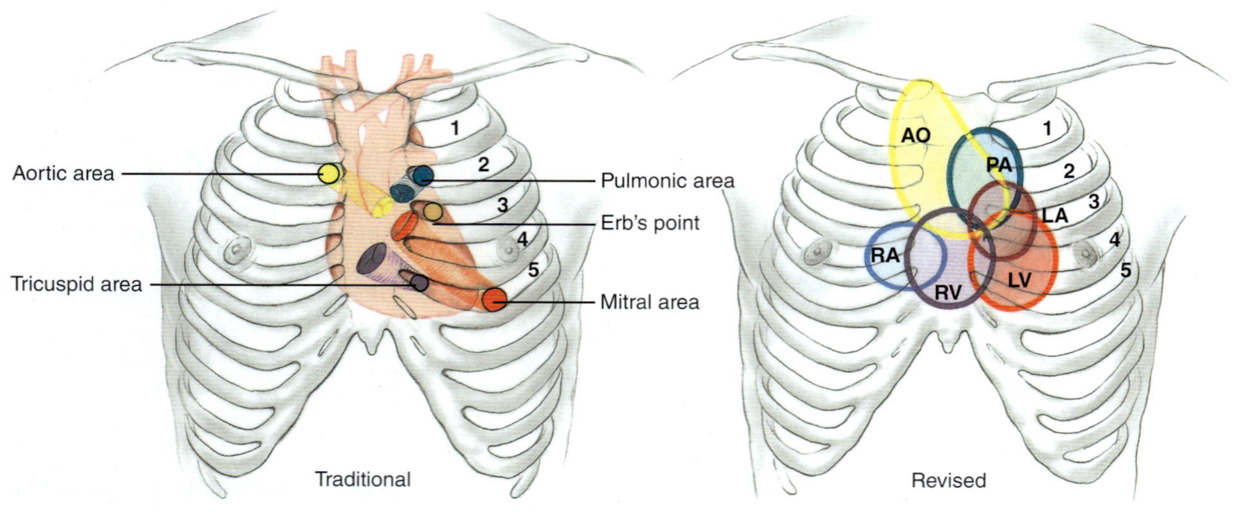

FIGURE 17.21 Positions for auscultation of the areas across the praecordium

A split S_1 is normal, but it occurs rarely. A split S_1 means you are hearing the mitral and tricuspid components separately. It is audible in the tricuspid valve area, the left lower sternal border. The split is very rapid, with the two components only 0.03 second apart.

Causes of accentuated or diminished S_1 (Table 17.5).

Both heart sounds are diminished with conditions that place an increased amount of tissue between the heart and your stethoscope: chronic obstructive pulmonary disease (hyperinflated lungs), obesity, pericardial fluid.

Splitting of S_2. A split S_2 is a normal phenomenon that occurs towards the end of inspiration in some people. Recall that closure of the aortic and pulmonic valves is nearly synchronous. Because of the effects of respiration on the heart described earlier, inspiration separates the timing of the two valves' closure, and the aortic valve closes 0.06 second before the pulmonic valve. Instead of one DUP, you hear a split sound—T-dup (Figure 17.22). During expiration, synchrony returns, and the aortic and pulmonic components fuse together. A split S_2 is heard only in the pulmonic valve area, the second left interspace.

Accentuated or diminished S_2 (Table 17.6).

PROCEDURES AND NORMAL FINDINGS	ABNORMAL FINDINGS AND CLINICAL ALERTS

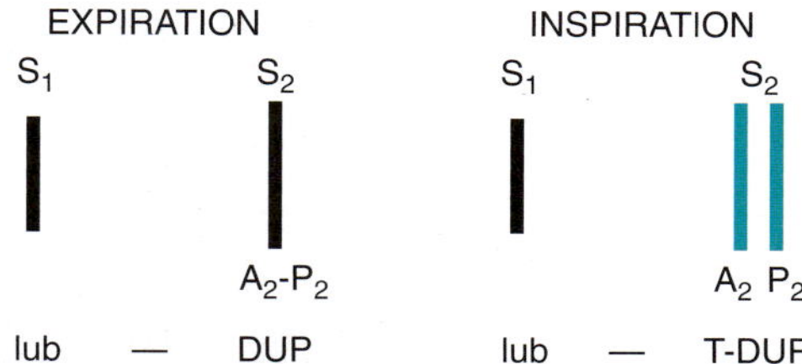

FIGURE 17.22 Diagrammatic representation of splitting of S_2

When you first hear the split $\mathbf{S_2}$, do *not* be tempted to ask the person to hold their breath so you can concentrate on the sounds. Breath holding will only equalise ejection times in the right and left sides of the heart and cause the split to go away. Instead, concentrate on the split as you watch the person's chest rise up and down with breathing. The split $\mathbf{S_2}$ occurs about every fourth heartbeat, fading in with inhalation and fading out with exhalation.

Focus on systole, then on diastole, and listen for any extra heart sounds. Listen with the diaphragm, then switch to the bell, covering all auscultatory areas (Figure 17.23). Usually, these are silent periods. When you do detect an extra heart sound, listen carefully to note its timing and characteristics. During systole, the **midsystolic click** (which is associated with mitral valve prolapse) is the most common extra sound (Table 17.7). $\mathbf{S_3}$ and $\mathbf{S_4}$ occur in diastole; either may be normal or abnormal (Table 17.8).

A **fixed split** is unaffected by respiration; the split is always there.

A **paradoxical split** is the opposite of what you would expect; the sounds fuse on inspiration and split on expiration (Table 17.7).

A pathological $\mathbf{S_3}$ (ventricular gallop) occurs with heart failure and volume overload; a pathological $\mathbf{S_4}$ (atrial gallop) occurs with coronary artery disease (see Table 17.9 for a full description).

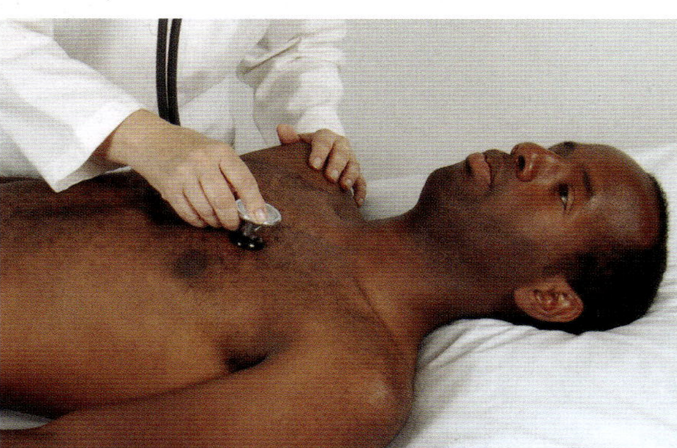

FIGURE 17.23 Auscultation of the praecordium using the bell of the stethoscope

PROCEDURES AND NORMAL FINDINGS

Listen for murmurs
A murmur is a blowing, swooshing sound that occurs with turbulent blood flow in the heart or great vessels. Except for the innocent murmurs described, murmurs are abnormal. If you hear a murmur, describe it by indicating these following characteristics:

Timing
It is crucial to define the murmur by its occurrence in systole or diastole. You must be able to identify $\mathbf{S_1}$ and $\mathbf{S_2}$ accurately to do this. Try to further describe the murmur as being in early, mid- or late systole or diastole; throughout the cardiac event (termed pansystolic or holosystolic/pandiastolic or holodiastolic); and whether it obscures or muffles the heart sounds.

Loudness
Describe the intensity in terms of six 'grades'. For example, record a grade ii murmur as 'ii/vi':

- *Grade i*—barely audible, heard only in a quiet room and then with difficulty
- *Grade ii*—clearly audible, but faint
- *Grade iii*—moderately loud, easy to hear
- *Grade iv*—loud, associated with a thrill palpable on the chest wall
- *Grade v*—very loud, heard with one corner of the stethoscope lifted off the chest wall
- *Grade vi*—loudest, still heard with entire stethoscope lifted just off the chest wall.

Pitch
Describe the pitch as high, medium or low. The pitch depends on the pressure and the rate of blood flow producing the murmur.

Pattern
The intensity may follow a pattern during the cardiac phase, growing louder (crescendo), tapering off (decrescendo) or increasing to a peak and then decreasing (crescendo–decrescendo or diamond-shaped). Because the whole murmur is just milliseconds long, it takes practice to diagnose any pattern.

ABNORMAL FINDINGS AND CLINICAL ALERTS

Murmurs may be due to congenital defects and acquired valvular defects. Study Tables 17.10 and 17.11 for a complete description.

A **systolic murmur** may occur with a normal heart or with heart disease; a **diastolic murmur** always indicates heart disease.

PROCEDURES AND NORMAL FINDINGS	ABNORMAL FINDINGS AND CLINICAL ALERTS
Quality Describe the quality as musical, blowing, harsh or rumbling. **Location** Describe the area of maximum intensity of the murmur (where it is best heard) by noting the valve area or intercostal spaces. **Radiation** The murmur may be transmitted downstream in the direction of blood flow and may be heard in another place on the praecordium, the neck, the back or the axilla. **Posture** Some murmurs disappear or are enhanced by a change in position. Some murmurs are common in healthy children or adolescents and are termed *innocent* or *functional*. **Innocent** indicates having no valvular or other pathological cause; **functional** is due to increased blood flow in the heart (e.g. in anaemia, fever, pregnancy, hyperthyroidism). The contractile force of the heart is greater in children. This increases blood flow velocity. The increased velocity plus a smaller chest measurement makes an audible murmur. The innocent murmur is generally soft (grade ii), midsystolic, short, crescendo–decrescendo and with a vibratory or musical quality ('vooot' sound like violin strings). Also, the innocent murmur is heard at the second or third left intercostal space and disappears with sitting, and the young person has no associated signs of cardiac dysfunction. Although it is important to distinguish innocent murmurs from pathological ones, it is best to suspect all murmurs as pathological until they are proved otherwise. Diagnostic tests such as ECG, phonocardiogram and echocardiogram are needed to establish an accurate diagnosis.	The murmur of mitral stenosis is rumbling, whereas that of aortic stenosis is harsh (Table 17.11).
Change position After auscultating in the supine position, roll the person towards their left side. Listen with the bell at the apex for the presence of any diastolic filling sounds (i.e. the $\mathbf{S_3}$ or $\mathbf{S_4}$) (Figure 17.24).	$\mathbf{S_3}$ and $\mathbf{S_4}$ and the murmur of mitral stenosis sometimes may be heard only when on the left side.

PROCEDURES AND NORMAL FINDINGS	ABNORMAL FINDINGS AND CLINICAL ALERTS

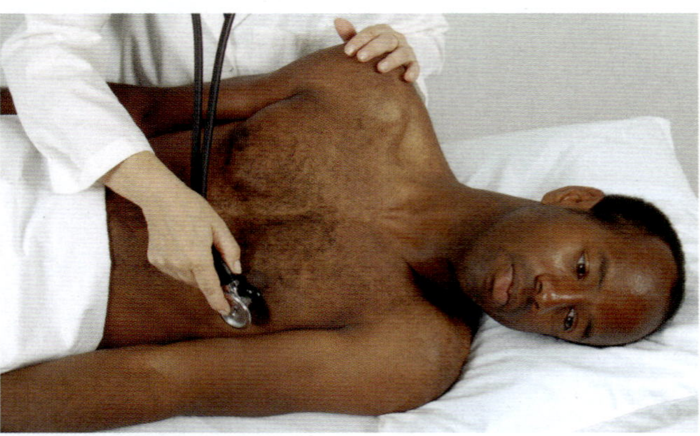

FIGURE 17.24 Change of position for auscultation of the praecordium

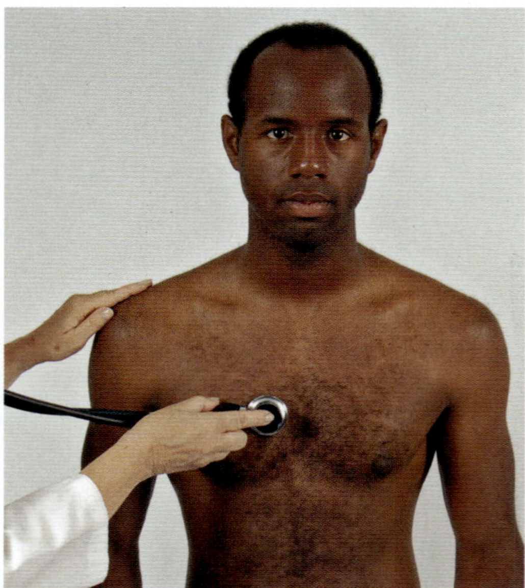

FIGURE 17.25 Auscultation of the praecordium in the upright position

Ask the person to sit up, lean forwards slightly and exhale. Listen with the diaphragm firmly pressed at the base, right and left sides. Check for the soft, high-pitched, early diastolic murmur of aortic or pulmonic regurgitation (Figure 17.25).

Murmur of aortic regurgitation sometimes may be heard only when the person is leaning forwards in the sitting position.

PROCEDURES AND NORMAL FINDINGS	ABNORMAL FINDINGS AND CLINICAL ALERTS
Additional objective data for infants	
The transition from fetal to pulmonic circulation occurs in the immediate newborn period. Fetal shunts normally close within 10 to 15 hours but may take up to 48 hours. Thus, you should assess the cardiovascular system during the first 24 hours and again in 2 to 3 days.	Failure of shunts to close (e.g. **patent ductus arteriosus (PDA)**, **atrial septal defect (ASD)**). See Table 17.10 for descriptions and clinical presentation.
Note any extra cardiac signs that may reflect cardiac status particularly in the skin, liver size and respiratory status. The skin colour should be pink to pinkish brown, depending on the infant's genetic heritage. If cyanosis occurs, determine its first appearance—at or shortly after birth versus after the neonatal period. Normally, the liver is not enlarged, and the respirations are not laboured. Also, note the expected parameters of weight gain throughout infancy.	Persistent cyanosis at or just after birth signals oxygen desaturation of congenital heart disease (Table 17.10). The most important signs of heart failure in an infant are persistent tachycardia, tachypnoea and liver enlargement. Engorged veins, gallop rhythm and pulsus alternans are also signs. Respiratory crackles are an important sign in adults but not in infants. Failure to thrive occurs with cardiac disease.
Palpate the apical impulse to determine the size and position of the heart. Because the infant's heart has a more horizontal placement, expect to palpate the apical impulse at the fourth intercostal space just lateral to the midclavicular line. It may or may not be visible.	The apex is displaced with: • cardiac enlargement—shifts to the left • **pneumothorax** (a collection of air outside the lungs but within the pleural cavity)—shifts away from the affected side • **diaphragmatic hernia** (herniation of part of the abdominal contents into the thoracic cavity)—shifts usually to the right because this hernia occurs more often on the left • **dextrocardia**—a rare anomaly in which the heart is located on the right side of the chest.
The heart rate is best auscultated because radial pulses are hard to count accurately. • Use the small (paediatric size) diaphragm and bell (Figure 17.26). • The heart rate may range from 70 to 190 per minute immediately after birth, then stabilise to an average of 120 per minute. • Infants normally have wide fluctuations with activity, from 170 per minute or more with crying or being active to 70 to 90 per minute with sleeping. Variations are greatest at birth and are even more so with premature babies (see Chapter 10—Table 10.1).	**Persistent tachycardia** is over 200 beats per minute in newborns or over 150 beats per minute in infants. **Bradycardia** is under 90 beats per minute in newborns or under 60 beats per minute in older infants or children. This causes a serious drop in cardiac output because the small muscle mass of their hearts cannot increase stroke volume significantly.

PROCEDURES AND NORMAL FINDINGS	ABNORMAL FINDINGS AND CLINICAL ALERTS

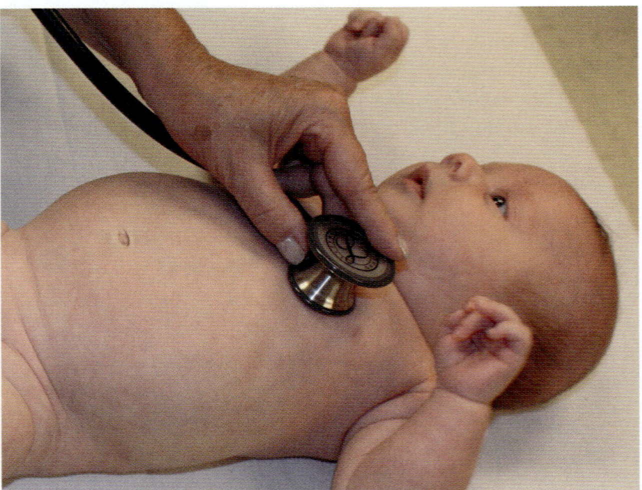

FIGURE 17.26 Auscultation of the infant heart to determine rate and rhythm

Expect the **heart rhythm** to have sinus arrhythmia, the phasic speeding up or slowing down with the respiratory cycle.

Rapid rates make it more challenging to evaluate heart sounds. Expect heart sounds to be louder in infants than in adults because of the infant's thinner chest wall. Also, $\mathbf{S_2}$ has a higher pitch and is sharper than $\mathbf{S_1}$. Splitting of $\mathbf{S_2}$ just after the height of inspiration is common, not at birth, but beginning a few hours after birth.

Investigate any irregularity except sinus arrhythmia.

Fixed split $\mathbf{S_2}$ indicates atrial septal defect (Table 17.10).

Murmurs in the immediate newborn period do not necessarily indicate congenital heart disease. Murmurs are relatively common in the first 2 or 3 days because of fetal shunt closure. These murmurs are usually grade i or ii, are systolic, accompany no other signs of cardiac disease and disappear in 2 to 3 days. The murmur of PDA is a continuous machinery murmur, which disappears by 2 or 3 days. On the other hand, absence of a murmur in the immediate newborn period does not ensure a perfect heart; congenital defects can be present that are not signalled by an early murmur. It is best to listen frequently and to note and describe any murmur according to the characteristics listed above.

Persistent murmur after 2 to 3 days, holosystolic murmurs or those that last into diastole, and those that are loud—all warrant further evaluation.

See Table 17.10 for descriptions and clinical presentation.

PROCEDURES AND NORMAL FINDINGS	ABNORMAL FINDINGS AND CLINICAL ALERTS
Additional objective data for children	
Note any **extracardiac or cardiac signs** that may indicate heart disease: poor weight gain, developmental delay, persistent tachycardia, tachypnoea, dyspnoea on exertion, cyanosis and clubbing. Note that clubbing of fingers and toes usually does not appear until late in the first year, even with severe cyanotic defects.	
The apical impulse is sometimes visible in children with thin chest walls. Note any obvious bulge or any heave—these are not normal.	A praecordial bulge to the left of the sternum with a hyperdynamic praecordium signals cardiac enlargement. The bulge occurs because the cartilaginous rib cage is more compliant. A substernal heave occurs with RV enlargement, and an apical heave occurs with LV hypertrophy.
Palpate the apical impulse In the fourth intercostal space to the left of the midclavicular line until age 4 years; at the fourth interspace at the midclavicular line from age 4 to 6 years; and in the fifth interspace to the right of the midclavicular line at age 7 years (Figure 17.27).	The apical impulse moves laterally with cardiac enlargement. Thrill (palpable vibration).

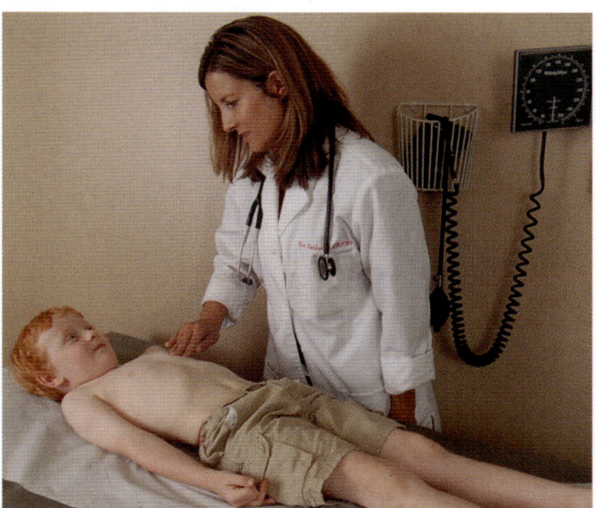

FIGURE 17.27 Palpation of the apical impulse in a child

PROCEDURES AND NORMAL FINDINGS	ABNORMAL FINDINGS AND CLINICAL ALERTS
The average heart rate slows as a child grows older, although it is still variable with rest or activity (see Chapter 10—Table 10.2). The heart rhythm remains characterised by sinus arrhythmia. Physiological $\mathbf{S_3}$ is common in children (Table 17.9). It occurs in early diastole, just after $\mathbf{S_2}$, and is a dull soft sound that is best heard at the apex. A **venous hum**—due to turbulence of blood flow in the jugular venous system—is common in healthy children and has no pathological significance. It is a continuous, low-pitched, soft hum that is heard throughout the cycle, although it is loudest in diastole. Listen with the bell over the supraclavicular fossa at the medial third of the clavicle, especially on the right or over the upper anterior chest.	
The venous hum is not usually affected by respiration, may sound louder when the child stands and is easily obliterated by occluding the jugular veins in the neck with your fingers.	This latter manoeuvre helps differentiate the venous hum from other cardiac murmurs (e.g. PDA).
Heart murmurs that are innocent (or functional) in origin are very common through childhood. Some authors say they have a 30% occurrence, and some authors say nearly all children may demonstrate a murmur at some time. Most innocent murmurs have these characteristics: soft, relatively short systolic ejection murmur; medium pitch; vibratory; best heard at the left lower sternal or midsternal border, with no radiation to the apex, base or back. For the child whose murmur has been shown to be innocent, it is very important that the parents understand this completely. They need to believe that this murmur is just a 'noise' and has no pathological significance. Otherwise, the parents may become overprotective and limit activity for the child, which may result in the child developing a negative self-concept.	Distinguish innocent murmurs from pathological ones. This may involve referral to another examiner or the performance of diagnostic tests such as an ECG or ultrasonography.
Additional objective data for pregnant women	
The **vital signs** usually yield an increase in resting pulse rate of 10 to 15 beats per minute and a drop in blood pressure from the normal pre-pregnancy level.[37] The blood pressure decreases to its lowest point during the second trimester and then slowly rises during the third trimester. The blood pressure varies with position.[37] It is usually lowest in left lateral recumbent position, a bit higher when supine and highest when sitting.	Suspect pregnancy-induced hypertension with a sustained rise of 30 mmHg systolic or 15 mmHg diastolic under resting conditions.

PROCEDURES AND NORMAL FINDINGS	ABNORMAL FINDINGS AND CLINICAL ALERTS
Inspection of the skin often shows a mild hyperaemia in light-skinned women because the increased cutaneous blood flow tries to eliminate the excess heat generated by the increased metabolism. Palpation of the apical impulse is higher and lateral compared with the normal position, as the enlarging uterus elevates the diaphragm and displaces the heart up and to the left and rotates it on its long axis. **Auscultation of the heart sounds** shows changes caused by the increased blood volume and workload: **Heart sounds.** There may be: • exaggerated splitting of $\mathbf{S_1}$ and increased loudness of $\mathbf{S_1}$ • a loud, easily heard $\mathbf{S_3}$. **The ECG** has no changes except for a slight left axis deviation and T wave inversion in the lateral leads and lead III due to the change in the heart's position, although this is very variable (upward movement of the diaphragm due to size of the uterus and fetus).[27]	

Abnormal findings for advanced practice

TABLE 17.5 Variations in S_1

The intensity of $\mathbf{S_1}$ depends on three factors: (1) position of AV valve at the start of systole, (2) structure of the valve leaflets and (3) how quickly pressure rises in the ventricle

	Factor	Examples
Loud (accentuated) S_1		
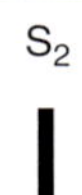	1. Position of AV valve at start of systole—wide open and no time to drift together 2. Change in valve structure—calcification of valve, needs increasing ventricular pressure to close the valve against increased atrial pressure	Hyperkinetic states where blood velocity is increased: exercise, fever, anaemia, hyperthyroidism. Mitral stenosis with leaflets still mobile

Continued

TABLE 17.5 Variations in S_1 cont'd

Faint (diminished) S_1		
S_1 S_2	1. Position of AV valve—delayed conduction from atria to ventricles. Mitral valve drifts shut before ventricular contraction closes it 2. Change in valve structure—extreme calcification, which limits mobility	First-degree heart block (prolonged PR interval) Mitral insufficiency
	3. More forceful atrial contraction into noncompliant ventricle; delays or diminishes ventricular contraction	Severe hypertension—systemic or pulmonary
Varying intensity of S_1		
S_1 S_2 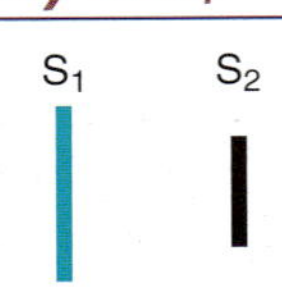	1. Position of AV valve varies before closing from beat to beat 2. Atria and ventricles beat independently	Atrial fibrillation—irregularly-irregular rhythm Complete heart block with changing PR interval
Split S_1		
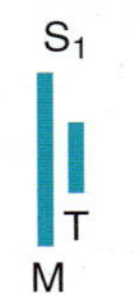 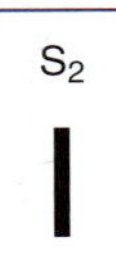 S_1 (M, T) S_2	Mitral and tricuspid components are heard separately	Normal but uncommon

TABLE 17.6 Variations in S_2

	Condition	Example
Accentuated S_2		
S_1 S_2	1. Higher closing pressure 2. Exercise and excitement increase pressure in aorta 3. Pulmonary hypertension 4. Semilunar valves calcified but still mobile	Systemic hypertension, ringing or booming $\mathbf{S_2}$ Mitral stenosis, heart failure Aortic or pulmonic stenosis
Diminished S_2		
S_1 S_2 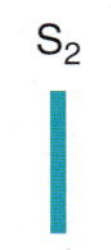	1. A fall in systemic blood pressure causes a decrease in valve strength 2. Semilunar valves thickened and calcified, with decreased mobility	Shock Aortic or pulmonic stenosis

TABLE 17.7 Variations in split S_2

Normal splitting

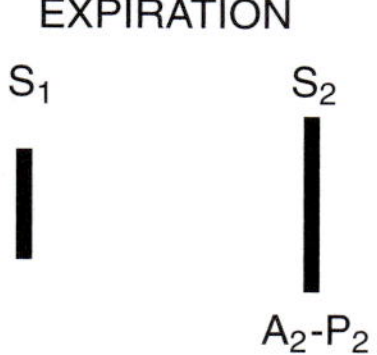

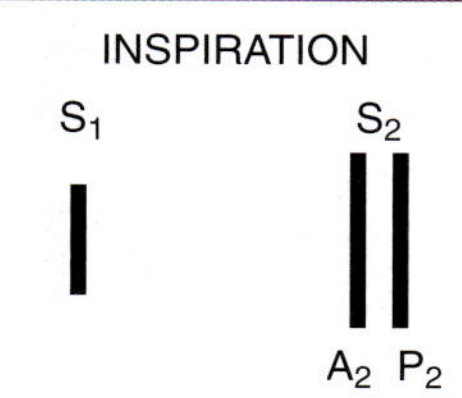

	Condition	Example

Fixed split

EXPIRATION
S_1
S_2
A_2 P_2

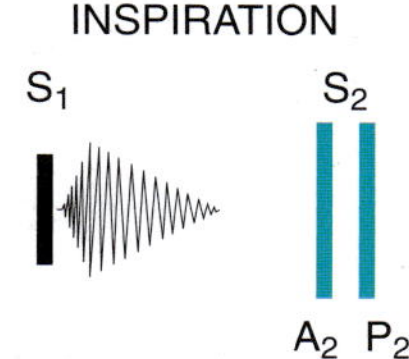

Condition: A fixed split is unaffected by respiration; the split is always there.

Example: Atrial septal defect; RV failure

Paradoxical split

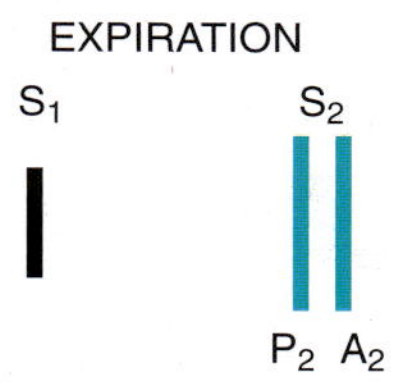

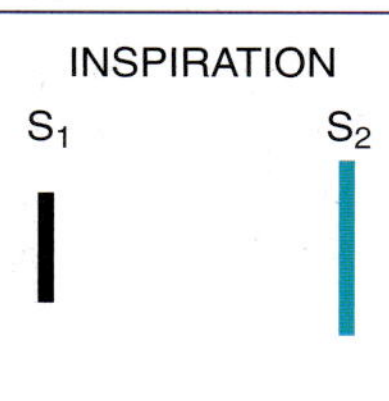

Condition: Conditions that delay aortic valve closure cause the opposite of a normal split. In inspiration, $\mathbf{P_2}$ is normally delayed, so with a paradoxical split the sounds fuse. In expiration you hear the split in the order of $\mathbf{P_2A_2}$.

Example: Aortic stenosis; Left bundle branch block; Patent ductus arteriosus

Wide split

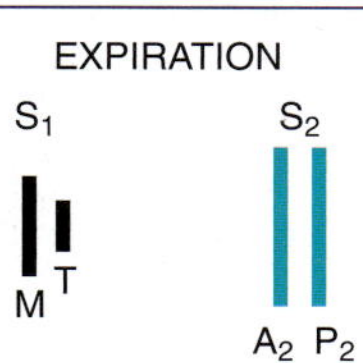

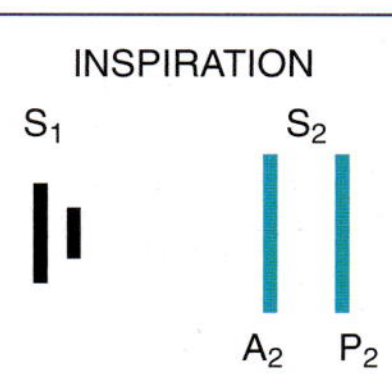

Condition: When the RV has delayed electrical activation, the split is very wide on inspiration and is still there on expiration.

Example: Right bundle branch block (which delays $\mathbf{P_2}$)

TABLE 17.8 Systolic extra sounds

Early systolic	Mid/late systolic
Ejection click	Midsystolic (mitral) click
Aortic prosthetic valve sounds	

Ejection click

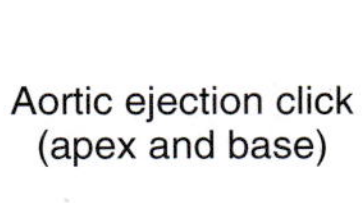

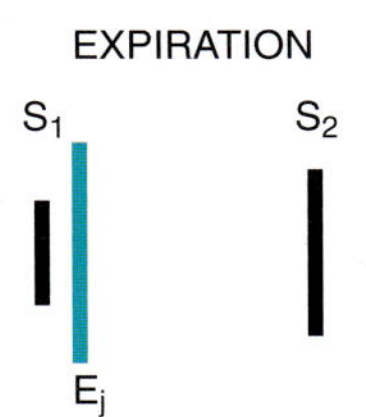

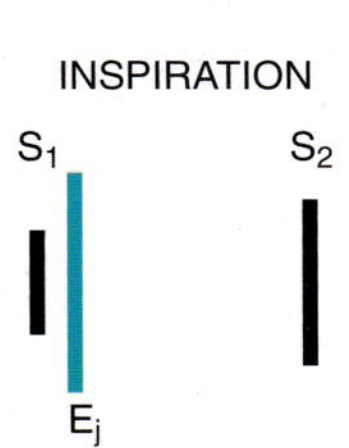

Continued

TABLE 17.8 Systolic extra sounds cont'd

The ejection click occurs early in systole at the start of ejection because it results from opening of the semilunar valves. Normally, the SL valves open silently, but in the presence of stenosis (e.g. aortic valve stenosis, pulmonary valve stenosis) their opening makes a sound. It is short and high pitched, with a click quality and is heard better with the diaphragm.
The aortic ejection click is heard at the second right interspace and apex and may be loudest at the apex. Its intensity does not change with respiration. The pulmonary valve ejection click is best heard in the second left interspace and often grows softer with inspiration.

Aortic prosthetic valve sounds

'Ball-in-cage'
AO = aortic opens
AC = aortic closes

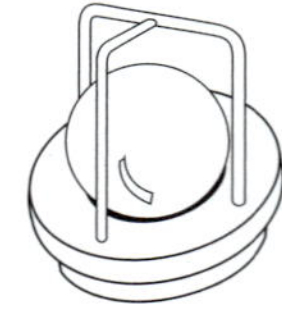

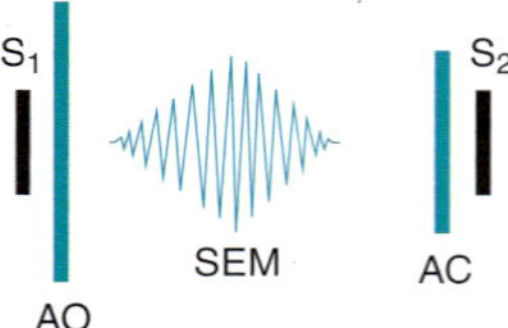

As a sequela of modern technological intervention for heart problems, some people now have *iatrogenically* induced heart sounds. The opening of an aortic ball-in-cage prosthesis (e.g. Starr-Edwards prosthesis) produces an early systolic sound. This sound is less intense with a tilting disk prosthesis (e.g. Bjork-Shiley prosthesis) and is absent with a tissue prosthesis (e.g. porcine).

Midsystolic click

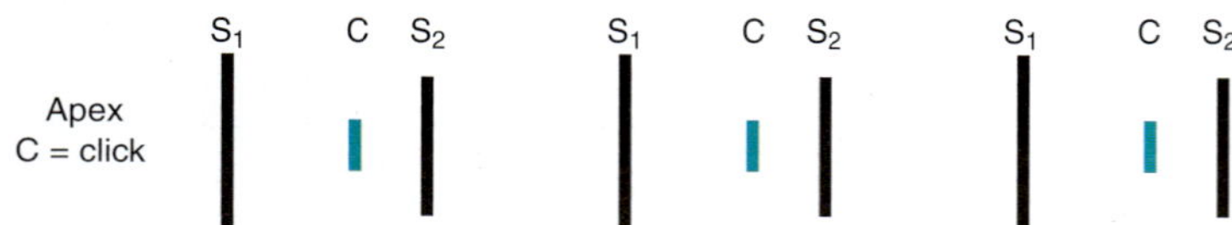

Although it is systolic, this is not an ejection click. It is associated with **mitral valve prolapse** in which the mitral valve leaflets not only close with contraction but balloon back up into the LA. During ballooning, the sudden tensing of the valve leaflets and the chordae tendineae creates the click.
The sound occurs in mid- to late systole and is short and high pitched, with a click quality. It is best heard with the diaphragm, at the apex, but also may be heard at the left lower sternal border. The click is usually followed by a systolic murmur. The click and murmur move with postural change; when the person assumes a squatting position, the click may move closer to $\mathbf{S_2}$, and the murmur may sound louder and delayed. The Valsalva manoeuvre also moves the click closer to $\mathbf{S_2}$.

TABLE 17.9 Diastolic extra sounds

Early diastole	Mid-diastole	Late diastole
Opening snap	Third heart sound	Fourth heart sound
Mitral prosthetic valve sound	Summation sound (S_3 + S_4)	Pacemaker-induced sound

Opening snap

EXPIRATION

S_1 S_2 OS

INSPIRATION

S_1 S_2 OS A_2 P_2

TABLE 17.9 Diastolic extra sounds cont'd

Normally the opening of the AV valves is silent. In the presence of stenosis, increasingly higher atrial pressure is required to open the valve. The deformed valve opens with a noise: the opening snap. It is sharp and high pitched, with a snapping quality. It sounds after **S_2** and is best heard with the diaphragm at the third or fourth left interspace at the sternal border, less well at the apex.

The opening snap is usually not an isolated sound. As a sign of mitral stenosis, the opening snap usually ushers in the low-pitched diastolic rumbling murmur of that condition.

Mitral prosthetic valve sound

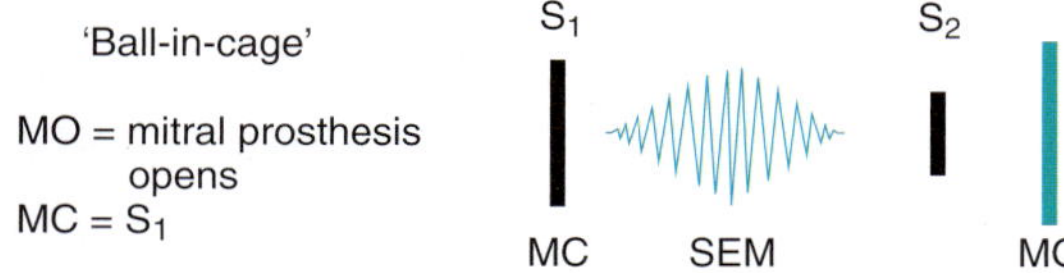

An iatrogenic sound, the opening of a ball-in-cage mitral prosthesis, gives an early diastolic sound: an opening click just after **S_2**. It is loud, is heard over the whole praecordium and is loudest at the apex and left lower sternal border.

Third heart sound

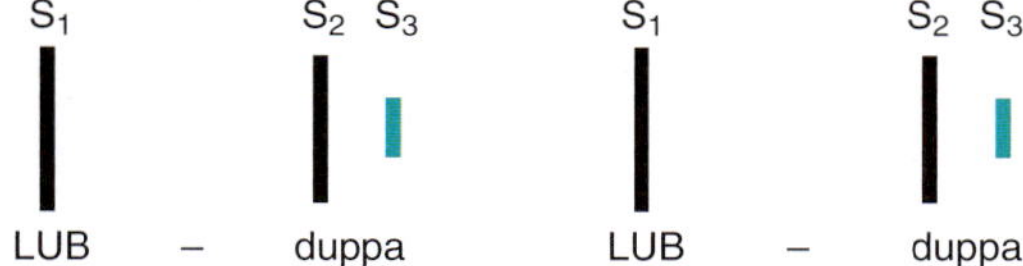

The **S_3** is a ventricular filling sound. It occurs in early diastole during the rapid filling phase. Your hearing quickly accommodates to the **S_3**, so it is best heard when you listen initially. It sounds after **S_2** but later than an opening snap would be. It is a dull, soft sound and it is low pitched, like 'distant thunder'. It is heard best in a quiet room, at the apex, with the bell held lightly (just enough to form a seal) and with the person in the left lateral position.

The **S_3** can be confused with a split **S_2**. Use these guidelines to distinguish the **S_3**:

- *location*—the **S_3** is heard at the apex or left lower sternal border; the split **S_2** at the base
- *respiratory variation*—the **S_3** does not vary in timing with respirations; the split **S_2** does
- *pitch*—the **S_3** is lower pitched; the pitch of the split **S_2** stays the same.

The **S_3** may be normal (physiological) or abnormal (pathological). The **physiological** S_3 is heard frequently in children and young adults; it occasionally may persist after age 40 years, especially in women. The normal **S_3** usually disappears when the person sits up.

In adults, the **S_3** is usually abnormal. The **pathological S_3** is also called a **ventricular gallop** or an **S_3** gallop and it persists when sitting up. The **S_3** indicates decreased compliance of the ventricles, as in heart failure. The **S_3** may be the earliest sign of heart failure. The **S_3** may originate from either the left or the RV; a left-sided **S_3** is heard at the apex in the left lateral position and a right-sided **S_3** is heard at the left lower sternal border with the person supine and is louder in inspiration.

The **S_3** occurs also with conditions of volume overload, such as mitral regurgitation and aortic or tricuspid regurgitation. The **S_3** is also found in high cardiac output states in the absence of heart disease, such as hyperthyroidism, anaemia and pregnancy. When the primary condition is corrected, the gallop disappears.

Continued

TABLE 17.9 Diastolic extra sounds cont'd

Fourth heart sound

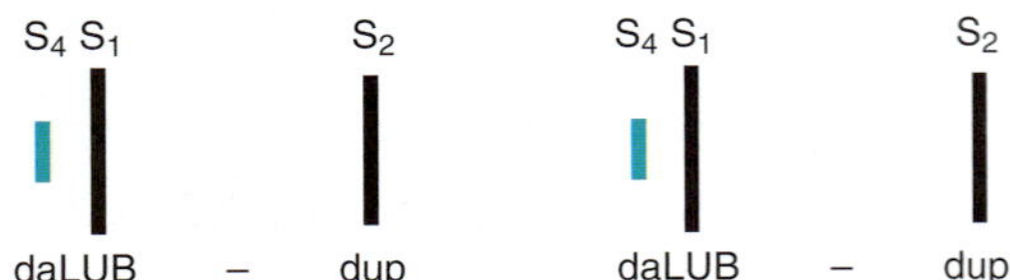

The S_4 is a ventricular filling sound. It occurs when the atria contract late in diastole. It is heard immediately before S_1. This is a very soft sound, of very low pitch. You need a good bell, and you must listen for it. It is heard best at the apex, with the person in left lateral position.

A **physiological S_4** may occur in adults older than 40 or 50 years with no evidence of cardiovascular disease, especially after exercise.

A **pathological S_4** is termed an **atrial gallop** or an S_4 gallop. It occurs with decreased compliance of the ventricle (e.g. coronary artery disease, cardiomyopathy) and with systolic overload (afterload), including outflow obstruction to the ventricle (aortic valve stenosis) and systemic hypertension. A left sided S_4 occurs with these conditions. It is heard best at the apex, in the left lateral position.

A right sided S_4 is less common. It is heard at the left lower sternal border and may increase with inspiration. It occurs with pulmonary valve stenosis or pulmonary hypertension.

Summation sound

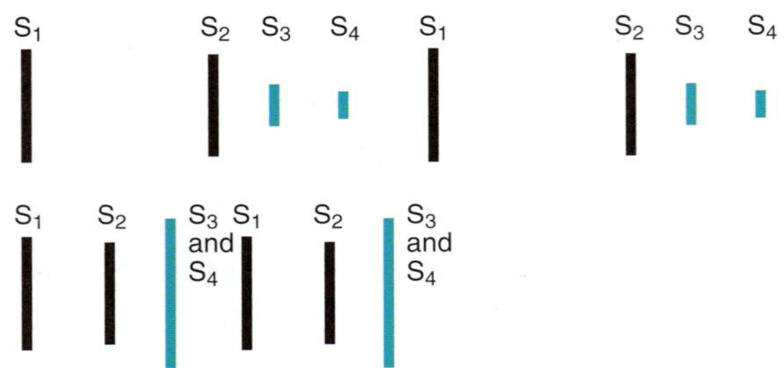

When both the pathological S_3 and S_4 are present, a quadruple rhythm is heard. Often, in cases of cardiac stress, one response is tachycardia. During rapid rates, the diastolic filling time shortens and the S_3 and S_4 move closer together. They sound superimposed in mid-diastole, and you hear one loud, prolonged, summated sound, often louder than either S_1 or S_2.

Extracardiac Sounds

Pericardial friction rub

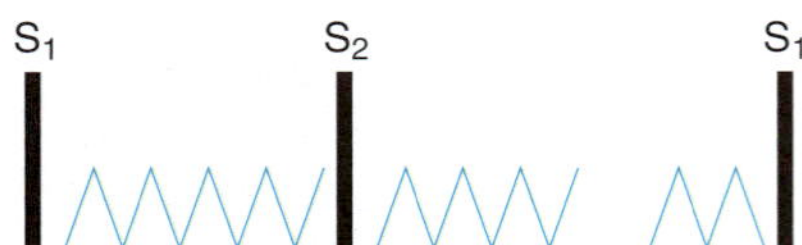

Inflammation of the praecordium gives rise to a friction rub. The sound is high pitched and scratchy, like sandpaper being rubbed. It is best heard with the diaphragm, with the person sitting up and leaning forwards and with the breath held in expiration.

A friction rub can be heard at any place on the praecordium but is usually best heard at the apex and left lower sternal border, places where the pericardium comes in close contact with the chest wall. Timing may be systolic and diastolic. The friction rub of pericarditis is common during the first week after an MI and may last only a few hours.

TABLE 17.10 Congenital heart defects

	Description	Clinical Data
Patent ductus arteriosus (PDA)		
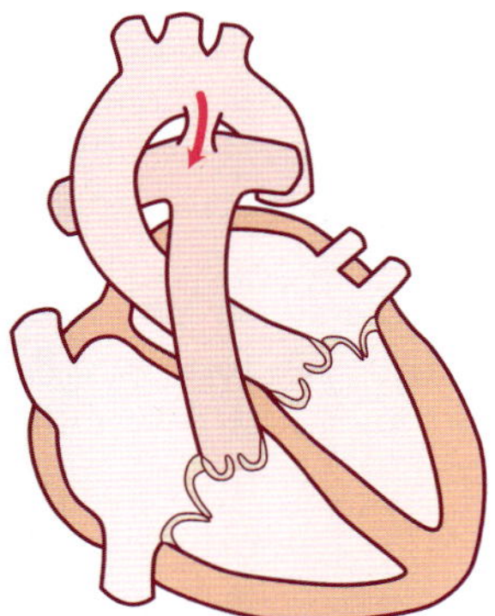	Persistence of the channel joining left pulmonary artery to aorta. This is normal in a fetus and usually closes spontaneously within hours of birth.	**Subjective data:** Usually no symptoms in early childhood; growth and development are normal. **Objective data:** Blood pressure has wide pulse pressure and bounding peripheral pulses from rapid runoff of blood into low-resistance pulmonary bed during diastole. The thrill is often palpable at the left upper sternal border. The continuous murmur heard in systole and diastole is called a machinery murmur.
Atrial septal defect (ASD)		
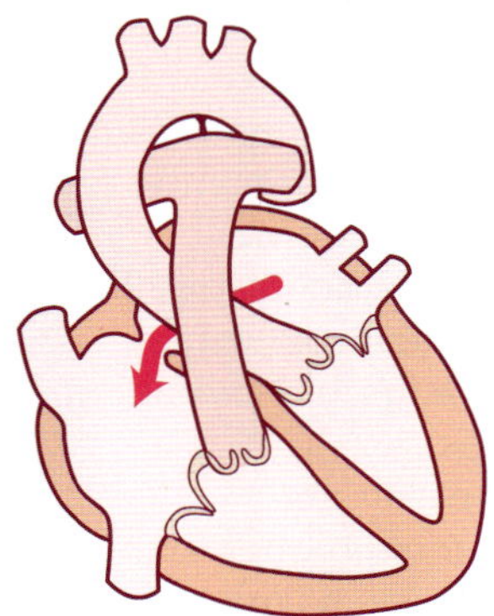	Abnormal opening in the atrial septum, resulting usually in a left-to-right shunt and causing a large increase in pulmonary blood flow.	**Subjective data:** Defect is remarkably well tolerated. Symptoms in infants are rare, growth and development normal. Children and young adults have mild fatigue and shortness of breath on exertion. **Objective data:** Sternal lift often present. S_2 has fixed split, with P_2 often louder than A_2. Murmur is systolic, ejection, medium pitch, best heard at the base in the second left interspace. Murmur caused not by the shunt itself but by increased blood flow through the pulmonic valve.
Ventricular septal defect (VSD)		
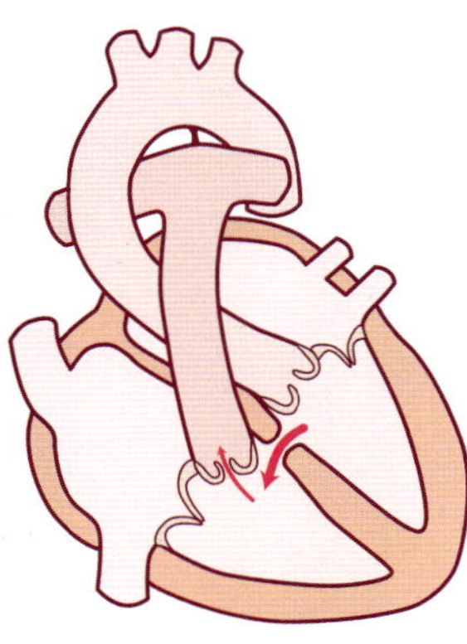	Abnormal opening in septum between the ventricles, usually subaortic area. The size and exact position vary considerably.	**Subjective data:** Small defects are asymptomatic. Infants with large defects have poor growth, slow weight gain; later look pale, thin and delicate. May have feeding problems; SOBOE; frequent respiratory infections; and, when the condition is severe, heart failure. **Objective data:** Loud, harsh holosystolic murmur, best heard at left lower sternal border, may be accompanied by thrill. Large defects also have a soft diastolic murmur at the apex (mitral flow murmur) due to increased blood flow through the mitral valve.

Continued

TABLE 17.10 Congenital heart defects cont'd

Tetralogy of Fallot

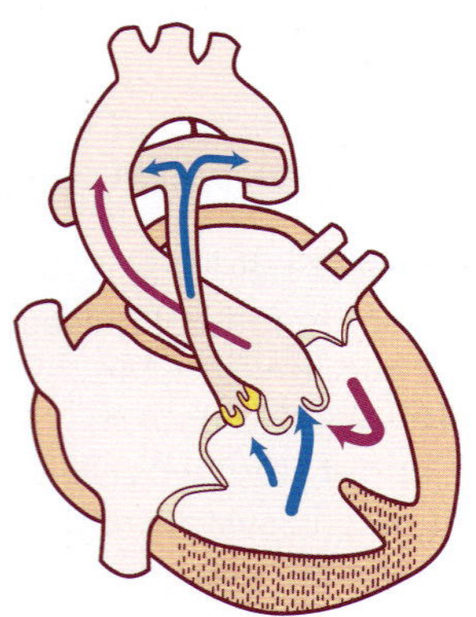

Four components:

- RV outflow stenosis
- VSD
- RV hypertrophy
- overriding aorta.

Result: Shunts a lot of venous blood directly into the aorta away from the pulmonary system, so blood never gets oxygenated.

Subjective data: Severe cyanosis, not in first months of life but develops as the infant grows and RV outflow (i.e. pulmonic) stenosis gets worse. Cyanosis with crying and exertion at first, then at rest. Uses squatting posture after starts walking. SOBOE common. Development is slowed.

Objective data: Thrill palpable at the left lower sternal border. $\mathbf{S_1}$ normal; $\mathbf{S_2}$ has $\mathbf{A_2}$ loud and $\mathbf{P_2}$ diminished or absent. Murmur is systolic, loud, crescendo–decrescendo.

Coarctation of the aorta

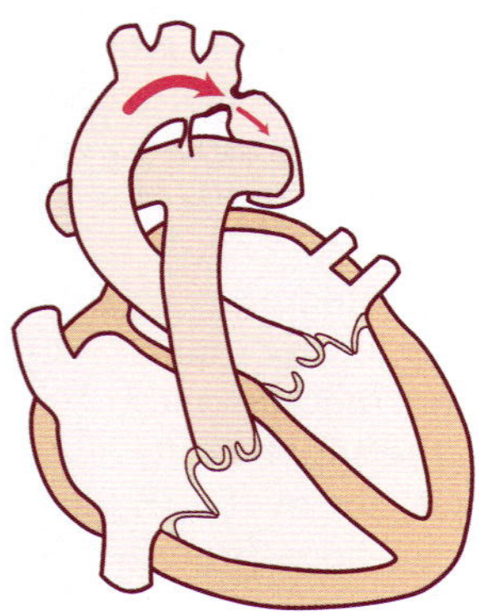

Severe narrowing of descending aorta, usually at the junction of the ductus arteriosus and the aortic arch, just distal to the origin of the left subclavian artery. Results in increased workload on the LV. Associated with defects of aortic valve in most cases, as well as associated patent ductus arteriosus; and associated ventricular septal defect.

Subjective data: In infants with associated lesions or symptoms; diagnosis occurs in first few months as symptoms of heart failure develop. For asymptomatic children and adolescents, growth and development are normal. Diagnosis usually accidental due to blood pressure findings. Adolescents may complain of vague lower extremity cramping that is worse with exercise.

Objective data: Upper extremity hypertension over 20 mmHg higher than lower extremity measures is a hallmark of coarctation. Another important sign is absent or greatly diminished femoral pulses. A systolic murmur is heard best at the left sternal border, radiating to the back.

TABLE 17.11 Murmurs due to valvular defects

Midsystolic ejection murmurs

Due to forward flow through semilunar valves

SYSTOLE DIASTOLE

S1 S2 S1 S2 S1 S2

TABLE 17.11 Murmurs due to valvular defects cont'd

	Description	Clinical Data
Aortic stenosis 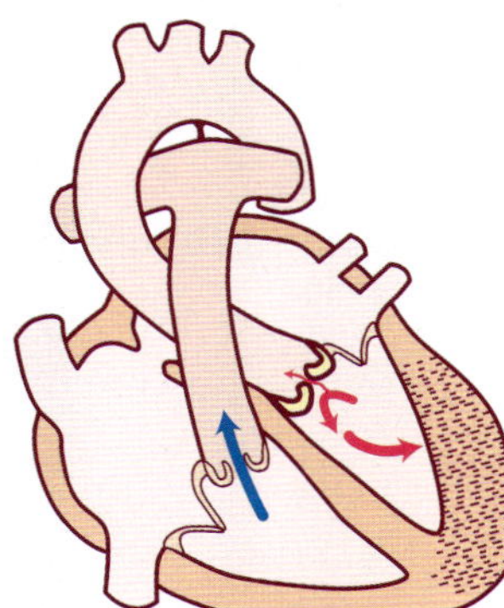	Calcification of aortic valve cusps restricts forward flow of blood during systole; LV hypertrophy develops.	**Subjective data:** Fatigue, shortness of breath and shortness of breath on exertion, palpitations, dizziness, fainting, anginal pain. **Objective data:** Pallor, slow diminished radial pulse, low blood pressure and auscultatory gap are common. Apical impulse sustained and displaced to left. Thrill in systole over second and third right interspaces and right side of neck. **S_1** normal, often ejection click present, often paradoxical split **S_2**, **S_4** present with LV hypertrophy. **Murmur:** Loud, harsh, midsystolic, crescendo–decrescendo, loudest at the second right interspace, radiates widely to the side of the neck, down the left sternal border or apex.
Pulmonic (pulmonary) valve stenosis 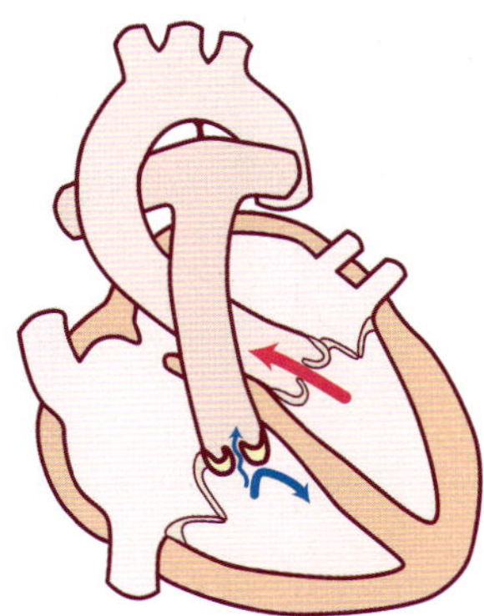	Calcification of pulmonic valve restricts forward flow of blood.	**Objective data:** Thrill in systole at the second and third left interspace, ejection click often present after **S_1**, diminished **S_2** and usually with wide split, **S_4** common with RV hypertrophy. **Murmur:** Systolic, medium pitch, coarse, crescendo–decrescendo (diamond shape), best heard at second left interspace, radiates to the left and neck.

Pansystolic regurgitant murmurs

Due to backward flow of blood from area of higher pressure to one of lower pressure.

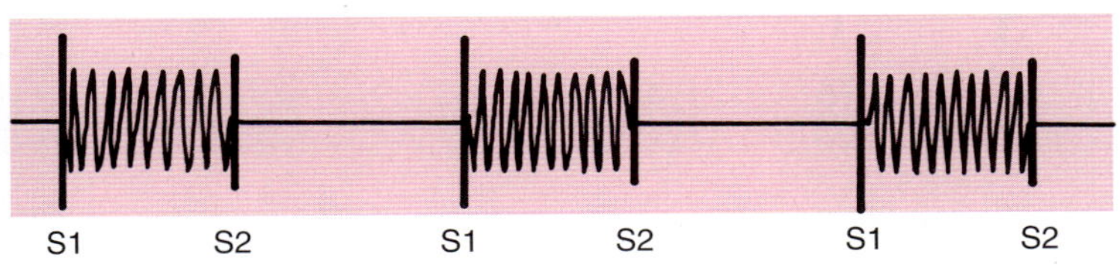

Continued

TABLE 17.11 Murmurs due to valvular defects cont'd

Mitral regurgitation

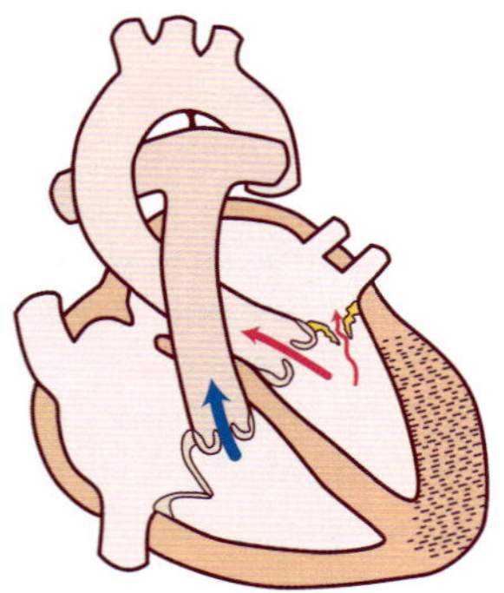

Stream of blood regurgitates back into LA during systole through incompetent mitral valve. In diastole, blood passes back into the LV again along with new flow; results in LV dilatation and hypertrophy.

Subjective data: Fatigue, palpitation, orthopnoea, PND. **Objective data:** Thrill in systole at the apex. Lift at the apex. Apical impulse displaced down and to the left. **S_1** diminished, **S_2** accentuated, **S_3** at apex often present.
Murmur: Pansystolic, often loud, blowing, best heard at the apex, radiates well to the left axilla.

Tricuspid regurgitation

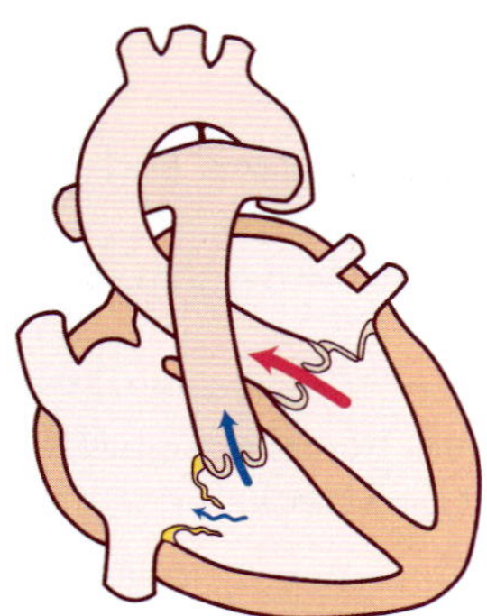

Backflow of blood through incompetent tricuspid valve into RA.

Objective data: Engorged pulsating neck veins, liver enlarged. Lift at the sternum if RV hypertrophy present, often thrill at the left lower sternal border.
Murmur: Soft, blowing, pansystolic, best heard at the left lower sternal border; increases with inspiration.

Diastolic rumbles of AV valves

Filling murmurs at low pressures, best heard with bell lightly touching skin.

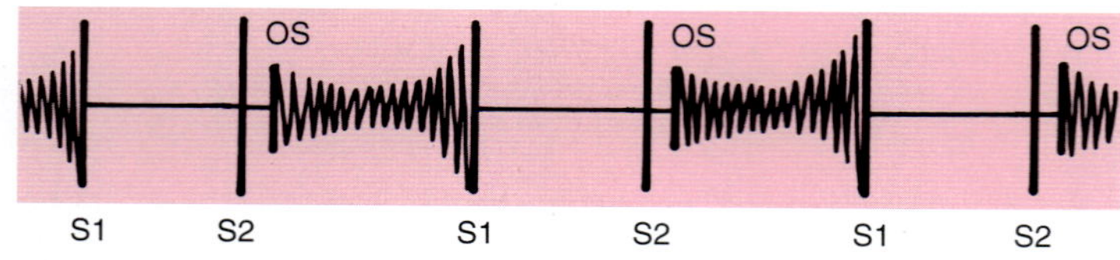

Mitral stenosis

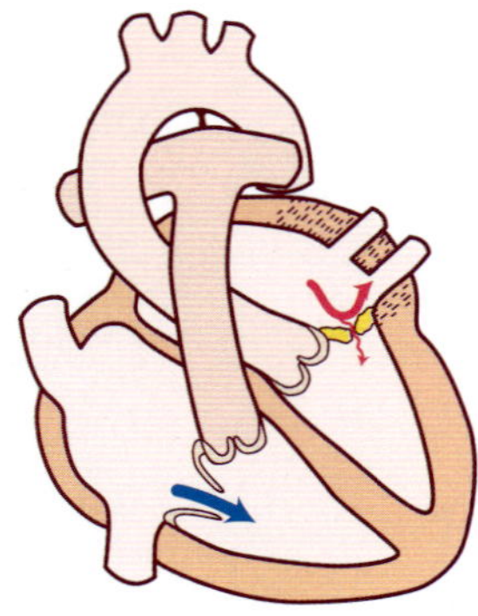

Calcified mitral valve will not open properly, impedes forward flow of blood into LV during diastole. Results in LA enlarged and LA pressure increased.

Subjective data: Fatigue, palpitations, SOBOE, orthopnoea, occasional PND or pulmonary oedema. **Objective data:** Diminished, often irregular arterial pulse. Lift at the apex, diastolic thrill common at the apex. **S_1** accentuated; opening snap after **S_2** heard over wide area of praecordium, followed by murmur.
Murmur: Low-pitched diastolic rumble, best heard at the apex, with the person in the left lateral position; does not radiate.

TABLE 17.11 Murmurs due to valvular defects cont'd

Tricuspid stenosis

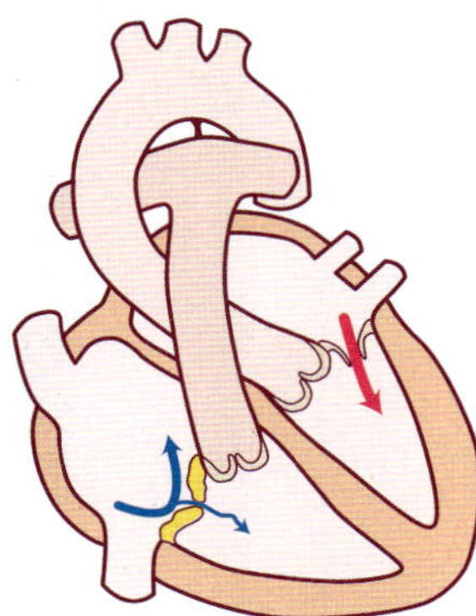

Calcification of tricuspid valve impedes forward flow into RV during diastole.

Objective data: Diminished arterial pulse, jugular venous pulse prominent.
Murmur: Diastolic rumble; best heard at the left lower sternal border; louder in inspiration.

Early diastolic murmurs

Due to SL valve incompetence.

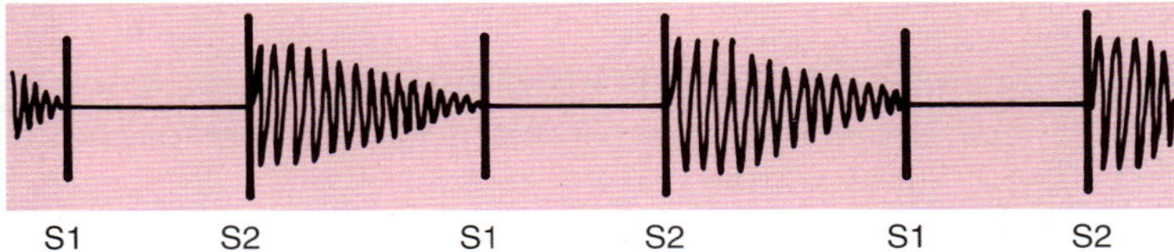

Aortic regurgitation

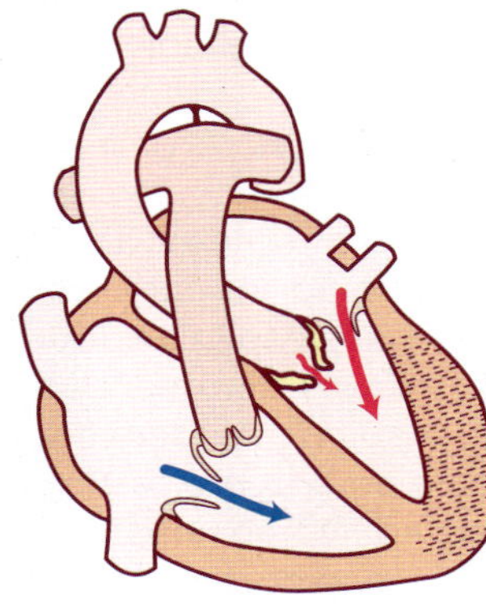

Stream of blood regurgitates back through incompetent aortic valve into LV during diastole. LV dilatation and hypertrophy due to increased LV stroke volume. Rapid ejection of large stroke volume into poorly filled aorta, then rapid runoff in diastole as part of blood pushed back into LV.

Subjective data: Only minor symptoms for many years, then rapid deterioration: SOBOE, PND, angina, dizziness.
Objective data: Bounding 'water-hammer' pulse in carotid, brachial and femoral arteries. Blood pressure has wide pulse pressure. Pulsations in cervical and suprasternal area, apical impulse displaced to left and down, apical impulse feels brief.
Murmur: Murmur' starts almost simultaneously with S_2: soft, high-pitched, blowing diastolic, decrescendo, best heard at the third left interspace at the base; as the person sits up and leans forwards, it radiates down.

Continued

TABLE 17.11 Murmurs due to valvular defects cont'd

Pulmonic regurgitation

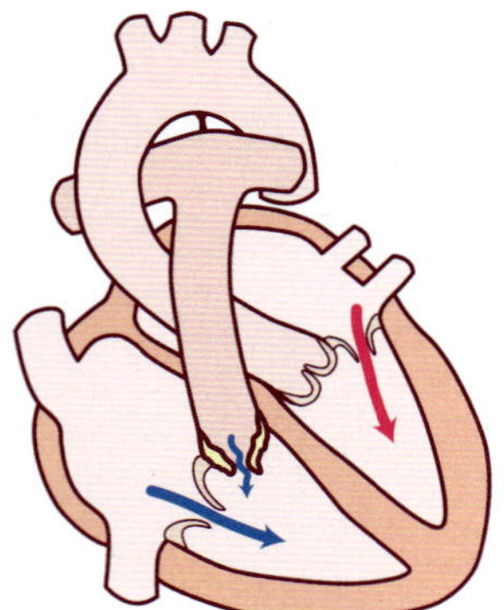	Backflow of blood through incompetent pulmonic valve, from pulmonary artery to RV.	Murmur has the same timing and characteristics as that of aortic regurgitation and is hard to distinguish on physical examination.

Clinical reasoning and documentation

The following is a continuation of the case study provided at the beginning of this chapter and the initial clinical reasoning process including problem/issue identification and documentation of clinical data. Consult a fundamentals of nursing or medical-surgical nursing text for information about goal setting, nursing interventions and evaluation.

Case study 1 (continued)—Cardiac chest pain

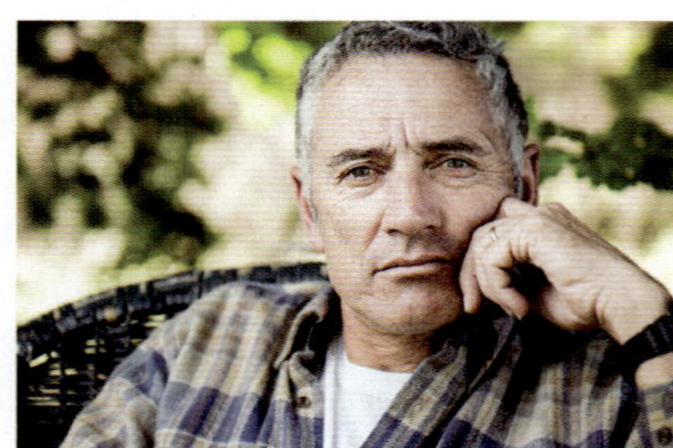

Context

You will recall from the case study described earlier in the chapter that you are on a clinical placement in a cardiac ward and are assisting the registered nurse to complete the admission assessment.

Consider the patient's situation

Mr Neil Andrews is a 53-year-old male who runs his own building company and was admitted to the cardiac ward with chest pain.

Collect cues/information

Your further assessment reveals the following information.

Subjective

One year ago: Mr Andrews was admitted to hospital with crushing substernal chest pain, radiating to the left shoulder, accompanied by nausea, vomiting and diaphoresis.

At that time, he was diagnosed as having an acute coronary syndrome, with no cardiac enzyme elevation and minor 12-lead ECG irregularities of T wave flattening in leads V5, V6, I and AVL. Mr Andrews was hospitalised for 4 days. During this time, he was commenced on antiplatelet therapy (aspirin), underwent serial 12-lead ECG and cardiac enzyme testing for 24 hours and scheduled for an inpatient percutaneous coronary angiogram. The angiogram identified a narrowing in his right coronary artery under 50% in diameter and he was started on medication to slow down his disease progression.

Since that hospital admission, Mr Andrews has continued to work. He had occasional fleeting episodes of chest pain with exercise, relieved by rest.

One day ago: Had increasing frequency of chest pain, about every 2 hours, lasting a few minutes and saw the change in pain pattern as a prompt to visit local doctor.

Clinical reasoning and documentation cont'd

Day of admission: Experiencing severe substernal chest pain ('*like someone sitting on my chest*') unrelieved by rest. Went to see his GP, where he had an episode of chest pain the same as last year, accompanied by diaphoresis, no nausea and vomiting or shortness of breath, relieved by two glyceryl trinitrate sprays. Transferred to hospital by ambulance. No further pain since presentation to the emergency department 4 hours ago. No new 12-lead ECG changes since last admission. He is booked for a cardiac angiogram as soon as possible.
Current chest pain: 2/10 central with no radiation.
Family history: Mother died of AMI at age 38 years.
Health and lifestyle management: Smoked 1½ pack cigarettes daily × 34 years, quit 1 year ago, does not drink alcohol, diet—trying to limit fat and fried food (eats takeaway food daily at work), still high in added salt.

Objective

General inspection: Appears anxious.
Height: 182 cm; **Weight:** 101 kg; **BMI:** 30.5 Abdominal obesity noted.
Extremities: Skin pink, no cyanosis. Upper extremities—capillary refill sluggish, no clubbing of fingertips. Lower extremities—no oedema, no hair growth 10 cm below knee bilaterally.
Pulses: carotid, brachial, radial, femoral − 2+; popliteal and posterior tibial − 0; dorsalis pedis − 1+. All equal bilaterally.
Blood pressure: R arm = L arm 104/66 mmHg
Praecordium: Inspection—Apical impulse visible 5th ICS, 7 cm left of midsternal line.
Palpation—Apical impulse palpable in 5th and 6th ICS.
Auscultation—Apical rate 92 regular. $\mathbf{S_1}$–$\mathbf{S_2}$ are normal, not diminished or accentuated.

Process information and identify problems/issues

Collaborative problems

Chest pain related to reduction in cardiac blood flow
Ineffective tissue perfusion related to interruption in cardiovascular blood flow
Decreased cardiac output related to reduction in stroke volume

Problem statements / nursing diagnoses

Chest pain related to reduction in cardiac blood flow
Fatigue related to reduced cardiac output
Anxiety and fear related to new cardiac episode and uncertainty about diagnosis
Knowledge deficit about reducing cardiac risk factors

ADDITIONAL RESOURCES

You can further develop your knowledge and skills relevant to cardiac assessment, related pathophysiology, common health issues and nursing interventions by:

- reading chapters of a fundamentals of nursing or medical-surgical nursing textbook
- answering chapter multiple choice questions online. Log onto ClinicalKey Student and search for the text 'Health Assessment, 4th edition'. Choose the section titled 'Teaching material'. In this section you will find question and answer documents for each chapter. Please check instructions on the inside cover of the book to access online resources.
- visiting websites:

  Australasian Cardiovascular Nursing College: www.acnc.net.au

ADDITIONAL RESOURCES cont'd

Cardiac Society of Australia & New Zealand: www.csanz.edu.au

Cardiomyopathy Association of Australia: www.cmaa.org.au

Heart Foundation (Australia): https://www.heartfoundation.org.au

Heart Foundation (New Zealand): www.heartfoundation.org.nz

Indigenous HeartInfoNet web resource: https://healthinfonet.ecu.edu.au/learn/health-topics/cardiovascular-health/

Pu Manawa—Rheumatic fever network: https://www.pumanawa.org.nz

Rheumatic Heart Disease Australia: https://www.rhdaustralia.org.au

Te Whatu Ora, Health New Zealand. Rheumatic fever: https://www.tewhatuora.govt.nz/for-the-health-sector/health-sector-guidance/communicable-disease-control-manual/rheumatic-fever/

REFERENCES

1. Amidei CB, Trevisan C, Dotto M, Ferroni E, Noale M, Maggi S, et al. Association of physical activity trajectories with major cardiovascular diseases in elderly people. Heart. 2022 Mar 1;108(5):360–366.
2. Brieger D, Amerena J, Attia JR, Bajorek B, Chan KH, Connell C, et al. National Heart Foundation of Australia and Cardiac Society of Australia and New Zealand: Australian clinical guidelines for the diagnosis and management of atrial fibrillation 2018. Medical Journal of Australia. 2018 Oct;209(8):356–362.
3. Australian Institute of Health and Welfare. Heart, stroke and vascular disease: Australian facts [Internet]. Canberra: Australian Institute of Health and Welfare, 2023. Available from: https://www.aihw.gov.au/reports/heart-stroke-vascular-disease/hsvd-facts
4. Sirochman M, Speight MK, Ro K, Mathur M, Perpetua EM. Ischaemic heart disease. In: Perpetua EM., Keegan P.A. (Eds). Cardiac nursing [electronic resource]: The red reference book for cardiac nurses. Wolters Kluwer; 2020. Available from: https://research.ebsco.com/linkprocessor/plink?id=714d2875-2868-38b1-b073-467f2824003b
5. Manfredi R, Verdoia M, Compagnucci P, Barbarossa A, Stronati G, Casella M, et al. Angina in 2022: Current Perspectives. Journal of Clinical Medicine. 2022 Nov 22;11(23):6891.
6. Heart Foundation New Zealand. Statistics. 2024. Available at: https://www.heartfoundation.org.nz/statistics
7. Figures NZ. New Zealand adults with ischaemic heart disease—June 2022. 2024. Available at: https://figure.nz/chart/MZK3hLTkW1XjQEK8-s34FUfi4TvwupDL7
8. Agostino JW, Wong D, Paige E, Wade V, Connell C, Davey ME, et al. Cardiovascular disease risk assessment for Aboriginal and Torres Strait Islander adults aged under 35 years: a consensus statement. Medical Journal of Australia. 2020 May; 212(9):422–427.
9. Ministry of Health, New Zealand. 2018. Cardiovascular disease risk assessment and management for primary care. Wellington: Ministry of Health. Available at: https://www.health.govt.nz/publication/cardiovascular-disease-risk-assessment-and-management-primary-care
10. Popovic D, Bjelobrk M, Tesic M, Seman S, Jayasinghe S, Hills AP, et al. Defining the importance of stress reduction in managing

cardiovascular disease—the role of exercise. Progress in Cardiovascular Diseases. 2022 Jan 1; 70:84–93.
11. Tortora GJ, Derrickson B, Burkett B, Cooke J, Di Pietro F, Diversi T, et al. Principles of Anatomy and Physiology, 3rd Asia-Pacific Edition. John Wiley & Sons; 2022.
12. Poznyak AV, Sadykhov NK, Kartuesov AG, Borisov EE, Melnichenko AA, Grechko AV, et al. Hypertension as a risk factor for atherosclerosis: Cardiovascular risk assessment. Frontiers in Cardiovascular Medicine. 2022 Aug 22;9: 959285.
13. Australian Bureau of Statistics. Hypertension and high measured blood pressure. Canberra: ABS; 2022. Available at: https://www.abs.gov.au/statistics/health/health-conditions-and-risks/hypertension-and-high-measured-blood-pressure/2022.statistics/health/health-conditions-and-risks/national-health-survey/latest-release
14. Australian Institute of Health and Welfare 2023. Aboriginal and Torres Strait Islander Health Performance Framework: summary report July 2023. Canberra: AIHW. Available at: https://www.indigenoushpf.gov.au/report-overview/overview/summary-report?ext=
15. Ministry of Health, New Zealand. 2023. Annual Data Explorer 2022/23: New Zealand Health Survey [Data File]. Available at: https://minhealthnz.shinyapps.io/nz-health-survey-2022-23-annual-data-explorer/
16. Chia J, Bhatia KS, Mihailidou AS, Kanagaratnam LB. The role of ambulatory blood pressure monitoring in current clinical practice. Heart, Lung and Circulation. 2022. 31(10): 1333–1340.
17. Benowitz, N.L. and Liakoni, E., 2022. Tobacco use disorder and cardiovascular health. Addiction, 117(4): 1128–1138.
18. World Health Organization. 2024. Obesity. Available at: https://www.who.int/health-topics/obesity#tab=tab_1
19. Zakir M, Ahuja N, Surksha MA, Sachdev R, Kalariya Y, Nasir M, et al. Cardiovascular complications of diabetes: from microvascular to macrovascular pathways. Cureus: Journal of Medical Science. 2023 Sep 24;15(9).
20. World Health Organization. 2024. Diabetes. Available at: https://www.who.int/health-topics/diabetes#tab=tab_1
21. Dooley LM, Ahmad TB, Pandey M, Good MF, Kotiw M. Rheumatic heart disease: a review of the current status of global research activity. Autoimmunity Reviews. 2021 Feb 1;20(2):102740.
22. Australian Institute of Health and Welfare. Acute rheumatic fever and rheumatic heart disease in Australia 2017–2021. Canberra: AIHW; 2023. https://www.aihw.gov.au/reports/indigenous-australians/arf-rhd/summary
23. Bennett J, Zhang J, Leung W, Jack S, Oliver J, Webb R, et al. Rising ethnic inequalities in acute rheumatic fever and rheumatic heart disease, New Zealand, 2000–2018. Emerging Infectious Diseases. 2021 Jan; 27(1):36.
24. The Australian Strep A Vaccine Initiative. 2024. Available at: https://www.asavi.org.au
25. Australian Bureau of Statistics. Causes of Death, Australia. Canberra: ABS; 2022. Available from: https://www.abs.gov.au/statistics/health/causes-death/causes-death-australia/latest-release
26. Te Whatu Ora, Health. Mortality web tool. New Zealand Government. 2023. Available at: https://www.tewhatuora.govt.nz/our-health-system/data-and-statistics/mortality-web-tool/#:,:text=For%20the%20total%20population%2C%20the,deaths%20per%20100%2C000%20population%20respectively
27. Heart Foundation (Australia). Key Statistics Heart Attack. 2024. Available at: https://www.heartfoundation.org.au/bundles/for-professionals/key-statistics-heart-attack
28. Dawson LP, Nehme E, Nehme Z, Davis E, Bloom J, Cox S, et al. Sex differences in epidemiology, care, and outcomes in patients with acute chest pain. Journal of the American College of Cardiology. 2023 Mar 14; 81(10):933–945.
29. Heart Foundation. Cardiovascular disease risk factors and heart attack warning signs in women. 2023. Available at: https://www.heartfoundation.org.au/Bundles/Your-heart/Risk-factors-for-women

30. Talley NJ, O'Connor S. Clinical examination: a systematic guide to physical diagnosis. 9th ed. Chatswood: Elsevier; 2021.
31. Chew DP, Scott IA, Cullen L, French JK, Briffa TG, Tideman PA, et al. National Heart Foundation of Australia and Cardiac Society of Australia and New Zealand: Australian clinical guidelines for the management of acute coronary syndromes 2016. Medical Journal of Australia. 2016 Aug; 205(3):128–133.
32. Santos P. History and physical examination. In Perpetua EM, Keegan P.A. (Eds). Cardiac nursing [electronic resource]: The red reference book for cardiac nurses. Wolters Kluwer; 2020. Available from: https://research.ebsco.com/linkprocessor/plink?id=714d2875-2868-38b1-b073-467f2824003b
33. Potter JM, Hickman PE, Cullen L 2022. Troponins in myocardial infarction and injury. Australian Prescriber, 45(2): 53.
34. Royal College of Pathologists Australia (RCPA). RCPA manual of use and interpretation of pathology tests. 2024. Available at: https://www.rcpa.edu.au/Manuals/RCPA-Manual
35. Australian Red Cross Life Blood. Anaemia. 2024. Available at: https://www.lifeblood.com.au/patients/reasons-for-a-transfusion/anaemia#:~:text=For%20men%2C%20the%20haemoglobin%20reference,that%20is%20testing%20the%20blood
36. Shah P, Louis MA. Physiology, central venous pressure. Stat Pearls. National Library of Medicine. 2023. Available at: https://www.ncbi.nlm.nih.gov/books/NBK519493/
37. Morton A. Physiological changes and cardiovascular investigations in pregnancy. Heart, Lung and Circulation. 2021 Jan 1;30(1): e6–e15
38. Zitkus BS. Take chest pain to heart, Nurse Practitioner, 35(9):41–47, 2010.

CHAPTER 18

Upper airways assessment

Written by Carolyn Jarvis
Adapted by Debbie Massey

INTRODUCTION

The upper airways, including the nose and throat, are especially important when considering a person's respiratory and olfactory function. You are advised to review the structure and function of the nose and throat and their relationships with each other and the primary digestive function of the mouth (Chapter 21).

Case study

The following case study gives an example of a typical situation involving upper airways assessment and the initial clinical reasoning process. It will help you identify your learning needs.

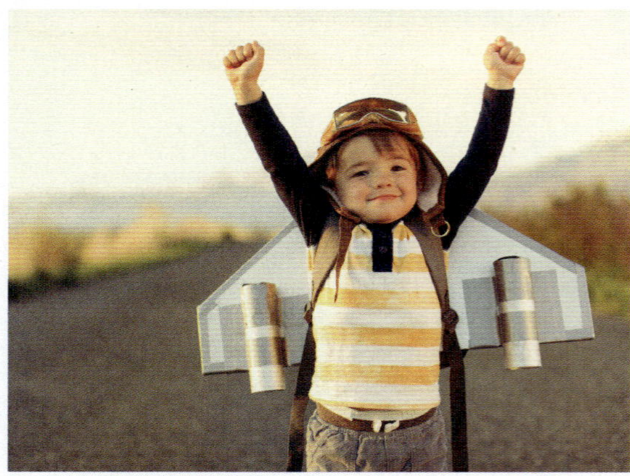

Context

You are a nurse practitioner working at a tertiary hospital in the emergency department. Your role includes assessing, treating, monitoring and evaluation of people with minor health issues and working collaboratively with the multidisciplinary healthcare team.

Consider the patient's situation

Liam Crawford, aged 3 years, has been brought to hospital by his distressed parents. Liam was observed pushing a small plastic bead up his nose this morning. His parents encouraged Liam to blow his nose but with no effect.

Questions to further your learning

- What are the possible things that might be going on with Liam and his parents?
- What knowledge do you need to be able to predict what might be going on?
- What approach to Liam's health assessment will you take?
- What questions (subjective data) will you ask Liam's parent to extend the health history and why?
- What physical examination (objective data) will you conduct and why?
- What resources are available to assist in your assessment of Liam?

Assessment plan

Assessment of the upper airways should include considering the impact of disease, trauma and/or alteration in the function of the intricate structures of the upper airways and the effect on the person's ability to breathe, eat and drink, undertake daily activities and exercise, sleep and undertake their role whether it be to work or attending school.

The main areas for subjective assessment are:

- presenting concern
- ear, nose or throat discharge
- blocked nose
- sinus pain
- trauma
- epistaxis
- allergies
- altered smell

- pain in mouth or throat
- sores or lesions
- hoarseness or change in voice
- lumps or swelling in the neck
- past history
- health and lifestyle management.

Following subjective data collection, you will get a sense of the areas needed to be examined for objective data. Only the relevant areas should be examined.

The main areas for physical examination, measurement and specimen screening are:

- general inspection
- inspecting and palpating the external nose
- inspecting the mouth
- inspecting the throat.

Resources available

You will find additional resources and the reference list at the end of this chapter.

Structure and function

Nose

The **nose** is the first segment of the respiratory system. It warms, moistens and filters the inhaled air and is a key sensory organ for chemical senses including smell. The external nose is shaped like a triangle, with one side attached to the face (Figure 18.1). On its leading edge, the superior part is the *bridge* and the free corner is the *tip*. The oval openings of the nose are the *nares* (nostrils); just inside, each naris widens into the *vestibule*. The *columella* divides the two nares and is continuous inside with the nasal septum. The *ala* is the lateral outside wing of the nose on either side. The support for the upper third of the external nose is made up of bone; the nasal bone, medially and the frontal processes of the maxillary bones laterally. The lower two-thirds of the support structure for the nose is made up of the septal and alar cartilages.

The space inside the **nasal cavity** is much larger than the external nose suggests (Figure 18.2). Nasal space extends back inside the skull over the roof of the mouth. The anterior edge of the cavity is lined with numerous coarse nasal hairs, or vibrissae. The cavity is lined with a blanket of ciliated mucous membrane. The nasal hairs filter the

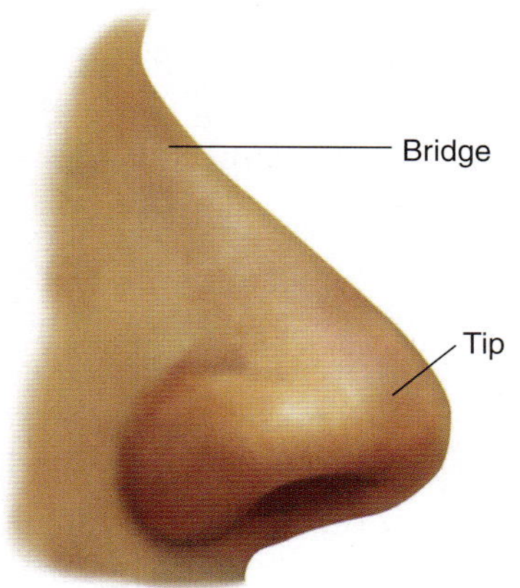

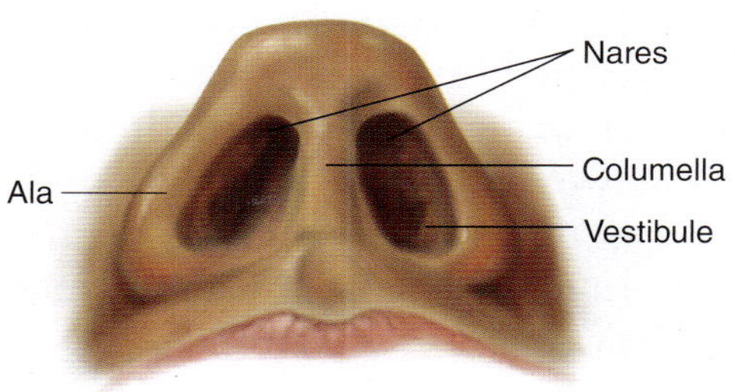

FIGURE 18.1 Nasal structures

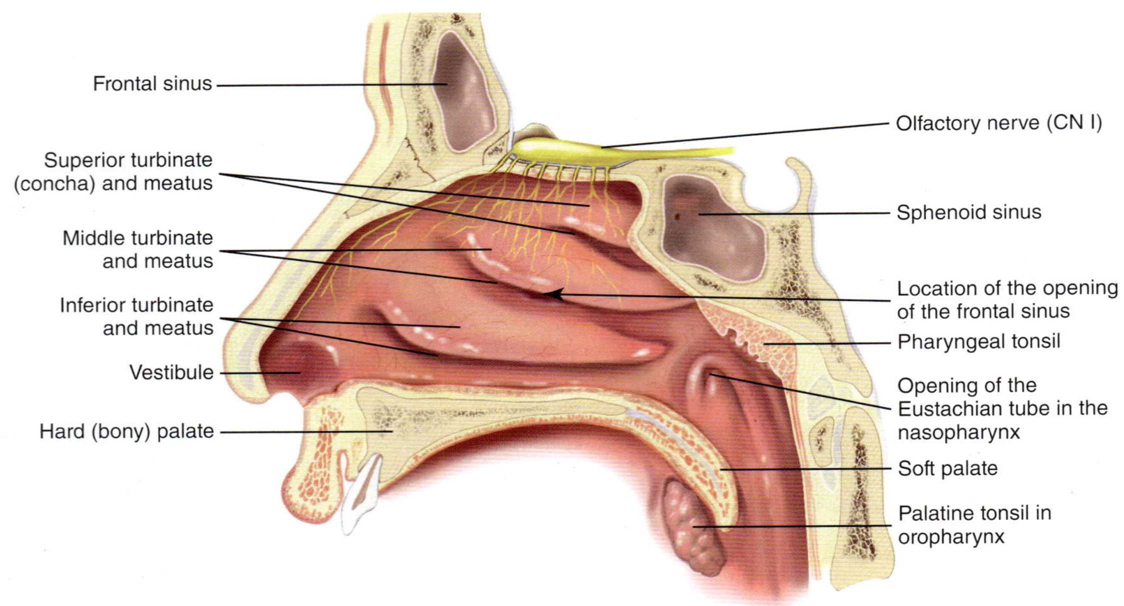

FIGURE 18.2 Right lateral wall nasal cavity

coarsest matter from inhaled air, including insects and other floating debris, helping to block the entry of very large particles into the airway. The ciliated mucous blanket, the respiratory mucosa, further inside the nasal space traps smaller particles such as dust and bacteria, enhancing air filtration to limit particle movement into the lower respiratory spaces. Nasal mucosa appears redder than oral mucosa because of the richer blood supply present. It warms and humidifies inhaled air and ensures ongoing mucous production.

The nasal cavity is divided medially by the **septum** into two slit-like air passages. The anterior part of the septum holds a rich vascular network, *Kiesselbach's plexus* or *Little's area*, the most common origin of nosebleeds. In many people, the nasal septum is not straight and may deviate towards one or the other passage. This deviation may contribute to poor airflow and snoring.

The lateral walls of each nasal cavity contain three parallel bony projections—the superior, middle and inferior **turbinates**. They increase the surface area inside the nasal passages so more blood vessels and ciliated mucous membranes are available to warm, humidify and filter the inhaled air. They also provide an area across which olfactory (smell) receptors can be located. Underlying each turbinate is a cleft, the **meatus**, which is named for the turbinate above. The sinuses drain into the middle meatus, and tears from the nasolacrimal duct drain into the inferior meatus.

The olfactory receptors lie embedded in the olfactory mucosa on the roof of the nasal cavity and in the upper one-third of the septum. The neurons associated with these receptors for smell merge to form the olfactory nerve, cranial nerve I, which moves through the sieve-like cribriform plate of the ethmoid bone and transmit to the temporal lobe of the brain. While smell is not considered necessary for human survival, loss of the sense of smell can decrease food enjoyment and potentially affect food choices and kilojoule intake.[1] Loss of smell was reported as a significant predictor of reduced quality of life post COVID-19.[1] Increasingly, smell is used as a marker of possible neural degeneration as it decays in people with many neurodegenerative conditions such as Alzheimer's disease and schizophrenia before the onset of other neurological symptoms.[2] Olfactory neurons are special in that in healthy people they regenerate throughout life. Stem cells that give rise to olfactory cells are present in the olfactory mucosa.[3]

The **paranasal sinuses** are air-filled pockets within the cranial bones of the skull (Figure 18.3). They communicate with the nasal cavity and are lined with the same type of ciliated mucous membrane. They lighten the weight of the skull bones, serve as resonators for sound production and provide mucus that drains into the nasal cavity. The sinus openings are narrow and easily occluded, which may cause pressure build-up, discomfort and enhanced/associated inflammation or sinusitis.

Two pairs of sinuses are accessible to examination: the **frontal** sinuses in the frontal bone above and medial to the orbits and the **maxillary** sinuses in the maxilla (cheekbone) along the side walls of the nasal

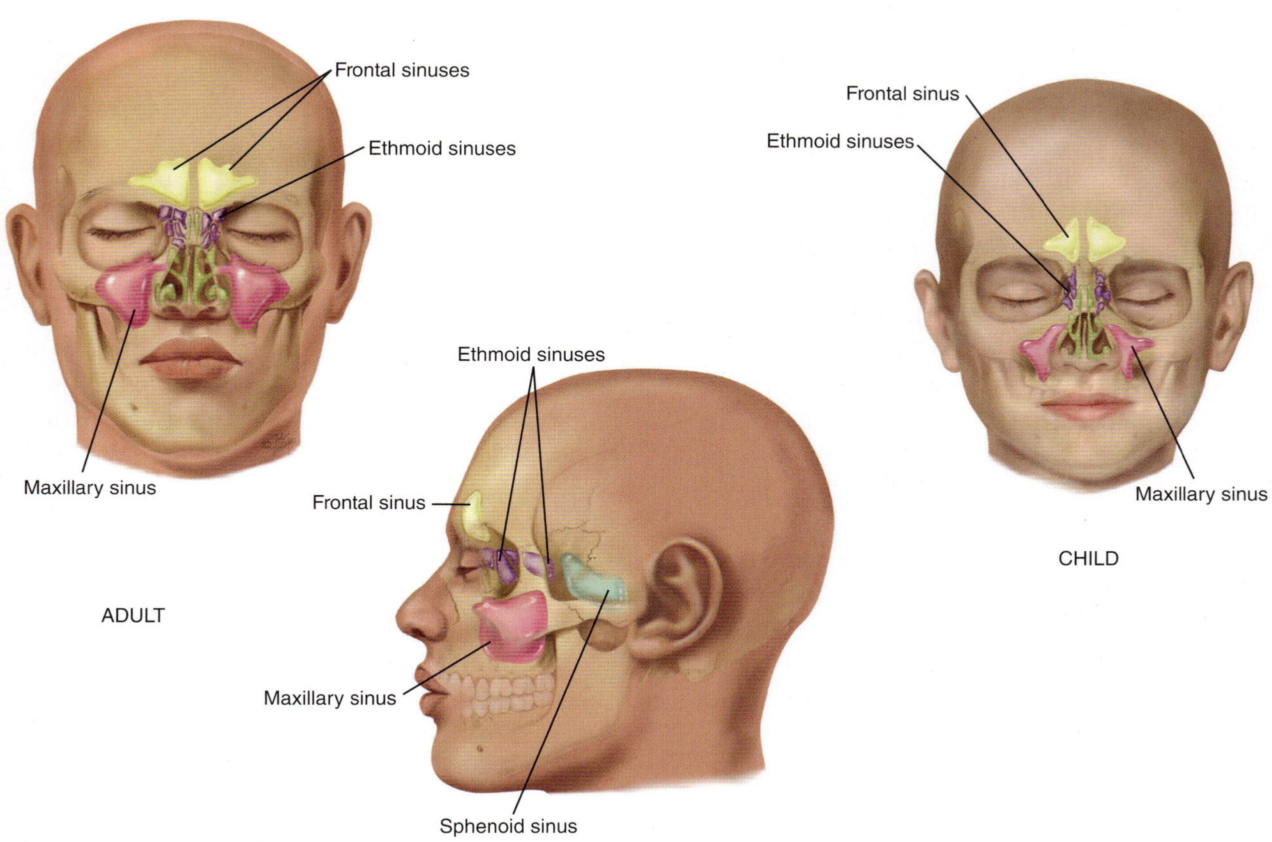

FIGURE 18.3 Paranasal sinuses

cavity. The other two sets are smaller and deeper: the **ethmoid** sinuses between the orbits and the **sphenoid** sinuses deep within the skull in the sphenoid bone. Sinuses support the humidification and warming of inspired air and the trapping of moisture and warmth in the body during exhalation.

Only the maxillary and ethmoid sinuses are present at birth. The maxillary sinuses reach full size after all permanent teeth have erupted. The ethmoid sinuses grow rapidly between 6 and 8 years of age and after puberty. The frontal sinuses are absent at birth, are fairly well developed between 7 and 8 years of age and reach full size after puberty. The sphenoid sinuses are minute at birth and develop after puberty.

Throat

The throat, or pharynx, is the area of the upper airway behind or posterior to the mouth and nose. The most superior section of the pharynx, directly behind the nose, is the nasopharynx. The pharyngeal tonsils (adenoids) and the pharyngotympanic (Eustachian) tube openings are in the nasopharyngeal region (Figure 18.2 and Figure 21.12, elsewhere in this book). Inferior to, but continuous with, the nasopharynx is the **oropharynx**. The **oropharynx** is separated from the mouth by a fold of tissue on each side, the anterior tonsillar pillar. Behind the folds are the palatine and lingual **tonsils**, each a mass of lymphoid tissue. The tonsils are the same colour as the surrounding mucous membrane, although they look more granular, and their surface shows deep crypts. Tonsillar tissue enlarges during childhood until puberty and then involutes. The posterior pharyngeal wall is seen behind these structures. Some small blood vessels may be visible.

The **nasopharynx** is continuous with the oropharynx, although it is above the oropharynx and behind the nasal cavity. The pharyngeal tonsils (adenoids) and the Eustachian tube openings are located here (Figure 18.2 and Figure 21.12). The section of the pharynx below the level of the epiglottis is known as the laryngopharyngeal region: the entry to the larynx (voice box) and the trachea (lower section of the upper airway).

Lymphatics

The lymphatic system is an extensive vessel system that is separate from the cardiovascular system. The lymphatics are a major part of the immune system, whose function is to detect and eliminate foreign substances from the body. The vessels allow the flow of clear, watery fluid (lymph) from the tissue spaces into the lymphatic and then back into the cardiovascular circulation. Lymph nodes are small, oval clusters of lymphatic tissue that are set at intervals along the lymph vessels like beads on a string (Figure 18.4). The nodes filter the lymph and engulf pathogens, limiting potentially harmful substances from entering the circulation. Nodes are located throughout the body but are accessible to palpation examination only in four areas: head and neck, arms, axillae and inguinal region. The oral cavity and throat have a rich lymphatic network (Figure 18.5). Although sources differ as to their nomenclature, one commonly used system is given here. Note that their labels correspond to adjacent structures.

- *preauricular*, in front of the ear
- *posterior auricular* (mastoid), superficial to the mastoid process
- *occipital*, at the base of the skull
- *submental*, midline, behind the tip of the mandible
- *submandibular*, halfway between the angle and the tip of the mandible
- *jugulodigastric*, under the angle of the mandible

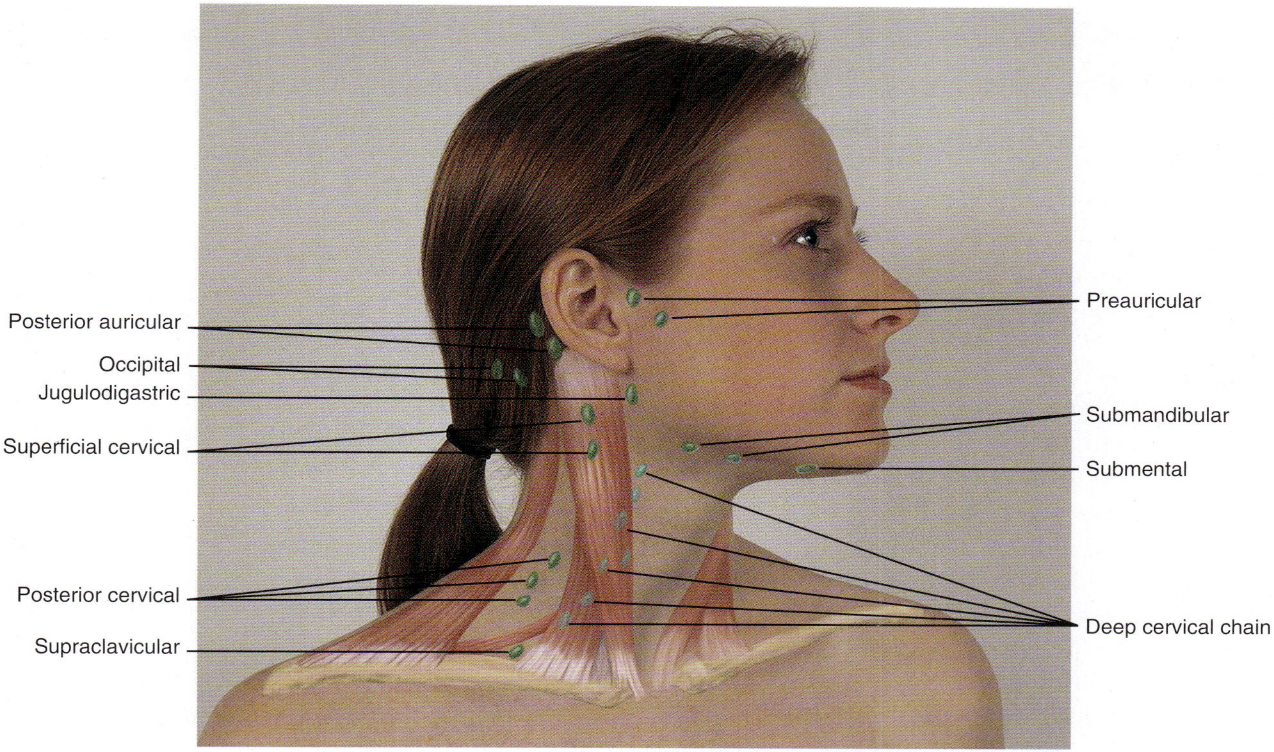

FIGURE 18.4 Lymph nodes of the head and neck

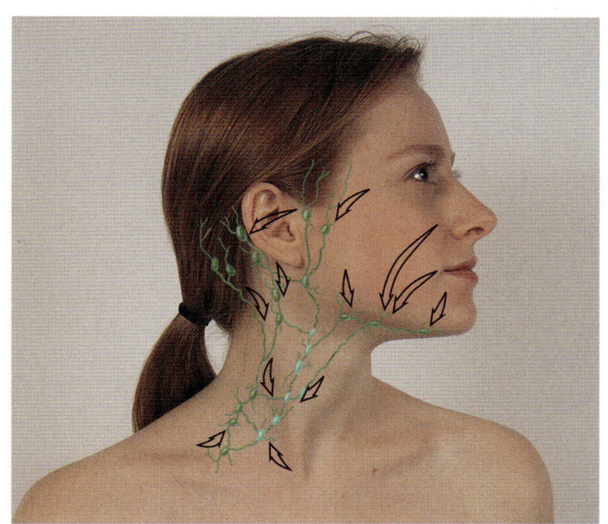

FIGURE 18.5 Lymphatic network—oral cavity and throat

- *superficial cervical*, overlying the sternocleidomastoid muscle
- *deep cervical*, deep under the sternocleidomastoid muscle
- *posterior cervical*, in the posterior triangle along the edge of the trapezius muscle
- *supraclavicular*, just above and behind the clavicle, at the sternocleidomastoid muscle.

Developmental considerations

Infants and children

Patent nasal passages are critical for a newborn baby because effective suckling (feeding) requires nasal breathing. The nose develops further during adolescence, along with other secondary sex characteristics. This growth starts at age 12 or 13 years, reaching full growth at age 16 years in females and age 21 years in males. The pharyngotympanic (Eustachian) tube opens in the nasopharyngeal region connecting the throat to the middle ear. This opening is proportionally smaller in young children and can easily become blocked or occluded, increasing the risk of middle ear pressure variation and difficulty resolving middle ear infections.

The upper sections of the trachea (subglottic region) tend to be proportionally narrower in young children with a very vascular and loosely attached mucosal lining. This increases the risks of partial and even total occlusion of the airway with infection and inflammation, particularly associated with high-risk conditions such as epiglottitis.

Pregnant women

Nasal stuffiness and epistaxis may occur during pregnancy because of increased vascularity in the upper respiratory tract. The gums may be hyperaemic and softened and may bleed with normal toothbrushing.

Late adulthood (65+ years)

A gradual loss of subcutaneous fat starts during the middle adult years, making the nose appear more prominent in some people. The nasal hairs grow coarser and stiffer and may not filter the air as well. The hairs may protrude and cause itching and sneezing. Many older people clip these hairs, thinking them unsightly, but this practice may increase the risk of infection and airway irritation. Olfaction, or the sense of smell, may diminish for many reasons, including underlying neurodegenerative disorders.

Cultural and social considerations

Ear, nose and throat infections remain almost twice as high in Aboriginal and Torres Strait Islander people as in the remainder of the population, contributing to the potentially preventable hospitalisation rates in Aboriginal and Torres Strait Islander people.[4] These infections contribute to burden of disease in First Nations populations.[5] The hearing impairment resulting from un/poorly treated otitis media has been recognised to reduce engagement with written and aural media, success in basic and higher education and ability to participate in many communal and social activities.[6] Ongoing multifactorial cycles of poverty, malnourishment, overcrowded inadequate housing, wider health ignorance and lack of access to or use of healthcare services, and therefore poor health and living standards, seem to increase the incidence of otitis media.[7]

Throat infections such as the group A streptococcal infections are also common in Māori and Pacific Islander populations in Aotearoa New Zealand. These impact directly on health outcomes and increase the risks of development of acute systemic conditions such as rheumatic fever. Thus, 'strep throat' forms the focus of several current Aotearoa New Zealand government health initiatives.[8]

HEALTH EDUCATION

Our amazing smelling ability: purpose and prediction

The sense of smell in humans is an important 'safety' sensory system, even though it may not be as well developed at detecting airborne chemicals as in other mammals. People use their sense of smell every day in many ways. For example, smell enables people to help determine the safety of food before they eat it, preventing gastric upset, nausea and vomiting that can occur by eating spoiled food. It also is an important contributor to food flavour, which is thought to increase kilojoule intake and so help maintain good nutritional status, particularly in older people. Smell can alert people to the presence of dangerous chemicals such as solvents like petrol or gas and to fire and smoke. Smell can alert people who are predisposed to skin and soft tissue ulceration and other peripheral wound formation, such as people with chronic diabetes, to the presence of poorly cared for or mismanaged wounds. Detecting and identifying smells is an essential part of many people's professional duties, including that of clinical nurses, alerting nurses to the presence of infection, gangrene and other disease states such as diabetic ketoacidosis. Finally, a functioning sense of smell can support and assist people in maintaining social connections by helping to ensure basic personal hygiene.

Tests of smell

With the re/introduction of school nurses and the increasing importance of nurses in clinics and GP practices to conduct basic health screening, it is increasingly important for nurses to be aware of the various tests of sensory function, including smell.[9] There are several specialist tests used to assess smell in adults. These are currently rarely used in standard clinical practice but can accurately detect smelling ability and loss of smelling ability. The Pennsylvania Scratch'n'Sniff test is a test in which small cards are impregnated with odours that are released when the surface is scratched.[9] When a person has scratched the card and smelt the odour, they are asked to identify the odour from one of four possible options written on the page, in a multiple-choice test. This test is easy to administer and has been shown to be an excellent test for identifying odours.

Other tests of smelling ability can be more detailed and time-consuming but are typically more informative. For example, the 'Sniffin' Sticks' test (Figure 18.6) requires people to sniff the barrel of a felt-tipped pen that contains different amounts (concentrations) of one of many different specific odourants.[9] These tests enable assessment of various aspects of our ability to smell including odour identification, discrimination (identifying the differences between smells) and detection threshold in various cultural groups and age groups. These tests come with 'picture' (visual) selection options for people with verbal dysfunction or reduced cognitive abilities.

The most objective test of smell requires an olfactometer, a machine that delivers warmed and humidified air together with specific concentrations of odour directly to a person's nose. Simultaneous EEG recordings enable clinicians to record brain activity associated with smell detection (Figure 18.7).

Why test for smell?

Smell is also a unique system because olfactory nerves (neurons), unlike those in any other human sensory system, continue to regenerate throughout life. Decrement or loss of smell often occurs before other clinical symptoms of such degenerative conditions, alerting clinicians to the need for medication or other

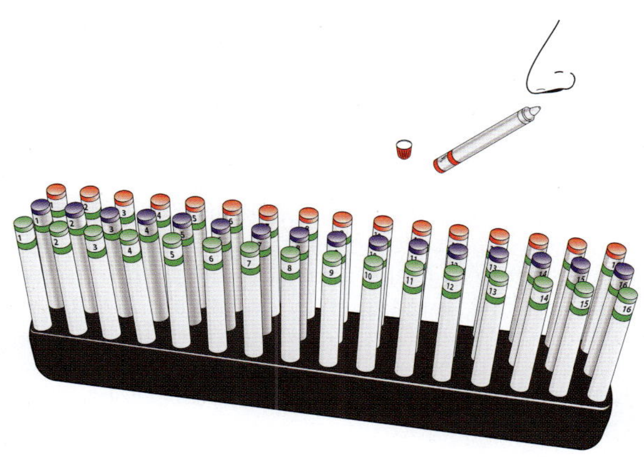

FIGURE 18.6 'Sniffin' Sticks' test

HEALTH EDUCATION cont'd

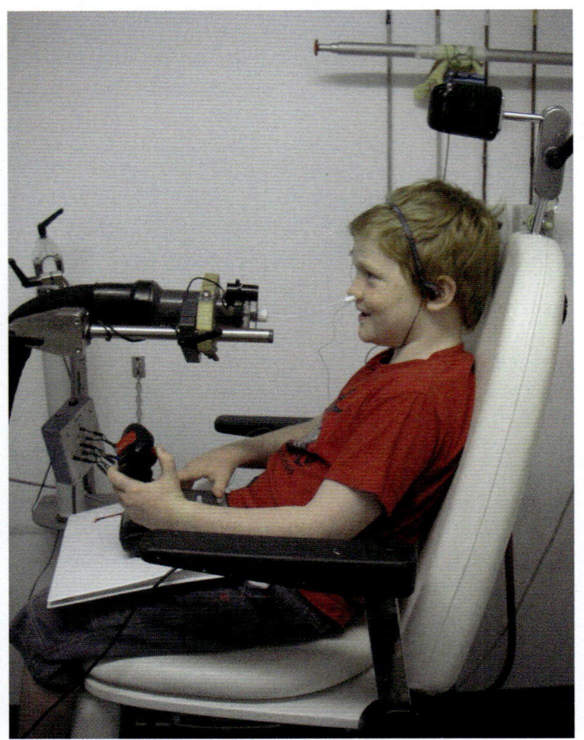

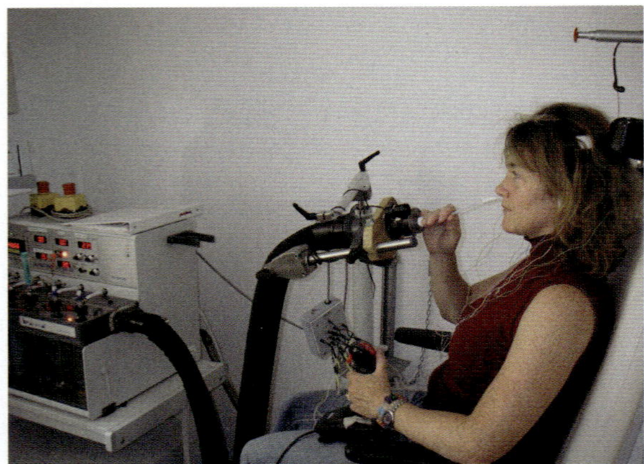

FIGURE 18.7 Use of olfactometry and EEG to assess smelling ability

clinical intervention. Thus, increasingly, loss of smell is being used as part of the screening tools applied to older people to detect neurological damage.[10,11] With increasingly aged populations, the need to screen effectively for neurodegeneration, often via relatively simple, nursing-applied tests, is also growing.

Exciting future possibilities

The presence of 'stem cells' ready to make new neurons in the adult brain offers hope of transplantation therapies to reduce the impact and severity of many neurological dysfunctions in the future.[3] Australian scientists are already harvesting stem cells from the olfactory mucosa of people to grow new nerve cells.[12] It has been shown that non-neural cells such as the heart, liver and kidney can also be grown from stem cells collected from the olfactory mucosa.[13]

Nurse's role

- Conduct a detailed assessment of history of anosmia (often accompanied by a loss of taste).
- Obtain a detailed medication history.
- Perform a comprehensive physical assessment that includes a neurological assessment (Chapter 12).
- Patient education should include:
  - reading food expiry dates carefully
  - making sure smoke alarms are working
  - checking cooking appliances are turned off properly.
- Refer the person to a medical practitioner for further assessment and management.

Subjective data

Disorders in the nose, mouth or throat cause pain, impaired function and, in extreme situations, could put the person at significant risk of airway obstruction. Subjective data collection should be done in conjunction with assessment of the lower airways (Chapter 1).

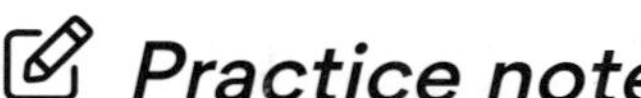

Practice note

Before you start the assessment, introduce yourself to the person, confirm the person's identity, discuss the purpose and scope of the assessment, clarify any questions the person may have and obtain verbal consent from the person to perform the assessment.

ASSESSMENT GUIDELINES	CLINICAL SIGNIFICANCE AND CLINICAL ALERTS
Presenting concern	
• *Is there a problem with your nose, mouth or throat?* It is important to ascertain the person's perception of their health of their upper airways. If a problem is perceived, ask: *Does this affect your quality of life? How?* (e.g. breathing, eating or drinking, sleep, performing daily activities, exercising, performing expected role)	
Ear, nose or throat discharge	
• *Do you have any nasal discharge or runny nose? Is it continuous?* • *Is the discharge watery, purulent, mucoid or bloody?* • *Can you describe any ear or throat discharge and frequency?*	**Rhinorrhoea** (discharge of thin mucus fluid from the nose) occurs with colds, allergies, sinus infection and trauma.
Blocked nose (upper respiratory infections / foreign body / common cold)	
• *Have you had any unusually frequent or severe colds (upper respiratory infections)?* • *How often do these occur?*	Most people have occasional colds, so asking this more precise question yields more meaningful data.
Sinus pain	
• *Do you have any sinus pain or sinusitis? How is this treated?* • *Do you have chronic postnasal drip?*	**Chronic postnasal drip** (mucus from nose or sinuses drips down the back of the throat) is a sign of sinusitis.
Trauma	
• *Have you ever had any injury to your nose?* • *Can you breathe through your nose? Are both sides obstructed, or one?*	Trauma may cause **deviated septum** (nasal septum is crooked making one nostril narrower than the other).
Epistaxis (nosebleeds)	
• *Have you experienced any nosebleeds? How often?* • *How much bleeding—a teaspoonful or does it pour out?* • *What is the colour of the blood—red or brown? Clots?*	**Epistaxis** (bleeding from the nose) occurs with trauma, vigorous nose blowing or foreign body.

ASSESSMENT GUIDELINES	CLINICAL SIGNIFICANCE AND CLINICAL ALERTS
• *Does it bleed from one nostril or both?* • *Is it aggravated by nose-picking or scratching?* • *How do you treat the nosebleeds? Are they difficult to stop?*	The person should sit up with their head tilted forwards and pinch the nose between the thumb and forefinger for 5 to 15 minutes.
Allergies	
• *Do you have any allergies or hay fever?* • *To what are you allergic (e.g. pollen, dust, pets)?* • *How was this determined?* • *What type of environment makes it worse?* • *Can you avoid exposure?*	**Seasonal rhinitis** (allergic response to pollens or other allergens causing sneezing, runny nose, watery, itchy eyes).
• *Do you use inhalers, nasal spray, nose drops? How often? Which type?* • *How long have you used this?*	Misuse of over-the-counter nasal medications may irritate the mucosa, causing rebound swelling, a common problem.
Altered smell	
• *Have you experienced any change in sense of smell or altered smelling ability?*	People are often poor at detecting changes in their smelling ability and often rely on reports from others. Sense of smell may deteriorate with chronic allergy, decreased nasal patency, prolonged cigarette smoking or the development of neurodegenerative conditions such as Alzheimer's, Parkinson's or motor neuron diseases.
Pain in mouth or throat	
• *Do you currently have a sore throat? When did it start? How frequently do you get them?* • *Is it associated with cough, fever, fatigue, decreased appetite, headache, postnasal drip or hoarseness?* • *Is it worse when rising? What is the humidity level in the room where you sleep? Any dust or smoke inhaled at work?* • *How have you treated this sore throat: medication, gargling? How effective are these? Have your tonsils or adenoids been taken out?*	Untreated **streptococcal infection (bacterial infection)** of the throat may lead to the complication of acute rheumatic fever if left untreated.
Sores or lesions	
• *Have you noticed any sores or ulcers in the mouth, tongue or gums?* • *How long have you had it?* • *Have you ever had this before?* • *Is it a single or are there multiple sores/ulcers?* • *Does it seem to be associated with stress, season change, food?* • *How have you treated the sore?* • *Have you applied any local medication?*	History helps determine whether oral lesions have infectious, traumatic, immunological or malignant aetiology.

ASSESSMENT GUIDELINES	CLINICAL SIGNIFICANCE AND CLINICAL ALERTS
Hoarseness or change in voice	
• *Do you have any hoarseness or voice change? For how long?* • *Do you feel like you must clear your throat? Or, like a 'lump in your throat'?* • *Do you use your voice a lot at work, recreation?* • *Does the hoarseness seem associated with a cold or sore throat?*	A disorder of the larynx with many causes such as overuse of the voice, upper respiratory infection, chronic inflammation, lesions or a neoplasm.
Lumps, swelling or sore areas in the neck, mouth or throat	
• *Do you have any lumps or swelling in the neck, mouth or throat?* • *Have you had any recent infection?* • *Do you have any tenderness?* For a lump that persists, ask: *How long have you had it? Has it changed in size?*	Tenderness suggests acute infection. A persistent lump arouses suspicion of malignancy. For those more than 40 years old, suspect malignancy until proven otherwise.
Past history	
• *Do you or a family member have a history of upper airways diseases?*	
Health and lifestyle management	
Medication use prescribed and recreational, including smoking. • *What medications are you taking? If so what and how often? Do you use recreational drugs? If so what and how often?* • *Do you smoke? Pipe or cigarettes? Nicotine vaporiser?* • *How many packs do you smoke per day?* • *How long have you smoked?*	Chronic tobacco use (smoking and/or chewing) is associated with significant oral and lung disease. Medications commonly used to treat conditions of the upper airways include antihistamines, steroids, antipyretics, antibiotics and paracetamol.
Additional subjective data for infants and children (questions for parents or guardians)	
• *Does the child have any mouth lesions or throat infections? How frequently do these occur?* • *Does the child have frequent sore throats, tonsillitis, ear or nasal infections?* • *How often do they occur?* • *How are these treated?* • *Has the child ever been diagnosed with a streptococcal infection?*	

Objective data

The purpose of the examination of the upper airways is to assess patterns of pain or any other abnormalities and the impact these have on the person's respiratory function. An objective examination should be done in conjunction with an assessment of the lower airways (Chapter 19).

Preparation

Position the person sitting up straight with their head at your eye level.

Equipment needed

Penlight
Two tongue blades
Hand hygiene solution
Gauze to invert and displace tongue

PROCEDURES AND NORMAL FINDINGS	ABNORMAL FINDINGS AND CLINICAL ALERTS
General inspection	
While collecting subjective data, you will have noticed the colour of the person's skin and mucous membranes, ease of breathing, tone of voice and general demeanour. All factors provide clues to the functioning of the upper respiratory system.	
Inspect and palpate the external nose	
Normally, the nose is symmetrical, in the midline and in proportion to other facial features (Figure 18.8A). Inspect for any deformity, asymmetry, deviated septum, inflammation or skin lesions. If an injury is reported or suspected, palpate gently for any pain or break in contour.	A **deviated septum** can cause the person difficulty with breathing through the nose (Figure 18.8B).
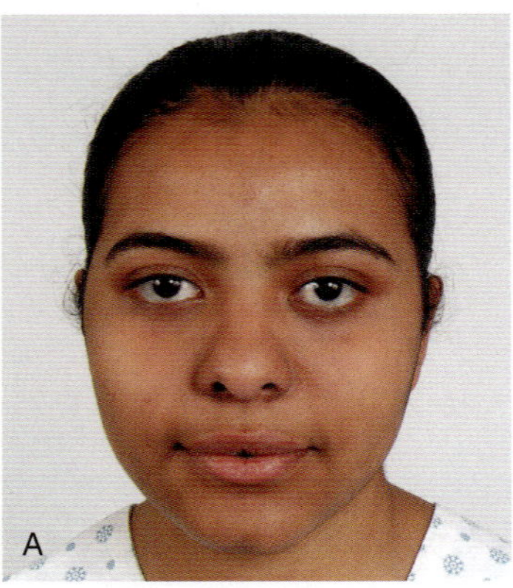 **FIGURE 18.8A** External nose	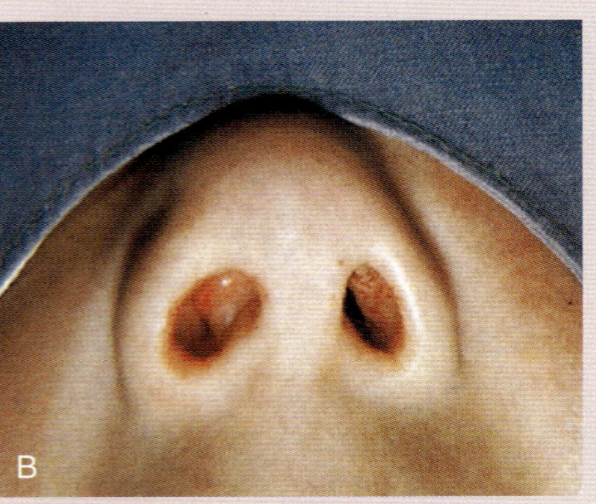 **FIGURE 18.8B** Deviated septum

PROCEDURES AND NORMAL FINDINGS	ABNORMAL FINDINGS AND CLINICAL ALERTS
Test the patency of the nostrils by pushing each nasal wing shut with your finger while asking the person to sniff inwards through the other naris. This may reveal an obstruction. The sense of smell, mediated by cranial nerve I, is usually not tested in a routine examination (Chapter 12).	Absence of sniff indicates obstruction (e.g. common cold, nasal polyps, rhinitis) (Table 18.1).
Inspect the mouth	
Lips and mouth	
Inspect the lips for colour and moisture. Retract the lips and note their inner surface as well (Figure 18.9). Inspect the anterior structures of the mouth and move posteriorly. Use a tongue blade to retract structures and a bright light for optimal visualisation. 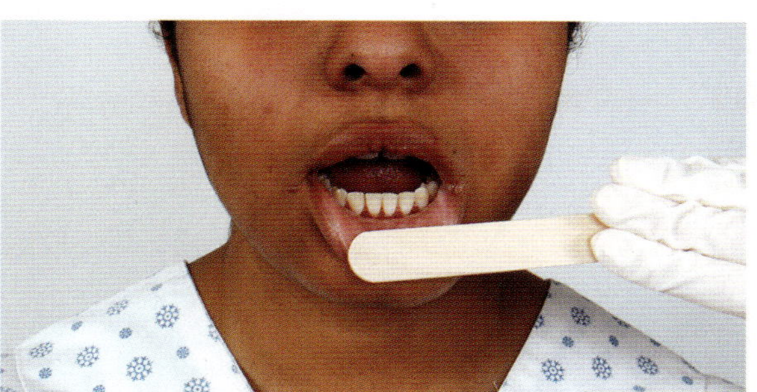 **FIGURE 18.9** Inspection of lips	**Circumoral pallor** occurs with shock and anaemia; **cyanosis** (blue tinge) with hypoxaemia and chilling; cherry red lips with carbon monoxide poisoning. ! ***Clinical alert:*** A significant change in the colour of the lips, such as cyanosis, indicates the need for immediate further assessment.
Tongue	
Inspect the tongue for presence of swelling.	! ***Clinical alert:*** When an **anaphylactic reaction** occurs with sudden onset of dyspnoea and/or dysphagia a medical practitioner must be notified immediately. This is an emergency.
Palate	
Inspect the **uvula**; it normally looks like a fleshy pendant hanging in the midline (Figure 18.10). Ask the person to say 'ahhh' and note the soft palate and uvula rise in the midline. This tests one function of cranial nerve X, the vagus nerve.	! ***Clinical alert:*** Significant oedema in the mouth and throat may indicate an increased risk of airway compromise and aspiration. Further assessment of swallow and airway patency is required. See Chapter 21 for further information on swallow assessment.

PROCEDURES AND NORMAL FINDINGS	ABNORMAL FINDINGS AND CLINICAL ALERTS

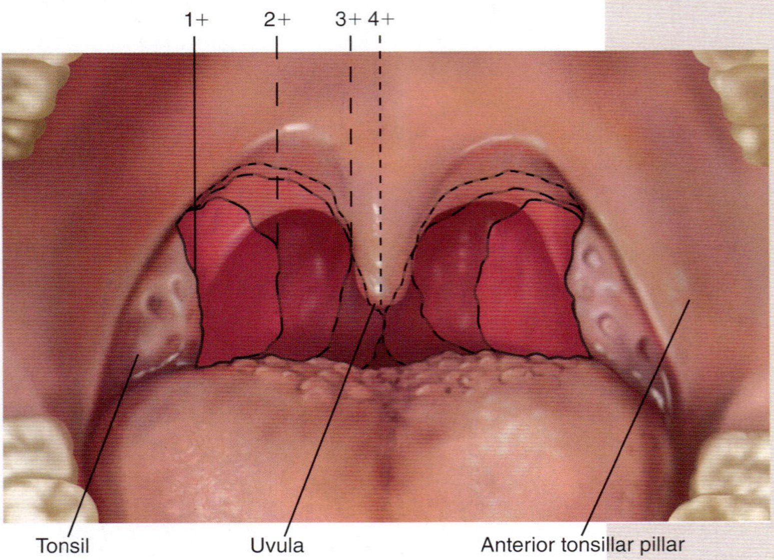

FIGURE 18.10 Inspection of the throat and uvula

Inspect the throat

With your torch, inspect the oval, rough-surfaced **tonsils** behind the anterior tonsillar pillar (Figure 18.10). Their colour is the same pink as the oral mucosa, and their surface is peppered with indentations or crypts. In some people the crypts collect small plugs of whitish cellular debris. This does not indicate infection. However, there should be no exudate on the tonsils. Tonsils are graded in size as follows:

- **1**+ Visible
- **2**+ Halfway between tonsillar pillars and uvula
- **3**+ Touching the uvula
- **4**+ Touching each other.

You may normally see 1+ or 2+ tonsils in healthy people, especially in children, because lymphoid tissue is proportionately enlarged until puberty.

Enlarge your view of the posterior pharyngeal wall by depressing the tongue with a tongue blade (Figure 18.11). Push down halfway back on the tongue. (Some people can lower their own tongue so the tongue blade is not needed.) Scan the posterior wall for colour, exudate or lesions. When finished, discard the tongue blade.

With an acute infection, tonsils are bright red, swollen and may have exudate or large white spots. See Table 18.2 for abnormalities of the oropharynx.

A white membrane covering the tonsils may accompany **infectious mononucleosis** (glandular fever), **leukaemias** (cancers of the white cells) and **diphtheria** (communicable bacterial disease that causes severe inflammation of the nose, throat and trachea).

Tonsils are enlarged to 2+, 3+ or 4+ with an acute infection.

PROCEDURES AND NORMAL FINDINGS	ABNORMAL FINDINGS AND CLINICAL ALERTS
FIGURE 18.11 Inspection of the throat	
During the examination, notice any breath odour. This is common and usually is due to a local cause such as poor oral hygiene or heavy smoking. Occasionally it may indicate a systemic disease.	A foul, fetid odour may be noticed as occurs in dental or respiratory infections.

Additional objective data for infants and children

Because oral examinations are intrusive for infants and young children, consider playing a game to help prepare the child. Encourage a preschool child to use a tongue blade to look into a puppet's mouth. Or place a mirror so the child can look into the mouth while you do. School-age children are usually cooperative and love to show off missing or new teeth. With some infants and toddlers, you need to be opportunistic with this examination. For example, take advantage of crying episodes to examine the open mouth and oropharynx. Ask the parent to help position the child. Place the infant supine on the table/bed, with the arms restrained (Figure 18.12). Older infants and toddlers may be held on the parent's lap with one of the parent's hands holding the arms down and the other hand securing the child's head against the parent's chest.	
Nose. There should be no nasal flaring or narrowing with breathing. It is essential to determine the patency of the nares in the immediate newborn period because most newborns are nose breathers.	**Nasal flaring** in an infant indicates respiratory distress and the need for further assessment. A transverse ridge across the nose occurs in a child with chronic allergy from wiping the nose upwards with palm. Nasal narrowing on inhalation is seen with chronic nasal obstruction and mouth breathing.

PROCEDURES AND NORMAL FINDINGS	ABNORMAL FINDINGS AND CLINICAL ALERTS

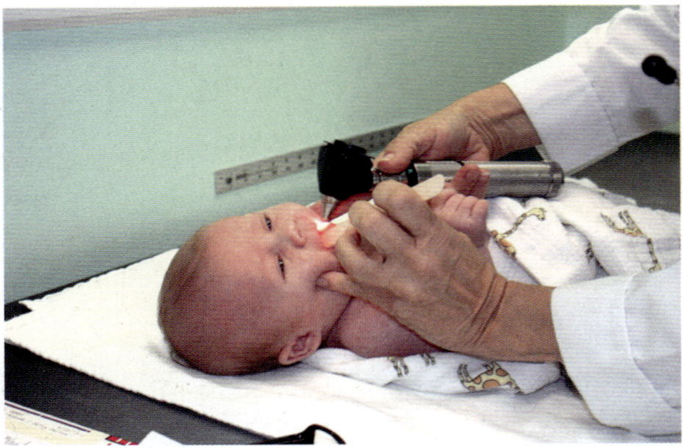

FIGURE 18.12 Position of infant for oral inspection

Inspect the palate

A high-arched palate is usually normal in a newborn. On the palate, **Epstein pearls** are a normal finding in newborns and infants (Figure 18.13). They are small, whitish, glistening, pearly papules along the median raphe of the hard palate and on the gums, where they look like teeth. They are small retention cysts and disappear in the first few weeks after birth.

A very narrow or high arch also occurs with:

- **Turner's syndrome** (occurs when one of the X chromosomes (sex chromosomes) is missing or partially missing)
- **Ehlers-Danlos syndrome** (a group of hereditary connective tissue disorders)
- **Marfan's syndrome** (inherited disorder that affects connective tissue)
- **Treacher Collins syndrome** (a genetic disorder that affects growth and development of the head).

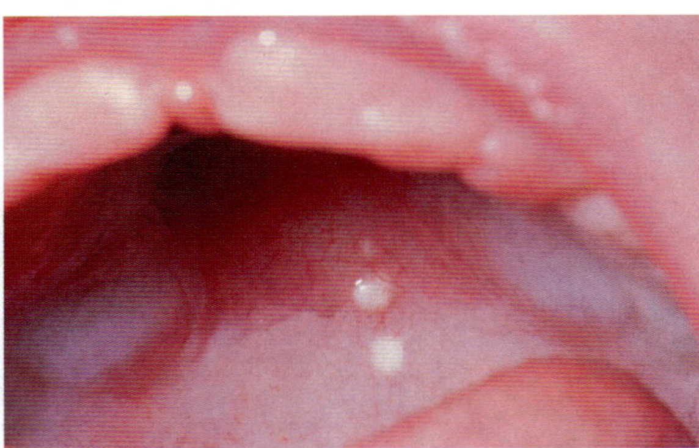

FIGURE 18.13 Epstein pearls

The tonsils are not visible in newborns. They gradually enlarge during childhood, remaining proportionately larger until puberty. Tonsils appear still larger if the infant is crying or gagging. Newborns can normally produce a strong, lusty cry.

Abnormal findings

TABLE 18.1 Abnormalities of the nose

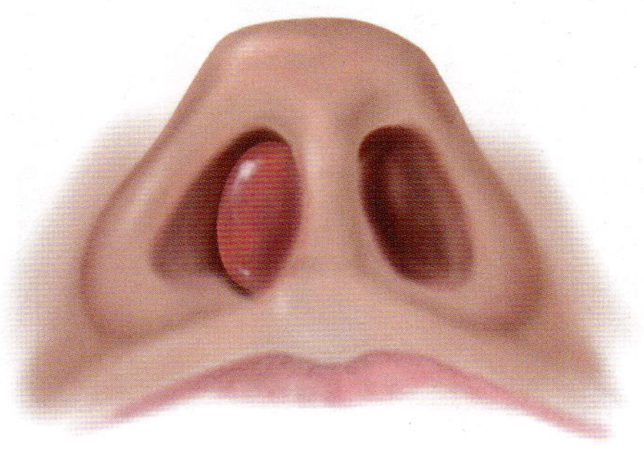

Furuncle

A small boil located in the skin or mucous membrane; appears red and swollen and is quite painful. Avoid any manipulation or trauma that may spread the infection.

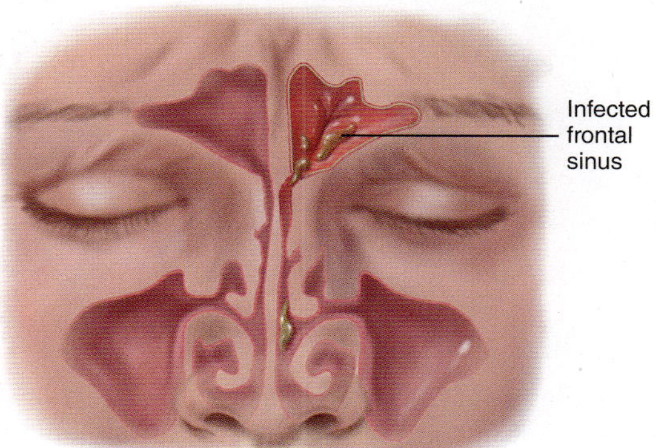

Sinusitis

Facial pain, after upper respiratory infection; signs include red swollen nasal mucosa, swollen turbinates and purulent discharge. Person also has fever, chills, malaise. With maxillary sinusitis, dull throbbing pain occurs in cheeks and teeth on the same side, and pain with palpation is present. With frontal sinusitis, pain is above the supraorbital ridge.

TABLE 18.2 Abnormalities of the oropharynx

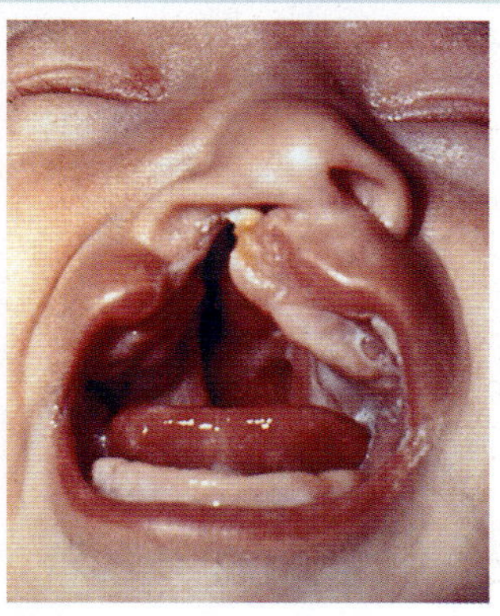

Cleft palate

A congenital defect, the failure of fusion of the maxillary processes. Wide variation occurs in the extent of cleft formation, from upper lip only, palate only, uvula only, to cleft of the nostril and the hard and soft palates.

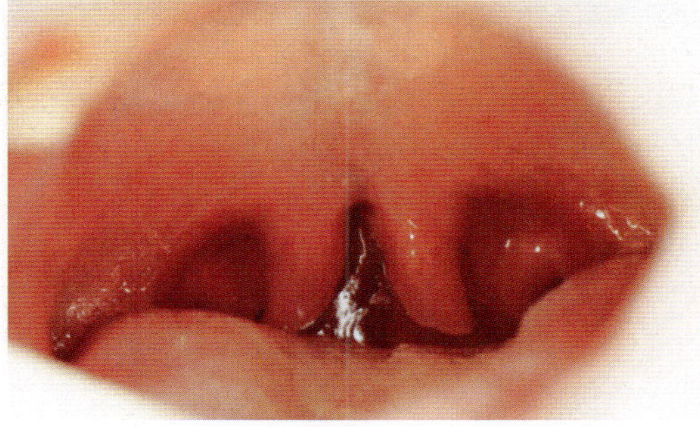

Bifid uvula

The uvula looks partly severed. May indicate a submucous cleft palate, which feels like a notch at the junction of the hard and soft palates. The submucous cleft palate may affect speech development because it prevents necessary air trapping.

Continued

TABLE 18.2 Abnormalities of the oropharynx cont'd

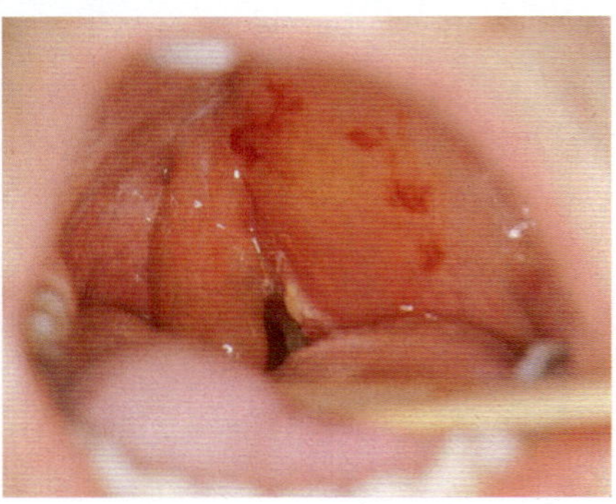

Peritonsillar abscess

A peritonsillar abscess (quinsy) is a collection of pus from an infection behind the tonsil (usually unilateral). It causes significant pain, fever and dysphagia. It can result in airway obstruction and requires urgent medical treatment.

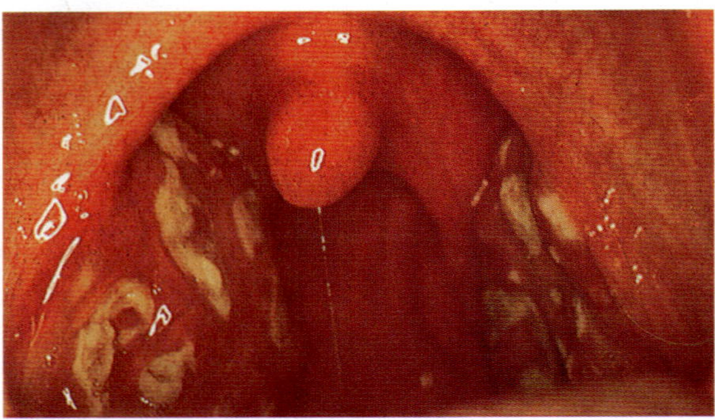

Acute tonsillitis and pharyngitis

Bright red throat; swollen tonsils; white or yellow exudates on tonsils and pharynx; swollen uvula; and enlarged, tender anterior cervical and tonsillar nodes. Accompanied by severe sore throat, painful swallowing, fever > 38°C of sudden onset. **Caution:** One cannot discriminate bacterial from viral infection on clinical data alone; all sore throats need a throat culture. Bacterial pharyngitis caused by group A β-haemolytic *Streptococcus*, if untreated, may lead to the complication of rheumatic fever. This is a serious complex illness characterised by fever, malaise, swollen joints, rash and scarring on the heart valves.

Advanced practice—additional data

The assessments that are described in the following sections require nurses to have advanced skill and scope of practice. Nurses working in specialist units and some community nurses need to develop these skills.

Equipment

Nasal speculum
Tongue blade
Torch

PROCEDURES AND NORMAL FINDINGS	ABNORMAL FINDINGS AND CLINICAL ALERTS
Inspect the nasal cavity	
Using the nasal speculum, inspect the turbinates, the bony ridges curving down from the lateral walls. The superior turbinate will not be in your view, but the middle and inferior turbinates appear the same light red colour as the nasal mucosa. Note any swelling but do not try to push the speculum past it. Turbinates are quite vascular and tender if touched.	Turbinates swell marginally in a cyclical manner, thus apparent abnormalities, particularly asymmetries, need to be repeatedly assessed over time (Table 18.3).

PROCEDURES AND NORMAL FINDINGS	ABNORMAL FINDINGS AND CLINICAL ALERTS
Note any polyps (benign growths) that accompany chronic allergy and distinguish them from the normal turbinates.	Polyps are smooth, pale grey, avascular, mobile and nontender (Table 18.3).

Palpate the sinus areas

Using your thumbs, press over the frontal sinuses below the eyebrows (Figure 18.14A) and over the maxillary sinuses below the cheekbones (Figure 18.14B). Take care not to press directly on the eyeballs. The person should feel firm pressure but no pain.

Sinus areas are tender to palpation in persons with chronic allergies and acute infection (**sinusitis**).

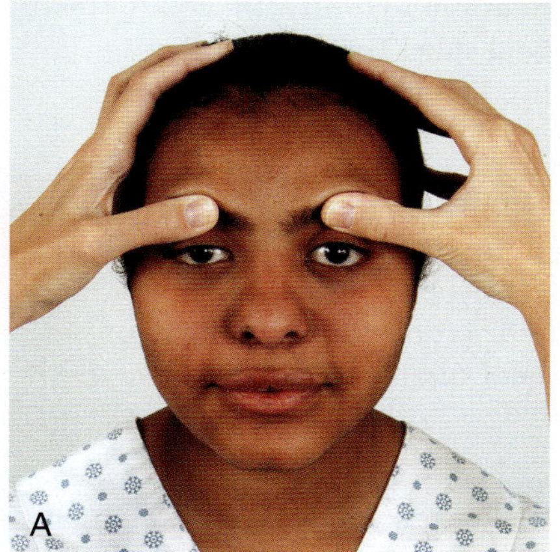

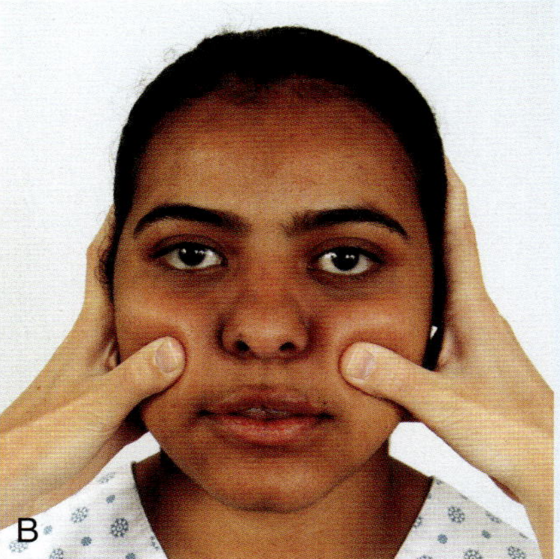

FIGURE 18.14 A, B Palpation of the sinuses

Palpate the trachea

Normally, the trachea is midline; palpate for any tracheal shift. Place your index finger on the trachea in the sternal notch and slip it off to each side (Figure 18.15). The space should be symmetrical on both sides. Note any deviation from the midline.

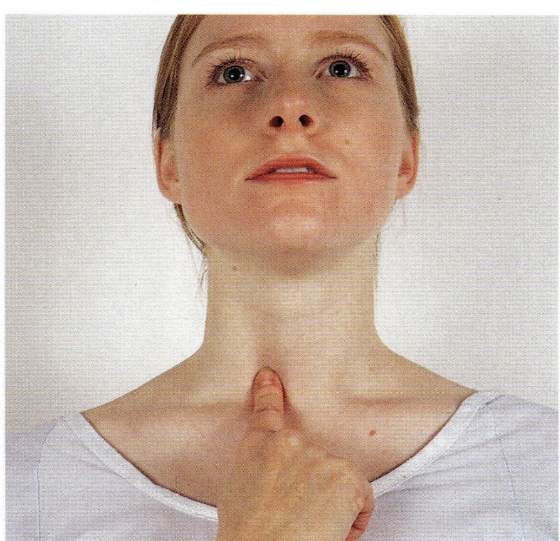

FIGURE 18.15 Palpate the trachea

PROCEDURES AND NORMAL FINDINGS	ABNORMAL FINDINGS AND CLINICAL ALERTS
Begin with anterior structures and move posteriorly. Use a tongue blade to retract structures and a bright light for optimal visualisation.	**Conditions of tracheal shift.** The trachea may be *pushed to the unaffected* (or healthy) side with any of: • **pneumothorax** (collection of air outside the lung but within the pleural cavity) • **aortic aneurysm** (a balloon-like bulge in the aorta) • **tumour** • **unilateral thyroid lobe enlargement.** **Tracheal shift:** The trachea is *pulled towards the affected* (diseased) side with significant atelectasis (collapse of part or all of a lung), pleural adhesions (formation of fibrotic bands that span the pleural space, between the parietal and visceral layers of the pleura) or fibrosis (thickening or scarring of the tissue). **Tracheal tug** is a rhythmic downwards pull that is synchronous with systole and occurs with aortic arch aneurysm.
Palpate the lymph nodes in the neck area	
Using a gentle circular motion of your fingerpads, palpate the lymph nodes (Figure 18.16). When symptoms warrant, check for parotid tenderness by palpating in a line from the outer corner of the eye to the lobule of the ear. Beginning with the preauricular lymph nodes in front of the ear, palpate the 10 groups of lymph nodes in a routine order. Many nodes are closely packed, so you must be systematic and thorough in your examination. Once you establish your sequence, do not vary or you may miss some small nodes.	The parotid gland is swollen with mumps (Table 21.12).

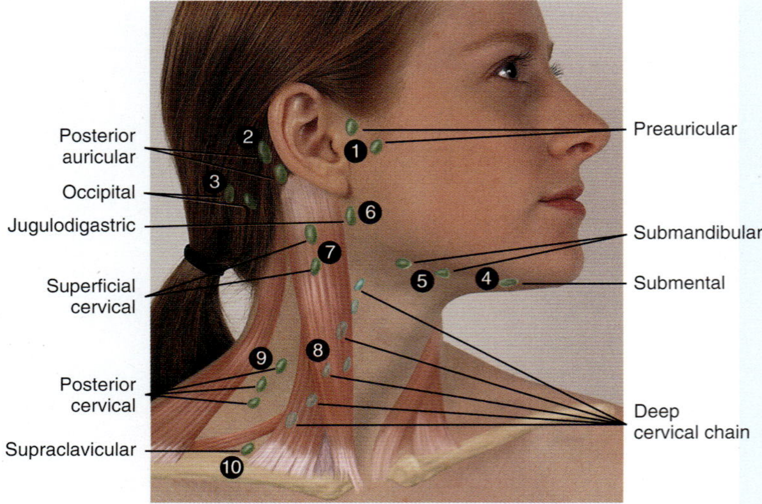

FIGURE 18.16 Palpate lymph nodes in the neck area

PROCEDURES AND NORMAL FINDINGS

Use gentle pressure because strong pressure could push the nodes into the neck muscles. It is usually most efficient to palpate with both hands, comparing the two sides symmetrically. However, the submental gland under the tip of the chin is easier to explore with one hand. When you palpate with one hand, use your other hand to position the person's head. For the deep cervical chain, tip the person's head towards the side being examined to relax the ipsilateral muscle (Figure 18.17). Then you can press your fingers under the muscle. Search for the supraclavicular node by having the person hunch the shoulders and elbows forwards (Figure 18.18); this relaxes the skin. The inferior belly of the omohyoid muscle crosses the posterior triangle here; do not mistake it for a lymph node.

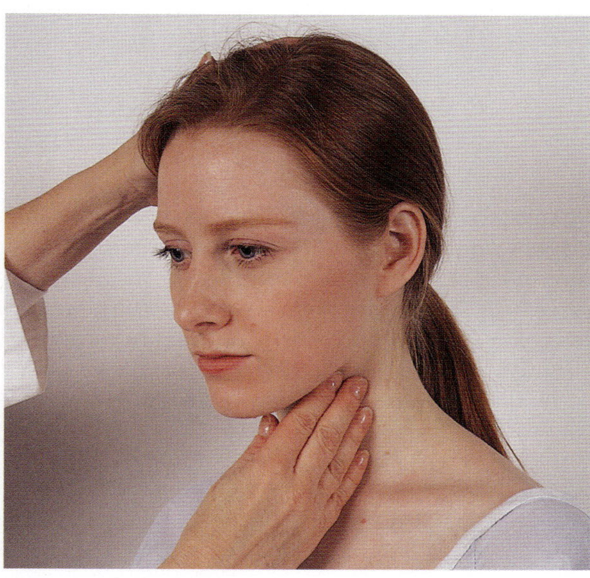

FIGURE 18.17 Palpate lymph nodes in the neck area

ABNORMAL FINDINGS AND CLINICAL ALERTS

PROCEDURES AND NORMAL FINDINGS	ABNORMAL FINDINGS AND CLINICAL ALERTS

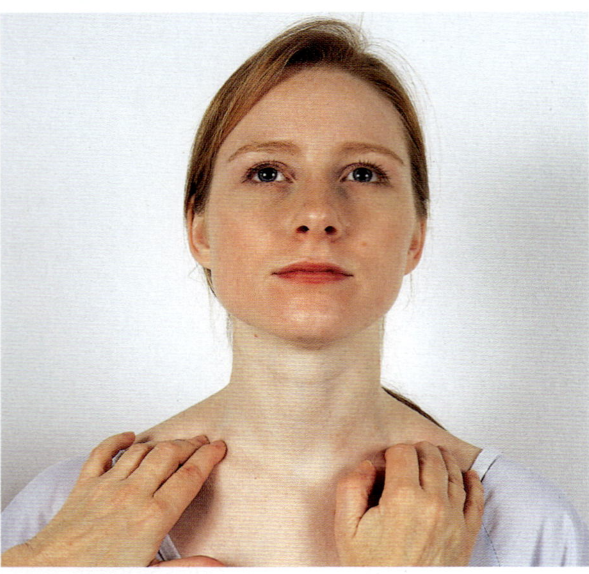

FIGURE 18.18 Palpate lymph nodes in the neck area

If nodes are enlarged or tender, check the area they drain for the source of the problem. For example, those in the upper cervical or submandibular area often relate to inflammation or a neoplasm in the head and neck. Follow up on or refer your findings. An enlarged lymph node, particularly when you cannot find the source of the problem, deserves prompt attention.

The following criteria are common clues but are not definitive in all circumstances.

Acute infection—nodes are bilateral, enlarged, warm, tender and firm but freely movable.

Chronic inflammation (e.g. in tuberculosis the nodes are clumped).

Cancerous nodes are hard, unilateral, nontender and fixed.

A single, enlarged, nontender, hard, left supraclavicular node (Virchow's node) may indicate neoplasm in thorax or abdomen.

Painless, rubbery, discrete nodes that gradually appear occur with **Hodgkin's lymphoma**.

Additional objective data for infants and children

Inspect the nose

When inspection of the nares of an infant is indicated, gently push up the tip of the nose with your thumb while using your other hand to shine the light into the naris. With a toddler, be alert for a possible foreign body lodged in the nasal cavity (Table 18.3).

Abnormal findings—advanced practice

TABLE 18.3 Abnormalities of the nose

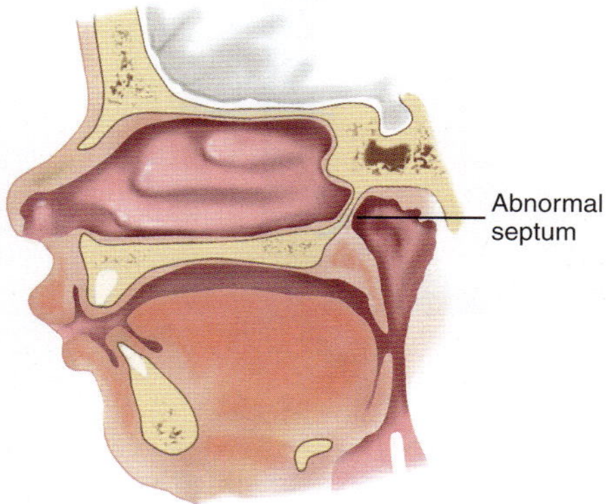

Choanal atresia

A bony or membranous septum between the nasal cavity and the pharynx of a newborn. When the condition is bilateral, it requires the immediate insertion of an oral airway to prevent asphyxia because most newborns are obligate nose-breathers. When the condition is unilateral, the infant may be asymptomatic until the onset of the first respiratory infection.

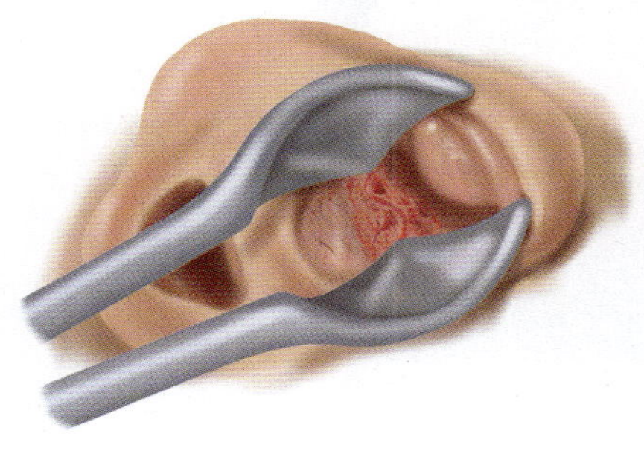

Foreign body

Children particularly are apt to put an object up the nose (here, yellow plastic foam), producing unilateral mucopurulent drainage and foul odour. Because some risk for aspiration exists, removal should be prompt.

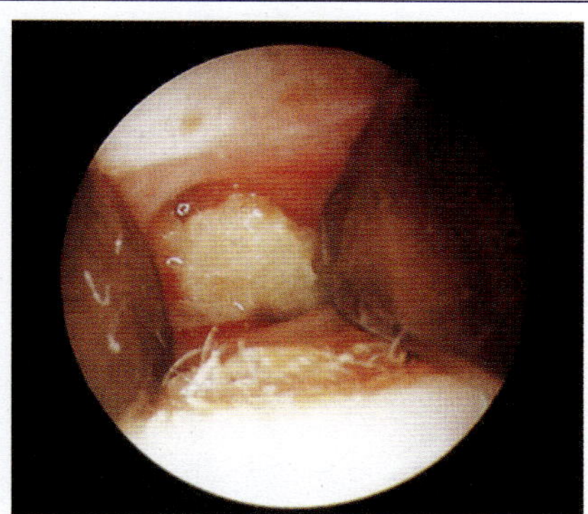

Epistaxis

The most common site of a nosebleed is Kiesselbach's plexus in the anterior septum. It may be spontaneous from a local cause or a sign of underlying illness. Causes include nose picking, forceful coughing or sneezing, fracture, foreign body, rhinitis, heavy exertion or a coagulation disorder. Bleeding from the anterior septum is easily controlled and rarely severe. A posterior haemorrhage is less common (<10%) but is more profuse, harder to manage and more serious.

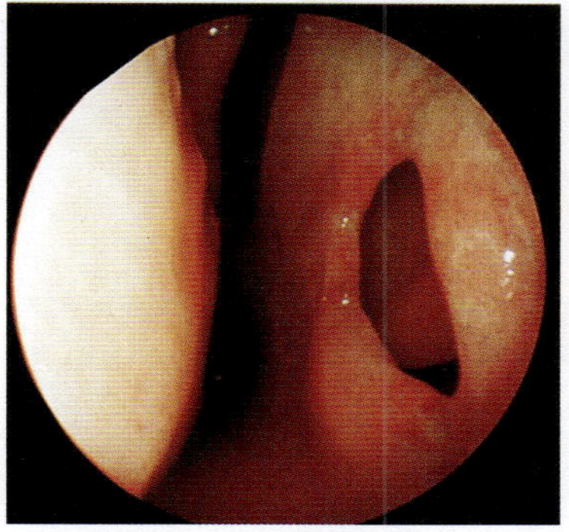

Perforated septum

A hole in the septum, usually in the cartilaginous part, may be caused by snorting cocaine, chronic infection, trauma from continual picking of crusts or nasal surgery. It is seen directly or as a spot of light when the penlight is directed into the other naris.

TABLE 18.3 Abnormalities of the nose cont'd

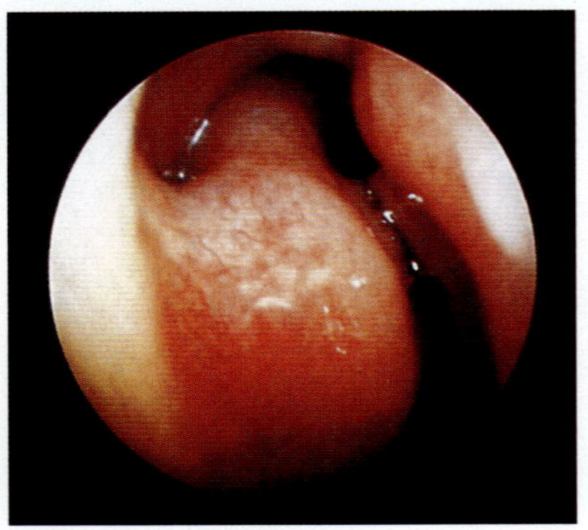

Acute rhinitis

The first sign is a clear, watery discharge, rhinorrhoea, which later becomes purulent. This is accompanied by sneezing and swollen mucosa, which causes nasal obstruction. Turbinates are dark red and swollen.

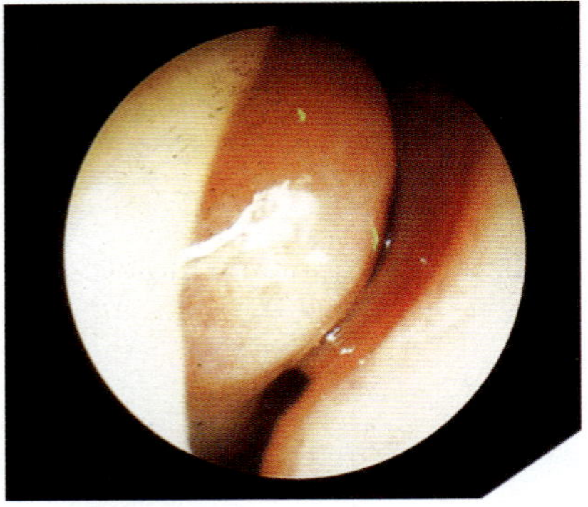

Allergic rhinitis

Rhinorrhoea, itching of nose and eyes, lacrimation, nasal congestion and sneezing are present. Note serous oedema and swelling of turbinates to fill the air space. Turbinates are usually pale (although may appear violet), and their surface looks smooth and glistening. May be seasonal or perennial, depending on allergen. The person has a strong family history of seasonal allergies.

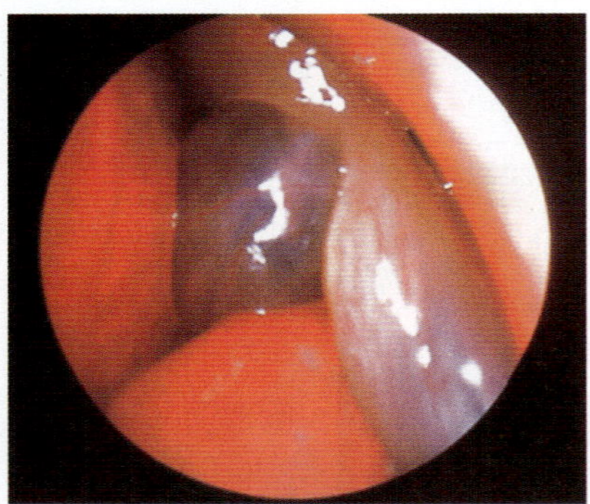

Nasal polyps

Smooth, pale grey nodules that are overgrowths of mucosa, mostly caused by chronic allergic rhinitis. May be stalked. A common site is protrusion from the middle meatus. Often multiple, they are mobile and nontender in contrast to turbinates. They may obstruct air passageways as they get larger. Symptoms include the absence of a sense of smell and a 'valve that moves' in the nose as the person breathes.

Clinical reasoning and documentation

The following is a continuation of the case study provided at the beginning of this chapter and the clinical reasoning process including problem/issue identification. You should consult a fundamentals of nursing or medical-surgical nursing text for information about goal setting, nursing interventions and evaluation.

Clinical case study (continued)—Foreign body in nose

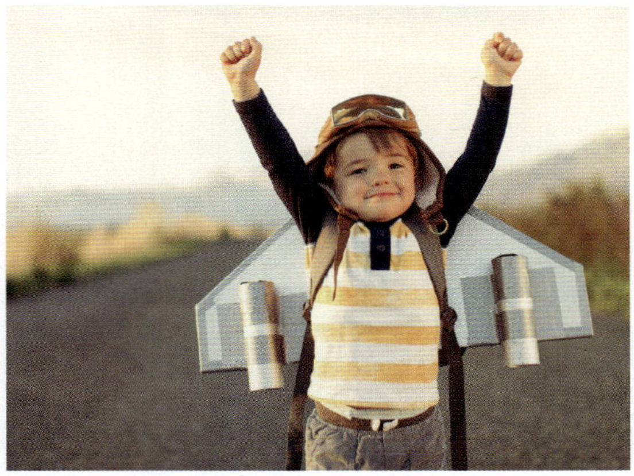

Context

You will recall from the case study described earlier in the chapter that you are working in an emergency department.

Consider the patient's situation

Three-year-old Liam has presented to the emergency department with what is thought to be a small plastic bead lodged in his nose.

Collect cues/information

Your further assessment reveals the following information.

Subjective data

Liam was brought to the emergency department by his distressed parent who observed him push the bead into his nose. They encouraged him to blow his nose, but the bead is still stuck. Liam has no other significant health problems.

Objective data

Liam is relaxed and cooperative but says his nose is sore and reports a lack of sense of smell (anosmia). Liam's parents are visibly anxious.
Nose: (L) naris patent. (R) naris: reddened distal mucosa with no nasal discharge observed. The foreign body is lodged high in the airway obstructing airflow. No pain with light palpation.

Process information and identify problems/issues

Collaborative problem

Foreign body in nose - refer to medical practitioner for further assessment

Problem statement/nursing diagnosis

Obstructed nasal airway related to presence of foreign body
Discomfort related to foreign body in the nose
Parental anxiety related to child's health

ADDITIONAL RESOURCES

You can further develop your knowledge and skills relevant to upper airways assessment, related pathophysiology, common health issues and nursing interventions by:

- reading chapters of a fundamentals of nursing or medical-surgical nursing textbook
- answering chapter multiple choice questions online. Log onto ClinicalKey Student and search for the text 'Health Assessment, 4th edition'. Choose the section titled 'Teaching material'. In this section you will find question and answer documents for each chapter. Please check instructions on the inside front cover of the book to access online resources.

ADDITIONAL RESOURCES cont'd

- visiting websites

Better Health Channel—Anosmia:

https://www.betterhealth.vic.gov.au/health/conditionsandtreatments/anosmia-loss-of-smell

Healthline—What is anosmia?: https://www.healthline.com/health/anosmia#causes

Melbourne ENT Group—Patient information on anosmia: https://melbentgroup.com.au/wp-content/uploads/2016/02/Anosmia.pdf

REFERENCES

1. Coelho DH, Reiter ER, Budd SG, Shin Y, Kons ZA, Costanzo RM. Quality of life and safety impact of COVID-19 associated smell and taste disturbances. American Journal of Otolaryngology. 2021 Jul 1;42(4):103001.
2. Bhatia-Dey N, Heinbockel T. The olfactory system as a marker of neurodegeneration in aging, neurological and neuropsychiatric disorders. International Journal of Environmental Research and Public Health. 2021 Jun 29; 18(13):6976.
3. Boody BS, Sharma R, Bronson WH, Russo G, Segar A, Vaccaro AR. Update on stem cell applications in spine surgery. Contemporary Spine Surgery, 2019;20(3):1–7.
4. Australian Institute of Health and Welfare. 2019. Potentially preventable hospitalisations in Australia by age groups and small geographic areas, 2017–18. Canberra: AIHW.
5. Jacups SP, Kinchin I (2021). A rapid review of evidence to inform an ear, nose and throat service delivery model in remote Australia. Rural and Remote Health, 21(1):1–12.
6. Graydon KC, Miller WH, Gunasekera H. Global burden of hearing impairment and ear disease. The Journal of Laryngology & Otology, 2019;133(1):18–25.
7. Banham D, Karnon J, Lynch J. Health related quality of life (HRQoL) among Aboriginal South Australians: a perspective using survey-based health utility estimates. Health and Quality of Life Outcomes 2019; 17(1):39.
8. Oliver J, Thielemans E, McMinn A, Baker C, Britton PN, Clark JE, et al. Invasive group A Streptococcus disease in Australian children: 2016 to 2018: a descriptive cohort study. BMC Public Health. 2019 Dec 30:1750.
9. Boesveldt S, Parma V. The importance of the olfactory system in human well-being, through nutrition and social behavior. Cell Tissue Research. 2021 Jan;383(1):559–567.
10. Marin C, Vilas D, Langdon C, Alobid I, López-Chacón M, Haehner A, et al. Olfactory dysfunction in neurodegenerative diseases. Current Allergy and Asthma Reports, 2018;18(2):42.
11. Hummel T, Whitcroft KL, Andrews P, Altundag A, Cinghi C, Costanzo RM, et al. Position paper on olfactory dysfunction. Rhinology. 2017;54:1–30.
12. Alizadeh R, Kamrava SK, Bagher Z, Farhadi M, Falah M, Moradi F, et al. Human olfactory stem cells: as a promising source of dopaminergic neuron-like cells for treatment of Parkinson's disease. Neuroscience Letters 2019;696:52–59.
13. Child KM, Herrick DB, Schwob JE, Holbrook EH, Jang W. The neuroregenerative capacity of olfactory stem cells is not limitless: implications for aging. Journal of Neuroscience 2018;38(31):6806–6824.

CHAPTER 19

Lower airways assessment

Written by Carolyn Jarvis
Adapted by Josh Allen

INTRODUCTION

The respiratory system is an important system responsible for supplying oxygen, removing carbon dioxide and maintaining the acid–base balance of arterial blood through hypoventilation and hyperventilation. To appreciate the impact of disease and trauma to this complex and dynamic system, you are advised to first review the structure and function of the thoracic cage, the lungs and tracheo-bronchial tree and the respiratory centre in the brainstem. Any changes to the respiratory system can have a serious impact on the person's functional capacity. For example, activity and exercise, body care, household maintenance, nutrition and metabolism, elimination, spiritual and social activities and roles and relationships are all affected to some degree.

Case study

The following case study gives an example of a typical situation involving assessing the lower airways and the initial clinical reasoning process.

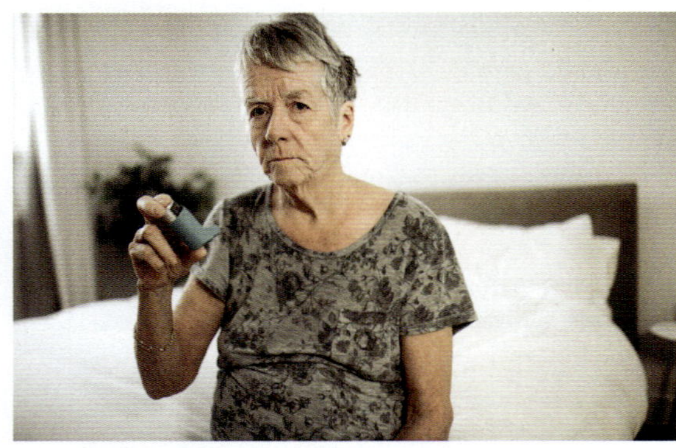

Context

You are a registered nurse working in the respiratory unit of a hospital.

Consider the patient's situation

Mrs Dorothy Smith is a 73-year-old woman who has been admitted for care in your clinical area with an infective exacerbation of chronic obstructive pulmonary disease (COPD). Mrs Smith reports a history of upper respiratory tract infections over the past 2 weeks.

Questions to further your learning

- What are the possible things that might be going on with Mrs Smith?
- What knowledge do you need to be able to predict what might be going on?
- What approach to Mrs Smith's health assessment will you take?
- What questions (subjective data) will you ask Mrs Smith to extend the health history and why?
- What physical examination (objective data) will you conduct and why?
- What resources are available to assist in your assessment of Mrs Smith?

Assessment plan

Subjective data relating to the respiratory system can give important clues as to a person's respiratory health and functional capacity as well as indicators of risk for developing lung disorders. Gathering information about respiratory function is also important in determining a person's ability to perform activities of daily living. The main areas for subjective data assessment are:

- presenting concern
- shortness of breath
- chest pain with breathing
- cough
- history of respiratory infections
- smoking history
- environmental exposure
- health and lifestyle management.

Following subjective data collection, you will get a sense of the areas needed to be examined for objective data. Only the relevant areas should be examined.

The main areas for physical examination are:

- general inspection
- inspection of the posterior chest wall
- palpation of the posterior chest wall
- auscultation of the posterior chest wall for breath sounds
- inspection of the anterior chest wall
- palpation of the anterior chest wall
- auscultation of the anterior chest wall for breath sounds
- measurement of pulmonary function.

Resources available

You will find additional resources and the reference list at the end of this chapter. This chapter also has a video available demonstrating objective data collection related to respiratory assessment. You will find a QR code in the objective data section, which enable you to access the video easily on your device.

Structure and function

Position and surface landmarks

The **thoracic cage** is a bony structure with a conical shape, which is narrower at the top (Figure 19.1). It is defined by the **sternum**, 12 pairs of **ribs** and 12 thoracic **vertebrae**. Its 'floor' is the **diaphragm**, a musculotendinous septum that separates the thoracic cavity from the abdomen. The first seven ribs attach directly to the sternum via their costal cartilages: ribs 8, 9 and 10 attach to the costal cartilage above, and ribs 11 and 12 are 'floating', with free palpable tips. The **costochondral junctions** are the points at which the ribs join their cartilages. They are not palpable.

ANTERIOR THORACIC LANDMARKS

Surface landmarks on the thorax are signposts for underlying respiratory structures. Knowledge of landmarks will help you localise a finding and will help communicate your findings to others.

Suprasternal notch. You can feel this hollow U-shaped depression just above the sternum, in between the clavicles.

Sternum. The 'breastbone' has three parts: the manubrium, the body and the xiphoid process. Walk your fingers down the manubrium a few centimetres until you feel a distinct bony ridge, the manubriosternal angle.

Manubriosternal angle. The manubriosternal angle is often called the

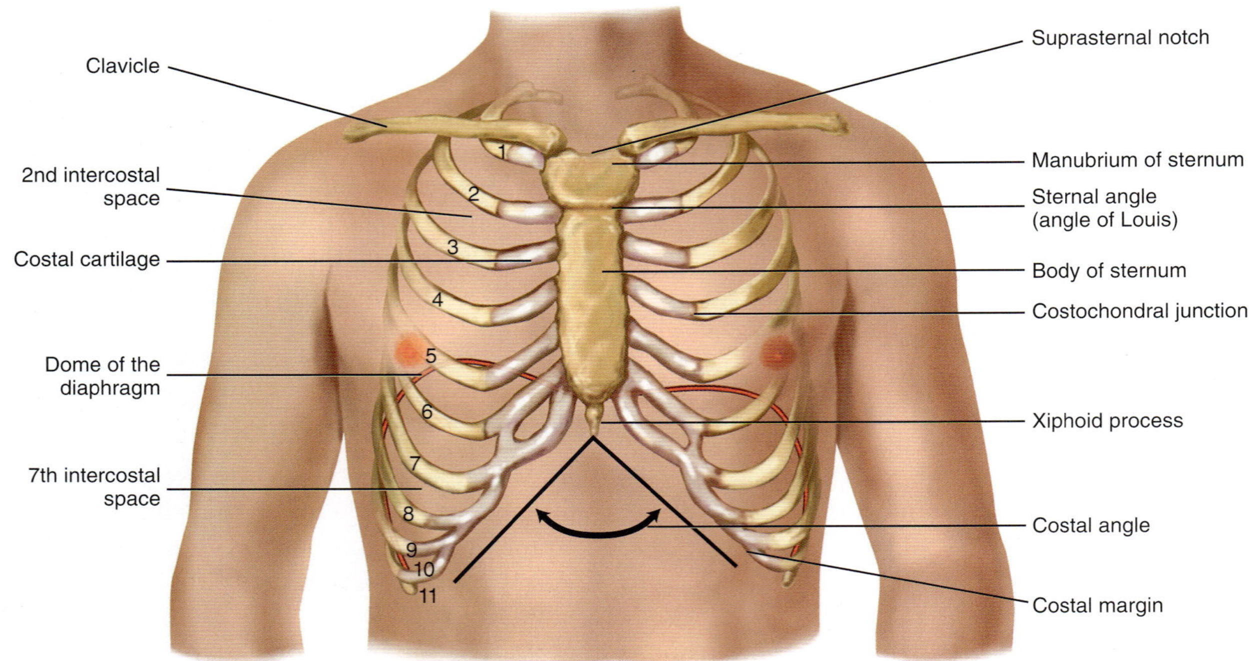

FIGURE 19.1 Anterior thoracic cage

sternal angle or the 'angle of Louis'. This is the articulation of the manubrium and body of the sternum, and it is continuous with the second rib. The angle of Louis is a useful place to start counting ribs, which helps localise a respiratory finding horizontally. Identify the angle of Louis, palpate lightly to the second rib and slide down to the second intercostal space. Each intercostal space is numbered by the rib above it. Continue counting down the ribs in the middle of the hemithorax, not close to the sternum where the costal cartilages lie too close together to count. You can palpate easily down to the 10th rib.

The angle of Louis also marks the site of tracheal bifurcation into the right and left main bronchi; it corresponds with the upper border of the atria of the heart, and it lies above the fourth thoracic vertebra on the back.

Costal angle. The right and left costal margins form an angle where they meet at the xiphoid process. Usually 90 degrees or less, this angle increases when the rib cage is chronically overinflated, as seen in people with emphysema.

POSTERIOR THORACIC LANDMARKS

Counting ribs and intercostal spaces on the back is a bit harder due to the muscles and soft tissue surrounding the ribs and spinal column (Figure 19.2). It is easiest to count down the spinous processes, starting with the vertebra prominens.

Vertebra prominens. Flex your head and feel for the most prominent bony spur protruding at the base of the neck. This is the spinous process of C7. If two bumps seem equally prominent, the upper one is C7 and the lower one is T1.

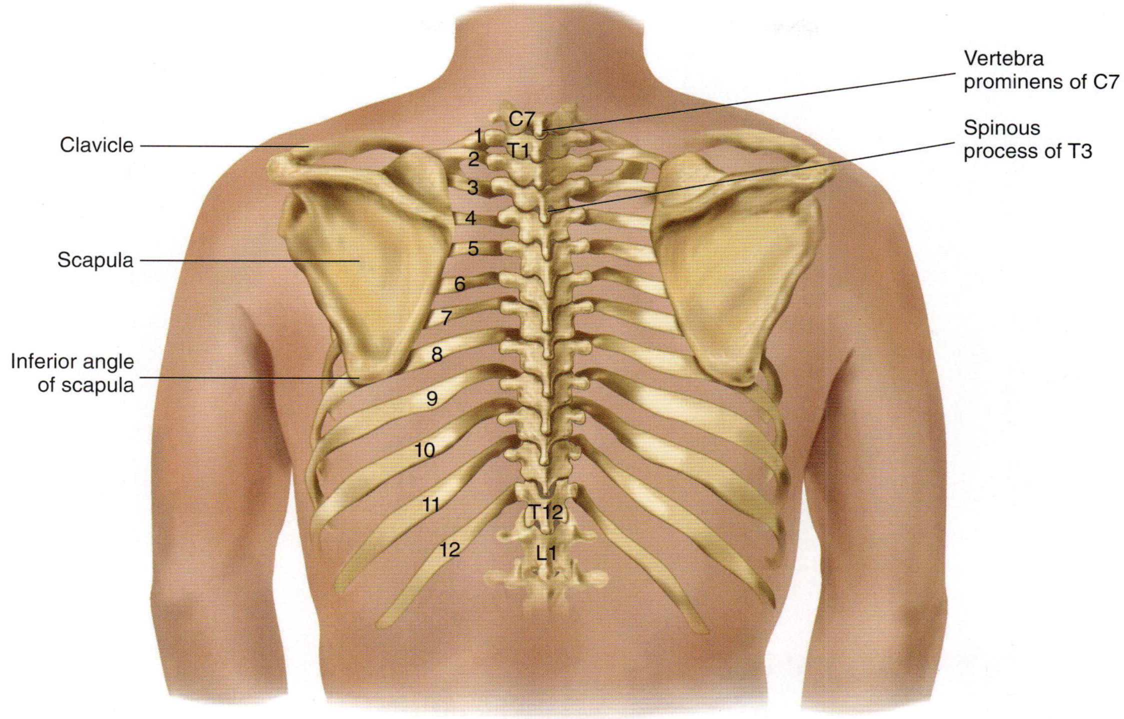

FIGURE 19.2 Posterior thoracic cage

Spinous processes. Count down these knobs on the vertebrae, which stack together to form the spinal column. Note that the spinous processes align with their same numbered ribs only down to T4. After T4, the spinous processes angle downwards from their vertebral body and overlie the vertebral body and rib below.

Inferior border of the scapula. The scapulae are located symmetrically in each hemithorax. The lower tip is usually at the seventh or eighth rib.

Twelfth rib. Palpate midway between the spine and the person's side to identify its free tip.

REFERENCE LINES

Use the reference lines to pinpoint a finding vertically on the chest. On the anterior chest, note the **midsternal** line and the **midclavicular** line. The midclavicular line bisects the centre of each clavicle at a point halfway between the palpated sternoclavicular and acromioclavicular joints (Figure 19.3).

The posterior chest wall has the **vertebral** (or midspinal) line and the **scapular** line, which extends through the inferior angle of the scapula when the arms are at the sides of the body (Figure 19.4).

Lift the person's arm up 90 degrees and divide the lateral chest by three lines: the **anterior axillary** line extends down from the anterior axillary fold where the pectoralis major muscle inserts; the **posterior axillary** line continues down from the posterior axillary fold where the latissimus dorsi muscle inserts; and the **midaxillary**

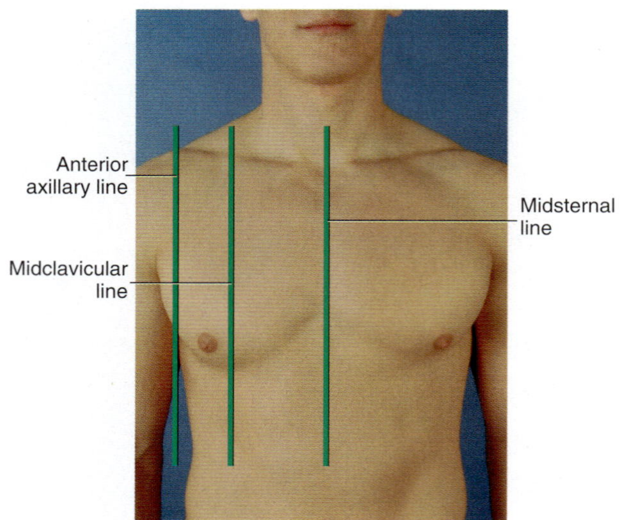

FIGURE 19.3 Reference lines—anterior chest

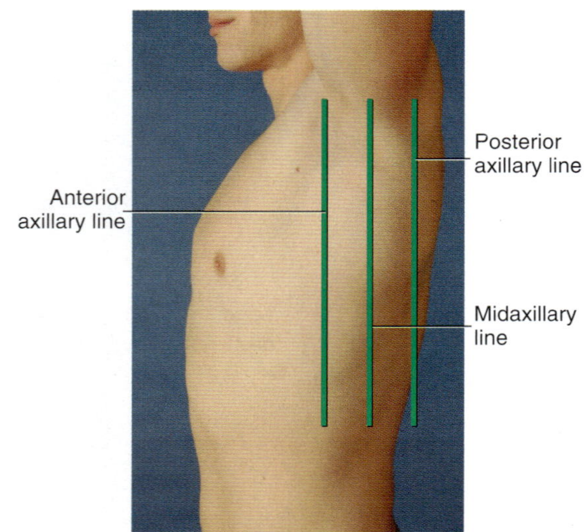

FIGURE 19.5 Anterior axillary line

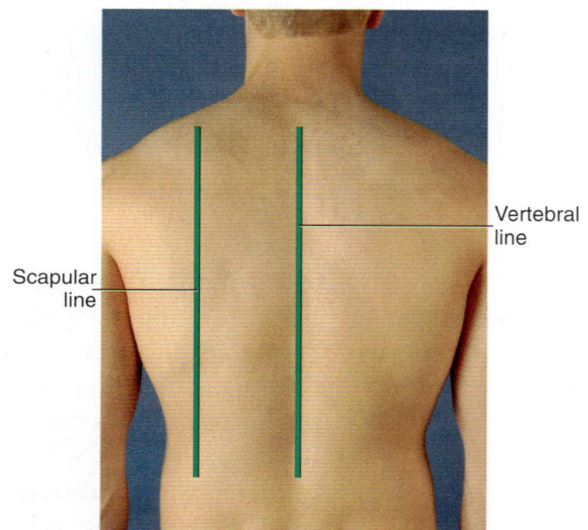

FIGURE 19.4 Reference lines—posterior chest

line runs down from the apex of the axilla and lies between and parallel to the other two (Figure 19.5).

The thoracic cavity

The **mediastinum** is the middle section of the thoracic cavity containing the oesophagus, trachea, heart and great vessels. The right and left **pleural cavities**, on either side of the mediastinum, contain the lungs.

Lung borders. In the anterior chest, the **apex**, or highest point, of lung tissue is 3 or 4 cm above the inner third of the clavicles. The **base**, or lower border, rests on the diaphragm at about the sixth rib in the midclavicular line. Laterally, lung tissue extends from the apex of the axilla down to the seventh or eighth rib. Posteriorly, the location of C7 marks the apex of lung tissue and T10 usually corresponds to the base. Deep inspiration expands the lungs, and their lower border drops to the level of T12.

LOBES OF THE LUNGS

The lungs are paired but not precisely symmetrical structures (Figure 19.6). The right lung is shorter than the left lung because of the underlying liver. The left lung is narrower than the right lung because the heart bulges to the left. The right lung has three lobes, and the left lung has two lobes. These lobes are not arranged in horizontal bands like dessert layers in a parfait glass.

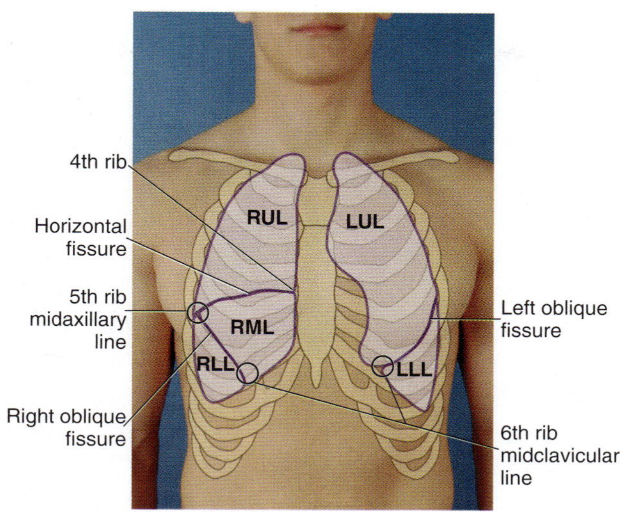

FIGURE 19.6 Midclavicular line

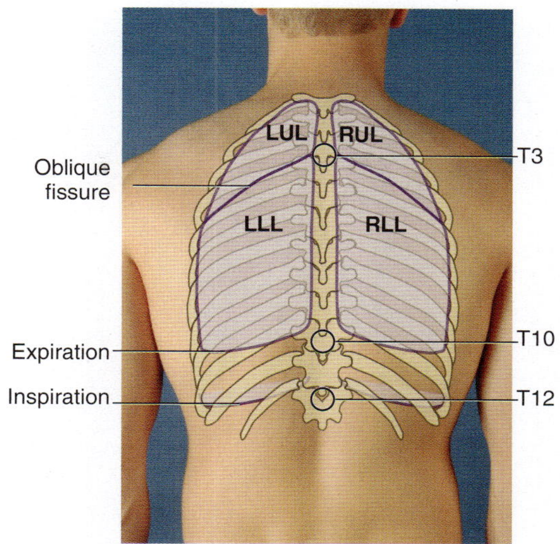

FIGURE 19.7 Lobes of the lung—posterior

Rather, they fit together in diagonal sloping segments and are separated by **fissures** that run obliquely through the chest.

Anterior. On the anterior chest, the **oblique** (the major or diagonal) fissure crosses the fifth rib in the midaxillary line and terminates at the sixth rib in the midclavicular line. The right lung also contains the **horizontal** (minor) fissure, which divides the right upper and middle lobes. This fissure extends from the fifth rib in the right midaxillary line to the third intercostal space or fourth rib at the right sternal border.

Posterior. The most remarkable point about the posterior chest is that it is almost all lower lobe (Figure 19.7). The upper lobes occupy a smaller band of tissue from their apices at T1 down to T3 or T4. At this level, the lower lobes begin, and their inferior border reaches down to the level of T10 on expiration and to T12 on inspiration. Note that the right middle lobe does not project onto the posterior chest at all. If the person abducts the arms and places the hands on the back of the head, the division between upper and lower lobes corresponds to the medial border of the scapulae.

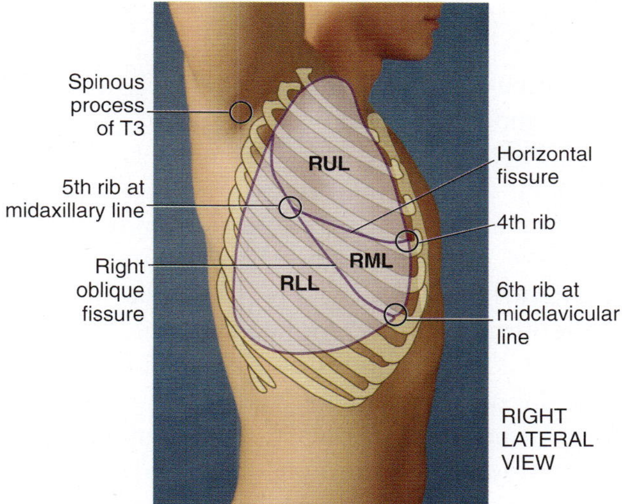

FIGURE 19.8 Right lateral or axillary view

Lateral. Laterally, lung tissue extends from the apex of the axilla down to the seventh or eighth rib. The right upper lobe extends from the apex of the axilla down to the horizontal fissure at the fifth rib (Figure 19.8). The right middle lobe extends from the horizontal fissure down and forwards to the sixth rib at the midclavicular line. The right lower lobe

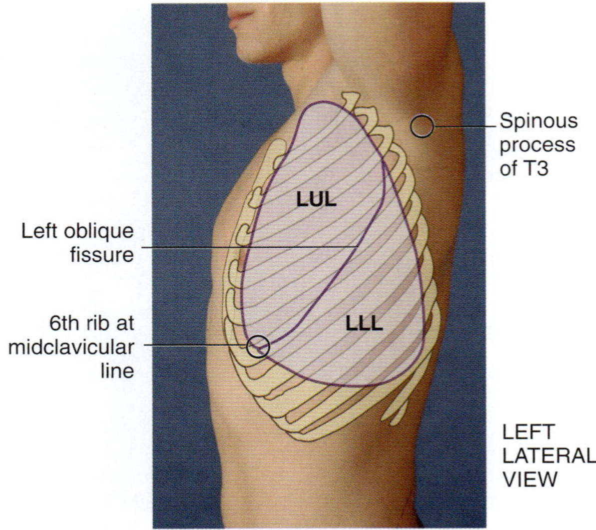

FIGURE 19.9 Left lateral or axillary view

continues from the fifth rib to the eighth rib in the midaxillary line.

The left lung contains only two lobes, upper and lower (Figure 19.9). These are seen laterally as two triangular areas separated by the oblique fissure. The left upper lobe extends from the apex of the axilla down to the fifth rib at the midaxillary line. The left lower lobe continues down to the eighth rib in the midaxillary line.

Using these landmarks, take a marker and try tracing the outline of each lobe on a willing partner. Take special note of the three points that commonly confuse novices:

1. The left lung has no middle lobe.
2. The anterior chest contains mostly upper and middle lobe with very little lower lobe.
3. The posterior chest contains almost all lower lobe.

PLEURAE

The thin, slippery **pleurae** form an envelope between the lungs and the chest wall (Figure 19.10). The **visceral** pleura lines the outside of the lungs, dipping down into the fissures. It is continuous, with the **parietal** pleura lining the inside of the chest wall and diaphragm.

The inside of the envelope, the pleural cavity, is a potential space filled with only a few millilitres of lubricating fluid. It normally has a vacuum, or negative pressure, which holds the lungs tightly against the chest wall. The lungs slide smoothly and noiselessly up and down during respiration, lubricated by a few millilitres of fluid. Think of this as similar to two glass slides with a drop of water between them; although it is difficult to separate the slides, they slide smoothly back and forth. The pleurae extend about 3 cm below the level of the lungs, forming the **costodiaphragmatic recess**. This is a potential space: when it abnormally fills with air or fluid, it compromises lung expansion.

TRACHEA AND BRONCHIAL TREE

The **trachea** lies anterior to the oesophagus and is 10 to 11 cm long in adults. It begins at the level of the cricoid cartilage in the neck and bifurcates just below the sternal angle into the right and left main bronchi. Posteriorly, tracheal bifurcation is at the level of T4 or T5. The right main bronchus is shorter, wider and more vertical than the left main bronchus.

The **trachea** and **bronchi** transport gases between the environment and the lung parenchyma. They constitute the *anatomical dead space*, or space that is filled with air but is not available for gaseous exchange. This is about 150 mL in adults. The goblet cells and cilia that line the bronchial tree also help to protect alveoli from small particulate matter in the inhaled air. The goblet cells secrete mucus that entraps the particles, while the cilia sweep particles upwards where they can be swallowed or expelled.

An **acinus** is a functional respiratory unit that consists of the bronchioles, alveolar ducts, alveolar sacs and the alveoli. Gaseous

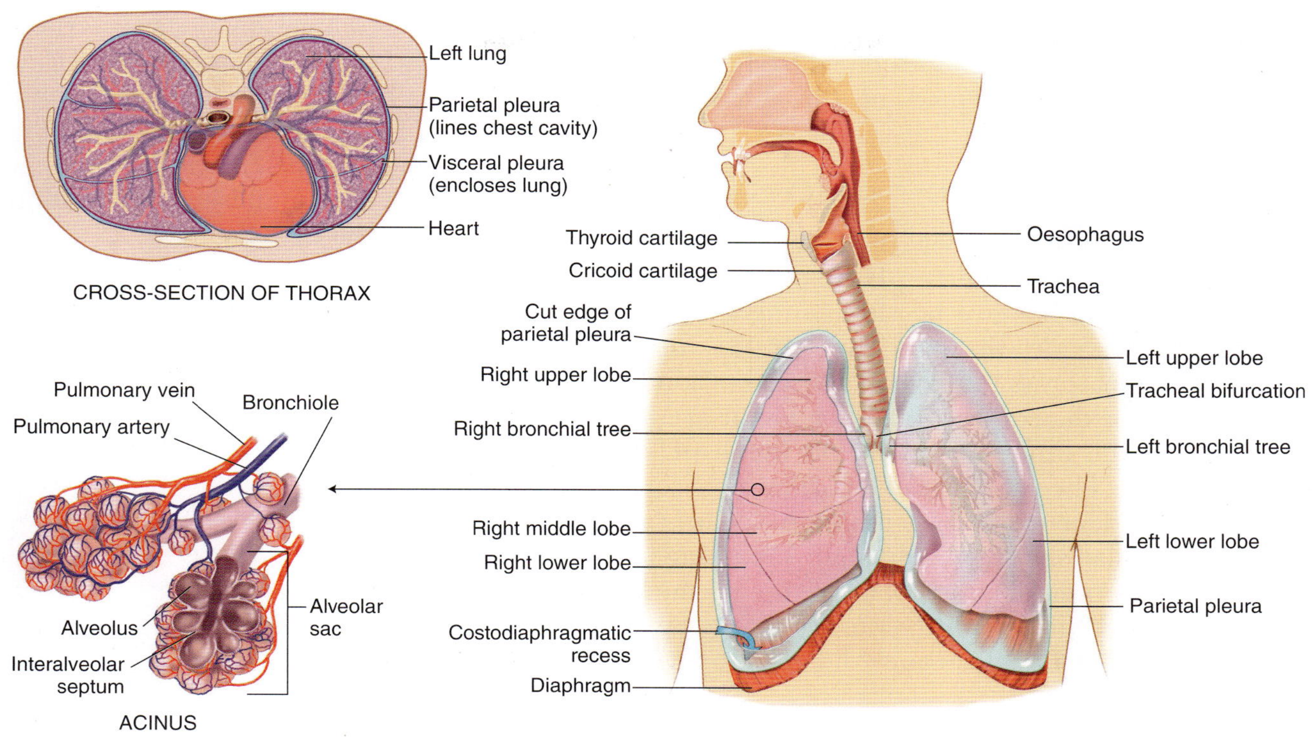

FIGURE 19.10 Pleurae and tracheobronchial tree

exchange occurs across the respiratory membrane in the alveolar duct and in the millions of alveoli. Note how the alveoli are clustered like grapes around each alveolar duct (Figure 19.10). This creates millions of interalveolar septa (walls) that increase tremendously the working space available for gas exchange. This bunched arrangement creates a total lung surface area for gas exchange that is as large as a tennis court.

Mechanics of ventilation and respiration

The respiratory system has two separate but related functions: (1) ventilation, the two-part process of moving air into and out of the lungs; and (2) respiration, the exchange of gases across the alveoli. Respiration can be divided into three further functions: (1) oxygenation, the supply of oxygen to the body for energy production; (2) removing carbon dioxide, a waste product of energy reactions; and (3) maintaining homeostasis (acid–base balance) of arterial blood. The respiratory system also plays a role in maintaining heat exchange, which is less important in humans than in some other animals.

The body tissues are bathed by blood that normally has a narrow acceptable range of pH. Unlike oxygen, which is predominantly transported by attaching to haemoglobin, carbon dioxide (CO_2) dissolves directly into the blood, where it combines with water (H_2O) to create carbonic acid (H_2CO_3), a relatively weak acid. Carbonic acid in turn dissociates into bicarbonate (HCO_3^-) and strongly acidic hydrogen ions (H^+). Thus, increased carbon dioxide in the blood increases acidity (decreases pH). The relationship between carbon dioxide and hydrogen is represented in the following equation:

$$CO_2 + H_2O \leftrightarrows H_2CO_3 \leftrightarrows HCO_3^- + H^+$$

Although a number of compensatory mechanisms regulate the pH, the lungs help maintain the balance by eliminating excess carbon dioxide through the process of respiration across the alveoli. When carbon dioxide is exhaled, the equation above moves back in the other direction and blood pH increases. The exchange of carbon dioxide is highly dependent on ventilation. That is, hypoventilation (slow, shallow breathing) causes carbon dioxide to build up in the blood, and hyperventilation (rapid, deep breathing) causes carbon dioxide to be blown off.

CONTROL OF BREATHING

Normally our breathing pattern changes without us being aware of it in response to cellular demands. This involuntary control of ventilation is mediated by the respiratory centre in the brainstem (pons and medulla). The major feedback loop is humoral regulation, or the change in carbon dioxide and oxygen levels in the blood and, less importantly, the hydrogen ion level. The *normal stimulus to breathe* for most of us is an increase of carbon dioxide in the blood, hypercarbia or **hypercapnia**. A decrease of oxygen in the blood (**hypoxaemia**) also increases respirations but is less effective than hypercapnia.

CHANGING CHEST SIZE

Ventilation is the physical act of breathing: air rushes into the lungs as the chest size increases (inspiration) and is expelled from the lungs as the chest recoils (expiration). The mechanical expansion and contraction of the chest cavity alters the size of the thoracic container in two dimensions: (1) the vertical diameter lengthens or shortens, which is accomplished by downwards or upwards movement of the diaphragm; and (2) the anteroposterior diameter increases or decreases, which is accomplished by elevation or depression of the ribs (Figure 19.11).

In inspiration, increasing the size of the thoracic container creates a slightly negative pressure relative to the atmosphere, so air rushes in to fill the partial vacuum. The major muscle responsible for this is the diaphragm. During inspiration, contraction of the bell-shaped diaphragm causes it to descend and flatten. This lengthens the vertical diameter of the thorax. Intercostal muscles lift the sternum and elevate the ribs, making them more horizontal. This increases the anteroposterior diameter.

Expiration is primarily passive. As the diaphragm relaxes, the elastic recoil of the lungs and rib cage cause it to return to its natural domed position. All this squeezing creates a relatively positive pressure within the alveoli, and the air flows out of the lungs. The volume of gas that moves in and out of the lungs during this ventilatory cycle is called the *tidal volume* (Figure 19.12).

Forced inspiration, such as that during and after heavy exercise or occurring pathologically with respiratory distress, commands the use of the accessory neck muscles to heave up the sternum and rib cage. These neck muscles are the sternocleidomastoids, the scaleni and the trapezii. In forced expiration, the abdominal muscles contract powerfully to push the abdominal viscera forcefully in and up against the diaphragm, making it dome upwards and squeeze against the lungs. Forced inspiration and expiration increases the volume of gas moving in and out of the lungs by tapping into the *inspiratory* and *expiratory reserve volumes.*

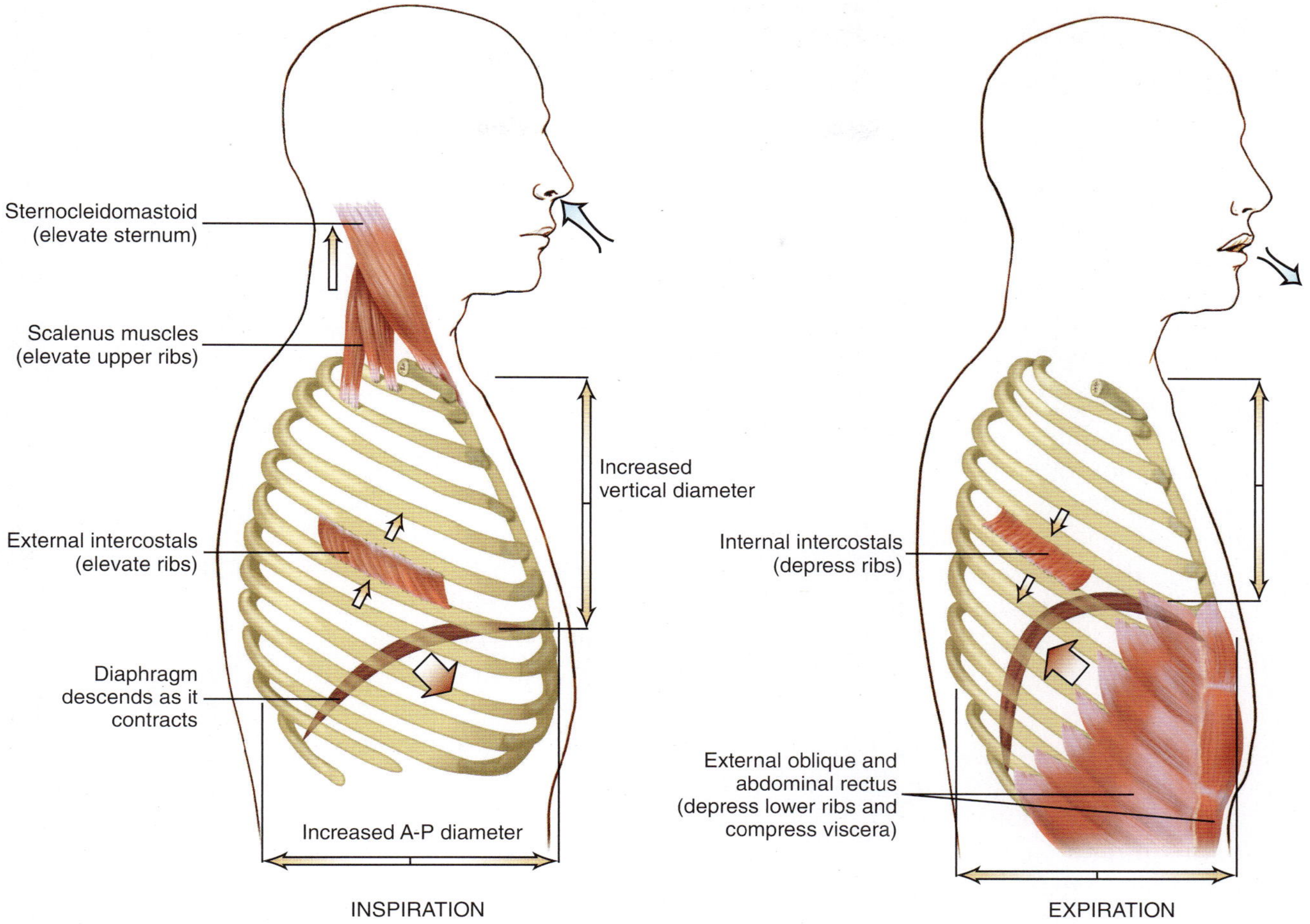

FIGURE 19.11 Inspiration and expiration

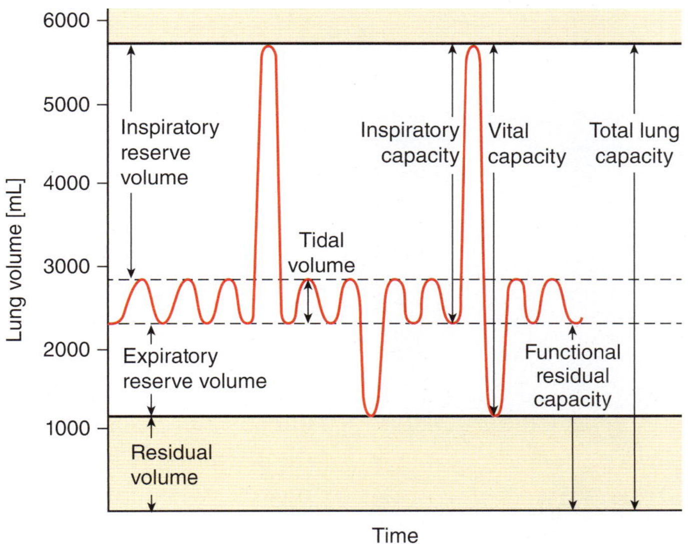

FIGURE 19.12 Inspiratory and expiratory reserve volumes
Source: https://cdn.clinicalkey.com/ck-thumbnails/C20130099677/B9780323287531000118/f011-023-9780323287531-t.gif

Developmental considerations

Infants and children

During the first 5 weeks of fetal life, the primitive lung bud emerges; by 16 weeks, the conducting airways reach the same number as in an adult; at 32 weeks, **surfactant**, the complex lipid substance needed for sustained inflation of the alveolar sacs, is present in adequate amounts; and by birth the lungs have 70 million primitive alveoli ready to start the job of respiration.

When the newborn inhales the first breath, the lusty cry that follows reassures straining parents that their baby is alright (Figure 19.13). The baby's body systems all develop in utero, but the respiratory system alone does not function until birth. Birth demands its instant performance.

When the umbilical cord is clamped and the blood flow between the baby and the placenta is disrupted, blood gushes into the baby's pulmonary circulation. Relatively less resistance exists in the pulmonary arteries than in the aorta, so the foramen ovale in the heart closes just after birth. (See the discussion of fetal circulation in Chapter 17.) The ductus arteriosus (linking the pulmonary artery and the aorta) contracts and closes some hours later, and pulmonary and systemic circulation are functional.

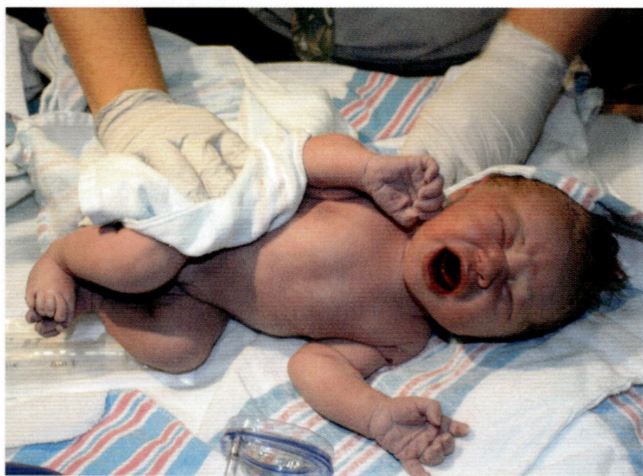

FIGURE 19.13 Newborn

Respiratory development continues throughout childhood, with increases in diameter and length of airways and increases in size and number of alveoli, reaching the adult range of 300 million by adolescence.

In the presence of older caregivers who smoke, the relatively smaller size and immaturity of children's pulmonary systems result in enormous vulnerability and increased risks to child health. Prenatal exposure results in chronic hypoxia and low birthweight. Postnatal exposure to environmental tobacco smoke is linked to increased rates of otitis media, respiratory tract infections and childhood asthma.[1] Other conditions associated with exposure to tobacco smoke include sudden infant death syndrome, negative behavioural and cognitive functioning and increased rates of adolescent smoking.

Pregnant women

The enlarging uterus elevates the diaphragm 4 cm during pregnancy. This decreases the vertical diameter of the thoracic cage, but this decrease is compensated for by an increase in the horizontal diameter. The increased production of the hormone relaxin relaxes the thoracic cage ligaments. This allows an increase in the transverse diameter of the thoracic cage by 2 cm, and the costal angle widens. The total circumference of the chest increases by 6 cm. Although the diaphragm is elevated, it is not fixed. It moves with breathing even more during pregnancy, which results in an increase in tidal volume.[2]

The growing fetus increases the oxygen demand on the mother's body. This is met easily by the increasing tidal volume (deeper breathing). Little change occurs in the respiratory rate. An increased awareness of the need to breathe develops, even early in pregnancy, and some pregnant women may experience dyspnoea although, structurally, nothing is wrong.

Late adulthood (65+ years)

In late adulthood, the costal cartilages become calcified, which produces a less mobile thorax. Respiratory muscle strength declines after age 50 years and continues to decrease into the 70s. A more significant change is the decrease in elastic properties within the lungs, making them less distensible and lessening their tendency to collapse and recoil. In all, the ageing lung is a more rigid structure that is harder to inflate.

These changes result in an increase in small airway collapse, and that yields a *decreased vital capacity* (the maximum amount of air that a person can expel from the lungs after first filling the lungs to maximum) and an *increased residual volume* (the amount of air remaining in the lungs even after the most forceful expiration) (Figure 19.12).

With ageing, histological changes (i.e. a gradual loss of intra-alveolar septa and a decreased number of alveoli) also occur, so less surface area is available for gas exchange. Also, the lung bases become less ventilated because of the closing off of a number of airways. This increases the older person's risk of dyspnoea, with exertion beyond their usual workload.

The histological changes also increase an older person's risk of postoperative pulmonary complications. That is, older people have a greater risk of postoperative atelectasis and infection from a decreased ability to cough, a loss of protective airway reflexes and increased secretions.

Cultural and social considerations

Respiratory diseases associated with exposure to harmful substances or infectious organisms disproportionately affect groups within Australian and Aotearoa New Zealand society. Lifestyle factors such as tobacco smoking, occupational exposure to asbestos or silica and environmental exposure to air pollutants or infectious diseases are each associated with particular groups in society.

Tobacco smoking is a major cause of preventable death and disease in Australia and Aotearoa New Zealand. There is a strong inverse relationship between tobacco use and socioeconomic indicators: around 21% of adults living in the most socioeconomic disadvantaged areas were current smokers, compared with 8% of adults in the least disadvantaged areas.[3] Men are more likely to be daily smokers than are women (16.5% vs 11.1%), and older Australians are more likely to be current or former smokers than younger Australians. Similar prevalence data is reported in Aotearoa New Zealand, with 8% of adults currently smoking. However, daily smoking rates for Māori (19.9%) and Pacific Islander people (18.2%) are significantly higher than for other New Zealanders.[4] In both Australia and Aotearoa New Zealand, socially and economically disadvantaged groups within the population are much more likely to smoke than the general population, placing them and those around them at higher risk of smoking-related disease.[3] This includes those living in rural and remote areas, Aboriginal and Torres Strait Islander populations in Australia and Māori populations in Aotearoa New Zealand.[3,4] Tobacco smoke contributes to a range of diseases including but not limited to lung cancer, emphysema, chronic bronchitis, chronic obstructive pulmonary disease, heart disease and other cancers.

Occupational exposure to harmful substances such as asbestos or silica disproportionately affects males working in manufacturing and construction industries. Mesothelioma is a form of cancer associated with exposure to asbestos fibres. Each year in Australia, between 700 and 800 new diagnoses of mesothelioma are made, with males 5 to 6 times more likely to be diagnosed than females.[5,6] Mesothelioma has a long latency period, and most people diagnosed are older than 60 years of age, despite exposure occurring many years earlier. The so-called 'third wave' of asbestos-related disease is expected to see a shift in source from industrial exposure to exposure that occurs from home renovations.[7] Similarly, silicosis arising from occupational exposure to the silica contained in manufactured stone products has increased with the rising popularity of home renovations.[8,9]

Finally, while both Australia and Aotearoa New Zealand have some of the lowest rates of tuberculosis (TB) in the world, migrant communities, particularly those from Southern, Central or Eastern Asia, are at much greater risk of being diagnosed with TB than the rest of the population. In Australia, 91% of all TB notifications were in foreign-born people, while in Aotearoa New Zealand, 78% of all TB notifications were in foreign-born people.[10,11]

HEALTH EDUCATION

Environmental tobacco smoke

Secondhand smoke, also referred to as environmental tobacco smoke, is a mixture of *sidestream smoke*, the smoke from the burning end of a cigarette, pipe or cigar, and *mainstream smoke*, the smoke exhaled from the lungs of a person who is smoking. The evidence indicates that there is no risk-free level of exposure to secondhand smoke. Exposure to secondhand smoke, which is primarily involuntary, increases our risk for adverse health effects. Further, the general public's exposure to secondhand smoke, regardless of whether they are smokers, is much higher than most people realise. The rapidly increasing use of e-cigarettes, 'vaping', and shisha especially among younger people, has raised new questions about the safety of exposure to secondhand vapour. Despite suggestions that these alternatives to traditional tobacco smoking are safer, emerging evidence suggests that e-cigarettes are likely to have harmful cardiovascular and respiratory effects.[12–14] Secondhand smoke is especially harmful to young children, increasing respiratory infection rates, inner ear infections and aggravation of asthma. There is a causal relationship between maternal smoking during pregnancy and:

- a persistent adverse lung function throughout childhood
- a small reduction in birthweight.

Following birth, infants and children exposed to environmental tobacco smoke face an increased risk of:

- sudden infant death syndrome
- lower level of lung function
- lower respiratory illness
- middle ear infections
- asthma, croup and bronchitis.[15]

According to the Australian Institute of Health and Welfare,[16] the number of children exposed to daily tobacco smoke in Australia is decreasing, falling from around 20% of children

HEALTH EDUCATION cont'd

in 2001 to just 2.1% in 2019. Similarly for adult Australians, in 2001 10.6% lived in households with at least one regular smoker who smoked indoors, down to 2.4% in 2019. Secondhand smoke contains hundreds of chemicals known to be toxic or carcinogenic including formaldehyde, benzene, vinyl chloride, arsenic and cyanide. Involuntarily inhaled by non-smokers, it can linger in the air for hours, long after the cigarette, cigar or pipe has been extinguished.

Exposure to secondhand smoke places non-smokers at risk for the same diseases as active smoking does. Non-smokers exposed to secondhand smoke are 25% more likely to have heart disease and 20% more likely to have lung cancer than are those non-smokers who are not exposed to smoke. Separating smokers from non-smokers, cleaning the air indoors and ventilating buildings do not eliminate the exposure risk to non-smokers. However, eliminating smoking from indoor spaces does fully protect non-smokers.

Nurse's role

- Assess the person's health literacy and readiness to stop smoking/vaping.
- Encourage adopting a healthy lifestyle such as not smoking, eating a healthy diet, drinking alcohol in moderation, exercising daily and losing weight where necessary.
- Help the person identify real or perceived barriers to quitting smoking/vaping.
- Offer information on nicotine replacement therapies such as nicotine patches, lozenges or gum.
- Provide information about online support services such as Quitline and support apps (e.g. Myquitbuddy) and smoking cessation literature.
- Refer to a GP for assessment regarding suitability for prescription medication such as bupropion (Zyban) and varenicline (Champix).

Further information

- Department of Health and Ageing. Quitting smoking. 2023 Australian Government. Available at: https://www.health.gov.au/topics/smoking-and-tobacco/how-to-quit-smoking/quitting-methods
- Department of Health and Ageing. Myquitbuddy app. 2023 Australian Government. Available at: https://www.health.gov.au/resources/apps-and-tools/my-quitbuddy-app
- Quit Victoria. E-cigarettes and teens: what you need to know. 2023. Available at: https://www.quit.org.au/articles/teenvaping

Subjective data

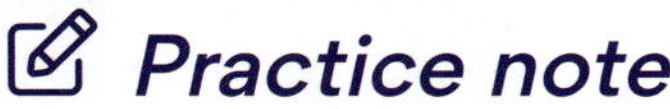

Practice note

Before you start the assessment, introduce yourself to the person, confirm the person's identity, discuss the purpose and scope of the assessment, clarify any questions the person may have and obtain verbal consent from the person to perform the assessment.

ASSESSMENT GUIDELINES	CLINICAL SIGNIFICANCE AND CLINICAL ALERTS
Presenting concern	
• *Do you have any problem with your lungs or your breathing?* It is important to ascertain the person's perception of the health of their lungs. If a problem is perceived, ask: *How does this affect your quality of life?*	
Shortness of breath	
• *Have you ever had any shortness of breath, difficulty breathing or difficulty catching your breath?* • *What brings it on? How severe is it? How long does it last?* • *How much activity precipitates shortness of breath—how many metres walked, what number of stairs?*	**Dyspnoea** (shortness of breath)
• *Is your breathing affected by position such as lying down?* • *How many pillows do you sleep on at night?*	**Orthopnoea** is difficulty breathing when lying down. Several pillows may be needed to achieve comfort (e.g. 'two-pillow orthopnoea'). This is a common symptom of pulmonary oedema, often because of heart failure. Changes in sleep pattern may affect activities of living due to fatigue during the day.
• *Does it occur at any specific time of day or night?*	**Paroxysmal nocturnal dyspnoea** is awakening from sleep with shortness of breath and needing to be upright to achieve comfort.
• *Do you experience shortness of breath episodes associated with night sweats?*	**Diaphoresis** is profuse sweating. Although associated with many conditions, nocturnal diaphoresis can indicate the presence of a respiratory infection or malignancy and should be investigated.
• *Is your shortness of breath associated with a cough or chest pain?* • *Have you had a bluish colour around lips or nails?* • *Have you had wheezing or other sound when breathing?*	**Cyanosis** is the bluish discolouration of the skin resulting from a lack of oxygen. **Peripheral cyanosis** (nails) is most often due to circulatory causes and should be investigated further. ! ***Clinical alert:*** **Central cyanosis (lips)** is always due to a gross lack of oxygen and should be considered an emergency. ! ***Clinical alert:*** Any **wheeze** (lower airway) or **stridor** (upper airway) that you can hear during the interview should prompt you to stop the interview and seek assistance.

ASSESSMENT GUIDELINES	CLINICAL SIGNIFICANCE AND CLINICAL ALERTS
• *Do your symptoms seem to be related to food, pollen, dust, animals, season or emotion?*	**Asthma** (swelling of the airways with inflammation, narrowing and production of additional mucus, making it difficult to breathe) attacks may be associated with a specific allergen, extreme cold or anxiety.
• *What do you do when having difficulty breathing?* • *Do you take a special position or use pursed-lip breathing?* • *Do you use oxygen, inhalers or medications for relief?* • *How does the shortness of breath affect your work or home activities?* • *Are you able to shower and dress yourself?* • *Is your breathing getting better or worse or staying about the same?*	
Chest pain with breathing	
• *Have you experienced any chest pain with breathing?* • *Can you point to the exact location?* • *When did it start? Is it constant or does it come and go?* • *Can you describe the pain?* • *Is it burning, stabbing or something else?* • *Was the pain brought on by respiratory infection, coughing or trauma?* • *Is the pain associated with fever or deep breathing?* • *What have you done to treat the pain?* • *Have you tried medication or applying heat?*	**Chest pain** with pulmonary origin may be a late sign of pulmonary disease.
Cough	
• *Do you have a cough?* • *When did it start?* • *Was it gradual or sudden?* • *How long have you had the cough?* • *How often do you cough?* • *Do you cough at any special time of day or just on rising?* • *Does your cough wake you up at night?*	Some conditions have a characteristic timing of a cough: • **continuous throughout day**—acute illness (e.g. respiratory infection) • **afternoon/evening**—may reflect exposure to irritants at work or during the day. • **night**—postnasal drip, sinusitis, asthma • **early morning**—chronic bronchial inflammation or smoking.

ASSESSMENT GUIDELINES	CLINICAL SIGNIFICANCE AND CLINICAL ALERTS
• *Do you cough up any phlegm or sputum? How much? What colour is it?*	**Chronic bronchitis** (inflammation of the bronchi) is characterised by a history of productive cough for 3 months of the year for 2 years in a row. Non-productive coughs are associated with upper respiratory tract infections or early heart failure.
• *Do you cough up any blood? Does this look like streaks or true red blood? Does the sputum have a foul odour?*	**Haemoptysis** (blood mixed in sputum). Some conditions have characteristic sputum production: • **white or clear mucoid**—colds, bronchitis, viral infections • **yellow or green**—bacterial infections • **rust-coloured**—TB, pneumococcal pneumonia • **pink, frothy**—pulmonary oedema, some sympathomimetic medications have a side effect of pink-tinged mucus.
• *How would you describe your cough: hacking, dry, barking, hoarse, congested, bubbling?*	Some conditions have a characteristic cough: • **mycoplasma pneumonia** (mild bacterial respiratory infection)—hacking • **heart failure** (heart fails to pump adequately)—dry • **croup** (upper airway infection, usually occurs in children)—barking • **colds, bronchitis, pneumonia** (alveoli filled with fluid in one or both lungs)—congested.
• *Does the cough seem to occur with activity, position (lying), fever, congestion, talking or anxiety?* • *Does the cough make activity better or worse?*	
• *Have you seen a medical practitioner?* • *What treatment was prescribed?* • *Have you used over-the-counter medications?* • *Have you tried complementary medicine?* • *Have you used a vaporiser or other strategies such as rest or a position change?* For people with a frequent productive cough and/or a long smoking history, use the following questionnaire (Figure 19.14). This is a simple, short tool to identify people who will need spirometry testing to confirm the diagnosis of COPD.	Coughs maybe attributed to adverse medication effects—for example, angiotensin-converting enzyme (ACE) inhibitors.

ASSESSMENT GUIDELINES	CLINICAL SIGNIFICANCE AND CLINICAL ALERTS

Lung Function Questionnaire

Do you suffer from breathing problems and/or frequent cough?

These questions ask about your breathing problems and/or frequent cough. As you answer these questions, think about how you feel physically when you experience these symptoms. For each question, choose the one answer that best describes your symptoms. Share the answers with your healthcare provider.

Step 1: Answer each question and write the score in the box next to it.

Step 2: Add together the scores in each box to get your total score.

Step 3: Take the test to your provider to talk about your score.

Question						SCORE
1. How often do you cough up mucus?	Never (5)	Rarely (4)	Sometimes (3)	Often (2)	Very often (1)	☐
2. How often does your chest sound noisy (wheezy, whistling, rattling) when you breathe?	Never (5)	Rarely (4)	Sometimes (3)	Often (2)	Very often (1)	☐
3. How often do you experience shortness of breath during physical activity (walking up a flight of stairs or walking up an incline without stopping to rest)?	Never (5)	Rarely (4)	Sometimes (3)	Often (2)	Very often (1)	☐
4. How many years have you smoked?	Never smoked (5)	10 years or less (4)	11-20 years (3)	21-30 years (2)	More than 30 years (1)	☐
5. What is your age?	Less than 40 years (5)	40-49 years (4)	50-59 years (3)	60-69 years (2)	70 years or older (1)	☐
						TOTAL ☐

Step 4: If your score is 18 or less, you may be at risk for Chronic Obstructive Pulmonary Disease (COPD). COPD includes chronic bronchitis, emphysema, or both.

FIGURE 19.14 Lung function questionnaire

- *Is the cough associated with any other symptoms such as chest or ear pain?*
- *Is it tiring?*
- *Are you concerned about it?*

History of respiratory infections

- *Do you have past history of breathing trouble or lung diseases such as bronchitis, emphysema, asthma or pneumonia?*
- *Does any other family member have a history of respiratory disease?*
- *Do you have any unusually frequent or unusually severe colds?*

Most people have had some colds. It is more meaningful to ask about excess number or severity.

- *Do you have any family history of allergies, tuberculosis or asthma?*

Smoking history

- *Do you smoke cigarettes, cigars or e-cigarettes?*
- *At what age did you start?*
- *How long have you smoked?*

ASSESSMENT GUIDELINES	CLINICAL SIGNIFICANCE AND CLINICAL ALERTS
• *Have you ever tried to quit? What helped? Why do you think it did not work?* • *What activities do you associate with smoking?* • *Would you like to speak to someone about trying to quit again now?* • *Do you live with someone who smokes?*	
Environmental exposure	
• *Are there any environmental conditions that may affect your breathing?* • *Where do you work? At a factory, chemical plant, coal mine, farming, outdoors in a heavy traffic area?* • *Have you travelled overseas recently?* • *Do you do anything to protect your lungs such as wear a mask or have the ventilatory system checked at work?* • *Do you do anything to monitor your exposure?* • *Do you have periodic examinations, pulmonary function tests or x-rays?*	Farmers may be at risk for grain or pesticide inhalation.
• *Do you know what specific symptoms to note that may signal breathing problems?*	General symptoms: cough, shortness of breath. Some gases produce specific symptoms: **carbon monoxide**—dizziness, headache, fatigue; **sulfur dioxide**—cough, congestion.
Health and lifestyle management	
• *What medications are you taking?* • *How are you coping with your illness?* • *What changes have you had to make to the way you live your life?* • *What impact has your illness had on your family members?*	**Respiratory depression** is a serious and life-threatening condition if it is not monitored and managed effectively. ***Clinical alert:*** **Respiratory depression** is slow and ineffective breathing. The following medications or combinations can significantly increase the risk of respiratory depression: benzodiazepines antipsychotics, anticonvulsants and opioids.
• *Are you up to date with COVID-19, flu and pneumococcal immunisations?*	
Additional subjective data for infants and children (questions for parents or guardians)	
• *Has the child had any frequent or very severe colds?*	Four to six uncomplicated upper respiratory infections per year is expected in early childhood.
• *Is there any history of allergy in the family?* (For a child under 2 years of age): • *At what age were new foods introduced?* • *Was the child breast fed or bottle fed?*	Consider new foods or formula as possible allergens.

ASSESSMENT GUIDELINES	CLINICAL SIGNIFICANCE AND CLINICAL ALERTS
• *Does the child have a cough?* • *Does the child seem to be congested?* • *Have you heard noisy breathing or wheezing?* (Further questions similar to those listed in the section on adults.) Screen for onset and follow a course of childhood chronic respiratory problems: asthma, bronchitis.	
• *What measures have you taken to child-proof your home and surrounding yards or balcony?* • *Is there any possibility of the child inhaling or swallowing toxic substances?* • *Are you familiar with emergency care measures in case of accidental choking?*	Young children are at risk for accidental aspiration, poisoning and injury.
• *Does anyone smoke in the home or in the car with the child?*	Environmental smoke increases the risk of ear and respiratory infections in children.
Additional subjective data for adults over 65 years	
Shortness of breath • *Have you noticed any shortness of breath or fatigue with your daily activities?*	Older adults have a less efficient respiratory system (decreased vital capacity, less surface area for gas exchange), so they have less tolerance for activity.
Physical activity • *Tell me about your usual amount of daily physical activity.*	May have reduced capacity to perform exercise because of pulmonary function deficits of ageing. Sedentary or bedridden people are at risk for respiratory dysfunction.
History of lung disease For those with a history of chronic obstructive pulmonary disease, lung cancer or TB: • *How are you getting along each day?* • *Has there been any weight change in the past 3 months?* • *How much have you lost/gained?*	People with chronic respiratory disease use large amounts of energy just breathing and may need nutritional support.
• *What is your energy level like?* • *Do you tire more easily?* • *How does your illness affect you at home?* • *How does your illness affect you at work?*	Activities may decrease because of increasing shortness of breath or pain.
Chest pain • *Do you have any chest pain with breathing?*	Some older adults feel **pleuritic pain** (sharp chest pain that worsens during breathing) less intensely than younger adults. Precisely localised sharp pain (points to it with one finger)—may be due to a fractured rib or muscle injury.

Objective data

Objective data collection begins at the first contact with the person (observation) for threats to the airway (partial or complete obstruction), difficulty breathing, a very rapid or very slow respiratory rate or other obvious abnormalities such as cyanosis. The presence of any of these abnormalities should prompt immediate intervention. A thorough assessment will involve collecting data through inspection, palpation and auscultation to evaluate lung function and respiratory health.

Preparation

Outline the process for respiratory assessment and ask the person for their consent to continue. Ask the person to sit upright. If they are comfortable doing so, ask them to disrobe to the waist. If they are not comfortable to do that, leave the gown on and open at the back. When examining the anterior chest, lift up the gown and drape it over the shoulders rather than removing it completely. This promotes comfort by giving the feeling of being somewhat clothed. These provisions will ensure further comfort: a warm room, a warm stethoscope diaphragm endpiece, adequate lighting and privacy.

Perform the inspection, palpation and auscultation on the posterior and lateral thorax. Then move to face the person and repeat the assessment on the anterior chest.

Finally, clean your stethoscope endpiece with antiseptic wipe. Because your stethoscope touches many people, it could be a possible vector for both aerobic and anaerobic bacteria. Cleaning your stethoscope is an essential measure to prevent cross-contamination.

Equipment needed

Hand hygiene solution
Stethoscope
Antiseptic wipe

PROCEDURES AND NORMAL FINDINGS	ABNORMAL FINDINGS AND CLINICAL ALERTS
A skills video (Respiratory assessment) is available to assist you in your skill development. Scan the QR code to access the videos (instructions on the inside front cover of the book to access multimedia resources)	
General inspection	
During subjective data collection you will have noticed the colour of the person's skin and mucous membranes, ease of breathing, tone of voice, height-to-weight ratio, level of hygiene and grooming and general demeanour. All these factors provide clues to the functioning of the lower respiratory system. Make note of your findings.	

PROCEDURES AND NORMAL FINDINGS	ABNORMAL FINDINGS AND CLINICAL ALERTS
Level of consciousness	
Assess the **level of consciousness**. A person who is alert and cooperative is conscious.	 ***Clinical alert:* Cerebral hypoxia** (reduced oxygen to the brain) may be reflected by excessive drowsiness or by anxiety, restlessness, confusion and irritability. These findings should trigger immediate intervention.
Skin, face, nailbeds, lips, earlobes, oral mucous membranes	
Inspect colour and condition of skin on face, nailbeds, lips, ear lobes and oral mucous membranes. The face, lips, nail beds and ear lobes are free of cyanosis or unusual pallor. The oral mucous membranes should be pink and moist. The nails are of normal configuration and pink. Explore any skin lesions (Chapter 22).	**Cyanosis** occurs due to lack of oxygenated blood supplying body tissues. Cyanosis can be **central**, meaning that there is a circulatory or ventilatory problem that leads to poor oxygenation in the lungs. **Peripheral cyanosis** occurs when there is an inadequate supply of oxygenated blood reaching the periphery. Peripheral cyanosis occurs as a consequence of arterial obstruction, venous obstruction, exposure to cold weather, reduced cardiac output or those related to the causes of central cyanosis. **Clubbing** of distal phalanx occurs with chronic respiratory disease.
Breathing effort	
Assess the quality of **breaths and breathing effort**. Normal relaxed breathing is automatic and effortless, regular and even and produces no noise. The chest expands symmetrically with each inspiration. Note any localised lag on inspiration.	Noisy breathing occurs with severe asthma or chronic bronchitis. Unequal chest expansion occurs when part of the lung is obstructed or collapsed, as with pneumonia or when guarding to avoid pain (Table 19.1).
Note the person's **facial expression.** The facial expression should be relaxed and benign, indicating an unconscious effort of breathing.	A person with COPD may look tense, strained and tired. They may purse the lips in a whistling position. By exhaling slowly and against a narrow opening, the pressure in the bronchial tree remains positive and fewer airways collapse (Table 19.2). **Cutaneous angiomas** (spider naevi) associated with liver disease or portal hypertension may be evident on the chest.
Inspect the posterior chest wall	
Note the **shape and configuration** of the chest wall. **Identify bony landmarks**—scapulae, ribs and spine. The spinous processes should appear in a straight line.	Skeletal deformities may limit thoracic cage excursion: scoliosis, kyphosis (Table 19.3).

PROCEDURES AND NORMAL FINDINGS	ABNORMAL FINDINGS AND CLINICAL ALERTS
The thorax is symmetrical, in an elliptical shape, with downward-sloping ribs, about 45 degrees relative to the spine. The scapulae are placed symmetrically in each hemithorax.	
The **anteroposterior diameter** should be less than the transverse diameter. The ratio of anteroposterior to transverse diameter is from 1:2 to 5:7.	Anteroposterior = transverse diameter or 'barrel chest'. Ribs are horizontal, chest appears as if held in continuous inspiration. This occurs in **chronic emphysema** from hyperinflation of the lungs (Table 19.3).
The **neck muscles and trapezius muscles** should be developed normally for age and occupation.	Neck muscles may be hypertrophied in COPD from aiding in forced inspiration and expiration.
Note the **position** the person takes to breathe. This includes a relaxed posture and the ability to support one's own weight with arms comfortably at the sides or in the lap. Take note of how freely the person can speak in between breaths. The person should be able to communicate in full sentences.	People with COPD often sit in a tripod position, leaning forwards with the arms braced against their knees, chair or bed. This gives them leverage so their accessory neck and shoulder muscles can aid in inspiration. A person who is short of breath may only be able to communicate in phrases or single words (Table 19.2).
Inspect **skin colour and condition of the chest wall**. Colour should be consistent with person's genetic background, with allowance for sun-exposed areas on the chest and the back. No cyanosis or pallor should be present. Note any lesions. Inquire as to any change in a naevus on the back—for example, where the person may have difficulty monitoring (Chapter 22).	Use the ABCD system when assessing lesions and naevi (A–asymmetry, B–border, C–colour, D–diameter) (Chapter 22). When assessing skin colour of a person with very dark skin, the ventral surface of the hand may be more useful than the dorsal when assessing for peripheral cyanosis or pallor. The oral mucosa may be most useful to assess for central cyanosis. **Cutaneous angiomas** (spider naevi) associated with liver disease or portal hypertension may be evident on the chest.
Palpate the posterior chest wall	
Confirm **symmetrical chest expansion** by placing your warmed hands on the posterolateral chest wall with thumbs at the level of T9 or T10. Slide your hands medially to pinch up a small fold of skin between your thumbs (Figure 19.15).	
Ask the person to take a deep breath. Your hands serve as mechanical amplifiers; as the person inhales deeply, your thumbs should move apart symmetrically. Note any lag in expansion.	Unequal chest expansion occurs with: • marked **atelectasis** (collapse of part or all of a lung, caused by a blockage of the bronchus or bronchioles) • **pneumonia** • **thoracic trauma**, such as fractured ribs, or • **pneumothorax** (abnormal collection of air in the pleural space). • Pain accompanies deep breathing when the **pleurae** are inflamed (Table 19.2).

PROCEDURES AND NORMAL FINDINGS	ABNORMAL FINDINGS AND CLINICAL ALERTS
FIGURE 19.15 Palpate symmetrical chest expansion—posterior	
Using the fingers, gently **palpate the entire chest wall**. This enables you to note any areas of tenderness, to note skin temperature and moisture, to detect any superficial lumps or masses and to explore any skin lesions noted on inspection.	**Crepitus** (coarse crackling sensation) palpable over the skin surface. It occurs in subcutaneous emphysema when air escapes from the lung and enters the subcutaneous tissue, as after open thoracic injury or surgery.
Auscultate the posterior chest wall for breath sounds	
The passage of air through the tracheobronchial tree creates a characteristic set of noises that are audible through the chest wall. These noises may also be modified by obstruction within the respiratory passageways or by changes in the lung parenchyma, the pleura or the chest wall.	
Auscultate breath sounds for quality. The person is sitting, leaning forwards slightly, with the arms resting comfortably across their lap. Instruct the person to breathe through the mouth, a little bit more deeply than usual, but to stop if they begin to feel dizzy. Be careful to monitor the breathing throughout the examination and offer times for the person to rest and breathe normally. Watch that they do not hyperventilate to the point of fainting.	See Table 19.4.
Use the flat diaphragm endpiece of the stethoscope and hold it firmly on the person's chest wall. Listen to at least one full breath in each location. Side-to-side comparison is most important.	

PROCEDURES AND NORMAL FINDINGS	ABNORMAL FINDINGS AND CLINICAL ALERTS
Do not confuse background noise with lung sounds. Become familiar with these extraneous noises that may be confused with lung pathology if not recognised.	Extraneous noise can be created by: • the examiner's breath on the stethoscope tubing • the stethoscope tubing bumping together • the person shivering • a man's hairy chest (movement of hairs under stethoscope sounds like crackles); noises caused by hair can be minimised by pressing harder or by wetting the hair with a damp cloth • rustling of the paper gown or paper drapes.
While standing behind the person, listen to the following lung areas—posterior from the apices at C7 to the bases (around T10) and laterally from the axilla down to the seventh or eighth rib. Use the sequence illustrated in Figure 19.16.	When assessing a person who is severely short of breath or physically tired and pathology is suspected in the bases or lower lobes, it may be necessary to commence listening at the bases and progress up towards the apices, as well as reduce the number of locations auscultated. This will ensure the adventitious sounds are heard while not exacerbating the person's dyspnoea.
Continue to visualise approximate locations of the lobes of each lung so you correlate your findings to anatomical areas. As you listen, think: • What *am* I hearing over this spot? • What should I *expect* to be hearing?	

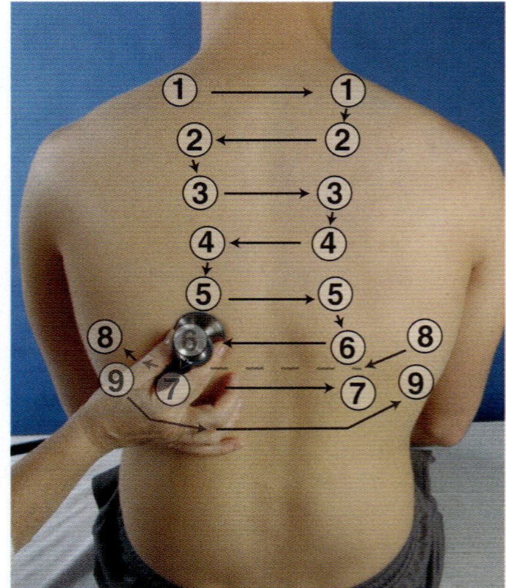

FIGURE 19.16 Auscultate posterior chest wall

PROCEDURES AND NORMAL FINDINGS	ABNORMAL FINDINGS AND CLINICAL ALERTS
You should expect to hear three types of normal breath sounds in an adult and older child: • **bronchial** (sometimes called tracheal or tubular) • **bronchovesicular** • **vesicular**. Study the description of the characteristics of these normal breath sounds in Table 19.4.	
Note the normal location of the three types of breath sounds on the chest wall of an adult and older child (Figures 19.16 and 19.17).	**Decreased or absent breath sounds occur:** When the bronchial tree is obstructed at some point by secretions, mucous plug or a foreign body. In emphysema, air movement is decreased because of loss of elasticity in the lung fibres and hyperinflation of the lungs, decreasing the force and noise of inspired air. When anything obstructs transmission of sound between the lung and your stethoscope, such as pleurisy or pleural thickening or air (pneumothorax) or fluid (**pleural effusion**) in the pleural space.

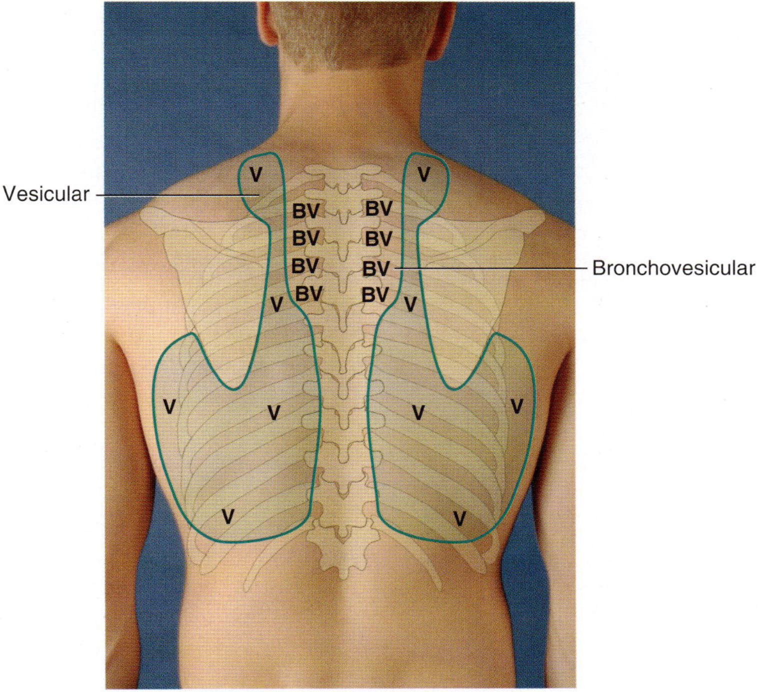

FIGURE 19.17 Location of normal breath sounds

PROCEDURES AND NORMAL FINDINGS	ABNORMAL FINDINGS AND CLINICAL ALERTS
	 ***Clinical alert:*** A silent chest means no air is moving in or out. This is an emergency. Report to a medical practitioner immediately.
	Increased breath sounds mean that sounds are louder than they should be (e.g. bronchial sounds are abnormal when they are heard over an abnormal location, the peripheral lung fields). They have a high-pitched tubular quality, with a prolonged expiratory phase and a distinct pause between inspiration and expiration. They sound very close to your stethoscope, as if they were right in the tubing close to your ear. They occur when consolidation (e.g. pneumonia) or compression (e.g. fluid in the intrapleural space) yields a dense lung area that enhances the transmission of sound from the bronchi. When the inspired air reaches the alveoli, it hits solid lung tissue that conducts sound more efficiently to the surface.
Abnormal (adventitious) sounds	
	Note the presence of any **abnormal (adventitious) sounds**. These are added sounds that are not normally heard in the lungs. If present, they are heard as being superimposed on the breath sounds. They are caused by moving air colliding with secretions in the tracheobronchial passageways or by the popping open of previously deflated airways. Sources differ as to the classification and nomenclature of these sounds (Table 19.5), but **crackles and wheezes** are terms most examiners use.
	One type of adventitious sound, **crackles**, is sometimes not pathological. These crackles are short, popping, crackling sounds that sound like fine crackles but do not last beyond a few breaths. When sections of alveoli are not fully aerated (as in people who are asleep or in the elderly), they deflate slightly and accumulate secretions. These physiologically 'normal' atelectatic crackles (Table 19.5) are heard when these sections are expanded by a few deep breaths. Crackles are heard only in the periphery, usually in dependent portions of the lungs and disappear after the first few breaths or after a cough. Crackles that persist beyond this should be considered pathological.
	During normal tidal flow, high-pitched wheeze occurs with asthma.

PROCEDURES AND NORMAL FINDINGS	ABNORMAL FINDINGS AND CLINICAL ALERTS
Inspect the anterior chest wall	
Note the **shape and configuration** of the chest wall. **Identify bony landmarks**—clavicles, sternum, ribs, costal angle. The ribs are sloping downwards with symmetrical intercostal spaces. The costal angle is within 90 degrees. Development of abdominal muscles is as expected for the person's age, weight and athletic condition.	**Barrel chest** has horizontal ribs and costal angle = 90 degrees. Hypertrophy of abdominal muscles occurs in chronic emphysema.
No retraction or bulging of the intercostal spaces should occur on inspiration.	**Retraction of the intercostal spaces** suggests obstruction of the respiratory tract or increased inspiratory effort is needed, as with atelectasis. **Bulging** indicates trapped air as in the forced expiration associated with emphysema or asthma.
Normally, accessory muscles are not used to augment respiratory effort. However, with very heavy exercise, the accessory neck muscles (scalene, sternocleidomastoid, trapezius) are used momentarily to enhance inspiration.	**Accessory muscles** are used in acute airway obstruction and massive atelectasis. Rectus abdominis and internal intercostal muscles are used to force expiration in COPD.
The respiratory rate is within normal limits for the person's age and the pattern of breathing is regular. Occasional sighs normally punctuate breathing.	Tachypnoea, bradypnoea, hyperventilation, hypoventilation, periodic breathing (Table 19.1).
Palpate the anterior chest	
Palpate **symmetrical chest expansion**. Place your hands on the anterolateral wall with the thumbs along the costal margins and pointing towards the xiphoid process (Figure 19.18).	An abnormally wide costal angle with little inspiratory variation occurs with emphysema.
Ask the person to take a deep breath. Watch your thumbs move apart symmetrically and note smooth chest expansion with your fingers. Any limitation in thoracic expansion is easier to detect on the anterior chest because greater range of motion exists with breathing here.	A lag in expansion occurs with atelectasis, pneumonia and postoperative guarding.
Palpate the anterior chest wall for any tenderness (normally none is present) and to detect any superficial lumps or masses (again, normally none are present). Note skin mobility and turgor and note skin temperature and moisture.	Tenderness, superficial lumps or masses.

PROCEDURES AND NORMAL FINDINGS	ABNORMAL FINDINGS AND CLINICAL ALERTS

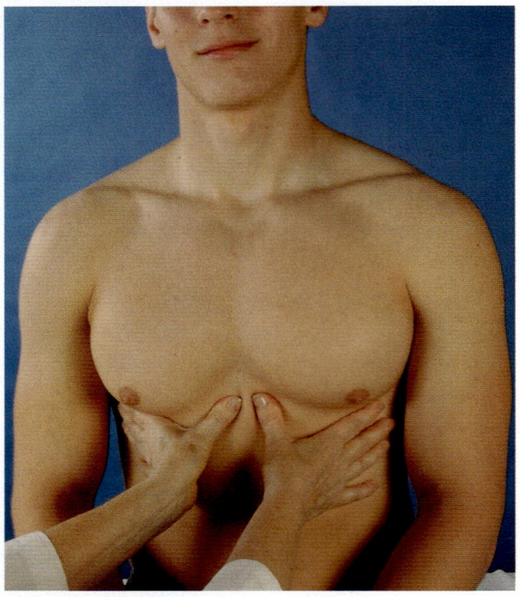

FIGURE 19.18 Palpate symmetrical chest expansion—anterior

Auscultate the anterior chest wall for breath sounds

Auscultate the lung fields over the anterior chest from the apices in the supraclavicular areas down to the sixth rib. Progress from side to side as you move downwards and listen to one full respiration in each location. Do not place your stethoscope directly over a female breast. Displace the breast and listen directly over the chest wall (under or to the side of the breast). Use the sequence illustrated in Figure 19.19.

Auscultate for normal breath sounds (Figure 19.20), noting any abnormal breath sounds and any adventitious sounds. If the situation warrants, assess the voice sounds on the anterior chest.

See Table 19.6 for a complete description of abnormal breath sounds.

Measure pulmonary function

The **forced expiratory time** is the number of seconds it takes for the person to exhale from total lung capacity to residual volume. It is a screening measure of airflow obstruction. Although the test is not usually performed in the respiratory assessment, it is useful when you wish to screen for pulmonary function.

PROCEDURES AND NORMAL FINDINGS	ABNORMAL FINDINGS AND CLINICAL ALERTS

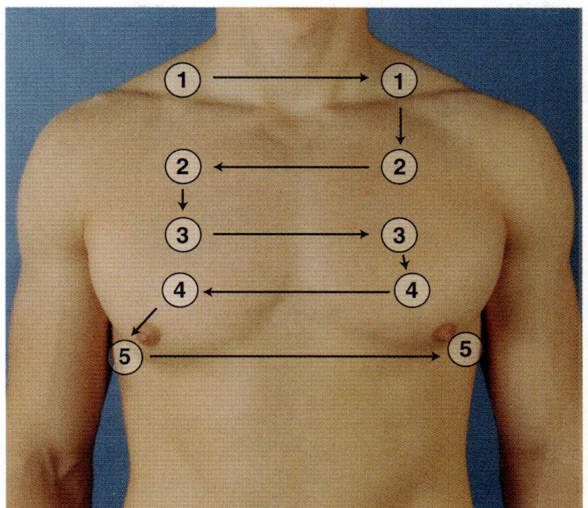

FIGURE 19.19 Auscultate the lung fields—anterior chest

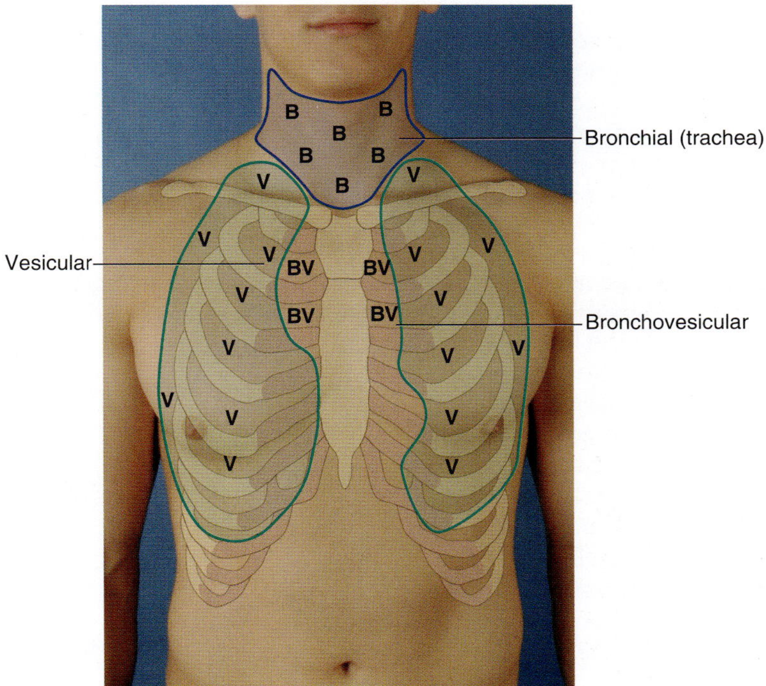

FIGURE 19.20 Palpation sites and normal breath sounds

PROCEDURES AND NORMAL FINDINGS	ABNORMAL FINDINGS AND CLINICAL ALERTS
Ask the person to inhale the deepest breath possible and then to blow it all out hard, as quickly as possible, with the mouth open. Listen with your stethoscope over the sternum. The normal time for full expiration is 4 seconds or less.	A forced expiration of 6 seconds or more occurs with obstructive lung disease. Refer this person for more precise pulmonary function studies.
The **pulse oximeter** is a noninvasive method to assess arterial oxygen saturation (SpO_2) and its use is described in Chapter 10. A healthy person with no lung disease and no anaemia normally has an SpO_2 of 95 to 98%. However, every SpO_2 result must be evaluated in the context of the person's haemoglobin level, acid–base balance and ventilatory status.	
The **6-minute distance (6MD) walk** is a safe, simple, inexpensive, clinical measure of functional status in ageing adults. The 6MD is used as an outcome measure for people in pulmonary rehabilitation because it mirrors conditions that are used in everyday life. Locate a flat-surfaced corridor that has little foot traffic, is wide enough to permit comfortable turns and has a controlled environment. Ensure the person is wearing comfortable shoes and equip them with a pulse oximeter to monitor oxygen saturation. Ask the person to set their own pace to cover as much ground as possible in 6 minutes and assure the person it is all right to slow down or to stop to rest at any time. Use a stopwatch to time the walk. A person who walks more than 300 m in 6 minutes is more likely to engage in activities of daily living.	Ask the person to stop the walk if you measure an SpO_2 below 88% or if extreme breathlessness occurs.
Additional objective data for infants and children	
To prepare, let the parent hold the infant supported against the parent's chest or shoulder (Figure 19.21). Do not let the usual sequence of the physical examination restrain you; seize the opportunity with a sleeping infant to inspect and then to listen to lung sounds next. This way you can concentrate on the breath sounds before the baby wakes up and possibly cries. Infant crying does not have to be a problem though because it enhances palpation of tactile fremitus and auscultation of breath sounds.	

PROCEDURES AND NORMAL FINDINGS	ABNORMAL FINDINGS AND CLINICAL ALERTS

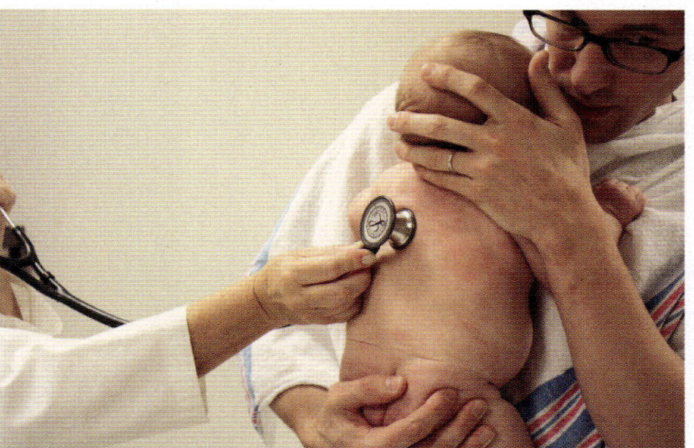

FIGURE 19.21 Auscultate posterior chest—infant

A child may sit upright on the parent's lap. Offer the stethoscope and let the child handle it. This reduces any fear of the equipment. Promote the child's participation; school-age children usually are delighted to hear their own breath sounds when you place the stethoscope properly. While listening to breath sounds, ask the young child to take a deep breath and 'blow out' your penlight while you hold the stethoscope with your other hand. Time your letting go of the penlight button so the light goes off after the child blows. Or ask the child to 'pant like a dog' while you auscultate.

Inspection

Infants have a rounded thorax with an equal anteroposterior-to-transverse chest diameter (Figure 19.22). By age 6 years, the thorax reaches the adult ratio of 1:2 (anteroposterior-to-transverse diameter). The newborn's chest circumference is 30 to 36 cm and is 2 cm smaller than the head circumference until 2 years of age. The chest wall is thin with little musculature. The ribs and the xiphoid are prominent; you can see as well as feel the sharp tip of the xiphoid process. The thoracic cage is soft and flexible.

Note a barrel shape persisting after age 6 years, which may develop with chronic asthma or cystic fibrosis.

In newborn males and females, the breasts may look enlarged by the second or third day from maternal estrogen. Occasionally a white fluid, sometimes referred to by the slang expression 'witch's milk', can be expressed. This resolves within a week.

PROCEDURES AND NORMAL FINDINGS	ABNORMAL FINDINGS AND CLINICAL ALERTS

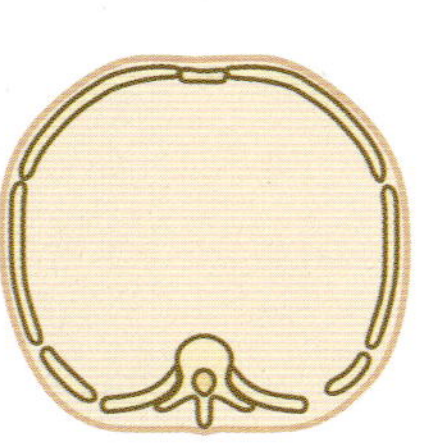
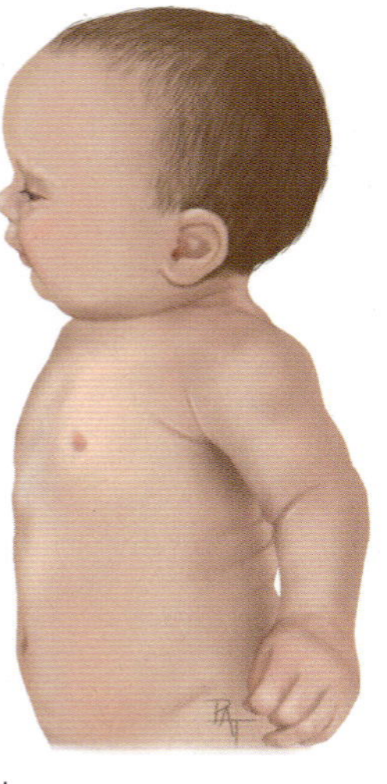

FIGURE 19.22 Thorax—infant

In some children, 'Harrison groove' occurs normally. This is a horizontal groove in the rib cage at the level of the insertion of the diaphragm, extending from the sternum to the midaxillary line.

Harrison groove also occurs with rickets from the pull of the diaphragm on weakened ribs.

A newborn's first respiratory assessment is part of the **Apgar scoring system** to measure the successful transition to extrauterine life (Table 19.7). The five standard parameters are scored at 1 minute and at 5 minutes after birth. A 1-minute Apgar with a total score of 7 to 10 indicates a newborn in good condition, needing only suctioning of the nose and mouth and otherwise routine care.
Apgar assesses skin colour, heart rate, respiration rate, muscle tone, reflexes and responsiveness. Each aspect is scored from 0 to 2, with 2 being the best score.

In the immediate newborn period, depressed respirations are due to maternal drugs, interruption of the uterine blood supply or obstruction of the tracheobronchial tree with mucus or fluid.

A 1-minute Apgar score with a total score of **3 to 6** indicates a moderately depressed newborn needing more resuscitation and subsequent close observation. **0 to 2** indicates a severely depressed newborn needing full resuscitation, ventilatory assistance and subsequent intensive care.

Infants breathe through the nose rather than the mouth and is an obligate nose breather until 3 months. Slight flaring of the lower costal margins may occur with respirations, but normally no flaring of the nostrils and no sternal retractions or intercostal retractions occur. The diaphragm is the newborn's major respiratory muscle. Intercostal muscles are not well developed. Thus, you observe the abdomen bulge with each inspiration but see little thoracic expansion.

Marked **retractions of sternum and intercostal muscles** indicate increased inspiratory effort, as in atelectasis, pneumonia, asthma and acute airway obstruction.

PROCEDURES AND NORMAL FINDINGS	ABNORMAL FINDINGS AND CLINICAL ALERTS
Count the respiratory rate for a full minute. Normal rates for the newborn are 30 to 40 breaths per minute but may spike up to 60 per minute. Obtain the most accurate respiratory rate by counting when the infant is asleep because infants reach rapid rates with very little excitation when awake. The respiratory pattern may be irregular when extremes in room temperature occur or with feeding or sleeping. Brief periods of apnoea less than 10 or 15 seconds are common. This periodic breathing is more common in premature infants.	**Rapid respiratory rates** accompany pneumonia, fever, pain, heart disease and anaemia. In an infant, tachypnoea of 50 to 100 per minute during sleep may be an early sign of heart failure.
Palpation Palpate symmetrical chest expansion by encircling the infant's thorax with both hands. Further palpation should yield no lumps, masses or crepitus, although you may feel the costochondral junctions in some normal infants.	**Asymmetrical expansion** occurs with diaphragmatic hernia or pneumothorax. **Crepitus** is palpable around a fractured clavicle, which may occur with difficult forceps delivery. **Rachitic rosary**—prominent round knobs at costochondral junctions—is seen in infants with rickets or scurvy.
Auscultation Auscultation normally yields bronchovesicular breath sounds in the peripheral lung fields of infants and young children up to age 5 or 6 years. Their relatively thin chest walls with underdeveloped musculature do not damp off the sound as do the thicker walls of adults, so breath sounds are louder and harsher.	**Diminished breath sounds** occur with pneumonia, atelectasis, pleural effusion or pneumothorax.
Fine crackles are the adventitious sounds commonly heard in the immediate newborn period from opening of the airways and clearing of fluid. Because the newborn's chest wall is so thin, transmission of sounds is enhanced and sound is heard easily all over the chest, making localisation of breath sounds a problem. Even bowel sounds are easily heard in the chest. Try using the smaller paediatric diaphragm endpiece or place the bell over the infant's intercostal spaces and not over the ribs. Use the paediatric diaphragm on an older infant or toddler.	Persistent **fine crackles** that are scattered over the chest occur with pneumonia, bronchiolitis or atelectasis. Crackles only in upper lung fields occur with cystic fibrosis; crackles only in lower lung fields occur with heart failure. **Expiratory wheezing** occurs with lower airway obstruction (e.g. asthma or bronchiolitis). When unilateral, it may be foreign body aspiration. Persistent peristaltic sounds with diminished breath sounds on the same side may indicate diaphragmatic hernia. **Stridor** is a high-pitched inspiratory crowing sound heard without the stethoscope, occurring with upper airway obstruction (e.g. croup, foreign body aspiration or acute epiglottitis).

PROCEDURES AND NORMAL FINDINGS	ABNORMAL FINDINGS AND CLINICAL ALERTS
Additional objective data for pregnant women	
The thoracic cage may appear wider, and the costal angle may feel wider than in the non-pregnant state. Respirations may be deeper, although this can be quantified only with pulmonary function tests.	
Additional objective data for adults over 65 years	
The rib cage commonly shows an increased anteroposterior diameter, giving a round barrel shape and **kyphosis** or an outward curvature of the thoracic spine (Table 19.3). The person compensates by holding the head extended and tilted back. You may palpate marked bony prominences because of decreased subcutaneous fat. Chest expansion may be somewhat decreased with the older person, although it should still be symmetrical. The costal cartilages become calcified with ageing, resulting in a less mobile thorax. The frail older person may tire easily, especially during auscultation when deep mouth breathing is required. Take care that this person does not hyperventilate and become dizzy. Allow brief rest periods or quiet breathing. If the person does feel faint, holding the breath for a few seconds will restore equilibrium.	
Common diagnostic tests	
Chest x-ray A chest x-ray is performed to assess for fractures of the bony thorax (sternum, ribcage, vertebrae) as well as the position and potential pathology associated with the contents of the thorax and mediastinum. An x-ray can highlight the presence of problems such as pneumonia, pulmonary oedema, pulmonary effusions, atelectasis, pneumothorax or malignancy.	An abnormal chest x-ray will be followed up with further diagnostic imaging such as a CT or VQ scan or an MRI.
Sputum microbiology, culture and sensitivity In the presence or suspected presence of a lower respiratory tract infection, a sputum sample will often be used to determine the presence of, type and antibiotic sensitivity of the culprit microorganism.	

PROCEDURES AND NORMAL FINDINGS	ABNORMAL FINDINGS AND CLINICAL ALERTS
Arterial blood gases Performed to evaluate the levels of oxygen and carbon dioxide, as well as the pH and oxygen-carrying capacity of arterial blood. Arterial blood gases are routinely used within critical care areas to guide oxygen therapy and ventilator support but may also be used in the diagnosis of respiratory failure in other areas of health care. Normal values: • pH: 7.35–7.45 • Oxygen saturation (SaO_2): 94.5–98.2% • PaO_2: 80–100 mmHg • $PaCO_2$: 35–45 mmHg **Venous blood gases** Used more commonly outside of the critical care areas to evaluate the level of carbon dioxide and pH of the venous blood. Unlike arterial blood gases, venous blood gases are not usually used to guide oxygen therapy. Pulmonary function testing is performed to evaluate the effectiveness of inspiration, expiration, lung capacity and the movement of gases (respiration) across the alveoli. Normal values: • pH: 7.32–7.43 • $PvCO_2$: 41–50 mmHg	

Abnormal findings

TABLE 19.1 Respiration patterns

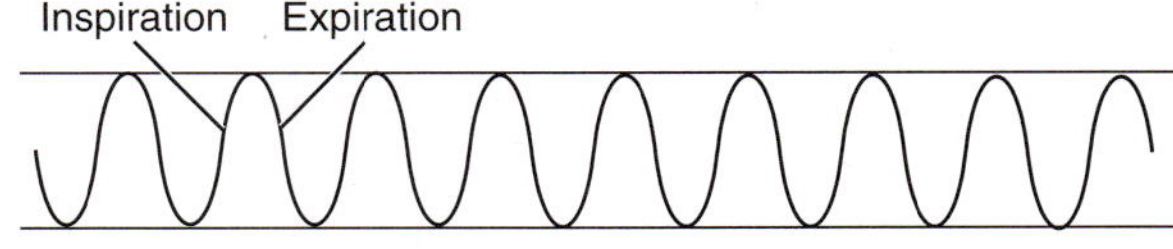

Normal adult (for comparison)

Rate: 10–20 breaths per minute
Depth: 500–800 mL
Pattern: regular
The ratio of pulse to respirations is fairly constant, about 4:1. Both values increase as a normal response to exercise, fear or fever.
Depth: air moving in and out with each respiration.

Tachypnoea

Rapid shallow breathing. This is a physiological response to fever, fear or exercise. Rate also increases with respiratory insufficiency, pneumonia, alkalosis, pleurisy and lesions in the pons. A rate of greater than 24 breaths per minute is a strong predictor of clinical deterioration.

Continued

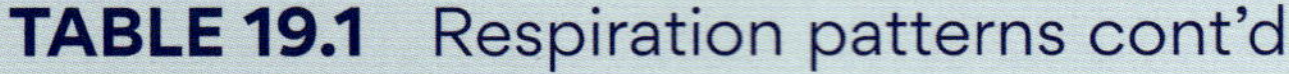

TABLE 19.1 Respiration patterns cont'd

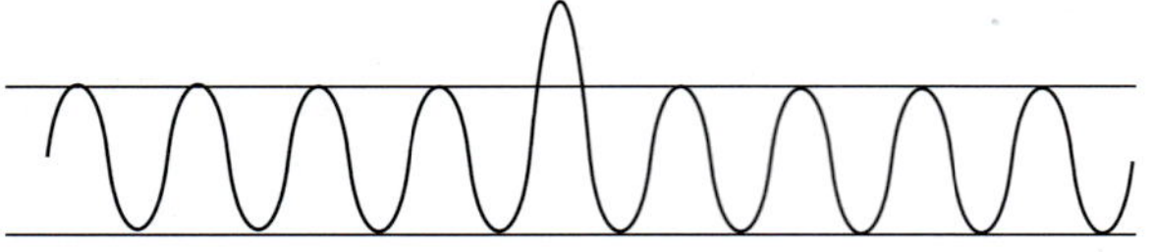

Sigh

Occasional sighs punctuate the normal breathing pattern and are purposeful to expand alveoli. Frequent sighs may indicate emotional dysfunction. Frequent sighs also may lead to hyperventilation and dizziness.

Hyperventilation

Increase in both rate and depth. Normally occurs with extreme exertion, fear or anxiety. Also occurs with diabetic ketoacidosis (Kussmaul's respirations), hepatic coma, salicylate overdose (producing a respiratory alkalosis to compensate for the metabolic acidosis), lesions of the midbrain and alteration in blood gas concentration (either an increase in carbon dioxide or decrease in oxygen). Hyperventilation blows off carbon dioxide, causing a decreased level in the blood (alkalosis).

Bradypnoea

Slow breathing. A decreased but regular rate (less than 10 per minute), as in drug-induced depression of the respiratory centre in the medulla, increased intracranial pressure and diabetic coma.

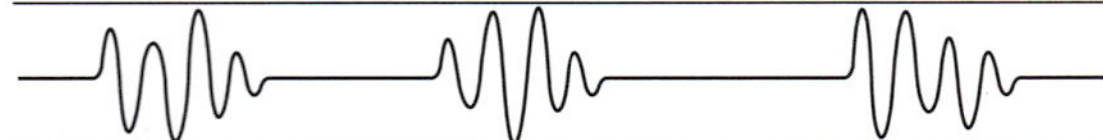

Biot's respiration

Similar to Cheyne-Stokes respiration, except that the pattern is irregular. A series of normal respirations (three to four) is followed by a period of apnoea. The cycle length is variable, lasting anywhere from 10 seconds to 1 minute. Seen with head trauma, brain abscess, heat stroke, spinal meningitis and encephalitis.

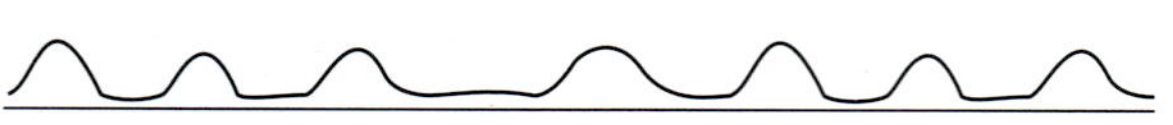

Hypoventilation

An irregular shallow pattern caused by an overdose of narcotics or anaesthetics. May also occur with prolonged bed rest or conscious splinting of the chest to avoid respiratory pain.

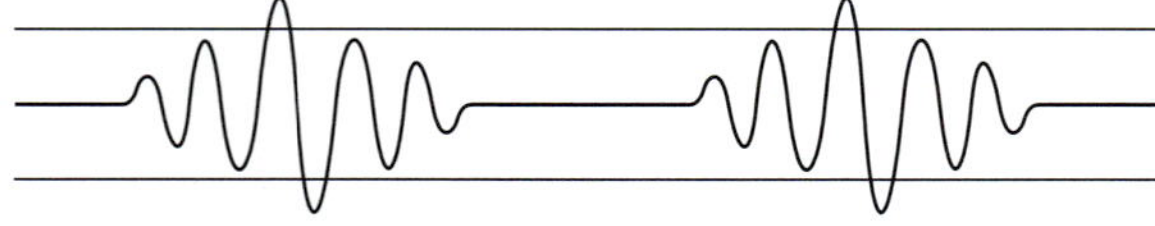

Chronic obstructive breathing

Normal inspiration and prolonged expiration to overcome increased airway resistance. In a person with COPD, any situation calling for increased heart rate (exercise) may lead to dyspnoeic episode (air trapping) because then the person does not have enough time for full expiration.

TABLE 19.1 Respiration patterns cont'd

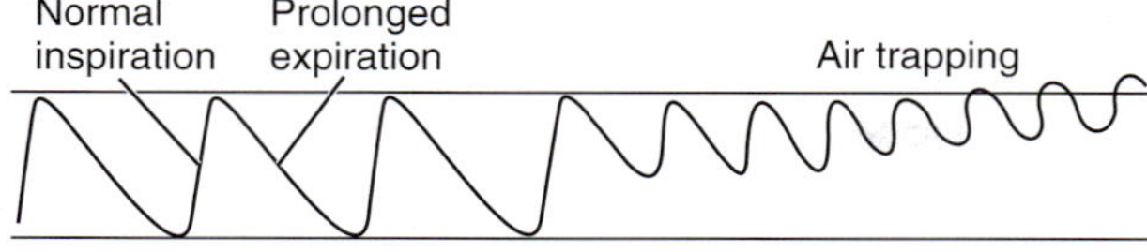

Cheyne-Stokes respiration

A cycle in which respirations gradually wax and wane in a regular pattern, increasing in rate and depth and then decreasing. The breathing periods last 30 to 45 seconds, with periods of apnoea (20 seconds) alternating the cycle. The most common cause is severe heart failure; other causes are renal failure, meningitis, drug overdose and increased intracranial pressure. Occurs normally in infants and ageing persons during sleep.

Note: Assess the (1) rate, (2) depth (tidal volume) and (3) pattern.

TABLE 19.2 Assessment of common respiratory conditions

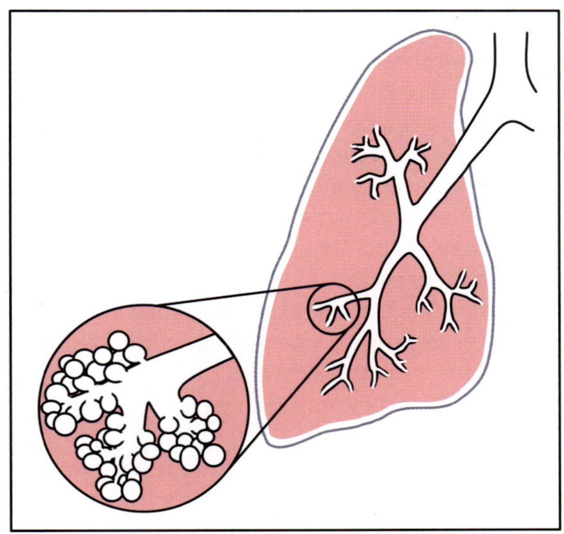

Normal lung (for comparison)

Inspection: Anteroposterior < transverse diameter, relaxed posture, normal musculature; rate 10 to 20 breaths per minute, regular, no cyanosis or pallor.
Palpation: Symmetrical chest expansion. No lumps, masses or tenderness.
Auscultation: Vesicular over peripheral fields. Bronchovesicular parasternally (anterior) and between scapulae (posterior). Infant and young child: bronchovesicular throughout.
Adventitious sounds: None.

Continued

TABLE 19.2 Assessment of common respiratory conditions cont'd

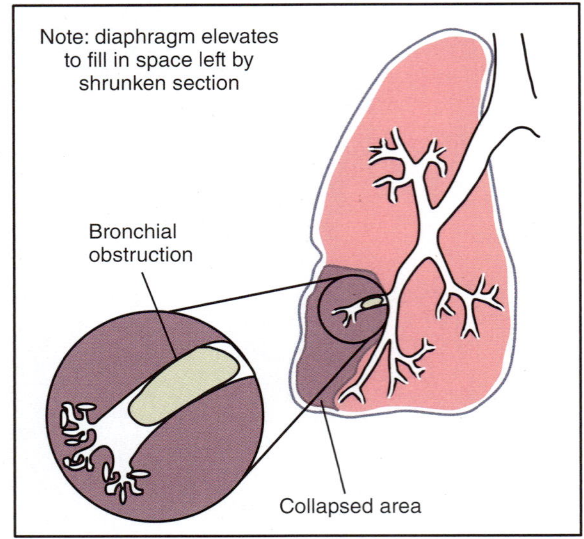

Atelectasis (collapse)

Condition: Collapsed shrunken section of alveoli or an entire lung, as a result of (1) airway obstruction (e.g. the bronchus is completely blocked by thick exudate, aspirated foreign body or tumour), the alveolar air beyond it is gradually absorbed by the pulmonary capillaries and the alveolar walls cave in; (2) compression on the lung; and (3) lack of surfactant (hyaline membrane disease).
Inspection: Cough. Lag on expansion on affected side. Increased respiratory rate and pulse. Possible cyanosis.
Palpation: Chest expansion decreased on affected side. With large collapse, tracheal shift towards affected side.
Auscultation: Breath sounds decreased vesicular or absent over area. Voice sounds variable, usually decreased or absent over affected area.
Adventitious sounds: None if bronchus is obstructed. Occasional fine crackles if bronchus is patent.

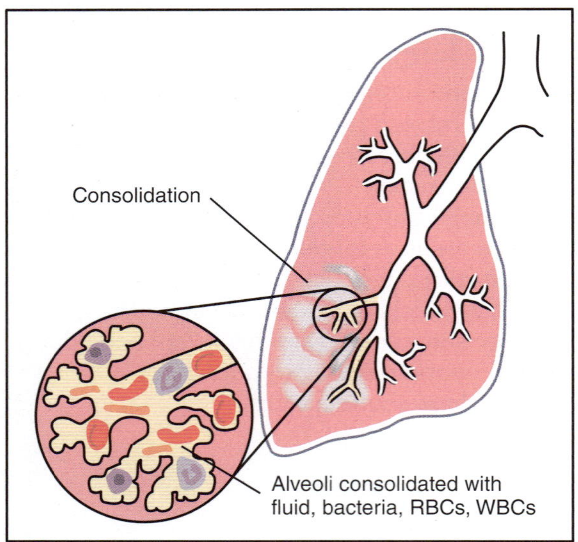

Lobar pneumonia

Condition: Infection in lung parenchyma leaves alveolar membrane oedematous and porous, so red blood cells and white blood cells pass from blood to alveoli. Alveoli progressively fill up (become consolidated) with bacteria, solid cellular debris, fluid and blood cells, all of which replace alveolar air. This results in decreased surface area of the respiratory membrane, which causes hypoxaemia.
Inspection: Increased respiratory rate. Guarding and lag on expansion on affected side. Children: sternal retraction, nasal flaring.
Palpation: Chest expansion decreased on affected side.
Auscultation: Breath sounds louder with patent bronchus, as if coming directly from larynx. Voice sounds have increased clarity, bronchophony, egophony, whispered pectoriloquy present. Children: diminished breath sounds may occur early in pneumonia.
Adventitious sounds: Crackles, fine to medium.

TABLE 19.2 Assessment of common respiratory conditions cont'd

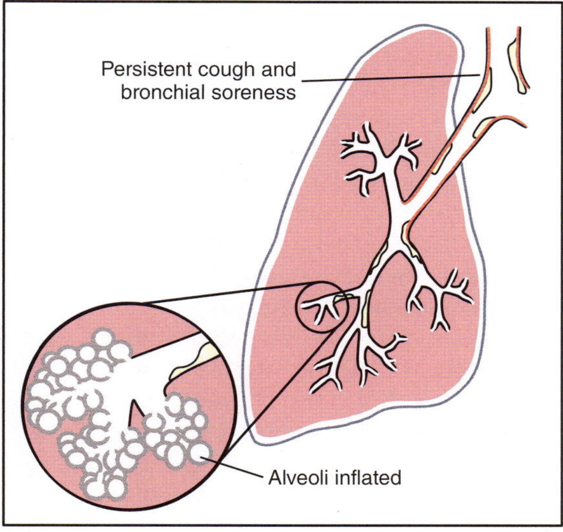

Bronchitis

Condition: Proliferation of mucous glands in the passageways, resulting in excessive mucus secretion. Inflammation of bronchi with partial obstruction of bronchi by secretions or constrictions. Sections of lung distal to obstruction may be deflated. Bronchitis may be acute or chronic with recurrent productive cough. Cigarette smoking usually causes chronic bronchitis.
Inspection: Hacking, rasping cough productive of thick mucoid sputum. Chronic: dyspnoea, fatigue, cyanosis, possible clubbing of fingers.
Auscultation: Normal vesicular. Voice sounds normal. Chronic: prolonged expiration.
Adventitious sounds Crackles over deflated areas. May have wheeze.

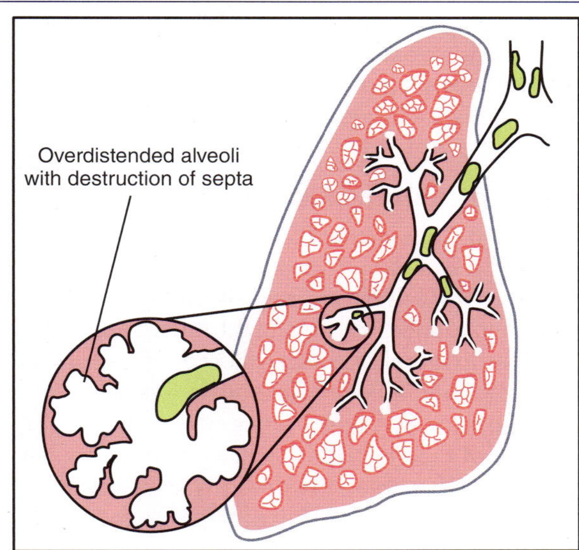

Emphysema

Condition: Caused by destruction of pulmonary connective tissue (elastin, collagen); characterised by permanent enlargement of air sacs distal to terminal bronchioles and rupture of interalveolar walls. This increases airway resistance, especially on expiration, producing a hyperinflated lung and an increase in lung volume. Cigarette smoking accounts for 80 to 90% of cases of emphysema.
Inspection: Increased anteroposterior diameter. Barrel chest. Use of accessory muscles to aid respiration. Tripod position. Shortness of breath, especially on exertion. Respiratory distress. Tachypnoea.
Auscultation: Decreased breath sounds. May have prolonged expiration. Muffled heart sounds resulting from overdistension of lungs.
Adventitious sounds Usually none; occasionally, wheeze.

Continued

TABLE 19.2 Assessment of common respiratory conditions cont'd

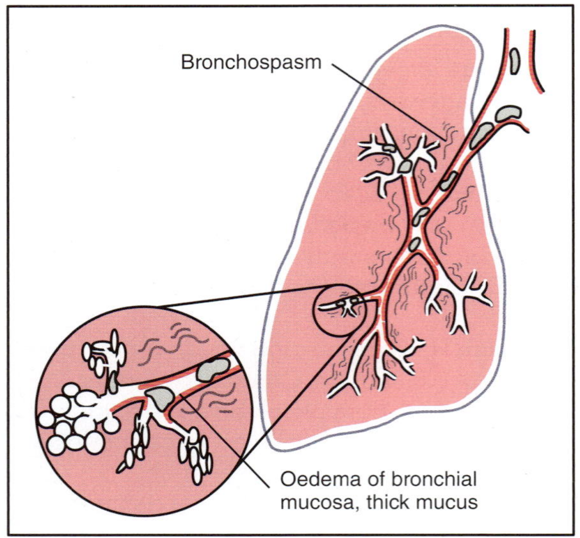

Asthma (reactive airway disease)

Condition: An allergic hypersensitivity to certain inhaled allergens (pollen), irritants (tobacco, ozone), microorganisms, stress or exercise that produces a complex response characterised by bronchospasm and inflammation, oedema in walls of bronchioles and secretion of highly viscous mucus into airways. These factors greatly increase airway resistance, especially during expiration and produce the symptoms of wheezing, dyspnoea and chest tightness.
Inspection: During severe attack: increased respiratory rate, shortness of breath with audible wheeze, use of accessory neck muscles, cyanosis, apprehension, retraction of intercostal spaces. Expiration laboured, prolonged. When chronic, may have barrel chest.
Auscultation: Diminished air movement. Breath sounds decreased, with prolonged expiration. Voice sounds decreased.
Adventitious sounds: Bilateral wheezing on expiration, sometimes inspiratory and expiratory wheezing.

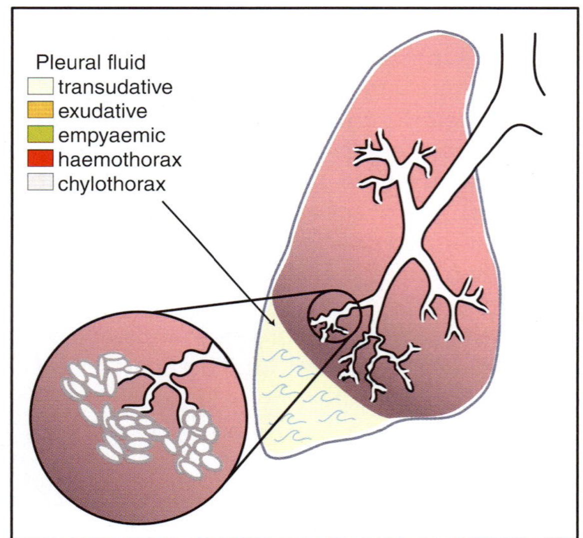

Pleural effusion (fluid) or thickening

Condition: Collection of excess fluid in the intrapleural space, with compression of overlying lung tissue. Effusion may contain watery capillary fluid (transudative), protein (exudative), purulent matter (empyaemic), blood (haemothorax) or milky lymphatic fluid (chylothorax). Gravity settles fluid in dependent areas of thorax. Presence of fluid subdues all lung sounds.
Inspection: Increased respirations, dyspnoea; may have dry cough, tachycardia, cyanosis, abdominal distension.
Auscultation: Breath sounds decreased or absent. Voice sounds decreased or absent. When remainder of lung is compressed near the effusion, may have bronchial breath sounds over the compression along with bronchophony, egophony, whispered pectoriloquy.
Adventitious sounds: None.

TABLE 19.2 Assessment of common respiratory conditions cont'd

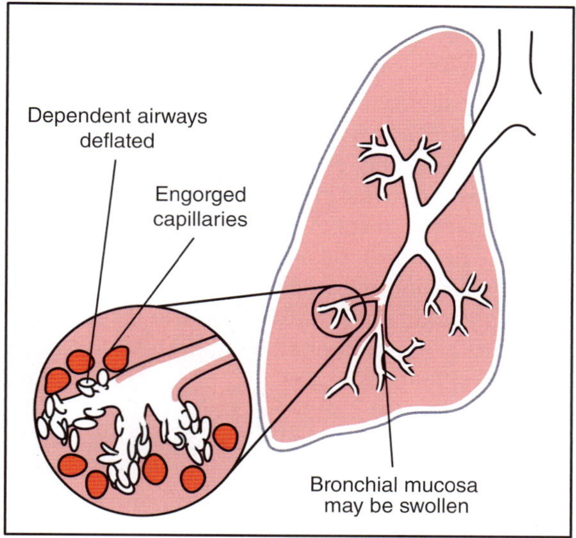

Heart failure

Condition: Pump failure with increasing pressure of cardiac overload causes pulmonary congestion or an increased amount of blood present in pulmonary capillaries. Dependent air sacs are deflated. Pulmonary capillaries engorged. Bronchial mucosa may be swollen.
Inspection: Increased respiratory rate, shortness of breath on exertion, orthopnoea, paroxysmal nocturnal dyspnoea, nocturia, ankle oedema, pallor in light-skinned people.
Auscultation: Normal vesicular. Heart sounds include S_3 gallop.
Adventitious sounds: Crackles at lung bases.

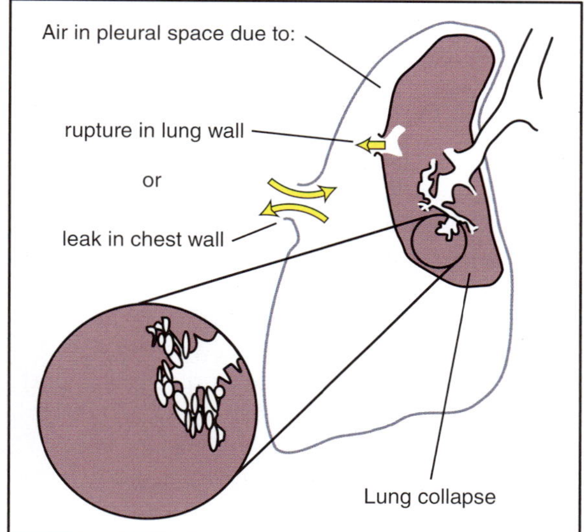

Pneumothorax

Condition: Free air in pleural space causes partial or complete lung collapse. Air in the pleural space neutralises the usual negative pressure present, so the lung collapses. Usually unilateral. Pneumothorax can be: (1) **spontaneous** (air enters pleural space through rupture in lung wall); (2) **traumatic** (air enters through opening or injury in chest wall); or (3) **tension** (trapped air in pleural space increases, compressing the lung and shifting mediastinum to the unaffected side).
Inspection: Unequal chest expansion. If large, tachypnoea, cyanosis, apprehension, bulging in intercostal spaces.
Palpation: Tracheal shift to opposite side (unaffected side). Chest expansion decreased on affected side. Tachycardia, decreased BP.
Auscultation: Breath sounds decreased or absent. Voice sounds decreased or absent.
Adventitious sounds: None.

Continued

TABLE 19.2 Assessment of common respiratory conditions cont'd

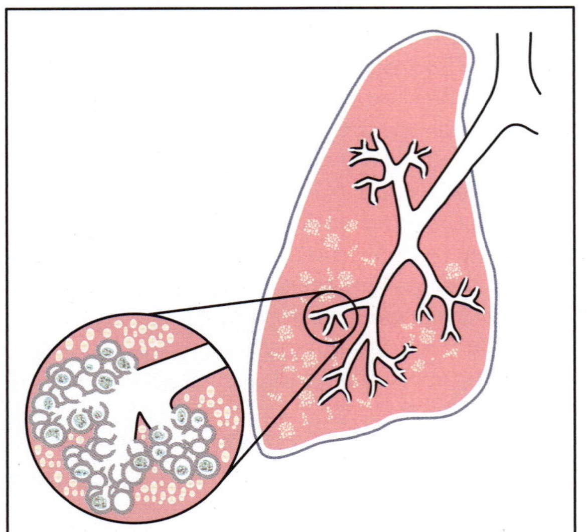

Pneumocystis jiroveci pneumonia

Condition: This virulent form of pneumonia is a protozoal infection associated with AIDS. The parasite *P. jiroveci* is common in the United States and relatively common in Australia and harmless to most people, except to the immunocompromised, in whom a diffuse interstitial pneumonitis ensues. Cysts containing the organism and macrophages form in alveolar spaces, alveolar walls thicken and the disease spreads to bilateral interstitial infiltrates of foamy, protein-rich fluid.
Inspection: Anxiety, shortness of breath, dyspnoea on exertion, malaise is common; also tachypnoea; fever; a dry, nonproductive cough; intercostal retractions in children; cyanosis.
Palpation: Decreased chest expansion.
Auscultation: Breath sounds may be diminished.
Adventitious sounds: Crackles may be present but are often absent.

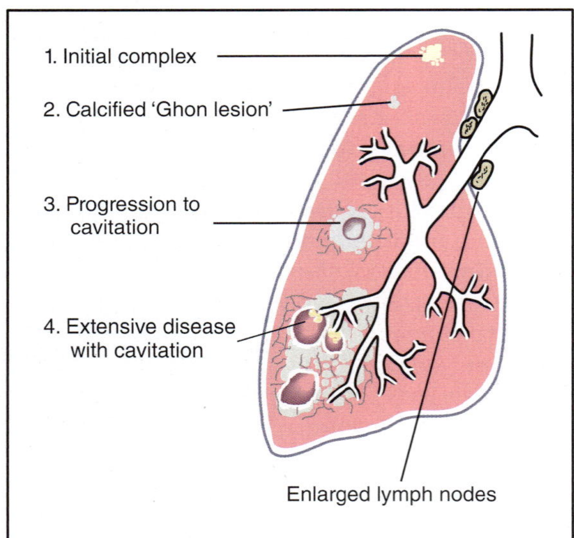

Tuberculosis

Condition: Inhalation of tubercle bacilli into the alveolar wall starts: (1) Initial complex is acute inflammatory response—macrophages engulf bacilli but do not kill them. Tubercle forms around bacilli; (2) scar tissue forms, lesion calcifies and shows on x-ray; (3) reactivation of previously healed lesion. Dormant bacilli now multiply, producing necrosis, cavitation and caseous lung tissue (cheese-like); (4) extensive destruction as lesion erodes into bronchus, forming air-filled cavity. Apex usually has the most damage.
Subjective: Initially asymptomatic, showing as positive skin test or on x-ray. Progressive TB involves weight loss, anorexia, easy fatiguability, low-grade afternoon fevers, night sweats. May have pleural effusion, recurrent lower respiratory infections.
Inspection: Cough initially nonproductive, later productive of purulent, yellow-green sputum, may be blood tinged. Dyspnoea, orthopnoea, fatigue, weakness.
Palpation: Skin moist at night from night sweats.
Auscultation: Normal or decreased vesicular breath sounds.
Adventitious sounds: Crackles over upper lobes common, persist following full expiration and cough.

TABLE 19.2 Assessment of common respiratory conditions cont'd

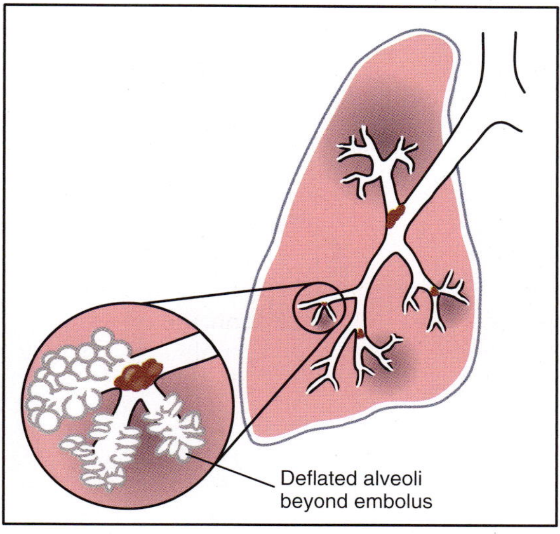

Pulmonary embolism

Condition: Pulmonary embolism is the occlusion of one or more pulmonary arteries. Undissolved materials (e.g. thrombus, air bubbles, fat globules) originating elsewhere in the body detach and travel through the venous system and right heart before lodging in the pulmonary artery(ies). Over 95% arise from deep vein thrombi in lower legs as a result of stasis of blood, vessel injury or hypercoagulability. Pulmonary embolism results in ischaemia of downstream lung tissue, increased pulmonary artery pressure, decreased cardiac output and hypoxia. Rarely, a saddle embolus in bifurcation of pulmonary arteries leads to sudden death from hypoxia. More often, small to medium pulmonary branches occlude, leading to dyspnoea. These may resolve naturally using the body's own fibrolytic activity or through the administration of fibrinolytics.
Subjective: Chest pain, worse on deep inspiration, dyspnoea.
Inspection: Apprehensive, restless, anxiety, mental status changes, cyanosis, tachypnoea, cough, haemoptysis, $PaO_2 < 80$ on pulse oximetry. Arterial blood gases show respiratory alkalosis.
Palpation: Diaphoresis, hypotension.
Auscultation: Tachycardia, accentuated pulmonic component of S_2 heart sound.
Adventitious sounds: Crackles, wheezes.

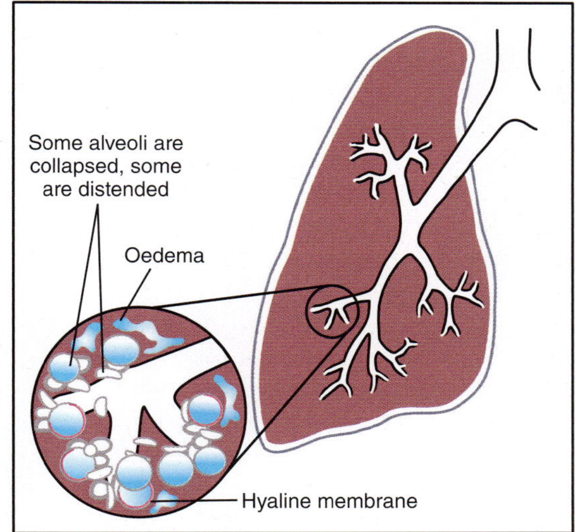

Acute respiratory distress syndrome

Condition: An acute pulmonary insult (trauma, gastric acid aspiration, shock, sepsis) damages alveolar capillary membrane, leading to increased permeability of pulmonary capillaries and alveolar epithelium and to pulmonary oedema. Gross examination (autopsy) would show dark red, firm, airless tissue, with some alveoli collapsed and hyaline membranes lining the distended alveoli.
Subjective: Acute onset of dyspnoea, apprehension.
Inspection: Restlessness, disorientation, rapid shallow breathing, productive cough, thin frothy sputum, retractions of intercostal spaces and sternum. Decreased PaO_2, blood gases show respiratory alkalosis, x-rays show diffuse pulmonary infiltrates, a late sign is cyanosis.
Palpation: Hypotension.
Auscultation: Tachycardia.
Adventitious sounds: Crackles, rhonchi.

TABLE 19.3 Configurations of the thorax

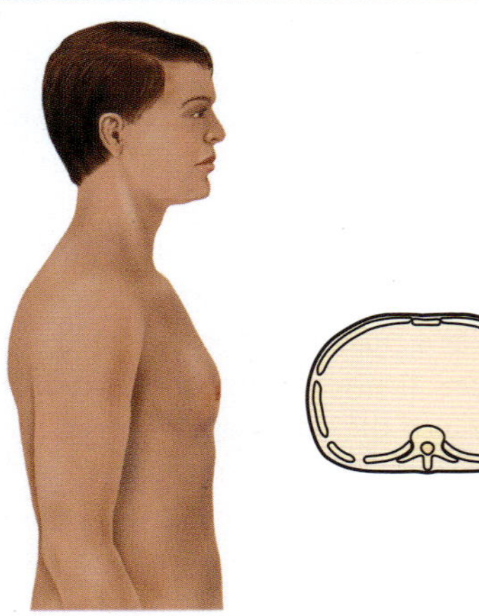

Normal adult (for comparison)

The thorax has an elliptical shape with an anteroposterior-to-transverse diameter of 1:2 or 5:7.

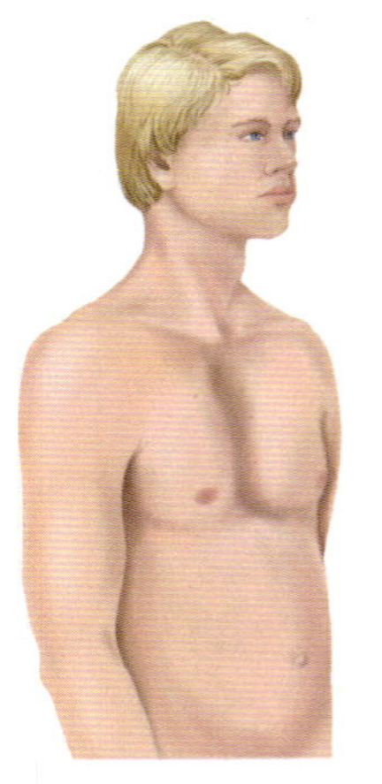
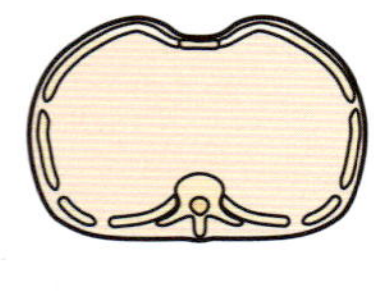

Pectus excavatum

A markedly sunken sternum and adjacent cartilages (also called funnel chest). Depression begins at second intercostal space, becoming depressed most at junction of xiphoid with body of sternum. More noticeable on inspiration. Congenital, usually not symptomatic. When severe, sternal depression may cause embarrassment and a negative self-concept. Surgery may be indicated.

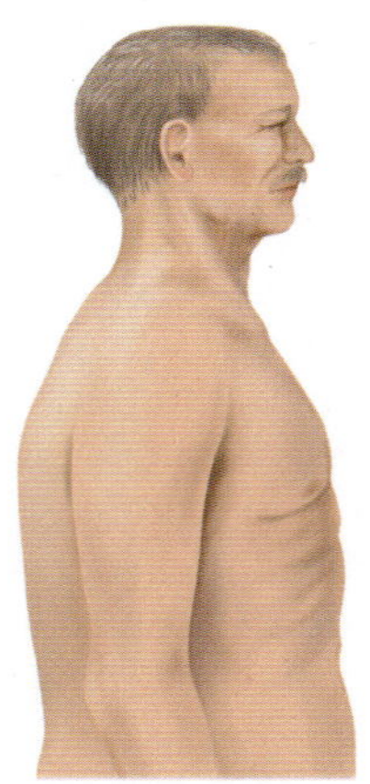
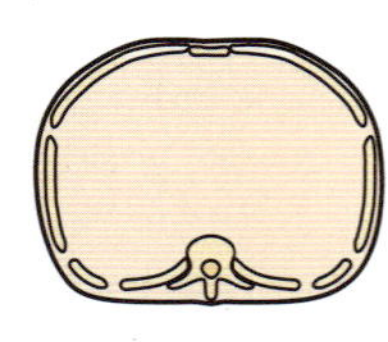

Barrel chest

Note equal anteroposterior-to-transverse diameter and that ribs are horizontal instead of the normal downward slope. This is associated with normal ageing and also with chronic emphysema and asthma as a result of hyperinflation of lungs.

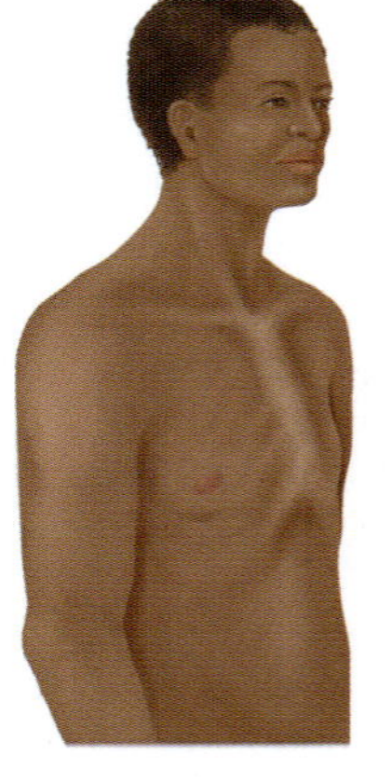
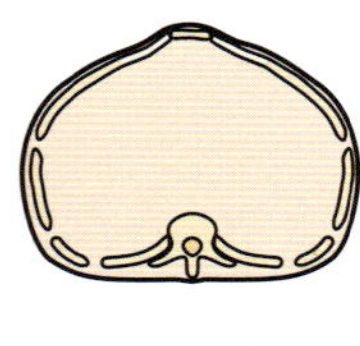

Pectus carinatum

A forward protrusion of the sternum, with ribs sloping back at either side and vertical depressions along costochondral junctions (pigeon chest). Less common than pectus excavatum, this minor deformity requires no treatment. If severe, surgery may be indicated.

TABLE 19.3 Configurations of the thorax cont'd

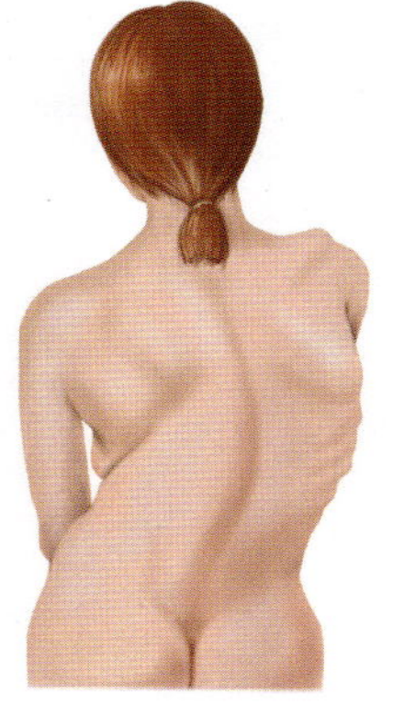
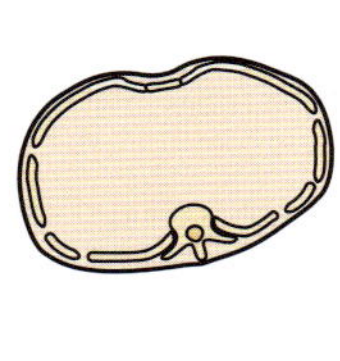

Scoliosis

A lateral S-shaped curvature of the thoracic and lumbar spine, usually with involved vertebrae rotation. Note unequal shoulder and scapular height and unequal hip levels, rib intercostal spaces flared on convex side. More prevalent in adolescent age groups, especially girls. Mild deformities are asymptomatic. If severe (> 45 degrees) deviation is present, scoliosis may reduce lung volume, then the person is at risk for impaired cardiopulmonary function. Primary impairment is cosmetic deformity, negatively affecting self-image. Refer early for treatment, often surgery.

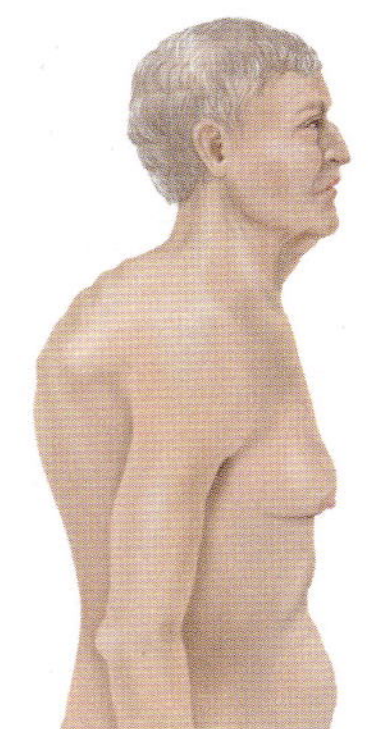
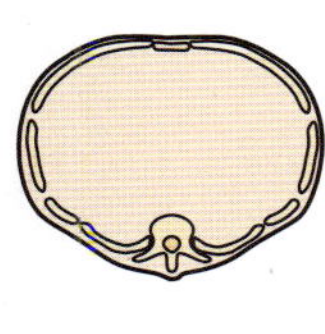

Kyphosis

An exaggerated posterior curvature of the thoracic spine (humpback) that causes significant back pain and limited mobility. Severe deformities impair cardiopulmonary function.
If the neck muscles are strong, compensation occurs by hyperextension of head to maintain level of vision.
Kyphosis has been associated with ageing, especially the familiar 'dowager's hump' of postmenopausal osteoporotic women. However, it is common well before menopause. It is related to physical fitness; women with adequate exercise habits are less likely to have kyphosis.

TABLE 19.4 Characteristics of normal breath sounds

	Pitch	Amplitude	Duration	Quality	Normal Location
Bronchial (tracheal)	High	Loud	Inspiration < expiration	Harsh, hollow tubular	Trachea and larynx
Broncho-vesicular 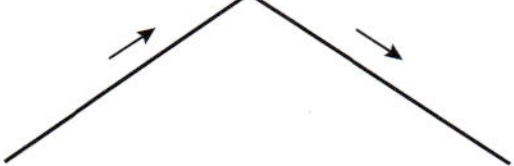	Moderate	Moderate	Inspiration = expiration	Mixed	Over major bronchi where fewer alveoli are located: posterior, between scapulae especially on right; anterior, around upper sternum in first and second intercostal spaces

Continued

TABLE 19.4 Characteristics of normal breath sounds cont'd

	Pitch	Amplitude	Duration	Quality	Normal Location
Vesicular 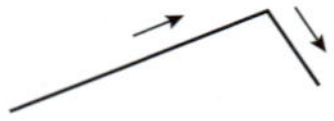	Low	Soft	Inspiration = expiration	Rustling, like the sound of the wind in the trees	Over peripheral lung fields where air flows through smaller bronchioles and alveoli

TABLE 19.5 Adventitious lung sounds

Sound	Description	Mechanism	Clinical Example
Discontinuous sounds **These are discrete, crackling sounds.**			
Crackles—fine Expiration Inspiration	Discontinuous, high-pitched, short crackling, popping sounds heard during inspiration that are not cleared by coughing; you can simulate this sound by rolling a strand of hair between your fingers near your ear or by moistening your thumb and index finger and separating them near your ear.	Inspiratory crackles: inhaled air collides with previously deflated airways; airways suddenly pop open, creating explosive crackling sound. Expiratory. crackles: sudden airway closing.	*Late inspiratory crackles* occur with restrictive disease: pneumonia, heart failure and interstitial fibrosis. *Early inspiratory crackles* occur with obstructive disease: chronic bronchitis, asthma and emphysema. *Posturally induced crackles* are fine crackles that appear with a change from sitting to the supine position or with a change from supine to supine with legs elevated.

TABLE 19.5 Adventitious lung sounds cont'd

Sound	Description	Mechanism	Clinical Example
Crackles—coarse	Loud, low-pitched, bubbling and gurgling sounds that start in early inspiration and may be present in expiration; may decrease somewhat by suctioning or coughing but will reappear shortly—sounds like opening a Velcro fastener.	Inhaled air collides with secretions in the trachea and large bronchi.	Pulmonary oedema, pneumonia, pulmonary fibrosis and the terminally ill who have a depressed cough reflex.
Atelectatic crackles	Sound like fine crackles but do not last and are not pathological; disappear after the first few breaths; heard in axillae and bases (usually dependent) of lungs.	When sections of alveoli are not fully aerated, they deflate and accumulate secretions. Crackles are heard when these sections re-expand with a few deep breaths.	In ageing adults, bedridden people or in people just aroused from sleep.
Pleural friction rub	A very superficial sound that is coarse and low pitched; it has a grating quality as if two pieces of leather are being rubbed together; sounds just like crackles, but *close* to the ear; sounds louder if you push the stethoscope harder onto the chest wall; sound is inspiratory and expiratory.	Caused when pleurae become inflamed and lose their normal lubricating fluid; their opposing roughened pleural surfaces rub together during respiration; heard best in anterolateral wall where greatest lung mobility exists.	Pleuritis, accompanied by pain with breathing (rub disappears after a few days if pleural fluid accumulates and separates pleurae).

Continued

TABLE 19.5 Adventitious lung sounds cont'd

Sound	Description	Mechanism	Clinical Example
Continuous sounds			
These are connected, musical sounds.			
Wheeze—high-pitched (sibilant)	High-pitched, musical squeaking sounds that sound polyphonic (multiple notes as in a musical chord); predominate in expiration but may occur in both expiration and inspiration.	Air squeezed or compressed through passageways narrowed almost to closure by collapsing, swelling, secretions or tumours; the passageway walls oscillate in apposition between the closed and barely open positions; the resulting sound is similar to a vibrating reed.	Diffuse airway obstruction from acute asthma or chronic emphysema.
Wheeze—low-pitched (sonorous rhonchi)	Low-pitched; monophonic single note, musical snoring, moaning sounds; they are heard throughout the cycle, although they are more prominent on expiration; may clear somewhat by coughing.	Airflow obstruction as described by the vibrating reed mechanism above; the pitch of the wheeze cannot be correlated to the size of the passageway that generates it.	Bronchitis, single bronchus obstruction from airway tumour.
Stridor	High-pitched, monophonic, inspiratory, crowing sound, louder in neck than over chest wall.	Originating in larynx or trachea, upper airway obstruction from swollen, inflamed tissues or lodged foreign body.	Croup and acute epiglottitis in children and foreign body inhalation, obstructed airway may be life threatening.

TABLE 19.6 Voice sounds

Technique	Normal Finding	Abnormal Finding
Bronchophony Ask the person to repeat 'ninety-nine' while you listen with the stethoscope over the chest wall; listen especially if you suspect pathology.	Normal voice transmission is soft, muffled and indistinct; you can hear sound through the stethoscope but cannot distinguish exactly what is being said.	Pathology that increases lung density will enhance transmission of voice sounds; you auscultate a clear 'ninety-nine'. The words are more distinct than normal and sound close to your ear.
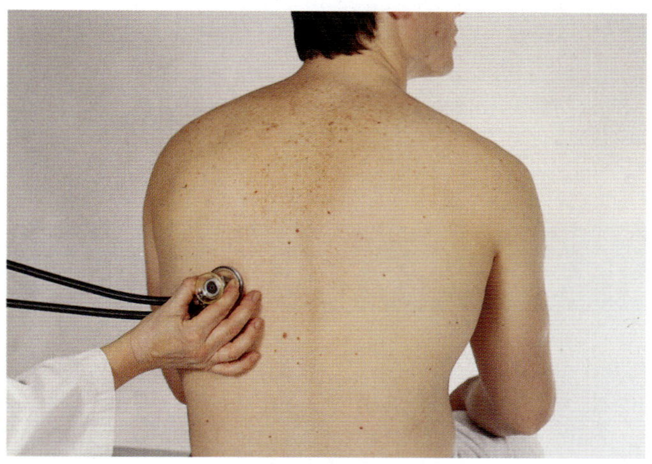		
Egophony (Greek: the voice of a goat) Auscultate the chest while the person phonates a long 'ee-ee-ee-ee' sound.	Normally, you should hear 'eeeeee' through your stethoscope.	Over area of consolidation or compression, the spoken 'eeeeee' sound changes to a bleating long 'aaaaaa' sound.
Whispered pectoriloquy Ask the person to whisper a phrase like 'one-two-three' as you auscultate.	The normal response is faint, muffled and almost inaudible.	With only small amounts of consolidation, the whispered voice is transmitted very clearly and distinctly, although still somewhat faint; it sounds as if the person is whispering right into your stethoscope, 'one-two-three'.

TABLE 19.7 Apgar scoring system

	2	1	0
Heart rate	Over 100	Slow (below 100)	Absent
Respiratory effort	Good, sustained cry; regular respirations	Slow, irregular, shallow	Absent
Muscle tone	Active motion, spontaneous flexion	Some flexion of extremities; some resistance to extension	Limp, flaccid
Reflex irritability (response to catheter nares)	Sneeze, cough, cry	Grimace, frown	No response
Colour	Completely pink	Body pink, extremities pale	Cyanotic, pale
			Total score

Further objective assessment for advanced practice

The assessments described in the following section require advanced knowledge, skill and scope of practice. Nurses working in specialist respiratory units, intensive care units and nurses working in community centres may need to develop these skills. Nurses who work in specialist respiratory units or are in specialist positions will be assessing people with chronic illness involving not only the respiratory system but the cardiac and neuromuscular systems, for example. See Tables 19.2 and 19.8.

Equipment

In addition to previously identified equipment: a centimetre ruler.

PROCEDURES AND NORMAL FINDINGS	ABNORMAL FINDINGS AND CLINICAL ALERTS
Palpate posterior chest wall for tactile fremitus	
Assess **tactile** (or **vocal**) **fremitus**. Fremitus is a palpable vibration. Sounds generated from the larynx are transmitted through patent bronchi and through the lung parenchyma to the chest wall, where you feel them as vibrations. Use either the palmar base (the ball) of the fingers or the ulnar edge of one hand and touch the person's chest while they repeat the words 'ninety-nine' or 'blue balloon'. These are resonant phrases that generate strong vibrations. Start over the lung apices and palpate from one side to another (Figure 19.23).	**Decreased fremitus** occurs when anything obstructs transmission of vibrations (e.g. obstructed bronchus, pleural effusion or thickening, pneumothorax or emphysema). Any barrier that comes between the sound and your palpating hand will decrease fremitus. **Increased fremitus** occurs with compression or consolidation of lung tissue (e.g. lobar pneumonia). This is present only when the bronchus is patent and when the consolidation extends to the lung surface. Note that only gross changes increase fremitus. Small areas of early pneumonia do not significantly affect fremitus.

PROCEDURES AND NORMAL FINDINGS

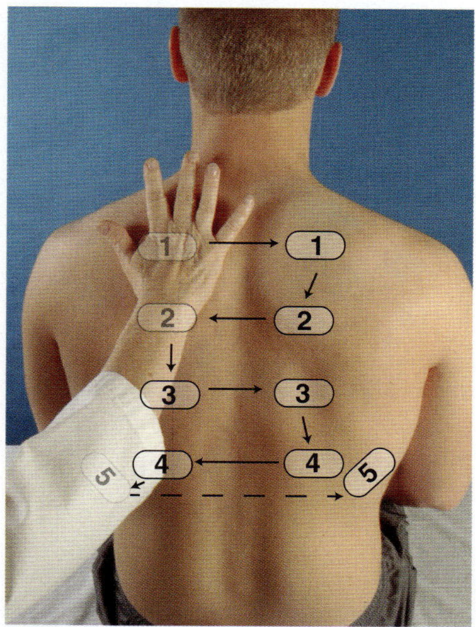

FIGURE 19.23 Palpate tactile fremitus—posterior chest

Fremitus varies among people, but symmetry is most important; the vibrations should feel the same in the corresponding area on each side. However, just between the scapulae, fremitus may feel stronger on the right side than on the left side because the right side is closer to the bronchial bifurcation. Avoid palpating over the scapulae because bone damps out sound transmission. The following factors affect the normal intensity of tactile fremitus:

Relative location of bronchi to the chest wall
Normally, fremitus is most prominent between the scapulae and around the sternum, sites where the major bronchi are closest to the chest wall. Fremitus normally decreases as you progress down because more and more tissue impedes sound transmission.

Thickness of the chest wall
Fremitus feels greater over a thin chest wall than over an obese or heavily muscular one where thick tissue damps the vibration.

ABNORMAL FINDINGS AND CLINICAL ALERTS

Rhonchal fremitus is palpable with thick bronchial secretions.

Pleural friction fremitus is palpable with inflammation of the pleura (Table 19.9).

PROCEDURES AND NORMAL FINDINGS	ABNORMAL FINDINGS AND CLINICAL ALERTS
Pitch and intensity A loud, low-pitched voice generates more fremitus than a soft, high-pitched one. Note any areas of abnormal fremitus. Sound is conducted better through a uniformly dense structure than through a porous one, which changes in shape and solidity (as does the lung tissue during normal respiration). Thus, conditions that increase the density of lung tissue make a better conducting medium for sound vibrations and increase tactile fremitus.	
Palpate the anterior chest wall for tactile fremitus	
Assess **tactile (vocal) fremitus**. Begin palpating over the lung apices in the supraclavicular areas (Figure 19.24). Compare vibrations from one side to the other as the person repeats 'ninety-nine'. Avoid palpating over female breast tissue because breast tissue normally damps the sound.	A palpable grating sensation with breathing indicates pleural friction fremitus (Table 19.9).
Percuss posterior lung fields	
Determine the **predominant note over the lung fields**. Start at the apices and percuss the band of normally resonant tissue across the tops of both shoulders (Figure 19.25). Then, percussing in the intercostal spaces, make a side-to-side comparison all the way down the lung region. Percuss at 5 cm intervals. Avoid the damping effect of the scapulae and ribs.	
Resonance is the low-pitched, clear, hollow sound that predominates in healthy lung tissue in adults (Figure 19.26). However, resonance is a relative term and has no constant standard. The resonant note may be modified somewhat in the athlete with a heavily muscular chest wall and in the heavily obese adult in whom subcutaneous fat produces scattered dullness. The depth of penetration of percussion has limits. Percussion sets into motion only the outer 5 to 7 cm of tissue. It will not penetrate to reveal any change in density deeper than that. Also, an abnormal finding must be 2 to 3 cm wide to yield an abnormal percussion note. Lesions smaller than that are not detectable by percussion.	**Hyperresonance** is a lower pitched, booming sound found when too much air is present, as in emphysema or pneumothorax. A **dull** note (soft, muffled thud) signals abnormal density in the lungs, as with pneumonia, pleural effusion, atelectasis or tumour.

PROCEDURES AND NORMAL FINDINGS

ABNORMAL FINDINGS AND CLINICAL ALERTS

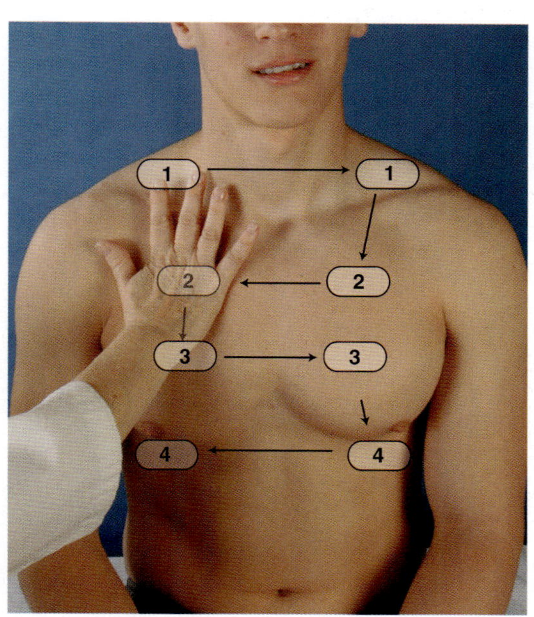

FIGURE 19.24 Palpate tactile (vocal) fremitus—anterior chest

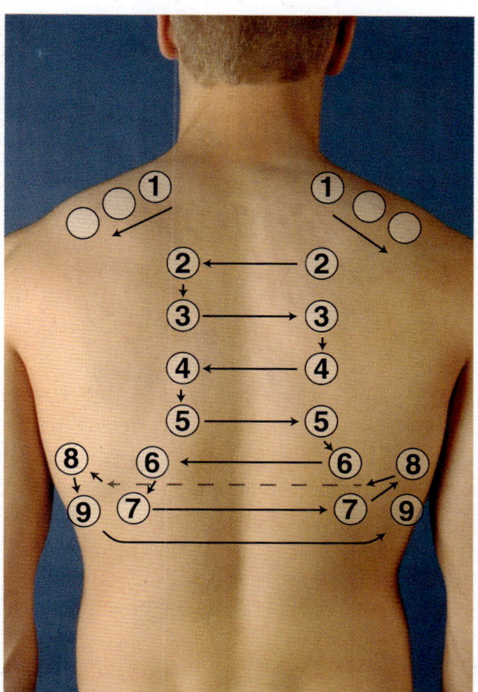

FIGURE 19.25 Percuss posterior lung fields

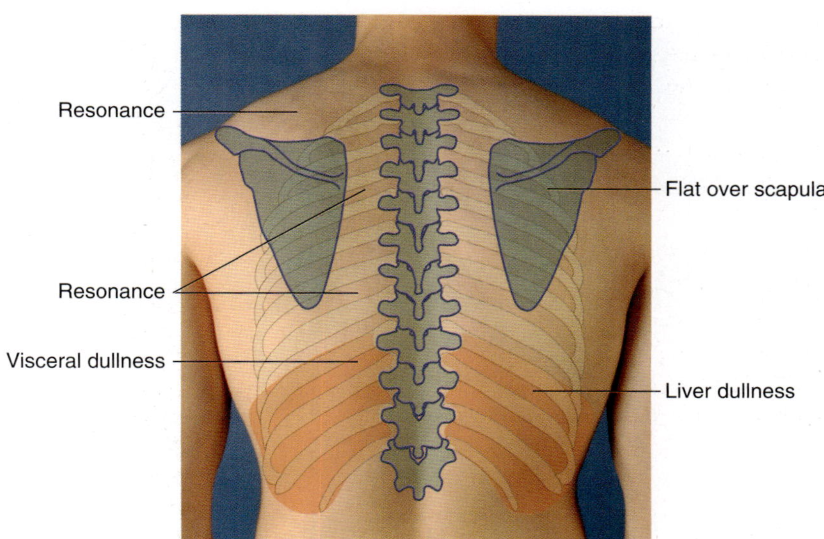

FIGURE 19.26 Percuss posterior chest for resonance

PROCEDURES AND NORMAL FINDINGS	ABNORMAL FINDINGS AND CLINICAL ALERTS
Diaphragmatic excursion	
Determine **diaphragmatic excursion** (Figure 19.27A). Percuss to map out the lower lung border, both in expiration and in inspiration. First, ask the person to 'exhale and hold it' briefly while you percuss down the scapular line until the sound changes from resonant to dull on each side. This estimates the level of the diaphragm separating the lungs from the abdominal viscera. It may be somewhat higher on the right side (1–2 cm) because of the presence of the liver. Mark the spot.	
Now ask the person to 'take a deep breath and hold it'. Continue percussing down from your first mark and mark the level where the sound changes to dull on this deep inspiration. Measure the difference. This diaphragmatic excursion should be equal bilaterally and measure about 3 to 5 cm in adults, although it may be up to 7 or 8 cm in well-conditioned people (Figure 19.27B).	Note an abnormally high level of dullness and absence of excursion. These occur with pleural effusion (fluid in the space between the visceral and parietal pleura) or atelectasis of the lower lobes.

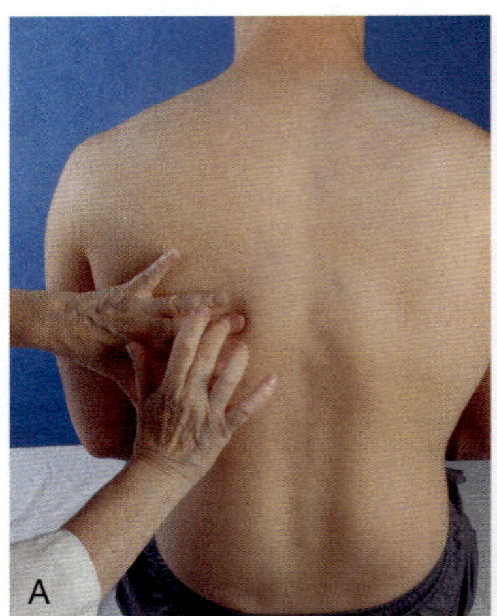

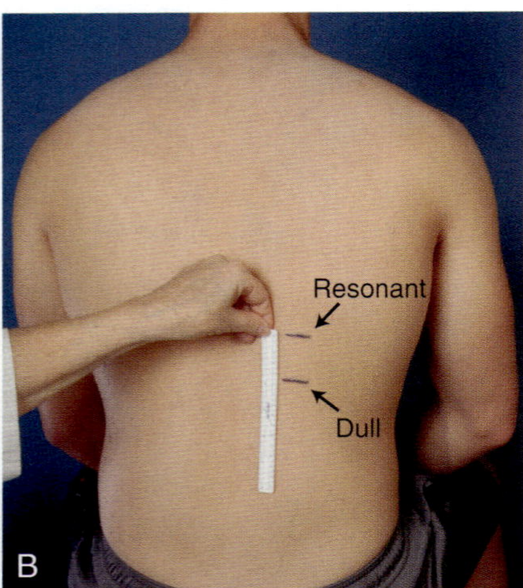

FIGURE 19.27A & B Determine diaphragmatic excursion

PROCEDURES AND NORMAL FINDINGS	ABNORMAL FINDINGS AND CLINICAL ALERTS
Percuss anterior lung fields	
Begin percussing the apices in the supraclavicular areas. Then, percussing the intercostal spaces and comparing one side to the other, move down the anterior chest. Intercostal spaces are easier to palpate on the anterior chest than on the back. Do not percuss directly over female breast tissue because this would produce a dull note. Shift the breast tissue over slightly using the edge of your stationary hand. In females with large breasts, percussion may yield little useful data. With all people, use the sequence illustrated in Figure 19.24.	
Sequence for percussion of anterior chest	
Note the borders of cardiac dullness normally found on the anterior chest and do not confuse these with suspected lung pathology (Figure 19.28). In the right hemithorax, the upper border of liver dullness is in the fifth intercostal space in the right midclavicular line. On the left, tympany is evident over the gastric space.	Lungs are hyperinflated with chronic emphysema, resulting in hyperresonance where you would expect cardiac dullness.

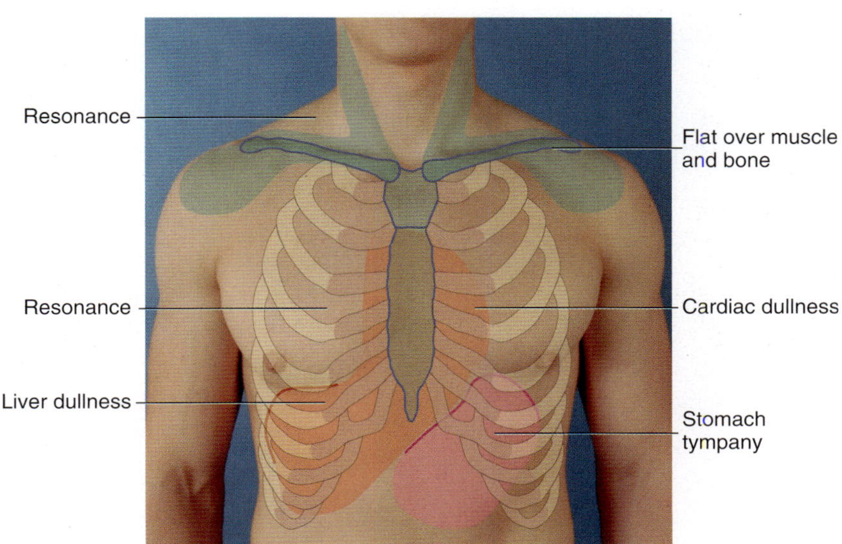

FIGURE 19.28 Percussion notes—anterior chest

PROCEDURES AND NORMAL FINDINGS	ABNORMAL FINDINGS AND CLINICAL ALERTS
Auscultate for vocal sounds	
Determine the quality of **voice sounds** or **vocal resonance.** The spoken voice can be auscultated over the chest wall just as it can be felt in tactile fremitus. Ask the person to repeat a phrase such as 'ninety-nine' while you listen over the chest wall. Normal voice transmission is soft, muffled and indistinct; you can hear sound through the stethoscope but cannot distinguish exactly what is being said. Pathology that increases lung density enhances transmission of voice sounds. Eliciting the voice sounds is not usually done in the routine examination. Rather, these are supplemental manoeuvres that may be used by nurses working in advanced practice roles. When they are performed, the advance practice nurse is assessing for possible presence of **bronchophony**, **egophony** and **whispered pectoriloquy** (Table 19.9).	Consolidation or compression of lung tissue will enhance the voice sounds, making the words more distinct.

Abnormal findings for advanced practice

TABLE 19.8 Diagnostic clues to chronic dyspnoea and associated systems

System/ Physiology	Example	History	Examination	Diagnostic Study
Pulmonary				
Alveolar	Chronic pneumonia	Fever, productive cough, shortness of breath	Fever, crackles, increased fremitus, bronchophony	Chest radiography, chest CT, bronchoscopy/ bronchoalveolar lavage, culture or biopsy
Interstitial	Idiopathic fibrosis	Exertional dyspnoea, dry cough, malignancy, prescription or illicit drug use, chemical exposures	Hypoxia, clubbing, persistent inspiratory crackles	Chest radiography (fibrosis, interstitial markings), chest CT, bronchoscopy/ biopsy

TABLE 19.8 Diagnostic clues to chronic dyspnoea and associated systems cont'd

System/ Physiology	Example	History	Examination	Diagnostic Study
Obstruction of air flow	Chronic obstructive pulmonary disease	Tobacco use, cough, relief with bronchodilator, increased sputum production, haemoptysis and weight loss with malignancy	Wheezing, barrel chest, decreased breath sounds, accessory muscle use, clubbing, paradoxical pulse	Peak flow, spirometry, chest radiography (hyperinflation), PFT
Restrictive	Pleural effusion	Pleuritic chest pain, dyspnoea not improved with oxygen	Decreased breath sounds, chest morphology, pleural rub, basal dullness	Chest radiography (effusion, anatomical abnormality), spirometry, pulmonary function testing
Vascular	Chronic pulmonary emboli	Fatigue, pleuritic chest pain, prior emboli/ deep venous thrombosis, syncope	Wheezing, lower extremity swelling, pleural rub, prominent P_2, murmur, right ventricular heave, jugular vein distension (JVD)	D-dimer, ventilation/ perfusion scan, CT angiography, echocardiography, right heart catheterisation
Cardiac				
Arrhythmia	Atrial fibrillation	Palpitations, syncope	Irregular rhythm, pauses	ECG, event recorder, Holter monitor, stress testing
Heart failure	Ischaemic cardiomyopathy	Dyspnoea on exertion, paroxysmal nocturnal dyspnoea, orthopnoea, chest pain or tightness, prior coronary artery disease or atrial fibrillation	Oedema, JVD, S_3, displaced cardiac apical impulse, hepatojugular reflex, murmur, crackles, wheezing, tachycardia, S_4	ECG, brain natriuretic peptide, echocardiography, stress testing, coronary angiography
Restrictive or constrictive pericardial disease	Metastatic tumour	Viral infection, malignancy, chest radiation, inflammatory diseases	Decreased heart sounds	Echocardiography

Continued

TABLE 19.8 Diagnostic clues to chronic dyspnoea and associated systems cont'd

System/ Physiology	Example	History	Examination	Diagnostic Study
Valvular	Aortic stenosis	Dyspnoea on exertion	Murmur, JVD	Echocardiography
Gastrointestinal				
Aspiration	Gastro-oesophageal reflux disease	Postprandial, night cough	Intermittent crackles, wheezes	Chest radiography, oesophagography, oesophageal pH
Neuromuscular				
Respiratory muscle weakness	Phrenic nerve palsy	Known neuromuscular disorders, weakness	Atrophy	Maximal inspiratory and expiratory pressures
Psychological				
	Anxiety	Anxiety, depression, history of trauma or abuse	Sighing	Normal

TABLE 19.9 Abnormal tactile fremitus

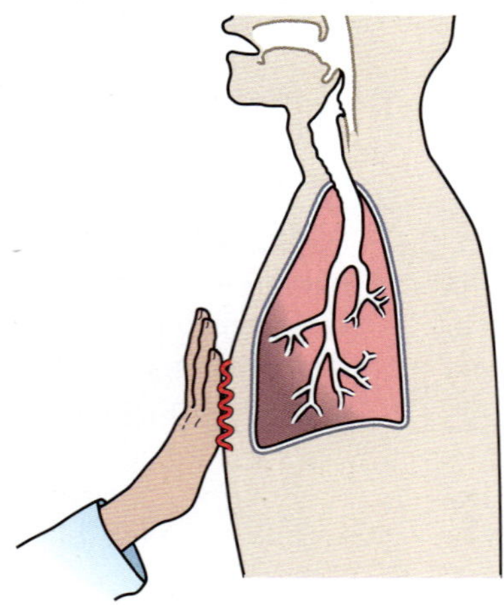

Increased tactile fremitus

Occurs with conditions that increase the density of lung tissue, thereby making a better conducting medium for vibrations (e.g. compression or consolidation [pneumonia]). There must be a patent bronchus and consolidation must extend to lung surface for increased fremitus to be apparent.

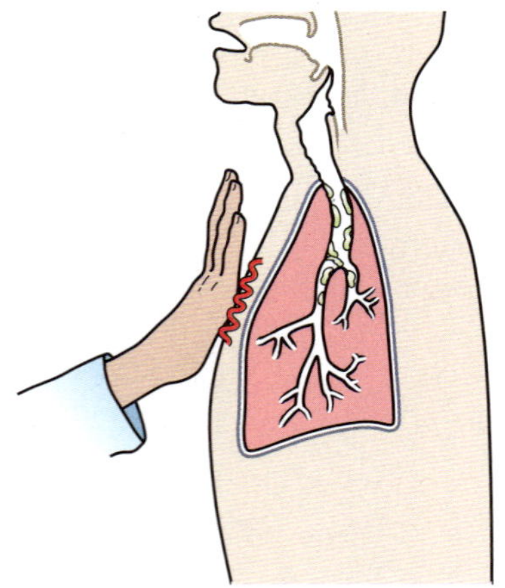

Rhonchal fremitus

Vibration felt when inhaled air passes through thick secretions in the larger bronchi. This may decrease somewhat by coughing.

TABLE 19.9 Abnormal tactile fremitus cont'd

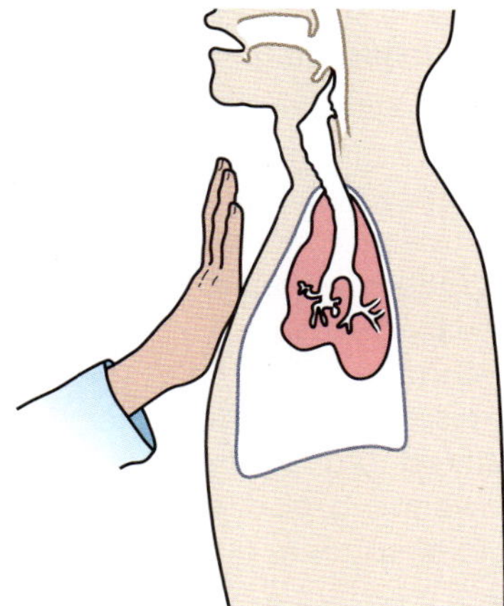

Decreased tactile fremitus

Occurs when anything obstructs transmission of vibrations (e.g. an obstructed bronchus, pleural effusion or thickening, pneumothorax and emphysema). Any barrier that gets in the way of the sound and your palpating hand decreases fremitus.

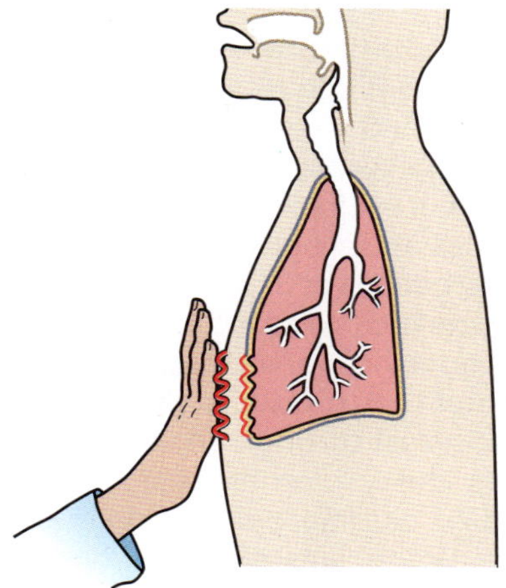

Pleural friction fremitus

Produced when inflammation of the parietal or visceral pleura causes a decrease in the normal lubricating fluid. Then the opposing surfaces make a coarse grating sound when rubbed together during breathing. Although this sound is best detected by auscultation, it may sometimes be palpable and feels like two pieces of leather grating together. It is synchronous with respiratory excursion. Also called a *palpable friction rub.*

Clinical reasoning and documentation

The following is a continuation of the case study provided at the beginning of this chapter and the clinical reasoning process including problem/issue identification. Consult a fundamentals of nursing or medical-surgical nursing text for information about goal setting, nursing interventions and evaluation.

Case study (continued)—Exacerbation of chronic obstructive pulmonary disease

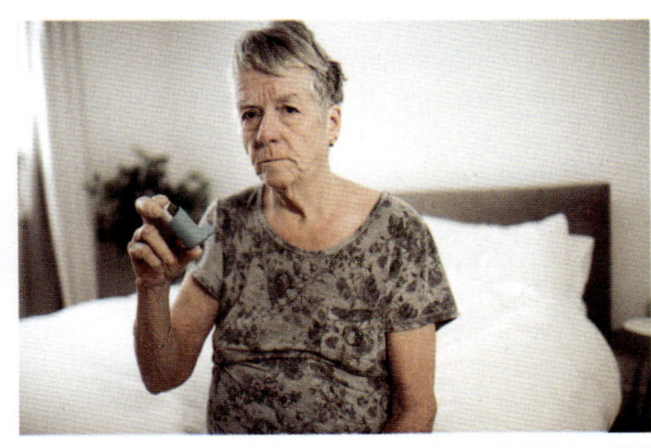

Context

You will recall from the case study described earlier in the chapter that you are a registered nurse working in the respiratory unit of a hospital.

Consider the patient's situation

Mrs Dorothy Smith is a 73-year-old woman who has been admitted for care in your clinical area with an infective exacerbation of chronic obstructive pulmonary disease (COPD). Mrs Smith reports a history of upper respiratory tract infections over the past 2 weeks.

Collect cues/information

Your further assessment reveals the following information.

Subjective data

Mrs Smith reports increased difficulty breathing and decreased ability to independently complete ADLs. Dyspnoea is significantly

Continued

Clinical reasoning and documentation cont'd

worse following any exertion. Mrs Smith tells you she hasn't been sleeping well and is feeling very tired. She reports no chest pain but has had a productive cough, worse in the mornings, producing sputum that is thick and brown in colour. Mrs Smith has had several other previous admissions for exacerbations of COPD.

She has never smoked tobacco, but her husband was a builder who worked extensively with asbestos-containing products. She was exposed to asbestos dust through shaking out and laundering his dusty clothes every day. Her husband died of cardiac disease several years ago, and Mrs Smith lives alone. She has two daughters, one of whom lives interstate. The other daughter has recently moved to be closer to her mother. Mrs Smith is on regular inhaled medications including long and short acting beta-agonists and inhaled corticosteroids.

Objective data

General inspection: Mrs Smith is sitting in bed, leaning forward with her arms braced against the tray table. She looks tired and appears anxious and agitated.

Vital signs: Temp 37.8° aurally, HR: 100 bpm, Resp. rate: 28/min, regular, shallow with a prolonged expiration time, BP: 110/60, SpO_2: 90%

Inspection: Alert and orientated but only able to speak in short phrases. She is in tripod position and using purse-lipped breathing. Her skin is pale, oral mucous membranes and tongue are dry. No audible wheeze or stridor. Accessory muscle use is noted including neck, shoulder and abdominal muscles. Her thorax is hyper inflated, the sternum is lifted and ribs flared to almost horizontal position.

Palpation: Her skin is cool to touch. Minimal but symmetrical chest expansion. No lumps, masses or tenderness on palpation.

Auscultation: Breath sounds diminished. Quiet continuous wheeze bilaterally, anterior and posterior. No crackles.

Process information and identify problems/issues

Collaborative problem

Probable acute exacerbation of COPD

Problem statements/nursing diagnoses

Impaired gas exchange related to chronic obstructive pulmonary disease

Potential ineffective airway clearance related to chronic obstructive pulmonary disease

Ineffective breathing pattern related to chronic obstructive pulmonary disease

Anxiety related to dyspnoea

Activity intolerance related to dyspnoea

Sleep disturbance related to dyspnoea, cough

Self-care deficit (showering, grooming, dressing, toileting) related to dyspnoea

Case study 2—Thunderstorm asthma

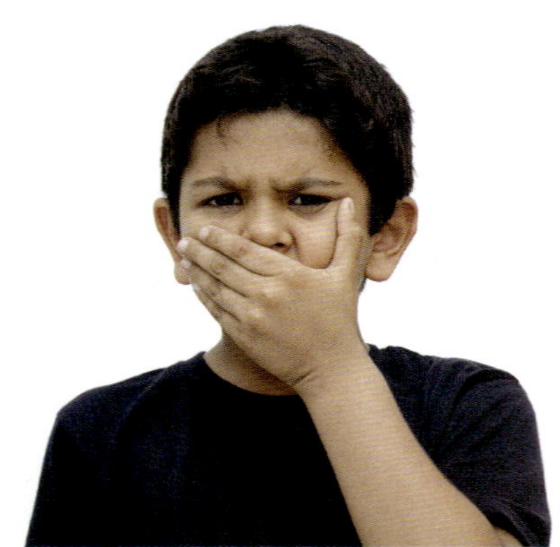

Context

You are a registered nurse working in the emergency department of a hospital.

Consider the patient's situation

Raj Patel, aged 8 years, has arrived at the emergency department with acute shortness of breath which has coincided with a spring-time thunderstorm which included high winds and a lot of pollen in the air.

Collect cues/information

Subjective data

Raj's parents, who have some English proficiency, explained that during the thunderstorm Raj experienced a sudden onset of wheezing, coughing and severe shortness of breath. They noticed his symptoms worsened quickly, and he became very anxious and agitated. Raj has never been diagnosed with asthma.

Clinical reasoning and documentation cont'd

Objective data

General inspection: Appears anxious, restless and frightened.
Vital signs: Temp 37.0° orally, HR 140 bpm, RR 32 rpm—shallow with audible wheeze BP 100/60, SpO2 92% on room air
Inspection: Alert and orientated but only able to speak in short phrases. Raj is sitting up straight and has flaring of the nares. His parents mention that he has been sitting up in bed at night to breathe comfortably. Raj's oral mucous membranes are pale. There is an audible wheeze. Raj is visibly using his sternocleidomastoid, intercostal and abdominal muscles when breathing. Accessory muscle use is noted including neck, shoulder and abdominal muscles.
Palpation: Skin is cool to touch. Minimal but symmetrical chest expansion is noted. No lumps, masses or tenderness on palpation.
Auscultation: Widespread wheezing is audible upon auscultation. No crackles are noted.

Process information and identify problems/issues

Collaborative problem

Probable first presentation of acute asthma triggered by thunderstorm—for medical review

Problem statements/nursing diagnoses

Ineffective airway clearance related to asthma
Ineffective breathing pattern related to asthma
Anxiety related to dyspnoea
Activity intolerance related to dyspnoea
Knowledge deficit (parents and Raj) related to first presentation of new diagnosis of asthma

ADDITIONAL RESOURCES

You can further develop your knowledge and skills relevant to respiratory assessment, related pathophysiology, common health issues and nursing interventions by:

- reading chapters of a fundamentals of nursing or medical-surgical nursing textbook
- answering chapter multiple choice questions online. Log onto ClinicalKey Student and search for the text 'Health Assessment, 4th edition'. Choose the section titled 'Teaching material'. In this section you will find question and answer documents for each chapter. Please check instructions on the inside front cover of the book to access online resources
- visiting websites

  Quit—Quit education (health professionals): https://www.quit.org.au/health-professional-resources

  Lung Foundation Australia: https://lungfoundation.com.au/patients-carers/lung-health/quitting-smoking/

  World Health Organization: https://apps.who.int/iris/bitstream/handle/10665/112835/9789241506953_eng.pdf?sequence=1.

REFERENCES

1. Zhang H, Yu L, Wang Q, Tao Y, Li J, Sun T, et al. In utero and postnatal exposure to environmental tobacco smoke, blood pressure, and hypertension in children: the Seven Northeastern Cities study. International Journal of Environmental Health Research, 2019 May 29:1–12. doi: 10.1080/09603123.2019.1612043
2. Carr B. *(Lower airways assessment)* In: Tomkins Z. Applied Anatomy & Physiology: An interdisciplinary approach. Elsevier Australia. 2020
3. Australian Institute of Health and Australian Government. Available at: https://www.aihw.gov.au/reports/alcohol/alcohol-tobacco-other-drugs-australia/contents/drug-types/tobacco
4. Ministry of Health NZ. Annual update of key results 2021/22: New Zealand health survey; 2022. Available at: https://www.health.govt.nz/publication/annual-update-key-results-2021-22-new-zealand-health-survey
5. Australian Institute of Health and Welfare. Mesothelioma in Australia 2021. Cat. no. CAN 152. Canberra: AIHW. 2023. Available at: https://www.aihw.gov.au/getmedia/034ebfb9-554f-4eb7-8f0f-ad56d9d3c5ae/aihw-can-152.pdf?v=20230605165739&inline=true
6. Kirby T. Australia reports on audit of silicosis for stonecutters. Lancet 2019;393(10174):861.
7. Soeberg M, Vallance DA, Keena V, Takahashi K, Leigh J. Australia's ongoing legacy of asbestos: significant challenges remain even after the complete banning of asbestos almost fifteen years ago. International Journal of Environmental Research and Public Health 2018;15(2):384.
8. Hoy RF, Baird T, Hammerschlag G, Hart D, Johnson AR, King P, et al. Artificial stone-associated silicosis: a rapidly emerging occupational lung disease. Occupational and Environmental Medicine 2018;75(1):3–5.
9. Leso V, Fontana L, Romano R, Gervetti P, Iavicoli I. Artificial stone associated silicosis: a systematic review. International Journal of Environmental Research and Public Health 2019;16(4):568. doi.org/10.3390/ijerph16040568.
10. Australian Government, Department of Health. The strategic plan for control of tuberculosis in Australia, 2021–2025. The national tuberculosis advisory committee for the communicable diseases network of Australia, Vol 46. 2022. Available at: https://www1.health.gov.au/internet/main/publishing.nsf/Content/2A15CD097063EF40CA2587CE008354F1/$File/the_strategic_plan_for_control_of_tuberculosis_in_australia_2021_2025.pdf
11. Ministry of Health NZ. Guidelines for tuberculosis control in New Zealand, 2019. Wellington: Ministry of Health; 2019b. Available at: https://www.health.govt.nz/publication/guidelines-tuberculosis-control-new-zealand-2019
12. Byrne S, Brindal E, Williams G, Anastasiou K, Tonkin A, Battams S, et al. E-cigarettes, smoking and health: a literature review update. CSIRO, Australia. 2018.
13. Gotts JE, Jordt S, McConnell R, Tarran R. What are the respiratory effects of e-cigarettes? BMJ 2019: 366:l5275 doi: 10.1136/bmj.l5275
14. Kennedy CD, van Schalkwyk MCI, McKee M, Pisinger C. The cardiovascular effects of electronic cigarettes: a systematic review of experimental studies. Preventive Medicine. 2019 Oct;127:105770. doi: 10.1016/j.ypmed.2019.105770. Epub 2019 Jul 22. PMID: 31344384.
15. Campbell MA, Winnall WR, Ford C, Winstanley MH. 4.17 Health effects of secondhand smoke for infants and children. In: Greenhalgh EM, Scollo MM, Winstanley MH [editors]. Tobacco in Australia: Facts and issues. Melbourne: Cancer Council Victoria; 2021. Available at: http://www.tobaccoinaustralia.org.au/chapter-4-secondhand/4-17-health-effects-of-secondhand-smoke-for-infants
16. Australian Institute of Health and Welfare (AIHW). National Drug Strategy Household Survey 2019. Drug Statistics series no. 32. PHE 270. Canberra: AIHW; 2020. Available at: https://www.aihw.gov.au/getmedia/77dbea6e-f071-495c-b71e-3a632237269d/aihw-phe-270.pdf?v=20230605184325&inline=true

CHAPTER 20

Musculoskeletal assessment

Written by Carolyn Jarvis
Adapted by Kate Schimmelbusch

INTRODUCTION

The musculoskeletal system is a vast organ system that provides locomotion and an upright posture and protection for the body. It comprises various forms of connective tissue including bones, skeletal muscle, cartilage, ligaments, tendons and joints. To appreciate the impact of disease and trauma to this complex and dynamic system, you are advised to first review the structure and function of bones, skeletal muscle, cartilage, ligaments, tendons and joints.

Case study

The following case study gives an example of a typical situation involving musculoskeletal assessment and the initial clinical reasoning process. It will help you to identify your learning needs.

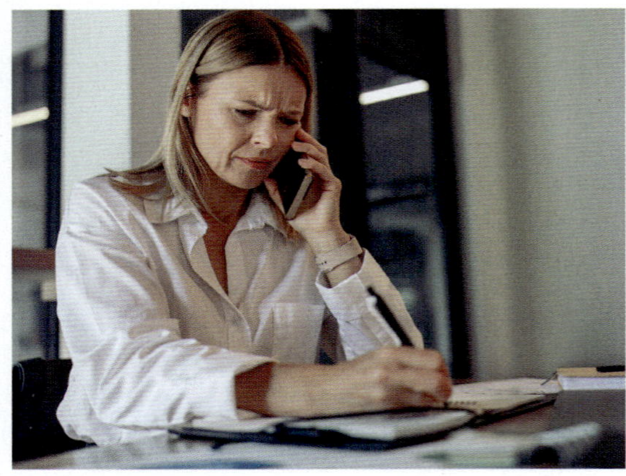

Context

You are working as an occupational health nurse in an onsite multidisciplinary health clinic that is part of a large company. The role includes providing first aid treatment, assessing workplace injuries, conducting audiometric assessments and providing occupational health and injury management advice.

Consider the patient's situation

Ms Mari Timms is a 45-year-old female office worker with a diagnosis of rheumatoid arthritis 3 years ago, who seeks care now for 'swelling and burning pain' in her hands for 1 day, which is affecting her ability to complete her normal work tasks and daily activities.

Questions to further your learning

- What are the possible things that might be going on with Ms Timms?
- What knowledge do you need to be able to plan a focused health assessment?
- What questions (subjective data) will you ask Ms Timms to extend the health history and why?
- What physical examination (objective data) will you conduct and why?
- What resources are available to assist in your assessment of Ms Timms?

Assessment plan

Musculoskeletal assessment is commonly performed in conjunction with assessing neurological, nutritional and metabolic function and pain. Collecting subjective and objective data will help you identify potential or actual health issues so you can plan care. A detailed knowledge of structure and function, developmental and cultural considerations are necessary before you start.

The focus of musculoskeletal assessment outlined in this chapter is the GALS framework (gait, arms, legs and spine). Through the process of questioning the person or family you may become aware of gaps in the person's knowledge about living a healthy lifestyle. The opportunity to provide health information is an important part of health assessment.

The main areas for subjective assessment are:

- presenting concern
- GALS screening assessment – questions
- joints
- muscles
- bones
- functional assessment (activities of daily living)
- general health history
- family history
- health and lifestyle management.

Following subjective data collection, the following sequence is used to collect objective data, inspection and palpation. The purpose of the musculoskeletal examination is to assess patterns of pain, joint abnormalities and the impact these have on the person's activities of daily living (ADLs) and psychosocial functioning:

- general inspection
- GALS screening assessment – physical examination
- laboratory studies.

Resources available

You will find additional resources and the reference list at the end of this chapter.

Structure and function

The musculoskeletal system has both structural and metabolic functions. Its structural function is essential for locomotion, respiration and the protection of internal organs and the central nervous system. The marrow within bones contains critical components of the haematopoietic and immune system. The bone marrow produces B cells, granulocytes and immature thymocytes, in addition to red blood cells and platelets.

The main metabolic function of bones is the homeostasis of calcium and phosphate, which is achieved through a combination of bone resorption and formation.[1] Its metabolic function is as a storehouse for calcium, phosphorus and carbonate and as a buffering system in hydrogen ion concentration. Calcium levels are regulated through the absorption from the digestive tract and resorption from the bone and the kidneys.[1] The enormous mineral surface of the skeleton can also bind toxins and heavy metals, minimising their ability to cause cellular damage.

Components of the musculoskeletal system

BONE

Bone is a mineralised connective tissue consisting of cells embedded in a protein matrix of collagen, alkaline phosphatase and osteopontin. This dynamic tissue responds to mechanical stresses through a complex process of remodelling. The remodelling process involves the resorption of micro-damaged bone by osteoclast cells followed by a phase of bone formation by osteoblast cells. In healthy adults, this process is coupled to ensure bone density remains stable.

Endocrine regulation of bone metabolism is controlled by subcategories of growth, gonadal and calciotropic hormones to promote bone mass accrual.[2]

When gradual degradation occurs, or the process becomes uncoupled, normal bone density is altered. This can be seen in diseases such as osteoporosis where reduced bone density and deterioration of osseous tissue leads to bone fragility.[3] Another example of disorganised bone formation can be seen in diseases such as Paget's.[4]

CARTILAGE

This connective tissue is a firm gel-like substance characterised by resilience and the ability to absorb mechanical forces. The human body contains three major types of cartilage: hyaline cartilage, elastic cartilage and fibrocartilage. Hyaline cartilage is the most common type of cartilage found in parts of the respiratory tract and on joint surfaces. Within joints, articular cartilage protects the joint by distributing applied loads and by providing a low-friction-bearing surface to maximise movement. Fibrocartilage is found in the intervertebral discs, menisci of the knee joint and the symphysis pubis. Its structure provides resistance to the compression and shearing forces within these joints. All types of cartilage are avascular and aneural, therefore tears in cartilage cannot heal.

LIGAMENTS AND TENDONS

Ligaments and tendons are connective tissues with complex biomechanical properties. Ligaments connect bone to bone and tendons connect muscles to bone. Injury to a ligament or tendon results in a drastic change in structure, resulting in the formation of scar tissue that is biomechanically inferior. For example, repairing the anterior cruciate ligament (ACL) in the knee requires a new piece of tissue graft from a hamstring muscle. The resultant graft does not possess the same qualities of strength and stability as the original ACL.

MUSCLES

There are three types of muscle in the human body: smooth, cardiac and skeletal muscle. Skeletal muscles are innervated by the motor nerve fibres of peripheral nerves. Conscious and subconscious contractions of muscles affect posture and locomotion and generate reflexes. The human body contains more than 400 skeletal muscles representing 40 to 50% of total bodyweight. A whole skeletal muscle is considered an organ of the muscular system. Skeletal muscle fibres have an abundant blood and nerve supply and are bundled together in a compartment wrapped in a tough fibrous connective tissue called fascia.

Diseases and disorders of the muscular system are diverse and include infections, hormonal, genetic and autoimmune disorders and malignancies. Minor traumatic injuries are the most common disorders of the muscular skeletal system. When major injury to muscles occurs as in limb trauma, intracompartmental tissue pressure can quickly rise. A rise in intracompartmental tissue pressure is known as compartment syndrome. This syndrome is characterised by muscle necrosis called rhabdomyolysis. Rhabdomyolysis ultimately leads to the release of cellular contents, including myoglobin, into the circulatory system. This may result in potentially life-threatening complications, most commonly myoglobinuric acute renal failure. Electrolyte imbalances such as hyperkalaemia and hyponatremia are also a high risk.[5]

Muscle mass and strength declines with age (sarcopenia) due to a diverse range of lifestyle factors often associated with ageing including a decrease in physical activity, dietary protein and calorie intake, an increased intracellular oxidative stress and age-related decreases in hormone concentrations.[6]

JOINTS

Joints are the functional units of the skeleton. Individual joints are described and classified by two qualities—the structure of the joint and the range of movement permitted by the joint.

Classification of joints by range of movement

Diarthroses—moveable joints
Synarthroses—immoveable joints
Amphiarthroses—'mixed' joints of limited movement

Classification of joints by structure

Fibrous (synarthrotic) joints. The articulating bones are joined by fibrous connective tissue—for example, the joints (sutures) of the skull bones.

Cartilaginous (amphiarthrotic) joints. The articulating bones are joined by cartilage—for example, the pubic symphysis.

Synovial (diarthrotic) joints. These are freely mobile joints characterised by a joint cavity lined with synovial tissue and supported by ligaments, tendons and bursae (Figure 20.1). Synovial joints may be also subclassified according to the type of movement that they permit—for example, the ball and socket joint of the hip and hinge joint of the knee.

Each joint reflects a compromise between stability and range of motion (ROM). The bones of the skull, for example, are stable but immobile, whereas the shoulder joint allows for a full ROM but is a relatively unstable joint.

Movement of joints involving muscle contraction produces the following patterns of motion (Figure 20.2):

- flexion—bending a limb at a joint
- extension—straightening a limb at a joint
- abduction—moving a limb away from the midline of the body
- adduction—moving a limb towards the midline of the body
- pronation—turning the forearm so that the palm is down
- supination—turning the forearm so that the palm is up
- circumduction—moving the arm in a circle around the shoulder
- inversion—moving the sole of the foot inwards at the ankle
- eversion—moving the sole of the foot outwards at the ankle
- rotation—moving the head around a central axis
- protraction—moving a body part forwards and parallel to the ground
- retraction—moving a body part backwards and parallel to the ground
- elevation—raising a body part
- depression—lowering a body part.

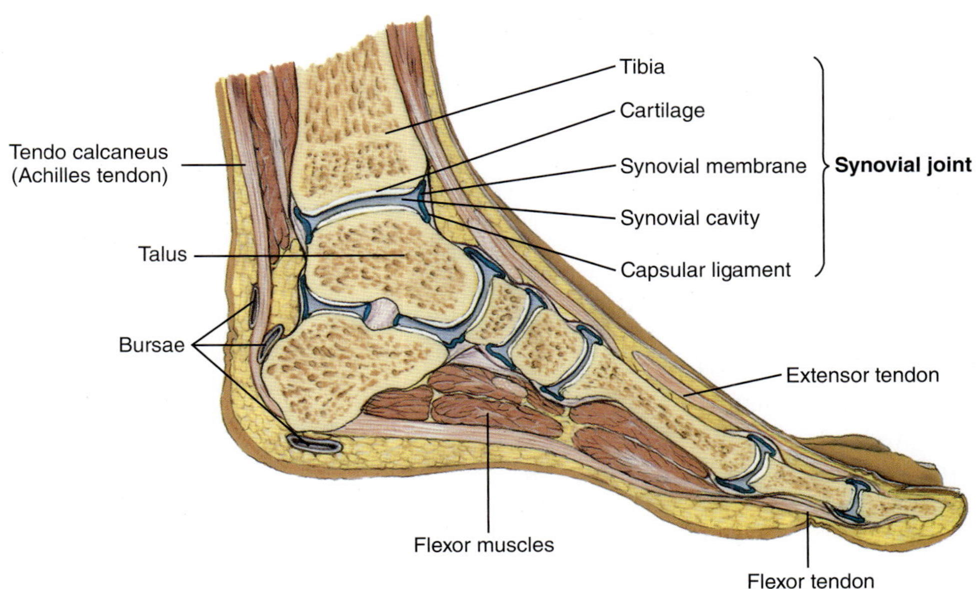

FIGURE 20.1 Anatomy of the foot

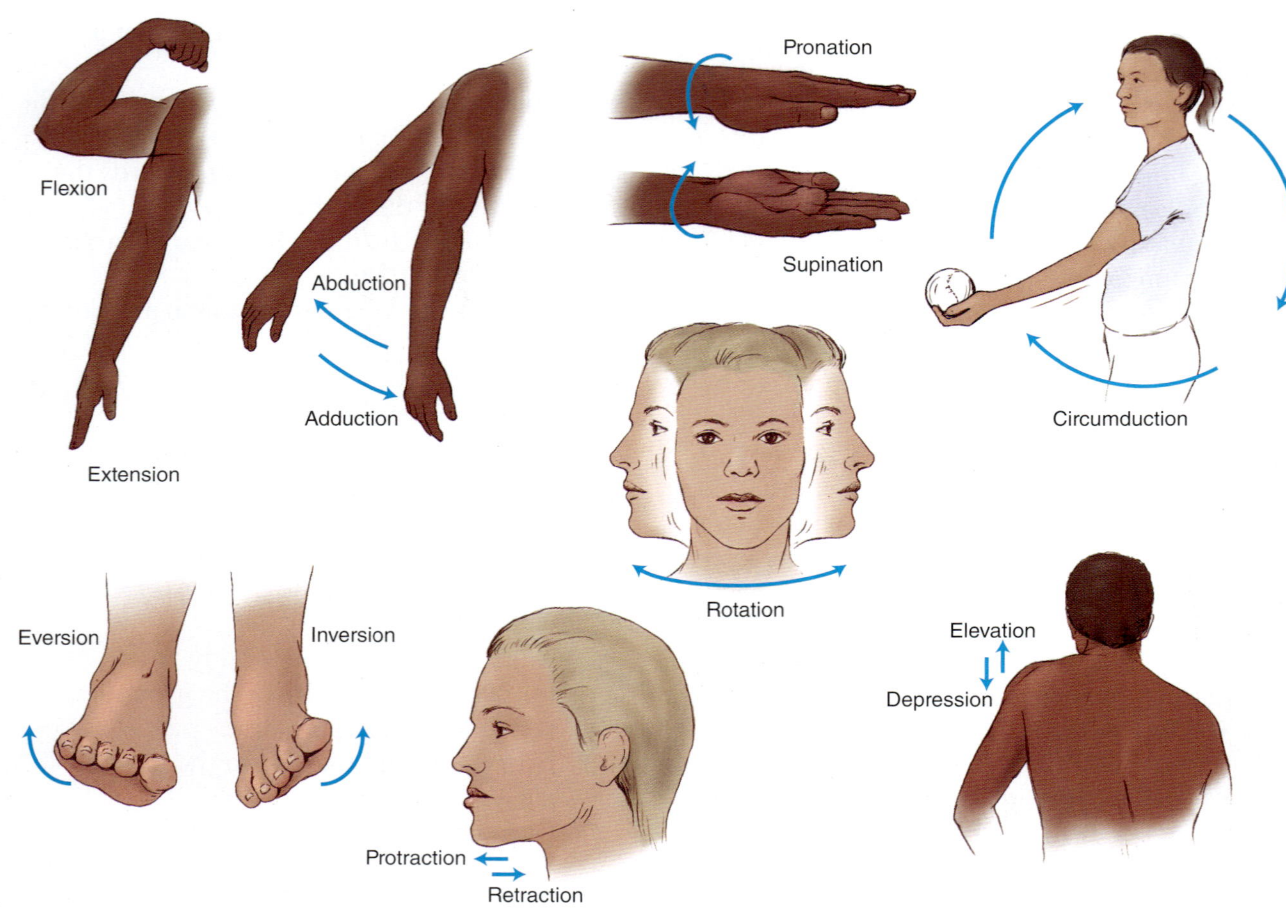

FIGURE 20.2 Terminology related to skeletal muscle movements

Joint anatomy

Temporomandibular joint

The temporomandibular joint (TMJ) is the articulation of the mandible and the temporal bone (Figure 20.3). The TMJ permits jaw function for speaking and chewing. The joint allows three motions: (1) hinge action to open and close the jaws; (2) gliding action for protrusion and retraction; and (3) gliding for side-to-side movement of the lower jaw.

Spinal column

The **vertebrae** are 33 connecting bones stacked in a vertical column (Figure 20.4). The spinous processes can be palpated as a furrow down the midline of the back. The furrow has paravertebral muscles mounded on either side down to the sacrum, where it flattens. Humans have 7 cervical, 12 thoracic, 5 lumbar, 5 sacral and 3 or 4 coccygeal vertebrae. The following surface landmarks will orient you to their levels:

- The spinous processes of C7 and T1 are prominent at the base of the neck.
- The inferior angle of the scapula normally is at the level of the interspace between T7 and T8.

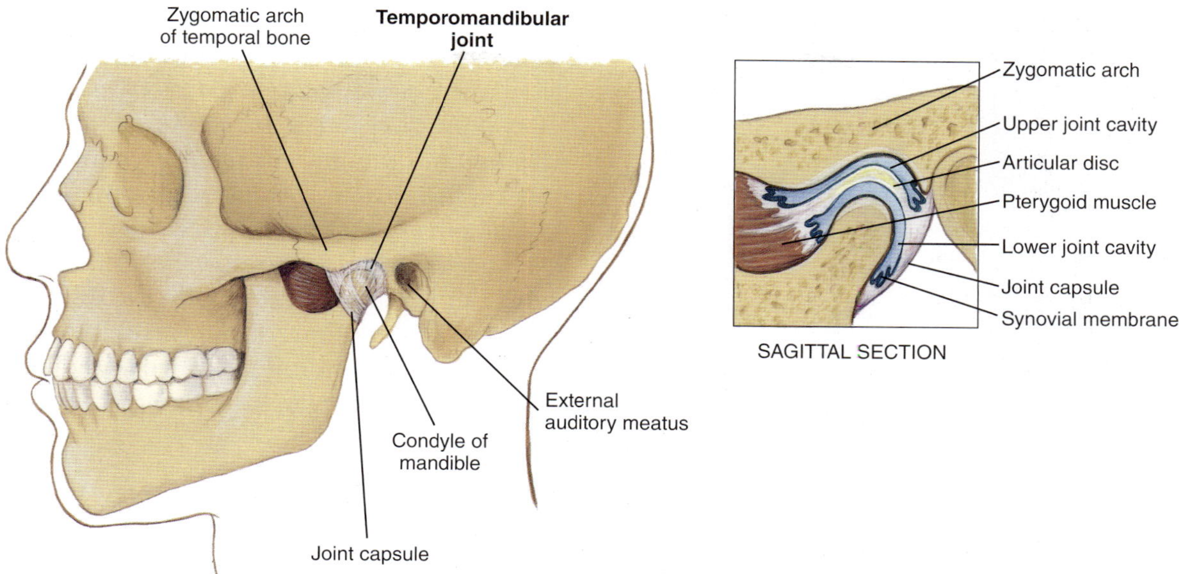

FIGURE 20.3 Anatomy of the temporomandibular joint

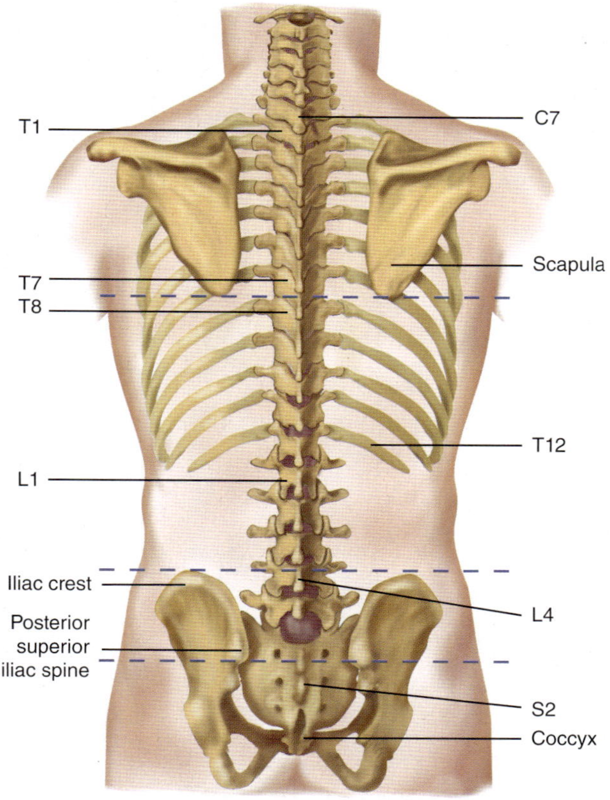

FIGURE 20.4 Bony landmarks of the back and posterior pelvis

- An imaginary line connecting the highest point on each iliac crest crosses L4.
- An imaginary line joining the two symmetric dimples that overlie the posterior superior iliac spines crosses the sacrum.

A lateral view shows that the vertebral column has four curves (a double-S shape) (Figure 20.5). The cervical and lumbar curves are concave (inwards or anterior), and the thoracic and sacrococcygeal curves are convex (outwards or posterior). The balanced or compensatory nature of these curves, together with the resilient intervertebral discs, allows the spine to absorb a great deal of shock.

The **intervertebral discs** are fibrocartilaginous plates that constitute a quarter of the length of the column (Figure 20.6). Each disc is made up of three basic structures: the nucleus pulposus, the annulus fibrosus and the vertebral end plates. The inner **nucleus pulposus** is the semi-fluid gel centre and has the consistency of toothpaste in a young adult. The main function of the intervertebral discs is to transfer the compression forces from one vertebra to another as loads are put on the spinal column

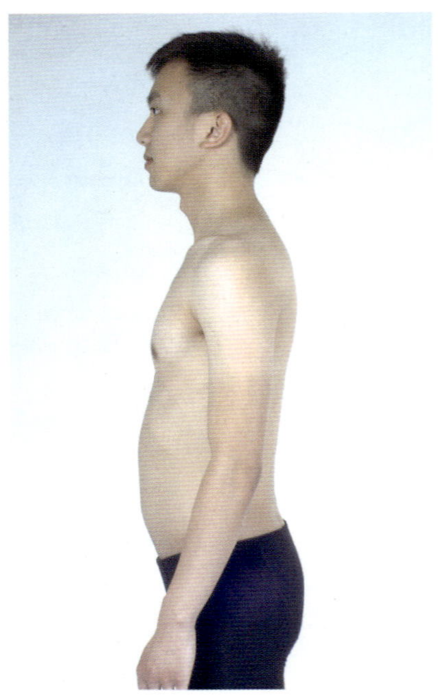

FIGURE 20.5 Normal curves of vertebral column

during daily activities. As the spine moves, the elasticity of the discs allows compression on one side, with compensatory expansion on the other. If compression forces are too great, a disc can rupture and the nucleus pulposus can herniate out of the vertebral column, compressing the spinal nerves and causing pain.

The unique structure of the spine enables both upright posture and flexibility for motion. The motions of the vertebral column are flexion (bending forwards), extension (bending back), abduction (to either side) and rotation.

Shoulder

The **glenohumeral joint** is the articulation of the humerus with the glenoid fossa of the scapula (Figure 20.7). Its ball-and-socket action allows great mobility of the arm on many axes. The joint is enclosed by a group of four powerful muscles and tendons that

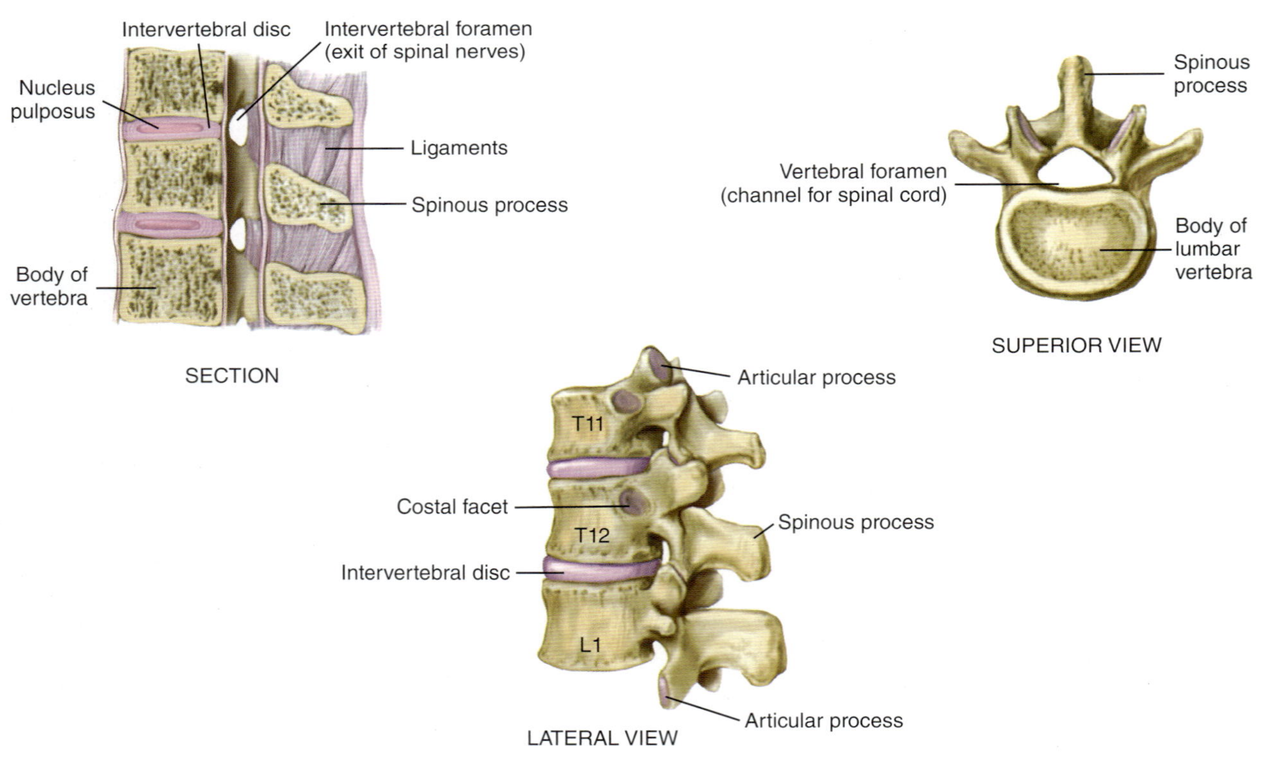

FIGURE 20.6 Anatomy of the spine

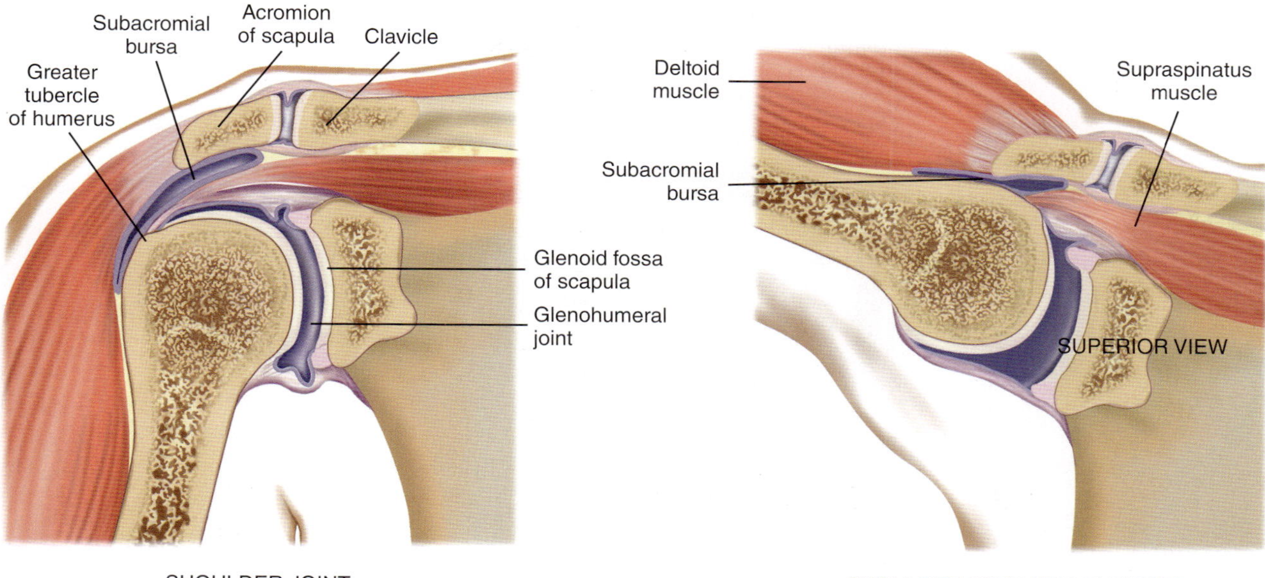

FIGURE 20.7 Anatomy of the shoulder

support and stabilise it. Together these are called the **rotator cuff** of the shoulder. The large **subacromial bursa** helps during abduction of the arm so the greater tubercle of the humerus moves easily under the acromion process of the scapula.

The bones of the shoulder have palpable landmarks to guide your examination (Figure 20.8). The scapula and the clavicle connect to form the shoulder girdle. You can palpate the bump of the scapula's **acromion process** at the very top of the shoulder. Move your fingers in a small circle outward, down and around. The next bump is the **greater tubercle** of the humerus a few centimetres down and laterally, and from that the **coracoid process** of the scapula is a few centimetres medially. These surround the deeply situated joint.

Elbow

The elbow joint contains the three bony articulations of the humerus, radius and ulna of the forearm (Figure 20.9). Its hinge action moves the forearm (radius and ulna) on one plane, allowing flexion and extension. The olecranon bursa lies between the olecranon process and the skin.

Palpable landmarks are the **medial** and **lateral epicondyles** of the humerus and the large **olecranon process** of the ulna in between them. The sensitive ulnar nerve runs between the olecranon process and the medial epicondyle.

The radius and ulna articulate with each other at two radioulnar joints, one at the elbow and one at the wrist. These move together to permit pronation and supination of the hand and forearm.

Wrist and carpals

Of the body's 206 bones, more than half are in the hands and feet. The wrist or **radiocarpal** joint is the articulation of the radius (on the thumb side) and a row of carpal bones (Figure 20.10). Its condyloid action permits movement in two planes at right angles: flexion and extension and side-to-side

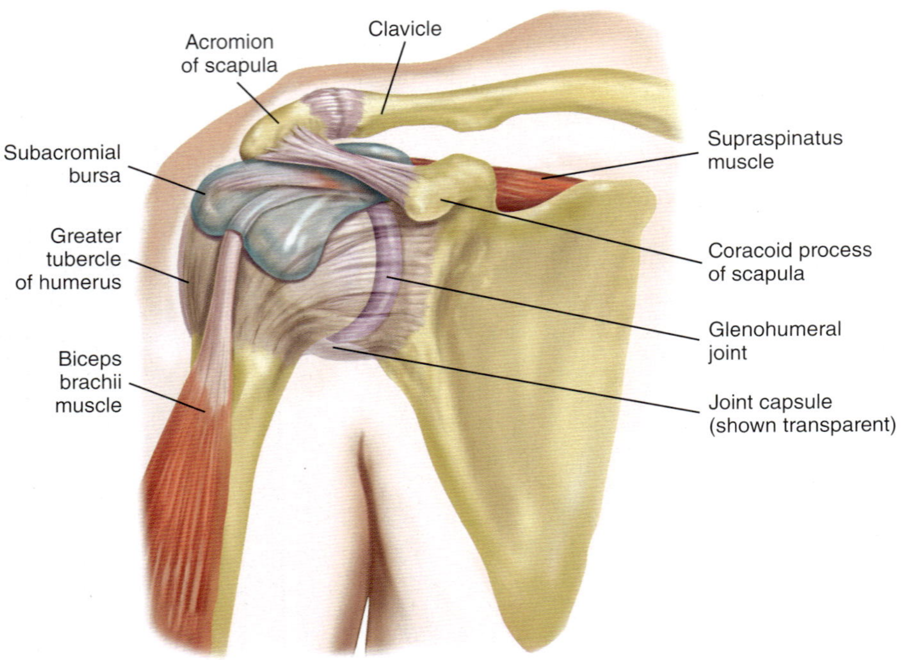

FIGURE 20.8 Bony landmarks of the anterior shoulder

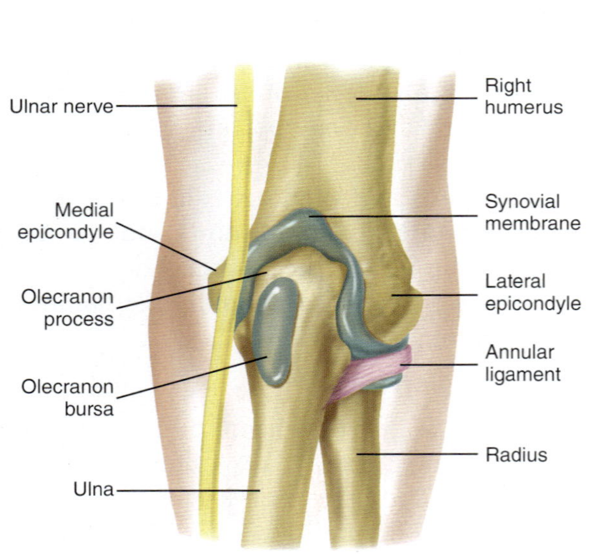

FIGURE 20.9 Anatomy of the posterior elbow

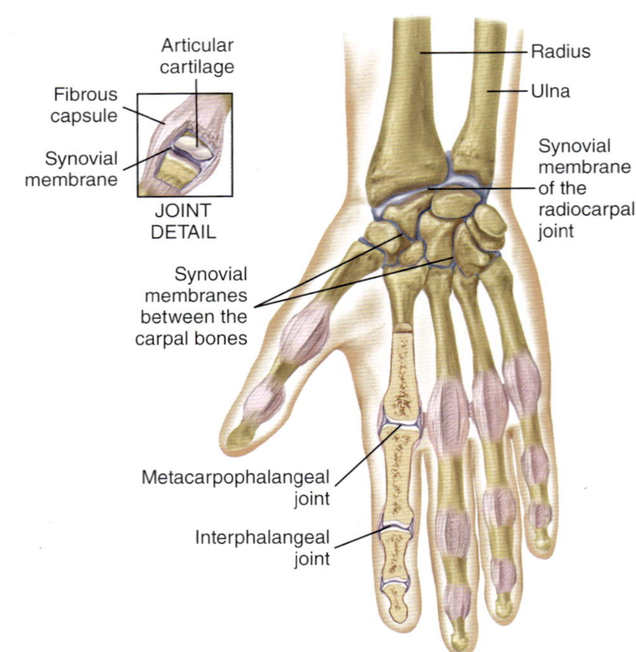

FIGURE 20.10 Anatomy of the hand—palmar view

deviation. The groove of this joint can be palpated on the dorsum of the wrist.

The **midcarpal** joint is the articulation between the two parallel rows of carpal bones. It allows flexion, extension and some rotation. The **metacarpophalangeal** and the **interphalangeal** joints permit finger flexion and extension. The flexor tendons of the wrist and hand are enclosed in synovial sheaths.

Hip

The hip joint is the articulation between the acetabulum and the head of the femur (Figure 20.11). As in the shoulder, ball-and-socket action permits a wide ROM on many axes. The hip has somewhat less ROM than the shoulder, but it has more stability as befits its weight-bearing function. Hip stability is due to powerful muscles that spread over the joint, a strong fibrous articular capsule and the very deep insertion of the head of the femur. Three bursae facilitate movement.

Palpation of these bony landmarks will guide your examination. You can feel the entire iliac crest, from the **anterior superior iliac spine** to the posterior. The **ischial tuberosity** lies under the gluteus maximus muscle and is palpable when the hip is flexed. The **greater trochanter** of the femur is normally the width of the person's palm below the iliac crest and halfway between the anterior superior iliac spine and the ischial tuberosity. This landmark is best palpated when the person is standing, in a flat depression on the upper lateral side of the thigh.

Knee

The knee joint is the articulation of three bones—the femur, the tibia and the patella (kneecap)—in one common articular cavity (Figure 20.12). It is the largest joint in the body and is complex. It is a hinge joint, permitting flexion and extension of the lower leg, as well as a slight medial and lateral rotation.

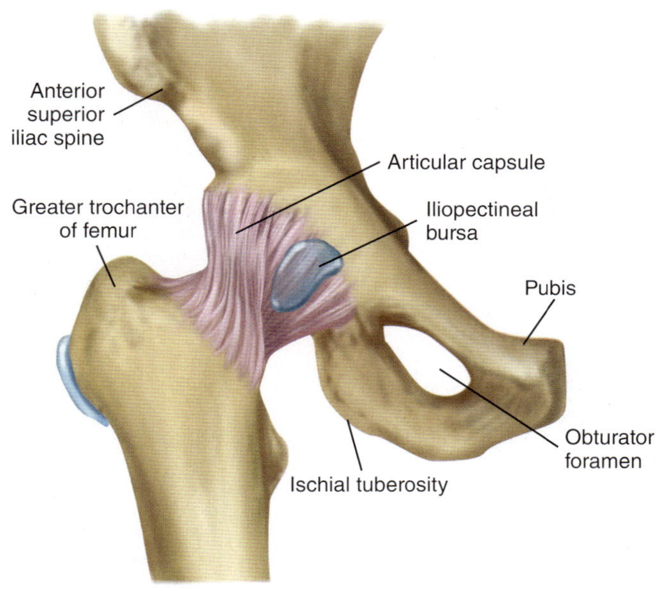

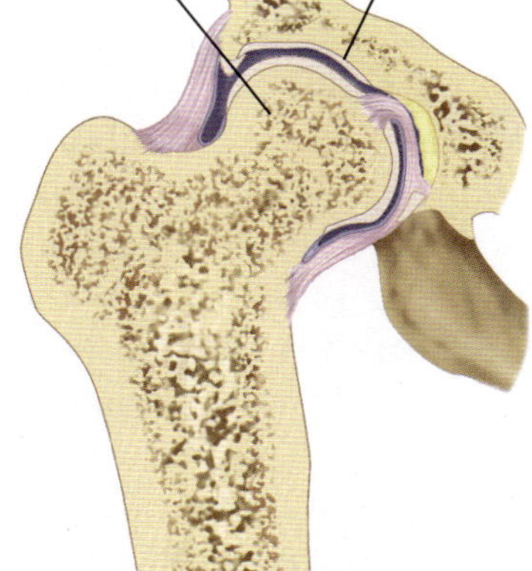

HIP JOINT

FIGURE 20.11 Anatomy of the hip joint

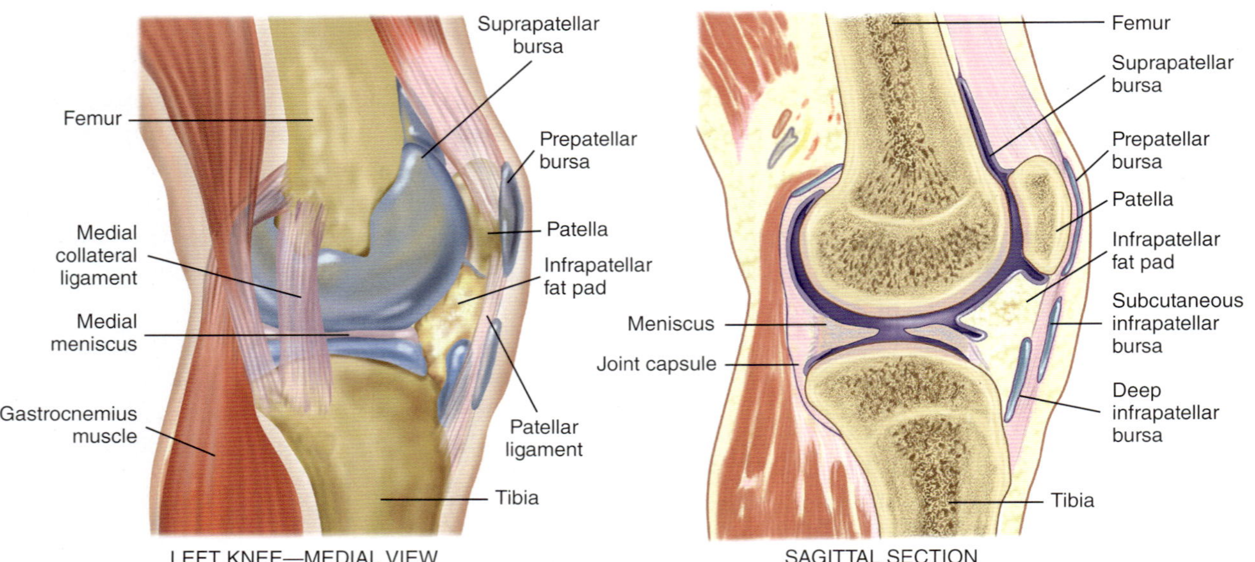

FIGURE 20.12 Anatomy of the knee

The knee's synovial membrane is the largest in the body. It forms a sac at the superior border of the patella, called the **suprapatellar pouch**, which extends up as much as 6 cm behind the quadriceps muscle. Two wedge-shaped cartilages, called the **medial** and **lateral menisci**, cushion the tibia and femur. The joint is stabilised by two sets of ligaments. The **cruciate ligaments** (not shown) crisscross within the knee; they give anterior and posterior stability and help control rotation. The **collateral ligaments** connect the joint at both sides; they give medial and lateral stability and prevent dislocation. Numerous bursae prevent friction. One, the **prepatellar bursa**, lies between the patella and the skin. The **infrapatellar fat pad** is a small, triangular fat pad below the patella behind the patellar ligament.

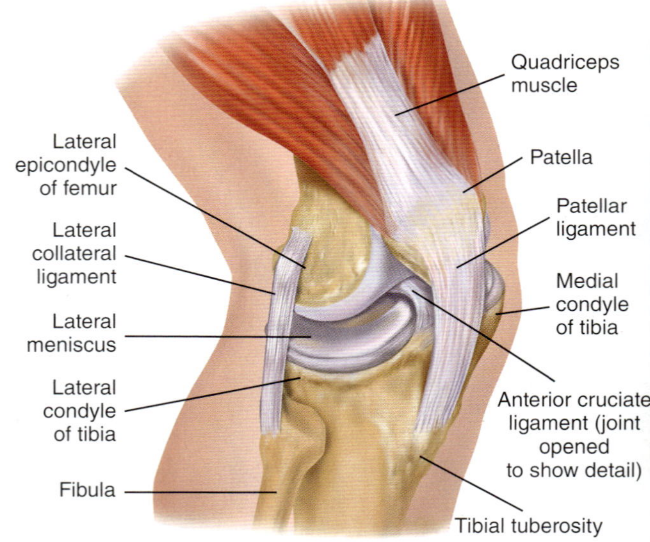

FIGURE 20.13 Landmarks of the knee

Landmarks of the knee joint start with the large **quadriceps** muscle, which is palpated on the anterior and lateral thigh (Figure 20.13). The muscle's four heads merge into a common tendon that continues down to enclose the round bony patella. Then the tendon inserts down on the **tibial tuberosity**, which is palpated as a bony prominence in the midline. Move to the sides and superiorly and note the lateral and

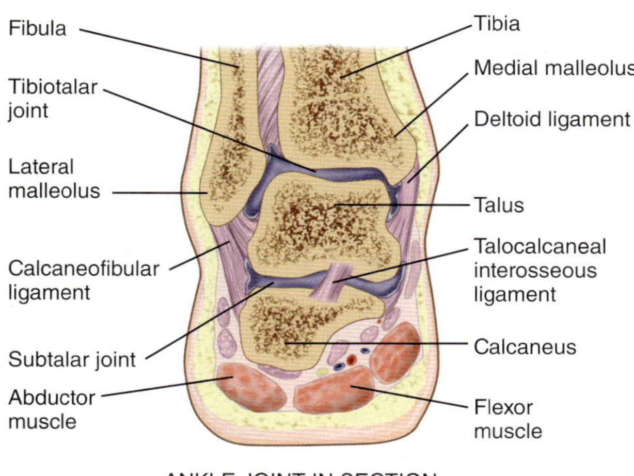

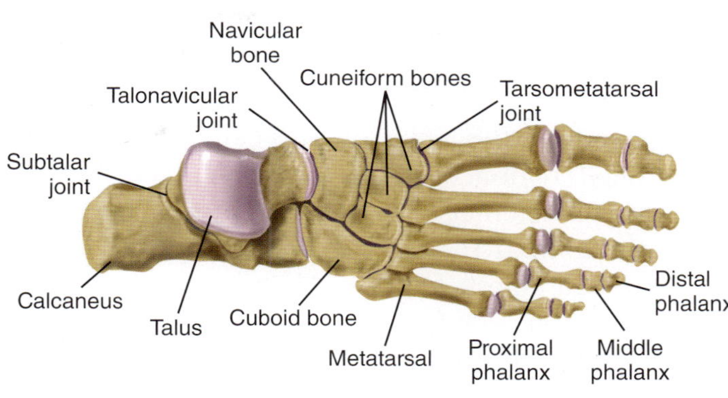

FIGURE 20.14 Anatomy of the ankle joint and foot

medial condyles of the tibia. Superior to these on either side of the patella are the medial and lateral epicondyles of the femur.

Ankle and foot

The ankle or tibiotalar joint is the articulation of the tibia, fibula and talus (Figure 20.14). It is a hinge joint, limited to flexion (dorsiflexion) and extension (plantar flexion) on one plane. Landmarks are two bony prominences on either side—the **medial malleolus** and the lateral **malleolus**. Strong, tight medial and lateral ligaments extend from each malleolus onto the foot. These help the lateral stability of the ankle joint, although they may be torn in eversion or inversion sprains of the ankle.

Joints distal to the ankle give additional mobility to the foot. The subtalar joint permits inversion and eversion of the foot. The foot has a longitudinal arch, with weight bearing distributed between the parts that touch the ground—the heads of the metatarsals and the calcaneus (heel).

Developmental considerations

Infants and children

By 3 months' gestation, the fetus has formed a 'scale model' of the skeleton that is made up of cartilage. During the following months in utero, the cartilage ossifies into true bone and starts to grow. Bone growth continues after birth—rapidly during infancy and then steadily during childhood—until adolescence, when both boys and girls undergo a rapid growth spurt.

Long bones grow in two dimensions. They increase in width or diameter by deposition of new bony tissue around the shafts. Lengthening occurs at the epiphyses or growth plates. These specialised growth centres are transverse discs located at the ends of long bone. Any trauma or infection at this location puts the growing child at risk for bone deformity. This longitudinal growth continues until closure of the epiphyses; the last closure occurs at about age 20 years.

Skeletal contour changes are apparent at the vertebral column. At birth the spine has a single C-shaped curve. At 3 to 4 months, raising the baby's head from prone position develops the anterior curve in the cervical neck region. From 1 year to 18 months, standing erect develops the anterior curve in the lumbar region.

Musculoskeletal conditions seen in the neonatal period include developmental dysplasia of the hip (DDH), talipes equinovarus (clubfoot) and upper and lower limb development deformities.

The term developmental DDH describes a wide range of hip abnormalities found within the neonatal period in which the femoral head has an abnormal relationship to the acetabulum. Variances in these disorders range from stable hips with acetabular dysplasia to complete displacement of the femoral head out of an abnormal acetabulum. The prevalence of DDH varies due to diagnostic criteria, examiner skills and disorder progress. Minor hip dysplasia often resolves spontaneously. The incidence is variable however estimated from 1 to 20 per every 1,000 births globally.[7] Clinical DDH screening programs within Australia using midwives, maternal child health nurses and primary care clinicians have been created to reduce the cases of 'late diagnosed' DDH. Late diagnosis (beyond 12 weeks of age) occurs at approximately 1.28 per 1,000 births. This can often be because of screening failures with variability in the assessment guidelines, progression of pathology, inappropriate swaddling/wrapping or lack of continued follow-up screening.[8] Untreated DDH has the potential to cause long-term hip dysplasia and early hip arthritis in adulthood.[7]

Musculoskeletal conditions, however, are evident throughout childhood, affecting up to 30% of children and adolescents. The majority are self-limiting and often trauma related. These conditions also include life-threatening disorders such as malignant disease and infection. Chronic musculoskeletal conditions include a spectrum of autoimmune/inflammatory joint and muscle disorders. Juvenile idiopathic arthritis (JIA) relates to the group of heterogeneous diseases that are a feature of chronic inflammatory arthritis of unknown cause lasting longer than 6 weeks with onset before 16 years of age. In Australia, the estimated overall prevalence of JIA is between 241 and 383 per 100,000 population aged between 0 and 24 years.[9] Juvenile arthritis affects the child's growth and musculoskeletal development. The associated disability, chronic pain and growth disturbances impact on all aspects of the child's life and family/social dynamics. JIA has an unpredictable pattern where there can be periods without symptoms, followed by sudden flares of unknown causes.

Pregnant women

Almost all women experience some degree of musculoskeletal discomfort during pregnancy, with a prevalence rate of 44% in the Australian population experiencing pregnancy related pelvic girdle pain.[10] Increased levels of circulating hormones (estrogen, relaxin from the corpus luteum and corticosteroids) cause increased mobility in the joints. Increased mobility in the sacroiliac, sacrococcygeal and symphysis pubis joints in the pelvis contributes to the noticeable changes in maternal posture. The most characteristic change is progressive lordosis, which compensates for the enlarging fetus; otherwise, the centre of balance would shift forwards. Lordosis compensates by shifting the weight further back on the lower extremities. This shift in balance in turn creates strain on the low back muscles, which some women experience as low back pain during late pregnancy.

Anterior flexion of the neck and slumping of the shoulder girdle are other postural changes that compensate for the lordosis. These upper back changes may put pressure on the ulnar and median nerves during the third trimester. Carpal tunnel syndrome in pregnancy is often bilateral and mostly present in the third trimester. The course of carpal tunnel syndrome found in association with pregnancy varies with most women having resolution of symptoms following the birth, although some women will have persistent symptoms.[11]

EFFECTS OF PREGNANCY ON PRE-EXISTING MUSCULOSKELETAL CONDITIONS

Pregnancy and the associated changes in circulating hormones and postural changes affect a diverse range of pre-existing musculoskeletal conditions. Examples include disease improvement in slightly more than half of women with pre-existing rheumatoid arthritis (RA) who become pregnant.[12] This, however, can be followed by an exacerbation of symptom flare-ups in the postpartum period.[13]

Some of the pharmacological treatment options of RA can affect fertility, along with increased risk of spontaneous abortion and embryotoxicity,[14] therefore health information and support are required. Knowledge of the effects of pregnancy on the musculoskeletal system is vital to ensure people with pre-existing conditions receive effective counselling and support during pregnancy.

Late adulthood (65+ years)

With ageing, loss of bone matrix (resorption) occurs more rapidly than new bone growth (deposition). The net effect is a loss of bone density, or **osteoporosis**. While the age-adjusted incidence of osteoporotic hip fracture in Australia appears to have decreased over recent years, the actual number of cases has increased in both sexes when population growth and the proportion of older people are considered. In Australia, 5.6% of people aged over 55 and 20.1% over 75 years of age have been diagnosed with osteoporosis or osteopenia.[15] Of the estimated 924,000 Australians with osteoporosis, it is more common in women than men.[16] As the population ages, the incidence is expected to increase. (See also 'Osteoporosis—the silent disease' below.)

Postural changes are evident with ageing in some people and decreased height is the most noticeable. Decreased height is due to shortening of the vertebral column caused by the gradual loss of water and associated thinning of the intervertebral discs. Both men and women can expect a progressive decrease in height beginning at age 40 years in males and age 43 years in females, although this decrease is not significant until age 60 years. A greater decrease may occur in the 70s and 80s because of osteoporotic collapse of the vertebrae. The result is a shortening of the trunk and comparatively long extremities. Other postural changes are kyphosis, a backwards head tilt to compensate for the kyphosis and a slight flexion of hips and knees.

The distribution of subcutaneous fat changes through life. Usually, men and women gain weight in their 40s and 50s. The contour is different, even if the weight is the same as when younger. They begin to lose fat in the face and deposit it in the abdomen and hips. In the 80s and 90s, fat further decreases in the periphery, which is especially noticeable in the forearms and becomes more apparent over the abdomen and hips. Loss of subcutaneous fat leaves bony prominences more marked (e.g. tips of the vertebrae, ribs, iliac crests) and body hollows deeper, for example, cheeks and axillae.

An absolute loss in muscle mass occurs with ageing; some muscles decrease in size and some atrophy, producing weakness, particularly in people with low physical activity levels. The contour of muscles becomes more prominent, and muscle bundles and tendons feel more distinct. This age-related loss of muscle mass and strength including loss of function (sarcopenia) is associated with increased risk of frailty and functional decline in some older people.[17]

It has become more apparent that lifestyle affects musculoskeletal changes. A sedentary lifestyle hastens the musculoskeletal changes of ageing. Multimodal exercise programs incorporating progressive resistance training, aerobic training, weight-bearing impact training with balance training several times per week has been shown to increase bone and muscle strength and reduce falls and potentially fractures in older people.[18]

The musculoskeletal changes and the associated musculoskeletal degenerative diseases have a major impact on an older person's safety. Gait pattern changes include slowing down and shorter stride length. Within Australia, falls are the leading cause of injury-related hospitalisations, representing 43% of admissions and 42% of injury deaths. In 2021–22, falls resulted in 233,000 hospitalisations.[19]

The impact of a fall may lead to a fear of falling, which spirals into physical, functional and psychological consequences for older adults.[20] Falls prevention programs are therefore widespread at both state and Commonwealth levels in Australia.

Cultural and social considerations

Musculoskeletal conditions are the most common chronic conditions in Australia, affecting 27% (or 6.9 million) of the Australian population. They represent some of the most common causes of pain and disability.[19] The most common musculoskeletal conditions affecting Australians are back pain (23% in the 45–65 age group), osteoarthritis (OA) (41% in the over-65 age group), other forms of arthritis and osteoporosis.[19] Musculoskeletal disease conditions were the leading contributors to the non-fatal health burden in 2022.[21]

In Australia, musculoskeletal injuries after road traffic accidents occur with differing levels of severity. Injury sequelae include not only functional impairments such as chronic pain and joint disorders or fractures but also a range of negative health outcomes including psychological, social and economic challenges. These often-profound injuries cause a ripple effect of loss and grief that affects families, friends and communities.[22]

Musculoskeletal diseases contribute to over 14.6% of the non-fatal disease burden in Indigenous Australians. In Australia the prevalence of OA among Aboriginal and Torres Strait Islander people is high and yet access to care and services is low. For a range of reasons, there is not always the same level of access to health services compared with non-Indigenous Australians.[23] Indigenous Australian males are twice as likely as other Australian males to have a hip fracture resulting from a fall. Indigenous females are 26% more likely to have a hip fracture than other Australian females. Indigenous Australians are on average much younger than other Australians at the time of their hip fracture, aged 65 years (compared with 81 years) for males and 74 years (compared with 83 years) for females.[24] The increased occurrence has been associated with a prevalence of chronic diseases that can contribute to an increased falls risk. Chronic musculoskeletal diseases and trauma statistics for Indigenous Australians are incomplete.

In Australia, there is an increasing trend for vitamin D deficiency. Although skin cancers impose a considerable health risk, protection from UV exposure has been linked to decreased vitamin D production. Vitamin D deficiency is directly linked to musculoskeletal health and increased risk of osteomalacia and osteoporosis.[25] An Australian study indicated that 32% of young adults were vitamin D deficient, higher than any other age group. The most significant bone health concerns have been highlighted for people born outside of Australia or living in the southern parts of Australia. Also, not being a healthy weight, smoking, having low physical activity levels, increased time spent indoors and not taking vitamin D supplements are contributing to widespread vitamin D deficiency.[26]

HEALTH EDUCATION

Osteoporosis—'the silent disease'

Bone is a dynamic tissue that responds to mechanical stresses through a complex process of remodelling. The remodelling process involves resorbing microdamaged bone by osteoclast cells followed by a phase of bone formation by osteoblast cells. In healthy adults, this process is coupled to ensure bone density remains stable. This process begins in childhood, with peak bone mass reached by the end of the second decade of life. Adolescence is a critical period for skeletal growth, particularly for females, who develop 40 to 50% of their total bone mass during early teen years.[27] There is also a direct association between good nutrition and exercise in developing bone health and bone mass in children and adolescence, emphasising the value of a healthy lifestyle and weight management from childhood through to adulthood to prevent osteopenia/osteoporosis.[28]

When this bone remodelling process becomes uncoupled, normal bone density is altered, leading to a change in the normal architecture of bone seen in diseases such as osteoporosis. Osteoporosis is a systemic skeletal disorder characterised by decreased bone mass and micro-architectural deterioration of bone tissue, leading to enhanced bone fragility and a consequent increase in fracture risk.[3] The loss of bone occurs 'silently' and progressively. Often there are no symptoms until the first fracture occurs. Fractures associated with osteoporosis are termed low trauma or fragility fractures and occur most frequently in the neck of femur, vertebrae, distal radius, ribs and sacrum, often resulting in reduced quality of life and increased morbidity and mortality.[29]

Around 924,000 Australians have osteoporosis. Twenty per cent of Australians aged 75 years or older have osteoporosis or osteopenia; females are four times as likely to have osteoporosis than males, but this varies with age.[16] As the population ages, these rates are expected to rise. Osteoporosis has a significant impact on the person in terms of risk of fracture, actual fracture, disability or even death. It also has a huge burden on the health system on the direct costs of treating fracture, rehabilitation and ongoing support.[30]

Risk factors for osteoporosis and fractures include both non-modifiable factors and modifiable factors:[31]

- **non-modifiable factors—**family history, especially maternal family history of osteoporotic fracture
- **modifiable and lifestyle factors—**early menopause, multiple falls, low physical activity or immobility, low bodyweight or obesity, low muscle mass and strength, poor balance, protein or calcium undernutrition, smoking, consuming more than two standard alcoholic drinks per day, vitamin D deficiency and/or lack of sunlight
- **medical conditions—**including malabsorption syndromes (coeliac disease and inflammatory bowel disease), chronic renal and liver diseases, rheumatoid arthritis, hyperthyroidism
- **medications—**including glucocorticoids, hormone therapy for breast and prostate cancers, antiepileptic therapy, antipsychotic, proton-pump inhibitors.

Continued

HEALTH EDUCATION cont'd

Nurse's role

Nurses should be actively promoting bone health with all people. This includes information concerning:[31,32]

- **bone health awareness—**including risk factors for osteoporosis, the need for screening of risk and the 'Know your bones' bone health assessment tool
- **diet and lifestyle—**adequate calcium and protein intake, adequate but safe exposure to sunlight (vitamin D), healthy bodyweight and BMI, cessation of smoking, following the national guidelines for alcohol consumption, exercise (high impact and strength training for increasing bone mineral density and improving balance 2–3 times per week)
- **promoting available resources—for example:**
  - Know Your Bones: www.knowyourbones.org.au
  - Healthy Bones Australia: https://healthybonesaustralia.org.au
  - Osteoporosis New Zealand: https://osteoporosis.org.nz

Subjective data

Musculoskeletal assessment can be challenging for nurses and the person. It often involves asking intimate questions as well as requiring the person to be partially undressed and therefore vulnerable. You need to ensure the privacy and comfort of the person during musculoskeletal assessment.

Practice note

Before you start the assessment, introduce yourself to the person, confirm the person's identity, discuss the purpose and scope of the assessment, clarify any questions the person may have and get verbal consent from the person to perform the assessment.

ASSESSMENT GUIDELINES	CLINICAL SIGNIFICANCE AND CLINICAL ALERTS
Presenting concern	
• *Do you have any problems with your joints, muscles, bones or walking and moving that affects your ability to exercise and go about your daily activities?* It is important to ascertain the person's perception of their musculoskeletal function. If they do perceive a problem, ask: *How does this affect your quality of life?*	The person's response to this question will guide you to areas to focus on in further subjective and objective data collection.
Gait, arms, legs and spine (GALS) screening questions	
A screening musculoskeletal examination can rapidly identify those people who need comprehensive musculoskeletal assessment. The GALS screening assessment is a highly sensitive, specific and well-validated screening assessment for detecting joint abnormalities.[33,34] Subjective data from this screening assessment involves three core questions: • *Have you any pain or stiffness in your muscles, joints or back?*	

ASSESSMENT GUIDELINES	CLINICAL SIGNIFICANCE AND CLINICAL ALERTS
• *Can you dress yourself completely without any difficulty?* • *Can you walk up and down stairs without any difficulty?* A positive response to the first question and/or a negative response to the second or third question indicates a detailed history should be taken. A paediatric-specific GALS assessment (pGALS) has also proved highly sensitive, specific and well validated.[34,35]	
Joints	
• *Do you have any problems with your joints? Tell me about your* pain.	**Joint pain and loss of function** are the most common musculoskeletal concerns that prompt a person to seek care.
Location • *Which joints are affected? On one side or both sides?*	**Rheumatoid arthritis (RA)** involves symmetrical joints; other musculoskeletal illnesses and trauma involve isolated or unilateral joints. **Osteoarthritis (OA)** (degenerative joint disease)—asymmetrical joint involvement commonly affects hands, knees, hips and lumbar, as well as cervical segments of the spine (Table 20.1).
Quality • *What does the pain feel like: aching, stiff, sharp, or dull, shooting?* **Severity** • *How strong is the pain?* **Onset** • *When did this pain start?*	**Exquisite tenderness** felt with acute inflammation. **Persistent** (chronic) **pain** is often associated with degenerative musculoskeletal disorders.
Timing • *What time of day does the pain occur?* • *How long does it last?* • *How often does it occur?*	**RA** pain is worse in the morning when arising; **OA** is worse later in the day; **tendonitis** (inflammation of a tendon caused by overuse or injury) is usually a dull but constant soreness and is often worse in the morning, improving during the day as the muscles get warmer.
• *Is the pain aggravated by movement, rest, position, weather?* • *Is the pain relieved by rest, medications, application of heat or ice?* • *Is there anything that assists in turning down the volume of the persistent (chronic) pain?*	Most joint pain is mechanical except in RA, when deformities restrict movement. Many people have tried prescribed medications, homeopathic remedies, over the counter medications or combination formulations. These need to be identified and included in your assessment.
• *Is the pain associated with chills, fever, recent sore throat, trauma or repetitive activity?*	Joint pain 10 to 14 days after an untreated streptococcal throat infection (strep throat) suggests rheumatic fever (Chapter 17). Joint injury occurs from trauma or repetitive motion.

ASSESSMENT GUIDELINES	CLINICAL SIGNIFICANCE AND CLINICAL ALERTS
• *Do you have any stiffness in your joints?*	**Stiffness** from RA or OA occurs in the morning and after rest periods.
• *Do you have any swelling, heat, redness in the joints?*	Suggests acute inflammation.
• *Do you have any limitation of movement in any joint? Which joint?* • *Which activities give you problems?* (See 'Functional assessment' below.)	**Decreased range of movement (ROM)** may be due to injury, joint disease or to muscle contracture.
Muscles	
• *Do you have any problems in the muscles such as any pain or cramping? Which muscles? What makes it worse or better?*	**Myalgia** (pain in one or more muscle) is usually felt as cramping or aching.
• If in calf muscles: *Is the pain with walking? Does it go away with rest?*	**Intermittent claudication** is pain in the leg muscles, usually the calf muscle, which occurs during exercise and is eased by rest. It is associated with peripheral vascular disease (Chapter 16).
• *Are your muscle aches associated with fever, chills or the flu?*	Viral illness often includes myalgia.
• *Do you have any weakness in any muscles?* **Location** • *Where is the weakness? How long have you noticed weakness?*	**Weakness** may also involve peripheral vascular system or neurological systems (Chapters 12 and 16).
• *Do the muscles look different there?*	Smaller, asymmetrical muscles may indicate **atrophy** (decrease in size of the muscle due to injury or disease) (Table 20.2). Swelling may indicate **haematoma** (a collection of blood outside of blood vessels), especially when there is a history of recent injury.
Bones	
• *Do you have any bone pain? Is the pain affected by movement?* • *Do you have any deformity of any bone or joint? Is the deformity due to injury or trauma? Does the deformity affect the amount of movement in the joint?* • *Have any accidents or trauma ever affected the bones or joints: fractures, joint strain, sprain, dislocation? Which ones?*	Trauma causes sharp pain that increases with movement. Other bone pain usually feels 'dull' and 'deep' and is unrelated to movement. Injury to ligaments affects joint kinematics such as whiplash trauma and may result in cervical ligament laxity and chronic pain syndromes.
• *When did this occur? What treatment was given? Any problems or limitations now as a result?*	Previous joint trauma increases risk of OA. Many people with back pain have sought treatments provided by physiotherapists, chiropractors, osteopaths or acupuncturists.

ASSESSMENT GUIDELINES	CLINICAL SIGNIFICANCE AND CLINICAL ALERTS
• *Do you have any back pain? In which part of your back? Is pain felt anywhere else, like shooting down your leg or arm?* • *How long have you had this pain?*	The aetiology of back pain is diverse such as degenerative or traumatic conditions of the **spine, fibrositis, inflammatory spondyloarthropathy** and metabolic bone conditions are also cited as causes.
• *Do you have any numbness and tingling? Any limping?*	Spinal nerve-root dysfunction is associated with altered sensory and motor function (Chapter 12).
Functional assessment	
• *Do your joint (muscle, bone) problems create any limits on your usual activities of daily living (ADLs)? Which ones?* (Note: Ask about each category; if the person answers 'yes', ask specifically about each activity in the category.)	**Functional assessment** screens the safety of independent living, the need for community supports and quality of life.
Bathing • *Do you have any difficulty getting in and out of the shower/bath or turning on taps?* • *Can you wash your back, legs, feet and hair?*	Degenerative lower limb joint dysfunction affects mobility and steppage and increases the risk of falls. Upper limb nerve compression affects precision and grip such as **carpal tunnel syndrome**.
Toileting • *Do you have any difficulty urinating or moving bowels? Can you get yourself on/off the toilet, undress, wipe yourself and redress after using the toilet?*	Altered bowel and bladder function may be an indication of **cauda equina syndrome**, which occurs when the nerve roots in the lumbar spine are compressed, cutting off sensation and movement.
Dressing • *Do you have any difficulty doing up buttons or a zip? Can you fasten the opening behind your neck, pull a dress or sweater overhead and pull up your pants? Do you have trouble tying your shoelaces or getting shoes that fit?*	Degenerative processes can lead to foot deformity, pain and disability. Foot deformities and ill-fitting shoes all increase falls risk.
Grooming • *Do you have any difficulty brushing your teeth, brushing or fixing your hair or applying make-up?*	
Eating • *Do you have any difficulty preparing meals, pouring liquids, cutting up foods, bringing food to your mouth or drinking?*	
Mobility • *Do you have any difficulty walking, getting up or down stairs, getting in/out of bed or getting out of the house?*	When a person has significant impairment of mobility a **falls risk screening** should be conducted.

ASSESSMENT GUIDELINES	CLINICAL SIGNIFICANCE AND CLINICAL ALERTS
Communicating • *Do you have any difficulty talking, using the phone, using a computer or writing?*	Chronic diseases can cause a decrease in independence with activities of daily living, social isolation and depression.
General health history	
• *Do you have any other medical/health conditions for which you are being treated?* • *Have you had treatment for fractures, muscle tears or a tendon or joint injury? If so, which areas and when did it occur? Was the treatment successful?*	A variety of endocrine/metabolic disorders, nutritional conditions and medications can affect bone health. Diseases such as hyperthyroidism, diabetes, renal disease, malabsorption syndromes and medications such as glucocorticoids and loop diuretics are the most common risk factors. Previous bone, muscle, tendon or joint injury can predispose the person to OA.
Family health history	
• *Do other members of your extended family have problems with their muscles, bones or joints?*	There is a strong genetic link associated with musculoskeletal health so the person should be asked to discuss any family history of fractures or arthritis.
Health and lifestyle management	
Work • *Do you have any occupational hazards that could affect your muscles and joints?* • *Does your work involve heavy lifting?* • *Is there any repetitive motion or chronic stress to joints in your work?* • *What measures have you used to alleviate these?*	Where the workplace is contributing to potential injuries, the person should undergo a formal workplace assessment.
Exercise • *Do you have any pain during exercise? How do you treat it?*	
Diet *Has your weight changed recently? Please describe your usual daily diet.* (Note the person's usual kilojoule intake, all four food groups, daily amount of protein, calcium.)	Weight affects joint function. Low calcium and vitamin D, together with smoking and excessive alcohol, are risk factors for osteoporosis.
Medications • *Are you taking any medications for musculoskeletal pain?* • *Are you taking any herbal supplements, vitamins or other natural remedies?*	Common medications for musculoskeletal pain include: aspirin, anti-inflammatory, muscle relaxant, other pain relievers. Over-the-counter medications are common first-line treatments for joint pain (glucosamine, fish oils). Complementary medications have iatrogenic effects and should be included in a health history. Persistent (chronic) pain sufferers often use multiple analgesia.

ASSESSMENT GUIDELINES	CLINICAL SIGNIFICANCE AND CLINICAL ALERTS
If the person has a chronic disability and/or severe musculoskeletal dysfunction, ask how the symptoms/illness affects: • their interactions with family and friends • their work and leisure activities • the way they view themselves • how they manage their health • their social life • their stress levels and coping ability.	Possible consequences include: • self-esteem disturbance • loss of independence • body image disturbance • role performance disturbance • social isolation/stress and coping • health management ability. Significant issues in any of these areas may indicate the need for further focused assessment.
Additional subjective data for infants and children (questions for parents or guardians)	
Children with musculoskeletal problems often present to primary care services with traumatic or non-traumatic injuries. Most problems are self-limiting, but the presentation of life-threatening illnesses such as **malignancy** or **septic arthritis** will require urgent referrals to specialty services. Chronic illnesses such as **juvenile arthritis** and the **muscular dystrophies** also require urgent referrals to improve care outcomes.	Children with 'growing pains' do not limp or experience morning stiffness. **Non-accidental injury** can present as unexplained fracture patterns or bruising with incongruity between the child's and the carer/parent's history. Ensuring the child's safety and completing detailed documentation are priorities. Refer to your local state and territory legislation on non-accidental injury and your local hospital/community guidelines for assessment and treatment plans (Chapter 5).
• *Were you told about any trauma to your child during labour and delivery?* • *Did the baby's head come first?* • *Was there a need for forceps?*	Traumatic delivery increases risk for fractures (e.g. humerus, clavicle) and **developmental dysplasia of the hip (DDH).**
• *Did the baby need resuscitation?*	A period of anoxia may result in hypotonia of muscles.
• *Were the baby's motor milestones achieved at about the same time as siblings or age mates?* • *Have any of the baby's milestones changed recently?*	Pain, joint dysfunction, malaise and fever all have an impact on activity and learning capacity, hence milestones may be affected. For example, a toddler may stop walking, develop enuresis or have sleep disturbances.
• *Has your child been well? Any weight loss, fever or malaise?*	A recent fever with pain and/or swelling of one joint or bone may indicate an infective or inflammatory process.
• *Has your child ever broken any bones?* • *Any bruising or dislocations? Where and how were these treated?*	Fractures of the epiphyseal plate may lead to deformity. Immediate pain, swelling and loss of function following traumatic injury may indicate a fracture or dislocation.

ASSESSMENT GUIDELINES	CLINICAL SIGNIFICANCE AND CLINICAL ALERTS
• *Have you ever noticed any bone deformity?* • *Head tilting or spinal curvature?* • *Unusual shape of toes or feet? At what age?* • *Have you ever sought treatment for any of these?*	Gait changes can indicate normal development or undiagnosed hip problems such as DDH, **Legg-Calvé-Perthes** disease and slipped upper femoral epiphysis. Spinal problems may present as asymmetrical ribs or waist and head tilting.
Additional subjective data for adolescents	
• *Are you involved in any sports at school or after school? How frequently?*	40% of bone mass accumulates during adolescence. This is achieved through exercise and a healthy diet.
• *Do you use any special equipment?*	Assess use of safety equipment (e.g. mouth guards, helmets) and safe sporting practices.
• *Is there any training program for your sport?*	Use of safety equipment and the presence of adult supervision decreases the risk of sports injuries.
• *What is the nature of your daily warm-up?*	Lack of adequate warm-up increases the risk of sports injury.
• *What do you do if you get hurt?*	Adolescents may not report injury or pain for fear of limiting participation in sport.
• *Have you ever noticed any bone deformity? Spinal curvature?*	Adolescents with **scoliosis** (abnormal lateral curvature of the spine) may report unilateral changes in the shoulders, rib cage, hip levels and an uneven waist.
Additional subjective data for adults over 65 years	
The questions you ask older adults should focus on functional abilities. The aim is to elicit any loss of function, self-care deficit or safety risk that may occur as a process of ageing or musculoskeletal illness. Ask questions only where relevant to the person's situation.	
• *Have you experienced any muscle weakness over the past months or years?*	Pain/joint dysfunction impacts on activity and increases weakness and lethargy.
• *Have you had any falls or stumbling over the past months or years?*	It is essential to focus on exploring all falls risks in a positive way. Numerous general health issues and prescribed medications for musculoskeletal function, such as chronic heart and lung disease, affect mobility. Visual deficits, hypotension, vitamin B12 deficiency and incontinence all increase falls risk.
• *Do you use any walking aids to help you get around inside or outside your home?* • *Where did you purchase these walking aids?*	All gait aids should be supplied as part of a comprehensive mobility assessment performed by a physiotherapist.

Objective data

The subjective data will assist in targeting your objective data collection and referral criteria. As you progress through the physical examination, observe the person's ability to complete activities of daily living as they go through the motions necessary for an examination: gait, posture, how the person sits in a chair, rises from a chair, takes off a jacket, manipulates a small object such as a pen and rises from the supine position. It is essential to identify painful joints in collecting the health history to ensure these are examined last. Ensure the privacy and comfort of the person during musculoskeletal assessment.

Preparation

All forms of musculoskeletal assessment require a systematic approach:

- head to toe
- proximal to distal
- compare the corresponding paired joint.

Expect symmetry of structure and function and normal parameters for that joint.

Also, a neurovascular assessment of upper and lower limbs is a mandatory component for all musculoskeletal assessments (Chapters 12 and 16).

As you approach this examination, focus on the principles of 'look, feel, move and listen':

- **look (inspect)**—asymmetry of joints, joint swelling, deformity, abnormalities of muscle and soft tissue bulk, erythema, ecchymosis, lesions and rashes, the general health of the person and their response/reaction to movement of muscles and joints
- **feel (palpate)**—soft tissue swelling, bony or crystal nodules, tenderness, joint warmth and pain; palpate and listen for crepitation (grating or crunching sensations/sounds) when moving the joints
- **move**—active movement first followed by passive movement; perform painful movements last.

PROCEDURES AND NORMAL FINDINGS	ABNORMAL FINDINGS AND CLINICAL ALERTS
General inspection	
While collecting subjective data, you will have noticed ease of movement and breathing, ability to sit and stand, height-to-weight ratio, level of hygiene and grooming and general demeanour. All these factors provide clues to the functioning of the musculoskeletal system.	
GALS screening assessment (inspection and palpation)	
Gait	
Observe the person walking, turning, then walking back. Observe for symmetry and smoothness of gait.	**Antalgic gait** is a symptom of pain with weight bearing. The stance phase of the gait is abnormally shortened relative to the swing phase.

PROCEDURES AND NORMAL FINDINGS	ABNORMAL FINDINGS AND CLINICAL ALERTS
Does the person limp? Observe for any reduced muscle bulk in the gluteals. Can the person turn quickly?	**Ataxia** is gross lack of coordination of muscle movement—for example, when walking the person may appear intoxicated. It is a neurological sign (Chapter 12).
Arms	
Shoulder movements (Figures 20.15A and 20.15B) Ask the person to place their hands behind their head, with their elbows back. This movement assesses abduction, external rotation of the shoulder and elbow flexion. Palpate each shoulder for symmetry in shape and strength of muscles. **Elbow movements and hands** Ask the person to extend their arms fully and turn their hands over so palms are down (Figure 20.15C). Following this ask the person to turn their hands over. Observe the elbow and hands for any joint/tissue swelling or deformities. **Grip strength** (Figure 20.15D) Ask the person to make a fist. Observe the hand and finger movements. Ask the person to grip your fingers and assess the degree of grip strength. **Observe for pain** Squeeze across the second to fifth metacarpal. Observe for pain (Figure 15.E). **Palpate (and listen) for cracking or crunching (crepitation)** As the person moves the joint, feel and listen for crepitation.	***Clinical alert:*** If the person has significantly restricted ROM of any joint, they should be referred for further assessment by a medical practitioner or physiotherapist, particularly if they are experiencing pain or a restriction in their ability to complete their ADLs. **Grip strength** is a measure of muscular strength and can be used as a screening tool for measuring upper body strength and overall body strength. A low grip strength is associated with a higher all-cause mortality rate in older people.[36] Common abnormalities include atrophy of muscles, a tear in a major muscle (e.g. rotator cuff in the shoulder), dislocation of a joint, inability to move a joint, bursitis (inflammation of the joint bursa), presence of nodules and pain (Tables 20.2, 20.3 and 20.4). **Crepitation** is a popping, cracking or grinding sound during movement of a joint which may sometimes be accompanied by pain. It can be caused by air within the joint (normal), tendons or ligaments moving over a joint or in a joint that has RA or OA (usually also accompanied by pain). It may be felt by the person or heard by the examiner (Figure 20.15).
Legs	
Position the person lying down with the upper torso covered. **Hip movement** • Hold the knee and hip flexed to 90 degrees. Assess the degree of internal rotation in each hip (Figure 20.15F). **Knee** • Observe: Look for any reduced muscle bulk, especially in the quadriceps. • Assess: Ask the person to flex and extend both knees.	**Pain** on movement is an abnormal finding. **Limited or reduced ROM** of the hips, knees, ankles or feet is an abnormal finding. Common abnormalities include inflammation of a joint or tendon, swelling, **bursitis**, presence of nodules and pain. **Crepitus** is any grinding, creaking, cracking, grinding or grating sensation felt by the person or the examiner (Tables 20.5 and 20.6).

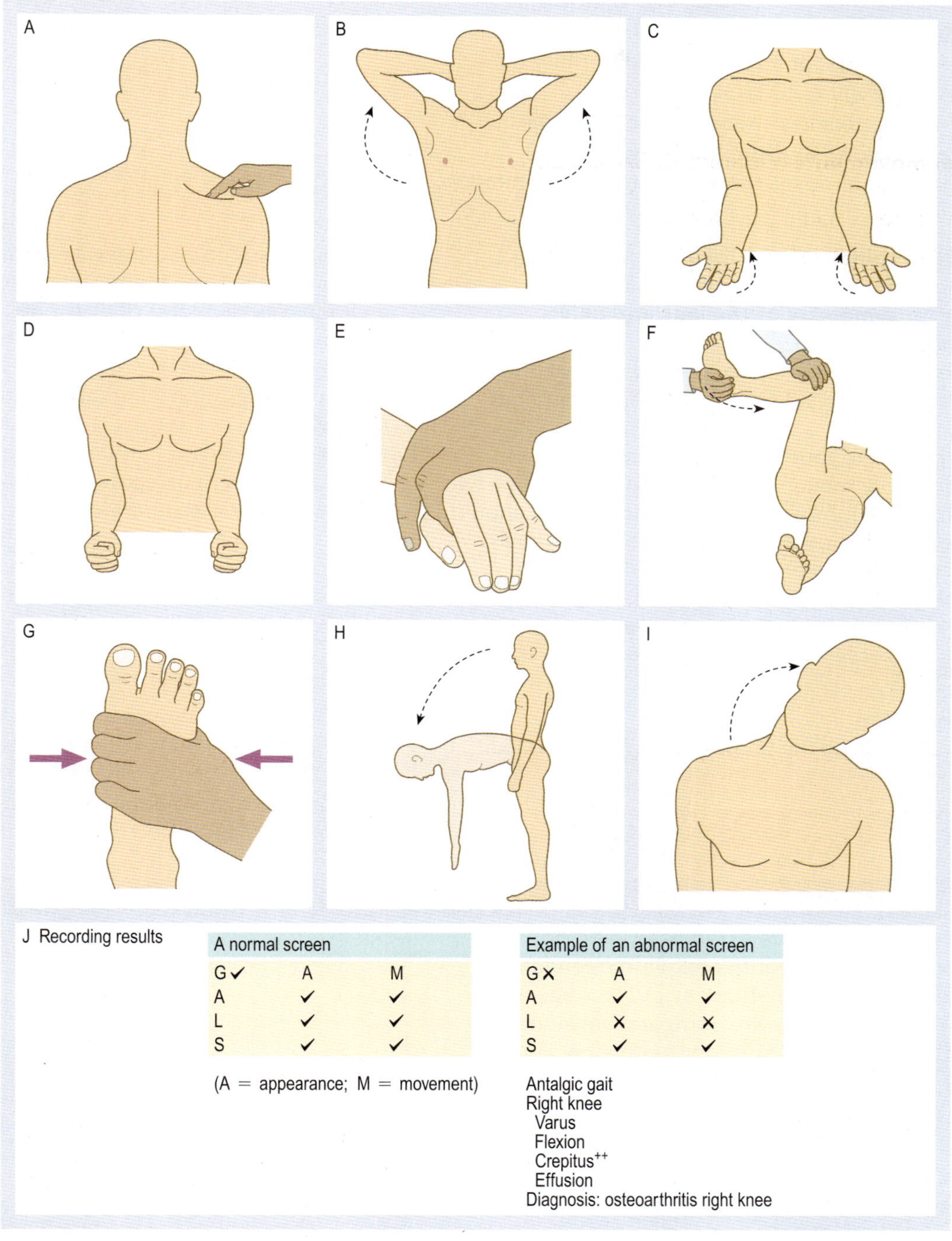

FIGURE 20.15 The GALS screening assessment

PROCEDURES AND NORMAL FINDINGS	ABNORMAL FINDINGS AND CLINICAL ALERTS
• Palpate the knee for crepitus and warmth. **Inspection of feet and shoes** • Inspect the feet for any swelling, deformity or callosities (Figure 20.15G). • Look at the person's shoes for unequal wear. **Listen for cracking or crunching (crepitation)** • As the person moves the joint, listen for crepitation.	
Spine	
Inspect the spinal column for any abnormalities including kyphosis, scoliosis or lordosis. Observe for **symmetry of the legs and pelvis**. **Thoracolumbar spine** Hold the person's pelvis from behind and ask them to turn from side to side—assesses thoracolumbar rotation. Ask the person to touch their toes. Palpate for the range of lumbar movement (Figure 20.15H). Place two fingers over the lumbar vertebrae. Your fingers should move apart as the person bend forwards—assess lumbar spine movement. **Cervical spine** Ask the person to bring their ear towards their shoulder—assesses lateral cervical flexion (Figure 20.15I).	**Kyphosis** is a spinal disorder where there is excessive curvature of the spine causing an abnormal rounding of the upper back. It can occur at any age but is more common in adolescence. **Scoliosis** is an abnormal lateral curvature of the spine. **Lordosis** is an increase in the natural curve of the lower (lumbar) spine (swayback). It can also occur in the cervical spine (Table 20.7).
Documentation Record results using the framework in Figure 20.15J.	When abnormal results are obtained on the screening GALS assessment refer to a medical practitioner or physiotherapist or complete a more detailed physical examination (described in the advanced practice section).
Additional objective data for adults over 65 years	
Postural changes include a decrease in height, more apparent in the eighth and ninth decades. 'Lengthening of the arm–trunk axis' describes this shortening of the trunk with comparatively long extremities. Kyphosis is common, with a backwards head tilt to compensate. This creates the outline of a figure 3 when you view this older adult from the left side. Slight flexion of hips and knees is also common. Contour changes include a decrease of fat in the body periphery and fat deposition over the abdomen and hips. The bony prominences become more marked.	

PROCEDURES AND NORMAL FINDINGS	ABNORMAL FINDINGS AND CLINICAL ALERTS
For most adults over 65, ROM testing proceeds as described earlier. ROM and muscle strength are much the same as with younger adults, provided no musculoskeletal illnesses or arthritic changes are present.	

Functional assessment

For those with advanced ageing changes, arthritic changes or musculoskeletal disability, perform a **functional assessment for ADLs**. You need to determine the adequate and safe performance of functions essential for independent home life.

Instructions to the person	Common adaptation for ageing changes
1. Walk (with shoes on).	Shuffling pattern; swaying; arms out to help balance; broader base of support; person may watch feet.
2. Climb up stairs.	Person holds handrail; may haul body up with it; may lead with favoured (stronger) leg.
3. Walk downstairs.	Holds handrail, sometimes with both hands. If the person is weak, they may descend sideways, lowering the weaker leg first. If the person is unsteady, they may watch feet.
4. Pick up an object from the floor.	The person may bend at the waist instead of bending the knees; holds furniture to support while bending and straightening.
5. Rise from sitting in a chair.	The person uses the arms to push off the chair arms, the upper trunk leans forwards before the body straightens, the feet are planted wide in broad base of support.

PROCEDURES AND NORMAL FINDINGS	ABNORMAL FINDINGS AND CLINICAL ALERTS
6. Rise from lying in bed. The person may roll to one side, push with the arms to lift the torso, grab the bedside table to increase leverage.	
Laboratory studies	
There are many relevant specialist laboratory tests done to assess musculoskeletal health. We have listed the most common tests.	
Vitamin D is essential for bone and muscle health and regulating the immune system and cell activity. Vitamin D is required for effective absorption of calcium. A serum 25-hydroxyvitamin D (25-OHD) level of ≥ 50 nmol/L at the end of winter (10–20 nmol/L higher at the end of summer).[37]	**Low vitamin D** is associated with rickets and bone and muscle pain.
Rheumatoid factor: Normal levels are under 30 IU/L.[37]	People who have RA and a positive rheumatoid factor tend to have more aggressive disease.
Calcium levels detect hyper- or hypocalcaemia. Corrected calcium rather than total calcium levels are used for clinical diagnosis. Reference levels for corrected calcium: 2.10–2.6 mmol/L; total calcium: 2.10–2.60 mmol/L.[37]	**Hypercalcaemia** is associated with hyperparathyroidism, malignancy, bony metastases, sarcoidosis and vitamin D or A toxicity. **Hypocalcaemia** is associated with hypopara-thyroidism, renal failure, osteomalacia or rickets.

Abnormal findings

TABLE 20.1 Abnormalities affecting multiple joints

Inflammatory Conditions

Articular cartilage
Joint capsule
Synovial membrane
NORMAL JOINT (joint space enlarged for clarity)

Inflamed synovial membrane
Cyst
Erosion
Fibrous formation
Swelling of soft tissue

Rheumatoid arthritis

RA is a chronic, systemic inflammatory disease of the joints and surrounding connective tissue. Inflammation of synovial membrane leads to thickening, then to fibrosis, which limits motion and finally to bony ankylosis. The disorder is symmetrical and bilateral and is characterised by heat, redness, swelling and painful motion of the affected joints. RA is associated with fatigue, weakness, anorexia, weight loss, low-grade fever and lymphadenopathy. Associated signs are described in the following tables, especially Table 20.4.

Degenerative Conditions

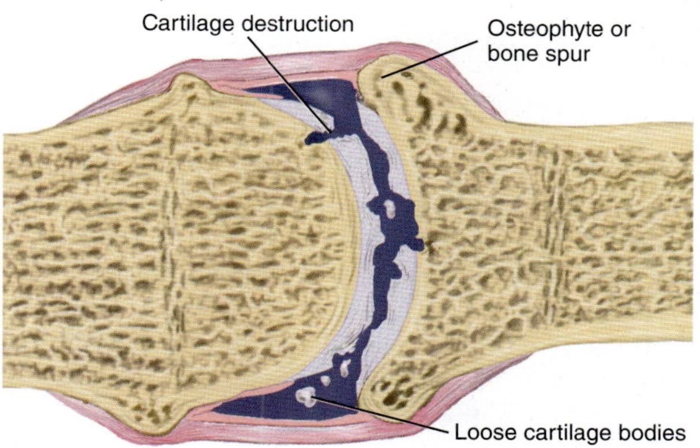

Osteoarthritis

Non-inflammatory, localised, progressive disorder involving deterioration of articular cartilages and subchondral bone and formation of new bone (osteophytes) at joint surfaces. Ageing increases incidence; nearly all adults over 60 years old have some radiographic signs of OA. Asymmetrical joint involvement commonly affects the hands, knees, hips and lumbar and cervical segments of the spine. Affected joints have stiffness, swelling with hard, bony protuberances, pain with motion and limitation of motion (Table 20.4).

Continued

TABLE 20.1 Abnormalities affecting multiple joints cont'd

Inflammatory Conditions

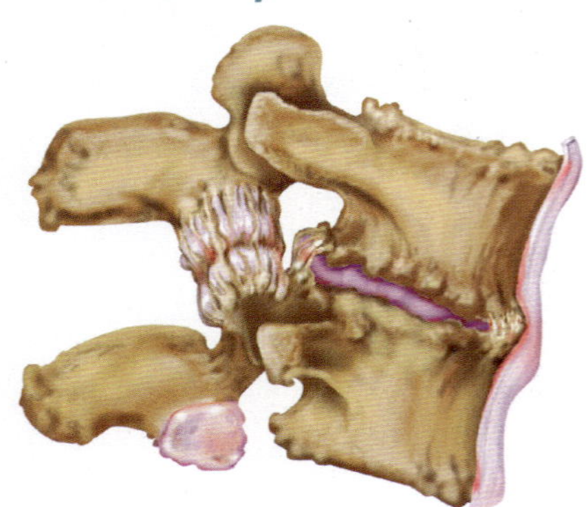

Ankylosing spondylitis

Chronic progressive inflammation of the spine, sacroiliac and larger joints of the extremities, leading to bony ankylosis and deformity. A form of RA, this affects primarily men by a 10:1 ratio, in late adolescence or early adulthood. Spasm of the paraspinal muscles pulls the spine into forward flexion, obliterating cervical and lumbar curves. The thoracic curve is exaggerated into single kyphotic rounding. Also includes flexion deformities of the hips and knees.

Degenerative Conditions

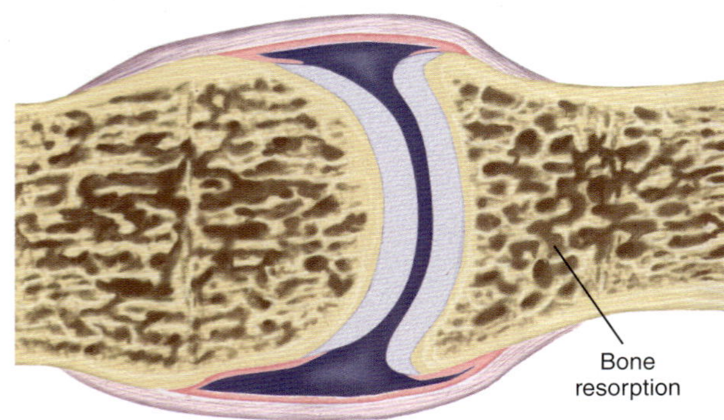

Osteoporosis

Osteoporosis occurs when there is a decrease in skeletal bone mass when the rate of bone resorption is greater than that of bone formation. The weakened bone state increases the risk for stress fractures, especially at the wrist, hip and vertebrae. For more information see the previous section on promoting a healthy lifestyle.

TABLE 20.2 Abnormalities of the shoulder

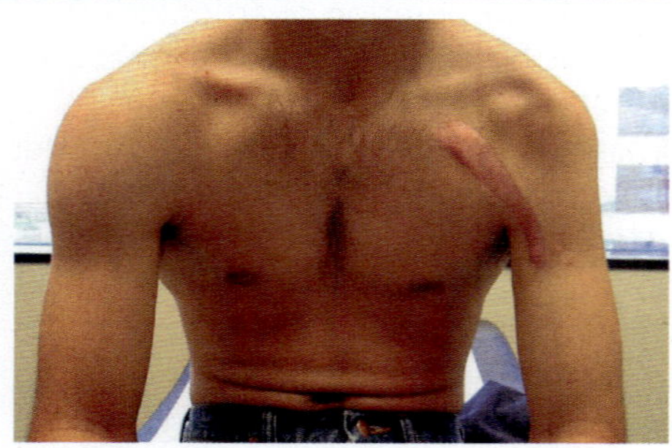

Atrophy

Loss of muscle mass is exhibited as a lack of fullness surrounding the deltoid muscle. In this case, atrophy is due to axillary nerve palsy. Atrophy also occurs from disuse, muscle tissue damage or motor nerve damage.

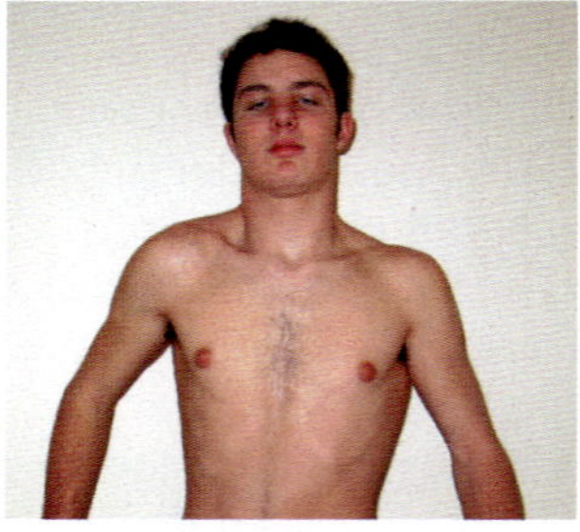

Tear of rotator cuff

Characteristic 'hunched' position and limited abduction of arm. Occurs from traumatic adduction while the arm is held in abduction, or from a fall on the shoulder, throwing or heavy lifting. Positive drop arm test: If the arm is passively abducted at the shoulder, the person cannot sustain the position and the arm falls to the side.

TABLE 20.2 Abnormalities of the shoulder cont'd

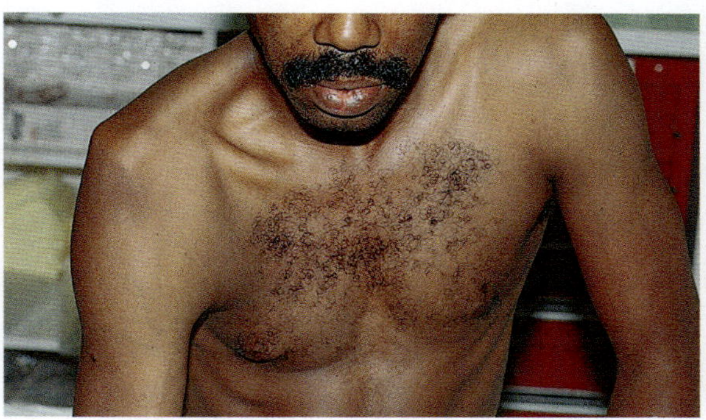

Dislocated shoulder

Anterior dislocation (95%) is exhibited when hunching the shoulder forward and the tip of the clavicle dislocates. It occurs with trauma involving abduction, extension and rotation (e.g. falling on an outstretched arm or diving into a pool).

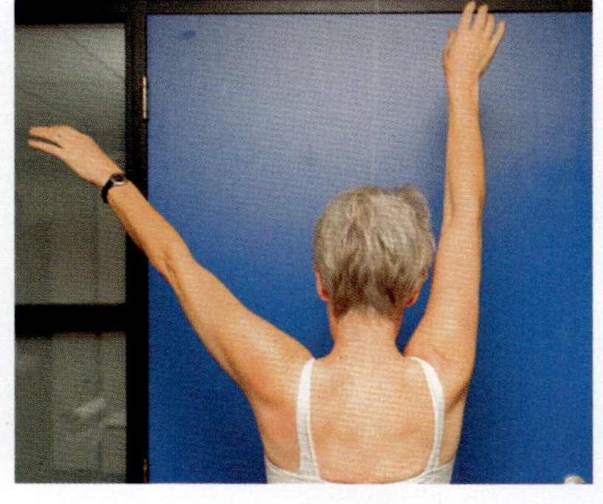

Frozen shoulder—adhesive capsulitis

Fibrous tissues form in the joint capsule, causing stiffness, progressive limitation of motion and pain. Motion limited in abduction and external rotation; unable to reach overhead. It may lead to atrophy of shoulder girdle muscles. Gradual onset; unknown cause. It is associated with prolonged bed rest or shoulder immobility. May resolve spontaneously.

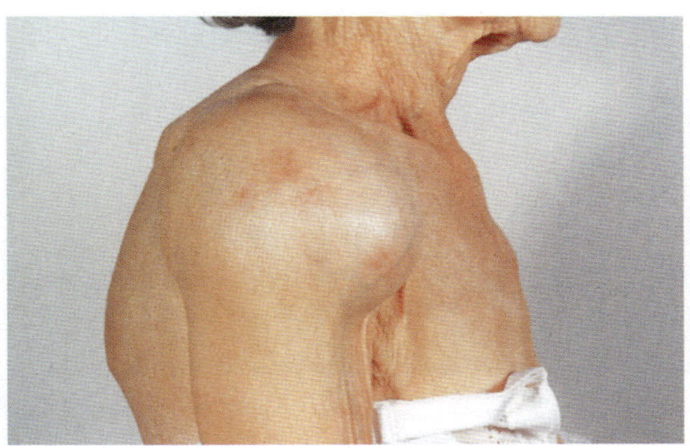

Joint effusion

Swelling from excess fluid in the joint capsule, here from RA. Best observed anteriorly. Fluctuant to palpation. Considerable fluid must be present to cause a visible distension because the capsule is normally so loose.

TABLE 20.3 Abnormalities of the elbow

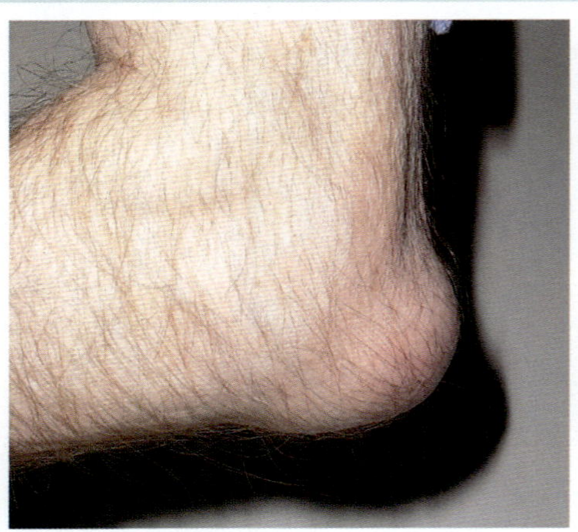

Olecranon bursitis

Large soft knob, or 'goose egg', and redness from inflammation of the olecranon bursa. Localised and easy to see because the bursa lies just under the skin.

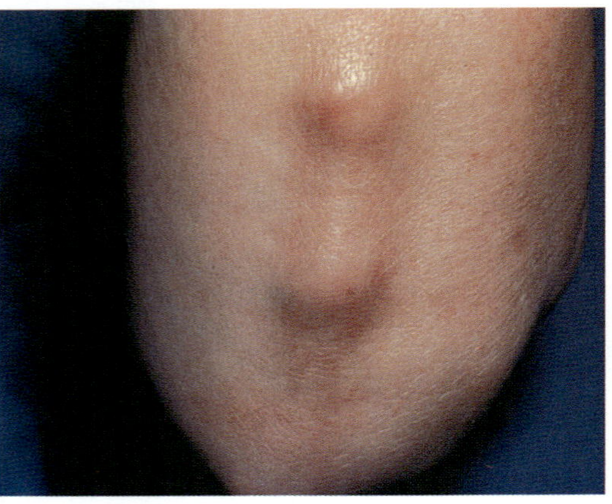

Subcutaneous nodules

Raised, firm, nontender nodules that occur with RA. Common sites are in the olecranon bursa and along the extensor surface of the arm. The skin slides freely over the nodules.

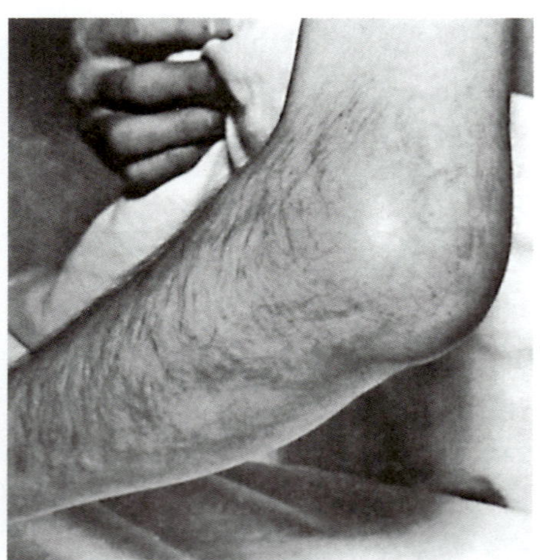

Arthritis of the elbow

Arthritis

Joint effusion or synovial thickening, seen first as a bulge or fullness in grooves on either side of olecranon process. Redness and heat can extend beyond the area of synovial membrane. Soft, boggy or fluctuant fullness to palpation. Limited extension of the elbow. Occurs with OA, RA, gout and trauma.

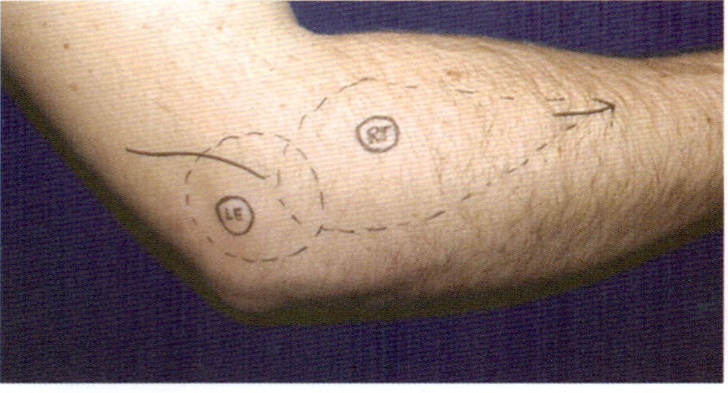

Epicondylitis—tennis elbow

Chronic disabling pain at the lateral epicondyle of the humerus; radiates down the extensor surface of the forearm. Pain can be located with one finger. Resisting extension of the hand will increase the pain. Occurs with activities combining excessive pronation and supination of the forearm with an extended wrist (e.g. racquet sports or using a screwdriver).
Medial epicondylitis is rarer and is due to activity of forced palmar flexion of the wrist against resistance.

TABLE 20.4 Abnormalities of the wrist and hand

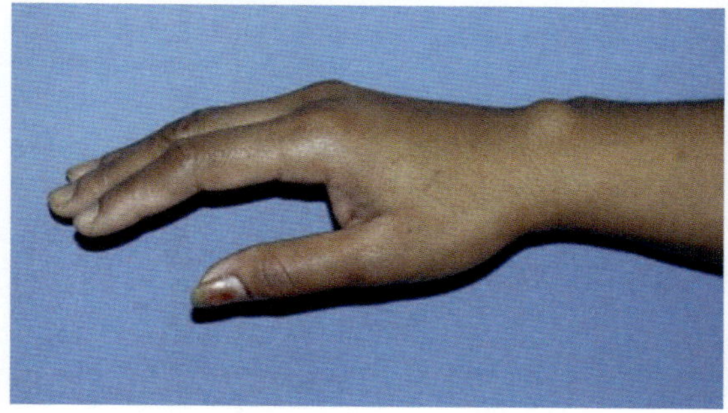

Ganglion cyst

Round, cystic, nontender nodule overlying a tendon sheath or joint capsule, usually on the dorsum of the wrist. Flexion makes it more prominent. A common benign tumour: it does not become malignant.

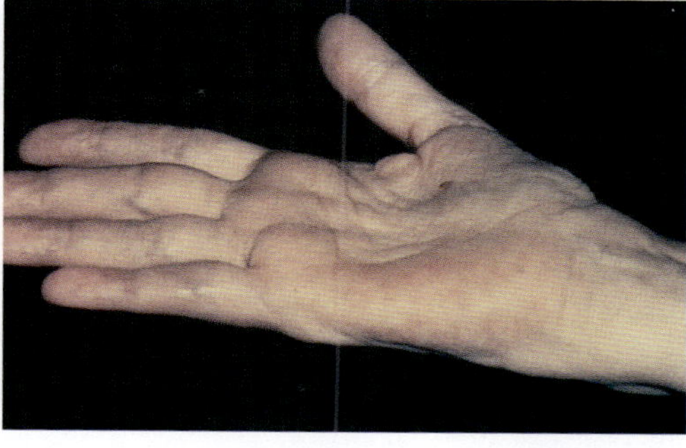

Carpal tunnel syndrome with atrophy of thenar eminence

Atrophy occurs from interference with motor function from compression of the median nerve inside the carpal tunnel. Caused by chronic repetitive motion; occurs between 30 and 60 years of age and is five times more common in women than in men. Symptoms of carpal tunnel syndrome include pain, burning and numbness, positive findings on a Phalen's test, positive indication of Tinel's sign and often atrophy of the thenar muscles.

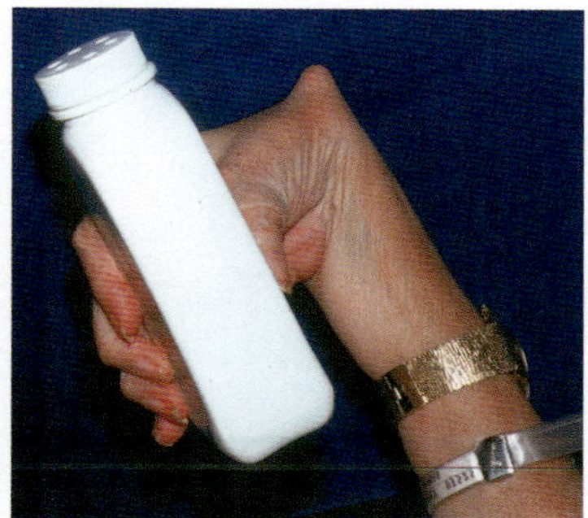

Ankylosis

Wrist in extreme flexion due to severe RA. This is a functionally useless hand because when the wrist is palmar flexed, a good deal of power is lost from the fingers, and the thumb cannot oppose the fingers.

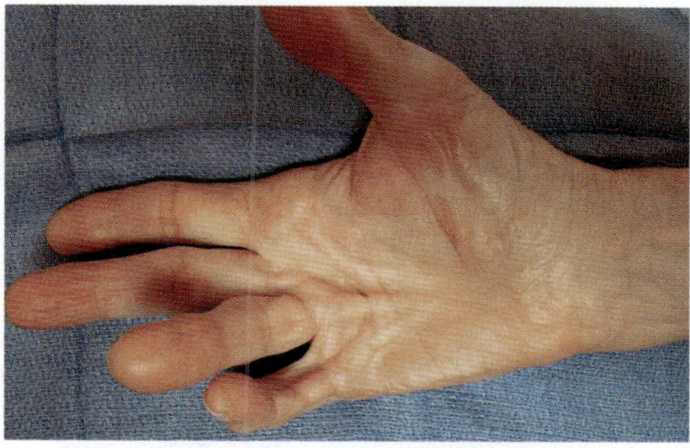

Dupuytren's contracture

Chronic hyperplasia of the palmar fascia causes flexion contractures of the digits, first in the fourth digit, then the fifth digit and then the third digit. Note the bands that extend from the midpalm to the digits and the puckering of palmar skin. The condition occurs commonly in men past 40 years of age and is usually bilateral. It occurs with diabetes, epilepsy and alcoholic liver disease and as an inherited trait. The contracture is painless but impairs hand function.

Continued

TABLE 20.4 Abnormalities of the wrist and hand cont'd

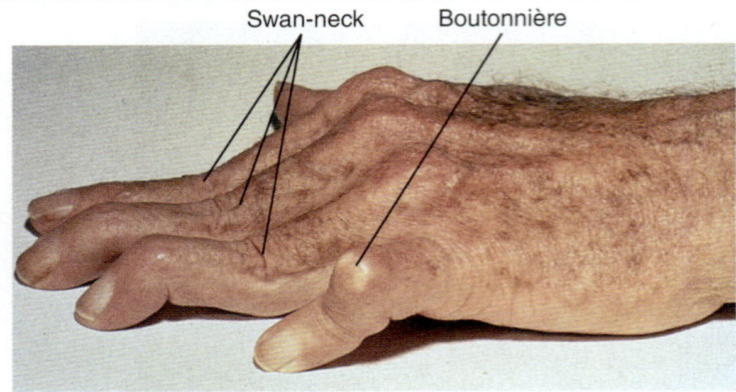

Swan-neck and boutonnière deformity

Flexion contracture resembles curve of a **swan's neck**. Note flexion contracture of the metacarpophalangeal joint, then hyperextension of the proximal interphalangeal joint and flexion of the distal interphalangeal joint. It occurs with chronic RA and is often accompanied by ulnar drift of the fingers.

In **boutonnière deformity**, the knuckle looks as if it is being pushed through a buttonhole. It is a relatively common deformity and includes flexion of the proximal interphalangeal joint with compensatory hyperextension of the distal interphalangeal joint.

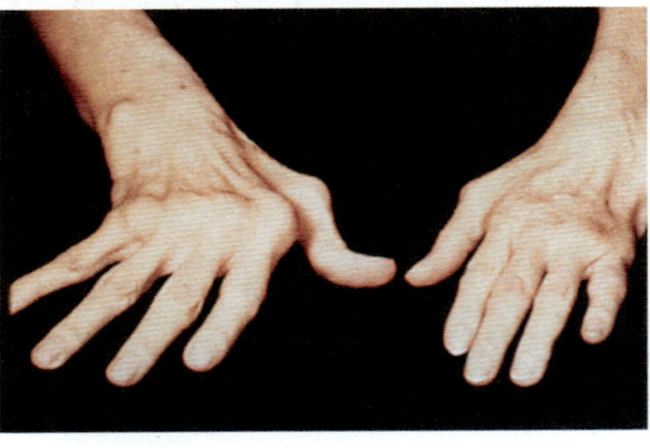

Ulnar deviation or drift

Fingers drift to the ulnar side because of stretching of the articular capsule and muscle imbalance. Also note subluxation and swelling in the joints and muscle atrophy on the dorsa of the hands. This is caused by chronic RA.

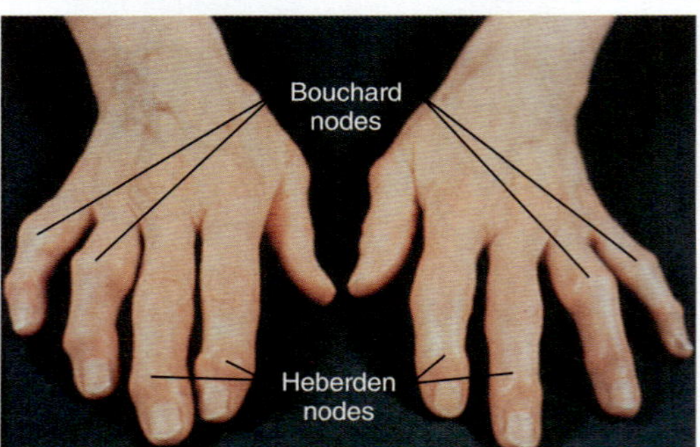

Osteoarthritis in the fingers

OA is characterised by hard, nontender nodules, 3 mm or more. These osteophytes (bony overgrowths) of the distal interphalangeal joints are called Heberden's nodes, and those of the proximal interphalangeal joints are called Bouchard's nodes.

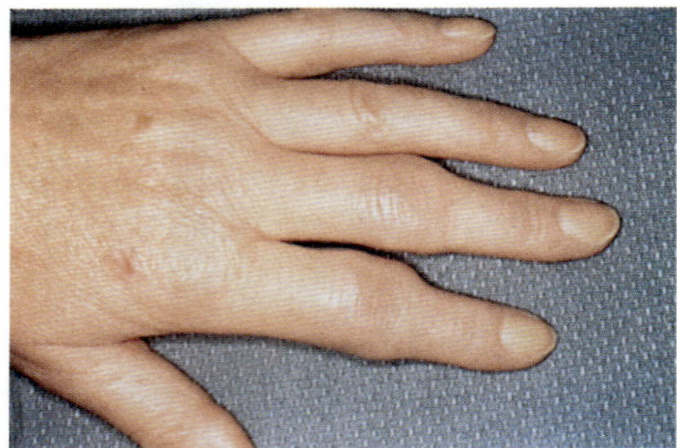

Acute rheumatoid arthritis in the fingers

Painful swelling and stiffness of joints, with fusiform or spindle-shaped swelling of the soft tissue of the proximal interphalangeal joints. Fusiform swelling is usually symmetrical, the hands are warm and the veins are engorged. The inflamed joints have a limited ROM.

TABLE 20.5 Abnormalities of the knee

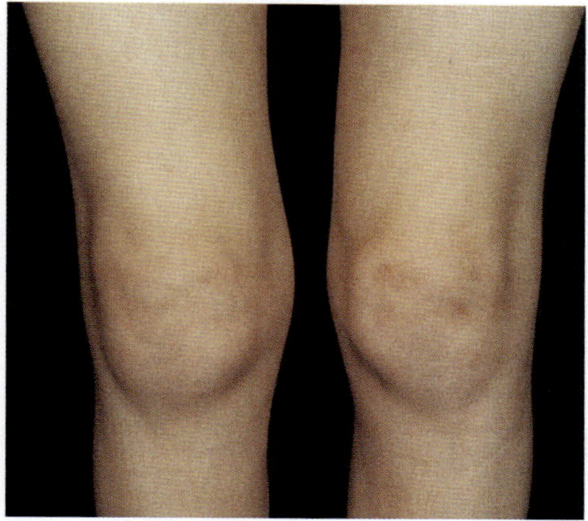

Mild synovitis

Loss of normal hollows on either side of the patella, which are replaced by mild distension. Occurs with synovial thickening or effusion (excess fluid). Also note mild distension of the suprapatellar pouch.

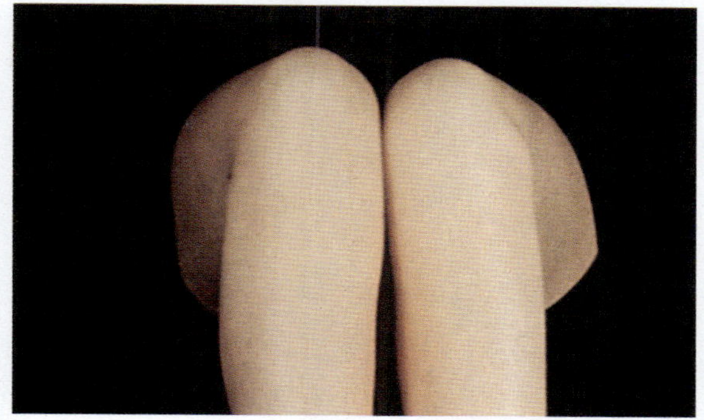

Swelling of menisci

Localised soft swelling from a cyst in the lateral meniscus shows at the midpoint of the anterolateral joint line. Semiflexion of the knee makes swelling more prominent.

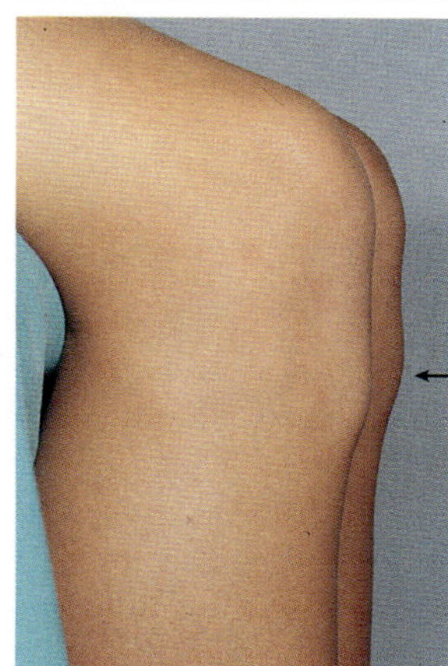

Osgood-Schlatter disease

Painful swelling of the tibial tubercle just below the knee, probably from repeated stress on the patellar tendon. Occurs most in puberty during rapid growth and most often in males. Pain increases with kicking, running, bike riding, stair climbing or kneeling. The condition is usually self-limited, and symptoms resolve with rest.

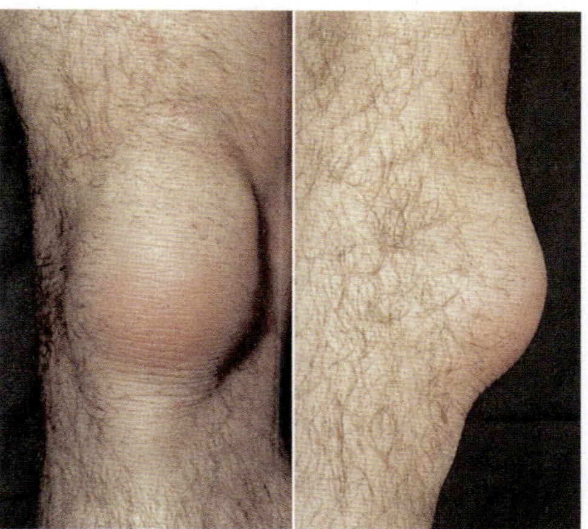

Prepatellar bursitis

Localised swelling on the anterior knee between the patella and the skin. A tender fluctuant mass indicates swelling; in some cases, infection spreads to the surrounding soft tissue. The condition is limited to the bursa, and the knee joint itself is not involved. Overlying skin may be red, shiny, atrophic or coarse and thickened.

TABLE 20.6 Abnormalities of the ankle and foot

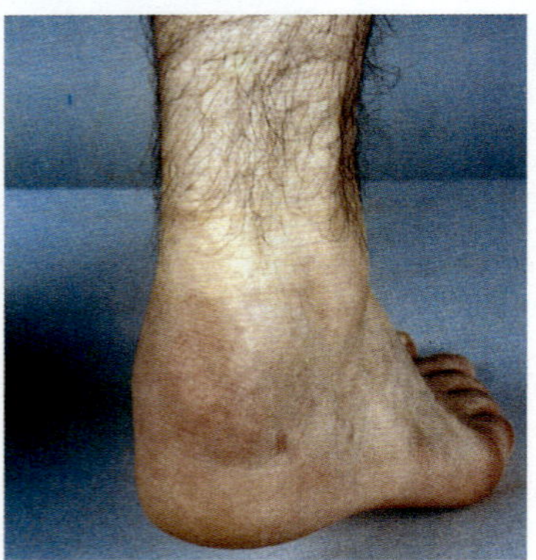

Achilles tenosynovitis

Inflammation of a tendon sheath near the ankle (here, the Achilles tendon) produces a superficial linear swelling and a localised tenderness along the route of the sheath. Movement of the involved tendon usually causes pain.

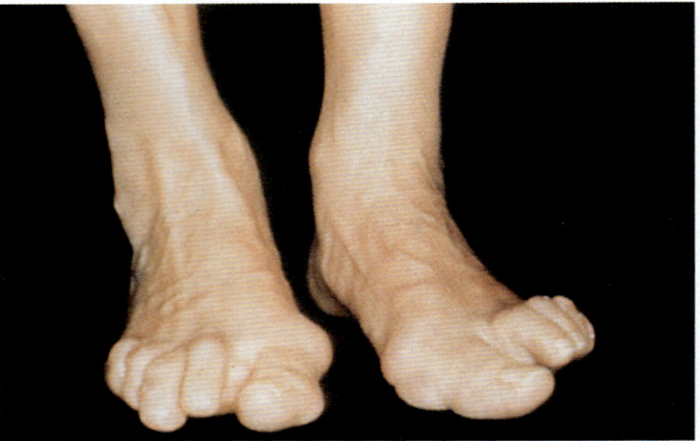

Hallux valgus with bunion and hammertoes

Hallux valgus is a common deformity from RA. It is a lateral or outward deviation of the great toe with medial prominence of the head of the first metatarsal. The bunion is the inflamed bursa that forms at the pressure point. The great toe loses power to push off while walking; this stresses the second and third metatarsal heads, and they develop calluses and pain. Note the hammertoe deformities in the second, third, fourth and fifth toes.

TABLE 20.6 Abnormalities of the ankle and foot cont'd

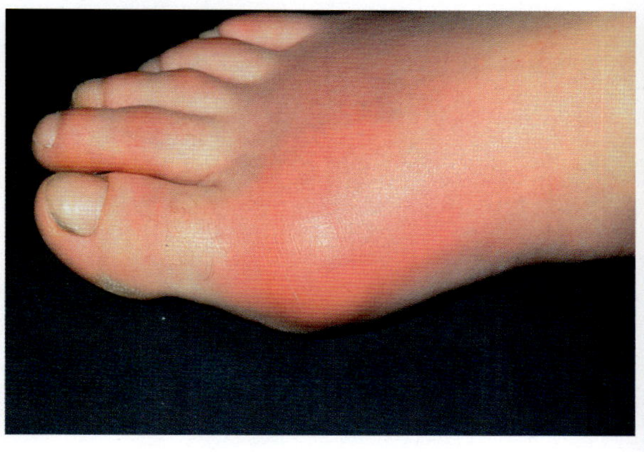

Acute gout

An acute episode of gout usually involves first the metatarso phalangeal joint. Clinical findings consist of redness, swelling, heat and extreme tenderness. Gout is a metabolic disorder of disturbed purine metabolism, associated with elevated serum uric acid and deposits of urate crystals in the joint space. There is increased risk of gout in obesity, metabolic syndrome, hypertension and hyperlipidaemia. Acute episodes can be triggered by trauma, acute stress and increased alcohol intake.

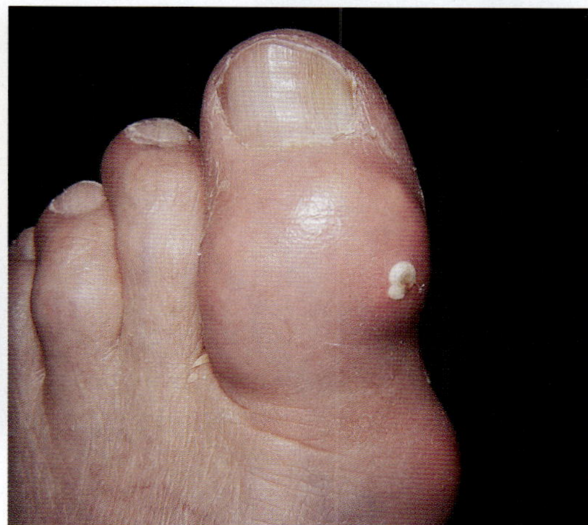

Tophi with chronic gout

Hard, painless nodule (tophi) over metatarsophalangeal joint of first toe. Tophi are collections of sodium urate crystals due to chronic gout in and around the joint that cause extreme swelling and joint deformity. They sometimes burst through the skin with a chalky discharge.

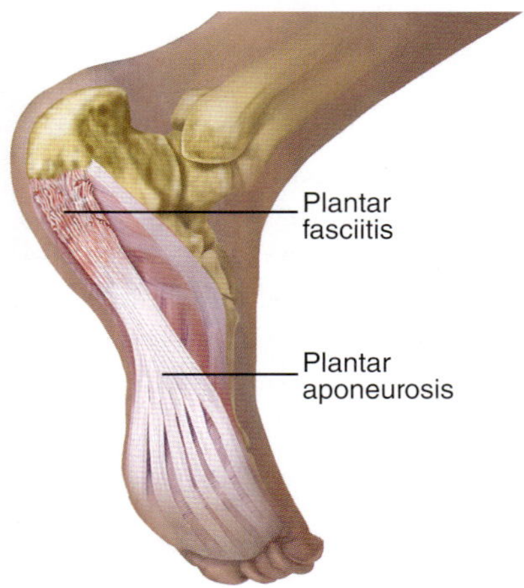

Plantar fasciitis

The plantar fascia is a band of connective tissue that extends lengthwise from the medial tubercle of the heel to the metatarsal heads and the five proximal phalanges of the toes. An inflammatory response to repetitive microtrauma to this fascia is the most frequent cause of heel pain. Risk factors include obesity, high-arched foot, running, standing for long periods on a hard floor, recent injury to the lower limbs or a change in activity. Pain is unilateral and described as throbbing, piercing or searing; the pain is worse in the morning or after periods of long rest.

TABLE 20.7 Abnormalities of the spine

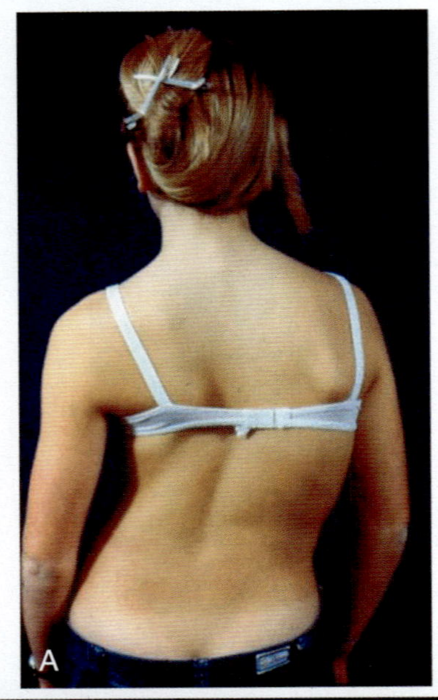

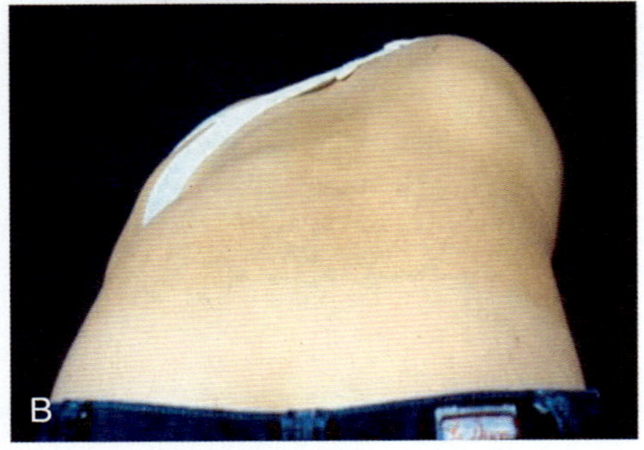

Scoliosis

Lateral curvature of thoracic and lumbar segments of the spine, usually with some rotation of involved vertebral bodies.

Functional scoliosis is flexible; it is apparent with standing and disappears with forward bending. It may be compensatory for other abnormalities such as leg length discrepancy.

Structural scoliosis is fixed; the curvature shows both on standing and on bending forwards. Note rib hump with forward flexion. When the person is standing, note unequal shoulder elevation, unequal scapulae, obvious curvature and unequal hip level. At greatest risk are females 10 years of age through adolescence, during the peak of the growth spurt.

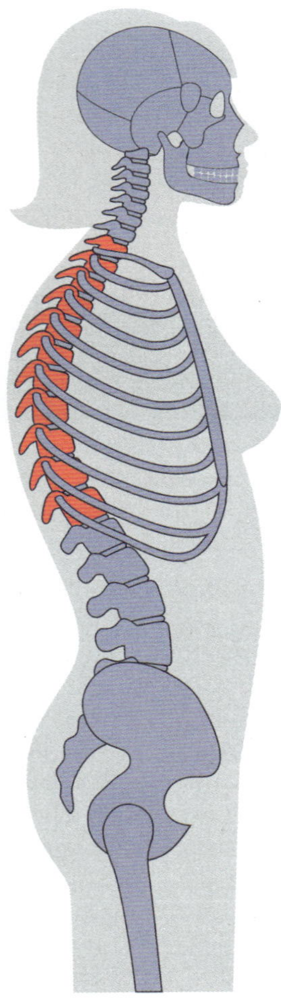

Kyphosis

Kyphosis is an excess curvature of the spine resulting in a hunchback type deformity. Kyphosis can be congenital, postural or acquired. In older people kyphosis is often due to vertebral compression, usually as a result of osteoporosis. Symptoms and signs include curvature of the spine of more than 50 degrees, back pain and, in severe cases, difficulty breathing.

Advanced practice—additional data

In addition to the GALS assessment described above, the assessments that are described in the following section require advanced skill and scope of practice. A complete musculoskeletal examination, as described in the following section, is appropriate for people with a positive musculoskeletal screening described previously.

Equipment

Goniometer

PROCEDURES AND NORMAL FINDINGS	ABNORMAL FINDINGS AND CLINICAL ALERTS
Inspection of joints	
Note the **size** and **contour** of the joint. Inspect the skin and tissues over the joints for **colour**, **swelling** and any **masses** or **deformity**. Presence of swelling is significant and signals joint irritation.	Swelling may be excess joint fluid (effusion), thickening of the synovial lining, inflammation of the surrounding soft tissue (bursae, tendons) or bony enlargement.
Palpation of joints	
Palpate each joint, including its skin for temperature, its muscles, bony articulations and the area of the joint capsule. Notice any heat, tenderness, crepitus, swelling or masses. Joints are not normally tender to palpation. If any tenderness does occur, try to localise it to specific anatomical structures (e.g. skin, muscles, bursae, ligaments, tendons, fat pads or joint capsule).	Deformities include dislocation (one or more bones in a joint being out of position), **subluxation** (partial dislocation of a joint), **contracture** (shortening of a muscle leading to limited ROM of the joint) or **ankylosis** (stiffness or fixation of a joint).
The synovial membrane is not normally palpable. When thickened, it feels 'doughy' or 'boggy'. A small amount of fluid is present in the normal joint, but it is not palpable.	Palpable fluid is abnormal. Because fluid is contained in an enclosed sac, if you push on one side of the sac, the fluid will shift and cause a visible bulging on another side.
Range of motion	
Ask for **active ROM** while stabilising the body area proximal to that being moved. Familiarise yourself with the type of each joint and its normal ROM so you can recognise limitations. If you see a limitation, gently attempt **passive motion**. Anchor the joint with one hand while your other hand slowly moves it to its limit. The normal ranges of active and passive motion should be the same.	
If any limitation or any increase in ROM occurs, use a goniometer to measure the angles precisely (Figure 20.16). First extend the joint to neutral or 0 degrees. Centre the 0 point of the goniometer on the joint. Keep the fixed arm of the goniometer on the 0 line and use the movable arm to measure; then flex the joint and measure through the goniometer to determine the angle of greatest flexion.	

PROCEDURES AND NORMAL FINDINGS	ABNORMAL FINDINGS AND CLINICAL ALERTS
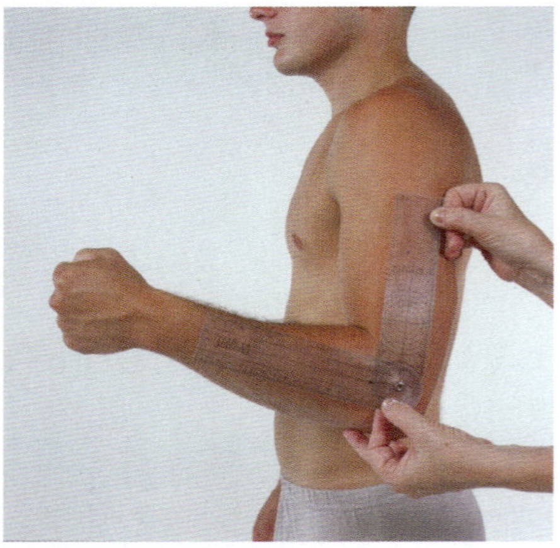 **FIGURE 20.16** Using a goniometer to measure range of motion Joint motion normally causes no tenderness, pain, or crepitation. Do not confuse crepitation with the normal discrete 'crack' heard as a tendon or ligament slips over bone during motion, such as when you do a knee bend.	
Muscle testing	
Test the strength of the prime mover muscle groups for each joint. Repeat the motions you elicited for active ROM. Now ask the person to flex and hold as you apply opposing force. Muscle strength should be equal bilaterally and should fully resist your opposing force. (Note: Muscle status and joint status are interdependent and should be interpreted together. Chapter 12 discusses the examination of muscles for size and development, tone and presence of tenderness.) A wide variability of strength exists among people. You may wish to use a grading system from no voluntary movement to full strength, as shown.	
Temporomandibular joint	
With the person seated, **inspect** the area just anterior to the ear. Place the tips of your first two fingers in front of each ear and ask the person to open and close the mouth. Drop your fingers into the depressed area over the joint and note smooth motion of the mandible. An audible and palpable snap or click occurs in many healthy people as the mouth opens (Figure 20.17).	Swelling looks like a round bulge over the joint, although it must be moderate or marked to be visible. Crepitus and pain occur with temporomandibular joint (TMJ) dysfunction.

PROCEDURES AND NORMAL FINDINGS		ABNORMAL FINDINGS AND CLINICAL ALERTS
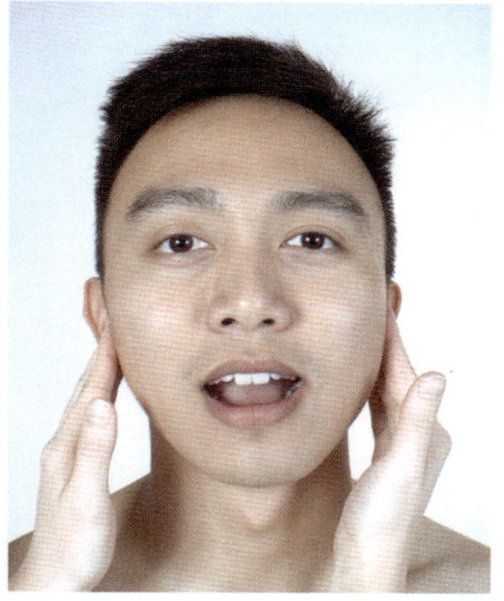 **FIGURE 20.17** Palpation of the temporomandibular joint movement	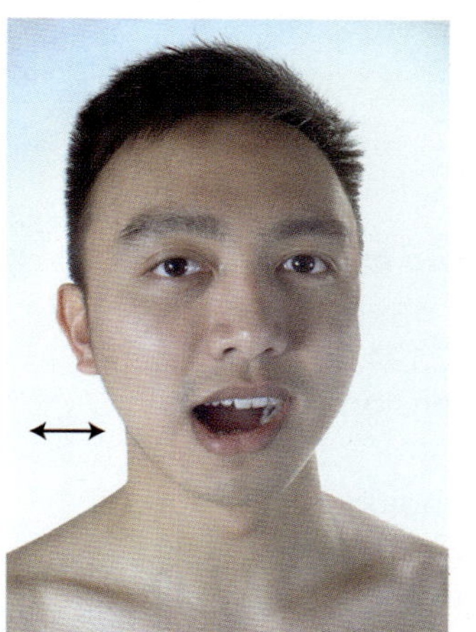 **FIGURE 20.18** Lateral movement of the temporomandibular joint	
Instructions to the person	***Motion and expected range***	Lateral motion may be lost earlier and more significantly than vertical.
Open mouth maximally.	Vertical motion. You can measure the space between the upper and lower incisors. Normal is 3 to 6 cm, or three fingers inserted sideways.	
Partially open mouth, side to side	Lateral motion. Normal extent is 1 to 2 cm. Protrude lower jaw and move it (Figure 20.18).	
Stick out lower jaw.	Protrude without deviation.	
Palpate the contracted temporalis and masseter muscles as the person clenches the teeth. Compare right and left sides for size, firmness and strength. Ask the person to move the jaw forwards and laterally against your resistance and to open mouth against your resistance. This also tests the integrity of **cranial nerve V (trigeminal)**.		
Cervical spine		
Inspect the alignment of head and neck. The spine should be straight and the head erect. **Palpate** the spinous processes and the sternocleidomastoid, trapezius and paravertebral muscles. They should feel firm, with no muscle spasm or tenderness.		Head tilted to one side. Asymmetry of muscles. Tenderness and hard muscles with muscle spasm.

PROCEDURES AND NORMAL FINDINGS

Ask the person to follow these motions (Figure 20.19):

Instructions to the person	*Motion and expected range*
Touch chin to chest.	Flexion of 45 degrees (Figure 20.19A). Hyperextension of 55 degrees.
Lift the chin towards the ceiling.	Lateral bending of 40 degrees (Figure 20.19B).
Touch each ear towards the corresponding shoulder.	Do not lift the shoulder.
Turn the chin towards each shoulder.	Rotation of 70 degrees (Figure 20.19C).

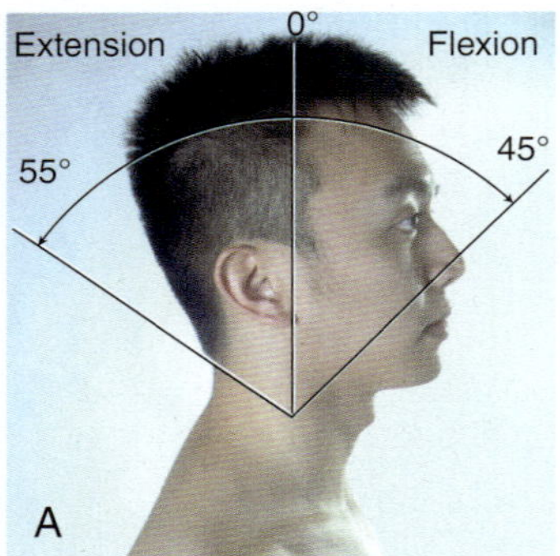

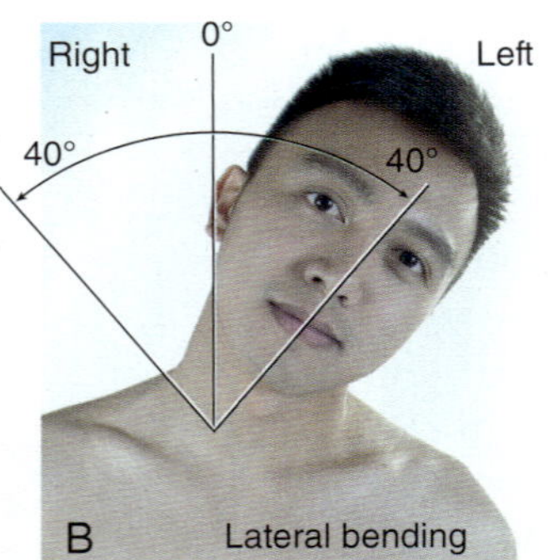

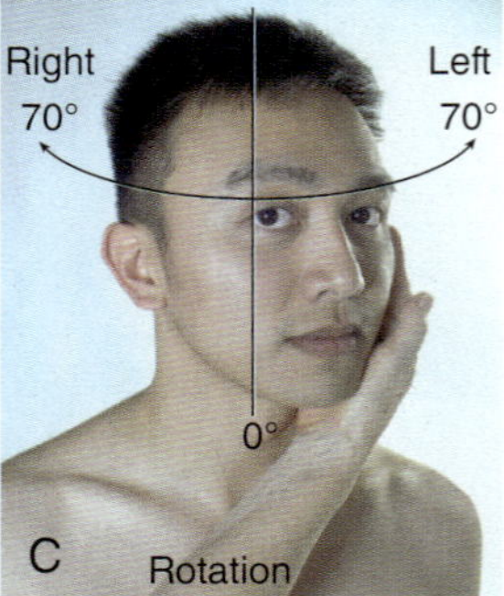

FIGURE 20.19 Range of motion of the cervical spine

ABNORMAL FINDINGS AND CLINICAL ALERTS

Clinical alert: Do not examine neck movement where there is any suspicion of neck trauma, limited ROM or pain with movement.

PROCEDURES AND NORMAL FINDINGS	ABNORMAL FINDINGS AND CLINICAL ALERTS
Repeat the motions while applying opposing force. The person normally can maintain flexion against your full resistance. This also tests integrity of **cranial nerve XI (spinal)**.	
Inspect and palpate the upper extremities	
Shoulder	
Inspect and compare both shoulders posteriorly and anteriorly. Check the size and contour of the joint and compare shoulders for equality of bony landmarks. Normally, no redness, muscular atrophy, deformity or swelling is present. Check the anterior aspect of the joint capsule and the subacromial bursa for abnormal swelling.	**Redness:** Inequality of bony landmarks. **Atrophy** shows as a lack of fullness. A dislocated shoulder loses the normal rounded shape and looks flattened laterally. **Swelling** from excess fluid is best seen anteriorly. Considerable fluid must be present to cause a visible distension because the capsule normally is so loose.
If the person reports any shoulder pain, ask that they point to the spot with the hand of the unaffected side.	Swelling of subacromial bursa is localised under the deltoid muscle and may be accentuated when the person tries to abduct the arm. Be aware that shoulder pain may be from local causes, or it may be referred pain from a hiatus hernia or a cardiac or pleural condition, which could be potentially serious. Pain from a local cause is reproducible during the examination by palpation or motion.
While standing in front of the person, **palpate** both shoulders, noting any muscular spasm or atrophy, swelling, heat or tenderness. Start at the clavicle and methodically explore the acromioclavicular joint, scapula, greater tubercle of the humerus, area of the subacromial bursa, the biceps groove and the anterior aspect of the glenohumeral joint. Palpate the pyramid-shaped axilla; no adenopathy or masses should be present.	Swelling. Hard muscles with muscle spasm. **Tenderness** or pain.
Test ROM by asking the person to perform four motions (Figure 20.20). Cup one hand over the shoulder during ROM to note any crepitation; normally none is present.	

PROCEDURES AND NORMAL FINDINGS	ABNORMAL FINDINGS AND CLINICAL ALERTS

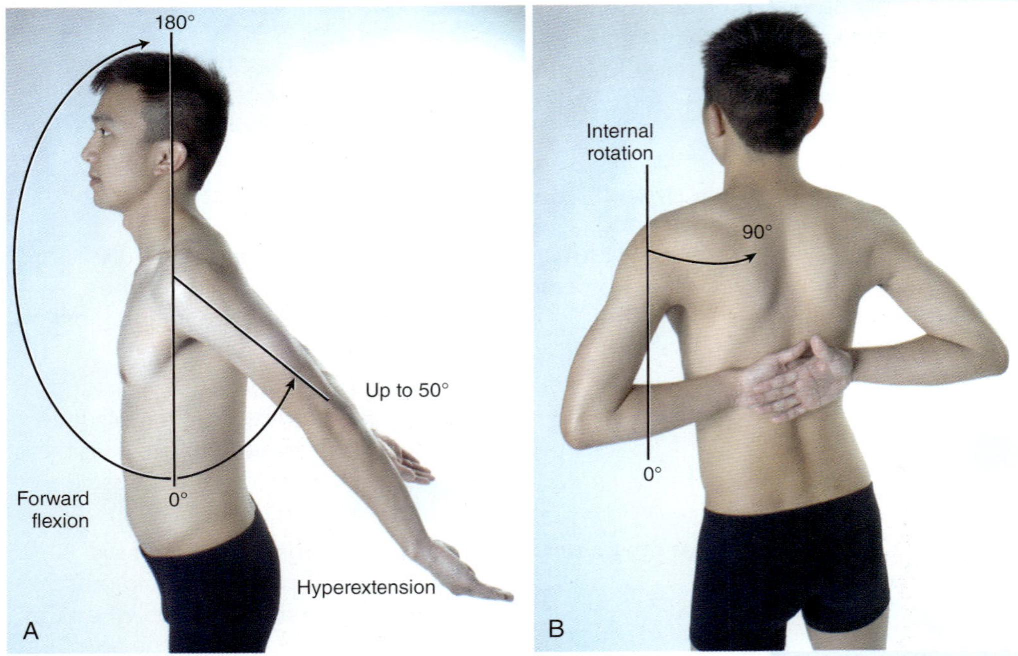

FIGURE 20.20 A Hyperextension of the shoulder B Internal rotation of the shoulder

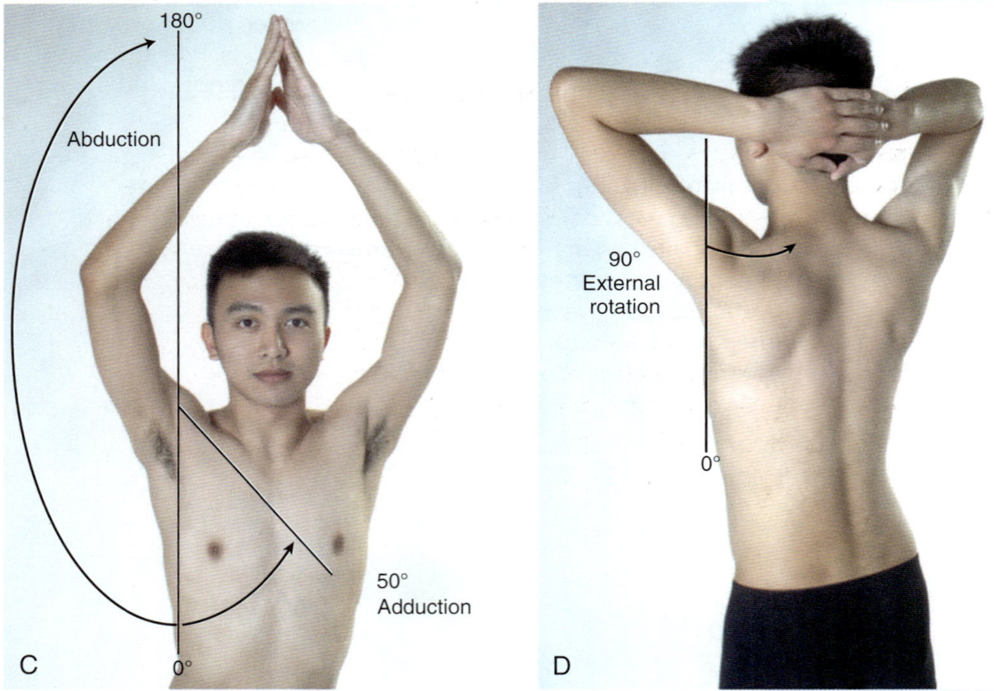

FIGURE 20.20 C Abduction of the shoulder D External rotation of the shoulder

PROCEDURES AND NORMAL FINDINGS		ABNORMAL FINDINGS AND CLINICAL ALERTS
Instructions to the person	***Motion and expected range***	**Limited ROM.** **Asymmetry.** Pain with motion. **Crepitus** with motion. Rotator cuff lesions may cause limited ROM, pain and muscle spasm during abduction, whereas forward flexion stays fairly normal.
With the arms at the sides and elbows extended, move both arms forwards and up in wide vertical arcs, then move them back.	Forward flexion of 180 degrees. Hyperextension up to 50 degrees (Figure 20.20A).	
Rotate the arms internally behind the back, place the back of the hands as high as possible towards the scapulae.	Internal rotation of 90 degrees (Figure 20.20B).	
With the arms at the sides and elbows extended, raise both arms in wide arcs in the coronal plane. Touch the palms together above the head.	Abduction of 180 degrees. Adduction of 50 degrees (Figure 20.20C).	
Touch both hands behind the head with the elbows flexed and rotated posteriorly.	External rotation of 90 degrees head (Figure 20.20D).	

Test the strength of the shoulder muscles by asking the person to shrug the shoulders, flex forwards and up and abduct against your resistance. The shoulder shrug also tests the integrity of cranial nerve XI, the spinal accessory.

Elbow

Inspect the size and contour of the elbow in both the flexed and the extended positions. Look for any deformity, redness or swelling. Check the olecranon bursa and the normally present hollows on either side of the olecranon process for abnormal swelling.

Subluxation of the elbow shows the forearm dislocated posteriorly.

Swelling and redness of olecranon bursa are localised and easy to observe because of the proximity of the bursa to the skin.

Effusion or synovial thickening shows first as a bulge or fullness in the groove on either side of the olecranon process, and it occurs with gouty arthritis.

Palpate with the elbow flexed about 70 degrees and as relaxed as possible (Figure 20.21). Use your left hand to support the person's left forearm and palpate the extensor surface of the elbow—the olecranon process and the medial and lateral epicondyles of humerus—with your right thumb and fingers.

PROCEDURES AND NORMAL FINDINGS	ABNORMAL FINDINGS AND CLINICAL ALERTS
With your thumb in the lateral groove and your index and middle fingers in the medial groove, palpate either side of the olecranon process using varying pressure. Normally, present tissues and fat pads feel solid. Check for any synovial thickening, swelling, nodules or tenderness.	Soft, boggy or fluctuant swelling in both grooves occurs with synovial thickening or effusion. Local heat or redness (signs of inflammation) can extend beyond synovial membrane.
Palpate the area of the olecranon bursa for heat, swelling, tenderness, consistency or nodules.	**Subcutaneous nodules** are raised, firm and nontender and the overlying skin moves freely. Common sites are in the olecranon bursa and along the extensor surface of the ulna. These nodules occur with RA.

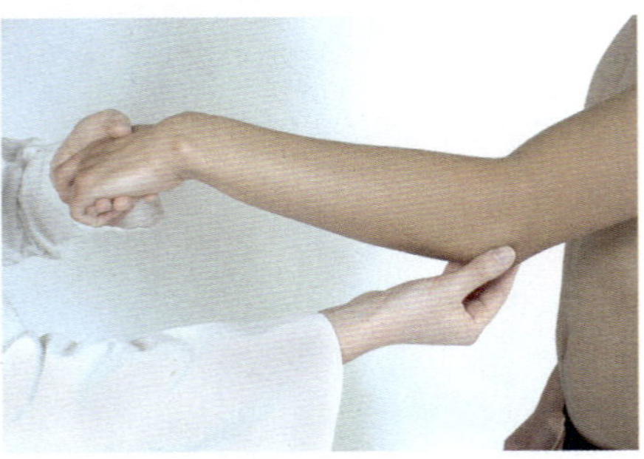

FIGURE 20.21 Epicondyles, head of radius and tendons are common sites of inflammation and local tenderness, or 'tennis elbow'

Test ROM by asking the person to:

Instructions to the person	***Motion and expected range***
Bend and straighten the elbow (Figure 20.22).	Flexion of 150–160 degrees; extension at 0. Some healthy people lack 5 to 10 degrees of full extension, and others have 5 to 10 degrees of hyperextension.
Move 90 degrees in pronation and supination.	Hold the hand midway; then touch the front and back sides of the hand to a table (Figure 20.23).

PROCEDURES AND NORMAL FINDINGS	ABNORMAL FINDINGS AND CLINICAL ALERTS

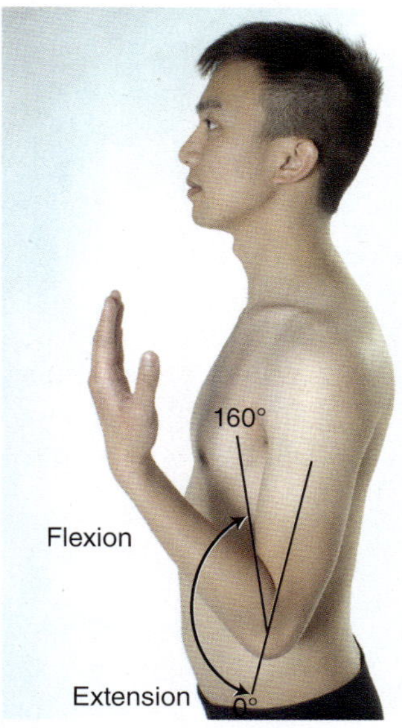

FIGURE 20.22 Flexion-extension of the elbow

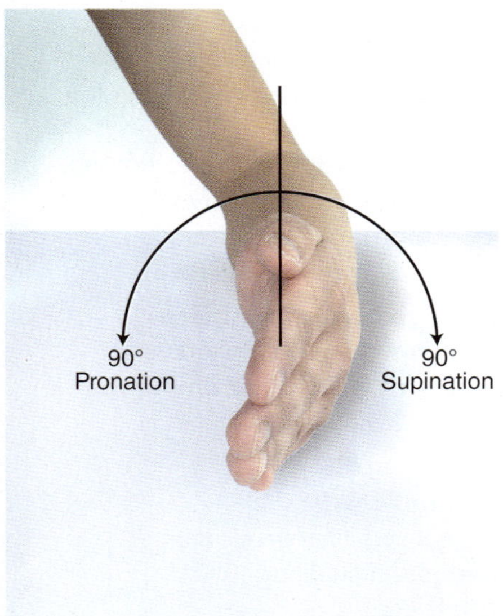

FIGURE 20.23 Pronation-supernation of the elbow and wrist

While testing **muscle strength**, stabilise the person's arm with one hand (Figure 20.24). Have the person flex the elbow against your resistance applied just proximal to the wrist. Then ask the person to extend the elbow against your resistance.

PROCEDURES AND NORMAL FINDINGS	ABNORMAL FINDINGS AND CLINICAL ALERTS

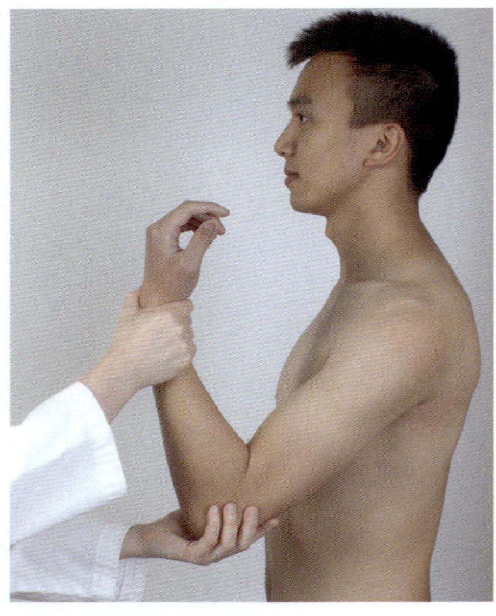

FIGURE 20.24 Hand position for testing elbow/arm muscle strength

Wrist and hand

Inspect the hands and wrists on the dorsal and palmar sides, noting the position, contour and shape. The normal functional position of the hand shows the wrist in slight extension. This way, the fingers can flex efficiently, and the thumb can oppose them for grip and manipulation. The fingers lie straight in the same axis as the forearm. Normally, no swelling or redness, deformity or nodules are present.

Subluxation of wrist.
Ulnar deviation: fingers list to ulnar side.
Ankylosis: wrist in extreme flexion.
Dupuytren's contracture: flexion contracture of finger(s).

The skin looks smooth with knuckle wrinkles present and no swelling or lesions. Muscles are full, with the palm showing a rounded mound proximal to the thumb (the **thenar eminence**) and a smaller rounded mound proximal to the little finger.

Swan-neck or boutonnière deformity in the fingers.
Atrophy of the thenar eminence (Table 20.4).

Palpate each joint in the wrist and hands. Facing the person, support the hand with your fingers under it and palpate the wrist firmly with both your thumbs on its dorsum (Figure 20.25). Make sure the person's wrist is relaxed and in straight alignment. Move your palpating thumbs side to side to identify the normal depressed areas that overlie the joint space. Use gentle but firm pressure. Normally, the joint surfaces feel smooth, with no swelling, bogginess, nodules or tenderness.

Ganglion in wrist.
Synovial swelling on dorsum.
Generalised swelling.
Tenderness.

Palpate the metacarpophalangeal joints with your thumbs, just distal to and on either side of the knuckle (Figure 20.26).

PROCEDURES AND NORMAL FINDINGS	ABNORMAL FINDINGS AND CLINICAL ALERTS

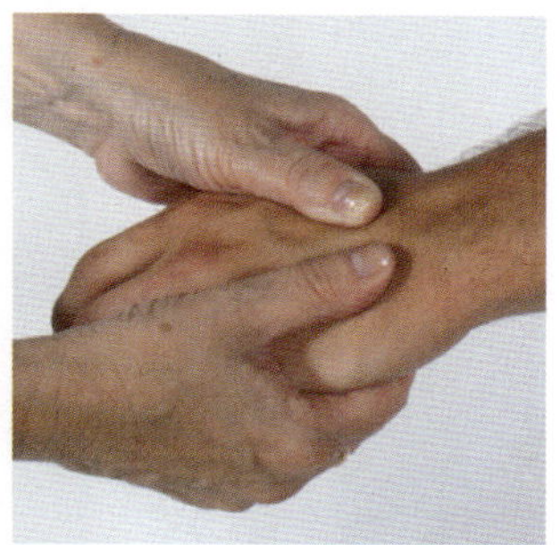

FIGURE 20.25 Palpation of the wrist

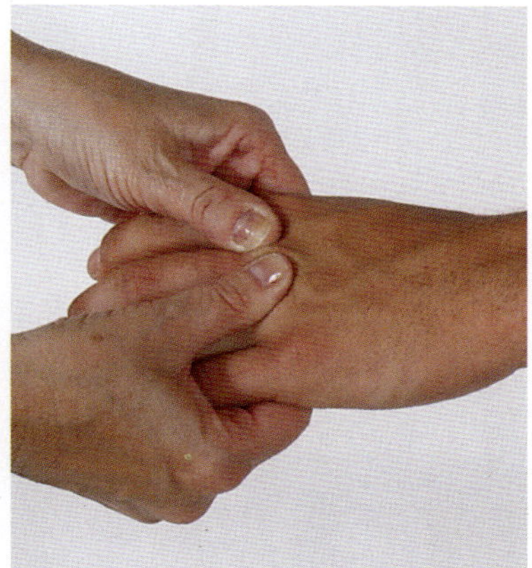

FIGURE 20.26 Palpation of the bones/joints of the hand

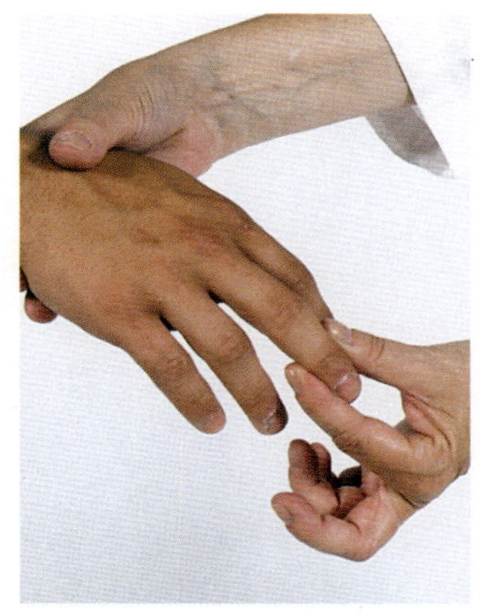

FIGURE 20.27 Palpation of the interphalangeal joints

Use your thumb and index finger in a pinching motion to palpate the sides of the interphalangeal joints (Figure 20.27). Normally, no synovial thickening, tenderness, warmth or nodules are present.

Heberden's and Bouchard's nodules are hard and nontender and occur with OA (Table 20.4).

PROCEDURES AND NORMAL FINDINGS	ABNORMAL FINDINGS AND CLINICAL ALERTS

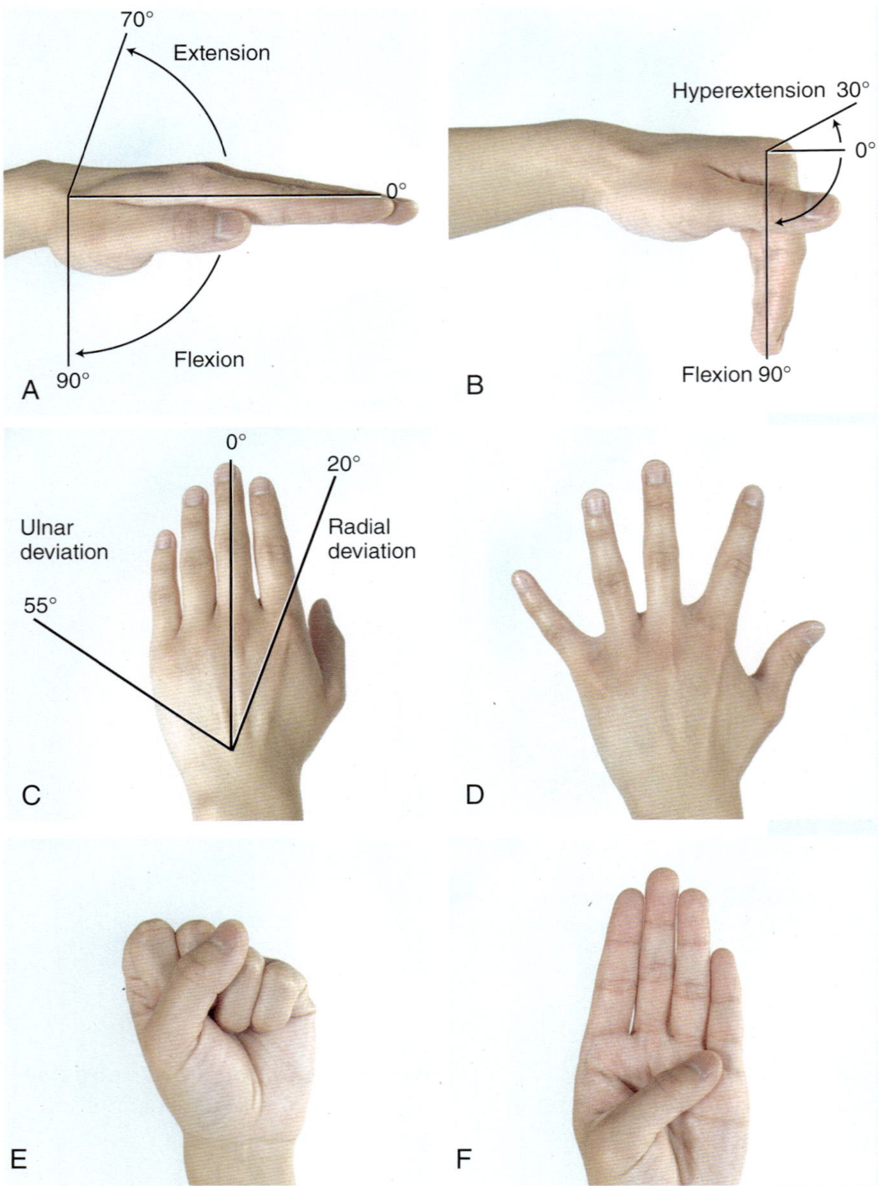

FIGURE 20.28 Testing range of motion of the hand and wrist

PROCEDURES AND NORMAL FINDINGS		ABNORMAL FINDINGS AND CLINICAL ALERTS
Test ROM (Figure 20.28):		**Loss of ROM** here is the most common and most significant functional loss of the wrist. Limited motion. Pain on movement.
Instructions to the person	***Motion and expected range***	
Bend the hand up at the wrist.	Hyperextension of 70 degrees (Figure 20.28A).	
Bend the hand down at the wrist.	Palmar flexion of 90 degrees.	
Bend the fingers up and down at the metacarpophalangeal joints.	Flexion of 90 degrees. Hyperextension of 30 degrees (Figure 20.28B).	
With palms flat on table, turn them outwards and in.	Ulnar deviation of 50 to 60 degrees and radial deviation of 20 degrees (Figure 20.28C).	
Spread the fingers apart; make a fist.	Abduction of 20 degrees; fist tight. The responses should be equal bilaterally (Figures 20.28D and E).	
Touch the thumb to each finger and to the base of the little finger.	The person can perform, and the responses are equal bilaterally (Figure 20.28F).	

For **muscle testing**, position the person's forearm supinated (palm up) and resting on a table (Figure 20.29). Stabilise by holding your hand at the person's mid-forearm. Ask the person to flex the wrist against your resistance at the palm.

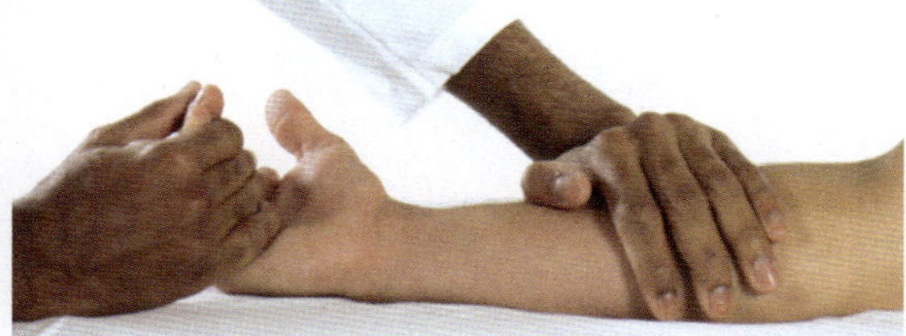

FIGURE 20.29 Position for testing muscle strength of the forearm and wrist

Phalen's test. Ask the person to hold both hands back-to-back while flexing the wrists 90 degrees. Acute flexion of the wrist for 60 seconds produces no symptoms in the normal hand (Figure 20.30).

Phalen's test reproduces numbness and burning in a person with carpal tunnel syndrome (Table 20.4).

PROCEDURES AND NORMAL FINDINGS	ABNORMAL FINDINGS AND CLINICAL ALERTS

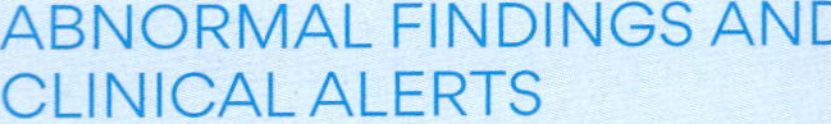

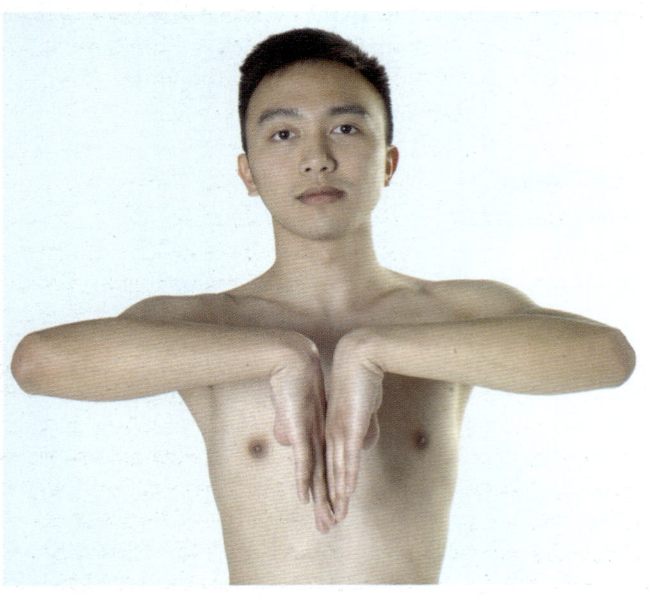

FIGURE 20.30 Phalen's test

Tinel's sign. Direct percussion of the location of the median nerve at the wrist produces no symptoms in a normal hand (Figure 20.31).

In carpal tunnel syndrome, percussion of the median nerve produces burning and tingling along its distribution, which is a positive Tinel's sign.

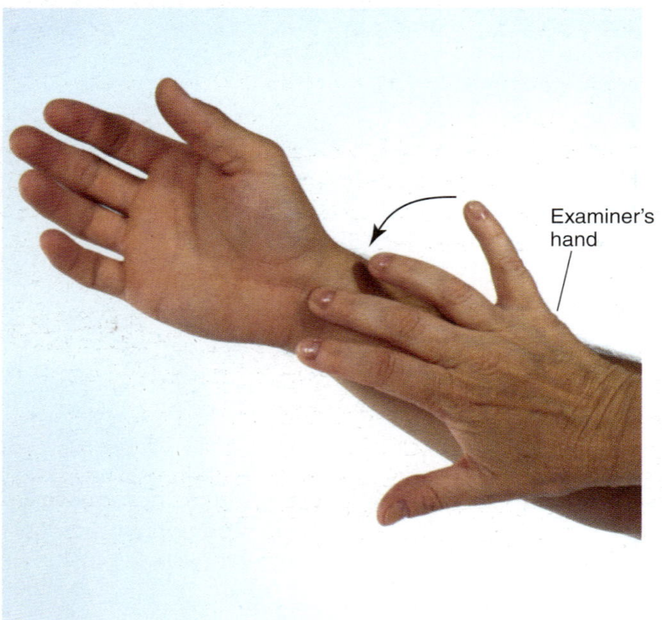

FIGURE 20.31 Tinel's sign

PROCEDURES AND NORMAL FINDINGS		ABNORMAL FINDINGS AND CLINICAL ALERTS
Inspect and palpate lower extremities		
Hip		
Wait to **inspect** the hip joint together with the spine a bit later in the examination as the person stands. At that time, note symmetrical levels of iliac crests, gluteal folds and equally sized buttocks. A smooth, even gait reflects equal leg lengths and functional hip motion.		
Help the person into a supine position and palpate the hip joints. The joints should feel stable and symmetrical, with no tenderness or crepitus.		Pain with palpation. Crepitation.
Assess ROM (Figure 20.32)		
Instructions to the person	***Motion and expected range***	Limited motion. Pain with motion.
Raise each leg with the knee extended.	Hip flexion of 90 degrees (Figure 20.32A).	
Bend each knee up to the chest while keeping the other leg straight.	Hip flexion of 120 degrees. The opposite thigh should remain on the table (Figure 20.32B).	Flexion flattens the lumbar spine; if this reveals a flexion deformity in the opposite hip, it represents a positive **Thomas test**.

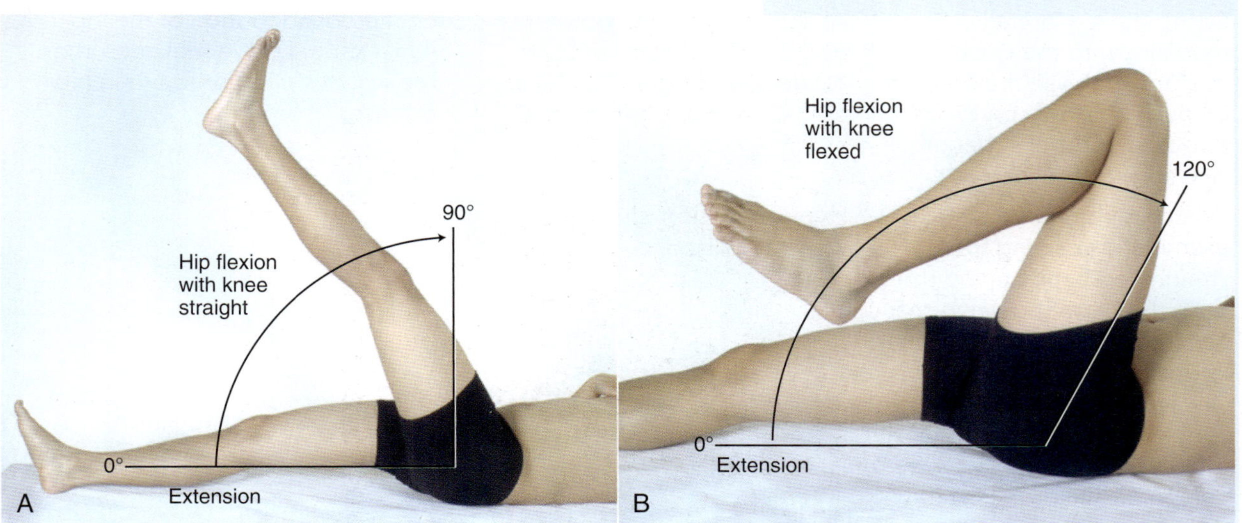

FIGURE 20.32 A, B Testing hip flexion and extension

PROCEDURES AND NORMAL FINDINGS		ABNORMAL FINDINGS AND CLINICAL ALERTS

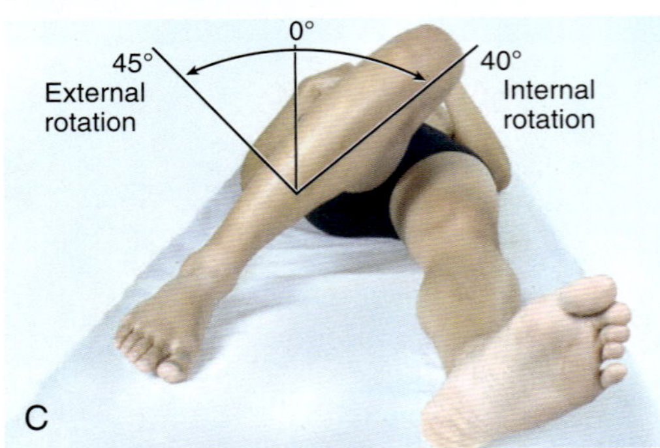

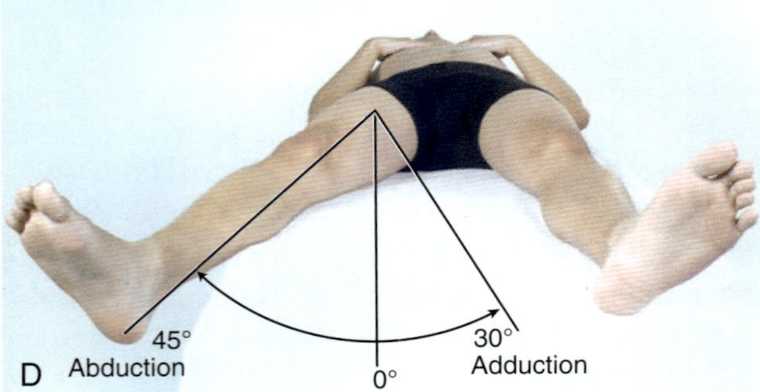

FIGURE 20.32 C Testing hip external and internal rotation D Testing hip abduction and adduction

Instructions to the person (cont'd)	***Motion and expected range (cont'd)***	
Flex the knee and hip to 90 degrees. Stabilise by holding the thigh with one hand and the ankle with the other hand. Swing the foot outwards. Swing the foot inwards. (Foot and thigh move in opposite directions.)	Internal rotation of 40 degrees. External rotation of 45 degrees (Figure 20.32C).	Limited internal rotation of hip is an early and reliable sign of hip disease.
Swing the leg laterally, then medially, with the knee straight. Stabilise the pelvis by pushing down on the opposite anterior superior iliac spine.	Abduction of 40 to 45 degrees. Adduction of 20 to 30 degrees (Figure 20.32D).	Limitation of abduction of the hip while supine is the most common motion dysfunction found in hip disease.
When standing (later in examination), swing the straight leg back behind the body. Stabilise the pelvis to eliminate exaggerated lumbar lordosis. The most efficient way is to ask person to bend over the table and to support the trunk on the table. Or the person can lie prone on the table.	Hyperextension of 15 degrees when stabilised.	

Knee

The person should remain supine with the legs extended, although some examiners prefer the knees to be flexed and dangling for **inspection.** The skin normally looks smooth, with even colouring and no lesions.	Shiny and atrophic skin. Swelling or inflammation (Table 20.5). Lesions (e.g. **psoriasis**).

PROCEDURES AND NORMAL FINDINGS	ABNORMAL FINDINGS AND CLINICAL ALERTS
Inspect the lower leg alignment. The lower leg should extend in the same axis as the thigh.	Angulation deformity: • **genu varum** (bowlegs) (see below) • **genu valgum** (knock knees) • **flexion contracture.**
Inspect the knee's shape and contour. Normally, distinct concavities, or hollows, are present on either side of the patella. Check them for any sign of fullness or swelling. Note other locations, such as the prepatellar bursa and the suprapatellar pouch, for any abnormal swelling.	Hollows disappear; then they may bulge with synovial thickening or effusion.
Check the quadriceps muscle in the anterior thigh for any atrophy. Because it is the prime mover of knee extension, this muscle is important for joint stability during weight bearing.	Atrophy occurs with disuse or chronic disorders. First, it appears in the medial part of the muscle, although it is difficult to note because the vastus medialis is relatively small.
Enhance **palpation** with the knee in the supine position with complete relaxation of the quadriceps muscle. Start high on the anterior thigh, about 10 cm above the patella. Palpate with your left thumb and fingers in a grasping fashion (Figure 20.33). Proceed down towards the knee, exploring the region of the suprapatellar pouch. Note the consistency of the tissues. The muscles and soft tissues should feel solid, and the joint should feel smooth, with no warmth, tenderness, thickening or nodularity.	Feels fluctuant or boggy with synovitis of suprapatellar pouch.

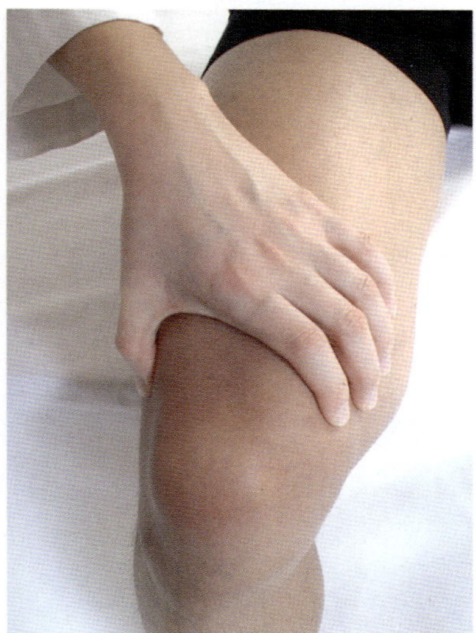

FIGURE 20.33 Position of the hand for palpation of the knee

PROCEDURES AND NORMAL FINDINGS

When swelling occurs, distinguish whether it is due to soft tissue swelling or increased fluid in the joint. The tests for the bulge sign and ballottement of the patella aid this assessment.

Bulge sign. For swelling in the suprapatellar pouch, the bulge sign confirms the presence of small amounts of fluid as you try to move the fluid from one side of the joint to the other. Firmly stroke up on the medial aspect of the knee two or three times to displace any fluid (Figure 20.34A). Tap the lateral aspect (Figure 20.34B). Watch the medial side in the hollow for a distinct bulge from a fluid wave. Normally, none is present.

Ballottement of the patella. This test is reliable when larger amounts of fluid are present. Use your left hand to compress the suprapatellar pouch to move any fluid into the knee joint. With your right hand, push the patella sharply against the femur. If no fluid is present, the patella is already snug against the femur (Figure 20.35A).

Continue palpation and explore the tibiofemoral joint (Figure 20.36). Note smooth joint margins and absence of pain. Palpate the infrapatellar fat pad and the patella. Check for **crepitus** by holding your hand on the patella as the knee is flexed and extended. Some crepitus in an otherwise asymptomatic knee is not uncommon.

ABNORMAL FINDINGS AND CLINICAL ALERTS

The bulge sign occurs with very small amounts of effusion, 4 to 8 mL, from fluid flowing across the joint (Figure 20.34C).

If fluid has collected, your tap on the patella moves it through the fluid, and you will hear a tap as the patella bumps up on the femoral condyles (Figure 20.35B).

Irregular bony margins occur with OA.

Pain at joint line.

Pronounced crepitus is significant and it occurs with degenerative diseases of the knee.

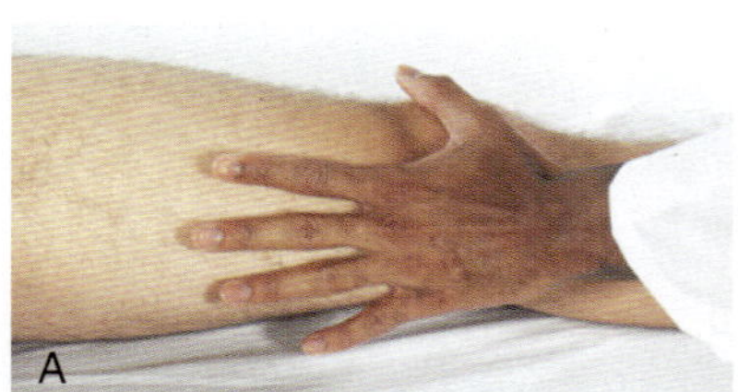
A

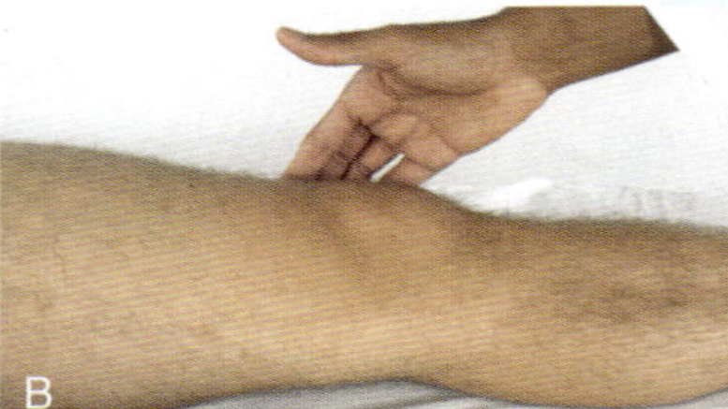
B

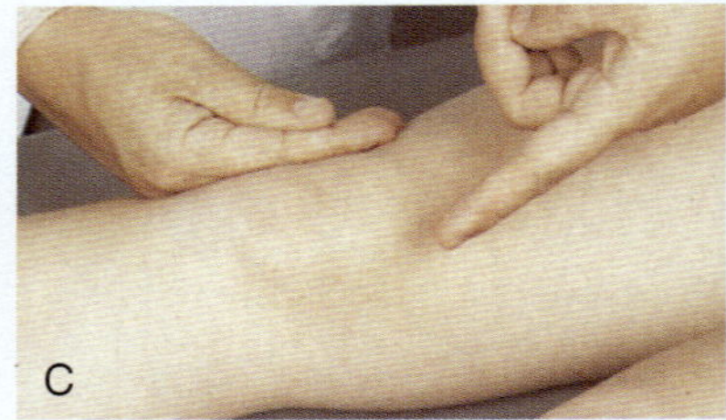
C

FIGURE 20.34 Bulge sign

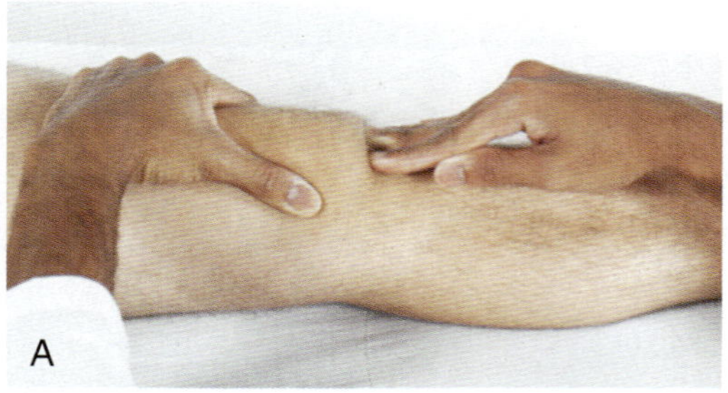
A

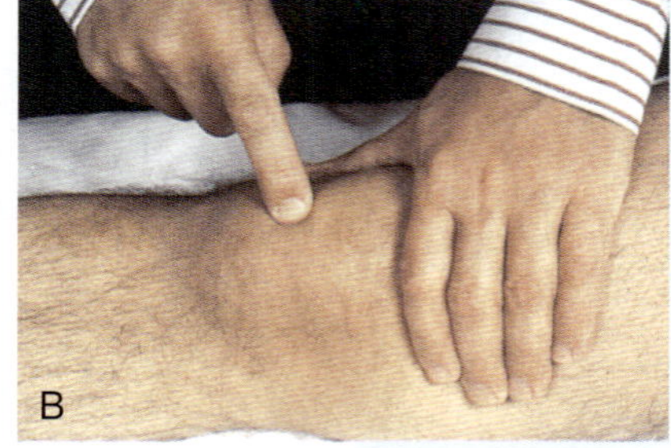
B

FIGURE 20.35 Ballottement of the knee joint

PROCEDURES AND NORMAL FINDINGS	ABNORMAL FINDINGS AND CLINICAL ALERTS
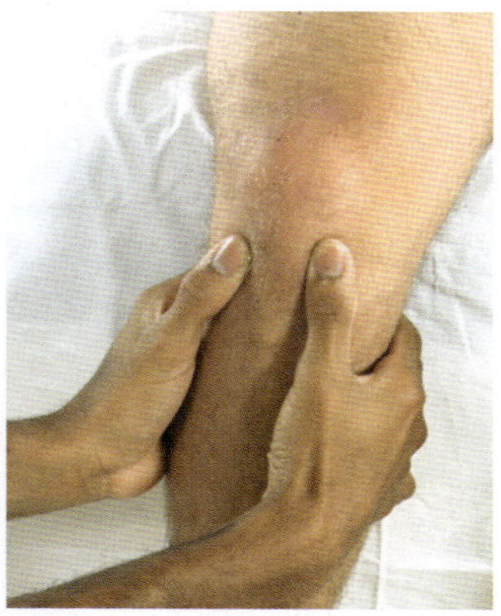 **FIGURE 20.36** Palpation of the tibiofemoral joint	
Check ROM (Figure 20.37):	Limited ROM. Contracture. Pain with motion. Limp. Sudden locking—the person is unable to extend the knee fully. This usually occurs with a painful and audible 'pop' or 'click'. Sudden buckling, or 'giving way', occurs with ligament injury, which causes weakness and instability.

Instructions to the person	***Motion and expected range***
Bend each knee.	Flexion of 130–150 degrees.
Extend each knee.	A straight line of 0 degrees in some people; a hyperextension of 15 degrees in others.

Check knee ROM during ambulation.

Check **muscle strength** by asking the person to maintain knee flexion while you oppose by trying to pull the leg forwards. Muscle extension is demonstrated by the person's success in rising from a seated position in a low chair or by rising from a squat without using the hands for support.

PROCEDURES AND NORMAL FINDINGS	ABNORMAL FINDINGS AND CLINICAL ALERTS

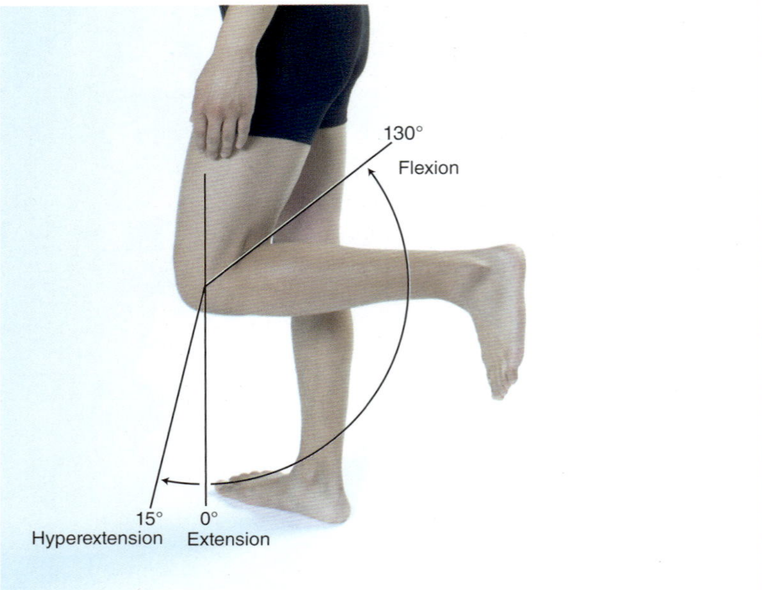

FIGURE 20.37 Testing range of motion of the knee joint

Special test for meniscal tears. *McMurray's test*. Perform this test when the person has reported a history of trauma followed by locking, giving way or local pain in the knee. Position the person supine as you stand on the affected side. Hold the heel and flex the knee and hip. Place your other hand on the knee with fingers on the medial side. Rotate the leg in and out to loosen the joint. Externally rotate the leg and push a valgus (inwards) stress on the knee. Then slowly extend the knee. Normally the leg extends smoothly with no pain.

If you hear or feel a 'click', McMurray's test is positive for a torn meniscus.

Ankle and foot

Inspect while the person is in a sitting, non-weight bearing position, as well as when standing and walking. Compare both feet, noting position of feet and toes, contour of joints and skin characteristics. The foot should align with the long axis of the lower leg; an imaginary line would fall from midpatella to between the first and second toes.

Weight bearing should fall on the middle of the foot, from the heel, along the midfoot, to between the second and third toes. Most feet have a longitudinal arch, although that can vary normally from 'flat feet' to a high instep.

PROCEDURES AND NORMAL FINDINGS	ABNORMAL FINDINGS AND CLINICAL ALERTS
The toes point straight forwards and lie flat. The ankles (malleoli) are smooth bony prominences. Normally the skin is smooth, with even colouring and no lesions. Note the locations of any calluses or bursal reactions because they reveal areas of abnormal friction. Examining well-worn shoes helps assess areas of wear and accommodation.	**Hallux valgus** (Table 20.6). Hammertoes. Claw toes. Swelling or inflammation. Calluses. Ulcers.
Support the ankle by grasping the heel with your fingers while palpating with your thumbs (Figure 20.38). Explore the joint spaces. They should feel smooth and depressed, with no fullness, swelling or tenderness.	Swelling or inflammation. Tenderness.
Palpate the metatarsophalangeal joints between your thumb on the dorsum and your fingers on the plantar surface (Figure 20.39).	Swelling or inflammation; tenderness.
Using a pinching motion of your thumb and forefinger, palpate the interphalangeal joints on the medial and lateral sides of the toes.	

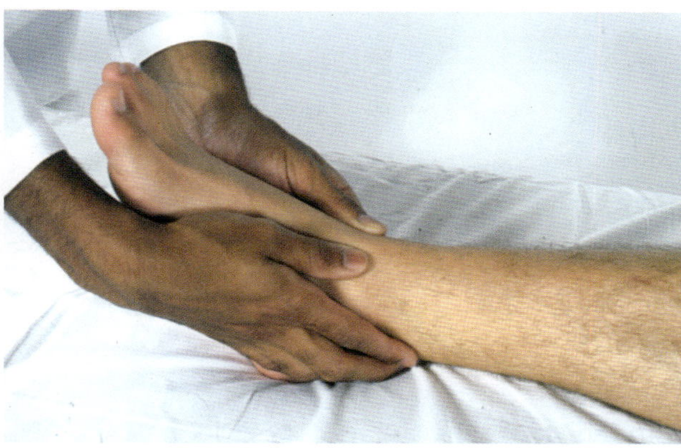

FIGURE 20.38 Palpation of the ankle joint

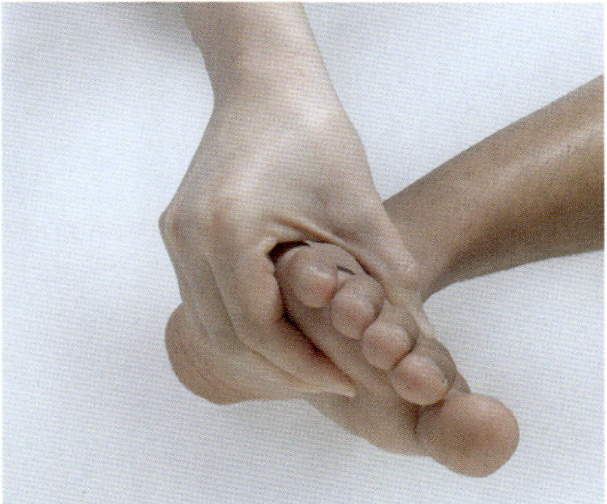

FIGURE 20.39 Palpation of the metatarsal phalangeal joints

PROCEDURES AND NORMAL FINDINGS	ABNORMAL FINDINGS AND CLINICAL ALERTS

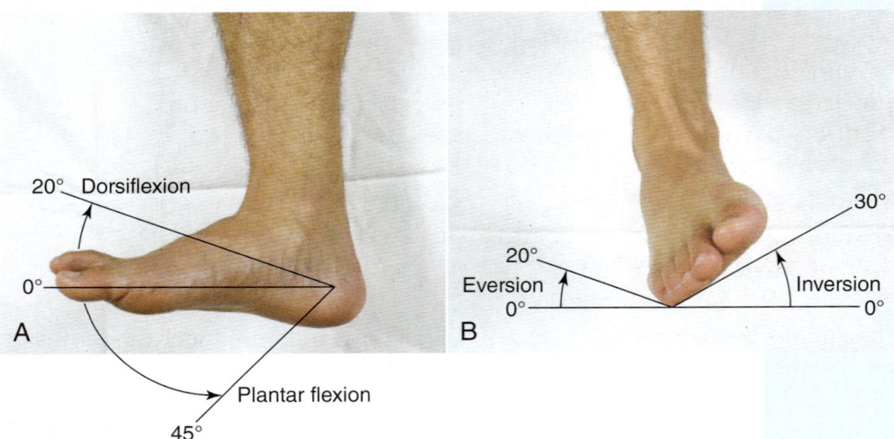

FIGURE 20.40 Testing the range of motion of the ankle joint

PROCEDURES AND NORMAL FINDINGS		ABNORMAL FINDINGS AND CLINICAL ALERTS
Test ROM (Figure 20.40):		Limited ROM. Pain with motion.
Instructions to the person	***Motion and expected range***	
Point the toes towards the floor.	Plantar flexion of 45 degrees.	
Point the toes towards your nose.	Dorsiflexion of 20 degrees (Figure 20.40A).	
Turn the soles of the feet out, then in.	Eversion of 20 degrees. (Stabilise the ankle with one hand, hold the heel with the other to test the subtalar joint.)	
Flex and straighten the toes.	Inversion of 30 degrees (Figure 20.40B).	
Assess **muscle strength** by asking the person to maintain dorsiflexion and plantar flexion against your resistance.		Unable to hold flexion.

Inspect and palpate the spine

The person should be standing, draped in a gown open at the back. Place yourself far enough back so you can see the entire back. **Inspect** and note whether the spine is straight by following an imaginary vertical line from the head through the spinous processes and down through the gluteal cleft, and by noting equal horizontal positions for the shoulders, scapulae, iliac crests and gluteal folds and equal spaces between arm and lateral thorax on the two sides (Figure 20.41A). The person's knees and feet should be aligned with the trunk and should be pointing forwards.	A difference in shoulder elevation and in level of scapulae and iliac crests occur with **scoliosis** (Table 20.7).

PROCEDURES AND NORMAL FINDINGS	ABNORMAL FINDINGS AND CLINICAL ALERTS
From the side, note the normal convex thoracic curve and concave lumbar curve (Figure 20.41B). An enhanced thoracic curve, or kyphosis, is common in people aged over 65 years. A pronounced lumbar curve, or lordosis, is common in obese people.	
Palpate the spinous processes. Normally they are straight and not tender. Palpate the paravertebral muscles; they should feel firm with no tenderness or spasm.	**Spinal curvature.** **Tenderness.** Spasm of paravertebral muscles.
Check **ROM** of the spine by asking the person to bend forwards and touch the toes (Figure 20.42). Look for flexion of 75 to 90 degrees and smoothness and symmetry of movement. Note that the concave lumbar curve should disappear with this motion, and the back should have a single convex C-shaped curve.	

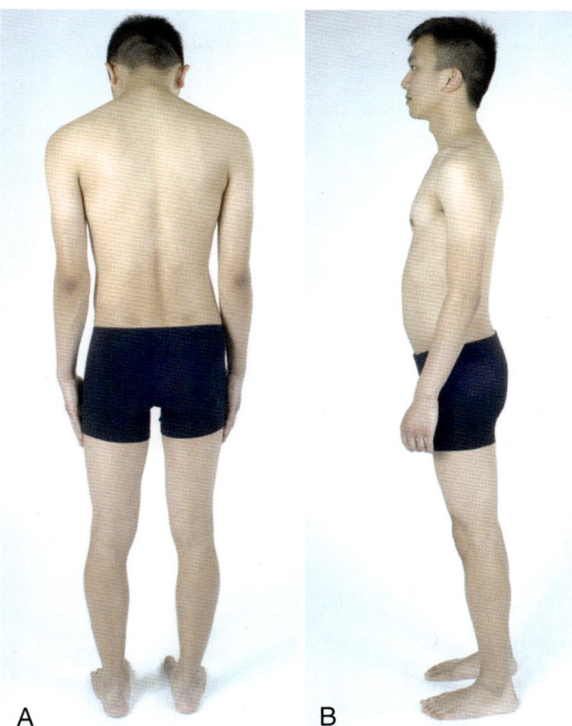

FIGURE 20.41 Posterior and lateral inspection of the spine

PROCEDURES AND NORMAL FINDINGS	ABNORMAL FINDINGS AND CLINICAL ALERTS

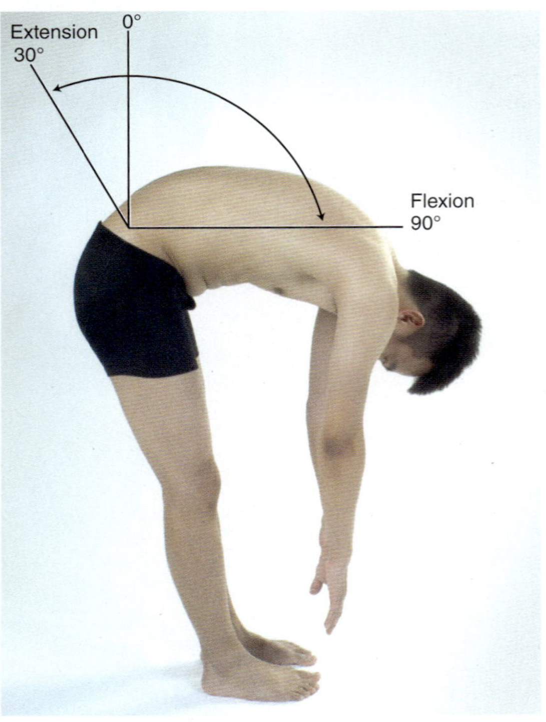

FIGURE 20.42 Testing extension-flexion of the spine

If you suspect a spinal curvature during inspection, this may be more clearly seen when the person touches the toes. While the person is bending over, mark a dot on each spinous process. When the person resumes standing, the dots should form a straight vertical line.

If the dots form a slight S-shape when the person stands, a spinal curve is present.

Stabilise the pelvis with your hands. Check ROM (Figure 20.43):

Instructions to the person	***Motion and expected range***
Bend sideways.	Lateral bending of 35 degrees (Figure 20.43A).
Bend backwards.	Hyperextension of 30 degrees.
Twist the shoulders to one side, bilaterally then the other.	Rotation of 30 degrees (Figure 20.43B).

These manoeuvres reveal only gross restriction. Movement is still possible even if some spinal fusion has occurred.

PROCEDURES AND NORMAL FINDINGS	ABNORMAL FINDINGS AND CLINICAL ALERTS

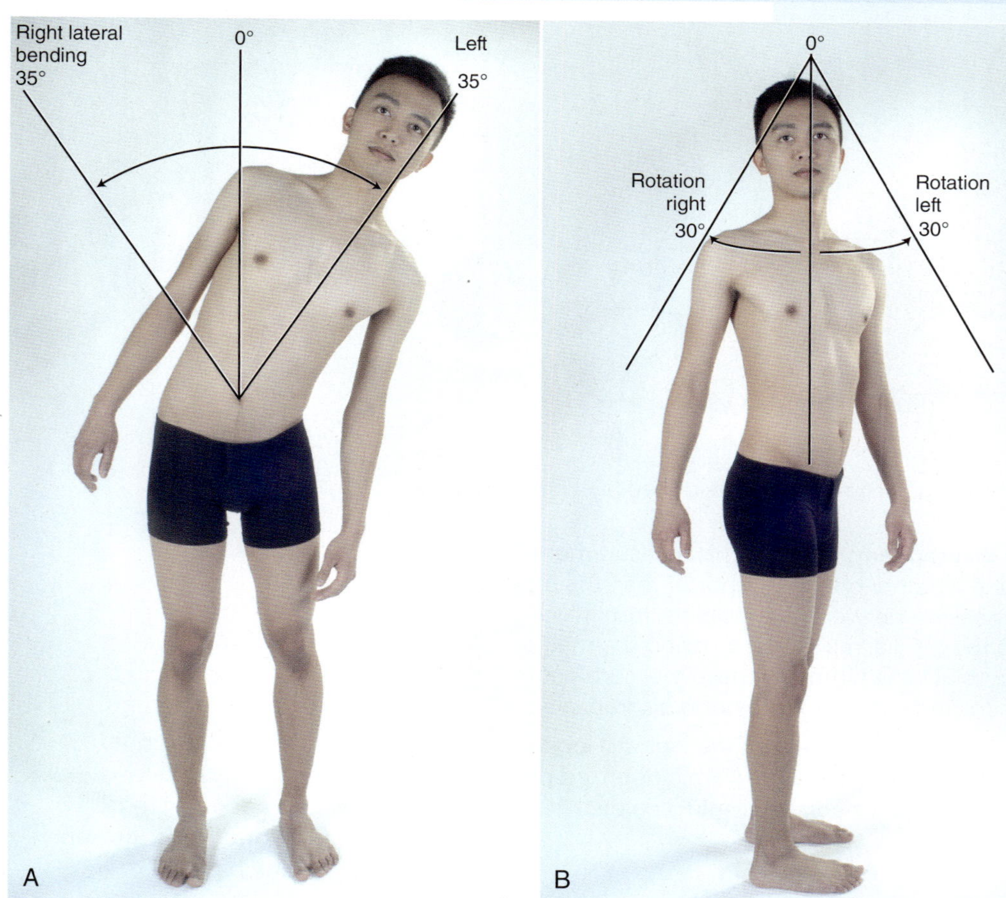

FIGURE 20.43 A Testing lateral movement of the spine B Testing rotation of the spine

Finally, ask the person to walk on their toes for a few steps; then return walking on the heels.

Straight leg raising or Lasègue's test. These manoeuvres reproduce back and leg pain and help confirm the presence of a herniated nucleus pulposus. Straight leg raising while keeping the knee extended normally produces no pain. Raise the affected leg just short of the point where it produces pain. Then dorsiflex the foot (Figure 20.44).

Lasègue's test is positive if it reproduces sciatic pain. If lifting the affected leg reproduces sciatic pain, it confirms the presence of a herniated nucleus pulposus.

Raise the unaffected leg while leaving the other leg flat. Enquire about the involved side.

If lifting the unaffected leg reproduces sciatic pain, it strongly suggests a herniated nucleus pulposus.

PROCEDURES AND NORMAL FINDINGS	ABNORMAL FINDINGS AND CLINICAL ALERTS

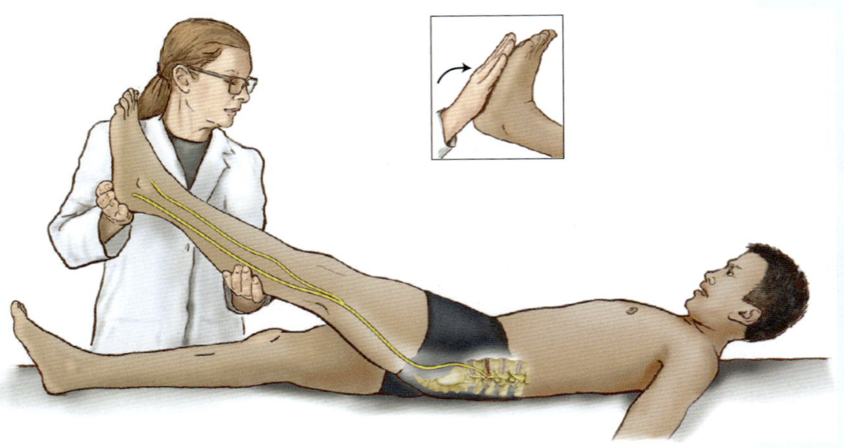

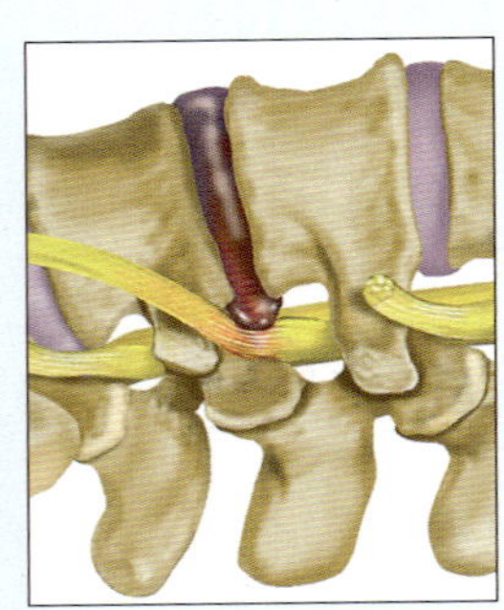

FIGURE 20.44 Testing straight leg raising for the presence of back or leg pain

Measure leg length discrepancy. Perform this measurement if you need to determine whether one leg is shorter than the other. For *true leg length*, measure between *fixed* points, from the anterior iliac spine to the medial malleolus, crossing the medial side of the knee (Figure 20.45). Normally these measurements are equal or within 1 cm, indicating no true bone discrepancy.

Unequal leg lengths.

Sometimes the true leg length is equal, but the legs still look unequal. For *apparent leg length*, measure from a nonfixed point (the umbilicus) to a fixed point (medial malleolus) on each leg.

True leg lengths are equal, but apparent leg lengths unequal—this condition occurs with pelvic obliquity or adduction or flexion deformity in the hip.

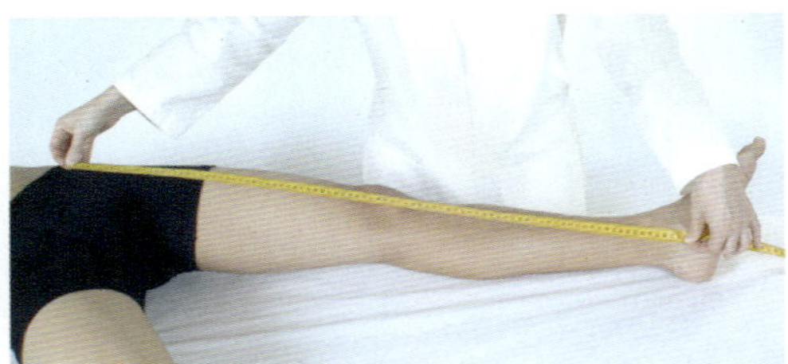

FIGURE 20.45 Measuring leg length

Additional objective data for infants

Review the developmental milestones discussed in Chapter 3. Keep handy a concise chart of the usual sequence of motor development so that you can refer to expected findings for the age of each child you are examining. Because some overlap exists between the musculoskeletal and neurological examinations, assessment of muscle tone, resting posture and motor activity are discussed in Chapter 12.

Examine the infant fully undressed and lying on the back. Take care to place the newborn on a warming table to maintain body temperature.

PROCEDURES AND NORMAL FINDINGS	ABNORMAL FINDINGS AND CLINICAL ALERTS
Feet and legs. Start with the feet and work your way up the extremities. Note any *positional deformities*, a residual of fetal positioning. Often the newborn's feet are not held straight but in a varus (apart) or valgus (together) position. It is important to distinguish whether this position is flexible (and thus usually self-correctable) or fixed. Scratch the outside of the bottom of the foot. If the deformity is self-correctable, the foot assumes a normal right angle to the lower leg. Or immobilise the heel with one hand and gently push the forefoot to the neutral position with the other hand. If you can move it to the neutral position, it is flexible.	A true deformity is fixed and assumes a right angle only with forced manipulation or not at all.
Note the relationship of the forefoot to the hindfoot. Commonly, the hindfoot aligns with the lower leg and just the forefoot angles inwards. This forefoot adduction is *metatarsus adductus.* It is usually present at birth and usually resolves spontaneously by age 3 years.	**Metatarsus varus**—adduction and inversion of forefoot. **Talipes equinovarus** (Table 20.8).
Check for *tibial torsion*, a twisting of the tibia. Place both feet flat on the table and push to flex up the knees. With the patella and the tibial tubercle in a straight line, place your fingers on the malleoli. In an infant, note that a line connecting the four malleoli is parallel to the table.	More than 20 degrees of deviation or if lateral malleolus is anterior to medial malleolus indicates tibial torsion.
Tibial torsion may originate from intrauterine positioning and then may be exacerbated at a later age by continuous sitting in a reverse tailor position, the 'TV squat'. This is sitting with the buttocks on the floor and the lower legs splayed back and out on either side.	
Hips. Check the hips for developmental hip dysplasia (DDH). The most reliable method is **Ortolani's manoeuvre**, which should be done at every professional visit until the infant is 1 year old. With the infant supine, flex the knees holding your thumbs on the inner mid-thighs and your fingers outside on the hips touching the greater trochanters. Adduct the legs until your thumbs touch (Figure 20.46A). Then gently lift and *abduct,* moving the knees apart and down so their lateral aspects touch the table (Figure 20.46B). This normally feels smooth and has no sound.	See developmental considerations section earlier in the chapter for definition and prevalence.

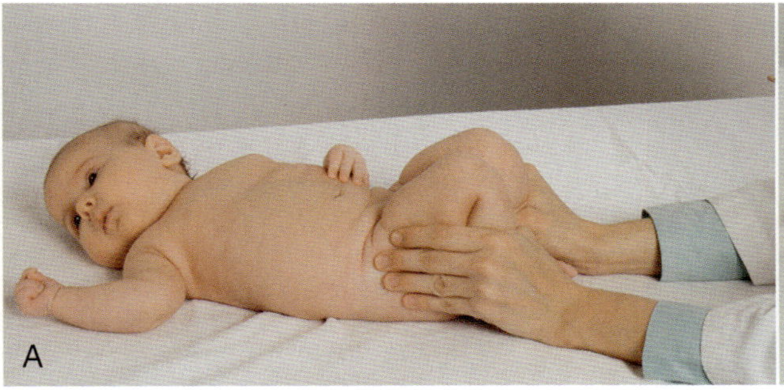

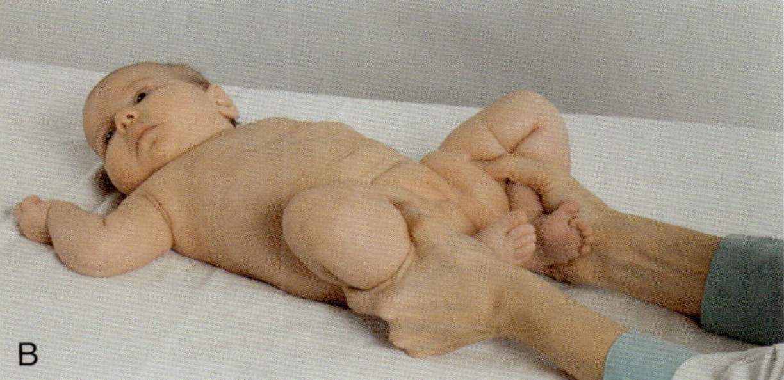

FIGURE 20.46 Ortolani's manoeuvre to test for developmental hip dysplasia

PROCEDURES AND NORMAL FINDINGS	ABNORMAL FINDINGS AND CLINICAL ALERTS
The **Allis test** is also used to check for hip dislocation by comparing leg lengths (Figure 20.47). Place the baby's feet flat on the table and flex the knees up. Scan the tops of the knees; normally they are at the same elevation. 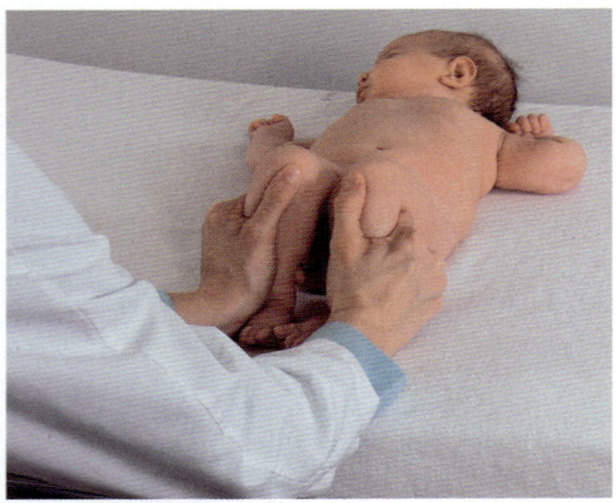 **FIGURE 20.47** Allis test—comparing leg length for hip dislocation	This test is usually performed by experienced midwives and maternal and child health nurses—not generalist nurses. Finding one knee significantly lower than the other is a *positive indication of Allis' sign* and suggests hip dislocation.
Note the gluteal folds. Normally they are equal on both sides. However, some asymmetry may occur in healthy children.	Unequal gluteal folds may accompany hip dislocation after 2 to 3 months of age.
Hands and arms. Inspect the hands, noting the shape, number and position of fingers and palmar creases.	**Polydactyly** is the presence of extra fingers or toes. Syndactyly is webbing between adjacent fingers or toes (Table 20.8). A **simian crease** is a single palmar crease that occurs with Down syndrome (trisomy 21), accompanied by short broad fingers, incurving of little fingers and low-set thumbs.
Palpate the length of the clavicles because the clavicle is the bone most frequently fractured during birth. The clavicles should feel smooth, regular and without crepitus. Also note equal ROM of arms during Moro's reflex.	Fractured clavicle: Note irregularity at the fracture site, crepitus and angulation. The site has rapid callus formation with a palpable lump within a few weeks. Observe limited arm ROM and unilateral response to Moro's reflex.

PROCEDURES AND NORMAL FINDINGS	ABNORMAL FINDINGS AND CLINICAL ALERTS
Back. Lift the infant and examine the back. Note the normal single C curve of the newborn's spine (Figure 20.48). By 2 months of age, the infant can lift the head while prone. This builds the concave cervical spinal curve and indicates normal forearm strength. Inspect the length of the spine for any tuft of hair, dimple in midline, cyst or mass. Normally, none are present.	A tuft of hair over a dimple in the midline may indicate spina bifida. A small dimple in the midline—anywhere from the head to the coccyx—suggests **dermoid sinus**. Mass, such as **meningocele** (Table 20.8).
Observe ROM through spontaneous movement of extremities.	
Test muscle strength by lifting the infant with your hands under the axillae (Figure 20.49). A baby with normal muscle strength wedges securely between your hands.	A baby who starts to 'slip' between your hands shows weakness of the shoulder muscles.

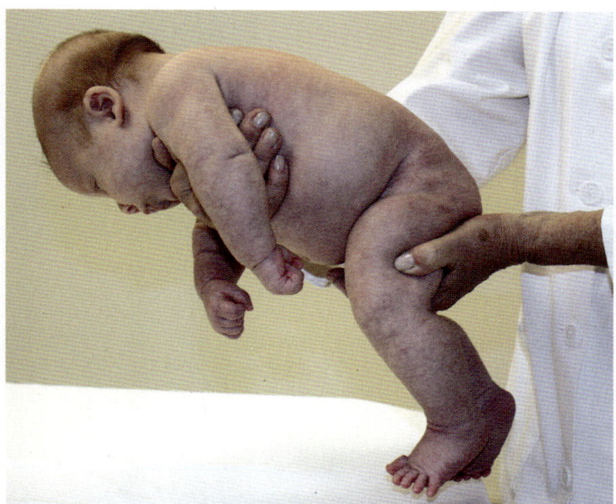

FIGURE 20.48 Inspecting an infant's spine

PROCEDURES AND NORMAL FINDINGS	ABNORMAL FINDINGS AND CLINICAL ALERTS

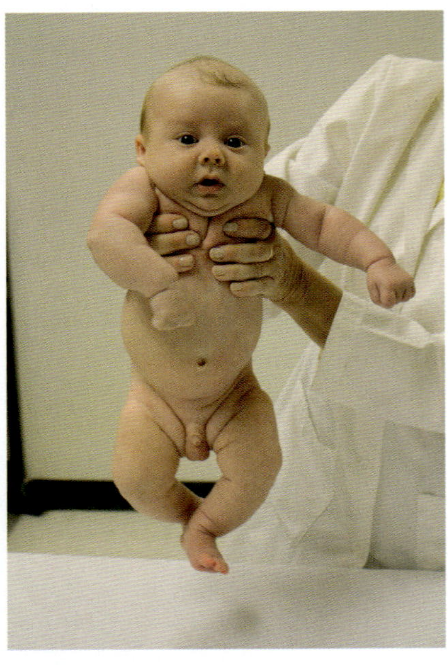

FIGURE 20.49 Testing infant muscle strength

Additional objective data for preschool and school-age children

Once an infant learns to crawl and then to walk, the waking hours show perpetual motion. This is convenient for your musculoskeletal assessment; you can observe the muscles and joints during spontaneous play before a table-top examination. Most young children enjoy showing off their physical accomplishments. For specific motions, coax the toddler: 'Show me how you can walk to Mummy' or 'Climb these steps'. Ask a preschooler to hop on one foot or to jump.

Back. While the child is standing, note the posture. From behind, note a 'plumb line' from the back of the head, along the spine, to the middle of the sacrum. Shoulders are level within 1 cm, and scapulae are symmetrical. From the side, lordosis is common throughout childhood, appearing more pronounced in children with a protuberant abdomen.

Lordosis is marked with muscular dystrophy and rickets.

Legs and feet. Anteriorly, note the leg position. A 'bowlegged' stance (genu varum) is a lateral bowing of the legs (Figure 20.50A). It is present when you measure a persistent space of more than 2.5 cm between the knees when the medial malleoli are together. Genu varum is normal for 1 year after a child begins walking. The child may walk with a waddling gait. This resolves with growth; no treatment is indicated.

Genu varum also occurs with rickets.

PROCEDURES AND NORMAL FINDINGS	ABNORMAL FINDINGS AND CLINICAL ALERTS

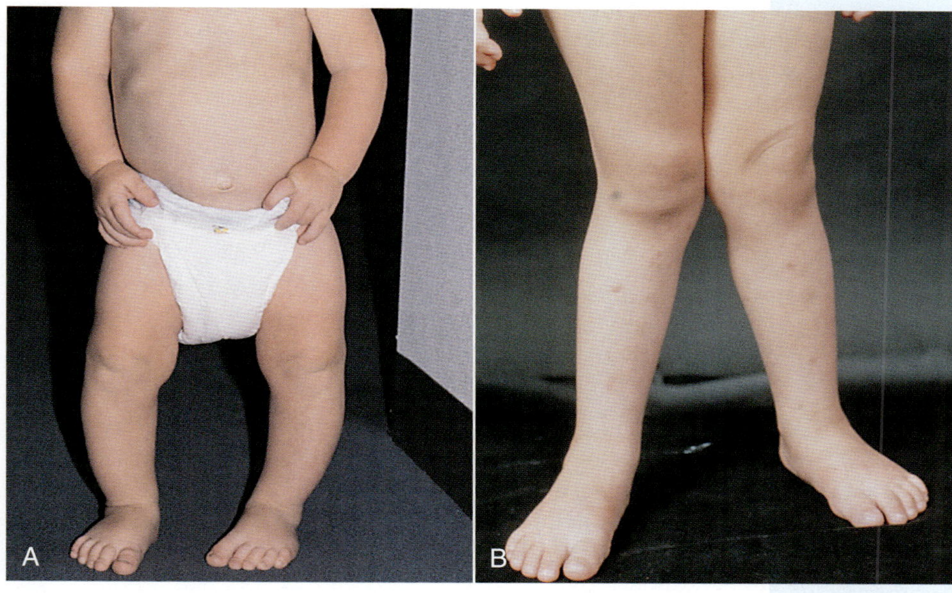

FIGURE 20.50 A Genu varum B Genu valgum

'Knock knees' (genu valgum) are present when there is more than 2.5 cm between the medial malleoli when the knees are together (Figure 20.50B). It occurs normally between 2 and 3½ years of age. Also, treatment is not indicated. (Note: To remember the two conditions, remember to link the Rs and Gs: genu va**r**um—knees apa**r**t; genu val**g**um—knees to**g**ether.)

Genu valgum also occurs with rickets, poliomyelitis and syphilis.

Often, parents tell you they are concerned about their child's foot development. The most common questions are about 'flatfeet' and 'pigeon toes'.

Flatfoot (pes planus) is pronation, or turning in, of the medial side of the foot. A young child may look flatfooted because the normal, longitudinal arch is concealed by a fat pad until age 3 years. When standing begins, the child takes a broad-based stance, which causes pronation. Thus, pronation is common between 12 and 30 months. You can see it best from behind the child, where the medial side of the foot drops down and in.

Pronation beyond 30 months.

Pigeon toes, or toeing in, are demonstrated when a child tends to walk on the lateral side of the foot, and the longitudinal arch looks higher than normal. It often starts as a forefoot adduction, which usually corrects spontaneously by age 3 years if the foot is flexible.

Toeing in from forefoot adduction that is fixed or lasts beyond age 3 years.

Toeing in from tibial torsion.

PROCEDURES AND NORMAL FINDINGS	ABNORMAL FINDINGS AND CLINICAL ALERTS
Check the child's gait while walking away from and returning to you. Let the child wear socks because a cold tile floor will distort the usual gait. From 1 to 2 years of age, expect a broad-based gait, with arms out for balance. Weight bearing falls on the inside of the foot. From 3 years of age, the base narrows and the arms are closer to the sides. Inspect the shoes for spots of greatest wear to aid your judgement of the gait. Normally the shoes wear more on the outside of the heel and the inside of the toe.	Limp, usually caused by trauma, fatigue or hip disease. Abnormal gait patterns (Chapter 12).
The child may sit for the rest of the examination. Start with the feet and hands of a child from 2 to 6 years of age because the child is happy to show these off and proceed through the examination described earlier.	
Particularly, check the arm for full ROM and presence of pain. Look for subluxation of the elbow (head of the radius). This occurs most often between 2 and 4 years of age because of forceful removal of clothing or dangling while adults suspend the child by the hands.	Inability to supinate the hand while the arm is flexed, together with pain in the elbow, indicates subluxation of the head of the radius.
Palpate the bones, joints and muscles of the extremities as described in the adult examination.	Pain or tenderness in extremities is usually caused by trauma or infection. Fractures are usually due to trauma and are exhibited as an inability to use the area, a deformity or an excess of motion in the involved bone with pain and crepitation. Enlargement of the tibial tubercles with tenderness suggests Osgood-Schlatter disease (Table 20.5).
Additional objective data for adolescents	
Proceed with the musculoskeletal examination you provide for the adult, except pay special note to spinal posture. Kyphosis is common during adolescence because of chronic poor posture. Be aware of the risk of sports-related injuries with the adolescent, because sports participation and competition often peak with this age group. **The National Self-Detection Program for Scoliosis.**[38] This program involves distributing a brochure for the target age group (girls 10–12 years of age) in which the physical signs of scoliosis are described. Advise the person to consult with their family doctor if they have any concerns. The program is endorsed by the Paediatrics and Child Health Division of the Royal Australasian College of Physicians.[37]	**Scoliosis** is most apparent during the preadolescent growth spurt. Asymmetry suggests scoliosis—ribs hump up on one side as child bends forwards and with unequal landmark elevation (Table 20.7).

PROCEDURES AND NORMAL FINDINGS

ABNORMAL FINDINGS AND CLINICAL ALERTS

Screen for scoliosis with the *forward bend test* (Figure 20.51). Seat yourself behind the standing child and ask the child to stand with the feet shoulder-width apart and bend forwards slowly to touch the toes. Expect a straight vertical spine while standing and while bending forwards. Posterior ribs should be symmetrical, with equal elevation of shoulders, scapulae and iliac crests. You may wish to mark each spinous process with a felt marker. The lineup of ink dots highlights even a subtle curve.

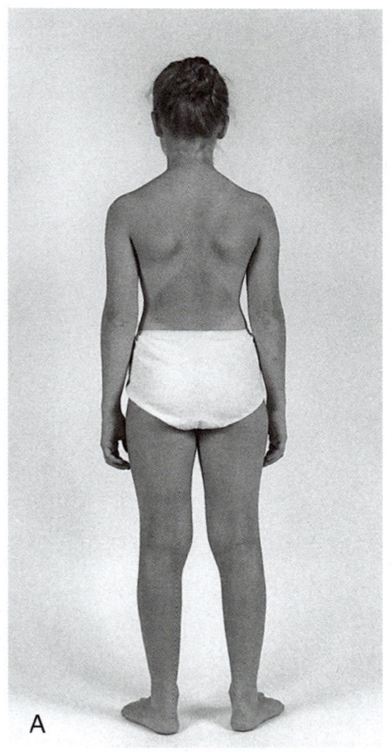

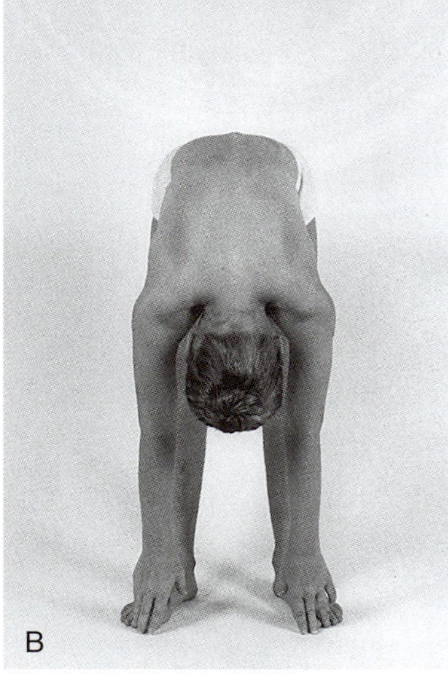

FIGURE 20.51 Screening for scoliosis

Additional objective data for pregnant women

Proceed through the examination described in the adult section. Expected postural changes in pregnancy include progressive lordosis and, towards the third trimester, anterior cervical flexion, kyphosis and slumped shoulders (Figure 20.52A). When the pregnancy is at term, the protuberant abdomen and the relaxed mobility in the joints create the characteristic 'waddling' gait (Figure 20.52B).

PROCEDURES AND NORMAL FINDINGS	ABNORMAL FINDINGS AND CLINICAL ALERTS

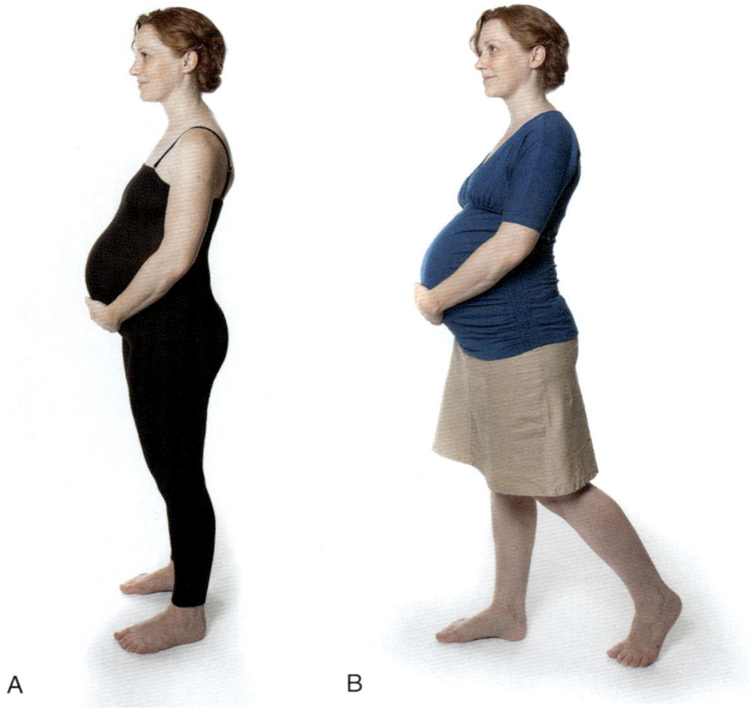

A B

FIGURE 20.52 Normal postural changes with pregnancy

Abnormal findings for advanced practice

TABLE 20.8 Congenital abnormalities of the feet, hands and spine

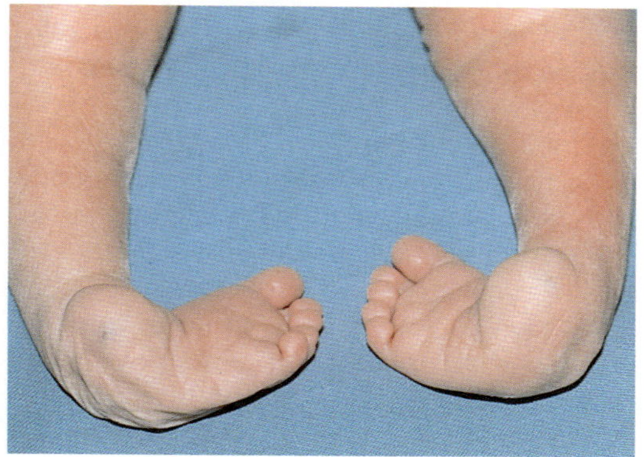

Talipes equinovarus (clubfoot)

Congenital, rigid and fixed malposition of the foot including (1) inversion, (2) forefoot adduction and (3) the foot pointing downwards (equinus). A common birth defect, with an incidence of 1 per 1,000 live births. Males are affected twice as frequently as females. There is no known cause of talipes although it can be common in some families. Talipes can be diagnosed in the prenatal ultrasound in 50% of cases. Treatment starts soon after birth and includes a series of plaster casts and surgery to correct the abnormality and restore function.

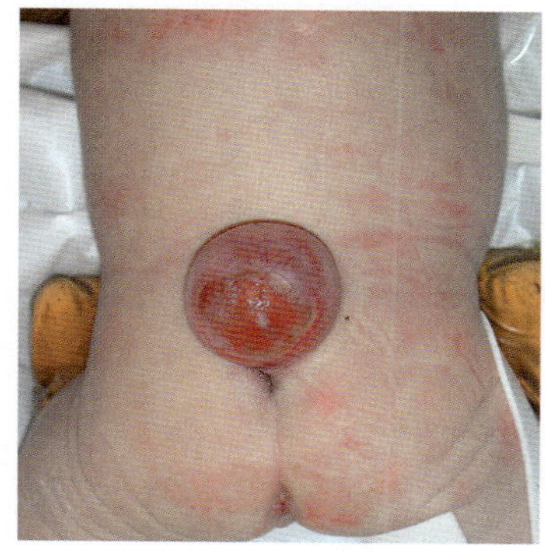

Spina bifida

Incomplete closure of the posterior part of the vertebrae results in a neural tube defect. Seriousness varies from a skin defect along the spine to protrusion of the sac containing meninges, spinal fluid or a malformed spinal cord. The most serious type is myelomeningocele (shown here), in which the meninges and neural tissue protrude. In these cases, the child is usually paralysed below the level of the lesion.

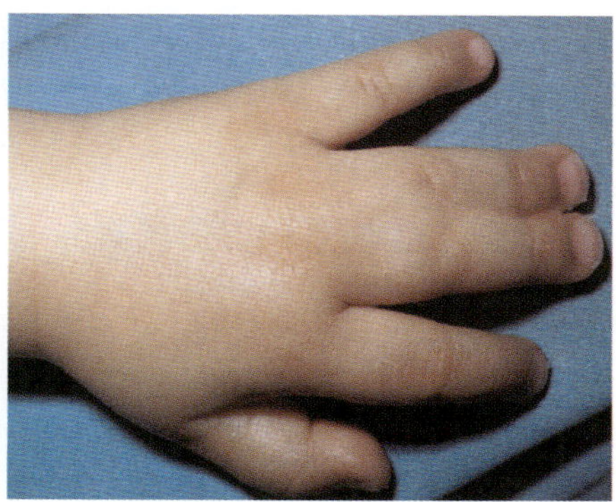

Syndactyly

Webbed fingers are a congenital deformity, usually requiring surgical separation. The metacarpals and phalanges of the webbed fingers are different lengths, and the joints do not line up. To leave the fingers fused would therefore limit their flexion and extension.

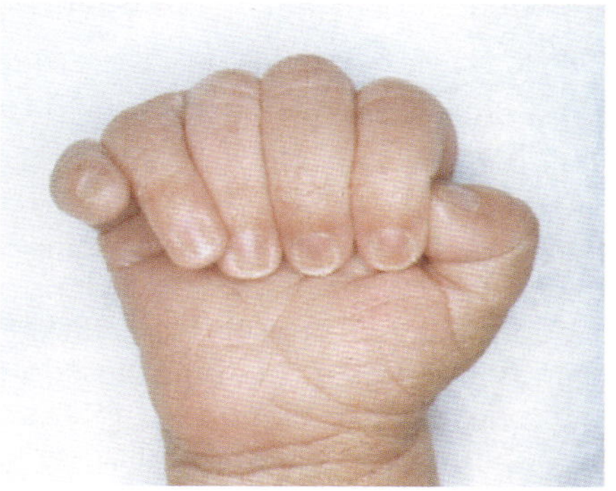

Polydactyly

Extra digits are a congenital deformity, usually occurring at the fifth finger or the thumb. Surgical removal is considered for cosmetic appearance. The sixth finger shown here was not removed because it had full ROM and sensation and a normal appearance.

Clinical reasoning and documentation

The following is a continuation of the case study provided at the beginning of this chapter and the clinical reasoning process including problem/issue identification. Consult a fundamentals of nursing or medical-surgical nursing text for information about goal setting, nursing interventions and evaluation.

Case study (continued)—Rheumatoid arthritis

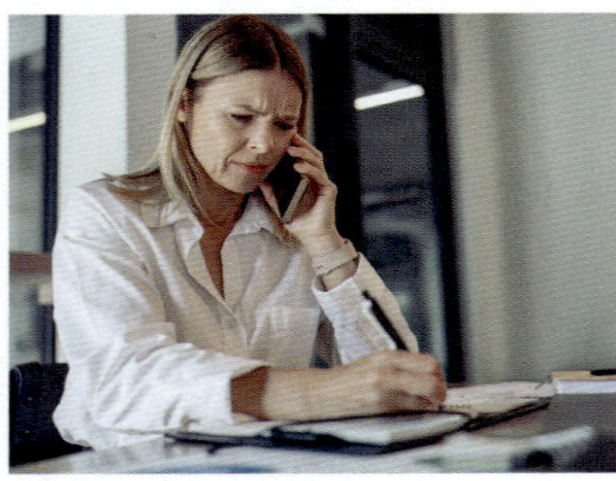

Context

You will recall from the case study described earlier in the chapter that you are working as an occupational health nurse in an onsite multidisciplinary health clinic that is part of a large company. The role includes providing first aid treatment, assessing workplace injuries, conducting audiometric assessments and providing occupational health and injury management advice.

Consider the patient's situation

Ms Mari Timms is a 45-year-old female office worker with a diagnosis of RA 3 years ago, who seeks care now for 'swelling and burning pain' in her hands for 1 day, which is affecting her ability to complete her normal work tasks and daily activities. She has not been assessed by a rheumatologist since diagnosis and is subsequently not on an effective disease-modifying treatment program.

Collect cues/information

Your further assessment reveals the following information.

Subjective data

Ms Timms was diagnosed as having RA at age 41 years by a rheumatologist. Since that time, her 'flare-ups' seem to come every 6 to 8 months. Acute episodes involve hand joints and are treated with aspirin, which gives relief. Typically experiences morning stiffness in all joints, lasting 30 minutes to 1 hour.

She can dress herself although has difficulty with buttons and zippers. Also has difficulty with heavy pots and pans. Avoids using stairs as this causes pain in her hips, knees and ankles. She manages all other activities of daily living herself.

Ms Timms says her joints feel warm, swollen and tender. She has had weight loss of 4 kg over past 4 years and feels fatigued much of the time. She states she should rest more, but 'I can't take the time'. Daily exercises have been prescribed but she doesn't do them regularly. When she has a flare up, she feels better in a few days and decreases aspirin dose by herself.

Objective data

Gait is smooth and symmetrical.

Joint ROM within normal limits with exception of joints of the wrist and hands. Radiocarpal, metacarpophalangeal and proximal interphalangeal joints are red, swollen and tender to palpation. Spindle-shaped swelling of proximal interphalangeal joints of third digit right hand and second digit left hand; ulnar deviation of metacarpophalangeal joints.

Difficulty in squeezing my hands. Grip strength reduced in both hands.

Process information and identify problems/issues

Collaborative problem

Acute joint pain (especially in hands) related to inflammation from arthritis—referral back to specialist via clinic medical practitioner

Problem statements/nursing diagnoses

Impaired physical mobility (in hands) related to arthritis

Acute joint pain (especially in hands) related to inflammation from arthritis

Fatigue related to systemic effects of arthritis and pain

Lack of knowledge about disease and symptom management and need for ongoing follow-up

ADDITIONAL RESOURCES

You can further develop your knowledge and skills relevant to musculoskeletal assessment, related pathophysiology, common health issues and nursing interventions by:

- reading chapters of a fundamentals of nursing or medical-surgical nursing textbook
- answering chapter multiple choice questions online. Log onto ClinicalKey Student and search for the text 'Health Assessment, 4th edition'. Choose the section titled 'Teaching material'. In this section you will find question and answer documents for each chapter. Please check instructions on the inside front cover of the book to access online resources
- visiting websites

Healthy Bones Australia: https://healthybonesaustralia.org.au

Arthritis Australia: https://arthritisaustralia.com.au

Osteoporosis NZ: https://osteoporosis.org.nz

Arthritis NZ: https://www.arthritis.org.nz

REFERENCES

1. Peake C, Shah K, Solan MC. Bone metabolism and the receptor activator of nuclear factor-κB ligand (RANKL) pathway: a comprehensive review. Orthopaedics and Trauma. 2021 Oct 1;35(5):297–304.
2. Hart NH, Newton RU, Tan J, Rantalainen T, Chivers P, Siafarikas A, et al. Biological basis of bone strength: anatomy, physiology and measurement. Journal of Musculoskeletal & Neuronal Interactions. 2020;20(3):347.
3. Joseph SY, Krishna NG, Fox MG, Blankenbaker DG, Frick MA, Jawetz ST, et al. ACR Appropriateness Criteria® osteoporosis and bone mineral density: 2022 update. Journal of the American College of Radiology. 2022 Nov 1;19(11):S417–S432.
4. Gendron E, Bouchard F, Singbo N, Brown JP, Michou L. Decline in clinical severity of Paget's disease of bone: comparison between a contemporary cohort and a historical cohort. Bone. 2023 May 1;170:116721
5. Cabral BM, Edding SN, Portocarrero JP, Lerma EV. Rhabdomyolysis. Disease-a-Month. 2020 Aug 1;66(8):101015.
6. Papadopoulou SK, Papadimitriou K, Voulgaridou G, Georgaki E, Tsotidou E, Zantidou O, et al. Exercise and nutrition impact on osteoporosis and Sarcopenia—The incidence of osteosarcopenia: a narrative review. Nutrients. 2021 Dec 16;13(12):4499.
7. Marriott E, Twomey S, Lee M, Williams N. Variability in Australian screening guidelines for developmental dysplasia of the hip. Journal of Paediatrics and Child Health. 2021 Dec;57(12):1857–1865.
8. Fludder CJ, Keil BG, Neave MJ. Case report: Morphological changes evident after manual therapy in two cases of late-diagnosed developmental dysplasia of the hip. Frontiers in Pediatrics. 2023 Jan 26;10:1045812.
9. Australian Institute of Health and Welfare. Chronic musculoskeletal conditions. Canberra: Australian Institute of Health and Welfare, 2023. Available at: https://www.aihw.gov.au/reports/chronic-musculoskeletal-conditions/musculoskeletal-conditions
10. Ceprnja D, Chipchase L, Liamputtong P, Gupta A. 'This is hard to cope with': the lived experience and coping strategies adopted amongst Australian women with pelvic girdle pain in pregnancy. BMC Pregnancy and Childbirth. 2022 Dec;22(1):96.
11. Australian Government, Department of Health and Aged Care. Pregnancy Care Guidelines. Australian Government Department of Health;

2020. Available at: https://www.health.gov.au/resources/pregnancy-care-guidelines
12. Castro-Gutierrez A, Young K, Bermas BL. Pregnancy and management in women with rheumatoid arthritis, systemic lupus erythematosus, and obstetric antiphospholipid syndrome. Medical Clinics. 2021 Mar 1;105(2):341–353.
13. Andreoli L, Chighizola CB, Iaccarino L, Botta A, Gerosa M, Ramoni V, et al. Immunology of pregnancy and reproductive health in autoimmune rheumatic diseases. Update from the 11th International Conference on Reproduction, Pregnancy and Rheumatic Diseases. Autoimmunity Reviews. 2022 Dec 20:103259.
14. Zanetti A, Zambon A, Scirè CA, Bortoluzzi A. Impact of rheumatoid arthritis and methotrexate on pregnancy outcomes: retrospective cohort study of the Italian Society for Rheumatology. RMD Open. 2022 Dec 1;8(2):e002412.
15. Australian Bureau of Statistics. Health Conditions Prevalence [Internet]. Canberra: ABS; 2020-21. Available at: https://www.abs.gov.au/statistics/health/health-conditions-and-risks/health-conditions-prevalence/2020-21
16. Australian Institute of Health and Welfare. Osteoporosis [Internet]. Canberra: Australian Institute of Health and Welfare, 2023 [cited 2023 Jul. 19]. Available at: https://www.aihw.gov.au/reports/chronic-musculoskeletal-conditions/osteoporosis-1
17. Coletta G, Phillips SM. An elusive consensus definition of sarcopenia impedes research and clinical treatment: a narrative review. Ageing Research Reviews. 2023 Feb 13:101883.
18. Izquierdo M, Singh MF. Promoting resilience in the face of ageing and disease: The central role of exercise and physical activity. Ageing Research Reviews. 2023 Apr 29:101940.
19. Australian Institute of Health and Welfare. Chronic conditions and multimorbidity [Internet]. Canberra: Australian Institute of Health and Welfare, 2023 [cited 2023 Jul. 11]. Available at: https://www.aihw.gov.au/reports/australias-health/chronic-conditions-and-multimorbidity
20. Baltes M, Herber OR, Meyer G, Stephan A. Fear of falling from the perspective of affected persons: a systematic review and qualitative meta-summary using Sandelowski and Barroso's method. International Journal of Older People Nursing. 2023 Jan;18(1):e12520.
21. Australian Institute of Health and Welfare (AIHW). Australia's Health in brief. 2022. Available at: https://www.aihw.gov.au/getmedia/c6c5dda9-4020-43b0-8ed6-a567cd660eaa/aihw-aus-421.pdf.aspx
22. Gane EM, Plinsinga ML, Brakenridge CL, Smits EJ, Aplin T, Johnston V. The impact of musculoskeletal injuries sustained in road traffic crashes on work-related outcomes: a systematic review. International Journal of Environmental Research and Public Health. 2021 Nov 1;18(21):11504.
23. O'Brien P, Thuraisingam S, Bunzli S, Lin I, Bessarab D, Coffin J, et al. Total joint replacement may be a valuable treatment for Aboriginal and Torres Strait Islander people with osteoarthritis, but uptake is low. ANZ Journal of Surgery. 2022 Oct;92(10):2676–2682.
24. Australian Institute of Health and Welfare. Indigenous Australians and the health system [Internet]. Canberra: Australian Institute of Health and Welfare, 2022 [cited 2023 Jul. 29]. Available at: https://www.aihw.gov.au/reports/australias-health/indigenous-australians-use-of-health-services
25. Tran V, Janda M, Lucas RM, McLeod DS, Thompson BS, Waterhouse M, et al. Vitamin D and sun exposure: a community survey in Australia. Current Oncology. 2023 Feb 18;30(2):2465–2481.
26. Horton-French K, Dunlop E, Lucas RM, Pereira G, Black LJ. Prevalence and predictors of vitamin D deficiency in a nationally representative sample of Australian adolescents and young adults. European Journal of Clinical Nutrition. 2021 Nov;75(11):1627–1636.
27. LeBoff MS, Greenspan SL, Insogna KL, Lewiecki EM, Saag KG, Singer AJ, et al. The clinician's guide to prevention and treatment of osteoporosis. Osteoporosis International. 2022 Oct;33(10):2049–2102.

28. Lopes KG, Rodrigues EL, da Silva Lopes MR, do Nascimento VA, Pott A, Guimarães RD, et al. Adiposity metabolic consequences for adolescent bone health. Nutrients. 2022 Aug 10;14(16):3260.
29. Lorentzon M, Johansson H, Harvey NC, Liu E, Vandenput L, McCloskey EV, et al. Osteoporosis and fractures in women: the burden of disease. Climacteric. 2022 Jan 2;25(1):4–10.
30. Tatangelo G, Watts J, Lim K, Connaughton C, Abimanyi-Ochom J, Borgström F, et al. The cost of osteoporosis, osteopenia, and associated fractures in Australia in 2017. Journal of Bone and Mineral Research, 2019;3(5):616–625.
31. Royal Australian College of General Practitioners (RACGP). Guideline for preventative activities in general practice: Osteoporosis. 2021. Available at: https://www.racgp.org.au/clinical-resources/clinical-guidelines/key-racgp-guidelines/view-all-racgp-guidelines/guidelines-for-preventive-activities-in-general-pr/osteoporosis
32. Rizzoli R. Diagnosis and clinical aspects of osteoporosis. In: Ferrari SL, Roux C, editors. Pocket reference to osteoporosis. Cham, Switzerland: Springer International Publishing; 2019. Pp. 31–42.
33. Doherty M, Dacre J, Dieppe P, Snaith M. The 'GALS' locomotor screen. Annals of the Rheumatic Diseases, 1992;51:1165–1169.
34. Dacre J. The GALS screen: the rapid rheumatological exam. Medical Journal of Australia 2019;210(9):396–397.
35. Purushe DA, Dhage PP, Phansopkar P, Arora SP. Orthopedic screening using pGALS assessment tools in children's between 5 and 12 years. Journal of Medical Pharmaceutical and Allied Sciences 2022;11(1, 1348):4405–4408.
36. Jeong W, Moon JY, Kim JH. Association of absolute and relative hand grip strength with all-cause mortality among middle-aged and old-aged people. BMC Geriatrics 23, 321 (2023). https://doi.org/10.1186/s12877-023-04008-8
37. Royal College of Pathologists of Australia (RCPA). RCPA manual. 2019. [internet]. Available at: https://www.rcpa.edu.au/Manuals/RCPA-Manual/Pathology-Tests
38. Scoliosis Australia. The National detection program for scoliosis. 2023. Available at: https://www.scoliosis-australia.org/policies-programs/the-national-scoliosis-detection-program/

CHAPTER 21

Nutritional and metabolic assessment

Written by Joyce K Keithly
Adapted by Trish Burton

INTRODUCTION

Nutrition plays an essential part in growth, development and general health and wellbeing and as such is becoming an increasing focus for health professionals. Nutritional status refers to the degree of balance between nutrient intake and nutrient requirements. This balance is affected by many factors, including physiological, psychosocial, developmental, cultural and economic.

A person is said to have an optimal nutritional status when enough nutrients are consumed to support day-to-day body needs and any increased metabolic demands due to growth, pregnancy or illness. People with an optimal nutritional status are more active, have fewer physical illnesses and live longer than people who are malnourished.

Case study

The following case study gives an example of a typical situation involving nutritional assessment and the initial clinical reasoning process. The following case study will help you identify your learning needs.

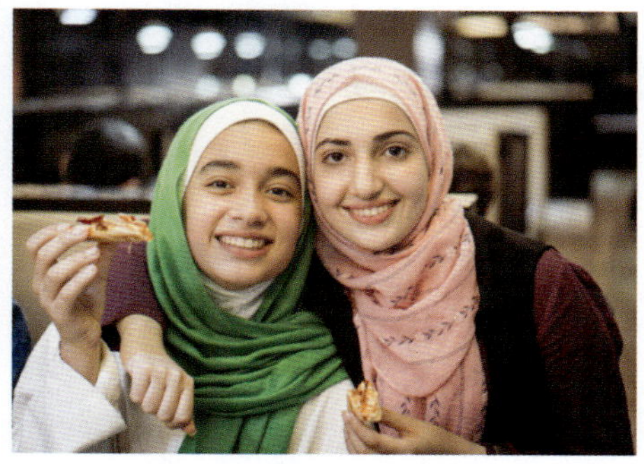

Context

You are the registered nurse working in a multidisciplinary health team in a general practice setting. Your role in the team is to conduct client assessments, assist with referrals to specialist services and help plan care for people with chronic illness.

Consider the patient's situation

Lisa Alfarsi is a 15-year-old girl with type 1 diabetes. She presents with her mother for the usual 3-monthly check-up. Her mother is concerned that Lisa has not been checking blood glucose levels regularly. Lisa says she forgets occasionally and asks what the 'big deal' is.

Questions to further your learning

- What are the possible things that might be going on with Lisa?
- What knowledge do you need to be able to predict what might be going on?
- What approach to Lisa's health assessment will you take?
- What questions (subjective data) will you ask Lisa to extend the health history and why?
- What physical examination (objective data) will you conduct and why?
- What resources are available to assist in your assessment of Lisa?

Assessment plan

Nursing assessment of a person's nutritional status and risk is necessary to avoid developing nutrition-associated complications such as cognitive dysfunction, fatigue, pressure injuries and an increased susceptibility to infection. Nutritional status can be determined by applying nutritional assessment techniques.

In general, these techniques are noninvasive, inexpensive and easy to perform and can be conducted in any healthcare setting.

The purposes of nutritional assessment are to:

- identify people who are malnourished or are at risk of developing malnutrition
- provide data for designing a nutrition plan of care that will prevent or minimise the development of malnutrition
- establish baseline data for evaluating the efficacy of nutritional care.

Nutrition screening is a quick and easy way to identify people at nutritional risk, such as those with weight loss, inadequate food intake or recent illness. A variety of valid tools are available for screening different populations. For example, the Malnutrition Universal Screening Tool (MUST) has been validated in many patient groups for use in the hospital setting and the community.[1,2] People identified at nutritional risk should undergo a comprehensive nutritional assessment.

The main areas for subjective assessment are:

- presenting concern
- eating patterns
- usual weight
- changes in appetite, taste, smell, chewing, swallowing
- teeth
- recent surgery, burns, trauma, infection
- chronic illness
- nausea, vomiting, diarrhoea, constipation
- food allergies or intolerances
- past history
- health and lifestyle management.

Following subjective data collection, you will get a sense of the areas needed to be examined for objective data. Only the relevant areas should be examined. The main areas for physical examination and measurement are:

- general inspection
- inspecting the skin
- inspecting the face
- inspecting the mouth
- inspecting the throat
- anthropometric measures
- blood glucose monitoring.

Resources available

You will find additional resources and the reference list at the end of this chapter.

Structure and function

Mouth

The mouth is the first segment of the digestive system and an airway for the respiratory system. The **oral cavity** is a short passage bordered by the lips, palate, cheeks and tongue. It contains the teeth and gums, tongue and salivary glands (Figure 21.1).

The lips are the anterior border of the oral cavity—the transition zone from the outer skin to the inner mucous membrane lining the oral cavity. The arching roof of the mouth is the palate; it is divided into two parts. The anterior **hard palate** is made up of bone and is a whitish colour. Posterior to this is the **soft palate**, an arch of muscle that is pinker in colour and mobile. The **uvula** is the free projection hanging down from the middle of the soft palate. The cheeks are the side walls of the oral cavity.

The floor of the mouth consists of the horseshoe-shaped mandible bone, the tongue and underlying muscles. The **tongue** is a mass of striated muscle arranged in a crosswise pattern so it can change shape and

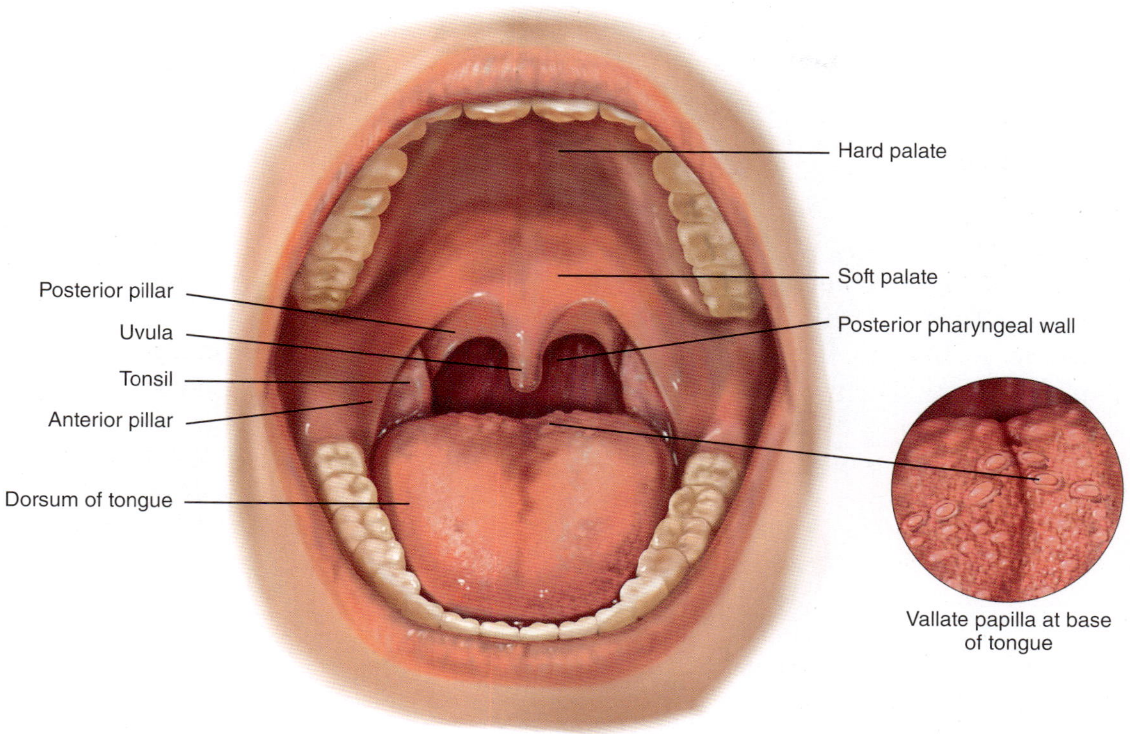

FIGURE 21.1 Oral cavity

position. The papillae are the rough, bumpy elevations on its dorsal surface. Note the larger vallate papillae in an inverted V shape across the posterior base of the tongue, and do not confuse them with abnormal growths. Underneath, the ventral surface of the tongue is smooth and shiny and has prominent veins. The **frenulum** is a midline fold of tissue that connects the tongue to the floor of the mouth.

The tongue's ability to change shape and position enhances its functions in mastication, swallowing, cleansing the teeth and the formation of speech. The tongue also functions in taste sensation. Microscopic taste buds are in the papillae at the back and along the sides of the tongue and on the soft palate.

The mouth contains three pairs of salivary glands (Figure 21.2). The largest, the **parotid** gland, lies within the cheeks in front of the ear extending from the zygomatic arch down to the angle of the jaw. Its duct, Stensen's duct, runs forwards to open on the buccal mucosa opposite the second molar. The **submandibular** gland is the size of a walnut. It lies beneath the mandible at the angle of the jaw. Wharton's duct runs up and forwards to the floor of the mouth and opens at either side of the frenulum. The smallest gland, the almond-shaped **sublingual** gland, lies within the floor of the mouth under the tongue. It has many small openings along the sublingual fold under the tongue. The glands secrete saliva, the clear fluid that moistens and lubricates the food bolus, starts digestion and cleans and protects the mucosa.

Adults have 32 **permanent** teeth—16 in each arch. Each tooth has three parts: the crown, the neck and the root (Figure 21.3). The gums (gingivae) collar the teeth. They

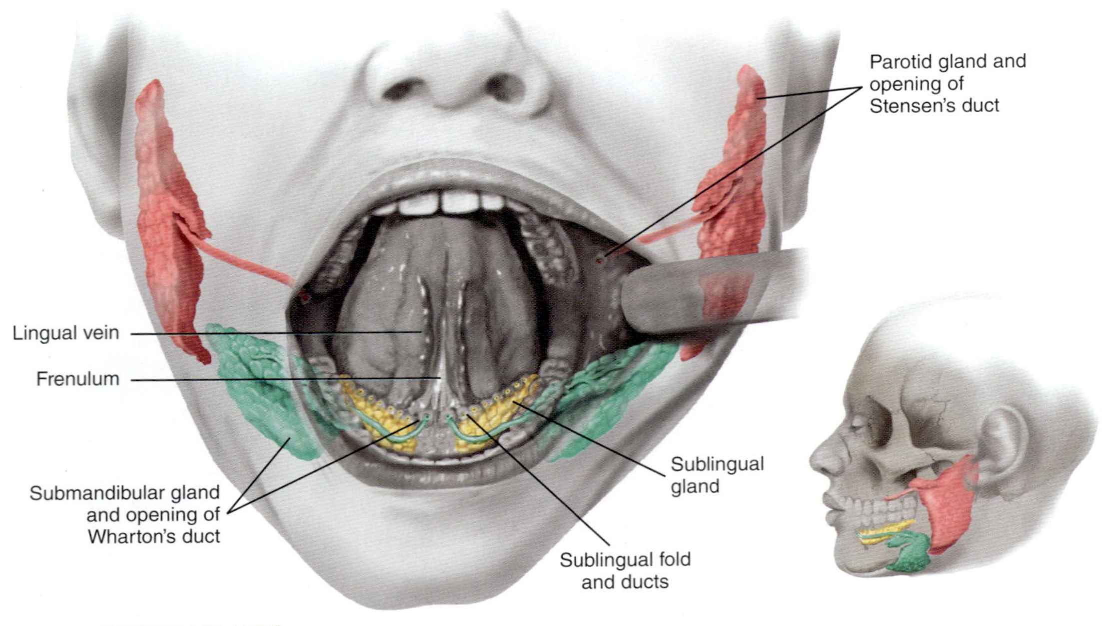

FIGURE 21.2 Salivary glands

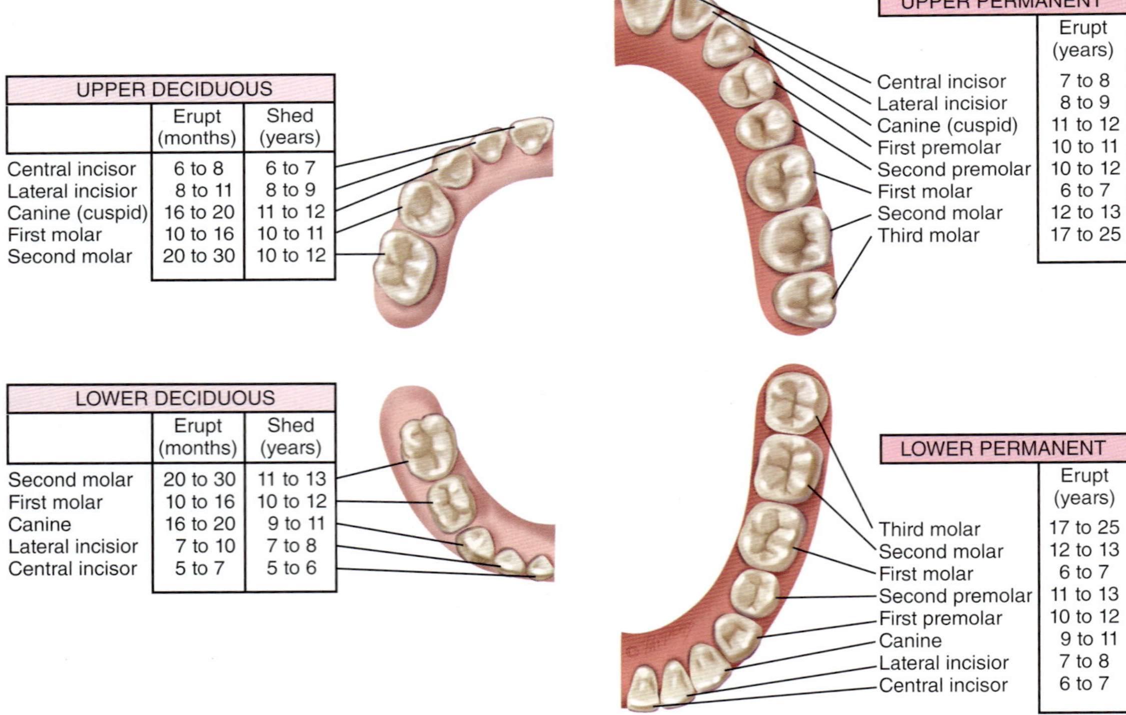

UPPER DECIDUOUS	Erupt (months)	Shed (years)
Central incisor	6 to 8	6 to 7
Lateral incisor	8 to 11	8 to 9
Canine (cuspid)	16 to 20	11 to 12
First molar	10 to 16	10 to 11
Second molar	20 to 30	10 to 12

LOWER DECIDUOUS	Erupt (months)	Shed (years)
Second molar	20 to 30	11 to 13
First molar	10 to 16	10 to 12
Canine	16 to 20	9 to 11
Lateral incisor	7 to 10	7 to 8
Central incisor	5 to 7	5 to 6

UPPER PERMANENT	Erupt (years)
Central incisor	7 to 8
Lateral incisor	8 to 9
Canine (cuspid)	11 to 12
First premolar	10 to 11
Second premolar	10 to 12
First molar	6 to 7
Second molar	12 to 13
Third molar	17 to 25

LOWER PERMANENT	Erupt (years)
Third molar	17 to 25
Second molar	12 to 13
First molar	6 to 7
Second premolar	11 to 13
First premolar	10 to 12
Canine	9 to 11
Lateral incisor	7 to 8
Central incisor	6 to 7

FIGURE 21.3 Deciduous and permanent teeth

are thick fibrous tissues covered with mucous membrane. The gums are different from the rest of the oral mucosa because of their pale pink colour and stippled surface. See Chapter 18 for information about the nose, oropharynx and throat.

Thyroid gland

The **thyroid gland** is an important endocrine gland with a rich blood supply. It straddles the trachea in the middle of the neck (Figure 21.4). This highly vascular endocrine gland synthesises and secretes thyroxine (T_4) and triiodothyronine (T_3), hormones that stimulate the rate of cellular metabolism. The gland has two lobes, both conical in shape, each curving posteriorly between the trachea and the sternocleidomastoid muscle. The lobes are connected in the middle by a thin isthmus lying over the second and third tracheal rings. (Sometimes a third lobe, the pyramidal lobe, is present. It is cone shaped, usually on the left and extends up towards the hyoid bone from the isthmus or from the neighbouring lobe.)

Just above the thyroid isthmus, within about 1 cm, is the **cricoid** cartilage or upper tracheal ring. The **thyroid** cartilage is above that, with a small palpable notch in its upper edge. This is the prominent 'Adam's apple' in males. The highest is the **hyoid** bone, palpated high in the neck at the level of the floor of the mouth.

Pancreas

The **pancreas** is a soft, lobulated gland located behind the stomach. It stretches obliquely across the posterior abdominal wall to the left upper quadrant. The pancreas has several important functions; the endocrine tissue (islets of Langerhans) regulates blood glucose levels by secreting glucagon and insulin. Exocrine cells produce digestive enzymes. See Chapter 23 for more information about the anatomical location of the pancreas in the abdominal cavity.

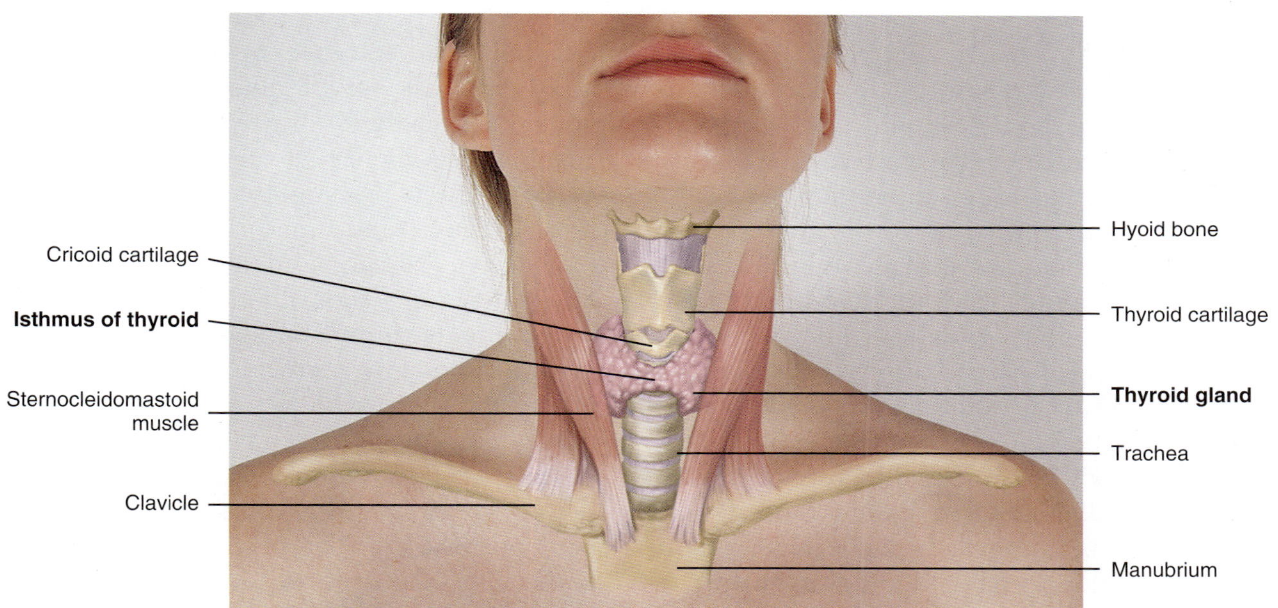

FIGURE 21.4 Thyroid gland

Developmental considerations

Infant to school-age child (birth to 12 years)

The time from birth to 4 months of age is the most rapid period of growth in the life cycle. Although infants lose weight during the first few days of life, birthweight is usually regained by the 7th to 10th day after birth. Thereafter, infants double their birthweight by 4 months and triple it by 1 year of age. Breastfeeding is recommended for full-term infants for the first year of life because breast milk is ideally formulated to promote normal infant growth and development and natural immunity. Although relatively few contraindications to breastfeeding exist, women who are human immunodeficiency virus (HIV)-positive should not breastfeed, since HIV can be transmitted through breast milk.

Infants increase their length by 50% during the first year of life and double it by 4 years of age. Brain size also increases very rapidly during infancy and childhood. By age 2 years, the brain has reached 50% of its adult size; by age 4, 75%; and by age 8, 100%. For this reason, infants and children younger than 2 years should not drink skim or low-fat milk or be placed on low-fat diets—fat (kilojoules and essential fatty acids) is required for proper growth and central nervous system development. Well-nourished infants are more likely to have appropriate physical and social growth and development.

In infants, salivation starts at 3 months. The baby will drool periodically for a few months before learning to swallow the saliva. This drooling does not herald the eruption of the first tooth, although many parents think it does.

The teeth, both sets, begin development in utero. Children have 20 **deciduous**, or temporary, teeth. These erupt between 6 months and 24 months of age. All 20 teeth should appear by 2½ years of age. The deciduous teeth are lost beginning at age 6 years through to age 12 years. They are replaced by permanent teeth, starting with the central incisors. Permanent teeth appear earlier in girls than in boys.

The preschool period is one of increasing growth and is the period when lifelong food habits form. Use of small portions, finger foods, simple meals and nutritious snacks are strategies to improve dietary intake.

Orofacial clefts describe the incomplete closure of the hard or soft palate of the mouth with or without midline clefting of the upper or lower lip. Clefts are congenital abnormalities arising during development of the oral region. Cleft palate is relatively rare in the Australian population, indicated by rates of around 1.5 per 1,000 births.[3]

Adolescent (12 or 13 years to 19 years)

Following a period of slow growth in late childhood, adolescence is characterised by rapid physical growth and endocrine and hormonal changes. Energy and protein requirements increase to meet this demand, and because of bone growth and increasing muscle mass (and, in girls, the onset of menarche), calcium and iron requirements also increase. Typically, these increased requirements cannot be met by three meals per day; therefore, nutritious snacks play an important role in achieving adequate nutrient intake.

In general, boys grow taller and have less body fat than girls. In adolescence, the percentage of body fat increases in females to about 25% and decreases in males (replaced by muscle mass) to about 12%. Typically, girls double their body weight between the ages of 8 and 14; boys double their body weight between the ages of 10 and 17 years.

Adulthood (20 to 64 years)

During adulthood, growth and nutrient needs stabilise. Most adults are in relatively good health. However, lifestyle factors such as cigarette smoking, stress, lack of exercise, excessive alcohol intake and diets high in saturated fat, cholesterol, salt and sugar and low in fibre can be factors in developing hypertension, obesity, atherosclerosis, cancer, osteoporosis and diabetes. The adult years, therefore, are an important time for education, to preserve health and to prevent or delay the onset of chronic disease.

For Australian adults, the statistics for obesity include:

- More than three in five Australian adults (63%) are overweight or obese.
- 71.6% of those over 18 years from low socioeconomic groups are overweight or obese compared with 61.5% in high socioeconomic groups.[4]

Late adulthood (65+ years)

As people age, many changes occur that make them prone to under-nutrition or over-nutrition. Poor physical or mental health, social isolation, alcoholism, limited functional ability, poverty and polypharmacy are the major risk factors for malnutrition in older adults.[5]

Normal physiological changes in late adulthood that directly affect nutritional status include poor dentition, decreased visual acuity, decreased saliva production, slowed gastrointestinal motility, decreased gastrointestinal absorption and diminished olfactory and taste sensitivity. Important nutritional features of the older years are a decrease in energy requirements due to loss of lean body mass, the most metabolically active tissue and an increase in fat mass.

Socioeconomic conditions frequently have a significant effect on the nutritional status of those in late adulthood. Decline of extended families and increased mobility of families reduce available support systems. Facilities for meal preparation and eating, transportation to grocery stores, physical limitations, income and social isolation are frequent problems and can obviously interfere with the acquisition of a balanced diet. Medications must also be considered because those in late adulthood frequently take multiple medications that have a potential for interaction with nutrients and with one another.

In the oral cavity, the soft tissues atrophy and the epithelium thins, especially in the cheek and tongue. This results in loss of taste buds, with about an 80% reduction in taste functioning. Further impairments to taste include a decrease in salivary secretion that is needed to dissolve flavouring agents and the presence of upper dentures that cover secondary taste sites. Atrophic tissues ulcerate easily, which places the older person at risk for infections such as oral moniliasis. An increased risk of malignant oral lesions is also present.

Many dental changes occur with ageing. The tooth surface is abraded. The gums begin to recede, and the teeth begin to erode at the gum line. A smooth V-shaped cavity forms around the neck of the tooth, exposing the nerve and making the tooth hypersensitive. Some tooth loss may occur from bone resorption (osteoporosis), which decreases the inner tooth structure and its outer support. Natural tooth loss is exacerbated by years of inadequate dental care, decay, poor oral hygiene and cigarette smoking.

If tooth loss occurs, the remaining teeth drift, causing **malocclusion**. The stress of chewing with malocclusion causes further problems: (1) excessive bone resorption with further tooth loss occurs; (2) muscle imbalance results from a mandible and maxilla now out of alignment, which produces muscle spasms, tenderness of muscles of mastication and chronic headaches; and (3) the temporomandibular joint is stressed, leading to osteoarthritis, pain and inability to fully open the mouth.

A diminished sense of taste and smell can decrease the ageing person's interest in food and may contribute to malnutrition. Saliva production decreases: saliva acts as a solvent for food flavours and helps move food around the mouth. Decreased saliva also reduces the mouth's self-cleaning property. The major cause of decreased saliva flow is not the ageing process itself but taking medications that have anticholinergic effects.

Reduction in or absence of teeth and trouble with mastication encourages older people to eat soft foods (usually high in carbohydrates) and to decrease meat and fresh vegetable intake. This may increase the risk of nutritional deficit for protein, vitamins and minerals.

Pregnancy and lactation

To support the nutritional requirements of the mother and fetus, sufficient kilojoules, protein, vitamins and minerals must be consumed. Weight gain will vary between people and can depend on the pre-pregnancy weight and body mass index (BMI) of the mother. Generally, if a woman's BMI is between 18.6 and 24.9 (kg/m^2) she is likely to gain 11 to 16 kg. If a woman is underweight (BMI < 18.5) she is likely to gain 12.5 to 18 kg and if she is overweight or obese, she is likely to gain 5 to 11.5 kg. To gain 1 or 2 kg in the first trimester is normal. Women should then gain approximately 400 g per week if in normal weight range, less than 300 g per week if overweight or obese and 500 g per week if underweight. However, the focus should remain on a healthy diet rather than specific weight gain. Also, dieting during pregnancy is not recommended because this may affect the development of the fetus.

Cultural and social considerations

As foods and eating customs are culturally distinct, each person has a unique cultural heritage that may affect nutritional status. Australia and Aotearoa New Zealand have had a continual influx of immigrants since the time of European settlement. Up until the second half of the 20th century, migrants to Australia and Aotearoa New Zealand were overwhelmingly from the British Isles. They brought with them traditional British and Irish diets. The large-scale arrival of non-British migrants saw new foods enter Australian and Aotearoa New Zealand menus. Migrants from the European continent brought wine, pasta and coffee. The variety of cuisines continued to diversify throughout the latter half of the 20th century with European, Asian, Middle Eastern and African cuisines commonly found in restaurants and homes, particularly in Australia. Since about 2005, the increased immigration of peoples from Islamic backgrounds, from the African continent, has seen a growing cultural awareness of religious food practices such as halal diets (Table 21.1).

Immigrants commonly maintain traditional eating customs (especially for holidays and observance of religious customs) long after the language and manner of dress of an adopted country have become routine. Occupation, class, religion, gender and health awareness all have a great bearing on eating customs.

TABLE 21.1 Typical religious dietary practices

Religious Group	Food Restrictions
Buddhism	All meat
Catholicism	Meat by some denominations on Ash Wednesday, Good Friday and other holy days Alcoholic beverages by some denominations
Hinduism	Beef, pork and some fowl Alcohol Garlic and onions by some Red-coloured foods (e.g. tomatoes) by some
Islam	All pork and pork products Meat not slaughtered according to ritual Alcoholic beverages and alcohol products (e.g. vanilla extract), coffee and tea Food and beverages before sunset during Ramadan
Mormon	Alcoholic beverages Caffeinated beverages (e.g. coffee, tea, soft drinks) and medicines containing caffeine, stimulants or alcohol (e.g. caffeine-based medications (e.g. NoDoz), some cold and flu medications) Food and beverages on first Sunday of each month
Orthodox Judaism	All pork and pork products Meat not slaughtered according to ritual All shellfish (e.g. crab, lobster, shrimp, oysters) Dairy products and meat at the same meal Leavened bread and cake during Passover Food and beverages on Yom Kippur
Seventh-Day Adventist	All pork and pork products Shellfish Meat, dairy products and eggs by some Alcoholic beverages, coffee and tea Highly seasoned foods

Newly arrived immigrants may be at nutritional risk for a variety of reasons. They have frequently emigrated from countries with limited food supplies—caused by poverty, poor sanitation, war or political strife. General under-nutrition, hypertension, diarrhoea, lactose intolerance, osteomalacia (soft bones), scurvy and dental caries are among the more common nutrition-related problems of new immigrants from developing countries. In addition, barriers such as language and cultural differences can further hinder the provision of nutritional information and health promotion among these groups.

The best way to learn about the eating patterns of a person is to ask about their dietary customs. The cultural factors that must be considered are the cultural definition of food, frequency and number of meals eaten away from home, form and content of ceremonial meals, amount and types of foods eaten and regularity of food consumption.

The 24-hours food history or 3-day food diaries, traditionally used for assessment, may be inadequate when dealing with people from culturally diverse backgrounds. Standard dietary handbooks may fail to provide culture-specific diet information because nutritional content is generally based on Western diets.

Cultural variation in diets can create confusion when completing a health assessment. For example, among Vietnamese migrants, the dietary intake of calcium may appear inadequate, particularly with the low consumption of dairy products common among members of this group.

Daily soups prepared by soaking bones in acidified broth or pickled or sweet and sour meats such as pork ribs (vinegar leaches calcium from the bones and makes it available to the body) are, however, commonly consumed, thus providing adequate quantities of calcium to meet daily requirements. Tofu is also a good source of calcium if calcium salts are used to precipitate the curd. In Middle Eastern countries, yoghurt and feta cheese are the major dietary sources of calcium since milk is not commonly consumed by adults. Food itself is only one part of eating. In some cultures, social contacts during meals are restricted to members of the immediate or extended family. For example, in some Middle Eastern cultures, men and women eat meals separately, or women may be permitted to eat with their husbands, but not with other males. Etiquette during meals, the use of hands, type of eating utensils (e.g. chopsticks, special flatware) and protocols governing the order in which foods are consumed during a meal all vary cross-culturally.

Australian and Aotearoa New Zealand children generally show good levels of dental health, but good oral health varies across the population. Australian children particularly appear to have good access to dental care enhancing their good oral health, with two in three Australian children visiting a dentist in each 12-month period.[6] The overall incidence of good oral health in children has increased due to factors such as having school dental care services, increased access to fluoridated toothpaste and drinking water and improved dental hygiene. However, nearly 50% of Australian children aged 12 years and above have decay in their permanent teeth. Children in remote and rural areas and those from the lowest socioeconomic groups show approximately twice the incidence of decayed, missing or filled teeth of their urban counterparts.[6]

Oral health of adults is also significantly impacted by location and age. Rural residents are twice as likely as city residents to be edentulous (no natural teeth), which can affect diet and nutritional status.[6] This percentage significantly increases with age; 5.5% of Australian adults between 45 and 64 years are likely to have no natural teeth, while about 21.1% of adults over 65 have no remaining natural teeth.[6] Compared with Australian adults, Aotearoa New Zealand adults had poorer oral health across a range of clinical oral health indicators and were also less likely to have visited a dental professional in the previous year.[7] The health of teeth and gums is clearly related to access to dental care, with about 49% of city dwellers visiting the dentist regularly compared with 31% of remote area dwellers. This is consistent with the Aotearoa New Zealand experience where poorer oral health and lower dental service attendance rates in adults were found among men, younger adults (aged 25–34 years), Māori, Pacific Islander peoples and people living in areas of socioeconomic deprivation.[7] Apparent lack of access to regular dental care, together with overall rates of dental decay, seems to affect levels of untreated dental decay. There are several initiatives that have been targeted at improving the oral health of Indigenous Australians—for example, offering full mouth fluoride varnishes, fissure sealants and clinical services in the Northern Territory.

Indigenous Australians

Before European settlement, Indigenous Australians lived on traditional diets of native plants and animals rich in nutrients and low in fat. Specific diets depended on the area in which the community lived and were affected by seasonal changes. While some groups held permanent settlements, in coastal and river areas, for example, others travelled vast distances seasonally to known food sources. The introduction of high energy and low nutrient modern diets has increased the risk of obesity, cardiovascular disease and diabetes in these and other population groups. Indigenous Australians are six times more likely to have diabetes than the general population, with poor nutrition contributing to morbidity and mortality among Indigenous populations. The persistently poor diet and health status is also attributed to their low socioeconomic status, as food purchases are often restricted to cheap, high-energy and nutrient-poor foods.[8]

Māori and Pacific Islanders

Like the Indigenous Australian population, the Māori and Pacific Islander people existed on a high nutrient, low–energy dense diet before colonisation. With the settlement of Europeans and urbanisation of Aotearoa New Zealand, the Māori diet and physical activity patterns changed. This led to reduced physical activity and a low-nutrient, high-energy diet. Māori and Pacific Islander people now have a diet higher in fat and lower in vegetables than the general population. Food has a central role in the cultural life of Māori and Pacific Islander people, and this must be considered when developing approaches to address obesity and nutrition. In addition to the cultural issues, healthy food choices in Aotearoa New Zealand are significantly tied to socioeconomic status. Māori and Pacific Islander peoples are over-represented in the low socioeconomic groups in Aotearoa New Zealand, and this must also be taken into consideration when addressing nutritional issues.

Dietary practices of selected cultural groups

It is necessary to avoid **cultural stereotyping**—the tendency to view people of common cultural backgrounds similarly and according to a preconceived notion of how they 'ought' to behave. For example, despite widely held stereotypes, there are of course Chinese people who do not like rice, Italian people who dislike spaghetti, Irish people who dislike corned beef and cabbage and so forth. Aggregate dietary preferences among people from certain cultural groups can, however, be described (e.g. characteristic ethnic dishes, methods of food preparation). Cultural food preferences are often interrelated with religious dietary beliefs and practices. Many religions use foods as symbols in celebrations and rituals.

Fasting and other religious observations may limit a person's food or liquid intake during specified times; for example, some Catholics fast and abstain from meat on Ash Wednesday and the Fridays of Lent. Muslims fast from dawn to sunset during the month of Ramadan in the Islamic calendar eating only twice a day—before dawn and after sunset; Jews observe a 24-hour fast on Yom Kippur.

Knowing the person's religious practices related to food enables you to suggest improvements or modifications that do not conflict with dietary laws. With widespread malnutrition in the hospital or supported care setting, it is imperative that people's cultural food preferences are assessed to support optimum nutrition in this unfamiliar environment (Table 21.1, earlier).

HEALTH EDUCATION

Obesity as a generational health issue

Intergenerational obesity has been identified as a health priority in Australia.[4] Early gestational weight gain is a predictor for developing intergenerational obesity.[9] Preventing intergenerational obesity begins in early life, with parent roles, their lifestyles and the context in which children live being seen to be important influences.[10]

As mentioned earlier in this chapter, for Australian adults, the statistics for obesity include:

- More than three in five Australian adults (63%) are overweight or obese.
- 71.6% of those over 18 years from low socioeconomic groups were overweight or obese. compared with 61.5% in high socioeconomic groups.[4]

The statistics for obesity in children include:[4]

- One in four (25%) children aged between 2 and 17 years are overweight or obese.
- 26% of children aged 15 to 17 years are overweight or obese.
- The highest prevalence of obesity (10.2%) for boys was at the age 15 to 17 years and 2 to 4 years for girls (10.8%).
- In low socioeconomic areas 28.1% of 2- to 17-year-olds are overweight or obese compared with 20.8% in high socioeconomic areas.

The statistics for obesity in Aotearoa New Zealand adults[7] show that approximately:

- One in three adults (aged 15 years or older) are obese (32%), and within this cohort are Māori adults (47%) and Pacific Islander adults (65%).
- Adults living in the most deprived areas are 1.6 times as likely to be obese as adults living in the least deprived areas.

The statistics for obesity in Aotearoa New Zealand children include:[7]

- One in eight children between ages 2 and 14 years are obese (12%).
- For Māori children, 17% identified as obese, and one in four Pacific Islander children are obese (27%).
- Children living in the most deprived areas are 2.1 times as likely to be obese as children living in the least deprived areas.

The keys to a healthy diet for adults are to:

- eat a variety of foods from all the basic food groups (Figure 21.5)
- consume the recommended amounts of fruits/vegetables, whole grains and fat-free or low-fat milk products or equivalents (Table 21.2)
- limit intake of foods high in saturated or trans fats, added sugars, starch, cholesterol, salt and alcohol
- match kilojoule intake with kilojoules expended
- be physically active for at least 30 minutes each day of the week
- follow food safety guidelines for handling, preparing and storing foods.

Nurse's role

Nurses in any setting can advise people about healthy eating by:

- promoting healthy eating guidelines
- providing nutritional information about healthy eating and the implications of obesity
- encouraging breast feeding for at least the first 6 months of life
- providing support and motivation for change in relation to healthcare beliefs
- referral to a dietitian and/or exercise physiologist for specific advice
- identifying the person's readiness to lose weight (where required) for their health care
- assisting people who are hospitalised with meal selection and feeding when needed.

Further information

- Better Health Channel—Healthy eating 2022: https://www.betterhealth.vic.gov.au/healthyliving/healthy-eating
- National Health and Medical Research Council—Australian Guide to healthy eating: https://www.eatforhealth.gov.au/guidelines/australian-guide-healthy-eating
- New Zealand Ministry of Health—Food and nutrition guidelines: https://www.tewhatuora.govt.nz/our-health-system/preventative-healthwellness/nutrition/eating-and-activity-guidelines

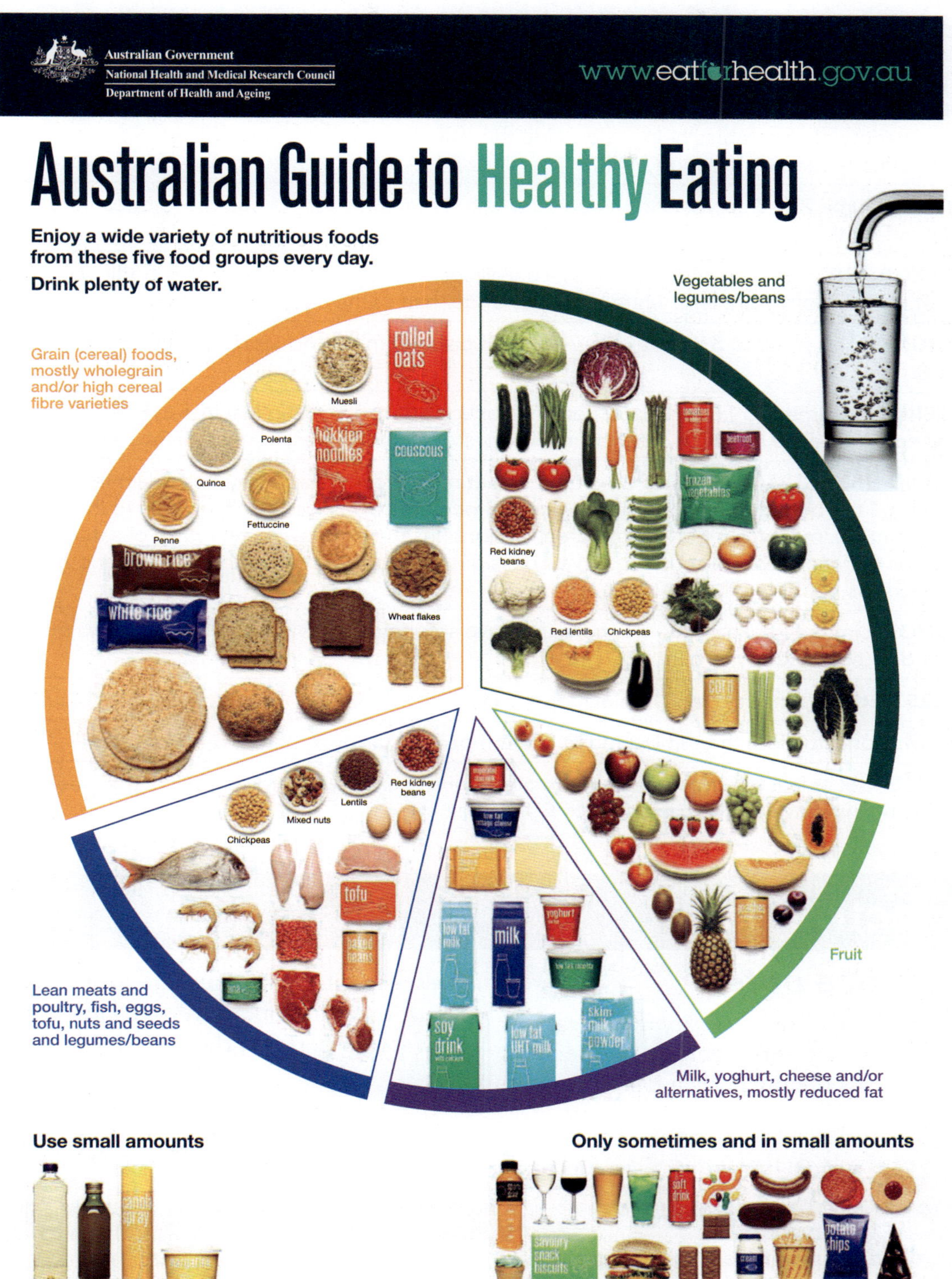

FIGURE 21.5 Australian Guide to Healthy Eating

TABLE 21.2 Summary of dietary guidelines for an adult (approx. 8,380 kJ per day)

VEGETABLES: Consume 4 to 7 serves of vegetables each day (e.g. 1 medium potato, 1 cup raw). Eating a variety of vegetables helps to provide the vitamins, minerals, antioxidants, fibre and carbohydrate necessary for good health.
FRUIT: Consume 2 to 3 serves of fruit each day (e.g. 1 medium piece, 1 cup diced or canned). Choose a variety of fruits.
WHOLEGRAINS: Consume 4 to 6 serves (e.g. 2 slices of bread, 1 cup rice pasta noodles) per day. Limit refined carbohydrate (e.g. white bread) to under half of the daily servings.
CALCIUM: Consume 2 to 3 serves of low-fat, high calcium milk products (e.g. 1 cup milk, 2 slices of cheese).
PROTEIN: Consume 1 to 1.5 serves of meat, fish or eggs (e.g. 65–100 g lean meat, 80–120 g fish, 2 small eggs). Choose meats or other sources of protein that are lean, low-fat, or fat-free.
FATS AND HIGH SUGAR FOODS: Consume sometimes and in small amounts and limited to 2½ serves (e.g. 1 tsp butter, 1 can soft drink, ½ small chocolate bar). Keep total fat intake to 20% to 35% of energy intake, most from polyunsaturated or monounsaturated fats. Limit intake of saturated fat. *Keep trans fatty acid consumption as low as possible.* Consume as little added sugar (or other low kJ sweeteners) as possible.
ALCOHOL: Limited intake. Men—no more than two standard drinks per day. Women—no more than one per day (e.g. 1 stubby of beer, 100 mL wine).
CHOLESTEROL: Consume less than 300 mg/day.
SODIUM: Consume less than 1,500 mg of sodium per day (approximately ½ tsp of salt).
EXERCISE: Get at least 30 minutes of moderate-intensity exercise on most days of the week; to lose weight or maintain weight loss, increase to 60–90 minutes.

Subjective data

Practice note

Before you start the assessment, introduce yourself to the person, confirm the person's identity, discuss the purpose and scope of the assessment, clarify any questions the person may have and obtain verbal consent from the person to perform the assessment.

ASSESSMENT GUIDELINES	CLINICAL SIGNIFICANCE AND CLINICAL ALERTS
Presenting concern	
• *Do you have any problems with your nutrition, ability to prepare food or eating food? Does this affect your energy or ability to carry out activities of daily living?*	The person's response to this question will guide areas to focus on in further subjective and objective data collection.

ASSESSMENT GUIDELINES	CLINICAL SIGNIFICANCE AND CLINICAL ALERTS
It is important to ascertain the person's perception of their nutritional and metabolic function. If the person does perceive a problem, ask: *How does this affect your quality of life?*	
Eating patterns	
• *How many meals/snacks do you have per day?* • *What kind and amount of food do you eat?* • *Are you on any special or alternative diets?* • *Where do you eat your meals?* • *Do you have any food preferences and dislikes?* • *Do you have any religious or cultural restrictions?* To obtain information about dietary intake, the **24-hours food diary is useful**. The person or family member completes a questionnaire or is interviewed and asked to recall everything eaten within the last 24 to 72 hours. A food diary is most complete and accurate if the person records information immediately after eating. **A food diary** relies on: • accurate recall of the type or amount of food eaten • inclusion of all snack items and use of gravies, sauces and condiments.	If there are misconceptions, begin gradual education to enact healthy eating habits. Ethnic/religious beliefs or feeding difficulties may affect intake of certain foods. Alternative diets, if not closely managed, may not be nutritionally adequate. Some people experience abdominal cramping after eating fermentable oligosaccharides, disaccharides, monosaccharides and polyols (short-chain carbohydrates) that the small intestine absorbs poorly. A low **FODMAP diet** reduces foods such as garlic, dairy, onions and apples to avoid symptoms.
Usual weight	
• *What is your usual weight?* • *Are you below or above desirable weight?* • *Recent weight change?* • *Over what time period?* • *How much lost or gained? Reason for loss or gain?*	People who have had a recent, **unintentional weight loss** or who are obese are at nutritional risk. **Underweight** people are vulnerable because their fuel reserves may be depleted. **Overweight** is associated with many health problems, ranging from hypertension to cancer.  ***Clinical alert:*** Protein and energy needs are often overlooked in acutely ill obese people.
Changes in appetite, taste, smell, chewing, swallowing	
• *What type of change have you experienced?* • *When did change occur?*	**Poor appetite, taste and smell alterations**, as well as chewing and swallowing difficulties, interfere with adequate nutrient intake and increase the likelihood of nutritional risk. **Dysphagia** (difficulty swallowing food or fluid) may occur with cancers in the mouth or oesophagus or neurological conditions such as stroke.

ASSESSMENT GUIDELINES	CLINICAL SIGNIFICANCE AND CLINICAL ALERTS
	Changes in appetite associated with weight loss may indicate an increase in metabolic activity such as thyrotoxicosis or diabetes. An increase in appetite with weight gain may indicate the effects of excessive glucocorticoids such as Cushing's syndrome or hypoglycaemia.[10]
Teeth	
• *How do you care for your teeth and gums? How often do you visit a dentist for a check-up?* • *Have you had any toothache? Are your teeth sensitive to heat or cold?* • *Have you lost any teeth?*	
Recent surgery, trauma, burns, infection	
• *When? Why?* • *Type?* • *How treated?* • *Conditions that increase nutrient loss (e.g. draining wounds, effusions, blood loss, dialysis and sepsis)?*	People who have had recent surgery, trauma, sepsis or conditions causing nutrient losses may have energy and nutrient needs that are two or three times greater than normal. **Under-nutrition** is commonly seen because of hospital admission and conditions such as cancer. **Malnutrition** in hospitals is associated with serious adverse effects of not responding to treatment to the desired level, poorer quality of life and higher mortality.[11]
Chronic illness	
• *What type of illness do you have?* • *When were you diagnosed?* • *What was/is the treatment?* • *Have you had to make any dietary modifications?* • *Have you had recent cancer chemotherapy or radiation therapy?*	People with chronic illnesses that affect nutrient use (e.g. **diabetes, pancreatitis, COPD or malabsorption**) or those receiving cancer treatment are twice as likely to have nutritional deficits.
Nausea, vomiting, diarrhoea, constipation	
• *Do you have any problems with nausea, vomiting, diarrhoea or constipation?* • *What do you think is the cause?* • *How long?*	**Gastrointestinal symptoms** such as nausea, vomiting, diarrhoea or constipation may interfere with nutrient intake or absorption. **Diarrhoea** may be associated with food intolerances, anxiety, bacterial infection, intestinal disease or hyperactive thyroid function. **Constipation** may be associated with dehydration, lack of dietary fibre, inactivity, medication side effects or an underactive thyroid function.

ASSESSMENT GUIDELINES	CLINICAL SIGNIFICANCE AND CLINICAL ALERTS
	 ***Clinical alert:*** Any significant changes in bowel function must be further investigated because of the link to bowel cancer (Chapter 25).
Food allergies or intolerances	
• *Are there any problematic foods?* • *What type of reaction have you had?* • *How long?* • *How are food allergies/intolerances managed?* **Food frequency questionnaires** may help identify problematic foods. The tool collects information on how many times per day, week or month the person eats particular foods. People may have dietary restrictions because of food intolerances (e.g. lactose intolerance, gluten intolerance, peanut or seafood allergies).	**Food allergies**, especially peanut allergies, are on the rise and a major health concern. Refer to published guidelines for more information on the management of food allergies. **Intolerances** may result in nutrient deficiencies (e.g. diarrhoea after milk ingestion). **The food frequency questionnaire:** • does not quantify amount of intake • relies on memory for how often a food was eaten.
Past history	
• *Do you or any family member have a history of heart disease, osteoporosis, cancer, gout, gastrointestinal disorders, obesity, thyroid disorders or diabetes?* • *What effect has there been on eating patterns?* • *What effect has there been on activity patterns?*	Early identification of nutritional alterations permits dietary and activity modifications to occur promptly—at a time when the body can recover more fully.
Health and lifestyle management	
Meals • *Do you have meal preparation facilities?* • *Do you have transportation for travel to the supermarket?* • *Do you have enough money to buy food?* • *Who prepares meals and does the shopping?* • *Describe your environment during mealtimes.*	Socioeconomic factors may interfere with the ability to purchase or access a range and amount of food necessary for an adequate diet.
Medications and/or nutritional supplements • *Are you taking any prescription medications?* • *Are you taking any nonprescription medications?* • *Describe use over a 24-hour period.*	Some medications interact with nutrients, impair digestion, absorption, metabolism or utilisation (e.g. analgesics, antacids, anticonvulsants, antibiotics, diuretics, laxatives, antineoplastic drugs, steroids and oral contraceptives).
Vitamin/mineral supplements • *What vitamins/minerals do you take?* • *What amount? For how long?* • *Do you take herbal and botanical products? What specific types/brands and where do you buy it?*	**Vitamin/mineral supplements** may cause harmful side effects if taken in large amounts. Complementary and alternative medicines can have interactions with other medications; for information refer to National Center for Complementary and Alternative Medicine website (see website list at end of chapter).

ASSESSMENT GUIDELINES	CLINICAL SIGNIFICANCE AND CLINICAL ALERTS
• *How often are they used? Who recommended that you take them?* • *Does it help you? Do you experience any problems?*	
Alcohol use • *Do you drink alcohol?* • *When was your last drink of alcohol?* • *How many drinks did you have?* • *How many drinks of alcohol do you have each day? Each week?* • *Duration of use?* See Chapter 6 for further detail. **Smoking/vaping** • *What do you smoke?* • *How many each day?* • *How long have you smoked/vaped?* • *Have you ever tried to give up smoking/vaping?* • *How long since you smoked?*	Alcohol and cigarettes/vapes are often substituted for nutritious foods and increase requirements for some nutrients. Pregnant women who smoke, drink alcohol or use non-prescription drugs give birth to a disproportionate number of infants with low birthweights, failure to thrive and other serious complications. Chronic tobacco use is associated with tooth loss and decay and periodontal disease. Chronic tobacco use combined with heavy alcohol consumption increases risk of **oral and pharyngeal cancers**.
Exercise and activity patterns • *How much exercise do you do?* • *What type?* • *How often do you exercise?* • *Do you experience lethargy or poor exercise tolerance?* • *Do you experience excessive sweating?* • *Can you complete your activities of daily living without assistance?*	Kilojoule and nutrient needs increase with increased activity and exercise, especially competitive sports and manual labour. Inactive or sedentary lifestyles often lead to excess weight gain. **Lethargy** is a common symptom of many health problems—for example, **hypothyroidism, diabetes, anaemia, cardiac or renal failure**.[10] Excessive sweating can indicate several metabolic disorders including hypothyroidism and hypoglycaemia.[10]
Additional subjective data for infants and children (questions for parents or guardians)	
Dietary histories of infants and children are generally obtained from the child's parents, guardian, babysitter or daycare centre. Usually, the person responsible for food preparation can provide a fairly accurate dietary history. Having the caregivers keep a thorough daily food diary or asking the caregiver to recall the nutritional intake over the previous 24 hours during clinic visits are the most employed techniques for this population group.	

ASSESSMENT GUIDELINES	CLINICAL SIGNIFICANCE AND CLINICAL ALERTS
Gestational nutrition • *Maternal history of alcohol or illicit drug use?* • *Any diet-related complications during gestation?* • *Infant's birthweight?* • *Any evidence of delayed physical or mental growth?*	**Low birthweight** (< 2,500 g) is a major factor in infant morbidity and mortality. Poor gestational nutrition, low maternal weight gain and maternal alcohol and drug use can lead to birth defects and delayed growth and development. Similarly, maternal history of gestational diabetes may affect the infant's blood glucose levels in the early neonatal period.
Infant feeding • *Describe type, frequency, amount and duration of feeding.* • *Any difficulties encountered?* • *Timing and method of weaning?*	Inexperienced mothers may have problems with breastfeeding or bottle-feeding or have questions about whether the infant is receiving adequate amounts of food.
Child's willingness to eat what you prepare • *Any special likes or dislikes?* • *How much will your child eat?* • *How do you control non-nutritious snack foods?*	For young children, avoid foods likely to be aspirated (e.g. nuts, grapes, round sweets and popcorn).
Teeth and gums • *Did the child's teeth erupt about on time?* • *Do the teeth seem straight to you?* • *Is the child using a bottle? How often during the day?* • *Does the child go to sleep with a bottle at night?* • *Have you noticed any thumb sucking after secondary teeth came in?* • *Have you noticed the child grinding their teeth?*	Delayed eruption may impair nutrition. Prolonged use of the bottle increases risk for tooth decay and middle ear infections. Prolonged thumb sucking (after age 6–7 years) may affect occlusion. **Bruxism** (grinding of teeth) usually occurs in sleep from dental problems, nervous tension.
Self-care behaviours • *Does the child use a toothbrush regularly?* • *How often does the child see a dentist?* • *Is the water where you live fluoridated?*	Evaluate child's self-care. Early self-care has best compliance.
Additional subjective data for adolescents	
Present weight • *How much do you weigh?* • *Do you diet to lose weight? If so, is it successful?* • *Do you have any specific strategies for losing weight such as intentionally vomiting or using laxatives or diuretics after eating?*	In adolescent girls, **obesity** may precipitate fad dieting. Increased body awareness and self-consciousness can make adolescents prone to eating disorders (**anorexia nervosa or bulimia**) (Chapter 11).

ASSESSMENT GUIDELINES	CLINICAL SIGNIFICANCE AND CLINICAL ALERTS
Use of anabolic steroids or other agents to increase muscle size and physical performance • *Do you take any agents to increase muscle size?* • *How much do you take?* • *How often?* • *Have you experienced any problems?* • *Do you drink caffeinated, energy-boosting drinks? When? Type? For how long?*	Adverse effects of anabolic steroids include personality disorders (aggressiveness), liver and other organ damage. Energy-boosting drinks (e.g. Red Bull, V Energy or XS Energy) contain large amounts of caffeine and may include other stimulants and/or herbal products. Side effects include dehydration, irritability, anxiety, dangerously high blood pressure, irregular heart rate and insomnia, nausea.
Snacks and fast foods • *What snacks or fast foods do you like to eat? What type? When? How much?*	An accurate dietary history may be difficult because of between-meal snacks and meals eaten on the run. These are often omitted or forgotten during the interview or in a food diary.
Menarche • *How old were you when you first started menstruating?* • *What is your menstrual flow like?* • *Are your periods regular?*	Menarche is usually delayed if malnutrition is present. Likewise, **amenorrhoea** (absence of periods) or scant menstrual flow is associated with nutritional deficiency.
Additional subjective data for pregnant women	
• *How many times have you been pregnant?* • *When?* • *Did you experience any problems during your pregnancies, like excessive vomiting, anaemia or gestational diabetes, constipation, indigestion or haemorrhoids?* • *Are you having any problems this pregnancy?*	A **multiparous** mother (having borne more than one child) with pregnancies occurring less than 1 year apart has an increased chance of depleted nutritional reserves. A history of a low-birthweight infant suggests past nutritional problems. Giving birth to an infant weighing 4.5 kg or more may signal *latent* diabetes in the mother.
Food preferences when pregnant • *What foods do you prefer when pregnant?* • *What foods do you avoid?* • *Do you crave any particular foods?*	Cravings for or aversions to some foods are common; evaluate for their potential contribution to, or interference with, dietary intake. There are certain foods that should be avoided; for more information see the Food Standards Australia and New Zealand website in the website list below.
Additional subjective data for middle adulthood (40–64 years)	
Menstrual history, menopausal symptoms • *Are your periods regular?* • *Do you have menopausal symptoms, like hot flushes, sleep disturbance or anxiety?* • *When did these symptoms begin?* • *How do you manage the symptoms?*	Normal changes to ovarian function can cause significant symptoms, which can affect quality of life (Chapter 26).

ASSESSMENT GUIDELINES	CLINICAL SIGNIFICANCE AND CLINICAL ALERTS
Additional subjective data for adults over 65 years	
Changes in diet • *How does your diet differ from when you were in your 40s and 50s?* • *What factors affect the way you eat?* • *What changes have you made to your diet?*	Note any physiological or psychological changes or socioeconomic changes that affect nutritional status. Malnutrition in older adults leads to frailty, delirium, decreased immunity, muscle wastage, hypothermia, osteoporosis, cognitive impairment, poorer quality of life and increased mortality.[12] 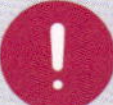 ***Clinical alert:*** Adults over 75 years of age and those with chronic health problems are particularly at risk of malnutrition.
Taste, smell and chewing • *Do you experience any dryness in the mouth? Are you taking any medications?* • *Have you lost any teeth? Can you chew all types of food?* • *Do you go for regular dental checkups?* • *Are you able to care for your own teeth or dentures?* • *Have you noticed a change in your sense of taste or smell?*	**Alterations in taste:** Some people add extra salt or sugar to enhance food. **Hyposmia** (diminished smell) may decrease a person's ability to detect food spoilage. **Xerostomia** (dry mouth) is a side effect of many drugs (antidepressants, anticholinergics, antihypertensives, antipsychotics, bronchodilators). Self-care may be decreased by disabilities such as arthritis, vision impairment, confusion or depression.

Objective data

Direct observation of the feeding and eating process can help detect problems not readily identified through standard nutrition interviews. For example, observing the typical feeding techniques used by a parent or caregiver and the interaction between the person and caregiver can be of value when assessing children whose height, weight and head circumference do not match standard growth charts or unintentional weight loss in older adults.

Preparation

Outline the process for assessment of the nutritional and metabolic status for the client and ask their consent to continue. The areas for assessment are detailed below.

Equipment needed

Measuring tape
Pen or pencil
Tongue blade
Pen torch
Nutritional assessment forms
Hand hygiene solution

PROCEDURES AND NORMAL FINDINGS	ABNORMAL FINDINGS AND CLINICAL ALERTS
General inspection	
During collection of subjective data, you will have noticed the condition of the person's skin, lips, hair and mucous membranes, breath odour, ease of breathing, height-to-weight ratio, body shape, level of hygiene and grooming and general demeanour. All these factors provide clues to the person's nutrition and metabolic health.	
Inspect the skin	
Inspect the skin for colour, texture, moisture and intactness. See Chapter 22.	Malnutrition is reflected in skin changes (Tables 21.3 and 21.4).
Inspect the face	
Note the facial expression and its appropriateness to behaviour or reported mood. Note any abnormal facial structures (coarse facial features, exophthalmos, changes in skin colour or pigmentation) or any abnormal swelling. Note any involuntary movements (tics) in the facial muscles. Normally none occur. Although the shape of facial structures may vary somewhat depending on ancestry, features always should be symmetrical. Expect symmetry of the eyebrows, palpebral fissures, nasolabial folds and sides of the mouth.	Anxiety is common in hospitalised and otherwise ill people. Tense, rigid muscles may indicate anxiety or pain. Exopthalmos (bulging eyeballs) occurs in hyperactive thyroid disorder where there is increased basal metabolic rate. Flat affect suggests depression, hypothyroidism or Parkinson's disease. Puffiness around the eyes suggests fluid retention (Table 21.5).
Inspect the mouth	
Begin with anterior structures and move posteriorly. Use a tongue blade to retract structures and a bright light for optimal visualisation.	
The lips	
Inspect the lips for colour, moisture, cracking or lesions. Retract the lips and note their inner surface as well (Figure 21.6).	**Cherry red lips** may be observed in ketoacidosis. **Cheilitis** (perlèche)—cracking at the corners (Tables 21.6 and 21.7).

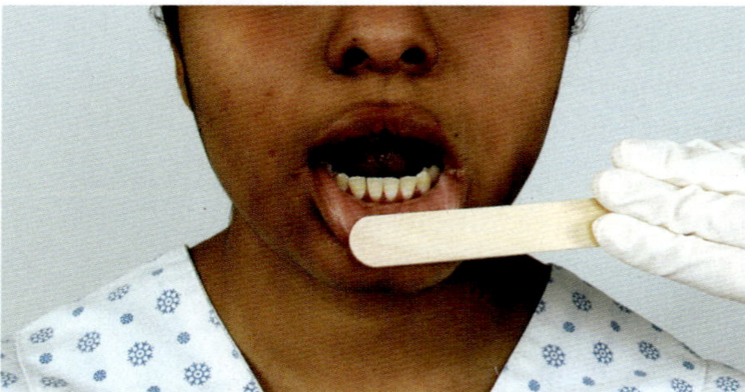

FIGURE 21.6 Inspecting the lips

PROCEDURES AND NORMAL FINDINGS	ABNORMAL FINDINGS AND CLINICAL ALERTS
The teeth and gums	
The condition of the teeth is an index of the person's general health. Your examination should not replace the regular dental examination, but note any diseased, absent, loose or abnormally positioned teeth. The teeth normally look white, straight and evenly spaced and clean and free of debris or decay.	Discoloured teeth appear brown with excessive fluoride use, yellow with tobacco use.
Compare the number of teeth with the number expected for the person's age. Ask the person to bite as if chewing something and note alignment of upper and lower jaw. Normal occlusion in the back is the upper teeth resting directly on the lowers; in the front, the upper incisors slightly override the lower incisors.	**Grinding** down of tooth surface. **Plaque**—soft debris. **Caries**—decay. **Malocclusion** (poor biting relationship), protrusion of upper or lower incisors (Table 21.8).
Normally, the gums look pink or coral with a stippled (dotted) surface. The gum margins at the teeth are tight and well defined. Check for swelling; retraction of gingival margins; and spongy, bleeding or discoloured gums. Dark-skinned people normally may have a dark melanotic line along the gingival margin.	**Gingival hypertrophy**, crevices between teeth and gums, pockets of debris. **Gingivitis** gums bleed with slight pressure (Table 21.8).
The tongue	
Inspect the tongue for colour, surface characteristics and moisture: • Colour is pink and even. • Dorsal surface is normally roughened from the papillae. • A thin white coating may be present. • Saliva is present. Ask the person to move their tongue so you can inspect the ventral and lateral surfaces: • Ventral surface looks smooth, glistening and shows veins. Inspect for any white patches or lesion: • Normally none are present. If any present, palpate the lesions for induration.	**Beefy red swollen tongue.** Smooth glossy areas (Table 21.9). **Enlarged tongue** occurs with hypothyroidism, acromegaly; a small tongue accompanies malnutrition. **Dry mouth** occurs with dehydration, fever; tongue has deep vertical fissures. **Saliva** is decreased while the person is taking anticholinergic and other medication. **Excess saliva** and drooling occur with gingivostomatitis and neurological dysfunction.
Test the cranial nerve XII (**hypoglossal nerve**) by asking the person to stick out their tongue. The tongue should protrude in the midline. Note any tremor, loss of movement or deviation to the side.	With cranial nerve XII damage, the tongue deviates towards the paralysed side.  ***Clinical alert:*** This finding may indicate a raised risk of potential airway compromise and aspiration. Further assessment of swallow and airway patency is required.

PROCEDURES AND NORMAL FINDINGS	ABNORMAL FINDINGS AND CLINICAL ALERTS
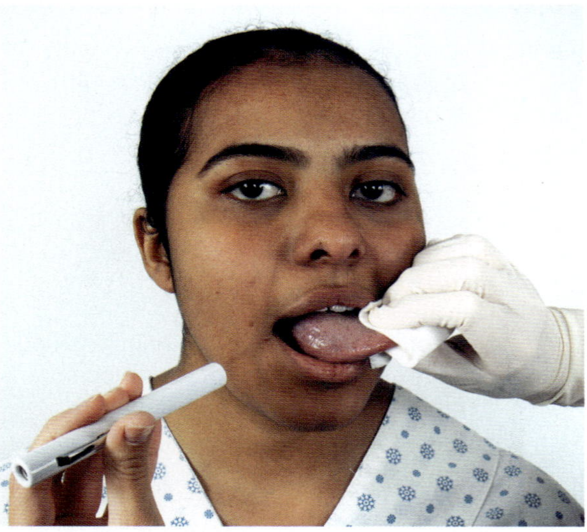 **FIGURE 21.7** Inspecting the tongue	
If the person is unconscious or otherwise unable to move their tongue on demand, with a gloved hand hold the tongue with a cotton gauze pad for traction and swing the tongue out and to each side (Figure 21.7).	
Inspect the entire U-shaped area under the tongue behind the teeth. Note any white patches, nodules or ulcerations. If lesions are present, or with any person over 50 years old or with a positive history of smoking or alcohol use, use your gloved hand to palpate the area. Place your other hand under the jaw to stabilise the tissue and to 'capture' any abnormality (Figure 21.8). Note any induration (thickened or hardened tissue).	Oral malignancies are most likely to develop in the U-shaped area under the tongue behind the teeth. ***Clinical alert:*** Any lesion or ulcer persisting for more than 2 weeks must be investigated. An indurated area may be a mass or **lymphadenopathy** (swelling of lymph glands) and must be investigated.
Buccal mucosa	
Hold the cheek open with a tongue blade and inspect the buccal mucosa for colour, nodules or lesions. Normal—pink, smooth and moist, although patchy. Hyperpigmentation is common and normal in dark-skinned people.	Dappled brown patches are present with **Addison's disease** (chronic adrenal insufficiency).

PROCEDURES AND NORMAL FINDINGS	ABNORMAL FINDINGS AND CLINICAL ALERTS
FIGURE 21.8 Inspecting under the tongue	
An expected finding is **Stensen's duct**, the opening of the parotid salivary gland. It looks like a small dimple opposite the upper second molar. You also may see a raised occlusion line on the buccal mucosa parallel with the level the teeth meet. This is caused by the teeth closing against the cheek.	**Orifice of Stensen's duct** looks red with mumps. **Koplik's spots**—early prodromal (early warning) sign of measles (Table 21.10).
A larger patch also may be present along the buccal mucosa. This is **leukoedema**, a benign greyish opaque area, more common in dark-skinned people. The patch disappears as you stretch the cheeks. The condition may increase with age, looking greyish white and thickened. The cause of the condition is unknown.	Do not mistake leukoedema for oral infections such as candidiasis (thrush).
Fordyce's granules are small, isolated white or yellow papules on the mucosa of cheek, tongue and lips (Figure 21.9). These little sebaceous cysts are painless and not significant.	**Leucoplakia** is a chalky white raised patch. It is abnormal and the person may have an increased risk of oral cancer (Table 21.10).

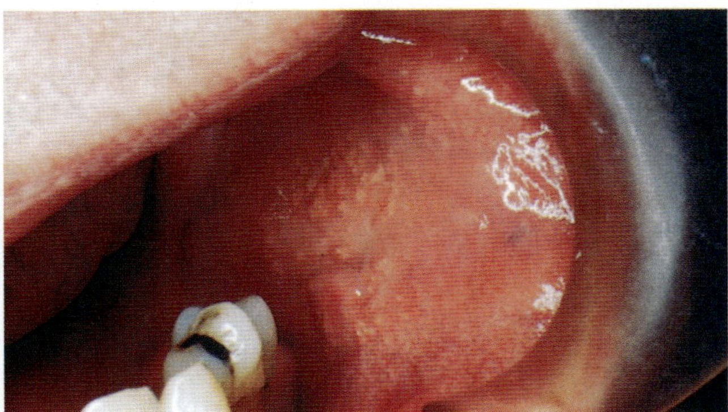

FIGURE 21.9 Fordyce's granule

PROCEDURES AND NORMAL FINDINGS	ABNORMAL FINDINGS AND CLINICAL ALERTS
The palate	
Shine your light up to the roof of the person's mouth. The more anterior hard palate should be white with irregular transverse rugae. The posterior soft palate should be pinker, smooth and upwardly movable. A normal variation is a nodular bony ridge down the middle of the hard palate, a **torus palatinus** (Figure 21.10). This benign growth arises after puberty in some people.	The hard palate appears yellow with jaundice. In dark-skinned people with jaundice, it may look yellow, muddy yellow or green-brown.
The **uvula** normally looks like a fleshy pendant hanging in the midline (Figure 21.11). Ask the person to say 'ahhh'. The soft palate and uvula will rise in the midline. This tests one function of the cranial nerve X and the vagus nerve. 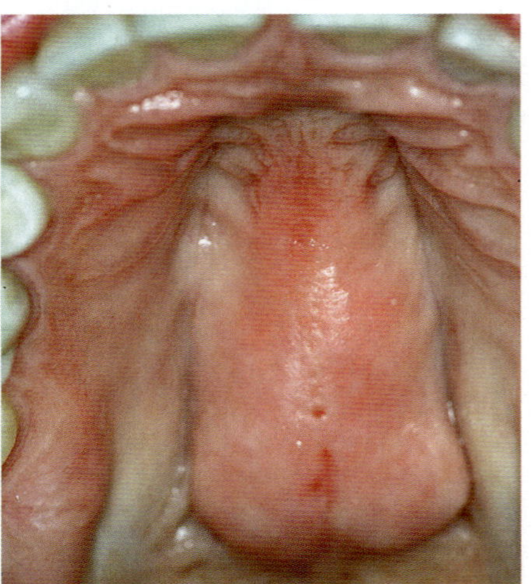 **FIGURE 21.10** Inspecting the palate showing torus palatinus	A **bifid** uvula looks like it is split in two. If the uvula deviates to one side or there is no movement, this indicates nerve damage, which might occur following a stroke or head injury. 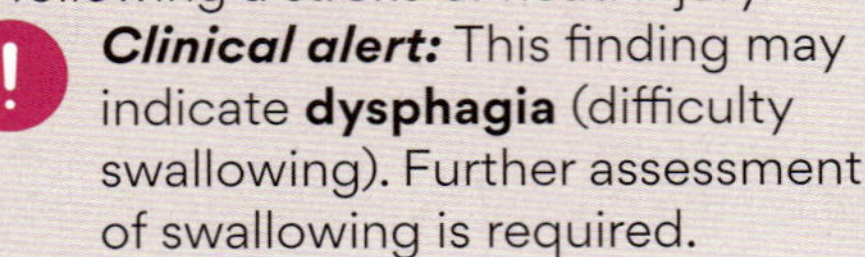 ***Clinical alert:*** This finding may indicate **dysphagia** (difficulty swallowing). Further assessment of swallowing is required.
Inspect the throat	
Enlarge your view of the posterior pharyngeal wall by depressing the tongue with a tongue blade (Figure 21.12). Push down halfway back on the tongue. Press slightly off centre to avoid eliciting the gag reflex. You can help the person whose gag reflex is easily triggered by offering a tongue blade to depress their own tongue.	**Acute tonsillitis** may affect appetite and nutritional intake.

PROCEDURES AND NORMAL FINDINGS	ABNORMAL FINDINGS AND CLINICAL ALERTS

FIGURE 21.11 Inspection of the oropharynx

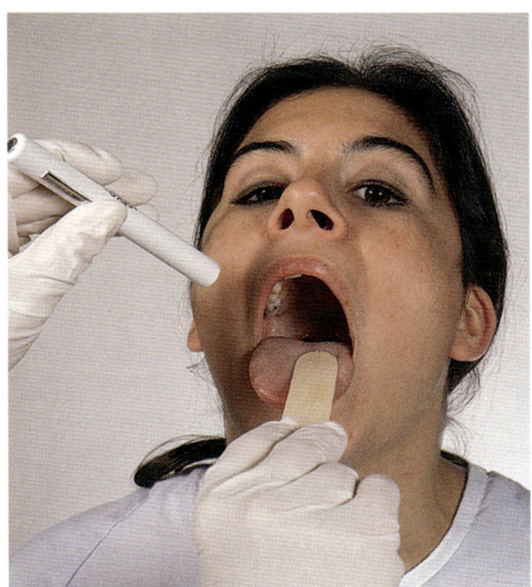

FIGURE 21.12 Inspecting the throat

Touching the posterior wall with the tongue blade should elicit the gag reflex. This tests **cranial nerves IX (glossopharyngeal) and X (vagus).**

Part of swallowing assessment.

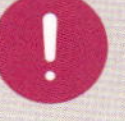

Clinical alert: Absence of a gag reflex means that the person would be a risk for respiratory aspiration. The person should be nil by mouth.

PROCEDURES AND NORMAL FINDINGS	ABNORMAL FINDINGS AND CLINICAL ALERTS
During the examination, notice any breath odour (**halitosis**). This is common and usually is due to a local cause such as poor oral hygiene, consumption of odoriferous foods, alcohol consumption, heavy smoking or dental infection. Occasionally, it may indicate a systemic disease.	**Diabetic ketoacidosis** has a sweet, fruity breath odour; this acetone smell also occurs in children with malnutrition or dehydration. Others are: • **uraemia—**ammonia breath odour • **liver disease—**musty odour • **dental or respiratory infections—** foul, fetid odour • **alcohol ingestion—**alcohol odour or chemicals.
Anthropometric measures	
Anthropometry is the measurement and evaluation of growth, development and body composition. The most used anthropometric measures for registered nurses are height, weight and waist-to-hip ratio. Measurement of height, weight and head circumference for children and infants is described in Chapter 10.	
Waist-to-hip ratio	
The **waist-to-hip ratio** assesses body fat distribution as an indicator of health risk. Obese people with a greater proportion of fat in the upper body, especially in the abdomen, are described as presenting with android obesity; obese people with most of their fat in the hips and thighs are described as presenting with gynoid obesity. The equation to calculate waist-to-hip ratio is: $$\text{Waist-to-hip} = \frac{\text{Waist circumference}}{\text{Hip circumference}}$$	A **waist-to-hip ratio** of ≥ 1.0 in men or ≥ 0.8 in women indicates **android (upper body) obesity** and increasing risk for obesity-related diseases and early mortality. Over-nutrition is caused by consuming nutrients—especially kilojoules, sodium and fat—more than the body needs. It can lead to obesity and is a risk factor for heart disease, type 2 diabetes, hypertension, stroke, gall bladder disease, sleep apnoea, certain cancers and osteoarthritis.[7] A waist circumference over 88 cm in women and over 102 cm in men increases risk of cardiovascular and metabolic diseases. For people of Asian or Aboriginal or Torres Strait Islander descent a circumference over 80 cm in women and over 90 cm in men increases risk of cardiovascular and metabolic diseases.[11]

PROCEDURES AND NORMAL FINDINGS	ABNORMAL FINDINGS AND CLINICAL ALERTS
Where **waist circumference** is measured in centimetres at the smallest circumference below the rib cage and above the umbilicus (Figure 21.13) and hip circumference is measured in centimetres at the largest circumference of the buttocks. In addition, waist circumference alone can be used to predict greater health risk. 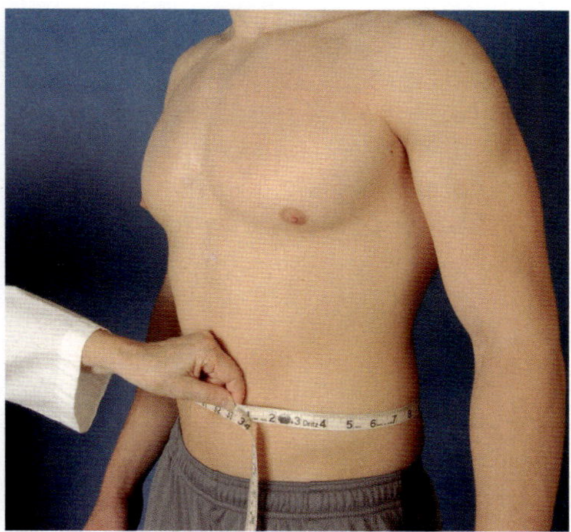 **FIGURE 21.13** Measuring waist circumference	
Derived weight measures	
Three derived weight measures are used to depict changes in body weight.	
Body weight as a percentage of ideal body weight is calculated using the following formula: $$\text{Percentage ideal body weight} = \frac{\text{Current weight}}{\text{Ideal weight}} \times 100$$	A current weight of 80 to 90% of ideal weight suggests mild malnutrition; 70 to 80%, moderate malnutrition; and under 70%, severe malnutrition.
The **percentage of usual body weight** is calculated as follows: $$\text{Percentage usual body weight} = \frac{\text{Current weight}}{\text{Ideal weight}} \times 100$$	A current weight of 85% to 95% of usual body weight indicates mild malnutrition; 75% to 84%, moderate malnutrition; and under 75%, severe malnutrition.
Recent weight change is calculated using the following formula: $$\frac{\text{Usual weight} - \text{current weight}}{\text{Usual weight}} \times 100$$	***Clinical alert:*** Unintentional loss of over 5% of body weight over 1 month, over 7.5% of body weight over 3 months or 10% of body weight over 6 months is clinically significant.

PROCEDURES AND NORMAL FINDINGS	ABNORMAL FINDINGS AND CLINICAL ALERTS
Body mass index	
BMI is a practical marker of optimal weight for height and an indicator of obesity or protein–kilojoule malnutrition. It is calculated by: $$\text{Body mass index} = \frac{\text{Weight (in kilograms)}}{\text{Height (in metres)}^2}$$	BMI interpretation for adults:[13] • < 18.5—Underweight • 18.5–24.99—Normal weight • ≥ 25.0—Overweight • ≥ 30.0—Obesity • ≥ 40—Obesity class III.
Blood glucose monitoring	
Blood glucose monitoring is a test to identify blood glucose concentration for people at risk of **hypoglycaemia** and **hyperglycaemia**. Test may also be used: • as a screening measure • to monitor the effectiveness of insulin therapy. The test is performed by a finger prick. The blood sample is applied to a disposable test-strip inserted into a testing monitor to calculate the level of glucose. Because of the wide range of technologies to perform this test, it is important to be familiar with how to use available equipment including how to calibrate the equipment. **Normal blood glucose levels** 4.0–6.0 mmol/L before meals 4.0–8.0 mmol/L 2 hours after meal *Fasting*: 3.0–5.4 mmol/L > 2 hours after eating (post-prandial) *Random*: 3.0–7.7 mmol/L	**Elevated blood glucose level (BGL)** reflects altered carbohydrate metabolism. ***Clinical alert: Random BGL*** over 7.7 mmol/L requires further investigation.
HbA_{1c}	
HbA_{1c} (glycated haemoglobin) is a blood test used to monitor blood glucose control for people with diabetes. The test determines the average blood glucose level over the past 2 to 3 months. Normal range for those who do not have diabetes is between 4% and 5.6% For people with diabetes the recommended general HbA_{1c} target is 7% (53 mmol/mol) or less	HbA_{1c} level between 5.7% and 6.4% may be an indication of pre-diabetes.
Additional objective data for infants, children and adolescents (birth to 19 years)	
Weight During infancy, childhood and adolescence, height and weight should be measured at regular intervals because longitudinal growth is one of the best indices of nutritional status over time.	

PROCEDURES AND NORMAL FINDINGS	ABNORMAL FINDINGS AND CLINICAL ALERTS
Body mass index Determination of BMI may be useful in evaluating childhood and teenage over- or under-nutrition. **Face, mouth and throat** Inspect the infant/child's face for the size of the eyes and upper lip and the shape of the nose. Inspect the infant/child's mouth. A normal finding in infants is the sucking tubercle, a small pad in the middle of the upper lip from friction of breast- or bottle-feeding. Note the number of teeth and whether it is appropriate for the child's age. Also note pattern of eruption, position, condition and hygiene. Use this guide for children under 2 years old; the child's age in months minus the number 6 should equal the expected number of deciduous teeth. Normally, all 20 deciduous teeth are evident by 2½ years. Saliva is present after 3 months of age and shows in excess with teething children.	**Fetal alcohol spectrum disorder** may be evident in newborn babies where the mother has abused alcohol during pregnancy. Damage ranges from mild to severe. Features include microcephaly, small eyes, short palpebral fissures, a short upturned nose and a thin upper lip. Deformities of joints, limbs and fingers and vision and hearing impairments are common. No teeth by age 1 year. Teeth can appear discoloured, with some antibiotics or where whose mothers took an antibiotic during the last trimester. Teeth may appear green or black with excessive iron ingestion, although this reverses when the iron is stopped. **Malocclusion:** upper or lower dental arches are out of alignment (Table 21.11).
Mobility should allow the tongue to extend at least as far as the alveolar ridge.	**Ankyloglossia**, a short lingual frenulum, can limit protrusion and impair speech development (Table 21.6).
Note any bruising or laceration on the buccal mucosa or gums of the infant or young child.	Trauma may indicate child abuse from forced feeding of bottle or spoon. **Bednar aphthae** are traumatic areas or ulcers on the posterior hard palate on either side of the midline. They result from abrasions while sucking.
Insert your gloved finger into the baby's mouth and palpate the hard and soft palate as the baby sucks. The sucking reflex can be elicited in infants up to 12 months old.	
Additional objective data for pregnant women	
Gum hypertrophy (surface looks smooth and stippling disappears) may occur normally at puberty or during pregnancy (pregnancy gingivitis).	
Weight Height and weight are measured on the first antenatal visit and BMI calculated. Further weight measurements are offered at subsequent visits (Chapter 29).	 ***Clinical alert:*** Pregnant women are at nutritional risk if their weight is 10% or more below ideal, or 20% or more above the norm for her height and age group.

PROCEDURES AND NORMAL FINDINGS	ABNORMAL FINDINGS AND CLINICAL ALERTS
Additional objective data for adults over 65 years	
In the edentulous (no natural teeth) person the mouth and lips fold in, giving a 'purse-string' appearance. The teeth may look slightly yellowed, although the colour is uniform.	Yellowing results from the dentin visible through worn enamel. The surface of the incisors may show vertical cracks from a lifetime of exposure to extreme temperatures. The teeth may look longer as the gum margins recede. Surfaces may look worn down or abraded. Old dental work deteriorates, especially at the gum margins. The teeth loosen with bone resorption and may move with palpation.
The tongue looks smoother because of papillary atrophy. An older adult's buccal mucosa is thinned and may look shinier, as though it were 'varnished'.	
Height With age, height declines in both men and women very slowly from the early 30s, leading to an average 2.9 cm loss in men and 4.9 cm loss in women. Height measures may not be accurate in people confined to a bed or wheelchair or those over 65 years of age (because of osteoporotic changes). Therefore, arm span (see below), which is correlated with height, may be a better measure for older people.	BMI and waist-to-hip ratio are better indicators of obesity in this age group.

Abnormal findings

TABLE 21.3 Clinical signs of malnutrition

Area of Examination	Normal Appearance	Signs Associated with Malnutrition	Nutrient Deficiency
Skin	Smooth, no signs of rashes, bruises, flaking	Dry, flaking, scaly	Vitamin A, vitamin B-complex, linoleic acid
		Petechiae/ecchymoses	Vitamins C and K
		Follicular hyperkeratosis (dry, bumpy skin)	Vitamin A, linoleic acid
		Cracks in skin, lesions on the hands, legs, face or neck	Niacin, tryptophan
		Pellagrous dermatosis (hyperpigmentation of skin exposed to sunlight)	Niacin

TABLE 21.3 Clinical signs of malnutrition cont'd

Area of Examination	Normal Appearance	Signs Associated with Malnutrition	Nutrient Deficiency
		Nasolabial seborrhoea	Riboflavin, vitamin B_6
		Acneiform forehead rash	Vitamin B_6
		Eczema	Linoleic acid
		Xanthomas (excessive deposits of cholesterol)	Excessive serum levels of LDLs or VLDLs
Hair	Shiny, firm, does not fall out easily, healthy scalp	Dull, dry, sparse	Protein, zinc, linoleic acid
		Colour changes	Copper or protein
		Corkscrew hair	Copper
Eyes	Corneas clear, shiny; membranes pink and moist; no sores at corners of eyelids	Foamy plaques (Bitot's spots)	Vitamin A
		Dryness (xerophthalmia)	Vitamin A
		Softening (keratomalacia)	Vitamin A
		Pale conjunctivae	Iron, vitamins B_6, B_{12}
		Red conjunctivae	Riboflavin
		Blepharitis	B-complex, biotin
Lips	Smooth, not chapped or swollen	Cheilosis (vertical cracks in lips)	Riboflavin, niacin
		Angular stomatitis (red cracks at sides of mouth)	Riboflavin, niacin, iron, vitamin B_6
Tongue	Appears red; not swollen or smooth, no lesions	Glossitis (beefy red)	Vitamin B-complex
		Pale	Iron
		Papillary atrophy	Niacin
		Papillary hypertrophy	Multiple nutrients
		Magenta/purplish coloured	Riboflavin
Gums	Reddish-pink, firm, no swelling or bleeding	Bleeding	Vitamin C
Nails	Smooth, pink	Brittle, ridged or spoon shaped (koilonychia)	Iron
		Splinter haemorrhages	Vitamin C

Continued

TABLE 21.3 Clinical signs of malnutrition cont'd

Area of Examination	Normal Appearance	Signs Associated with Malnutrition	Nutrient Deficiency
Musculoskeletal	Erect posture, no malformations, firm muscle tone, can walk or run without pain	Pain in calves, thighs	Thiamine
		Osteomalacia	Vitamin D, calcium
		Rickets	Vitamin D, calcium
		Joint pain	Vitamin C
		Muscle wasting	Protein, carbohydrate, fat
Neurological	Normal reflexes, appropriate affect	Peripheral neuropathy Hyporeflexia Disorientation or irritability	Thiamine, vitamin B_6, vitamin B_{12}

Source: World Health Organization 2023[13]

TABLE 21.4 Classification of malnutrition

Type/Aetiology	Clinical Features	Anthropometric Measures	Laboratory Findings
Obesity • Refers to weight more than 20% above ideal body weight • Morbidly obese—100% or more above ideal body weight • Causes—complex and multifaceted (e.g. genetic, social, cultural, pathological, psychological and physiological factors have all been implicated) • Usually the result of an imbalance of kilojoule intake and kilojoule expenditure • Visceral protein levels and immunocompetence are generally normal in obese people; anthropometric measures are above normal	Obese appearance	• Weight >120% standard for height • BMI > 30 • Triceps skinfold (TSF) > 10% standard • Waist-to-hip ratio > 1.0 (men) or > 0.8 (women)	• Serum cholesterol > 4.0 mmol/L • Serum triglycerides > 2 mmol/L

TABLE 21.4 Classification of malnutrition cont'd

Marasmus (protein–kilojoule malnutrition) • Due to inadequate intake of protein, kilojoules or prolonged starvation • Associated clinical conditions—anorexia, bowel obstruction, cancer cachexia and chronic illness • Can result from multifaceted factors—genetic, social, cultural, pathological, psychological and physiological • Characterised by decreased anthropometric measures—weight loss and subcutaneous fat and muscle wasting • Visceral protein levels may remain within normal ranges	Starved appearance 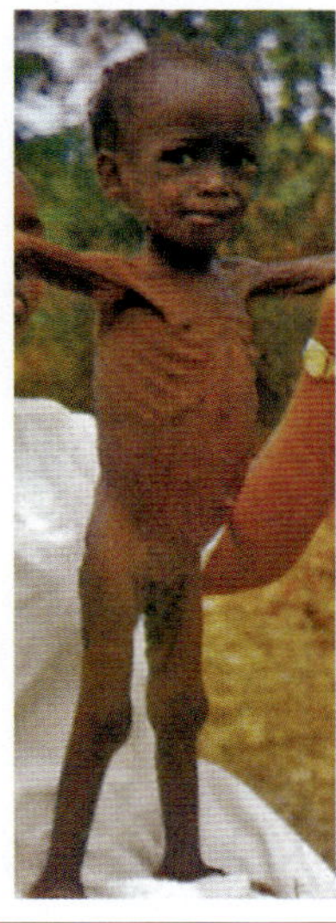	• Weight $<$ 80% standard for height • TSF $<$ 90% standard • Mid-arm muscle circumference (MAMC) $\leq$ 90% standard	Creatinine-height index $<$ 80%
Kwashiorkor (protein malnutrition) • Due to diets that may be high in kilojoules but contain little or no protein (e.g. low-protein liquid diets, fad diets and long-term use of dextrose-containing intravenous fluids) • Have decreased visceral protein levels and depressed immune function, but generally have adequate anthropometric measures • May appear well-nourished or even obese	• Well-nourished appearance • Oedematous	Weight $>$ 100% standard for height TSF > 100% standard	• Serum albumin $<$ 35 g/L • Serum transferrin $<$ 1.5 g/L • Lymphocytes $<$ 1,500 mm^3 • Anergen (absence of normal immune response to a particular allergen or antigen)
Marasmus/kwashiorkor mix • Due to prolonged inadequate intake of protein and kilojoules (e.g. severe starvation, severe catabolic states) • Combines elements of marasmus and kwashiorkor • Nutritional assessment findings include muscle, fat and visceral protein wasting, immune-incompetence • People have usually undergone acute catabolic stress such as major surgery, trauma or burns in combination with prolonged starvation • Without nutritional support, this type of malnutrition is associated with highest risk of morbidity and mortality	Emaciated appearance	• Weight $<$ 70% standard • TSF $<$ 80% standard • MAMC $<$ 60% standard	• Serum albumin $<$ 28 g/L • Serum transferrin $<$ 1.0 g/L • Lymphocytes $<$ 900 mm^3 • Anergy • Creatinine-height index $<$ 60% standard

TABLE 21.5 Abnormal facial appearances with thyroid disorders

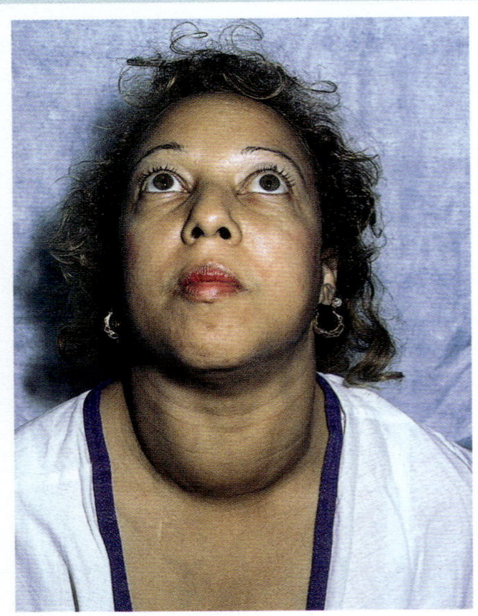

Hyperthyroidism

Goitre is an increase in the size of the thyroid gland and occurs with hyperthyroidism, Hashimoto's thyroiditis and hypothyroidism. Graves' disease (shown here) is the most common cause of hyperthyroidism, manifested by goitre and exophthalmos (bulging eyeballs). Symptoms include nervousness, fatigue, weight loss, muscle cramps and heat intolerance; signs include tachycardia, shortness of breath, excessive sweating, fine muscle tremor, thin silky hair and skin, infrequent blinking and a staring appearance.

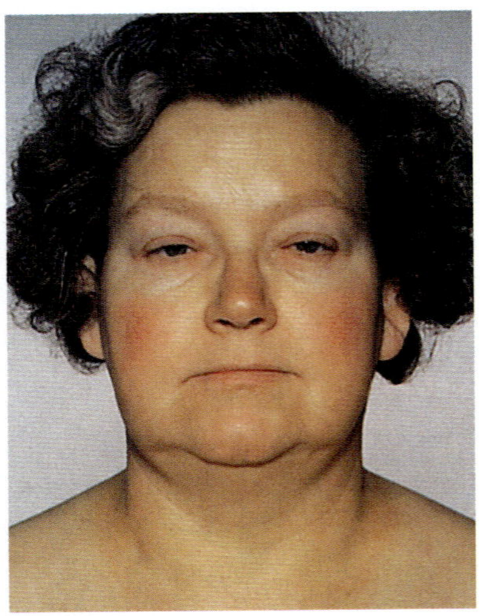

Myxoedema (hypothyroidism)

A deficiency of thyroid hormone, when severe, causes a non-pitting oedema or myxoedema. Note puffy oedematous face, especially around eyes (periorbital oedema), coarse facial features, dry skin and dry coarse hair and eyebrows.

TABLE 21.6 Abnormalities caused by nutritional deficiencies

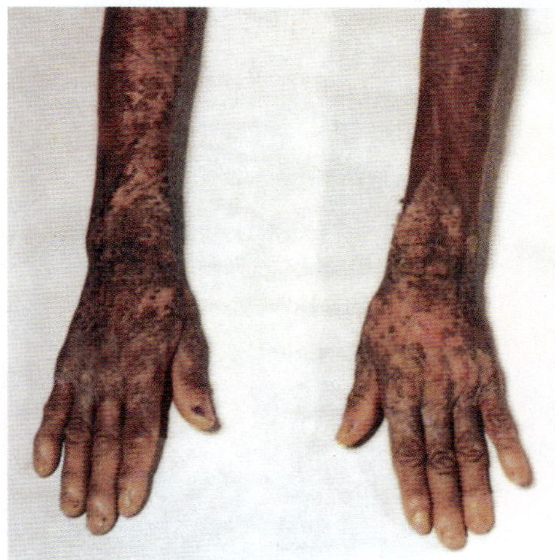

Pellagra

Pigmented keratotic scaling lesions resulting from a deficiency of niacin. These lesions are especially prominent in areas exposed to the sun, such as hands, forearms, neck and legs.

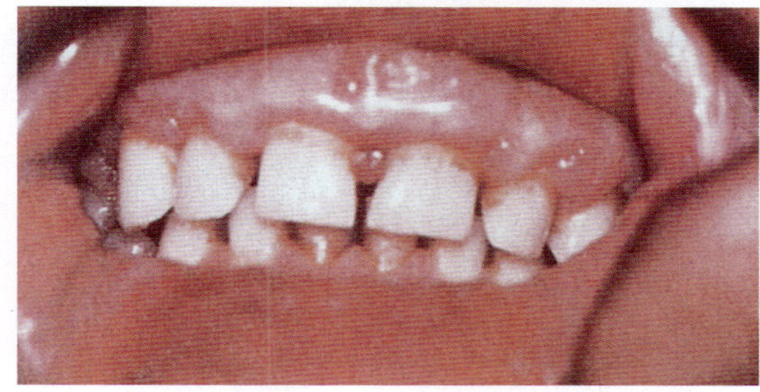

Scorbutic gums

Deficiency of vitamin C. Gums are swollen, ulcerated and bleeding due to vitamin C-induced defects in oral epithelial basement membrane and periodontal collagen fibre synthesis.

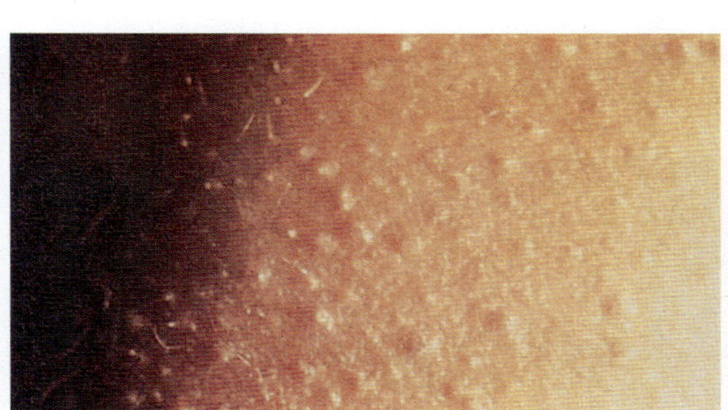

Follicular hyperkeratosis

Dry, bumpy skin associated with vitamin A and/or linoleic acid (essential fatty acid) deficiency. Linoleic acid deficiency may also result in eczematous skin, especially in infants.

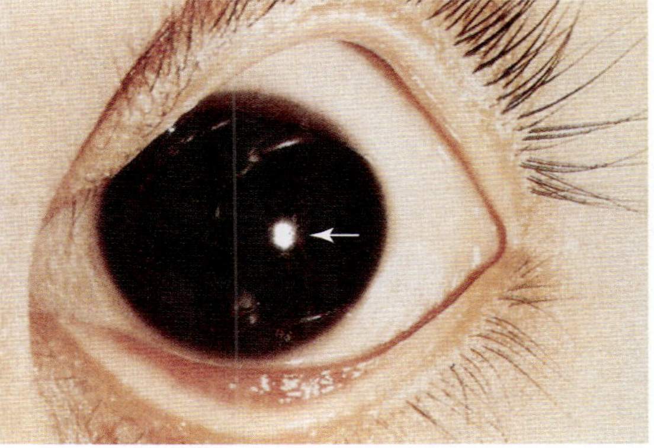

Bitot's spots

Foamy plaques of the cornea that signify a vitamin A deficiency. Severe depletion may result in conjunctival xerosis (drying) and progress to corneal ulceration and finally destruction of the eye (keratomalacia).

Continued

TABLE 21.6 Abnormalities caused by nutritional deficiencies cont'd

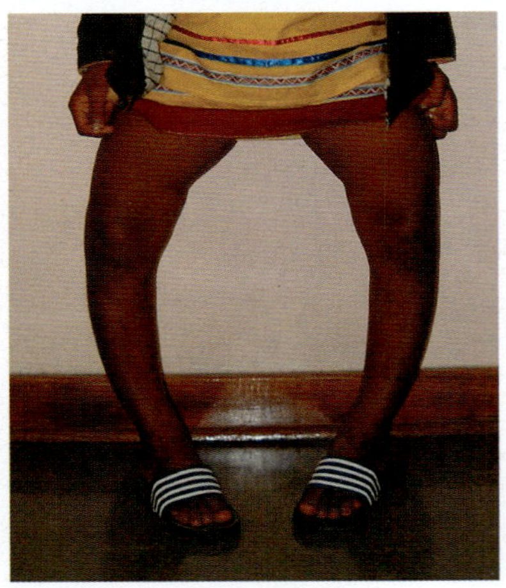

Rickets

Sign of vitamin D and calcium deficiencies in children (disorders of cartilage cell growth, enlargement of epiphyseal growth plates) and adults (osteomalacia).

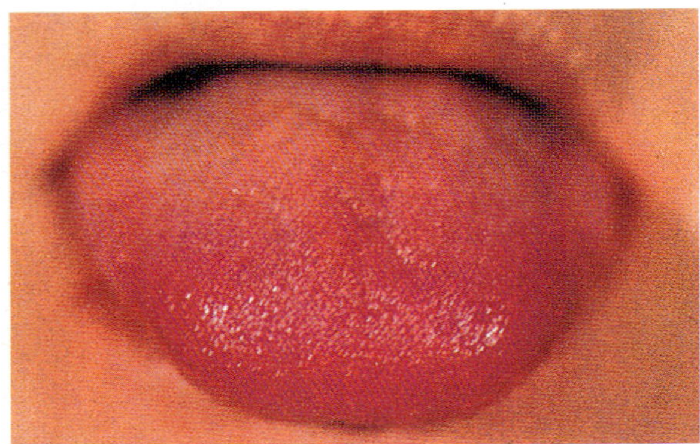

Magenta tongue

'Magenta tongue' is a sign of riboflavin deficiency. In contrast, a pale tongue is probably due to iron deficiency; a beefy red-coloured tongue is caused by vitamin B-complex deficiency.

TABLE 21.7 Abnormalities of the lips

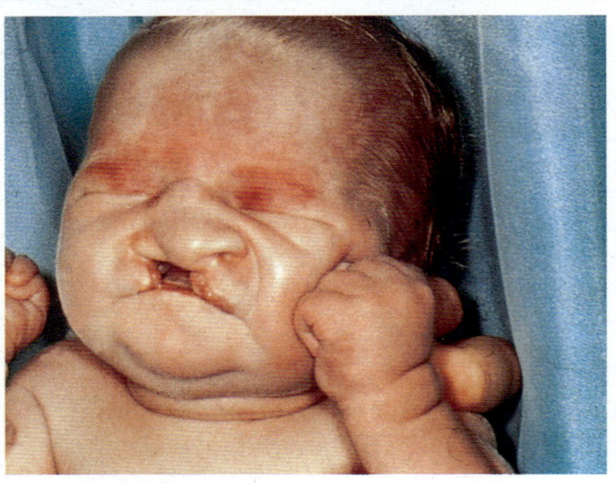

Cleft lip

Orofacial clefts are the most common congenital deformities of the head and neck. Early treatment preserves the functions of speech and language formation and swallowing.

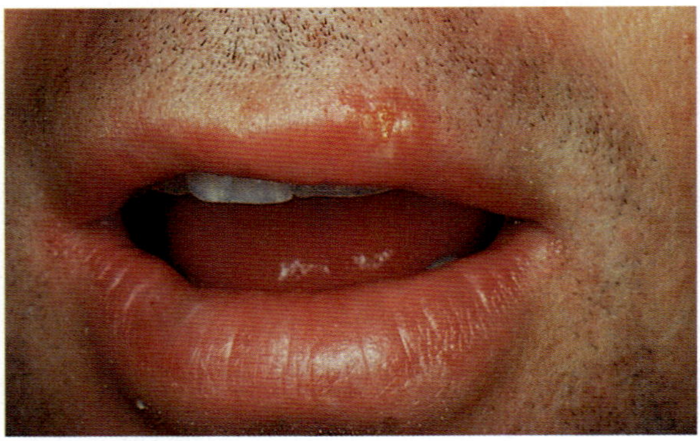

Herpes simplex 1

Cold sores are groups of clear vesicles with a surrounding indurated erythematous base. These evolve into pustules, which rupture, weep and crust and heal in 4 to 10 days. The most likely site is the lip–skin junction; infection often recurs in same site. Caused by the herpes simplex virus (HSV-1), the lesion is highly contagious and is spread by direct contact. Recurrent herpes infections may be precipitated by sunlight, fever, colds or an allergy. It is a very common lesion, affecting 50% of adults.

TABLE 21.7 Abnormalities of the lips cont'd

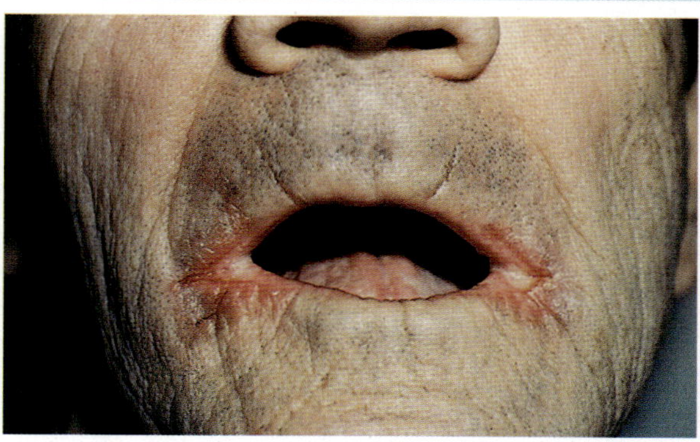

Angular cheilitis (stomatitis, perlèche)

Erythema, scaling, shallow and painful fissures at the corners of the mouth occur with excess salivation and *Candida* infection. It is often seen in edentulous people and in those with poorly fitting dentures causing folding in of corners of mouth, creating a warm and moist environment favouring the growth of yeast.

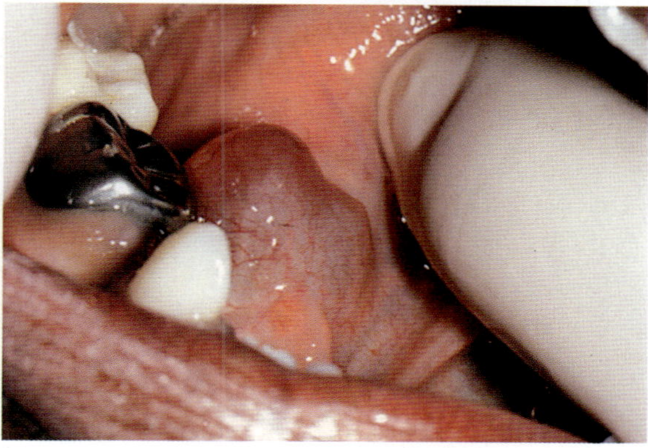

Retention 'cyst' (mucocoele)

A round, well-defined translucent nodule that may be very small or up to 1 or 2 cm. It is a pocket of mucus that forms when a duct of a minor salivary gland ruptures. The benign lesion also may occur on the buccal mucosa, on the floor of the mouth or under the tip of the tongue.

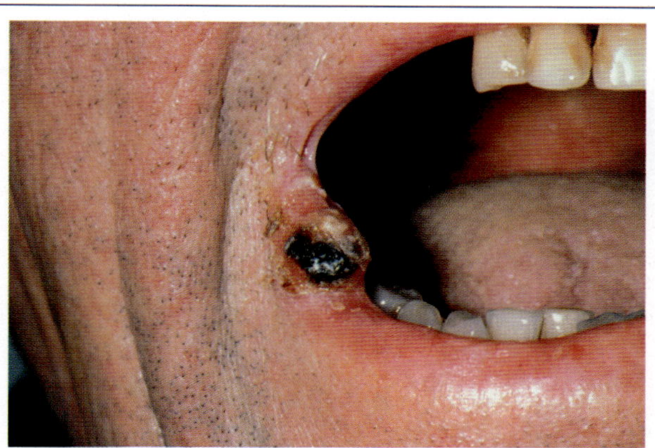

Carcinoma

The initial lesion is round and indurated, then it becomes crusted and ulcerated with an elevated border. The majority occur between the outer and middle thirds of the lip. Any lesion that is still unhealed after 2 weeks should be referred.

TABLE 21.8 Abnormalities of the teeth and gums

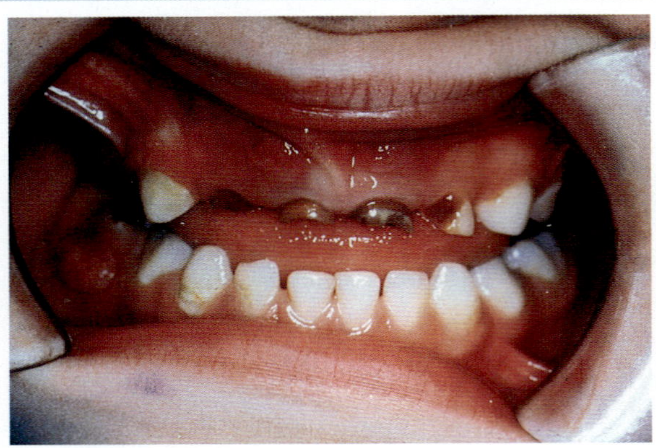

Baby bottle tooth decay

Destruction of numerous deciduous teeth may occur in older infants and toddlers who take a bottle of milk, juice or sweetened drink to bed and prolong bottle feeding past the age of 1 year. Liquid pools around the upper front teeth. Mouth bacteria act on carbohydrates in the liquid, especially sucrose, forming metabolic acids. Acids break down tooth enamel and destroy its protein.

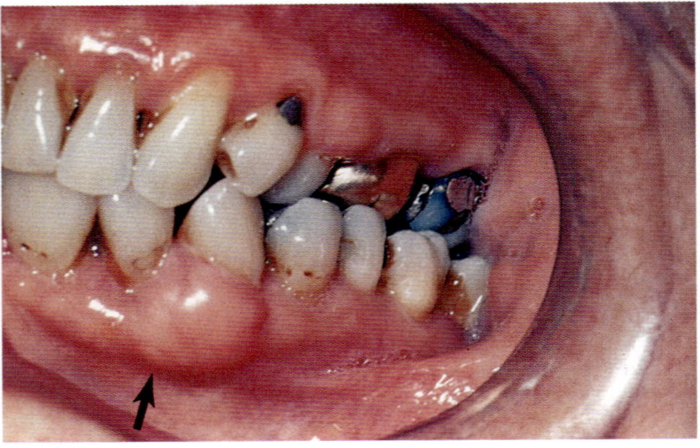

Epulis

A nontender, fibrous nodule of the gum, seen emerging between the teeth; an inflammatory response to injury or haemorrhage.

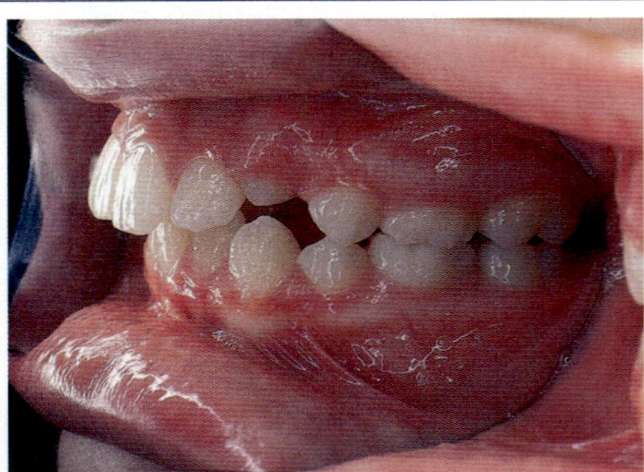

Malocclusion

Upper or lower dental arches are not in alignment and incisors protrude from developmental problem of mandible or maxilla, or incompatibility between jaw size and tooth size. The condition increases risk of facial deformity, negative body image, chewing problems or speech dysfluency.

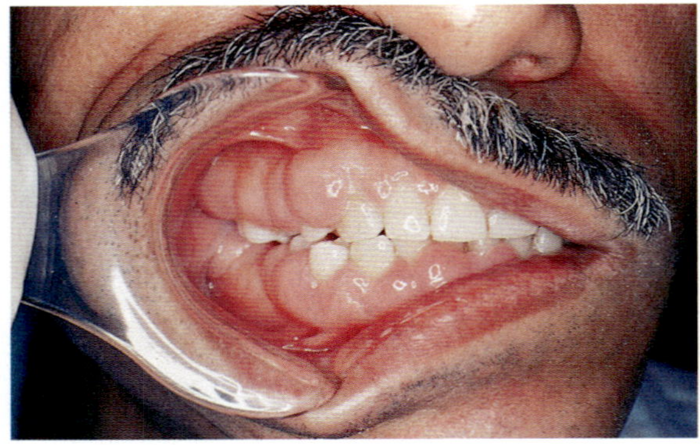

Gingival hyperplasia

Painless enlargement of the gums, sometimes overreaching the teeth. This occurs with puberty, pregnancy, leukaemia and with long-term therapeutic use of phenytoin (Dilantin).

TABLE 21.8 Abnormalities of the teeth and gums cont'd

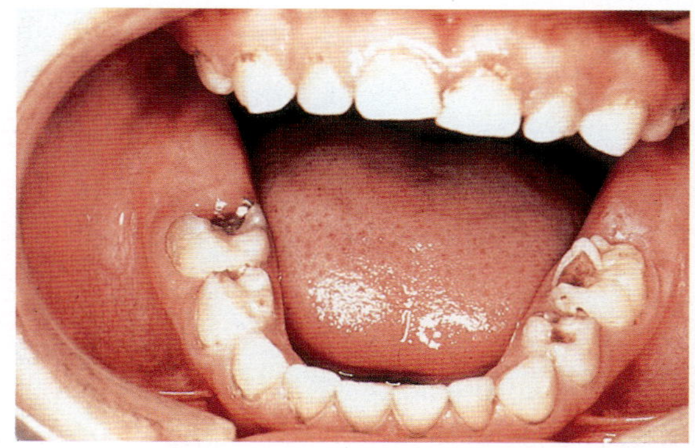

Dental caries

Progressive destruction of tooth. Decay initially looks chalky white. Later, it turns brown or black and forms a cavity. Early decay is apparent only on x-ray study. Susceptible sites are tooth surfaces where food debris, bacterial plaque and saliva collect.

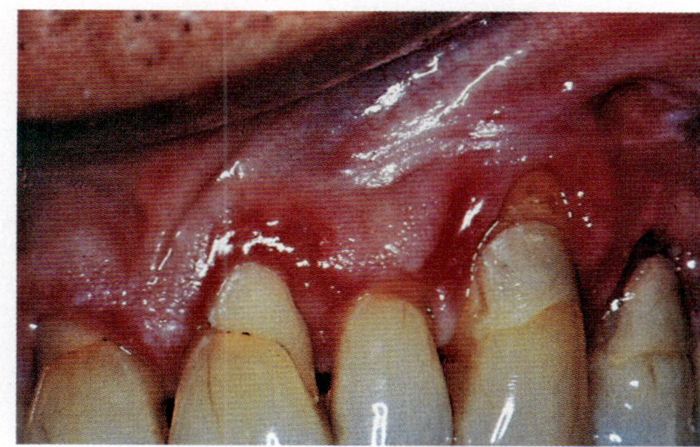

Gingivitis

Gum margins are red, swollen and bleed easily. This case is severe; gingival tissue has desquamated, exposing roots of teeth. Inflammation is usually due to poor dental hygiene or vitamin C deficiency. The condition may occur in pregnancy and puberty because of changing hormonal balance.

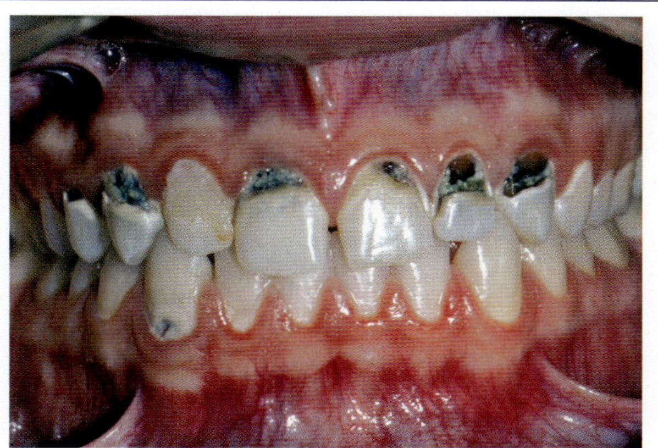

Meth mouth

Illicit methamphetamine abuse (crystal meth, meth ice) leads to extensive dental caries, gingivitis, tooth cracking and edentulism. Methamphetamine causes vasoconstriction and decreased saliva, and its use increases the urge to consume sugars and starches and to give up oral hygiene. Absence of the buffering saliva leads to increased acidity in the mouth and the increased plaque encourages bacterial growth. These conditions and the presence of carbohydrates set up an oral environment prone to caries, cracking of enamel and the damage seen here.

TABLE 21.9 Abnormalities of the tongue

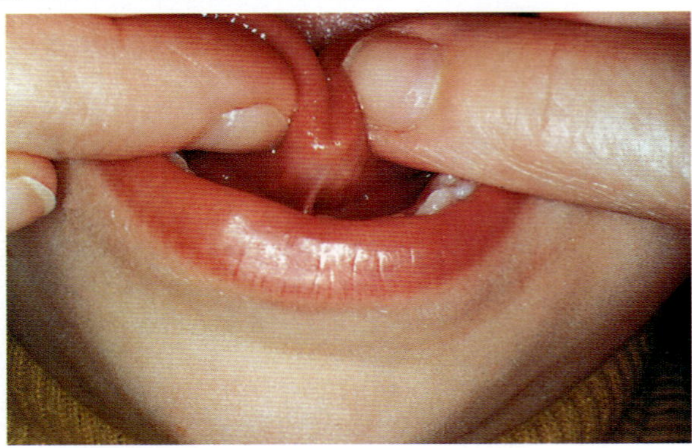

Ankyloglossia

(Tongue-tie.) A short lingual frenulum, here fixing the tongue tip to the floor of the mouth and gums. This limits mobility and will affect speech (pronunciation of a, d and n) if the tongue tip cannot be elevated to the alveolar ridge. A congenital defect.

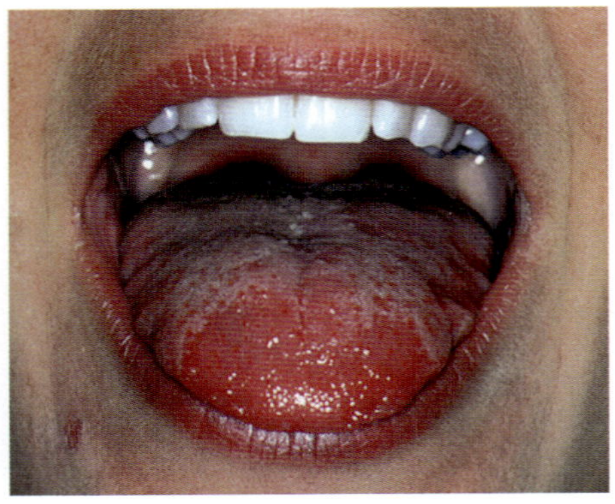

Geographic tongue (migratory glossitis)

Pattern of normal coating interspersed with bright red, shiny, circular bald areas with raised pearly borders. Pattern resembles a map and changes in a few days. Not significant, and its cause is not known.

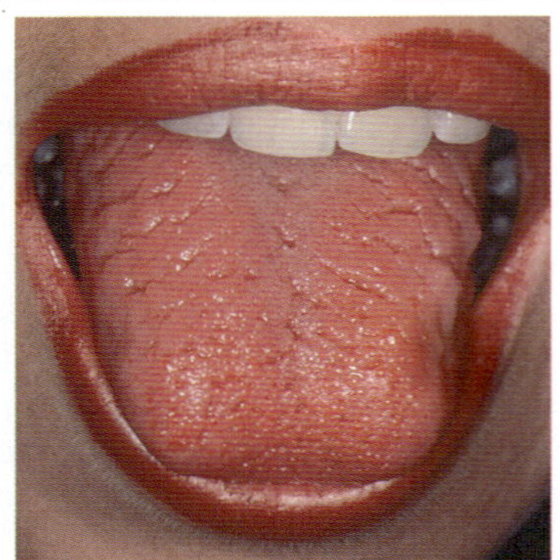

Fissured or scrotal tongue

Deep furrows divide the papillae into small irregular rows. The condition occurs in 5% of the general population and in trisomy 21 (Down syndrome). The incidence increases with age. (Vertical, or longitudinal, fissures also occur with dehydration because of reduced volume of the tongue.)

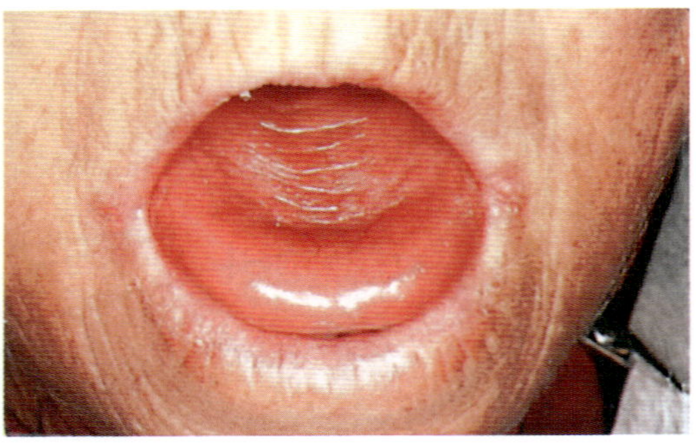

Smooth, glossy tongue (atrophic glossitis)

The surface is slick and shiny; the mucosa thins and looks red from decreased papillae. Accompanied by dryness of tongue and burning. Occurs with vitamin B_{12} deficiency (pernicious anaemia), folic acid deficiency and iron deficiency anaemia. Here, also note angular cheilitis.

TABLE 21.9 Abnormalities of the tongue cont'd

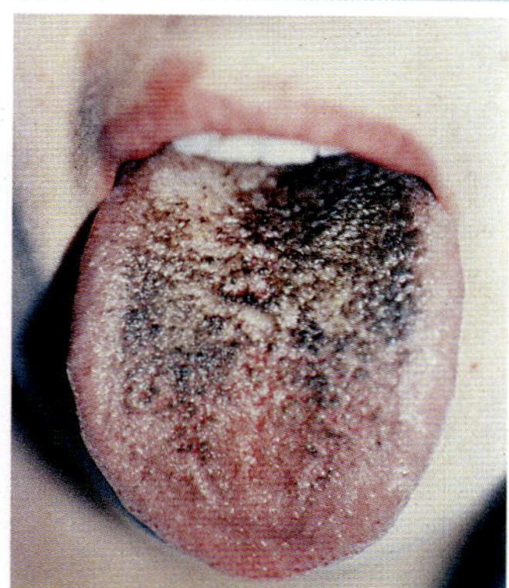

Black hairy tongue

This is not really hair but the elongation of filiform papillae and painless overgrowth of mycelial threads of fungus infection on the tongue. Colour varies from black-brown to yellow. It occurs after use of antibiotics, which inhibit normal bacteria and allow proliferation of fungus.

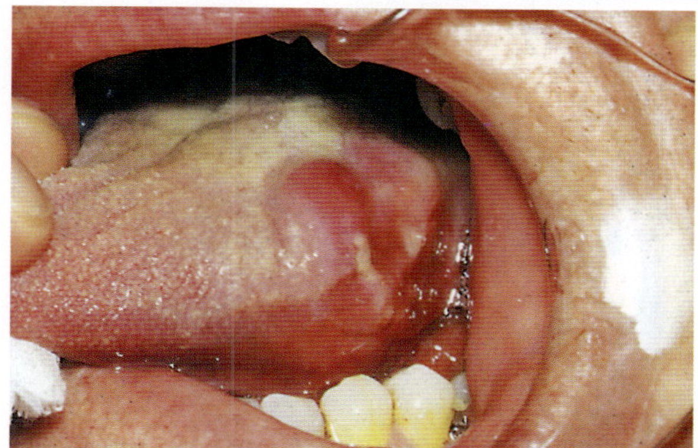

Carcinoma

An ulcer with rolled edges; indurated. Occurs particularly at the sides, base and under the tongue. When it is in the floor of mouth, it may cause painful movement or limited movement of tongue. Risk of early metastasis is present because of rich lymphatic drainage. Heavy smoking and heavy alcohol use place people at greater risk.

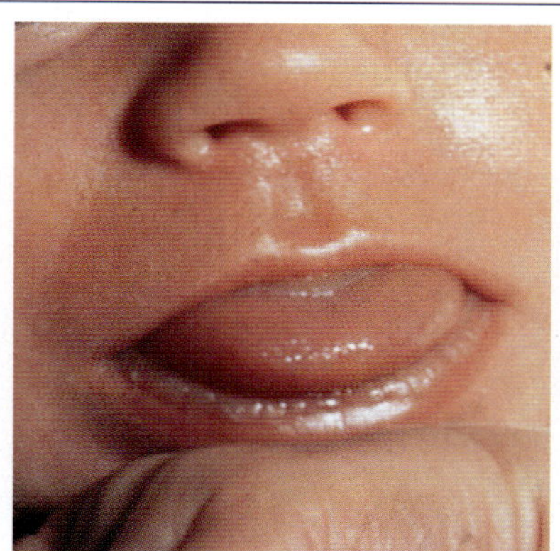

Enlarged tongue (macroglossia)

The tongue is enlarged and may protrude from the mouth. The condition is not painful but may impair speech development. Here, it occurs with trisomy 21 (Down syndrome), cretinism, myxoedema and acromegaly. A transient swelling occurs with local infections.

TABLE 21.10 Abnormalities of the buccal mucosa

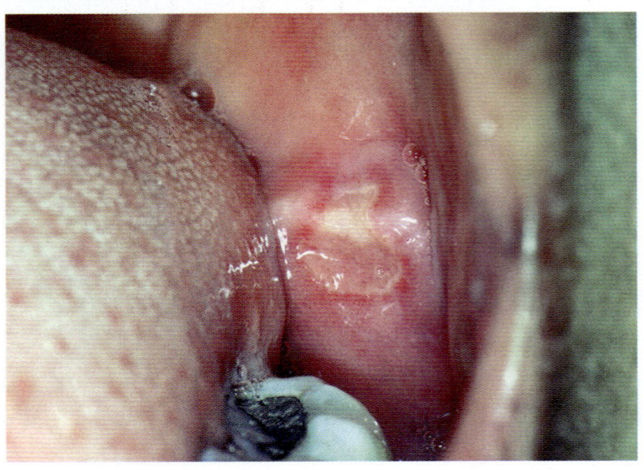

Aphthous ulcers

A 'canker sore' is a vesicle at first, then a small, round, 'punched-out' ulcer with white base surrounded by a red halo. It is quite painful and lasts for 1 to 2 weeks. The cause is unknown, although it is associated with stress, fatigue and food allergy. It is common, affecting 20 to 60% of the population.

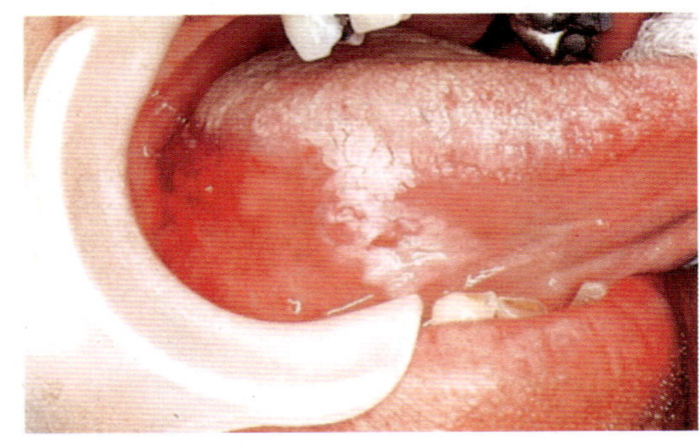

Leucoplakia

Chalky white, thick, raised patch with well-defined borders. The lesion is firmly attached and does not scrape off. It may occur on the lateral edges of tongue. It is due to chronic irritation and occurs more frequently with heavy smoking and heavy alcohol use. Lesions are precancerous, and the person should be referred. (Here, the lesion is associated with squamous carcinoma.)

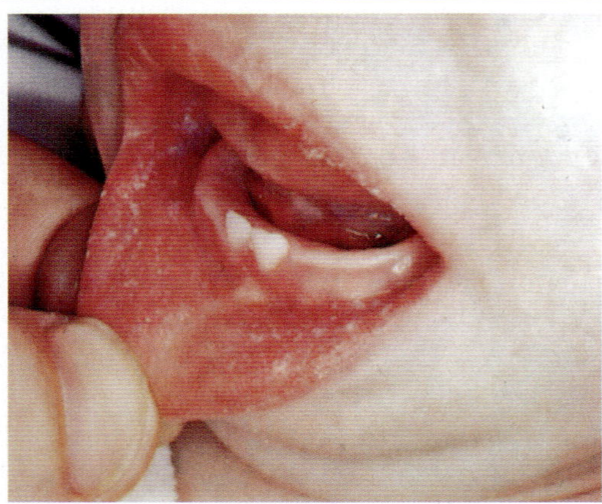

Koplik's spots

Small blue-white spots with irregular red halo scattered over mucosa opposite the molars. An early sign of measles.

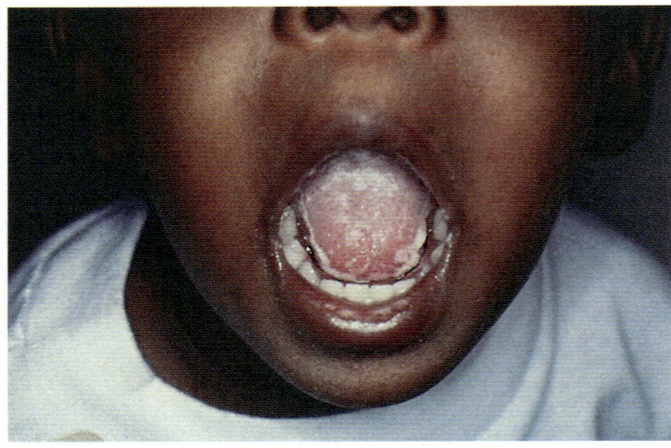

Candidiasis or monilial infection

A white, cheesy, curd-like patch on the buccal mucosa and tongue. It scrapes off, leaving raw, red surface that bleeds easily. Termed 'thrush' in the newborn. It is an opportunistic infection that occurs after the use of antibiotics, corticosteroids and in immunosuppressed people.

TABLE 21.11 Paediatric facial abnormalities

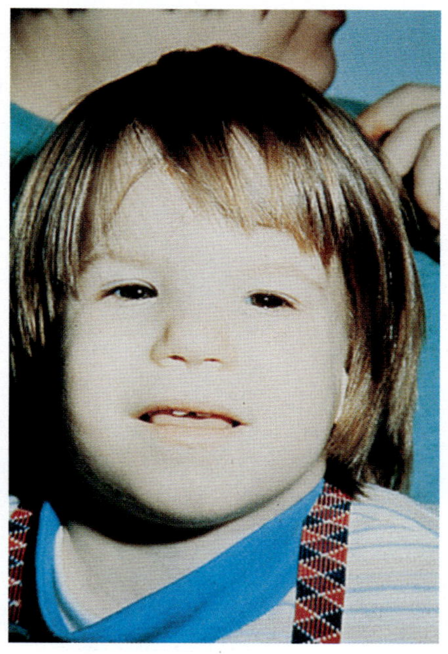

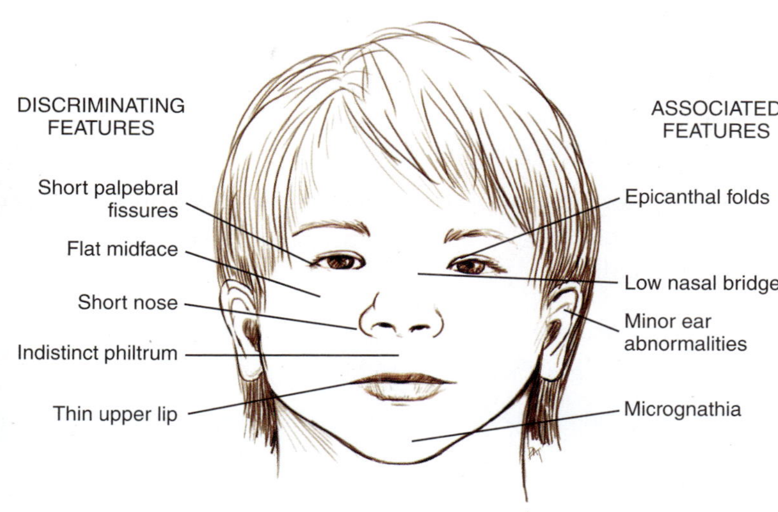

Fetal alcohol syndrome

Pregnant women who abuse alcohol are at great risk of producing a baby with a wide range of growth and development abnormalities. Facial malformations may be recognisable at birth. Characteristic facies include narrow palpebral fissures, epicanthal folds and midfacial hypoplasia.

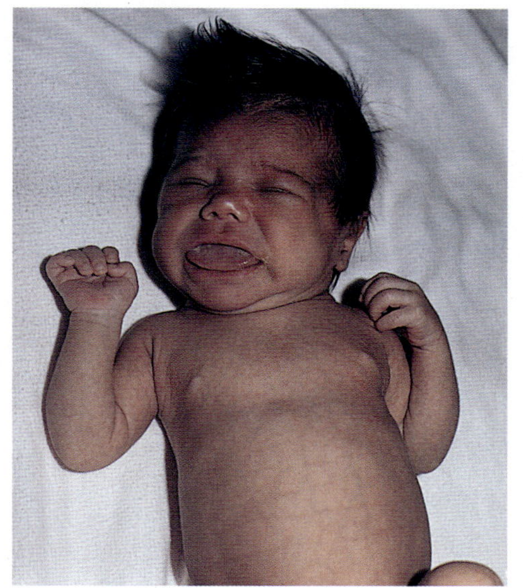

Congenital hypothyroidism

Thyroid deficiency at an early age produces impaired growth and neurological deficit. Without neonatal screening, characteristic facies develop by 3 to 6 months of age: low hairline, hirsute forehead, swollen eyelids, narrow palpebral fissures, widely spaced eyes, depressed nasal bridge, puffy face, thick tongue protruding through an open mouth and a dull expression. Head size is normal, but the anterior and posterior fontanels are wide open.

Advanced practice—additional data

In addition to the previous objective data, assessments described in the following section require nurses to have advanced skill and scope of practice. Nurses working in community settings and specialised clinics may need to develop these skills.

Equipment needed

In addition to the equipment listed previously you will require:

- anthropometer
- skinfold calipers.

PROCEDURES AND NORMAL FINDINGS	ABNORMAL FINDINGS AND CLINICAL ALERTS
Additional anthropometric measures	
In addition to measures of height and weight, advanced assessment includes triceps skinfold thickness, ulnar length, elbow breadth and arm circumferences.	
Skinfold thickness	
Skinfold thickness measurements provide an estimate of body fat stores or the extent of obesity or under-nutrition. Although other sites can be used (biceps, subscapular or suprailiac skinfolds), **the triceps skinfold (TSF)** is most selected because of its easy accessibility and because standards and techniques are most developed for this site. To measure TSF thickness: • Have the ambulatory person stand with arms hanging freely at the sides and back to the examiner. (Non-ambulatory people should lie on one side. The uppermost arm should be fully extended, with the palm of the hand resting on the thigh.) • Using the thumb and forefinger of your left hand, gently grasp a fold of skin and fat on the posterior aspect of the person's left upper arm, midway between the acromion process of the scapula and the olecranon process (the tip of the elbow). Gently pull the skinfold away from the underlying muscle (Figure 21.14).	

PROCEDURES AND NORMAL FINDINGS	ABNORMAL FINDINGS AND CLINICAL ALERTS

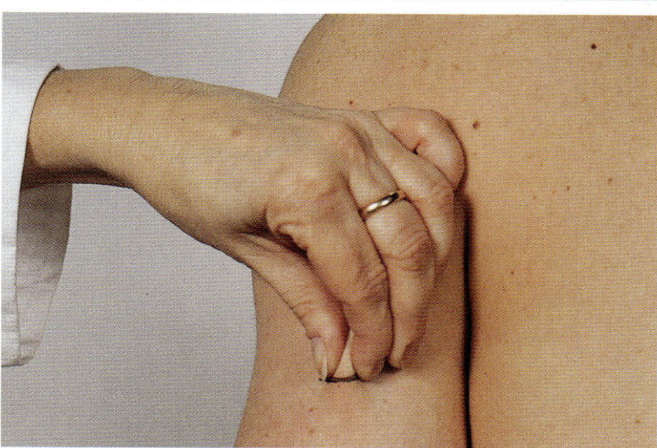

FIGURE 21.14 Measuring skinfold thickness

While grasping the skinfold, pick up the calipers with your right hand and depress the spring-loaded lever. Apply caliper jaws horizontally to the fat fold. Release the lever of the calipers while holding the skinfold. Wait 3 seconds, then take a reading. Repeat three times and average the three skinfold measurements (Figure 21.15).

TSF values 10% below or above standard suggest under-nutrition and over-nutrition, respectively.

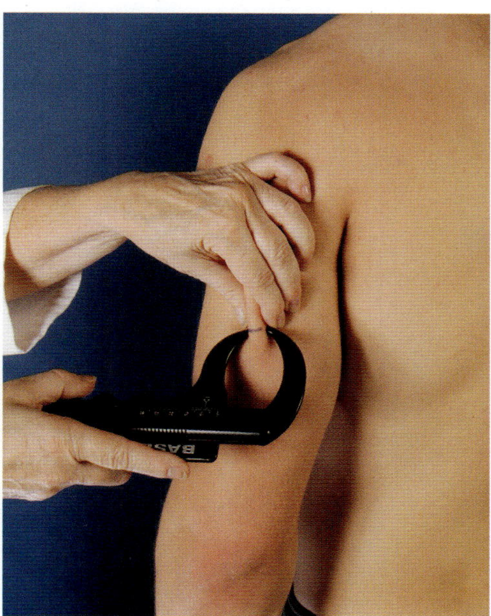

FIGURE 21.15 Measuring skinfold thickness—the caliper method

PROCEDURES AND NORMAL FINDINGS	ABNORMAL FINDINGS AND CLINICAL ALERTS
Record measurements to the nearest 5 mm (0.5 cm) on the nutritional assessment data form. Compare the person's measurements with standards by age, sex and body frame size.	Non-reproducible readings may be due to instrument malfunctions, use of plastic calipers (which are less accurate) or examiner error. Oedema may produce falsely high readings.
Other techniques to measure body composition	
Tests include **bioelectrical impedance analysis (BIA)** and **dual-energy x-ray absorptiometry (DEXA)**. Both BIA and DEXA measure fat and lean body mass; in addition, DEXA measures bone mineral density.	
Arm span or total arm length	
Measuring the arm span is useful for those situations in which height is difficult to measure, such as in children with cerebral palsy or scoliosis or in people in late adulthood with spinal curvature. Arm span, which is nearly equivalent to height, is sometimes used clinically instead of height.[14] Measure the distance from the sternal notch to the tip of the longest finger on one hand and multiply the number by 2.8.[15]	
Inspect and palpate the thyroid gland	
The thyroid gland is difficult to palpate; arrange your setting to maximise your likelihood of success. Position a standing lamp to shine tangentially across the neck to highlight any possible swelling. Give the person a glass of water and first inspect the neck as the person takes a sip and swallows. Thyroid tissue moves up with a swallow.	Diffuse enlargement or a nodular lump.
Posterior approach. To palpate, move behind the person (Figure 21.16A & B). Ask the person to sit up very straight and then to bend the head slightly forwards and to the right. This will relax the neck muscles. Use the fingers of your left hand to push the trachea slightly to the right.	See Table 21.11.

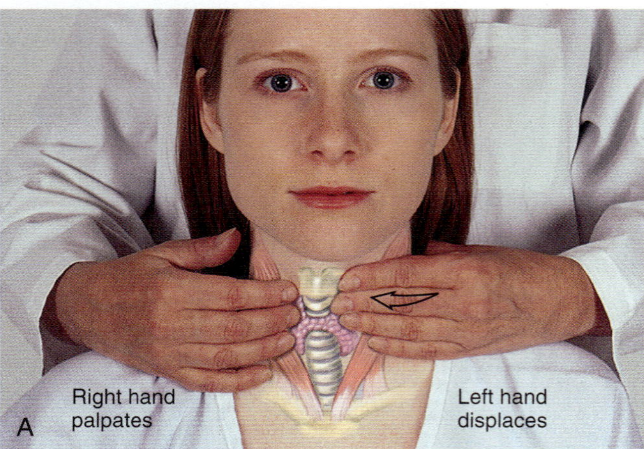

FIGURE 21.16A Palpating the thyroid gland

PROCEDURES AND NORMAL FINDINGS	ABNORMAL FINDINGS AND CLINICAL ALERTS
Then curve your right fingers between the trachea and the sternocleidomastoid muscle, retracting it slightly, and ask the person to take a sip of water. The thyroid moves up under your fingers with the trachea and larynx as the person swallows. Reverse the procedure for the left side.	
Usually, you cannot palpate the normal adult thyroid. If the person has a long, thin neck, you will sometimes feel the isthmus over the tracheal rings. The lateral lobes are not usually palpable; check them for enlargement, consistency, symmetry and the presence of nodules.	Enlarged lobes that are easily palpated before swallowing or are tender to palpation; or the presence of nodules or lumps (Figure 21.16B and Table 21.12).

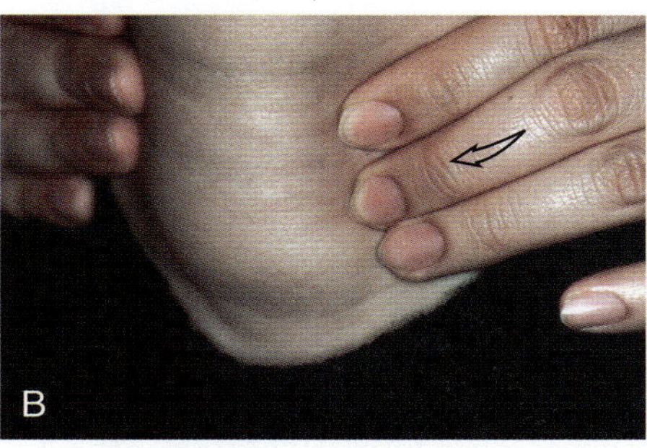

FIGURE 21.16B Palpating the thyroid gland for the presence of nodules or lumps

Anterior approach. This is an alternative method of palpating the thyroid, but it is more awkward to perform, especially for a beginning examiner.

Stand facing the person. Ask them to tip the head forwards and to the right. Use your right thumb to displace the trachea slightly to the person's right. Hook your left thumb and fingers around the sternocleidomastoid muscle. Feel for lobe enlargement as the person swallows (Figure 21.17).

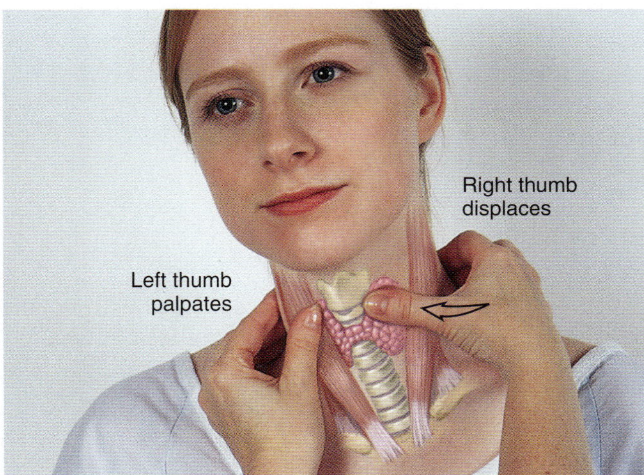

FIGURE 21.17 Anterior approach to palpating the thyroid gland

PROCEDURES AND NORMAL FINDINGS	ABNORMAL FINDINGS AND CLINICAL ALERTS

Laboratory studies

Routine laboratory tests are objective, can detect preclinical nutritional deficiencies and can be used to confirm subjective findings. Use caution, however, when interpreting test results that may be outside normal ranges, because they do not always reflect a nutritional problem and because standards for people in late adulthood have not yet been firmly established.

Haemoglobin. This test is used to detect iron deficiency anaemia.

Normal values are as follows:

- **infants**, 1 to 3 days—145 to 225 g/L, 2 months—90 to 140 g/L
- **children**, 6 to 12 years—115 to 155 g/L
- **adults**, males—140 to 180 g/L, females—120 to 160 g/L.

Increased haemoglobin levels suggest haemoconcentration due to polycythaemia vera or dehydration.

Decreased haemoglobin levels may indicate anaemia, recent haemorrhage or haemodilution caused by fluid retention.

Haematocrit is a measure of cell volume and an indicator of iron status.

Normal values are as follows:

- **infants**, 1 to 3 days—44% to 72%; 2 months—28% to 42%
- **children**, 6 to 12 years—35% to 45%
- **adults**, males—37% to 49%, females—36% to 46%.

A high **haematocrit** can indicate dehydration and subsequent concentration of the blood. A low value indicates insufficient haemoglobin formation; thus haematocrit and haemoglobin values should be interpreted together.

Cholesterol

Total cholesterol is measured to evaluate fat metabolism and to assess the risk of cardiovascular disease. Normal cholesterol concentrations vary with age and gender. **Normal cholesterol** is below 4.0 mmol/L, while the ratio between low density lipoproteins and high-density lipoproteins should be less than 4 (i.e. LDL:HDL = < 4 mmol/L).

Coronary artery disease risk steadily increases as serum cholesterol rises.

Serum cholesterol levels of 5.5 to 6.5 mmol/L (borderline high)—associated with moderate risk of coronary artery disease, heart attack, stroke and peripheral vascular disease.

Levels of 6.5 mmol/L or more (high) are associated with high risk.

Triglycerides

Serum triglycerides (TGs) are used to screen for hyperlipidaemia and to determine the risk of coronary artery disease. Triglyceride values are age related. Some controversy exists over the most appropriate normal ranges, but the following are widely accepted:

- **ages 0 to 19**—0.11 to 1.13 mmol/L
- **ages 20 to 65**—0.45 to 2.26 mmol/L.

Serum TG levels are also associated with coronary artery disease and are categorised as *borderline* (0.5–1.7 mmol/L) or *high* (> 1.7 mmol/L) (Tables 21.13 and 21.14).

Vitamin D is essential for bone and muscle health and regulating the immune system and cell activity. Vitamin D is required for effective absorption of calcium.

Normal level: 50 to 200 mmol/L

Low vitamin D: associated with rickets and osteoporosis, bone and muscle pain.

PROCEDURES AND NORMAL FINDINGS

Total lymphocyte count. The most used tests of immune function are total lymphocyte count (TLC) and skin testing, also called delayed cutaneous hypersensitivity testing. TLC is an important indicator of visceral protein status and therefore of cellular immune function.

The TLC is derived from the white blood cell count and the differential count:

$$\text{TLC} = \frac{\text{Number of lymphocytes in differential}}{\text{100 cells}}$$

TLC is calculated in cells per cubic millimetre.
Normal values for all age categories are between 1,800 and 3,000 cells/mm^3.

Skin testing. Adequate immunity can also be demonstrated by a positive reaction to multiple skin test antigens. In these tests of immune function, at least six antigens are injected intradermally in the forearm area and the response (redness and/or induration) is noted at 24 and 48 hours. A 5 mm or greater response to more than one antigen is generally considered to be a positive reaction (e.g. indicative of adequate immunity).
Commonly used antigens include *Candida*, tetanus toxoid, diphtheria toxoid, streptococcus, old tuberculin, proteus and trichophyton.

Serum proteins
Serum albumin is another common measurement of visceral protein status. Because of its relatively long half-life (17–20 days) and large body pool (4.0–5.0 g/kg), albumin is not an early indicator of protein malnutrition.
Normal serum albumin concentration in infants and children older than 6 months and adults ranges from 32 to 45 g/L.

Levels of **serum transferrin**, an iron-transport protein, can be measured directly or by an indirect measurement of total iron-binding capacity. Serum transferrin, with a half-life of 8 to 10 days, may be a more sensitive indicator of visceral protein status than albumin.
The most widely used formula for computing serum transferrin is:
Serum transferrin = (0.8 × Total iron-binding capacity) − 43
Normal: 1.7 to 2.5 g/L.

ABNORMAL FINDINGS AND CLINICAL ALERTS

Non-nutritional factors that affect TLC include hypoalbuminaemia, metabolic stress (e.g. major surgery, trauma and sepsis), infection, cancer and chronic diseases.

Total lymphocyte counts of 1,500 to 1,800: mild depletion; 900–1,500: moderate depletion; < 900: severe depletion.

A response of less than 5 mm indicates anergy or immune-incompetence.
Anergy occurs with malnutrition, hepatic failure, infection and immunosuppressive drugs (e.g. chemotherapy agents, steroids).
Lymphocytopenia and the lack of a positive response to skin test antigens increase the risk of infection and sepsis.

Low serum albumin levels occur with protein–kilojoule malnutrition, altered hydration status and decreased liver function.
A serum albumin level of 28–35 g/L represents moderate visceral protein depletion and < 28 g/L denotes severe depletion.[14]

Levels of 1.5 to 1.7 g/L—mild protein deficiency; 1.0 to 1.5 g/L—moderate deficiency; < 1.0 g/L—severe deficiency.
Because many clinical conditions can alter serum albumin and transferrin levels, consider the person's history in conjunction with these values for accurate interpretation.

PROCEDURES AND NORMAL FINDINGS	ABNORMAL FINDINGS AND CLINICAL ALERTS
Prealbumin, or thyroxin-binding prealbumin, serves as a transport protein for thyroxine (T_4) and retinol-binding protein. With a shorter half-life (48 hours) than either albumin or transferrin, prealbumin is sensitive to acute changes in protein status and sudden demands on protein synthesis. Normal level: 150 to 250 mg/L.	**Prealbumin levels** elevated in renal disease and reduced by surgery, trauma, burns and infection. Prealbumin levels of 100–150 mg/L—mild depletion; 50–100 mg/L—moderate depletion; < 50 mg/L—severe depletion.
C-reactive protein (CRP), a plasma protein marker of inflammatory status produced by the liver, is used to monitor generalised inflammation, metabolic stress (e.g. trauma, surgery, burns) and as an indicator of when to begin nutritional support in critically ill patients. CRP is generally not detectable in the blood (< 6 mg/L) of healthy people.	Detectable levels of **CRP** are associated with increased risk of atherosclerosis and may be seen in other inflammatory conditions (e.g. infections, rheumatoid arthritis or tuberculosis). The use of oral contraceptives and the last 4 to 5 months of pregnancy may also produce detectable CRP levels.
Nitrogen balance Nitrogen balance is also used as an index of protein nutritional status. Nitrogen is released with the catabolism of amino acids (proteins) and is excreted in the urine as urea. Nitrogen balance therefore indicates whether the person is anabolic (using the normal energy stores and therefore pooling proteins and nitrogen creating a positive nitrogen balance) or catabolic (breaking down proteins in tissues for energy and therefore excreting nitrogen and creating a negative nitrogen balance within the body). Nitrogen balance is estimated by a formula based on urine urea nitrogen (UUN) excreted during the previous 24 hours: Nitrogen balance is the difference between nitrogen intake and loss reflecting gain or loss of total body protein. The formula to calculate nitrogen balance is as follows: Nitrogen balance = Nitrogen intake – Nitrogen excretion = Protein intake/6.25 − 24 hours UNNg + 4 To interpret the formula: Nitrogen balance is measured in grams Daily protein intake in grams divided by 6.25 24 hours UNN (grams) 4 = non-urea nitrogen losses via faeces, skin, sweat and lungs	In response to stress and increased protein demand, the body rapidly mobilises its protein compartments, resulting in increased production of urea and excretion of urea in the urine. With infection, an estimated loss of 9 to 11 g/day of urinary urea nitrogen (UNN) can be expected. In patients with major burns, 12 to 18 g/day of urea nitrogen may be expected in the urine.[14]

PROCEDURES AND NORMAL FINDINGS	ABNORMAL FINDINGS AND CLINICAL ALERTS
The **creatinine-height index** (CHI) is a method of estimating the amount of skeletal muscle mass. Creatinine is derived from the breakdown of creatine, an energy-containing complex found in muscle. Creatinine is excreted unchanged in the urine at a constant rate in proportion to the amount of body muscle.	
Creatinine height index is calculated by first measuring urinary creatinine using a 24-hours urine collection specimen. This value is then compared with ideal urinary creatinine levels from a creatinine-for-height-standard table, by means of the following equation: $$CHI = \frac{\text{Actual 24-hours urine creatinine}}{\text{Ideal 24-hours urine creatinine for height}} \times 100$$ The person's CHI is then compared with a CHI standard table to determine the degree of skeletal muscle depletion.	The validities of CHI and nitrogen balance studies depend on the accuracy of the 24-hours urine collection. Failure to obtain an accurate sample and abnormal renal function result in underestimation of creatinine and nitrogen losses. Assuming an accurate 24-hours urine specimen, a CHI of 60 to 80% of standard indicates a moderate deficit in body mass. A value of under 60% indicates a severe deficit of body muscle mass. Stress, fever and trauma can increase urinary creatinine excretion.
Developmental considerations in laboratory testing	
In **infancy and childhood**, laboratory tests are performed only when under-nutrition is suspected or if the child has acute or chronic illnesses that affect nutritional status.	
During **adolescence**, unless overt disease is suspected, laboratory evaluation of haemoglobin and haematocrit levels and urinalysis for glucose and protein levels are adequate.	See Table 21.14.
In **pregnancy**, haemoglobin and haematocrit values can be used to detect deficiencies of protein, folic acid, vitamin B_{12} and iron. Urine is frequently tested for glucose and protein (albumin), which can signal diabetes, pre-eclampsia and renal disease. **Serum ferritin:** Normal level: ≥ 30 microg/L health iron stores.	Serum ferritin concentrations typically fall in the last 4 weeks of normal pregnancy. This reflects transfer of organic iron from mother to fetus, rather than any change in iron metabolism. However, a ferritin concentration under 30 microg/L is still considered diagnostic of iron deficiency at any stage of pregnancy.
In **late adulthood**, all serum and urine data must be interpreted with an understanding of declining renal efficiency and a tendency for people to be over-hydrated or under-hydrated.	

PROCEDURES AND NORMAL FINDINGS	ABNORMAL FINDINGS AND CLINICAL ALERTS
Serial nutritional assessment	
To monitor nutritional status in malnourished people or in those at risk for malnutrition, serial measurements of nutritional assessment parameters are made at routine intervals. At a minimum, weight and dietary intake should be evaluated weekly. Because the other nutritional assessment parameters change more slowly, data on these indicators may be collected every two weeks or monthly.	Based on the findings of the nutritional assessment, the type of malnutrition can be diagnosed. The four major types of malnutrition are: • obesity • marasmus • kwashiorkor • marasmus–kwashiorkor mix. See Tables 21.3, 21.4, 21.13 and 21.14. Each type of malnutrition has characteristic clinical and laboratory findings and a distinct cause.

Abnormal findings for advanced practice

TABLE 21.12 Swellings on the neck

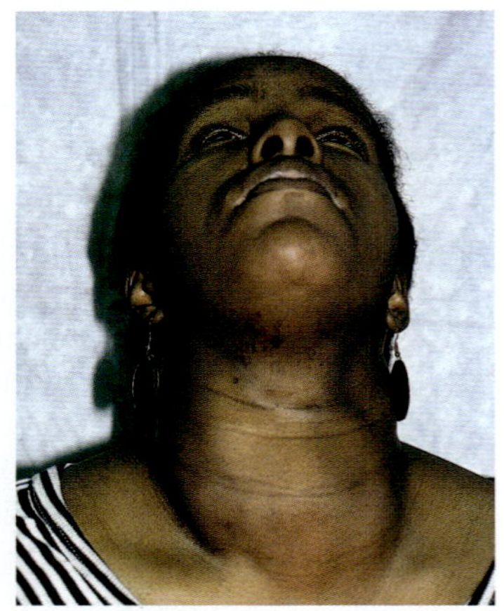

Thyroid—multiple nodules

Multiple nodules usually indicate inflammation or a multi-nodular goitre rather than a neoplasm. However, suspect any rapidly enlarging or firm nodule.

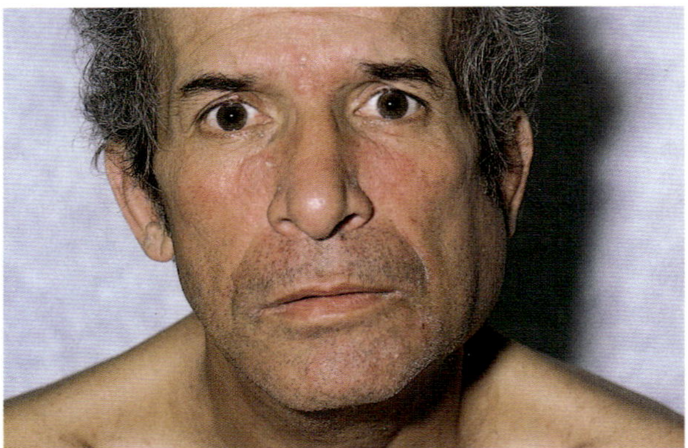

Parotid gland enlargement

Rapid painful inflammation of the parotid occurs with mumps. Parotid swelling also occurs with blockage of a duct, abscess or tumour. Note swelling anterior to lower ear lobe. Stensen's duct obstruction can occur in ageing adults dehydrated from diuretics or anticholinergics.

TABLE 21.13 Metabolic syndrome

MetS criteria—16 years or older

Metabolic syndrome (MetS) is a group of conditions that increase the risk of stroke, diabetes and heart disease syndrome. Signs include hypertension, hyperglycaemia, excess fat around the waist and abnormal cholesterol levels. Having three of these five biomarkers signifies MetS.

Its prevalence is estimated to be nearly 20% in adults aged 20 to 39 years, nearly 40% in adults aged 40 to 59 years and more than 48% in people older than 60 years of age.

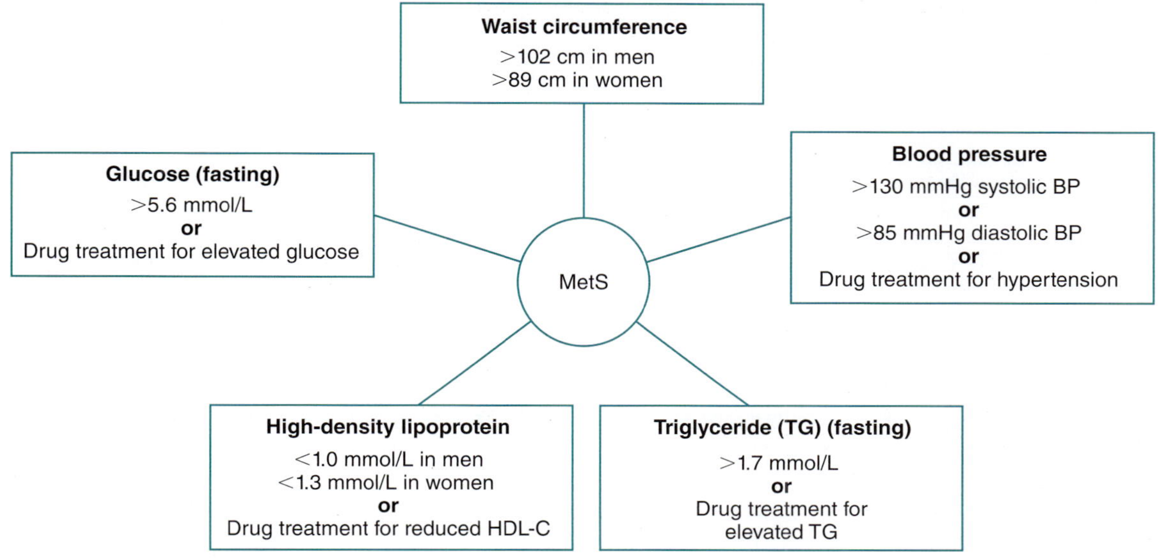

Source: Grodner et al. 2022[15]

TABLE 21.14 Paediatric Metabolic syndrome (PMetS) (6–16 years)

A standard definition of PMetS has not been adopted, but the International Diabetes Foundation recommends using the criteria in the diagram below for the diagnosis of PMetS in children aged 10 years to younger than 16 years. There is no recommendation for diagnosing PMetS in children under 10 years of age. Instead, healthcare providers must educate on the risk of PMetS and encourage lifestyle changes in young children. Having three or more of the biomarkers signifies PMetS in children 10 years of age to younger than 16 years of age.

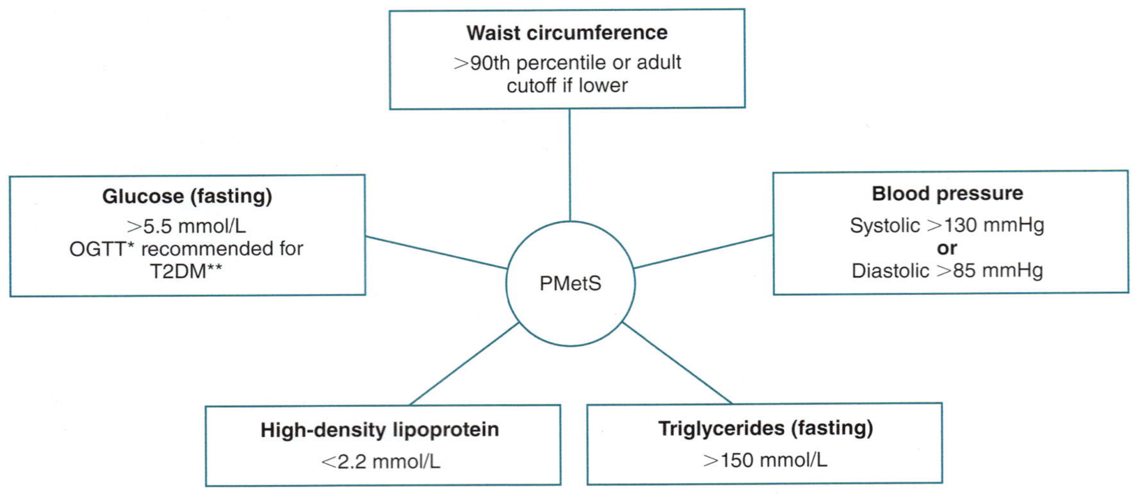

*OGTT = oral glucose tolerance test; *T2DM = type 2 diabetes

Sources: Detsky et al. 1987[16], Mancini 2009[17] and Xi et al. 2020[18]

Clinical reasoning and documentation

The following is a continuation of the case study provided at the beginning of this chapter and the initial clinical reasoning process including problem/issue identification and documentation of clinical data. Consult a fundamentals of nursing or medical-surgical nursing text for information about goal setting, nursing interventions and evaluation.

Case study (continued)—Type 1 diabetes

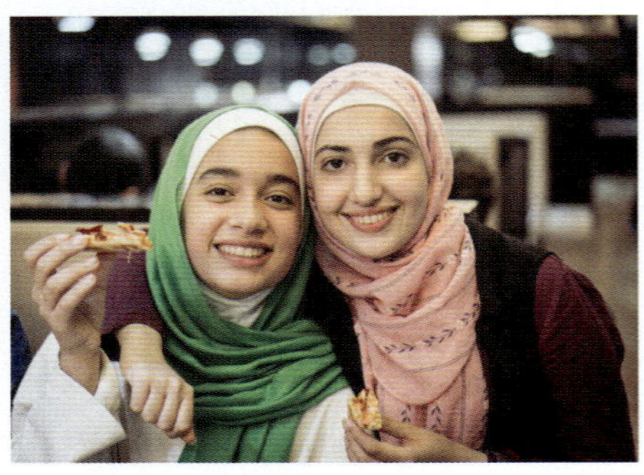

Context

You will recall from earlier in the chapter you are the registered nurse working within a multidisciplinary health team in a general practice setting. As previously stated, your responsibilities include assessing people with chronic health problems and reviewing the plan of care.

Consider the patient's situation

Lisa, aged 15 years, was diagnosed with type 1 diabetes when she was 13 years old. Her parents are divorced and they co-parent. She is an only child and spends quite a lot of time alone because both parents have jobs that have them working after hours. Her mother is not only concerned that Lisa has not been checking blood glucose levels regularly but that she skips school sometimes.

Collection cues/information

Your further assessment reveals the following information.

Clinical reasoning and documentation cont'd

Subjective data

Lisa states that she has lots of friends and she catches up with them after school and frequents a local fast-food restaurant. She often must cook her own evening meals and states that she doesn't have time to do frequent blood glucose checks.

Objective data

General appearance is a well-looking teenager.
Height is 166.4 cm. Current weight is 50.9 kg. BMI: 18.
HbA_{1c} 8% (10.2 mmol) which is slightly elevated.
Lisa's insulin administration technique and blood glucose checks were performed accurately.

Process information and identify problems/issues

Collaborative problem

Altered health maintenance type 1 diabetes related to elevated HbA_{1c} level.

Problem statement/nursing diagnoses

Ineffective health maintenance related to incomplete diabetes management.
Risk for unstable blood glucose levels related to incomplete diabetes management.
Risk for altered nutrition: eating less than body needs.

ADDITIONAL RESOURCES

You can further develop your knowledge and skills relevant to nutrition and metabolic assessment, related pathophysiology, common health issues and nursing interventions by:

- reading chapters of a fundamentals of nursing or medical-surgical nursing textbook
- answering chapter multiple choice questions online. Log onto ClinicalKey Student and search for the text 'Health Assessment, 4th edition'. Choose the section titled 'Teaching material'. In this section you will find question and answer documents for each chapter. Please check instructions on the inside front cover of the book to access online resources
- visiting websites

  Dietitians Australia: https://dietitiansaustralia.org.au/

  Food Standards Australia and New Zealand: https://www.foodstandards.gov.au/industry/npc/Pages/nutrition-panel-calculator.aspx

  National Center for Complementary and Alternative Medicine: http://nccih.nih.gov/

  National Institute of Diabetes and Digestive and Kidney Diseases: https://www.niddk.nih.gov/health-information/digestive-diseases

  Nutrition Australia: https://nutritionaustralia.org/

REFERENCES

1. Malnutrition Advisory Group, British Association for Parenteral and Enteral Nutrition. Malnutrition universal screening tool. 2013. Available at: https://www.bapen.org.uk/pdfs/must/must_full.pdf
2. Morris NF, Stewart S, Riley MD, Maguire GP. A comparison of two malnutrition screening tools in acute medical inpatients and validation of a screening tool among adult Indigenous Australian patients. Asia Pacific Journal of Clinical Nutrition 2018;27(6):1198–1206. doi: 10.6133/apjcn.201811_27(6).0005
3. Australian Institute of Health and Welfare (AIHW). Congenital abnormalities in Australia. 2023. Available at: https://www.aihw.gov.au/reports/mothers-babies/congenital-anomalies-in-australia/contents/at-a-glance
4. Australian Institute of Health and Welfare (AIHW). Overweight and obesity. 2023. Available at: https://www.aihw.gov.au/reports-data/behaviours-risk-factors/overweight-obesity/overview
5. Jaul E, Barron J, Rosenzweig JP, Menczel J. An overview of co-morbidities and the development of pressure ulcers among older adults. BMC Geriatrics 2018;18:305–315. doi: 10.1186/s12877-018-0997-7
6. Australian Institute of Health and Welfare (AIHW). Oral health and dental care in Australia. Canberra: AIHW; 2023. Available at: https://www.aihw.gov.au/reports/dental-oral-health/oral-health-and-dental-care-in-australia/contents/dental-care
7. Ministry of Health New Zealand. Annual update of key findings 2021/22: New Zealand Health Survey. Wellington: Ministry of Health; 2022. Available at: https://www.health.govt.nz/publication/annual-update-key-results-2021-22-new-zealand-health-survey
8. Lee A, Rainbow S, Tregenza J, Tregenza L, Balmer L, Bryce S, et al. Nutrition in remote Aboriginal communities: lessons from Mai Wiru and the Anangu Pitjantjatjara Yankunytjatjara Lands. Australian and New Zealand Journal of Public Health 2016;40(Suppl.1):S81–S88. doi: 10.1111/1753-6405.12419
9. Cheney K, Berkemeier S, Sim KA, Gordon A, Black K. Prevalence and predictors of early gestational weight gain associated with obesity risk in a diverse Australian antenatal population: a cross-sectional study. BMC Pregnancy Childbirth 2017;17:296. doi: 10.1186/s12884-017-1482-6
10. Talley NJ, O'Connor S. Clinical examination. 9th ed. Chatswood, NSW: Elsevier; 2021.
11. Kiss N, Loeliger J, Findlay M, Isenring E, Baguley BJ, Boltong A, et al. Clinical Oncology Society of Australia: Position statement on cancer-related malnutrition and sarcopenia. Nutrition and Dietetics 2020;77(4):416–425. Doi: 10.1111/17470080.12631
12. Dent E, Wright O, Woo J, Hoogendijk EO. Malnutrition in older adults. The Lancet 2023;41:951–966. doi: 10.1016/S0140-6736(22)02612-5
13. World Health Organization (WHO) 2023. Obesity and Overweight. Available at: https://www.who.int/data/gho/data/themes/topics/topic-details/GHO/body-mass-index
14. Cameron AJ, Magliano DJ, Zimmet PZ, Welborn T, Shaw JE. The metabolic syndrome in Australia: prevalence using four definitions. Diabetes research and clinical practice. 2007 Sep 1;77(3):471–478.
15. Grodner MS, Escott-Stump S, Dorner S. Nutritional foundations and clinical applications. 8th ed. Chatswood, NSW: Elsevier; 2022
16. Detsky AJ, McLaughlin JR, Baker JP, Johnston N, Whittaker S, Mendelson RA, et al. What is subjective global assessment of nutritional status? Journal of Parenteral and Enteral Nutrition, 1987, 11 (1):8–13. doi: 10.1177/014860718701100108
17. Mancini MC. Metabolic syndrome in children and adolescents: criteria for diagnosis. Diabetology & Metabolic Syndrome, 1, 20 (2009). https://doi.org/10.1186/1758-5996-1-20
18. Xi B, Zong XN, Kelishadi R, Litwin M, Hong YM, Poh BK, et al. International waist circumference percentile cutoffs for central obesity in children and adolescents aged 6 to 18 years. The Journal of Clinical Endocrinology & Metabolism. 2020 Apr;105(4):e1569– e1583.

CHAPTER 22

Skin, hair and nails assessment

Written by Carolyn Jarvis
Adapted by Trish Burton

INTRODUCTION

Think of the skin as the body's largest organ system—it covers 6.01 m^2 of surface area in an average adult. The skin is the sentry that guards the body from environmental stresses (e.g. trauma, pathogens, dirt) and adapts it to other environmental influences (e.g. heat, cold). We assess the skin in nearly every area of health assessment. Because nutrition is very important to the health of the skin, hair and nails, please also refer to Chapter 21. Assessing the skin, hair and nails is an important part of health assessment. Skin integrity refers to intact structure and function and relies on adequate perfusion by oxygenated blood and adequate nutrition and hydration.

Case study

The following case study gives an example of a typical situation involving a skin, nails and hair assessment and the initial clinical reasoning process. The case study will help you identify your learning needs.

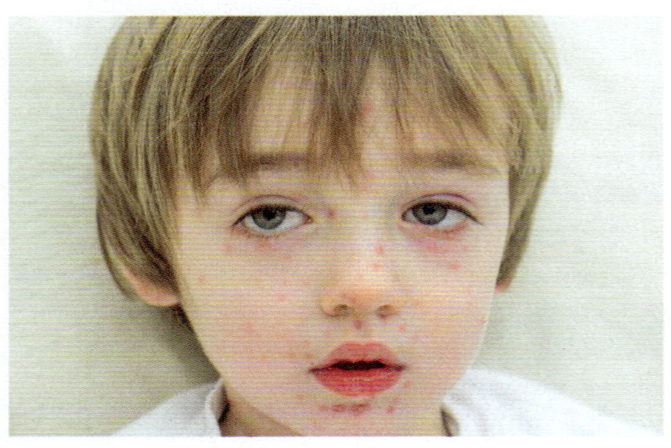

Context

You are a registered nurse in a general practice clinic performing an initial health assessment before consulting with a GP.

Consider the patient's situation

Ethan Evans, aged 3 years, attends the clinic with his mother Janet. Janet is worried because Ethan has had a fever, fatigue and a rash for the past 3 days.

Questions to further your learning

- What are the possible things that might be going on with Ethan?
- What knowledge do you need to be able to predict what might be going on?
- What approach to Ethan's health assessment will you take?
- What questions (subjective data) will you ask Janet and Ethan to extend the health history and why?
- What physical examination (objective data) will you conduct and why?
- What resources are available to assist in your assessment of Ethan?

Assessment plan

Changes in skin integrity may indicate alterations in perfusion and oxygenation, nutrition and hydration. Altered skin integrity can also occur because of reduced mobility, mechanical or chemical factors, extremes of temperature, bodily excretions or secretions and humidity or exposure to bacterial and viral infections. The main areas for subjective data are:

- presenting concern
- previous history of skin disease
- change in pigmentation

- change in a mole
- excessive dryness or moisture
- presence of pruritus
- presence of excessive bruising
- presence of a rash or lesion
- hair loss
- change in the nails
- environmental or occupational hazards
- health and lifestyle management.

Following subjective data collection, you will get a sense of the areas needed to be examined for objective data. Only the relevant areas should be examined. The main areas for physical examination and measurement are:

- general inspection
- inspecting and palpating the skin
- assessing for pressure injuries
- wound assessment
- inspecting and palpating the hair and scalp
- inspecting and palpating the nails.

Resources available

You will find additional resources and the reference list at the end of this chapter.

Structure and function

Skin

The skin has two layers: the outer highly differentiated *epidermis* and the inner supportive *dermis* (Figure 22.1). Beneath these layers is a third layer: the *subcutaneous* layer of adipose tissue.

The *epidermis* is thin but tough. Its cells are bound tightly together into sheets that form a rugged protective barrier. It is stratified into several zones. The inner **stratum germinativum**, or basal cell layer, forms new skin cells. Their major ingredient is the tough, fibrous protein *keratin*. The melanocytes interspersed along this layer produce the pigment *melanin*, which gives brown tones to the skin and hair. All people have the same number of melanocytes, but the amount of melanin they produce varies with genetic, hormonal and environmental influences.

From the basal layer, the new cells migrate up and flatten into the **stratum corneum**. This outer horny cell layer consists of dead keratinised cells that are interwoven and closely packed. The cells are constantly being shed or desquamated and are replaced with new cells from below. The epidermis is completely replaced every 4 weeks. In fact, each person sheds about half a kilogram of skin each year.

The epidermis is uniformly thin except on the surfaces that are exposed to friction, such as the palms and the soles. On these surfaces, skin is thicker because of work and weight bearing. The epidermis is avascular; it is nourished by blood vessels in the dermis below.

Skin colour is derived from three sources: (1) mainly from the brown pigment melanin, (2) also from the yellow-orange tones of the pigment carotene and (3) from the red-purple tones in the underlying vascular bed. All people have skin of varying shades of brown, yellow and red; the relative proportion of these shades affects the prevailing colour. Skin colour is further modified by the thickness of the skin and by the presence of oedema.

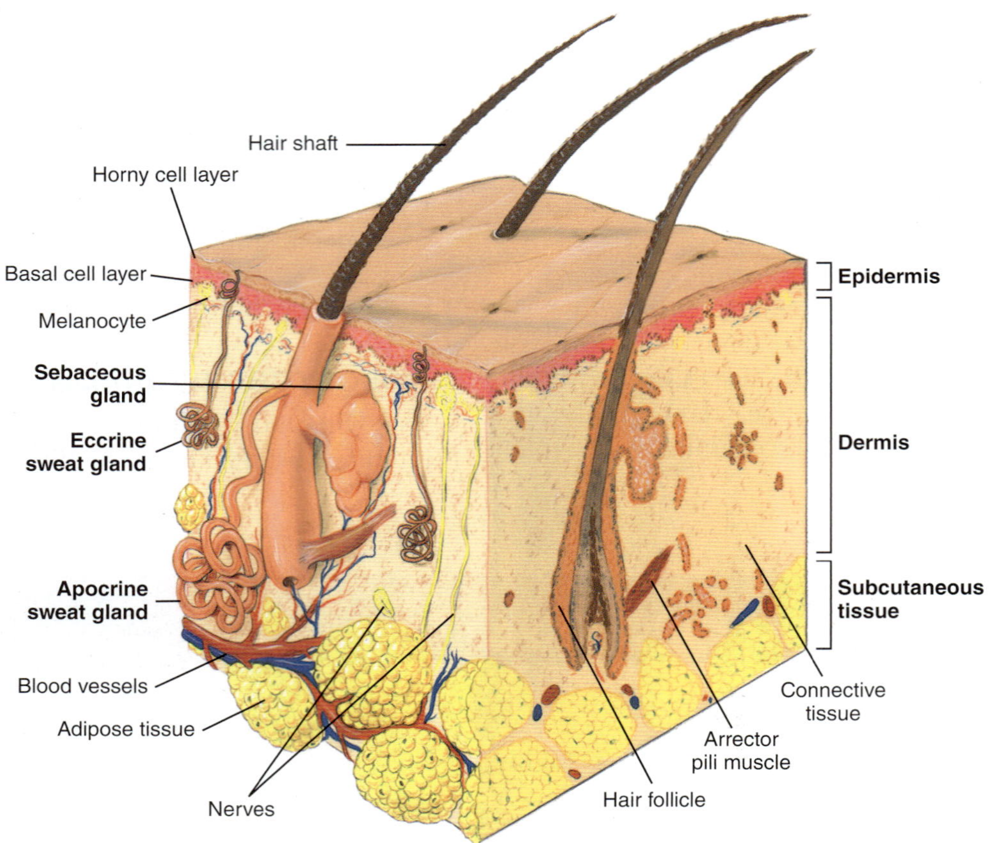

FIGURE 22.1 The two layers of the skin.

DERMIS

The *dermis* is the inner supportive layer consisting mostly of connective tissue, or *collagen.* This is the tough, fibrous protein that enables the skin to resist tearing. The dermis also has resilient elastic tissue that allows the skin to stretch with body movements. The nerves, sensory receptors, blood vessels and lymphatics lie in the dermis. Also, appendages from the epidermis—such as the hair follicles, sebaceous glands and sweat glands—are embedded in the dermis.

SUBCUTANEOUS LAYER

The *subcutaneous layer* is adipose tissue, which is made up of lobules of fat cells. The subcutaneous tissue stores fat for energy, provides insulation for temperature control and aids in protection by its soft, cushioning effect. Also, the loose subcutaneous layer gives skin its increased mobility over structures underneath.

Epidermal appendages

These structures are formed by a tubular invagination of the epidermis down into the underlying dermis.

HAIR

Hair is *vestigial* for humans; it is no longer needed for protection from cold or trauma. However, hair is highly significant in most cultures for its cosmetic and psychological meaning (see 'Cultural and social considerations' below).

Hairs are threads of keratin. The hair *shaft* is the visible projecting part, and the *root* is below the surface embedded in the follicle. At the root the *bulb matrix* is the expanded area where new cells are produced at a high rate. Hair growth is cyclical, with active and resting phases. Each follicle functions independently, so that while some hairs are resting, others are growing. Around the hair follicle are the muscular *arrector pili*, which contract and elevate the hair so it resembles 'goose flesh' when the skin is exposed to cold or in emotional states.

People have two types of hair. Fine, faint **vellus hair** covers most of the body (except the palms and soles, the dorsa of the distal parts of the fingers, the umbilicus, the glans penis and inside the labia). The other type is **terminal hair**, the darker thicker hair that grows on the scalp and eyebrows and, after puberty, on the axillae and the pubic area in both males and females and on the face and chest in males.

NAILS

The nails are hard plates of keratin on the dorsal edges of the fingers and toes (Figure 22.2). The nail plate is clear, with fine longitudinal ridges that become prominent in ageing. Nails take their pink colour from the underlying nail bed of highly vascular epithelial cells. The lunula is the white opaque semilunar area at the proximal end of the nail. It lies over the nail matrix where new keratinised cells are formed. The nail folds overlap the posterior and lateral borders. The cuticle works like a gasket to cover and protect the nail matrix.

SEBACEOUS GLANDS

These glands produce a protective lipid substance, *sebum*, which is secreted through the hair follicles. Sebum oils and lubricates the skin and hair and forms an emulsion with water that retards water loss from the skin. (Dry skin results from loss of water, not directly from loss of oil.) Sebaceous glands are everywhere except on the palms and soles. They are most abundant in the scalp, forehead, face and chin.

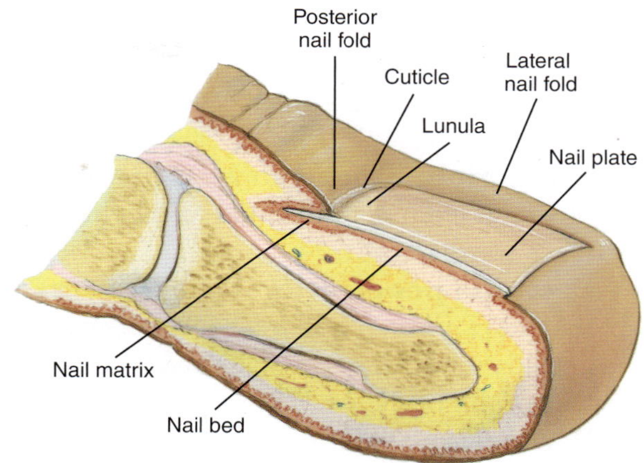

FIGURE 22.2 The nails

SWEAT GLANDS

There are two types. The **eccrine** glands are coiled tubules that open directly onto the skin surface and produce a dilute saline solution—*sweat*. The evaporation of sweat reduces body temperature. Eccrine glands are widely distributed through the body and are mature in infants at 2 months old.

The **apocrine** glands produce a thick, milky secretion and open into the hair follicles. They are located mainly in the axillae, anogenital area, nipples and navel and are vestigial in humans. They become active during puberty and secretion occurs with emotional and sexual stimulation. Bacterial flora living on the skin's surface react with apocrine sweat to produce a characteristic musky body odour. The functioning of apocrine glands decreases in older adults.

Function of the skin

The skin is a waterproof, almost indestructible covering that has protective and adaptive properties:

- **Protection.** Skin minimises injury from physical, chemical, thermal and light wave sources.
- **Prevents penetration.** Skin is a barrier that stops invasion of microorganisms and loss of water and electrolytes from within the body.
- **Perception.** Skin is a vast sensory surface holding the neurosensory end-organs for touch, pain, temperature and pressure.
- **Temperature regulation.** Skin allows heat dissipation through sweat glands and heat storage through subcutaneous insulation.
- **Identification.** People identify one another by unique combinations of facial characteristics, hair, skin colour and even fingerprints. Self-image is often enhanced or deterred by the way society's standards of beauty measure up to each person's perceived characteristics.
- **Communication.** Emotions are expressed in the sign language of the face and in the body posture. Vascular mechanisms such as blushing or blanching also signal emotional states.
- **Wound repair.** Skin allows cell replacement of surface wounds.
- **Absorption and excretion.** Skin allows limited excretion of some metabolic wastes, by-products of cellular decomposition such as minerals, sugars, amino acids, cholesterol, uric acid and urea.
- **Production of vitamin D.** The skin is the surface on which ultraviolet (UV) light converts cholesterol into vitamin D.

Developmental considerations

Infancy to adolescence (birth to 19 years)

The hair follicles develop in a fetus at 3 months' gestation; by mid-gestation most of the skin is covered with **lanugo**, the fine downy hair of a newborn infant. In the first few months after birth, this is replaced by fine vellus hair. Terminal hair on the scalp, if present at birth, tends to be soft and to suffer a patchy loss, especially at the temples and occiput. Also present at birth is **vernix caseosa**: the thick, cheesy substance made up of sebum and shed epithelial cells.

A newborn's skin is similar in structure to an adult's, but many of its functions are not fully developed. A newborn's skin is thin, smooth and elastic and is relatively more permeable than that of adults, so infants are at greater risk for fluid loss. Sebum, which holds water in the skin, is present for the first few weeks of life, producing milia and cradle cap in some babies. Then sebaceous glands decrease in size and production and do not resume functioning until puberty. Temperature regulation is ineffective. Eccrine sweat glands do not secrete in response to heat until the first few months of life and then only minimally throughout childhood. The skin cannot protect much against cold because it cannot contract and shiver and because the subcutaneous layer is inefficient. Also, the pigment system is inefficient at birth.

As a child grows, the epidermis thickens, toughens and darkens and the skin becomes better lubricated. Hair growth accelerates. At puberty, secretion from apocrine sweat glands increases in response to heat and emotional stimuli, producing body odour. Sebaceous glands become more active—the skin looks oily, and acne develops. Subcutaneous fat deposits increase, especially in females.

Secondary sex characteristics that appear during adolescence are evident in the integument (i.e. skin). In females, the diameter of the areola enlarges and darkens, and breast tissue develops. Coarse pubic hair develops in males and females, then axillary hair, then coarse facial hair in males.

Pregnant women

The change in hormone levels results in increased pigment in the areolae and nipples, vulva and sometimes in the midline of the abdomen (**linea nigra**) or in the face (**chloasma**). Hyperestrogenaemia probably also causes the common vascular spiders and palmar erythema. Connective tissue develops increased fragility, resulting in **striae gravidarum**, which may develop in the skin of the abdomen, breasts or thighs. Metabolism is increased in pregnancy; to dissipate heat, the peripheral vasculature dilates, and the sweat and sebaceous glands increase secretion. Fat deposits are laid down, particularly in the buttocks and hips, as maternal reserves for nursing a baby. For more information see Chapter 29.

Late adulthood (65+ years)

The skin is a mirror that reflects ageing changes that proceed in *all* our organ systems; it just happens to be the one organ we can view directly. The ageing process carries a slow atrophy of skin structures. The ageing skin loses its elasticity; it folds and sags. By the 70s to 80s, it looks parchment thin, lax, dry and wrinkled.

The epidermis's outer layer, the *stratum corneum*, thins and flattens. This allows chemicals easier access into the body. Wrinkling occurs because the underlying dermis thins and flattens. A loss of elastin, collagen and subcutaneous fat occurs as well as a reduction in muscle tone. The loss of collagen increases the risk for shearing, tearing injuries.

Sweat glands and sebaceous glands decrease in number and function, leaving dry skin. Decreased response of the sweat glands to thermoregulatory demand also puts older people at greater risk for heat stroke. The vascularity of the skin diminishes while the vascular fragility increases; a minor trauma may produce dark red, discoloured areas, or **senile purpura**.

Sun exposure and, to a lesser extent, cigarette smoking further accentuate ageing changes in the skin. Coarse wrinkling, decreased elasticity, atrophy, speckled and uneven colouring, more pigment changes and a yellowed, leathery texture occur. Chronic sun damage is even more prominent in pale or light-skinned people.

An accumulation of factors put older people at risk for skin disease and breakdown: the thinning of the skin, the decrease in vascularity and nutrients, the loss of protective cushioning of the subcutaneous layer, a lifetime of environmental trauma to skin, the social changes of ageing (e.g. less nutrition, limited financial resources), the increasingly sedentary lifestyle and the chance of immobility. When skin breakdown does occur, subsequent cell replacement is slower, and wound healing is delayed.

In the ageing hair matrix, the number of functioning melanocytes decreases, so the hair looks grey or white and feels thin and fine. A person's genetic script determines the onset of greying and the number of grey hairs. Hair distribution changes. Males may have a symmetrical W-shaped balding in the frontal areas. Some testosterone is present in both males and females; as it decreases with age, axillary and pubic hair decrease. As a female's estrogen also decreases, testosterone is unopposed, and females may develop some bristly facial hairs. Nails grow more slowly. Their surface is lustreless and is characterised by longitudinal ridges resulting from local trauma at the nail matrix.

Because ageing changes in the skin and hair can be viewed directly, they carry a profound psychological impact. For many people, self-esteem is linked to a youthful appearance. This view is compounded by media advertising in Western society. Although sagging and wrinkling skin and greying and thinning hair are usual processes of ageing, they prompt a loss of self-esteem for many adults.

Cultural and social considerations

Awareness of biocultural differences and the ability to recognise the unique clinical manifestations of disease are especially important when dealing with people with dark-pigmented skin. As described earlier, melanin is responsible for the various colours and tones of skin observed among people from culturally diverse backgrounds. Melanin protects the skin against harmful UV rays, a genetic advantage accounting for the lower incidence of skin cancer in people with dark-pigmented skin. The incidence of melanoma is higher among Caucasians than among people with dark-pigmented skin.

Areas of the skin affected by hormones and, in some cases, differing for culturally diverse people are the sexual skin areas such as the nipples, areola, scrotum and labia majora. In general, these areas are darker than other parts of the skin in both adults and children.

The apocrine and eccrine sweat glands are important for fluid balance and for thermoregulation. When apocrine gland secretions are contaminated by normal skin flora, odour results. The amount of chloride excreted by sweat glands varies widely.

While the characteristics of hair vary widely between people, hair condition is significant in diagnosing and treating certain disease states. For example, hair texture becomes dry, brittle and lacking in lustre with inadequate nutrition.

HEALTH EDUCATION

Artificial tanning and skin cancer risk

There are many documented adverse effects of skin tanning, whether it is by exposure to UV rays from sunlight or from sunbeds/tanning beds. It is well known that prolonged sun exposure can lead to skin cancer. Exposure to UV rays on the skin causes suppression of cutaneous DNA repair and immune functioning, ocular disorders and increased risk of skin cancer, specifically squamous/basal cell carcinoma and melanoma. Also, the amount of UVA light received in a tanning salon may be two to three times more than the UVA light received from the sun and is a known risk factor for melanoma. Before the national ban of commercial solariums in 2015, the Cancer Council of Australia reported that there were approximately 281 melanoma cases and 43 melanoma-related deaths each year.[1] While it is illegal to operate commercial solariums (sunbeds and tanning beds) in Australia, Aotearoa New Zealand has implemented age restrictions where anyone under 18 years cannot be given access to a

HEALTH EDUCATION cont'd

solarium. The Aotearoa New Zealand regulations do not control the proportion of UVB emitted, however. Most tanning salons promote their devices as emitting UVA light, which is thought to be 'safer' than UVB light, but this is not the case. UVA light penetrates the skin more deeply and is strongly linked to melanoma.[1]

While Australian melanoma rates have been decreasing for people under 40 years, rates for those 50 years or older continue to rise. There has been an overall increase from 54 cases per 100,000 people in 2000 to an estimated 69 cases per 100,000 people in 2023. In 2023 the estimated age-adjusted mortality rate was five deaths per 100,000 people.[2] Aotearoa New Zealand melanoma rates are also unacceptably high, with Aotearoa New Zealand having approximately 35 to 40 people per 100,000 population diagnosed annually.[3]

Although one of the sources of vitamin D is exposure to UV light, an adequate level of vitamin D is typically attained through incidental exposure to the sun and normal dietary intake of vitamin D. Sources of vitamin D that do not carry an increased risk of skin cancer include vitamin D supplements or food sources supplemented with vitamin D.

Nurse's role: Teach skin protection and self-examination

Nurses are in an ideal position to educate people about the dangers of excessive UV exposure. As you examine a person's skin:

- ask about sun exposure, tanning practices and sun-protective precautions
- show how to examine skin using the ABCDE rules (Figure 22.3) to identify suspicious lesions, in good light with appropriate mirrors

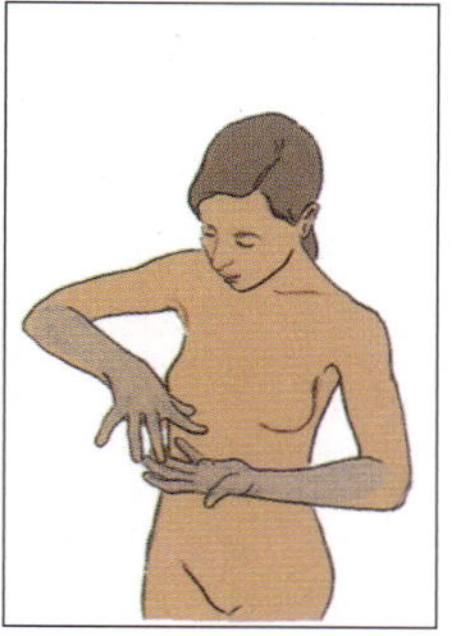

1. Undress completely. Check forearms, palms, space between fingers. Turn over hands and study the backs.

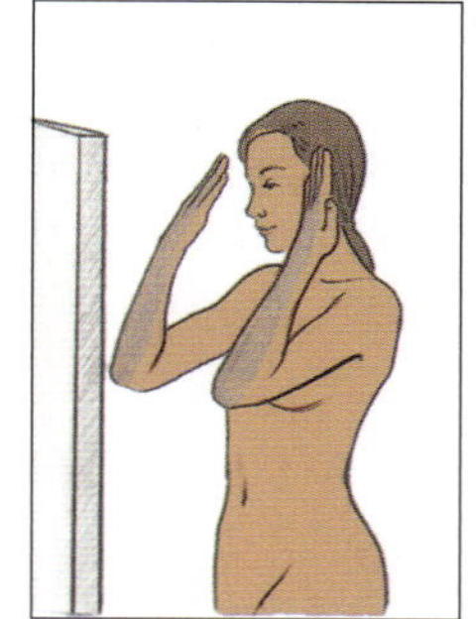

2. Face mirror; bend arms at elbow. Study arms in mirror.

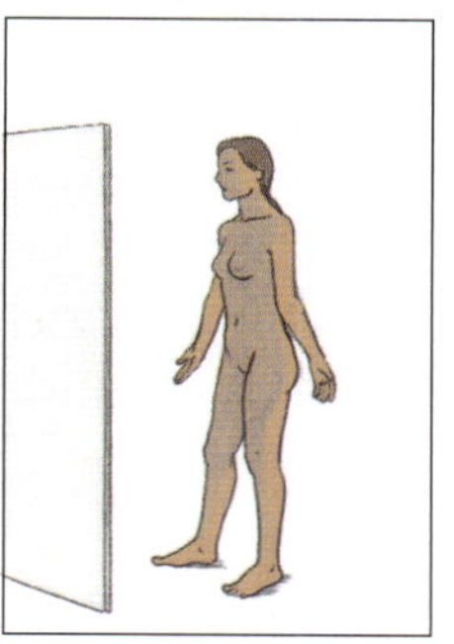

3. Face mirror and study entire front of body. Start at face, neck, torso, working down to lower legs.

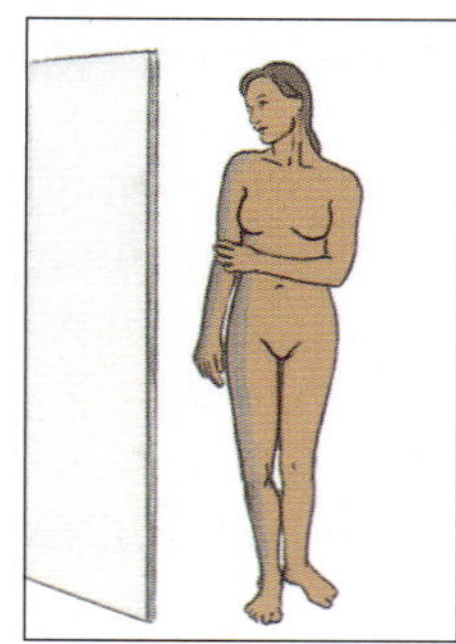

4. Pivot to right side facing mirror. Study sides of upper arms, working down to ankles. Repeat with left side.

5. With back to mirror, study buttocks, thighs, lower legs.

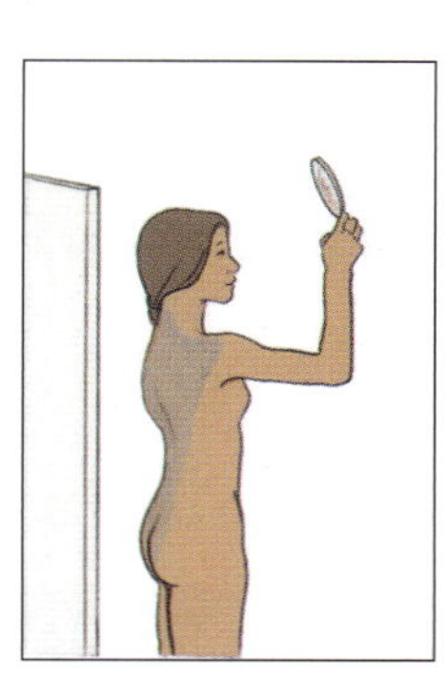

6. Use the handheld mirror to study upper back.

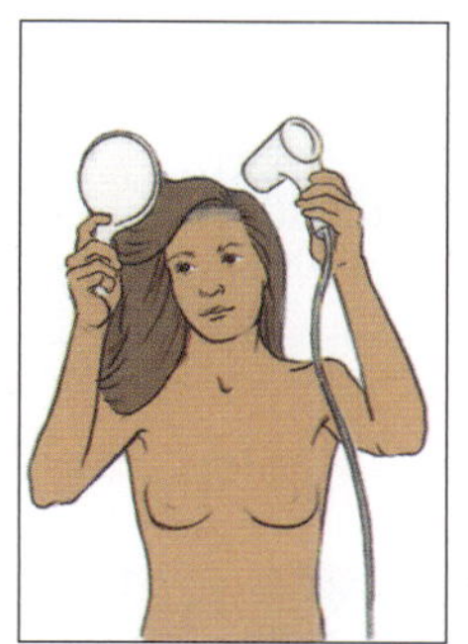

7. Use the handheld mirror to study scalp, lifting the hair. A blow-dryer on a cool setting helps to lift hair.

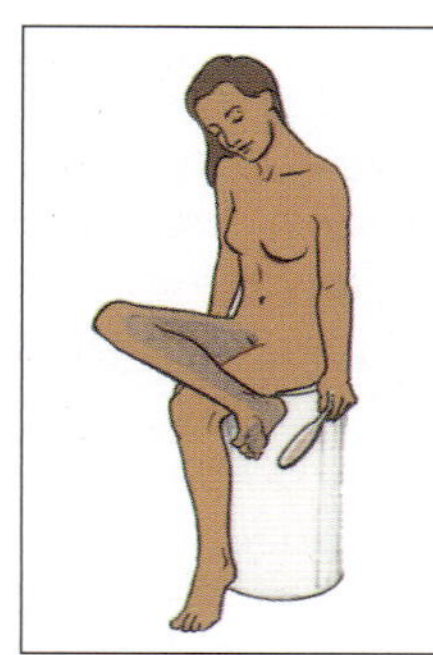

8. Sit on chair or bed. Study insides of each leg and soles of feet. Use the small mirror to help.

FIGURE 22.3 Teaching skin self-examination

HEALTH EDUCATION cont'd

- get help from another person to examine difficult areas (e.g. behind the ears, the back of the neck, the back)
- report any suspicious lesions promptly to their GP or practice nurse
- remind the person about sun protection using Slip, Slop, Slap
- refer people to the following websites:
  - Australian Skin and Skin Cancer Research Institute—balancing the harms and benefits of sun exposure: https://www.assc.org.au/wp-content/uploads/2023/01/Sun-Exposure-Summit-PositionStatement_V1.9.pdf
  - Cancer Council Australia—sun exposure and vitamin D: risks and benefits: https://www.cancer.org.au/about-us/policy-and-advocacy/position-statements/sunsmart#jump_3
  - Cancer Council Australia—sun safety: https://www.cancer.org.au/cancer-information/causes-and-prevention/sun-safety
  - Ministry of Health New Zealand—sunbeds: https://www.tewhatuora.govt.nz/our-health-system/environmental-health/sunbeds
  - Melanoma New Zealand—protect your skin year-round: https://melanoma.org.nz/

Subjective data

Altered skin integrity often results in pain and discomfort, putting the person at risk of infection. Altered skin integrity can also affect the person's coping and stress tolerance as well as affecting the ability to undertake daily activities including exercise, their sleep and rest, self-concept and self-perception, roles and relationships and sexuality.

Practice note

Before you start the assessment, introduce yourself to the person, confirm the person's identity, discuss the purpose and scope of the assessment, clarify any questions the person may have and get verbal consent from the person to perform the assessment.

ASSESSMENT GUIDELINES	CLINICAL SIGNIFICANCE AND CLINICAL ALERTS
Presenting concern	
• *Do you have any problems with your skin, hair or nails?* It is important to ascertain the person's perception of the health of their skin, hair and nails. If they do perceive a problem, ask: *How does this affect your quality of life?*	The person's response to this question will guide areas to focus on in further subjective and objective data collection.
Previous history of skin disease	
• *Have you had any previous skin disease or problem? How was this treated? Is there any family history of allergies or allergic skin problem?*	Some skin disorders have genetic or familial links such as allergies, **hay fever, psoriasis, atopic dermatitis** (eczema) and **acne.**

ASSESSMENT GUIDELINES	CLINICAL SIGNIFICANCE AND CLINICAL ALERTS
• *Do you have any allergies to drugs, plants, animals or foods?*	Identify offending allergens. Allergic reactions may result in skin symptoms such as redness, swelling and **pruritus**.
• *Do you have any birthmarks, tattoos or piercings?*	Using nonsterile equipment to apply tattoos increases the risk of **hepatitis C**.
Change in pigmentation	
• *Have you noticed any change in skin colour or pigmentation?*	Skin colour will vary from pink to dark brown. Exposed areas are often darker than non-exposed areas. **Hypopigmentation** is loss of pigmentation. **Hyperpigmentation** (increase in colour) such as freckles on the face and arms is common in people with pale skin.
• *Is the change in pigmentation generalised (all over) or localised?*	Generalised change suggests systemic illness: • **Pallor** (pale colour) may be caused by anaemia or vasoconstriction. • **Erythema** (red colour). Local redness of the skin indicates local inflammation, whereas generalised erythema is often related to systemic vasodilatation. • **Cyanosis** (blue colour) of the oral mucous membranes and lips results from hypoxaemia. Cyanosis of the extremities results from reduced peripheral blood flow. • **Jaundice** (yellow colour) is caused by changes in metabolism of bilirubin.
Change in a mole	
• *Have you noticed any change in a mole: colour, size, shape, sudden appearance of tenderness, bleeding, itching?* • *Do you have any 'sores' that do not heal?*	The person may be unaware of changes in a mole, especially if it is in an area that they cannot see such as on their back, buttocks, scalp, soles of the feet or between toes. ! ***Clinical alert:*** Any changes in the colour, size or edges or development of itchiness or bleeding could be signs of malignancy and should be referred to a medical practitioner for further assessment.[4]

ASSESSMENT GUIDELINES	CLINICAL SIGNIFICANCE AND CLINICAL ALERTS
Excessive dryness or moisture	
• *Has there been any change in the feel of your skin: temperature, moisture, texture?*	**Seborrhoea**—oily skin.
• *Have you noticed excess dryness? Is this seasonal or constant?*	**Xerosis**—dry skin.
Pruritus	
• *Have you had any skin itching? Is this mild (prickling, tingling) or intense (intolerable)?* • *Does it awaken you from sleep?*	**Pruritus** is the most common of skin symptoms. It occurs with dry skin, ageing, drug reactions, allergy, obstructive jaundice, uraemia, lice or other skin infestations.
• *Where is the itching? When did it start?*	The presence or absence of pruritus may be significant for diagnosis. Scratching may cause excoriation of a primary lesion.
• *Do you have any other skin pain or soreness? Where?*	
Excessive bruising	
• *Do you have any excess bruising? Where are the bruises?* • *How did this happen?* • *How long have you had it?*	With multiple cuts and bruises, bruises in various stages of healing, bruises above the knees and elbows and illogical explanation—consider the possibility of abuse. Frequent falls may be due to dizziness of neurological or cardiovascular origin. Also, frequent minor trauma may be a side effect of alcoholism or other drug abuse.
Rashes or lesions	
• *Have you had a skin rash or lesion?* **Onset** • *When did you first notice it?*	Rashes are a common reason for seeking health care. A careful history is important; it may be an accurate predictor of the type of lesion you will see in the examination and its cause.[5]
Location • *Where did it start?*	Identify the primary site—it may give clues as to the cause. Migration pattern, evolution.
Character or quality • *Describe the colour. Is it raised or flat? Any crust or odour? Does it feel tender or warm?* **Duration** • *How long have you had it?* **Setting**	
• *Anyone at home or work with a similar rash? Have you been camping, acquired a new pet, tried a new food or drug? Does the rash seem to come with stress?*	Identify new or relevant exposure and any household or social contacts with similar symptoms.

ASSESSMENT GUIDELINES	CLINICAL SIGNIFICANCE AND CLINICAL ALERTS
Alleviating and aggravating factors • *What home care have you tried? Bath, lotions, heat, cold? Do they help or make it worse?*	Myriad over-the-counter remedies are available. Many people try them and seek professional help only when they do not see improvement.
Associated symptoms • *Is it itchy? Have you had a fever?*	
• *What do you think the rash/lesion means?*	Assess person's perception of cause: fear of cancer, tick-borne illnesses or sexually transmitted diseases.
• *How has the rash/lesion affected your self-care, hygiene and ability to function at work/home/socially?*	Assess the effectiveness of coping strategies. Chronic skin diseases may increase the risk of loss of self-esteem, social isolation and anxiety.
• *Are there any new or increased stressors in your life?*	Stress can exacerbate chronic skin illness.
Hair loss	
• *Have you had any recent hair loss? Was it a gradual or sudden onset? Was the hair loss symmetrical? Was it associated with fever, illness or increased stress?*	**Alopecia** is a significant loss of hair. A full head of hair equates with vitality in many cultures. If treated as a trivial problem, the person may seek alternative, unproven methods of treatment.
• *Has there been any unusual hair growth?*	**Hirsutism** is shaggy or excessive hair.
• *Has there been a recent change in texture or appearance of your hair?*	
Change in nails	
• *Have there been any changes in the shape, colour or brittleness of your nails? Do you tend to bite or chew your nails?*	
Environmental or occupational hazards	
• *Have you been exposed to any environmental or occupational hazards?*	Most skin neoplasms result from occupational or environmental agents.
• *Are there any hazard-related problems with your occupation such as exposure to dyes, toxic chemicals or radiation?* • *What are your hobbies? Do you perform any household or furniture repair work that involves using paints or glues?*	People at risk include outdoor sports enthusiasts, farmers, sailors, outdoor workers; also creosote workers, tilers and coal workers.
• *How much sun exposure do you get from outdoor work, leisure activities and sunbaking?*	**Vitamin D** forms in the skin because of exposure to sunlight—in particular the UVB component of sunlight—and is important for strong healthy bones.[6] Cancer Council Australia recommends exposing the face, arms and hands or the equivalent area of skin to a few minutes of sunlight on either side of the peak UV periods on most days of the week.[7]

ASSESSMENT GUIDELINES	CLINICAL SIGNIFICANCE AND CLINICAL ALERTS
	People at risk of **vitamin D deficiency** include those who cover their skin, those with naturally very dark skin, elderly people, those who are housebound or are in institutional care and babies of vitamin D–deficient mothers. Overexposure during peak UV radiation periods (10 am to 3 pm) accelerates ageing of the skin and produces lesions. Those at high risk are light-skinned people, those over 40 years old and those regularly in the sun.[7] Using protection to prevent skin cancer when the UV index is moderate or above (i.e. UV index is 3 or higher) is recommended. Sun protection includes wearing a hat, using sunscreen and covering the skin.
• *Have you recently been bitten by an insect: bee, wasp, tick, mosquito or spider?* • *Have you had any recent exposure to plants or animals or been camping?*	Identify contactants that produce lesions or **contact dermatitis**. People with chronic recurrent **urticaria (hives)** can benefit by keeping a diary of meals and environmental contacts to identify precipitating factors.
Health and lifestyle management	
• *What do you do to care for your skin, hair and nails? What cosmetics, soaps and chemicals do you use?* • *Do you clip the cuticles on your nails or use adhesive for false fingernails?* • *If you have known allergies, how do you control your environment to minimise exposure?* • *Do you perform a skin self-examination?*	
Medications • *What medications are you taking?* • *How long have you been taking the medication?*	Drugs may: • produce allergic skin eruption: aspirin, antibiotics, barbiturates, some tonics • increase sunlight sensitivity and give a burn response: sulfonamides, thiazide diuretics, oral hypoglycaemic agents and tetracycline • cause hyperpigmentation: antimalarials, antineoplastic agents, hormones, metals and tetracycline. Even after a taking a medication for a long time, a person may develop a sensitivity to it.

ASSESSMENT GUIDELINES	CLINICAL SIGNIFICANCE AND CLINICAL ALERTS
Additional subjective data for infants and children (questions for parents or guardians)	
• *Does the child have any birthmarks?* • *Was there any change in their skin colour as a newborn?* • *Was there any jaundice? On which day after birth did it occur?* • *Has there been any cyanosis? What were the circumstances?*	
• *Have you noted any rash or sores? What seems to bring it on?*	Generalised rash—consider an allergic reaction to new food.
• *Have you introduced a new food or formula? When? Does your child eat chocolate, cow's milk or eggs?*	Irritability and general fussiness may indicate the presence of pruritus.
• *Does the child have nappy rash? How do you care for this? Do you use disposable nappies? If not, how do you wash their nappies? How often do you change their nappies? How do you clean their skin?*	Infrequent nappy changing may cause a rash. An infant may be allergic to a certain detergent or to disposable wipes.[8]
• *Does the child have any burns or bruises? Where? How did they happen?*	A careful history is important to distinguish expected childhood bumps and bruises from any lesion that may indicate child abuse or neglect: cigarette burns; excessive bruising, especially above knees or elbows; linear whip marks. With abuse, the history often will not coincide with the physical appearance and location of the lesion (Chapter 5).
• *Has the child had any exposure to contagious skin conditions: scabies, impetigo, lice? Or to communicable diseases: measles, chickenpox, scarlet fever?* • *Are the child's vaccinations up to date?*	
• *Does the child have any habits or habitual movements such as nail-biting, twisting their hair or rubbing their head on their mattress?*	
• *What steps are taken to protect the child from sun exposure? Do you use sunscreen? How do you treat sunburn?*	Excessive sun exposure, especially severe or blistering sunburns in childhood, increases the risk for melanoma in later life.
Additional subjective data for adolescents	
• *Have you noticed any skin problems such as pimples or blackheads?* • *How long have you had them? How do you feel about it?* • *How do you treat this? Have you sought medical advice? If so, what was the advice?* • *How do you look after your skin?*	About 70% of teenagers will have acne, and the psychological effect is often more significant than the physical effect. Self-treatment is common. Many myths surround the cause of acne. The cause is unknown; acne is not caused by poor diet, oily complexion or contagion.

ASSESSMENT GUIDELINES	CLINICAL SIGNIFICANCE AND CLINICAL ALERTS
Additional subjective data for adults over 65 years	
• *What changes have you noticed in your skin in the past few years?*	Assess the impact of ageing on self-concept. Common ageing changes may cause distress. Many changes attributed to ageing are due to chronic sun damage. Most skin cancers appear in older people, although sun damage often begins decades earlier.
• *Have you experienced a delay in wound healing?* • *Do you have skin itching?*	**Pruritus** is very common with ageing. Consider the side effects of medicine or systemic disease (e.g. liver or kidney disease, cancer, lymphoma), but senile pruritus is usually due to dry skin (**xerosis**) exacerbated by too-frequent bathing or use of soap. Scratching with dirty, jagged fingernails produces excoriations.
• *Do you have any skin pain?*	Some diseases, such as **herpes zoster (shingles)**, produce more intense sensations of pain and itching in older people. Other diseases (e.g. diabetes) may reduce pain sensation in the extremities. Also, some older people tolerate chronic pain as 'part of growing old' and hesitate to 'complain'.
• *Have you noticed any changes in your feet or toenails? Do you have any bunions? Are you able to wear shoes comfortably?* • *How often do you clip your nails?*	Some older people cannot reach down to care for their feet/nails.
• *Have you experienced any falls in the past 6 months?*	Note multiple bruises, trauma from falls.
• *Do you have a history of diabetes or peripheral vascular disease?*	Risk for skin lesions in the feet or ankles.
• *How do you care for your skin?*	Application of bland lotions is important to retain moisture in ageing skin. Dermatitis may ensue from certain cosmetics, creams, ointments and dyes applied to achieve a youthful appearance. Ageing skin has a delayed inflammatory response when exposed to irritants. If the person is not alerted by warning signs (e.g. pruritus, redness), exposure may continue and dermatitis may ensue.

Objective data

On admission to healthcare services, it is expected that nurses will perform a skin assessment to identify the risk of or presence of a pressure injury. Furthermore, skin assessment is done in an opportunistic way in which the skin is examined when performing other health assessments or nursing care activities. For example, assisting the person with activities of daily living or assisting the person to move and reposition may prompt the need for a more comprehensive assessment of a particular area of the skin. Nurses also assess the colour and moisture level of a person's skin, especially the face, lips, nose, ear lobes and periphery every time they interact with the person. Changes in skin colour and moisture along with variations in vital signs and conscious state may indicate clinical deterioration for which immediate further assessment and action is required. To help you focus, pay attention to the person's skin characteristics—the skin holds information about the body's circulation, nutritional status and signs of systemic diseases, as well as topical data on the integument itself. Baseline knowledge is important to assess colour or pigment changes.

Preparation

When performing a skin assessment, ensure the room is warm and that there is adequate lighting and privacy. Assist the person into a position of comfort and expose only those areas of the body being assessed.

Equipment needed

Small centimetre paper ruler
Penlight
Hand hygiene solution
Disposable gloves

PROCEDURES AND NORMAL FINDINGS	ABNORMAL FINDINGS AND CLINICAL ALERTS
General inspection	
While collecting subjective data, you will have noticed the colour, smoothness and moisture of the face, in particular the lips, nose and earlobes, the periphery, height-to-weight ratio, the level of hygiene and grooming and general demeanour. All these factors provide clues to the condition of the integument.	The condition of the skin can be an indicator of a person's general health and wellbeing. Interpretation should be guided by whether the person's skin indicates a health problem or puts the person at risk of a health problem or whether personal choices have been made (Tables 22.1 and 22.2).
Inspecting and palpating the skin	
Note the presence of scars, wounds, bruises, piercings, tattoos, enlarged veins and general hygiene and skin condition. Any bruising (**ecchymosis**) should be consistent with stage of life. For example, it is not uncommon for young children to have bruises on their legs because of vigorous play activities. For a frail, older person, the skin is easily bruised because of minor day-to-day bumps. There are normally no venous dilatations or varicosities.	**Varicosities** are enlarged or swollen veins. Bruises usually occur because of trauma, bleeding disorders or liver dysfunction.

PROCEDURES AND NORMAL FINDINGS	ABNORMAL FINDINGS AND CLINICAL ALERTS

Colour

General pigmentation

Observe the skin tone. Normally it is consistent with genetic background and varies from pinkish or from light to dark brown (Figure 22.4A and B). People who have dark-pigmented skin normally have areas of lighter pigmentation on the palms, nail beds and lips.

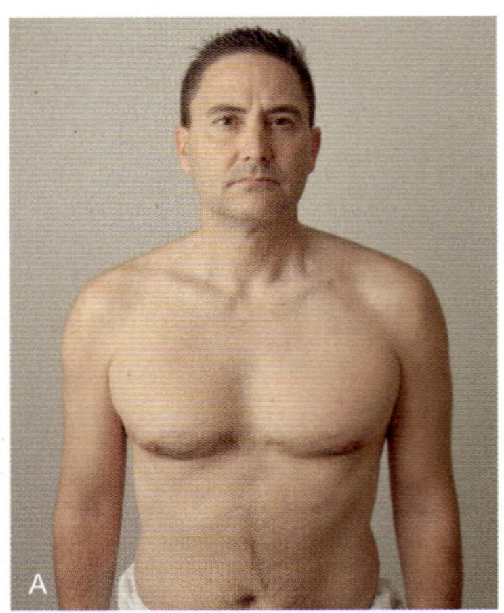

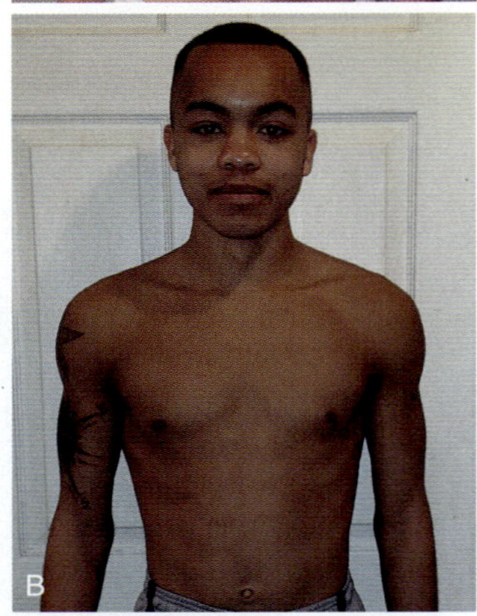

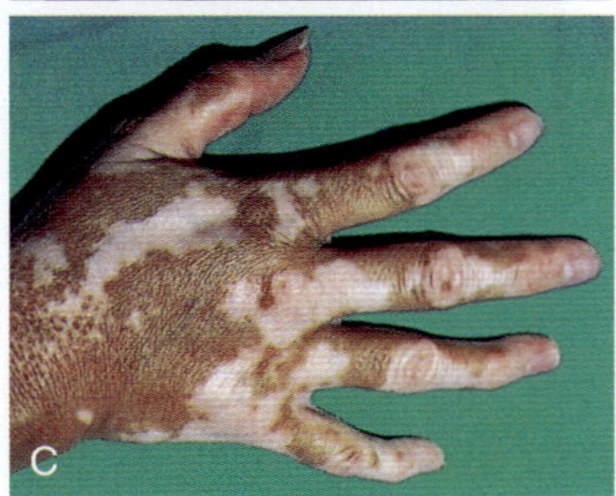

FIGURE 22.4 A, B Skin tone and C Vitiglio

Clinical alert: Any reddening of the skin over bony prominences is a pressure injury. Careful management is critical to avoid the injury progressing. See section - assessing for pressure injuries.

General pigmentation is darker in sun-exposed areas. Common (benign) pigmented areas also occur.

An acquired condition is **vitiligo** (complete absence of melanin pigment in patchy areas of white or light skin) on the face, neck, hands, feet, body folds and around orifices (Figure 22.4C). Vitiligo can occur in any person, although dark-skinned people are more severely affected and potentially suffer a greater threat to their body image (Tables 22.1 and 22.2).

PROCEDURES AND NORMAL FINDINGS	ABNORMAL FINDINGS AND CLINICAL ALERTS

- **Freckles** (ephelides)—small, flat macules of brown melanin pigment that occur on sun-exposed skin (Figure 22.5A).
- **Mole** (naevus)—a proliferation of melanocytes, tan to brown colour, flat or raised. Acquired naevi are characterised by their symmetry, small size (6 mm or smaller), smooth borders and uniform pigmentation. A **junctional naevus** (Figure 22.5B) is macular only and occurs in children and adolescents. It progresses to a **compound naevi** in young adults (Figure 22.5C) that are macular and papular. The intradermal naevus (mainly in older age) has naevus cells in the dermis only.
- **Birthmarks**—may be red or tan to brown in colour.

See also Tables 22.3 and 22.4.

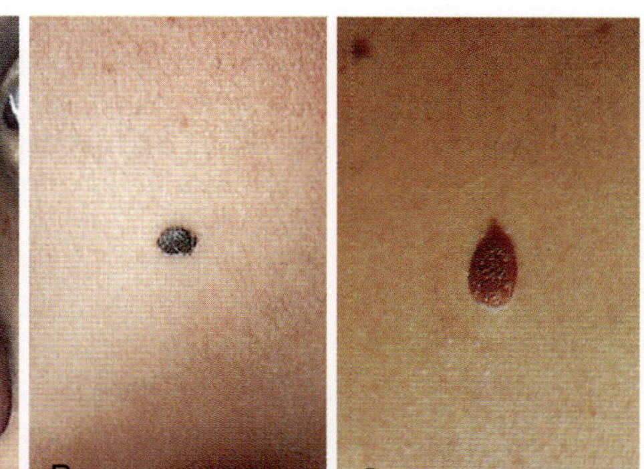

FIGURE 22.5 ABC A. Freckles; B. Junctional naevus; C. Compound naevus

Note any **skin colour change** over the entire body, such as **pallor** (whitish tone), **erythema** (red), cyanosis (blue) and **jaundice** (yellow). Note whether the colour change is transient and expected or if it is due to pathology.

In people who have dark-pigmented skin, the amount of pigment may mask colour changes. Lips and nail beds show some colour change, but they vary with the person's skin colour and may not always be accurate signs. The more reliable sites are those with the least pigmentation such as under the tongue, the buccal mucosa, the palpebral conjunctiva and the sclera. See Table 22.2 for specific clues to assessment.

Ashen grey colour in a person with dark skin or marked pallor in a person with light-coloured skin occurs with anaemia, shock and arterial insufficiency (Table 22.2).

PROCEDURES AND NORMAL FINDINGS	ABNORMAL FINDINGS AND CLINICAL ALERTS
Look for **pallor** in people with dark skin by the absence of the underlying red tones that normally give brown- or dark-coloured skin its lustre. Generalised pallor can be observed in the mucous membranes, lips and nail beds. The palpebral conjunctiva and nail beds are preferred sites for assessing the pallor of anaemia. When inspecting the conjunctiva, lower the lid sufficiently to visualise the conjunctiva near the outer canthus as well as the inner canthus. The colouration is often lighter near the inner canthus.	**Pallor.** When the red-pink tones from the oxygenated haemoglobin in the blood are lost, the skin takes on the colour of connective tissue (collagen), which is mostly white. Pallor is common in acute high-stress states, such as anxiety or fear, because of the powerful peripheral vasoconstriction from sympathetic nervous system stimulation. The skin also looks pale, with vasoconstriction from exposure to cold and cigarette smoking and in the presence of oedema. **Anaemias—chronic iron deficiency anaemia** may show 'spoon' nails, with a concave shape. **Pernicious anaemia** (autoimmune condition that prevents the body from absorbing vitamin B12)—lemon-yellow tint of the face and slightly yellow sclera, neurological deficits and a red, painful tongue. Fatigue, exertional dyspnoea, rapid pulse, dizziness and impaired mental function accompany most severe anaemias. ***Clinical alert:*** The pallor of impending shock is accompanied by other subtle manifestations such as increasing pulse rate, oliguria, apprehension and restlessness. Report changes such as this to a medical practitioner immediately.
Erythema is an intense redness of the skin from excess blood (**hyperaemia**) in the dilated superficial capillaries. This sign is expected with fever, local inflammation or with emotional reactions such as blushing in vascular flush areas (cheeks, neck and upper chest).	**Erythema** occurs with **polycythaemia** (an increase in all blood cells, particularly red blood cells), venous stasis, carbon monoxide poisoning and the extravascular presence of red blood cells **(petechiae, ecchymoses, haematoma)** (Table 22.2). When erythema is associated with fever or localised inflammation, it is characterised by increased skin temperature (increased rate of blood flow).

PROCEDURES AND NORMAL FINDINGS	ABNORMAL FINDINGS AND CLINICAL ALERTS
Cyanosis is a bluish, mottled colour that signifies that the tissues are not adequately perfused with oxygenated blood (Figure 22.6). Be aware that cyanosis can be a nonspecific sign. A person who is anaemic could have hypoxaemia without ever looking cyanosed because not enough haemoglobin is present (either oxygenated or reduced) to colour the skin. On the other hand, a person with polycythaemia (an increase in the number of red blood cells) always looks ruddy blue and may not necessarily be hypoxaemic. This person is just unable to fully oxygenate the massive numbers of red blood cells.	**Cyanosis** indicates hypoxaemia and occurs with shock, heart failure, chronic bronchitis and congenital heart disease.
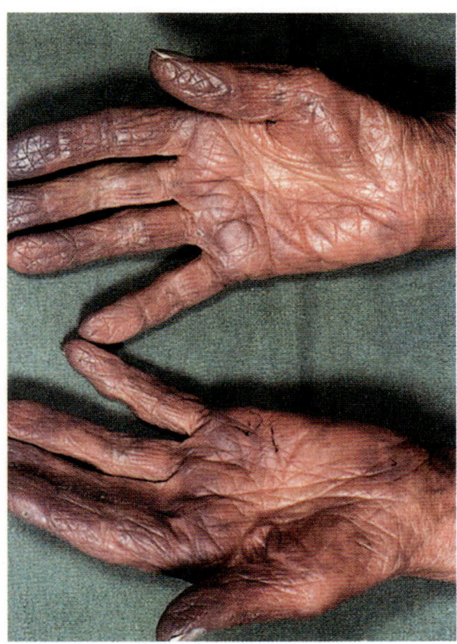 **FIGURE 22.6** Cyanosis	Cyanosis is difficult to observe in people with dark skin (Table 22.2). Given that most conditions causing cyanosis also cause decreased oxygenation of the brain, other clinical signs—such as changes in the level of consciousness and signs of respiratory distress—will be evident.
Jaundice is exhibited by a yellow colour, indicating rising amounts of bilirubin in the blood. Except for physiological jaundice in a newborn (see below), jaundice does not occur normally. Jaundice is *first* noted in the junction of the hard and soft palate in the mouth and in the sclera. But do not confuse scleral jaundice with the normal yellow subconjunctival fatty deposits that are common in the outer sclera of people with dark skin. The scleral yellow of jaundice extends up to the edge of the iris.	**Jaundice** occurs with hepatitis, cirrhosis, sickle-cell disease, transfusion reaction and haemolytic disease of newborns (Table 22.2).
As levels of serum bilirubin rise, jaundice is evident in the skin over the rest of the body. This is best assessed in direct natural daylight. Common calluses on the palms and soles often look yellow—do not interpret these as jaundice.	Light or clay-coloured stools and dark golden urine often accompany jaundice.

PROCEDURES AND NORMAL FINDINGS	ABNORMAL FINDINGS AND CLINICAL ALERTS
Temperature	
Note the temperature of your own hands. Use the backs (dorsa) of your hands to palpate the person bilaterally. The skin should be warm, and the temperature should be equal bilaterally; warmth suggests normal circulatory status. Hands and feet may be slightly cooler in a cool environment.	**Hypothermia** may be induced for surgery or high fever. **Localised coolness** is expected with an immobilised extremity, as when a limb is in a cast or with an intravenous infusion. **Localised hypothermia** occurs in peripheral arterial insufficiency and **Raynaud's disease** (decreased blood flow to fingers). **Generalised hyperthermia** occurs with an increased metabolic rate such as fever or after heavy exercise. **Localised hyperthermia** occurs with trauma, infection or sunburn. **General hypothermia** accompanies a central circulatory problem such as shock. **Localised hypothermia** occurs in peripheral arterial insufficiency and Raynaud's disease. **Hyperthyroidism** has an increased metabolic rate, causing warm, moist skin.
Moisture	
Perspiration appears normally on the face, hands, axillae and skinfolds in response to activity, a warm environment, fever or anxiety.	**Diaphoresis**, or profuse perspiration, accompanies an increased metabolic rate, such as occurs in heavy activity or fever. Diaphoresis occurs with thyrotoxicosis and with stimulation of the nervous system with anxiety or pain.
Inspect the oral mucous membranes and elasticity of the skin for dehydration. Normally the mucous membranes look smooth and moist, and the skin is elastic.	With **dehydration**, the mucous membranes look dry, and the lips look parched and cracked. With extreme dryness, the skin is fissured, resembling cracks in a dry lake-bed and does not recoil quickly when lightly pinched.
Texture	
Normal skin feels smooth and firm, with an even surface.	**Hyperthyroidism**—the skin feels smoother and softer, like velvet. **Hypothyroidism**—the skin feels rough, dry and flaky (Table 22.4).

PROCEDURES AND NORMAL FINDINGS	ABNORMAL FINDINGS AND CLINICAL ALERTS
Thickness	
The epidermis is uniformly thin over most of the body, although thickened callus areas are normal on the palms and soles. A callus is a circumscribed overgrowth of epidermis and is an adaptation to excessive pressure from the friction of work and weight bearing.	Very thin, shiny skin (atrophic) occurs with **arterial insufficiency**.
Oedema	
Oedema is fluid accumulating in the intercellular spaces; it is not present normally. To check for oedema, imprint your thumbs firmly against the ankle malleolus or the tibia. Normally, the skin surface stays smooth. If your pressure leaves a dent in the skin, 'pitting' oedema is present. Its presence is graded on a four-point scale: • 1+ **Mild pitting,** slight indentation, no perceptible swelling of the leg • 2+ **Moderate pitting,** indentation subsides rapidly • 3+ **Deep pitting,** indentation remains for a short time, leg looks swollen • 4+ **Very deep pitting,** indentation lasts a long time, leg is very swollen. This scale is somewhat subjective; outcomes vary among examiners (see further content on grading scale in Chapters 16 and 17). Oedema masks normal skin colour and obscures pathological conditions such as jaundice or cyanosis because the fluid lies between the surface and the pigmented and vascular layers. It makes skin look lighter.	**Dependent oedema** is most evident in dependent parts of the body (feet, ankles and sacral areas), where the skin looks puffy and tight. Oedema makes the hair follicles more prominent, so you note a pigskin or orange-peel look (called *peau d'orange*). **Unilateral oedema** is usually related to a local or peripheral cause. **Bilateral oedema** or oedema that is generalised over the whole body **(anasarca)** is usually related to a central problem such as heart failure or kidney failure because of increased capillary hydrostatic pressure.[9,10]
Mobility and turgor	
Pinch a large fold of skin on the anterior chest under the clavicle (Figure 22.7). Mobility is the skin's ease of rising, and turgor is its ability to return to place promptly when released. This reflects the elasticity of the skin. 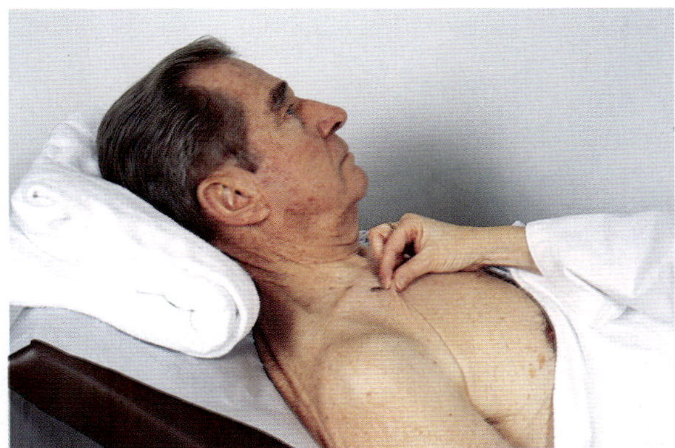 **FIGURE 22.7** Skin turgor	**Mobility and turgor** are decreased when oedema is present. **Poor turgor** is evident in severe dehydration or extreme weight loss; the pinched skin recedes slowly or 'tents' and stands by itself. **Scleroderma**, literally 'hard skin', is a chronic connective tissue disorder associated with decreased mobility.

PROCEDURES AND NORMAL FINDINGS	ABNORMAL FINDINGS AND CLINICAL ALERTS
Lesions	
If any lesions are present, note the: • **colour** • **elevation:** flat, raised or pedunculated • **pattern or shape:** the grouping or distinctness of each lesion—for example, annular, grouped, confluent, linear—the pattern may be characteristic of a certain disease • **size** in centimetres: use a ruler to measure; avoid household descriptions such as 'pea sized' • **location and distribution** on the body: is it generalised or localised to area of a specific irritant; around jewellery, watchband, around eyes? • any **exudate:** note its colour and any odour	**Macule:** small pigmented spot on the skin that is neither raised nor depressed **Papule:** a small hard round protuberance on the skin **Naevi:** moles **Danger signs:** abnormal characteristics of pigmented lesions are summarised in the mnemonic **ABCDE**: • **A**symmetry (not regularly round or oval, two halves of lesion do not look the same) • **B**order irregularity (notching, scalloping, ragged edges or poorly defined margins) • **C**olour variation (areas of brown, tan, black, blue, red, white or combination) • **D**iameter over 6 mm (i.e. the size of a small fingernail), although early melanomas may be diagnosed at a smaller size • **E**levation/**E**nlargement. See Tables 22.4 to 22.8.
Palpate lesions Wear a glove if you anticipate contact with blood, mucosa, body fluid or a skin lesion. Roll a nodule between the thumb and index finger to assess depth.	 ***Clinical alert:*** Change in a mole's size, a new pigmented lesion and development of itching, burning or bleeding in a mole. Any of these signs should raise suspicion of malignant melanoma and warrant referral to medical practitioner.[4]
Does the lesion blanch with pressure or stretch? Stretching the area of skin between your thumb and index finger decreases (blanches) the normal underlying red tones, thus providing more contrast and brightening the macules. Red macules from dilated blood vessels *will* blanch momentarily, whereas those from extravasated blood (petechiae) do not. Blanching also helps identify a macular rash in people with dark-pigmented skin. **Cherry angiomas** are small (1 to 5 mm), smooth, slightly raised bright red dots that commonly appear on the trunk in all adults over 30 years old (Figure 22.8). They normally increase in size and number with ageing and are not significant.	

PROCEDURES AND NORMAL FINDINGS	ABNORMAL FINDINGS AND CLINICAL ALERTS

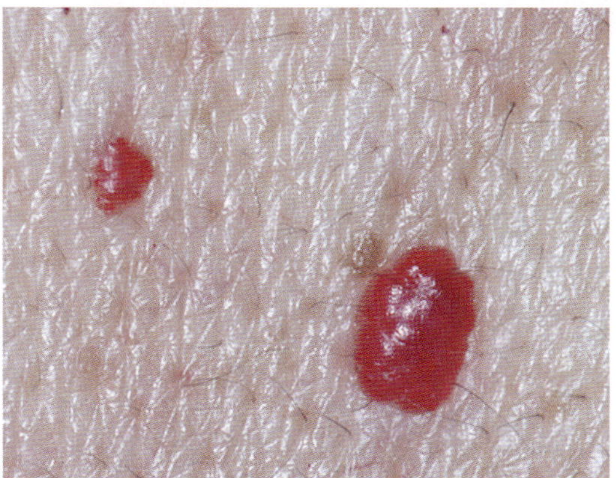

FIGURE 22.8 Cherry angioma

Assessing for pressure injuries

Assessment is an important aspect of a nurse's role in preventing pressure injuries.

Risk factors include:

- impaired mobility or reduced activity
- impaired sensory perception
- poor oxygenation
- incontinence
- malnutrition or obesity
- compromised skin integrity
- increasing age and frailty
- compromised or reduced blood supply to pressure points
- severely compromised status of health.
- friction/shear.

Ensure thorough and regular assessment of bony prominences, skin folds that trap moisture and areas that come in contact with tubing; for example, a patient may require oxygen or tube feeding and the nares or ears are vulnerable to pressure from this equipment.[11]

Pressure injury grading

Grade 1: non-blanchable erythema

Grade 2: partial thickness skin loss (damage to epidermis and/or dermis—including abrasion, blisters)

Grade 3: full thickness skin loss (damage or necrosis of subcutaneous tissues; does not include underlying fascia or underlying structures)

Grade 4: full thickness skin loss with extensive destruction and tissue necrosis extending to underlying bone, tendon or joint capsule (Table 22.6).

PROCEDURES AND NORMAL FINDINGS	ABNORMAL FINDINGS AND CLINICAL ALERTS
Wound assessment	
Wound assessment is usually conducted over time. It is important to use objective measures as described above to monitor healing or deterioration. It is important to note that many healthcare organisations have a specific wound assessment and care chart. Note and describe: • **anatomical location**—may use a body map • **size** (length, width, depth, undermining—wound extends underneath the skin edges); use a disposable ruler to measure and take a photograph if possible • **colour and type of wound tissue** (e.g. granulation, slough, necrotic) • **exudate or drainage**—amount and type (described at the time of a dressing change, number of dressing changes required) • **odour** (offensive, non-offensive) • **periwound skin condition**—colour and temperature • **wound margins**—colour and condition of skin • **pain**—presence or absence and type of pain.[12]	
Inspecting and palpating the hair and scalp	
Colour	
Hair colour comes from melanin production and may vary from pale blonde to total black. Greying begins as early as the third decade of life because of reduced melanin production in the follicles. Genetic factors affect the age of onset of greying.	
Texture	
Scalp hair may be fine or thick and may look straight, curly or kinky. It should look shiny, although this characteristic may be lost with the use of some beauty products such as dyes, rinses or other hair treatments.	Note dull, coarse or brittle scalp hair. Grey, scaly, well-defined areas with broken hairs accompany tinea capitis, a fungal infection that is found mostly in school-age children (Table 22.10).
Distribution	
Fine vellus hair coats the body, whereas coarser terminal hairs grow at the eyebrows, eyelashes and scalp. During puberty, distribution conforms to normal male and female patterns. At first, coarse curly hairs develop in the pubic area, then in the axillae and last in the facial area in boys. In the genital area, the female pattern is an inverted triangle; the male pattern is an upright triangle with pubic hair extending up to the umbilicus. The amount of hair varies from person to person.	Absent or abnormally configured pubic hair suggests endocrine abnormalities. **Hirsutism** is excess body hair. In females, this forms a male pattern of hair distribution on the face and chest and indicates endocrine abnormalities (Table 22.10).

PROCEDURES AND NORMAL FINDINGS	ABNORMAL FINDINGS AND CLINICAL ALERTS
Lesions	
Separate the hair into sections and lift it, observing the scalp. With a history of itching, inspect the hair behind the ears and in the occipital area as well. All areas should be clean and free of any lesions or pest inhabitants. Many people normally have seborrhoea (dandruff), which is indicated by loose white flakes on the scalp and hair.	Distinguish dandruff from nits (eggs) of lice, which are oval, adhere to the hair shaft and cause intense itching (Table 22.10).
Inspecting and palpating the nails	
Shape and contour	
The nail surface is normally slightly curved or flat, and the posterior and lateral nail folds are smooth and rounded. Nail edges are smooth, rounded and clean, suggesting adequate self-care.	Jagged nails bitten to the quick or traumatised nail folds from chronic nervous picking suggest nervous habits. Chronically dirty nails suggest poor self-care or some occupations in which it is impossible to keep them clean.
The profile sign View the index finger at its profile and note the angle of the nail base; it should be about 160 degrees (Figure 22.9). The nail base is firm to palpation. Curved nails are a variation of normal with a convex profile. They may look like clubbed nails, but notice that the angle between nail base and nail is normal (e.g. 160 degrees or less).	**Clubbing** of nails occurs with congenital chronic cyanotic heart disease and with emphysema and chronic bronchitis. In early clubbing, the angle straightens out to 180 degrees and the nail base feels spongy to palpation.

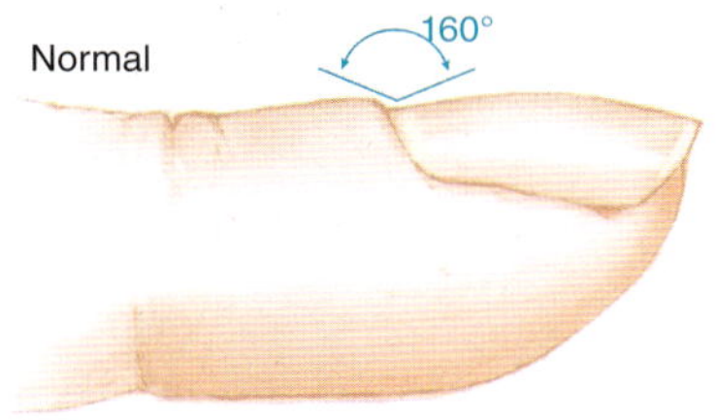

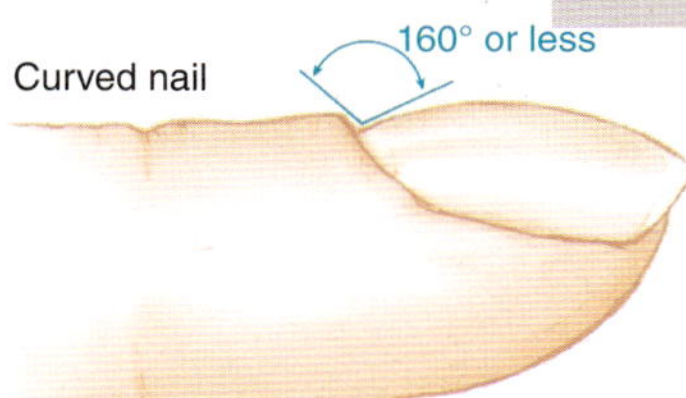

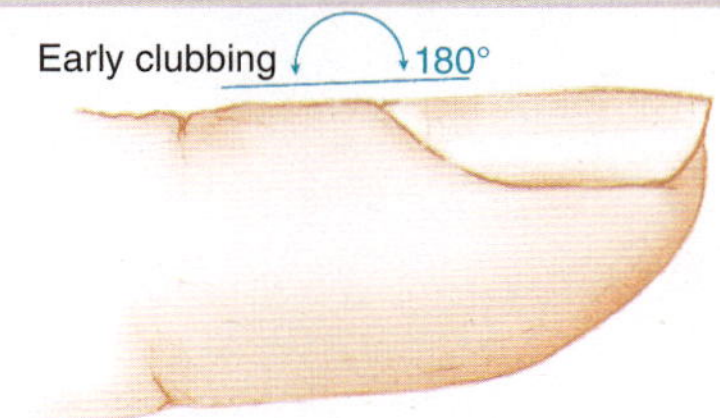

FIGURE 22.9 Nail profile

PROCEDURES AND NORMAL FINDINGS	ABNORMAL FINDINGS AND CLINICAL ALERTS
Consistency	
The surface is smooth and regular, not brittle or splitting.	Pits, transverse grooves or lines may indicate a nutrient deficiency or may accompany acute illness in which nail growth is disturbed (Table 22.11).
Nail thickness is uniform.	Nails are thickened and ridged with arterial insufficiency.

PROCEDURES AND NORMAL FINDINGS	ABNORMAL FINDINGS AND CLINICAL ALERTS
The nail is firmly adherent to the nail bed, and the nail base is firm to palpation.	A spongy nail base accompanies clubbing.
Colour	
The translucent nail plate is a window to the even, pink nail bed underneath. People with dark skin may have brown-black pigmented areas or linear bands or streaks along the nail edge (Figure 22.10). All people may normally have white hairline linear markings from trauma or picking at the cuticle (Figure 22.11). Note any abnormal marking in the nail beds.	**Cyanosis** or marked pallor. **Brown linear streaks** (especially sudden appearance) are abnormal in light-skinned people and may indicate melanoma. Splinter haemorrhages, transverse ridges or **Beau's lines** (Table 22.11).
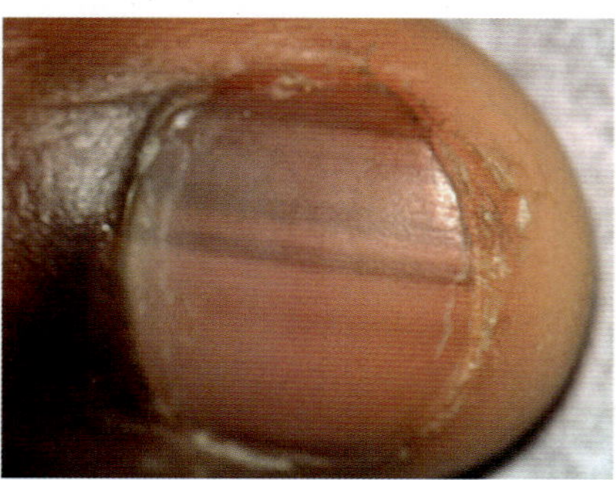 **FIGURE 22.10** Linear pigmentation 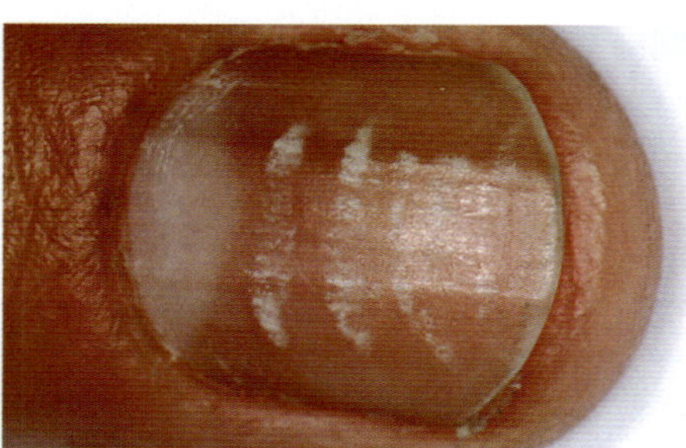 **FIGURE 22.11** Leuconchia pigmentation	
Capillary refill Depress the nail edge to blanch and then release, noting the return of colour. Normally, colour return is instant or at least within a few seconds in a cold environment. This indicates the status of the peripheral circulation. A sluggish colour return takes longer than 1 or 2 seconds. Inspect the toenails. Separate the toes and note the smooth skin in between.	**Cyanotic** nail beds or sluggish colour return: may be related to cardiovascular or respiratory dysfunction.

PROCEDURES AND NORMAL FINDINGS	ABNORMAL FINDINGS AND CLINICAL ALERTS

Additional objective data for infants or children

When inspecting the skin of infants, toddlers and school-aged children, pay particular attention to the 'nappy area', face, nose and skin folds.

Nappy rash is red, moist and painful.

Impetigo is a contagious skin infection common in infants and children. Sores form around the nose and mouth.

Thrush (Candida) is another red, moist rash irritated by urine, faeces and heat and is found in the inguinal and gluteal folds (Table 12.12).

Multiple bruises in various stages of healing or pattern injury suggest child abuse (Table 22.13).

Additional objective data for adolescents

The increase in sebaceous gland activity creates increased oiliness and **acne**. Acne is the most common skin problem of adolescence. Almost all teens have some acne, even if it is the milder form of open comedones (blackheads) (Figure 22.12A) and closed comedones (whiteheads). Severe acne includes papules, pustules and nodules (Figure 22.12B). Acne lesions usually appear on the face and sometimes on the chest, back and shoulders. Acne may appear in children as early as 7 or 8 years of age; then the lesions increase in number and severity and peak at 14 to 16 years in girls and at 16 to 19 years in boys.

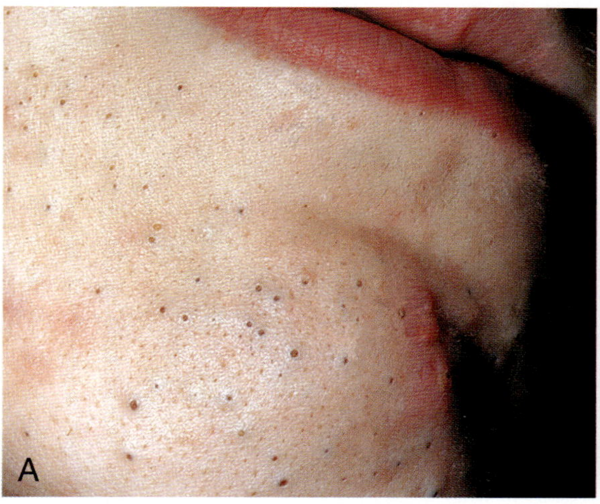

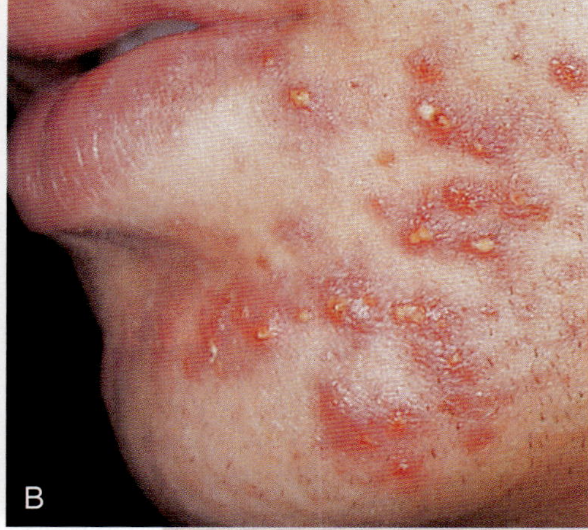

FIGURES 22.12 A. Open comedones; B. Acne

PROCEDURES AND NORMAL FINDINGS	ABNORMAL FINDINGS AND CLINICAL ALERTS

Additional objective data for adults over 65 years

Skin colour and pigmentation

Common variations of hyperpigmentation are:

Lentigines

Commonly called liver spots, these are small, flat, brown macules (Figure 22.13). These circumscribed areas are clusters of melanocytes that appear after extensive sun exposure. They appear on the forearms and dorsa of the hands. They are not malignant and require no treatment.

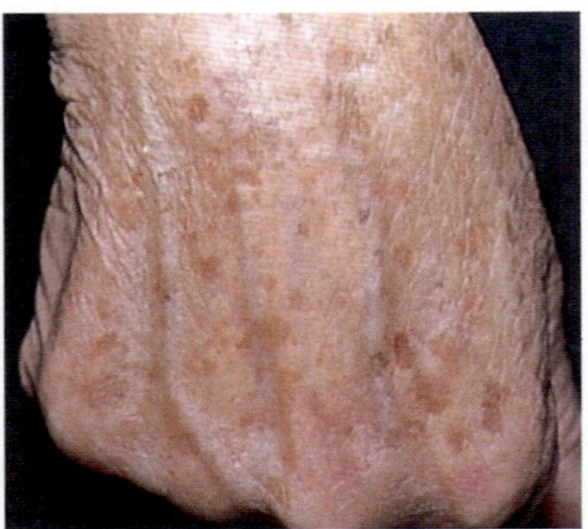

FIGURE 22.13 Lentigines

Keratoses

These lesions are raised, thickened areas of pigmentation that look crusted, scaly and warty. One type, **seborrhoeic keratosis**, looks dark, greasy and 'stuck on' (Figure 22.14). They develop mostly on the trunk but also on the face and hands and on unexposed as well as on sun-exposed areas. They do not become cancerous.

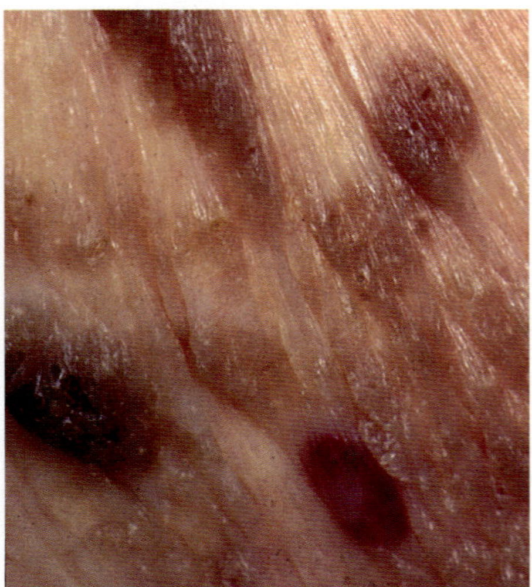

FIGURE 22.14 Serborrhoeic keratosis

PROCEDURES AND NORMAL FINDINGS	ABNORMAL FINDINGS AND CLINICAL ALERTS

Another type, **actinic (solar) keratosis**, is less common (Figure 22.15). These lesions are red-tan scaly plaques that increase over the years to become raised and roughened. They may have a silvery-white scale adherent to the plaque. They occur on sun-exposed surfaces and are directly related to sun exposure. They are premalignant and may develop into squamous cell carcinoma.

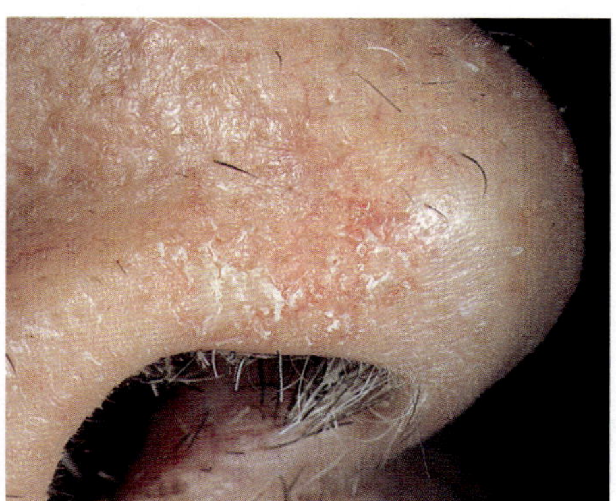

FIGURE 22.15 Actinic keratosis

Moisture
Dry skin (xerosis) is common in older people because of a decline in the size, number and output of the sweat glands and sebaceous glands. The skin itches and looks flaky and loose.

Texture
Common variations occurring in older adults are **acrochordons**, or 'skin tags', which are overgrowths of normal skin that form a stalk and are polyp-like (Figure 22.16). They occur frequently on the eyelids, cheeks, neck, axillae and trunk.

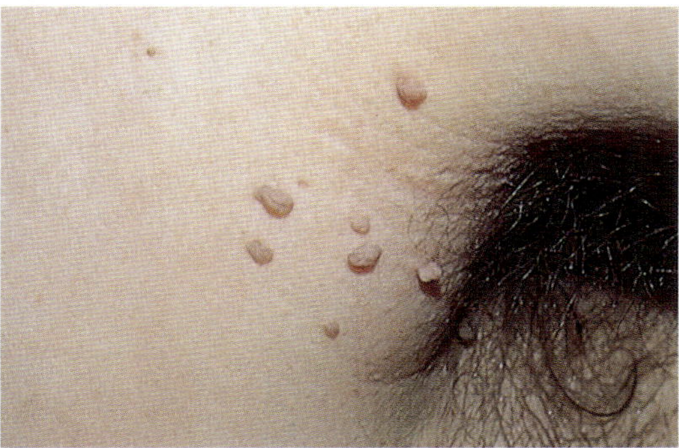

FIGURE 22.16 Acrochordons

PROCEDURES AND NORMAL FINDINGS	ABNORMAL FINDINGS AND CLINICAL ALERTS

Sebaceous hyperplasia consists of raised yellow papules with a central depression. They are more common in men, occurring over the forehead, nose or cheeks. They have a pebbly look (Figure 22.17).

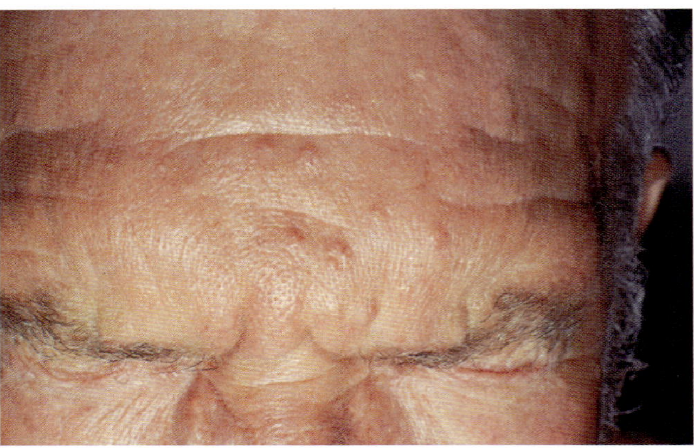

FIGURE 22.17 Sebaceous hyperplasia

Thickness

With ageing, the skin looks as thin as parchment and the subcutaneous fat diminishes. Thinner skin is evident over the dorsa of the hands, forearms, lower legs, dorsa of feet and over bony prominences. The skin may feel thicker over the abdomen and chest.

Mobility and turgor

The turgor is decreased (less elasticity), and the skin recedes slowly or 'tents' and stands by itself (Figure 22.18).

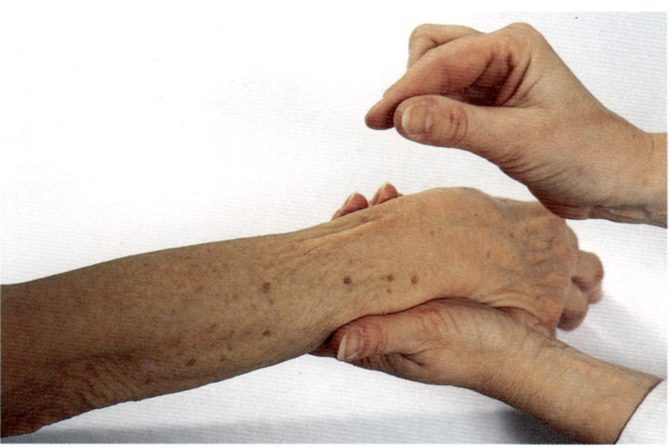

FIGURE 22.18 Testing skin turgor on the hand

PROCEDURES AND NORMAL FINDINGS	ABNORMAL FINDINGS AND CLINICAL ALERTS
Hair With ageing, the hair growth decreases, and the amount decreases in the axillae and pubic areas. After menopause, some women may develop bristly hairs on the chin or upper lip resulting from unopposed androgens. In men, coarse terminal hairs develop in the ears, nose and eyebrows, although the beard is unchanged. Male-pattern balding, or alopecia, is a genetic trait. It is usually a gradual receding of the anterior hairline in a symmetrical W shape. In men and women, scalp hair gradually turns grey because of the decrease in melanocyte function.	
Nails With ageing, the nail growth rate decreases, and local injuries in the nail matrix may produce longitudinal ridges. The surface may be brittle or peeling and sometimes yellowed. Toenails are also thickened and may grow misshapen, almost grotesque. The thickening may be a process of ageing, or it may be due to chronic peripheral vascular disease.	Fungal infections are common in ageing, with thickened crumbling toenails and erythematous scaling on contiguous skin surfaces.[13]

Abnormal findings

TABLE 22.1 External variables influencing skin colour

Variable	Causes	Misleading Outcome
Emotions		
Fear, anger	Peripheral vasoconstriction	False pallor
Embarrassment	Flushing in face and neck	False erythema
Environment		
Hot room	Vasodilatation	False erythema
Chilly or air-conditioned room	Vasoconstriction	False pallor, coolness
Cigarette smoking	Vasoconstriction	False pallor
Physical		
Prolonged elevation	Decreased arterial perfusion	Pallor, coolness
Dependent position	Venous pooling	Redness, warmth, distended veins
Immobilisation, prolonged inactivity	Slowed circulation	Pallor, coolness, nail beds pale, prolonged capillary filling time

TABLE 22.2 Detecting colour changes in light and dark skin

Aetiology	Light Skin	Dark Skin
Pallor		
Anaemia—decreased haematocrit **Shock**—decreased perfusion, vasoconstriction	Generalised pallor	Brown skin appears yellow-brown, dull; dark-coloured skin appears ashen grey, dull; skin loses its healthy glow—check areas with the least pigmentation, such as conjunctivae and mucous membranes
Local arterial insufficiency	Marked localised pallor (e.g. lower extremities, especially when elevated)	Ashen grey, dull; cool to palpitation
Albinism—total absence of pigment melanin throughout the integument	Whitish pink	Tan, cream, white
Vitiligo—patchy depigmentation from destruction of melanocytes	Patchy milky white spots, often symmetrical bilaterally	Same
Cyanosis		
Increased amount of unoxygenated haemoglobin **Central**—chronic heart and lung disease cause arterial desaturation	Dusky blue	Dark but dull, lifeless; only severe cyanosis is apparent in the skin—check conjunctivae, oral mucosa and nail beds
Peripheral—exposure to cold, anxiety	Nail beds dusky	
Erythema		
Hyperaemia—increased blood flow through engorged arterioles, such as in inflammation, fever, alcohol intake and blushing	Red, bright pink	Purplish tinge, but difficult to see; palpate for increased warmth with inflammation, taut skin and hardening of deep tissues
Polycythaemia—increased red blood cells, capillary stasis	Ruddy blue in face, oral mucosa, conjunctiva, hands and feet	Well-concealed by pigment—check for redness in the lips
Carbon monoxide poisoning	Bright cherry red in face and upper torso	Cherry-red colour in nail beds, lips and oral mucosa
Venous stasis—decreased blood flow from area, engorged venules	Dusky rubor of dependent extremities; a prelude to necrosis with pressure sore	Easily masked; use palpation for warmth or oedema

TABLE 22.2 Detecting colour changes in light and dark skin cont'd		
Aetiology	**Light Skin**	**Dark Skin**
Jaundice		
Increased serum bilirubin, more than 2 to 3 mg/100 mL from liver inflammation or haemolytic disease, such as after severe burns, some infections	Yellow in sclera, hard palate, mucous membranes, then progress to generalised yellow colouring of skin	Check sclera for yellow near the limbus; do not mistake normal yellowish fatty deposits in the periphery under the eyelids for jaundice—jaundice best noted in junction of hard and soft palate and palms
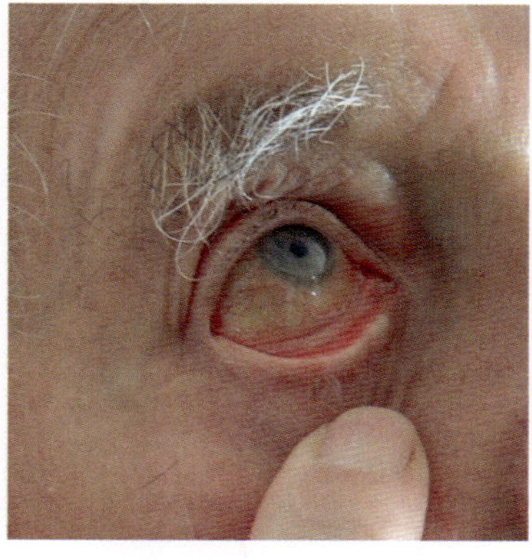	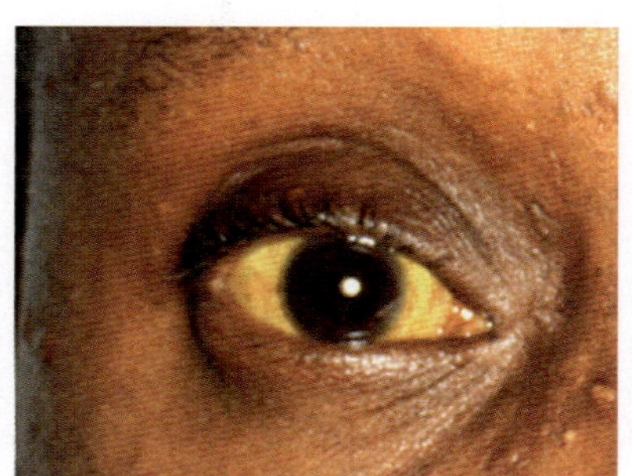	
Carotenaemia—increased serum carotene from ingestion of large amounts of carotene-rich foods	Yellow-orange in forehead, palms and soles, nasolabial folds, but no yellowing in sclera or mucous membranes	Yellow-orange tinge in the palms and soles
Uraemia—renal failure causes retained urochrome pigments in the blood	Orange-green or grey overlying pallor of anaemia; may also have ecchymoses and purpura	Easily masked; rely on laboratory and clinical findings
Brown-tan		
Addison's disease—cortisol deficiency stimulates increased melanin production	Bronzed appearance, an 'eternal tan', most apparent around nipples, perineum, genitalia and pressure points (inner thighs, buttocks, elbows, axillae)	Easily masked; rely on laboratory and clinical findings
Café au lait spots—caused by increased melanin pigment in the basal cell layer	Tan to light brown, irregularly shaped, oval patch with well-defined borders	

TABLE 22.3 Common lesions

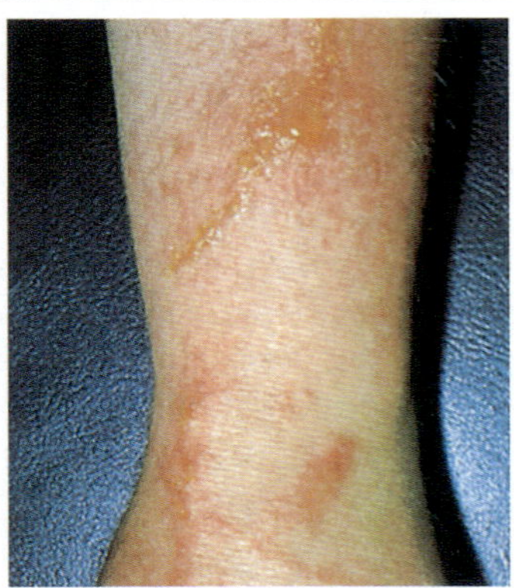

Primary contact dermatitis

Local inflammatory reaction to an irritant in the environment or an allergy. Characteristic location of the lesions is often a clue. Often erythema shows first, followed by swelling, wheals (or urticaria) or maculopapular vesicles and scales. Frequently accompanied by intense pruritus.

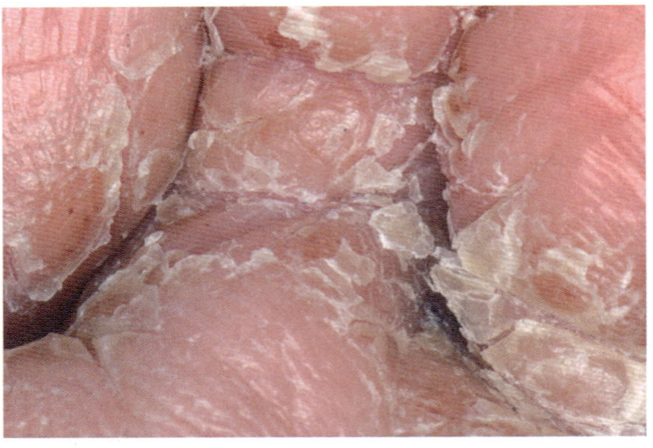

Tinea pedis

'Athlete's foot', a fungal infection, first appears as small vesicles between the toes, sides of feet and soles. Then grows scaly and hard. Found in chronically warm, moist feet: children after gym activities, athletes, ageing adults who cannot dry their feet well.

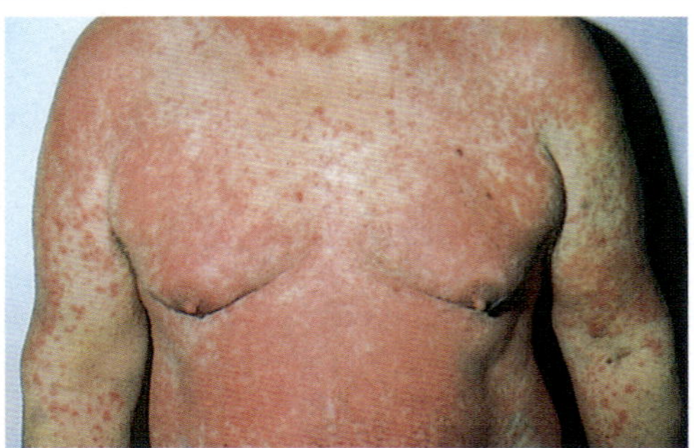

Allergic drug reaction

Erythematous and symmetric rash, usually generalised. Some drugs produce an urticarial rash or vesicles and bullae. History of drug ingestion.

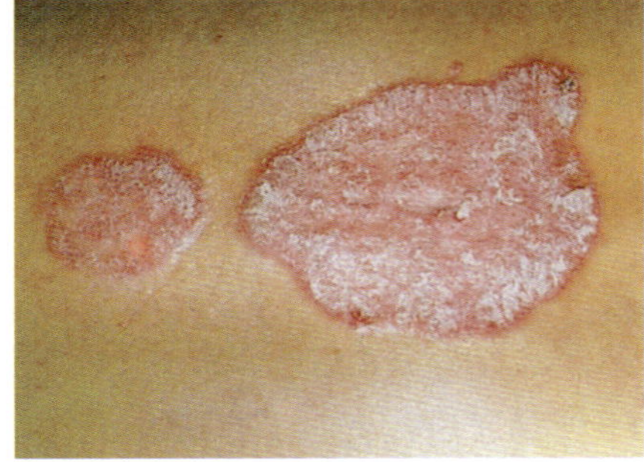

Psoriasis

Scaly erythematous patch with silvery scales on top. Usually on the scalp, outside of elbows and knees, low back and anogenital area.

TABLE 22.3 Common lesions cont'd

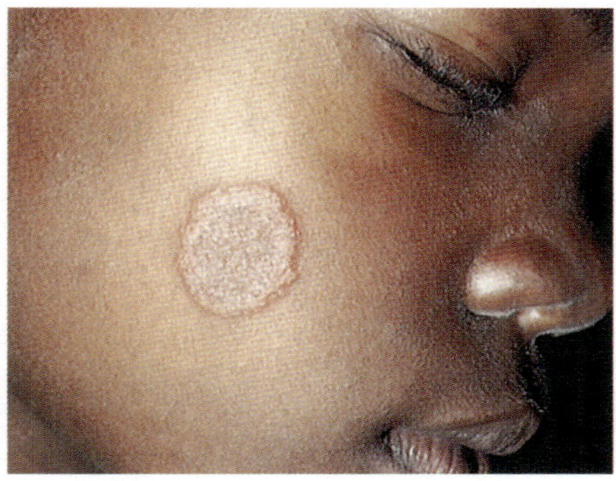

Tinea corporis

Scales—hyperpigmented in light-skinned people, depigmented in dark-skinned people—on the chest, abdomen and back of arms, forming multiple circular lesions with clear centres.

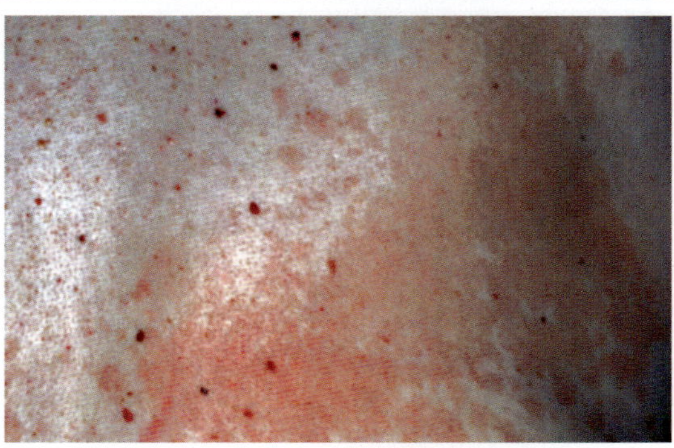

Tinea versicolor

Fine, scaling, round patches of pink, tan or white that (hence the name) do not tan in sunlight, caused by a superficial fungal infection. Usual distribution is on the neck, trunk and upper arms—a short-sleeved turtleneck sweater area. Most common in otherwise healthy young adults.

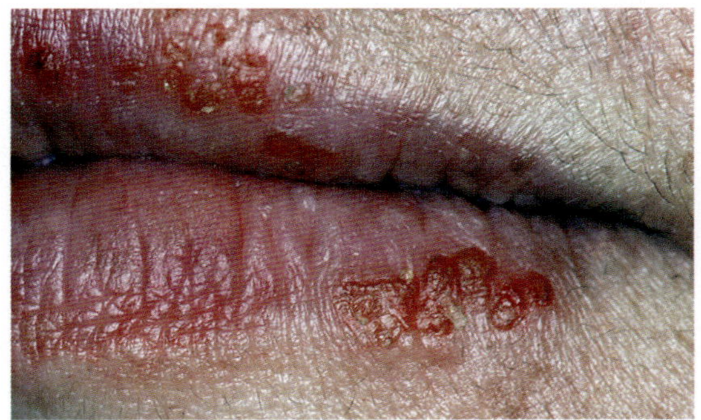

Herpes simplex (cold sores)

Herpes simplex virus infection has a prodrome of skin tingling and sensitivity. The lesion then erupts with tight vesicles followed by pustules and then produces acute gingivostomatitis with many shallow, painful ulcers. Common location is upper lip, also in oral mucosa and tongue.

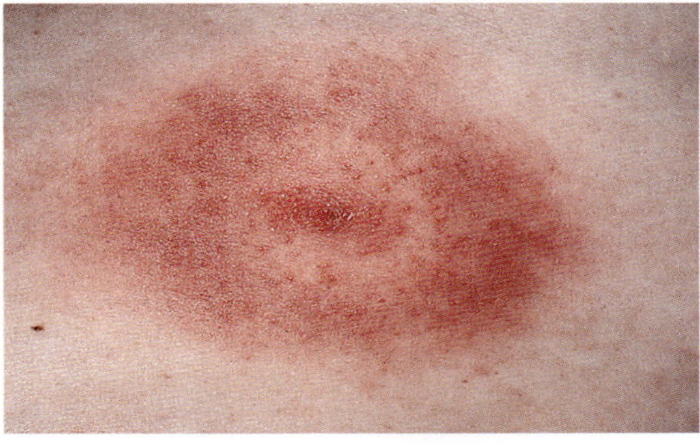

Lyme disease

Lyme disease is not fatal but may have serious arthritic, cardiac or neurological sequelae. It is caused by a spirochaete bacterium carried by ticks.

The first stage (early localised Lyme disease) has the distinctive bull's eye, red macular or papular rash (shown above) in 50% of cases. The rash radiates from the site of the tick bite (5 cm or larger) with some central clearing; it is usually located in axillae, midriff, inguinal region or behind the knees, with regional lymphadenopathy. Rash fades in 4 weeks; untreated people may then have disseminated disease with fatigue, anorexia, fever, chills or joint or muscle aches. Antibiotic treatment shortens symptoms and decreases risk for sequelae.[14]

Continued

TABLE 22.3 Common lesions cont'd

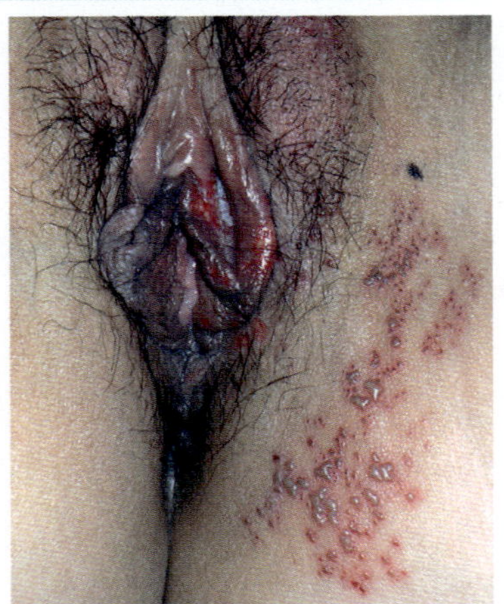

Herpes zoster (shingles)

Small, grouped vesicles emerge along the route of the cutaneous sensory nerve, then pustules, then crusts. Caused by the varicella zoster virus, a reactivation of the dormant virus of chickenpox. Acute appearance, unilateral, does not cross the midline. Commonly on the trunk; can be anywhere. If on the ophthalmic branch of cranial nerve V, it poses a risk to the eyes. Most common in adults over 50 years old. Pain is often severe and long-lasting in ageing adults; called *postherpetic neuralgia.*

Note: Be observant! The photo above is not genital herpes. This is herpes zoster with a linear lesion on only one side.

TABLE 22.4 Common shapes and configurations of lesions

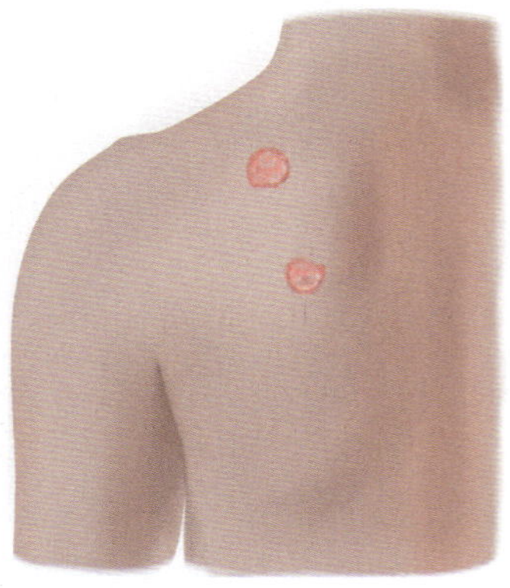

Annular, or circular, begins in centre and spreads to periphery (e.g. tinea corporis, tinea versicolor, pityriasis rosea)

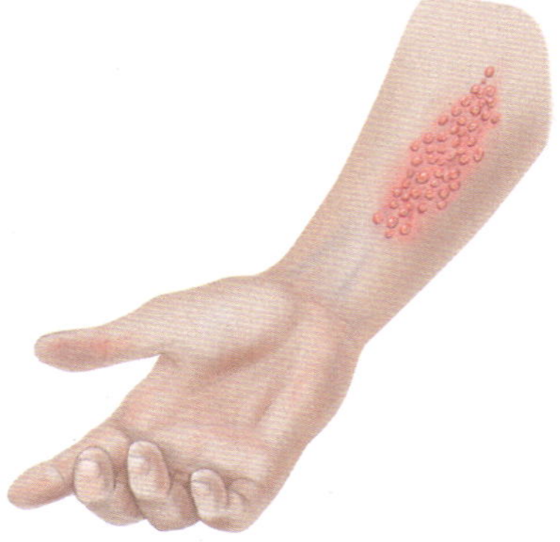

Grouped, clusters of lesions (e.g. vesicles of contact dermatitis)

TABLE 22.4 Common shapes and configurations of lesions cont'd

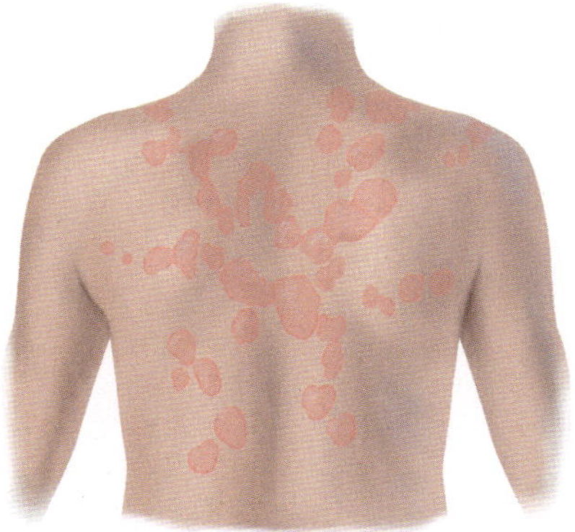

Confluent, lesions run together (e.g. urticaria, or hives)

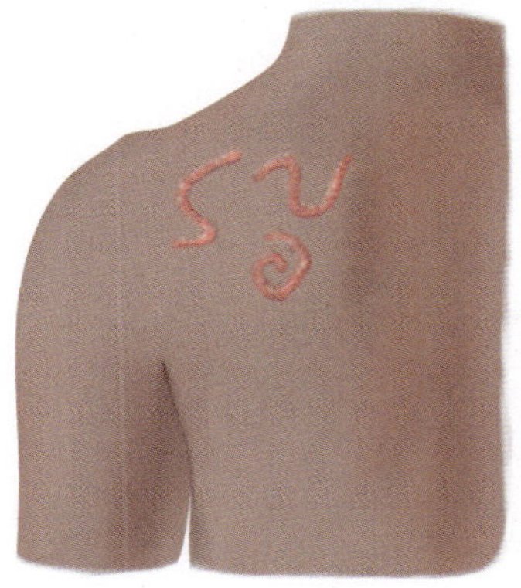

Gyrate, twisted, coiled spiral, snake-like

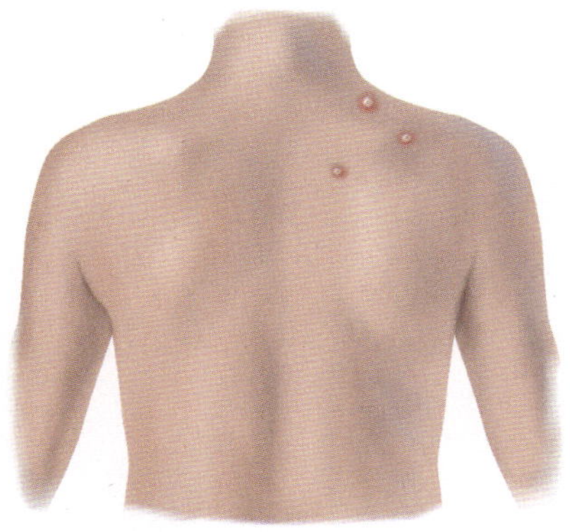

Discrete, distinct, individual lesions that remain separate (e.g. molluscum)

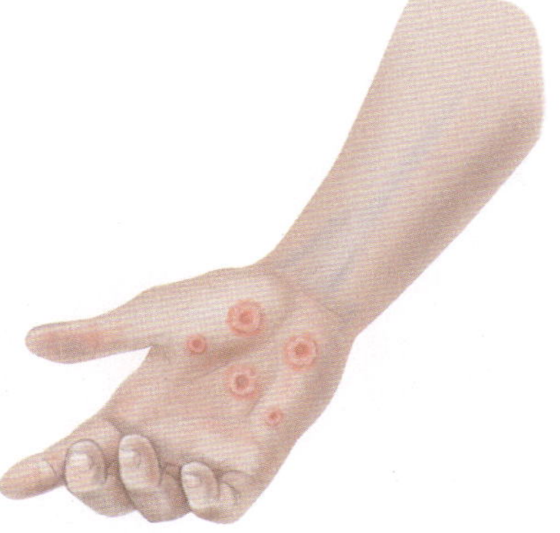

Target, or iris, resembles the iris of the eye, concentric rings of colour in the lesions (e.g. erythema multiforme)

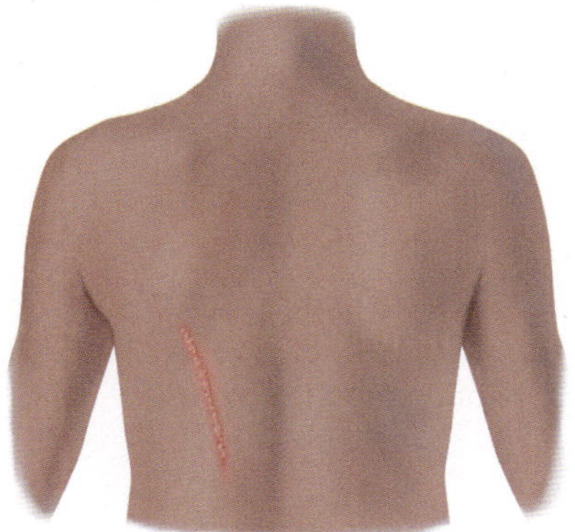

Linear, a scratch, streak, line or stripe

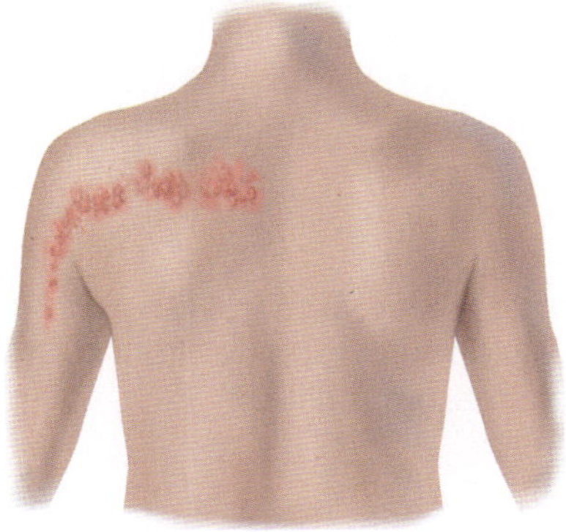

Zosteriform, linear arrangement along a nerve route (e.g. herpes zoster)

Continued

TABLE 22.4 Common shapes and configurations of lesions cont'd

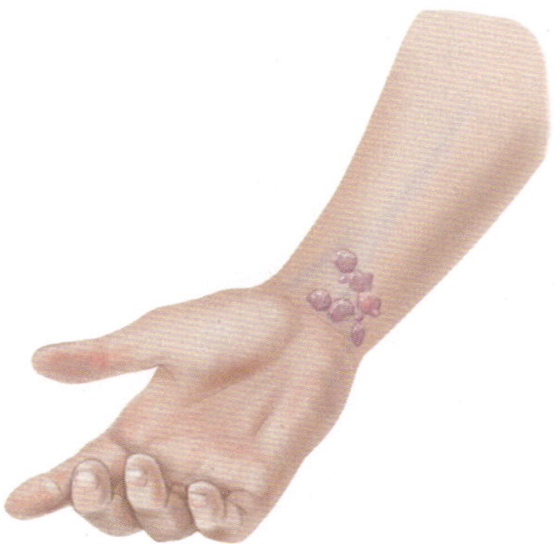

Polycyclic, annular lesions grow together (e.g. lichen planus, psoriasis)

TABLE 22.5 Primary skin lesions

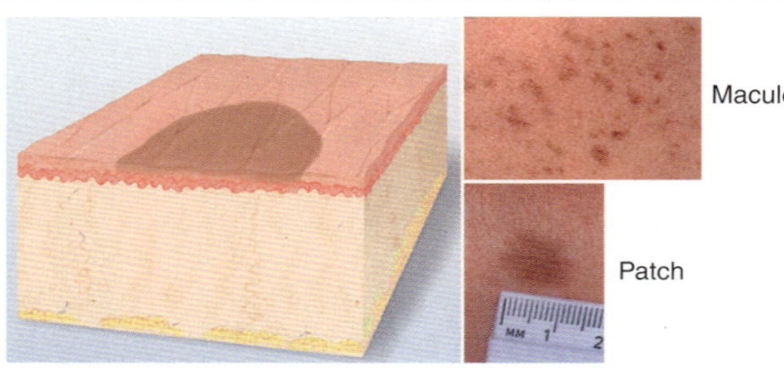

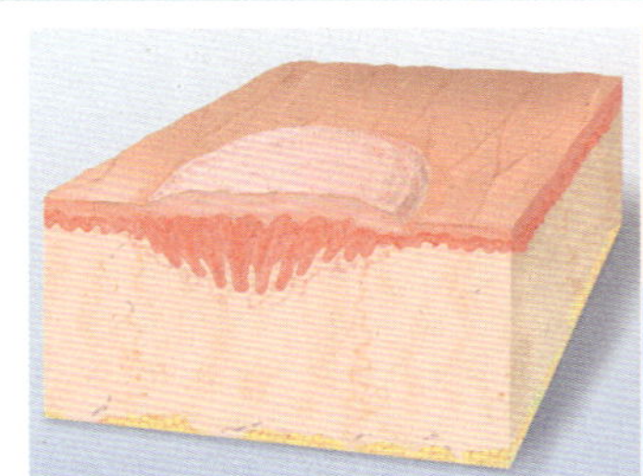

Macule

Solely a colour change, flat and circumscribed, of less than 1 cm
Examples: freckles, flat naevi, hypopigmentation, petechiae, measles, scarlet fever

Patch

Macules that are larger than 1 cm
Examples: Mongolian spot, vitiligo, café au lait spot, chloasma, measles rash

Papule

Something you can feel (i.e. solid, elevated, circumscribed, less than 1 cm diameter) caused by superficial thickening in the epidermis
Examples: elevated naevus (mole), lichen planus, molluscum, wart (verruca)

Plaque

Papules coalesce to form surface elevation wider than 1 cm; a plateau-like, disc-shaped lesion
Examples: psoriasis, lichen planus

TABLE 22.5 Primary skin lesions cont'd

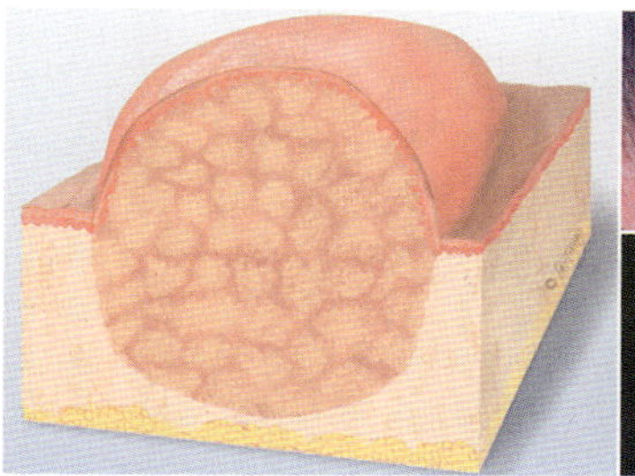

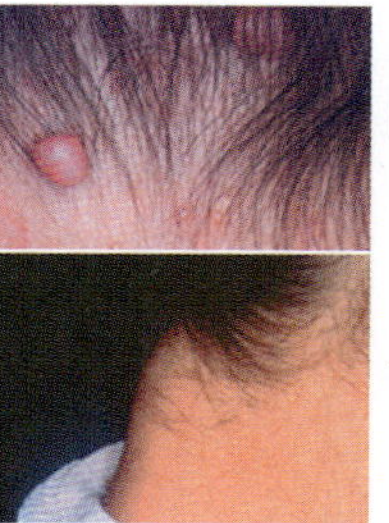

Nodule

Solid, elevated, hard or soft, larger than 1 cm; may extend deeper into dermis than papule
Examples: xanthoma, fibroma, intradermal naevi

Tumour

Larger than a few centimetres in diameter, firm or soft, deeper into dermis; may be benign or malignant, although 'tumour' implies 'cancer' to most people
Examples: lipoma, haemangioma

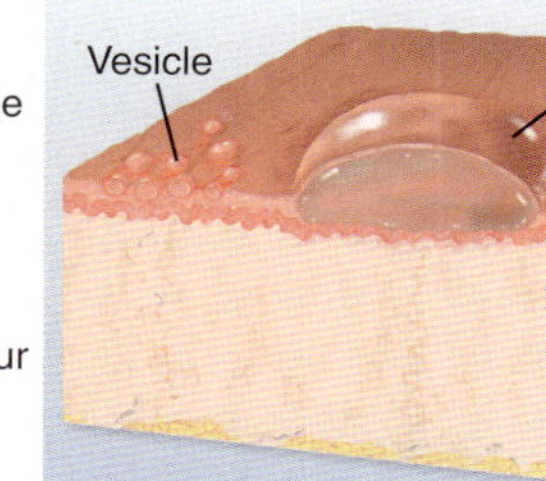

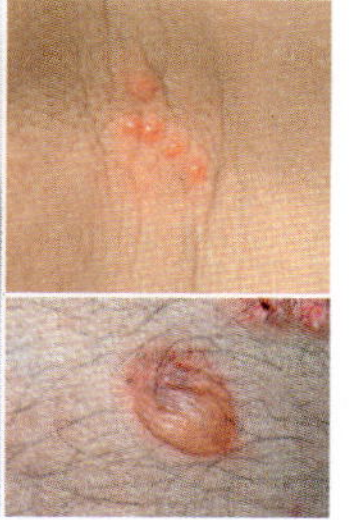

Vesicle

Elevated cavity containing free fluid, up to 1 cm; a 'blister'; clear serum flows if wall is ruptured
Examples: herpes simplex, early varicella (chickenpox), herpes zoster (shingles), contact dermatitis

Bulla

Larger than 1 cm diameter; usually single chambered (unilocular); superficial in epidermis; it is thin walled, so it ruptures easily
Examples: friction blister, pemphigus, burns, contact dermatitis

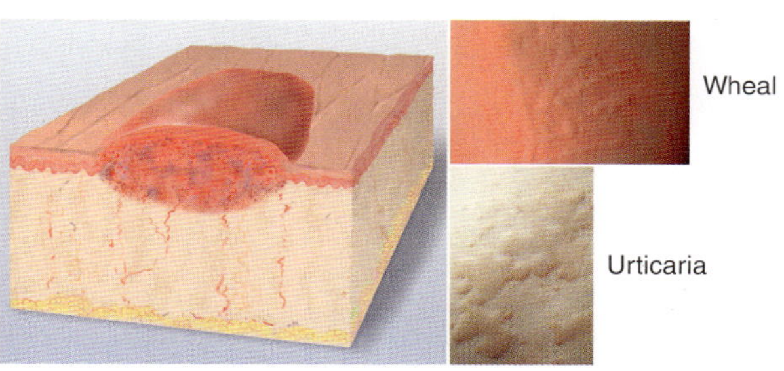

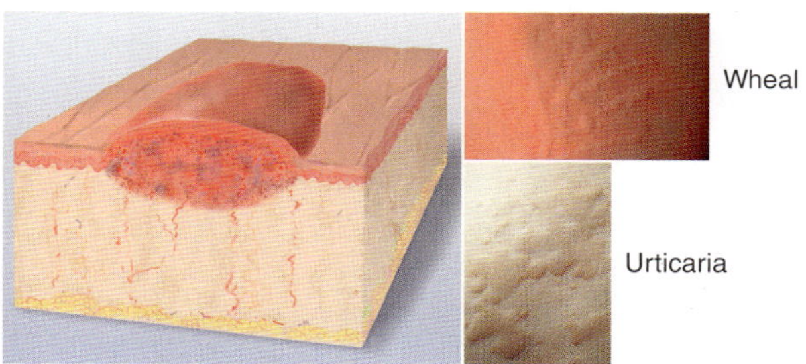

Wheal

Superficial, raised, transient and erythematous; slightly irregular shape due to oedema (fluid held diffusely in the tissues)
Examples: mosquito bite, allergic reaction, dermographism

Urticaria (hives)

Wheals coalesce to form extensive reaction, intensely pruritic

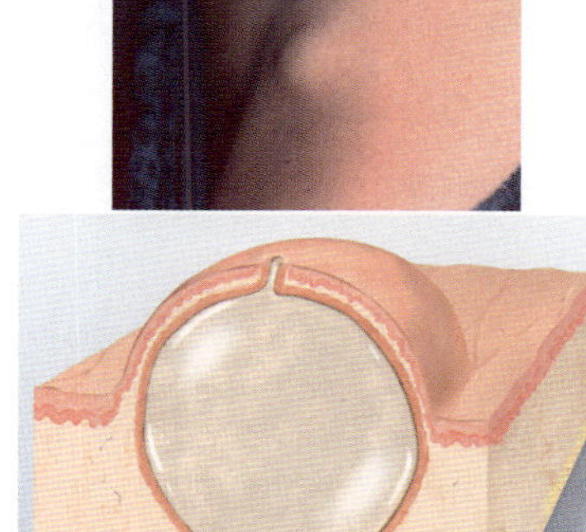

Cyst

Encapsulated fluid-filled cavity in dermis or subcutaneous layer, tensely elevating skin
Examples: sebaceous cyst, wen

Continued

TABLE 22.5 Primary skin lesions cont'd

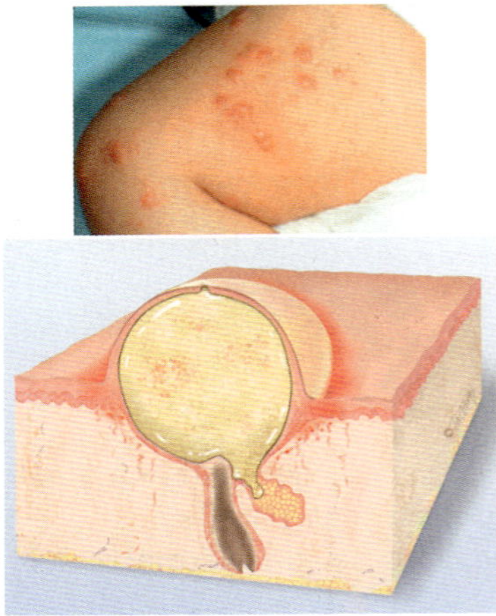

Pustule

Turbid fluid (pus) in the cavity; circumscribed and elevated
Examples: impetigo, acne

Note: Primary skin lesions are the immediate result of a specific causative factor; they develop on previously unaltered skin.

TABLE 22.6 Secondary skin lesions

Debris on Skin Surface

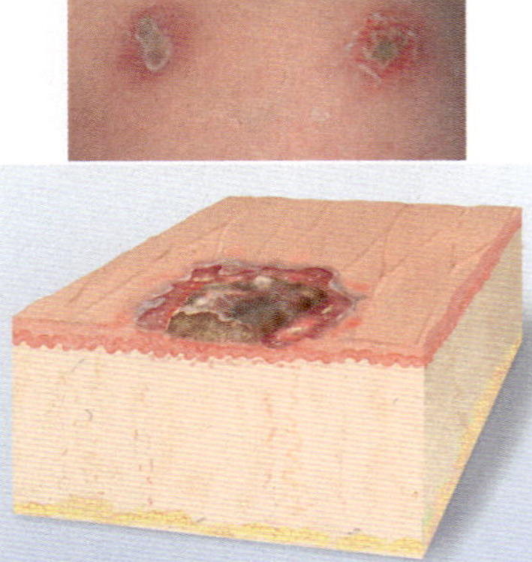

Crust

The thickened, dried-out exudate left when vesicles/pustules burst or dry up; colour can be red-brown, honey or yellow, depending on the fluid's ingredients (blood, serum, pus)
Examples: impetigo (dry, honey coloured), weeping eczematous dermatitis, scab after abrasion

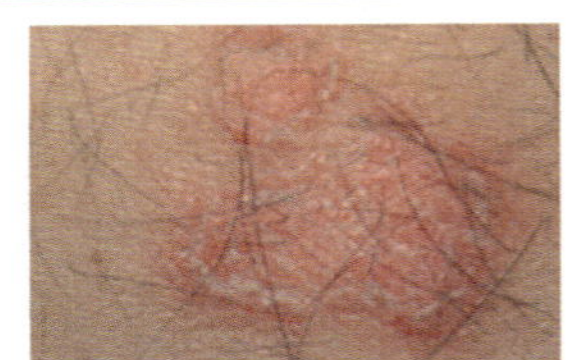

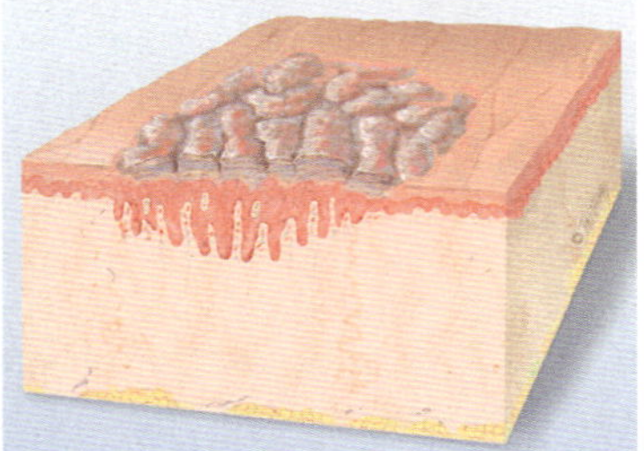

Scale

Compact, desiccated flakes of skin, dry or greasy, silvery or white, from shedding of dead excess keratin cells
Examples: after scarlet fever or drug reaction (laminated sheets), psoriasis (silver, mica-like), seborrhoeic dermatitis (yellow, greasy), eczema, ichthyosis (large, adherent, laminated), dry skin

TABLE 22.6 Secondary skin lesions cont'd

Break in Continuity of Surface

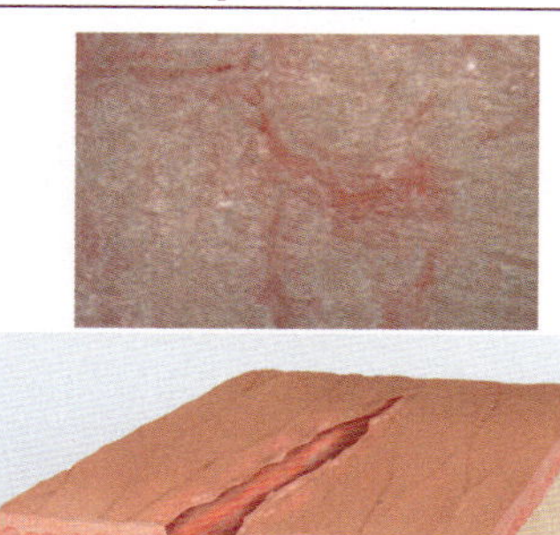

Fissure

Linear crack with abrupt edges, extends into dermis, dry or moist

Examples: cheilosis—at corners of the mouth due to excess moisture; athlete's foot

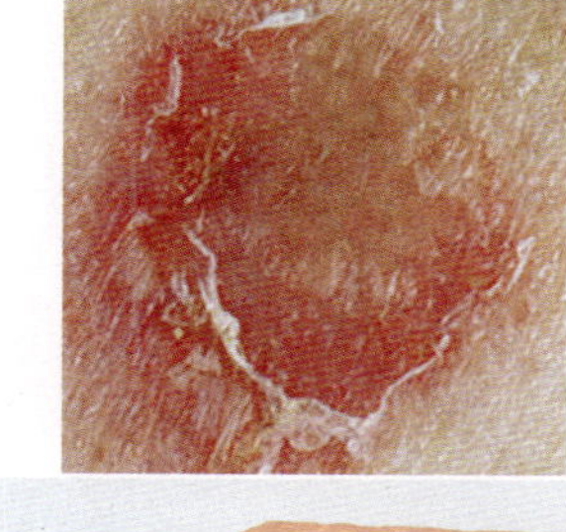

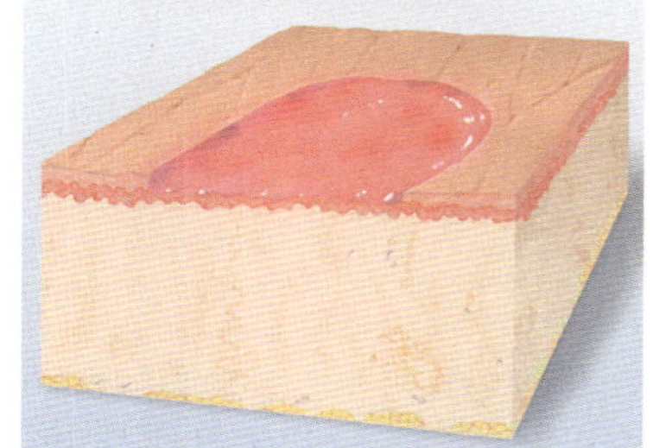

Erosion

Scooped out but shallow depression; superficial; epidermis lost; moist but no bleeding; heals without scar because erosion does not extend into dermis

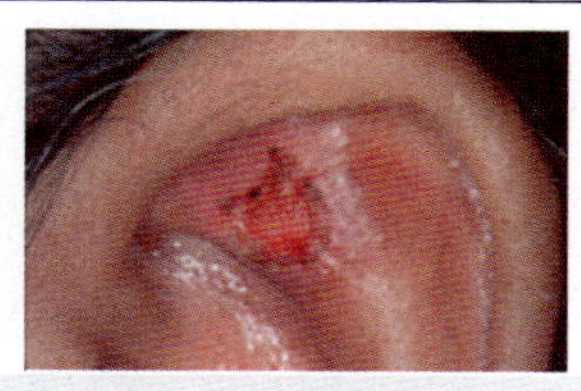

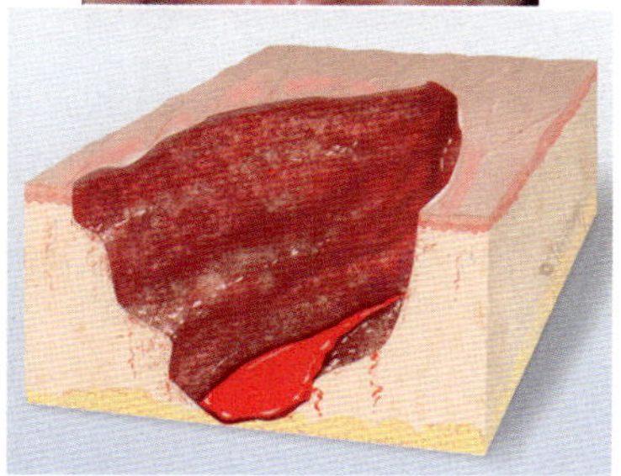

Ulcer

Deeper depression extending into the dermis, irregular shape; may bleed; leaves scar when heals

Examples: stasis ulcer, pressure injury, chancre

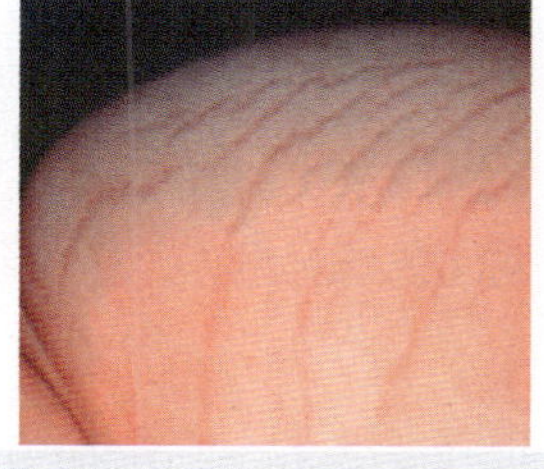

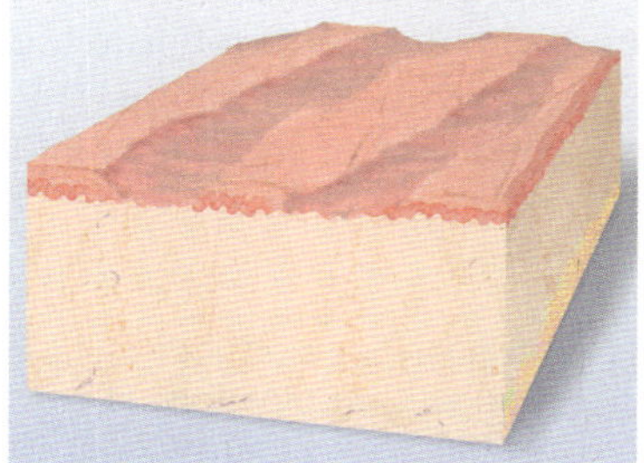

Atrophic scar

Resulting skin level depressed with loss of tissue; a thinning of the epidermis

Example: striae

Continued

TABLE 22.6 Secondary skin lesions cont'd

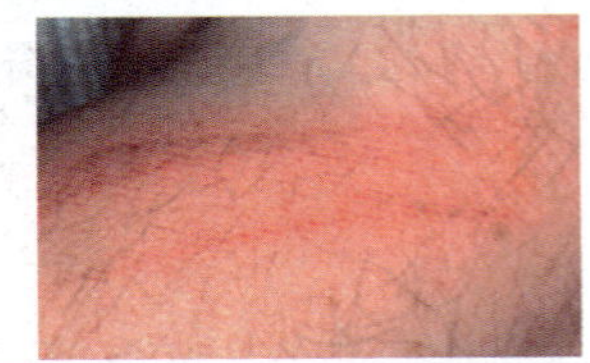

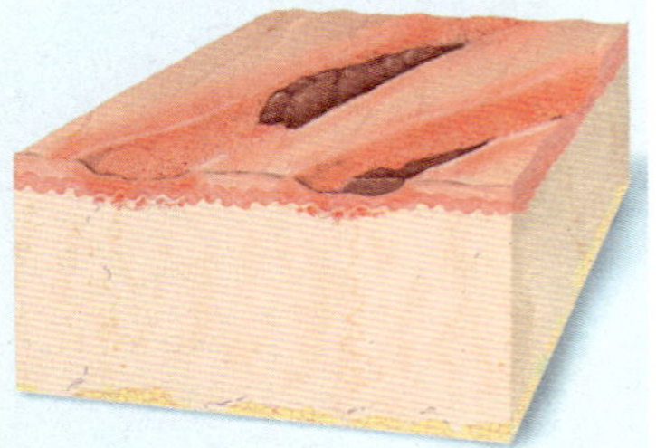

Excoriation

Self-inflicted abrasion; superficial; sometimes crusted; scratches from intense itching
Examples: insect bites, scabies, dermatitis, varicella

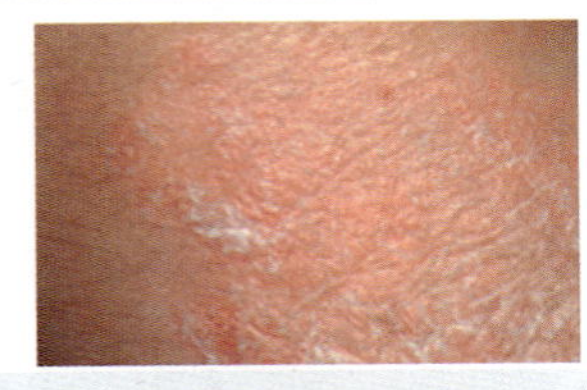

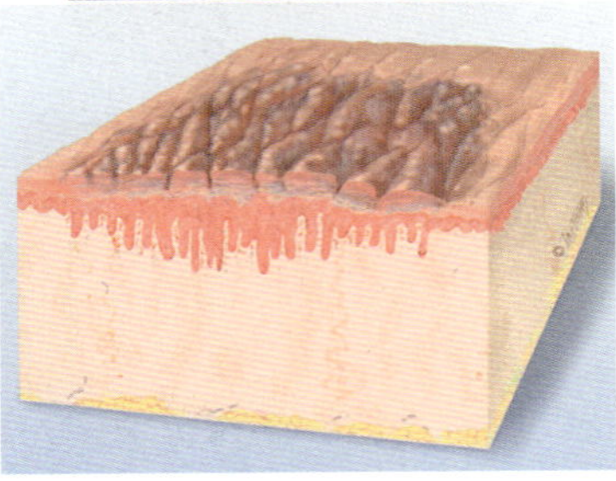

Lichenification

Prolonged intense scratching eventually thickens the skin and produces tightly packed sets of papules; looks like the surface of moss (or lichen)

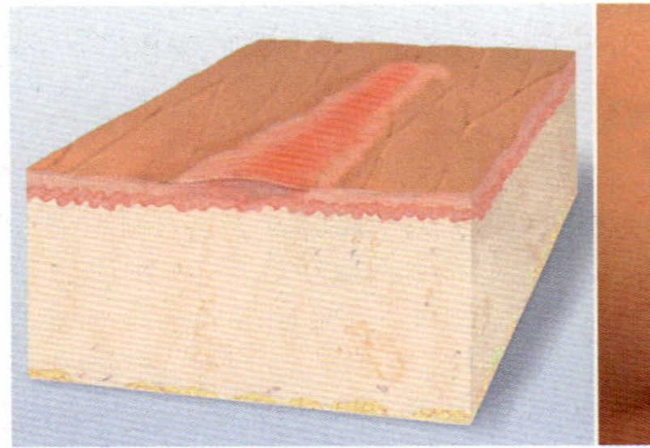

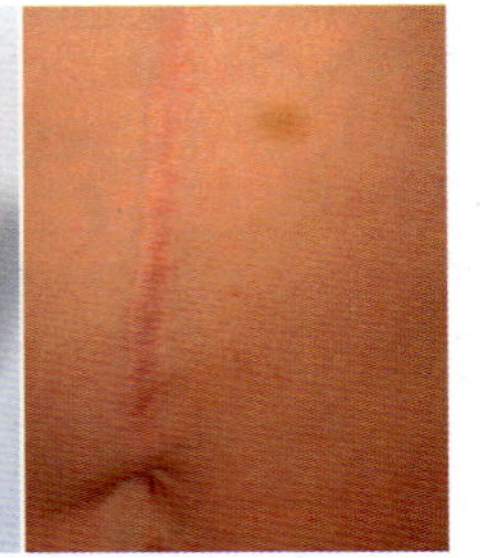

Scar

After a skin lesion is repaired, normal tissue is lost and replaced with connective tissue (collagen); this is a permanent fibrotic change
Examples: healed area of surgery or injury, acne

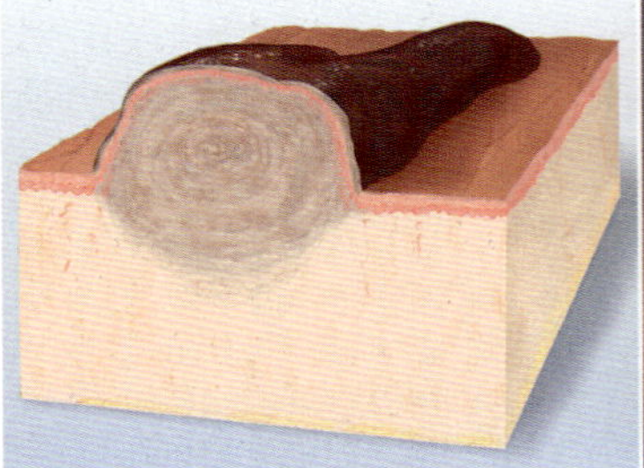

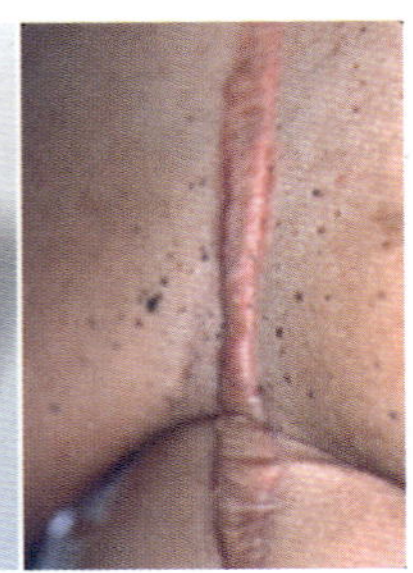

Keloid

A hypertrophic scar; the resulting skin level is elevated by excess scar tissue, which is invasive beyond the site of original injury
May increase long after healing occurs; looks smooth, rubbery, 'claw-like' and has a higher incidence among dark-skinned people

Note: Secondary skin lesions are those resulting from a change in a primary lesion from the passage of time; an evolutionary change. Combinations of primary and secondary lesions may coexist in the same person. Such combined designations may be termed papulosquamous, maculopapular, vesiculopustular or papulovesicular.

TABLE 22.7 Malignant skin lesions

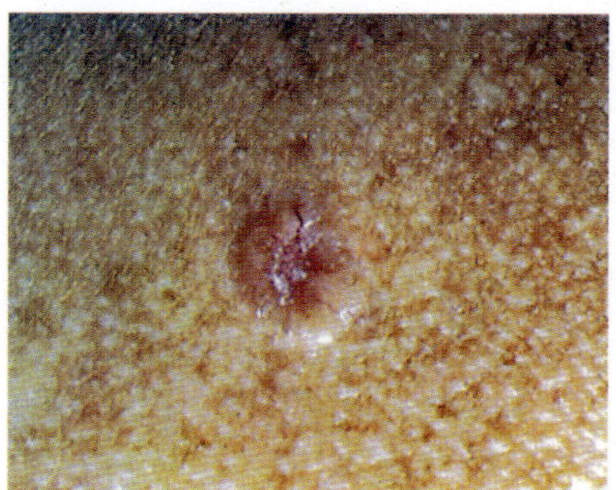

Basal cell carcinoma

Usually starts as a skin-coloured papule (may be deeply pigmented) with a translucent top and overlying telangiectasia. Then develops rounded pearly borders with a central red ulcer or looks like a large, open pore with central yellowing. Most common form of skin cancer; slow but inexorable growth.

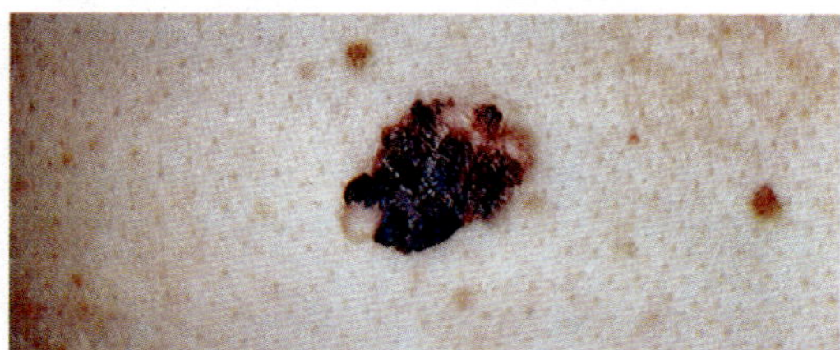

Malignant melanoma

Half of the occurrences of these lesions arise from pre-existing naevi. Usually brown; can be tan, black, pink-red, purple or mixed pigmentation. Often irregular or notched borders. May have scaling, flaking, oozing texture. Common locations are on the trunk and back in men and women, on the legs in women and on the palms, soles of the feet and the nails in dark-skinned people.

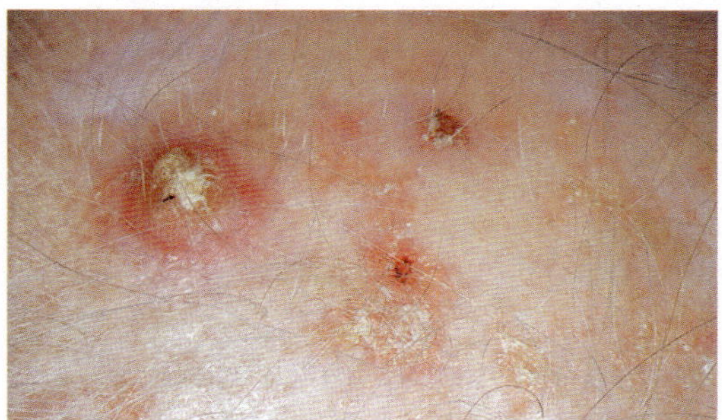

Squamous cell carcinoma

Erythematous scaly patch with sharp margins, 1 cm or more. Develops a central ulcer and surrounding erythema. Usually on the hands or head—areas exposed to solar radiation. Less common than basal cell carcinoma but grows rapidly.

TABLE 22.8 Vascular lesions

Haemangiomas

Caused by a benign proliferation of blood vessels in the dermis.

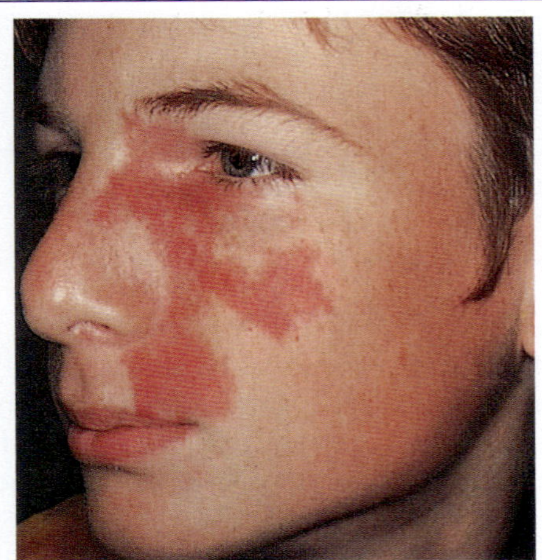

Port-wine stain (naevus flammeus)

A large, flat macular patch covering the scalp or face, frequently along the distribution of cranial nerve V. The colour is dark red, bluish or purplish and intensifies with crying, exertion or exposure to heat or cold. The marking consists of mature capillaries. It is present at birth and usually does not fade. The use of yellow light lasers now makes photoablation of the lesion possible, with minimal adverse effects.

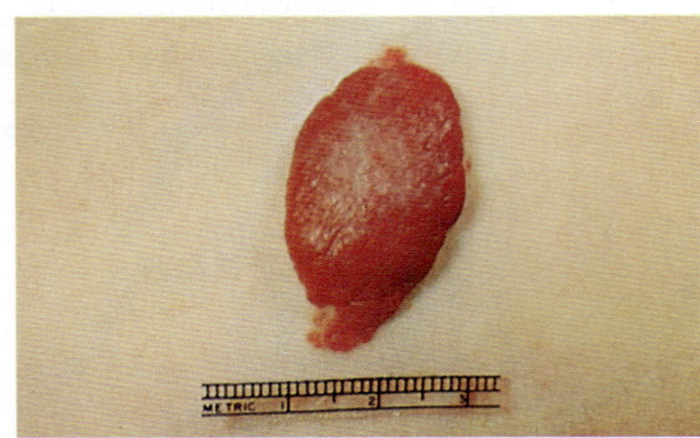

Strawberry mark (immature haemangioma)

A raised bright red area with well-defined borders 2 to 3 cm in diameter. It does not blanch with pressure. It consists of immature capillaries, is present at birth or develops in the first few months and usually disappears by age 5 to 7 years. Requires no treatment, although parental and peer pressure may prompt treatment.

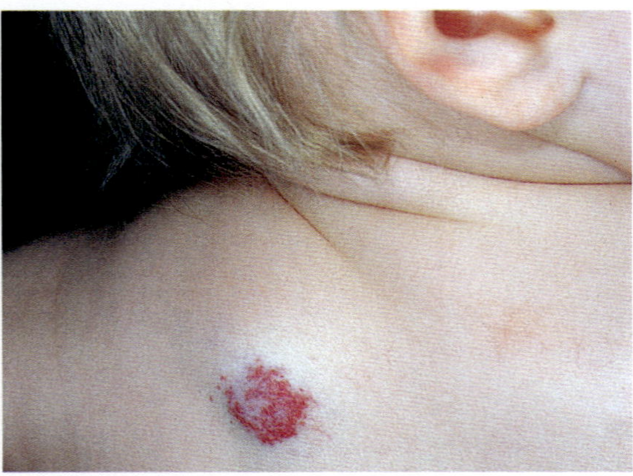

Cavernous haemangioma (mature)

A reddish-blue, irregularly shaped, solid and spongy mass of blood vessels. It may be present at birth, may enlarge during the first 10 to 15 months and will not involute spontaneously.

TABLE 22.8 Vascular lesions cont'd

Telangiectases

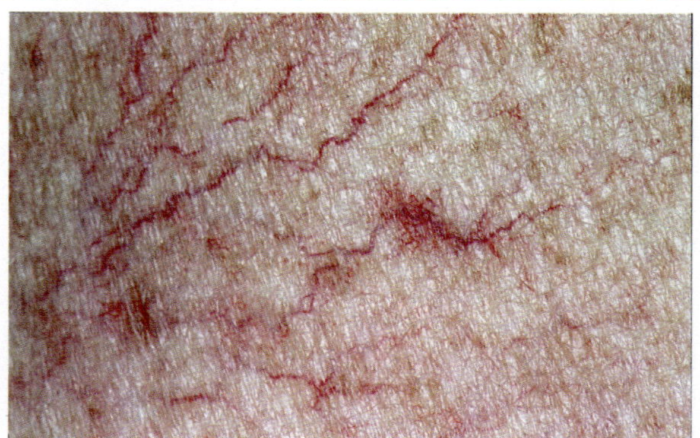

Telangiectasia

Caused by vascular dilatation; permanently enlarged and dilated blood vessels that are visible on the skin surface.

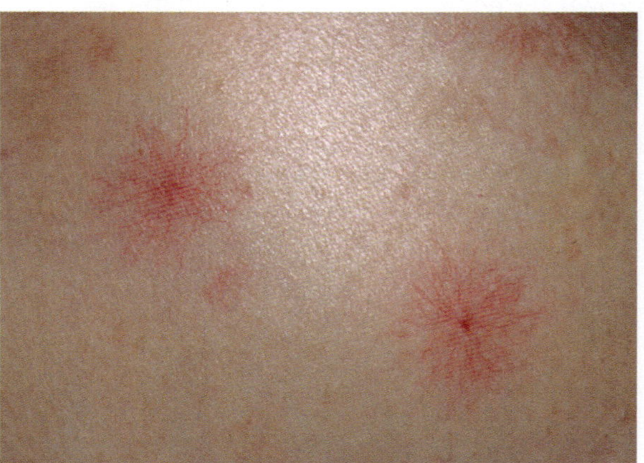

Spider or star angioma

A fiery red, star-shaped marking with a solid circular centre. Capillary radiations extend from the central arterial body. With pressure, note a central pulsating body and blanching of extended legs. Develops on the face, neck or chest; may be associated with pregnancy, chronic liver disease or estrogen therapy or may be normal.

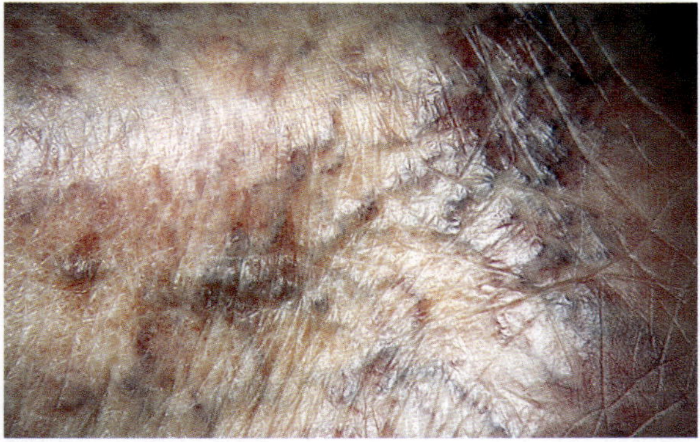

Venous lake

A blue-purple dilatation of venules and capillaries in a star-shaped, linear or flaring pattern. Pressure causes them to empty or disappear. Located on the legs near varicose veins and on the face, lips, ears and chest.

Continued

TABLE 22.8 Vascular lesions cont'd

Purpuric lesions

Caused by blood flowing out of breaks in the vessels. Red blood cells and blood pigments are deposited in the tissues (extravascular). Difficult to see in dark-skinned people.

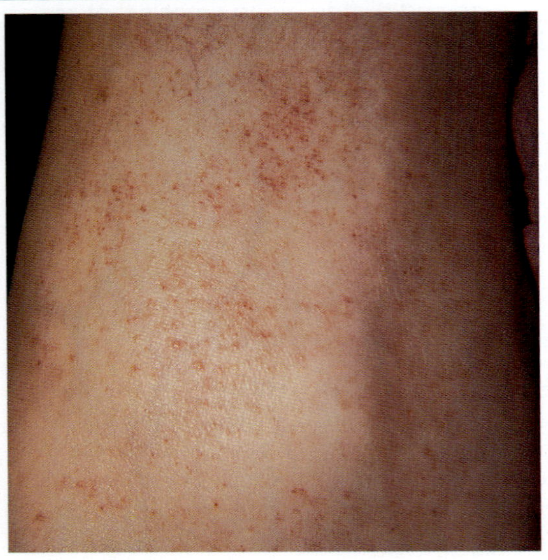

Petechiae

Tiny punctate haemorrhages, 1 to 3 mm, round and discrete, dark red, purple or brown in colour. Caused by bleeding from superficial capillaries; will not blanch. May indicate abnormal clotting factors. In dark-skinned people, petechiae are best visualised in the areas of lighter melanisation (e.g. the abdomen, buttocks and volar surface of the forearm). When the skin is black or very dark brown, petechiae cannot be seen in the skin. Most of the diseases that cause bleeding and microembolism formation—such as thrombocytopenia, subacute bacterial endocarditis and other septicaemias—are characterised by petechiae in the mucous membranes as well as on the skin. Thus, you should inspect for petechiae in the mouth, particularly the buccal mucosa and in the conjunctivae.

Ecchymosis

A purplish patch resulting from extravasation of blood into the skin, larger than 3 mm in diameter.

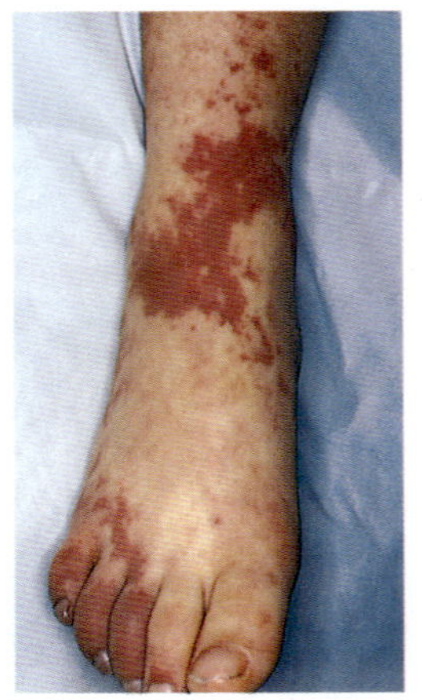

Purpura

Confluent and extensive patch of petechiae and ecchymoses, larger than 3 mm, flat, red to purple, macular haemorrhage. Seen in generalised disorders such as thrombocytopenia and scurvy. Also occurs in old age as blood leaks from capillaries in response to minor trauma and diffuses through the dermis.

TABLE 22.9 Pressure injury

Pressure injuries develop over a bony prominence when circulation is impaired, usually because of immobility. Immobility impedes delivery of blood-carrying oxygen and nutrients to the skin, and it impedes venous drainage carrying metabolic wastes away from the skin. This results in ischaemia and cell death. Common sites for pressure injuries are on the back (heel, ischium, sacrum, elbow, scapula, vertebra, head) or the side (ankle, knee, hip, rib, shoulder, ear).

Risk factors for pressure injuries include:

- impaired mobility
- the thin, fragile skin of ageing
- decreased sensory perception (unable to respond to pain accompanying prolonged pressure); impaired level of consciousness
- moisture from urine or stool incontinence
- excessive perspiration or wound drainage
- shearing injury (being pulled down or across in bed)
- poor nutrition
- infection.

Preventing pressure injuries is far more easily accomplished than is treating existing pressure injuries. However, once pressure injuries occur, they are assessed by stage, depending on the pressure injury depth:

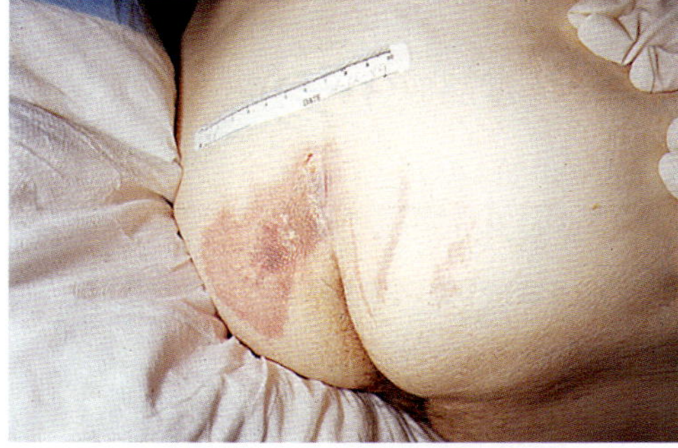

Stage I

Intact skin appears red but unbroken. Localised redness in lightly pigmented skin does not blanch (turn light with fingertip pressure). Dark skin appears darker but does not blanch.

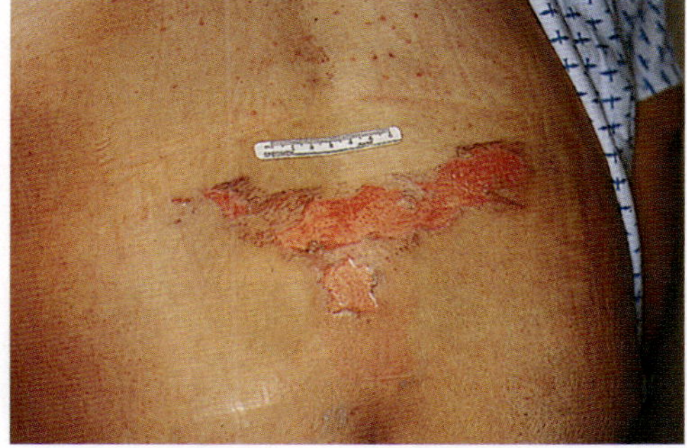

Stage II

Partial-thickness skin erosion with loss of epidermis or also the dermis. Superficial injury looks shallow, like an abrasion or open blister with a red-pink wound bed.

Continued

TABLE 22.9 Pressure injury cont'd

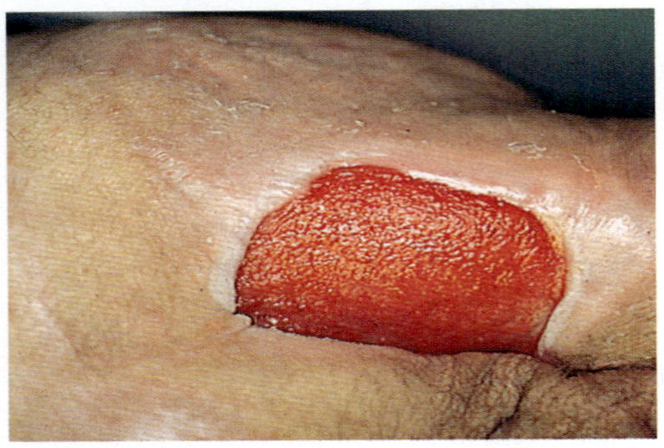

Stage III

Full-thickness pressure injury extending into the subcutaneous tissue and resembling a crater. May see subcutaneous fat but not muscle, bone or tendon.

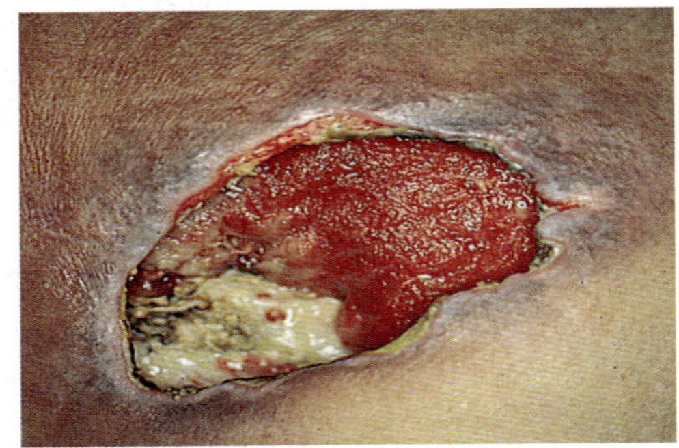

Stage IV

Full-thickness pressure injury involves all skin layers and extends into supporting tissue. Exposes muscle, tendon or bone and may show slough (stringy matter attached to wound bed) or eschar (black or brown necrotic tissue).

Once stage III or IV injuries occur, wound size must be measured weekly to provide quantifiable data for wound healing. Use disposable rulers with mm and cm markings and measure the greatest overall wound length.

TABLE 22.10 Abnormal conditions of the hair and scalp

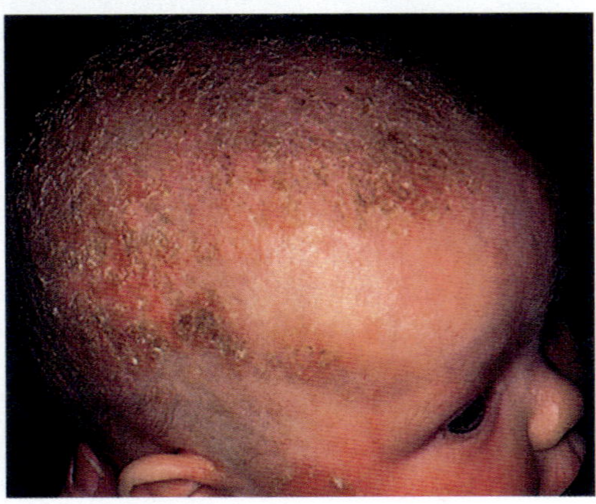

Seborrhoeic dermatitis

Thick, yellow to white, greasy, adherent scales with mild erythema on the scalp and forehead; very common in early infancy. Resembles eczema lesions except cradle cap is distinguished by the absence of pruritus, 'greasy' yellow-pink lesions and negative family history of allergy.

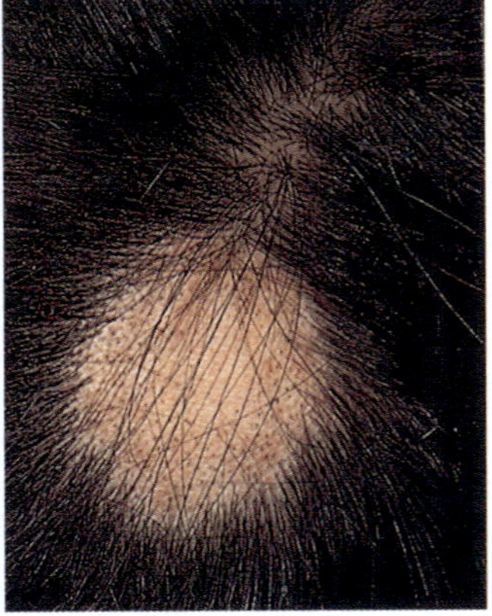

Alopecia areata

Sudden appearance of a sharply circumscribed, round or oval balding patch, usually with smooth, soft, hairless skin underneath. Unknown cause; when limited to a few patches, the person usually has complete regrowth.

TABLE 22.10 Abnormal conditions of the hair and scalp cont'd

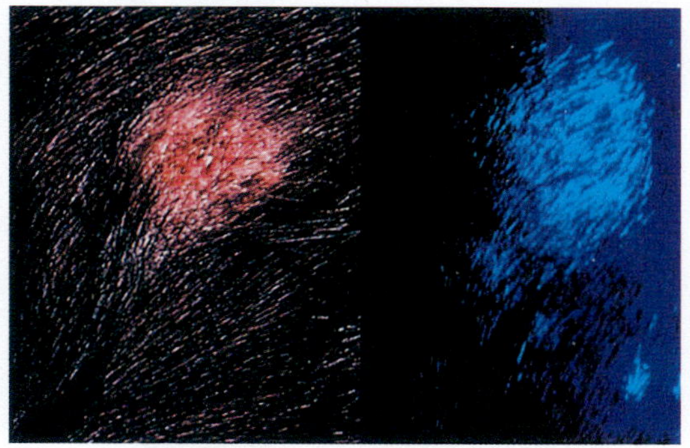

Tinea capitis

Rounded patchy hair loss on the scalp, leaving broken-off hairs, pustules and scales on the skin. Caused by fungal infection; lesions may fluoresce blue-green under Wood's light. Usually seen in children and farmers; highly contagious, may be transmitted by another person, by domestic animals or from soil.

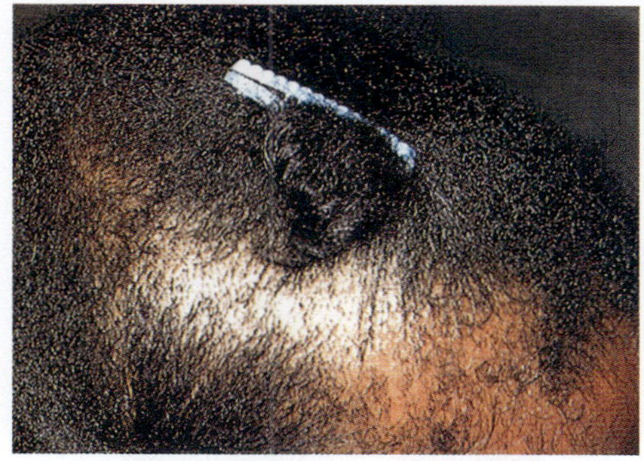

Traumatic alopecia: traction alopecia

Linear or oval patch of hair loss along the hair line, a part or scattered distribution; caused by trauma from hair rollers, tight braiding, tight ponytails or hair clips.

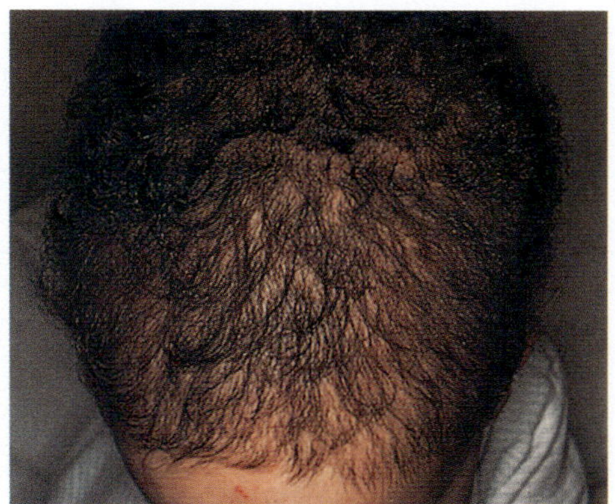

Toxic alopecia

Patchy, asymmetric balding that accompanies severe illness or use of chemotherapy where growing hairs are lost and resting hairs are spared. Regrowth occurs after illness or discontinuation of toxin.

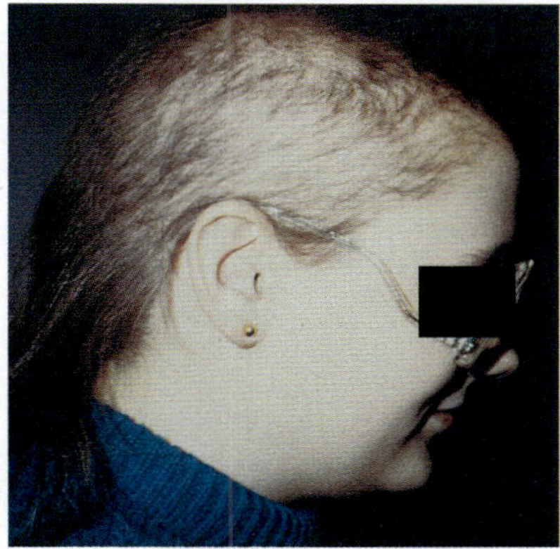

Trichotillomania

Traumatic self-induced hair loss, usually the result of compulsive twisting or plucking. Forms irregularly shaped patch, with broken-off, stub-like hairs of varying lengths; the person is never completely bald. Occurs as a child rubs or twists the area absently while falling asleep, reading or watching television. In adults, it can be a serious problem and is usually a sign of a personality disorder.

Continued

TABLE 22.10 Abnormal conditions of the hair and scalp cont'd

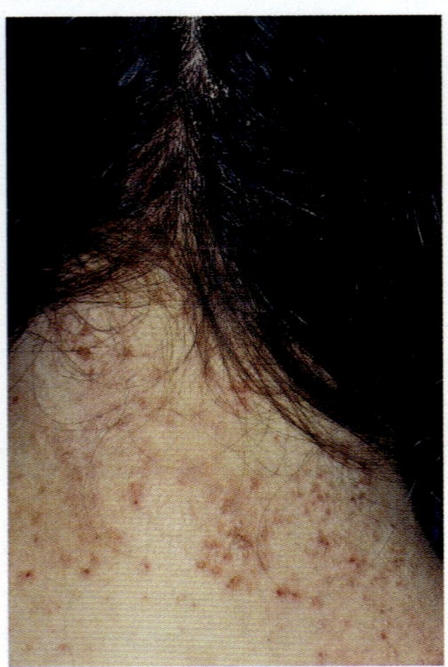

Pediculosis capitis

History includes intense itching of the scalp, especially the occiput. The nits (eggs) of lice are easier to see in the occipital area and around the ears, appearing as 2- to 3-mm oval translucent bodies, adherent to the hair shafts. Common among school-age children. Over-the-counter pediculicide shampoos are available, but nit removal by daily combing of wet hair with a fine-tooth metal comb is especially important.

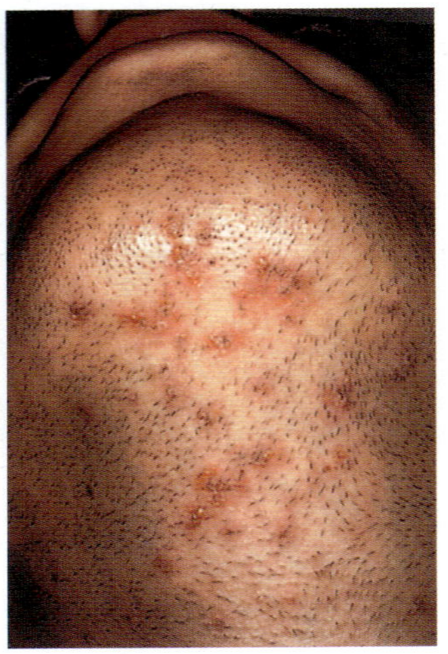

Folliculitis

Superficial infection of hair follicles. Multiple pustules ('whiteheads'), with hair visible at the centre and erythematous base. Usually on the arms, legs, face and buttocks.

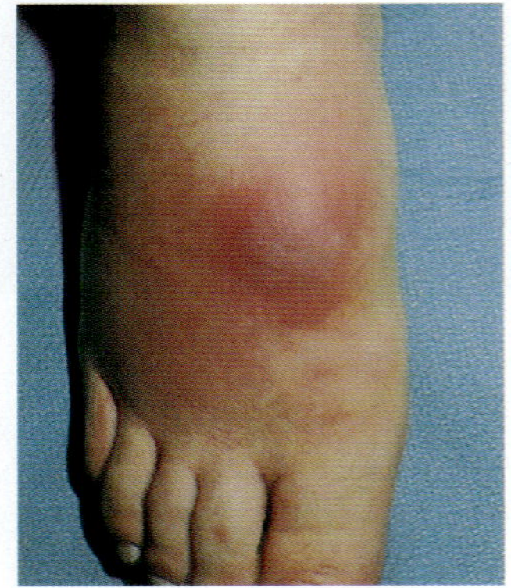

Furuncle and abscess

Red, swollen, hard, tender, pus-filled lesion caused by acute localised bacterial (usually staphylococcal) infection; usually on the back of the neck, buttocks, occasionally on wrists or ankles. Furuncles are due to infected hair follicles, whereas abscesses are due to the traumatic introduction of bacteria into the skin. Abscesses are usually larger and deeper than furuncles.

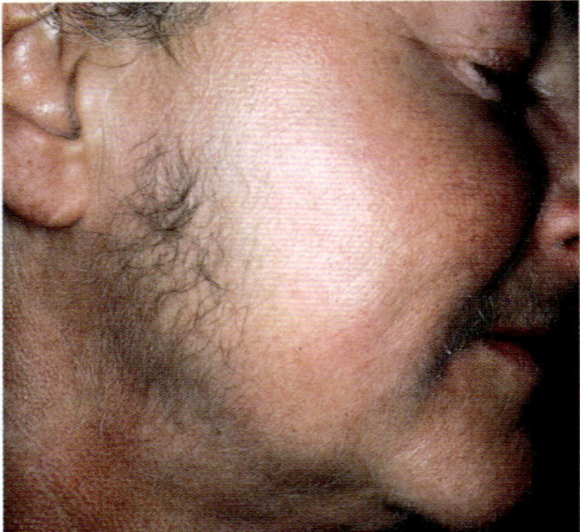

Hirsutism

Excess body hair in females forming a male sexual pattern (upper lip, face, chest, abdomen, arms, legs); caused by endocrine or metabolic dysfunction or occasionally is idiopathic.

TABLE 22.11 Abnormal conditions of the nails and hands

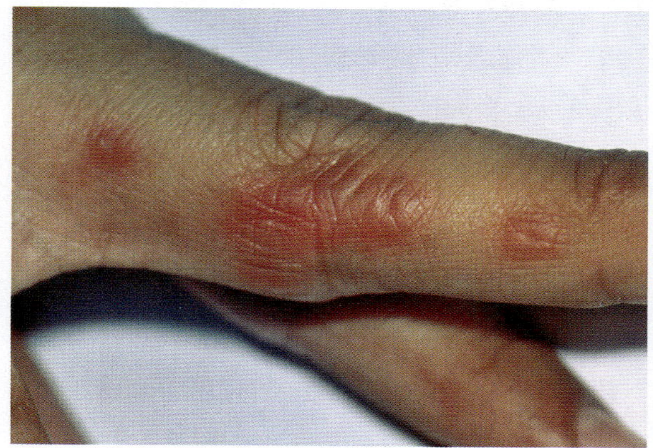

Scabies

An intensely pruritic contagion caused by the scabies mite. Mites form a linear or curved elevated burrow on the fingers, web spaces of the hands and wrists. Other family members are usually infected. The affected person cannot stop scratching.

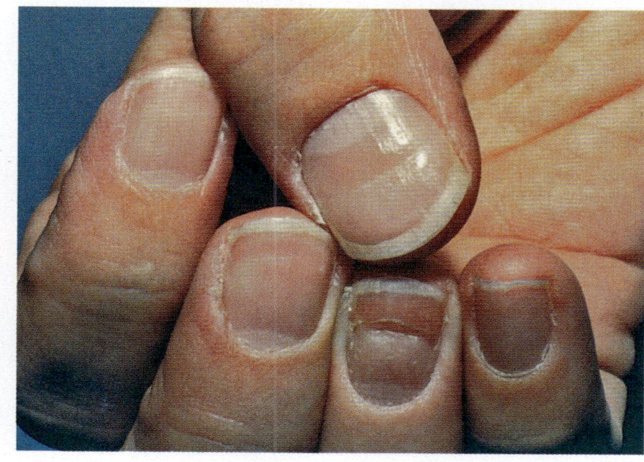

Beau's line

Transverse furrow or groove. A depression across the nail that extends down to the nail bed. Occurs with any trauma that temporarily impairs nail formation such as acute illness, toxic reaction or local trauma. Dent appears first at the cuticle and moves forward as the nail grows.

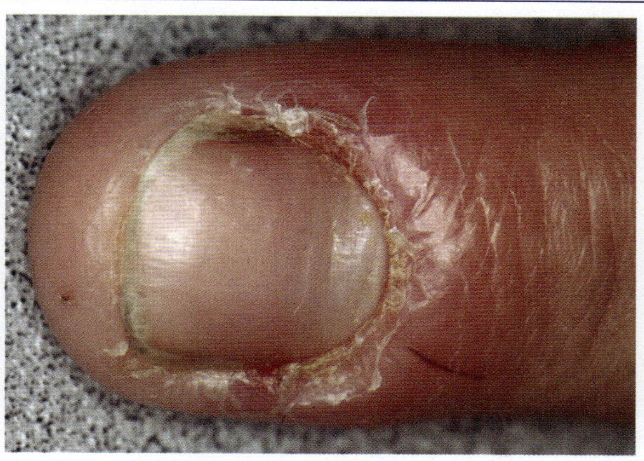

Paronychia

Red, swollen, tender inflammation of the nail folds. Acute paronychia is usually a bacterial infection; chronic paronychia is most often a fungal infection from a break in the cuticle in those who perform 'wet' work.

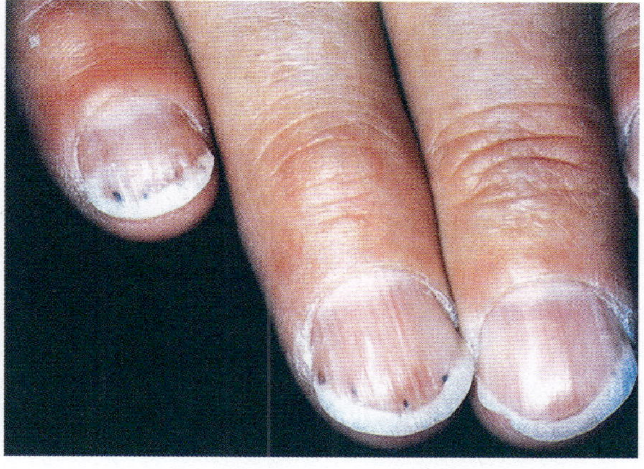

Splinter haemorrhages

Red-brown linear streaks, embolic lesions, occur with subacute bacterial endocarditis; may also occur with minor trauma.

Continued

TABLE 22.11 Abnormal conditions of the nails and hands cont'd

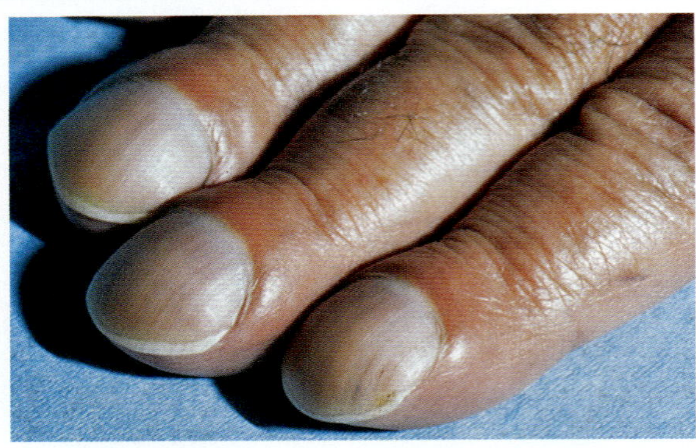

Late clubbing

The proximal edge of the nail elevates; the angle is greater than 180 degrees. The distal phalanx looks rounder and wider. Seen with chronic obstructive pulmonary disease and congenital heart disease with cyanosis. Occurs first in the thumb and index finger.

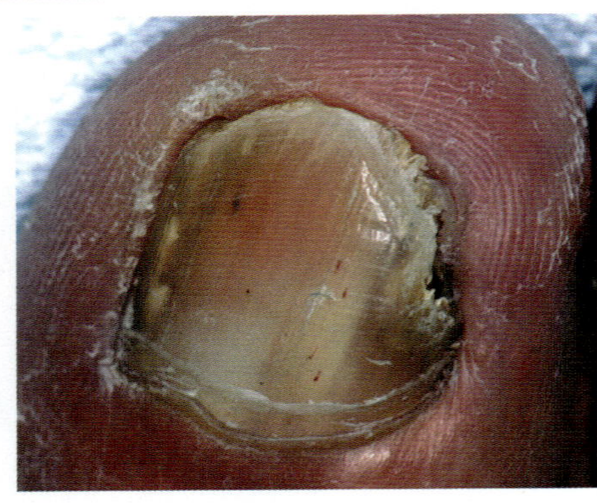

Onycholysis

This is a slow, persistent fungal infection of the fingernails and, more often, toenails, common in older adults. Fungus causes a change in colour (green where the nail plate separates from the bed), texture, thickness, with the nail crumbling or breaking and loosening of the nail plate, usually beginning at the distal edge and progressing proximally.

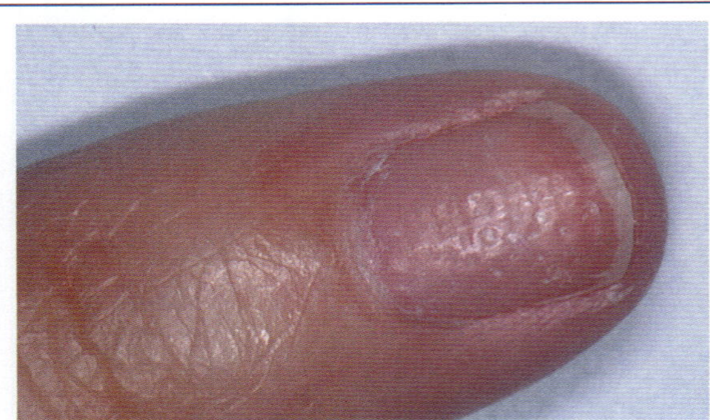

Pitting

Sharply defined pitting and crumbling of the nails with distal detachment; often occurs with psoriasis.

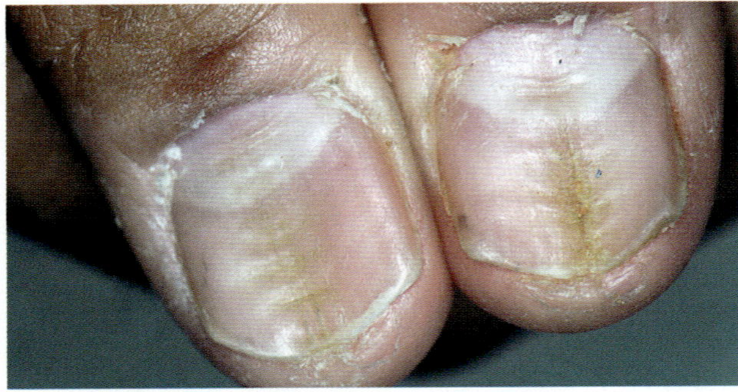

Habit-tic dystrophy

Depression down the middle of the nail or multiple horizontal ridges, caused by continuous picking of the cuticle by another finger on the same hand, which injures the nail base and nail matrix.

TABLE 22.12 Common skin lesions in children

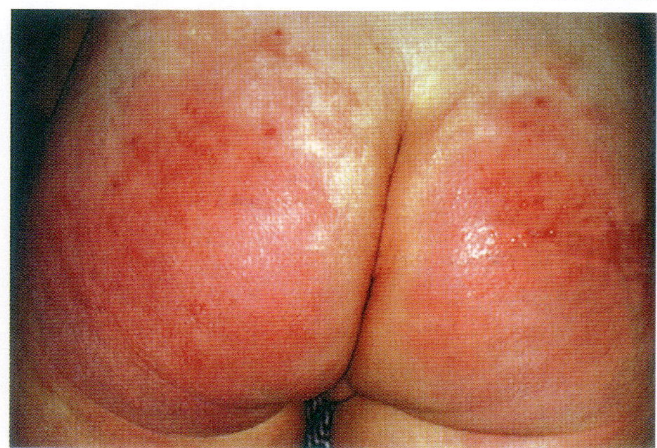

Nappy dermatitis

Red, moist maculopapular patch with poorly defined borders in the nappy area, extending along the inguinal and gluteal folds. History of infrequent nappy changes or occlusive coverings. Inflammatory disease caused by skin irritation from ammonia, heat and moisture occlusive nappies.

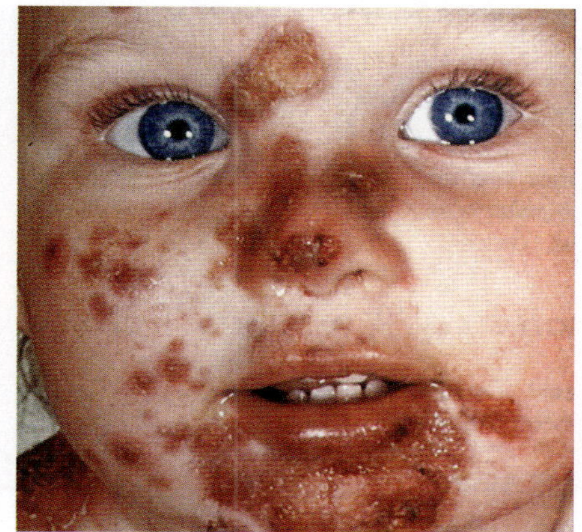

Impetigo

Moist, thin-roofed vesicles with a thin, erythematous base. Rupture to form thick, honey-coloured crusts. Contagious bacterial infection of the skin; most common in infants and children.

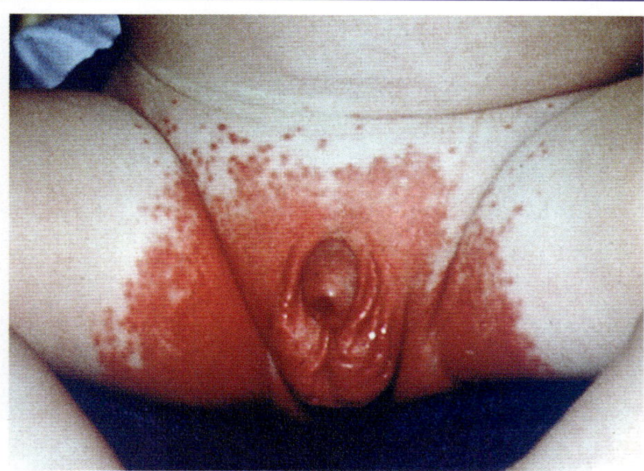

Intertrigo (candidiasis)

Scalding red, moist patches with sharply demarcated borders, some loose scales. Usually in the genital area extending along the inguinal and gluteal folds. Aggravated by urine, faeces, heat and moisture, the *Candida* fungus infects the superficial skin layers.

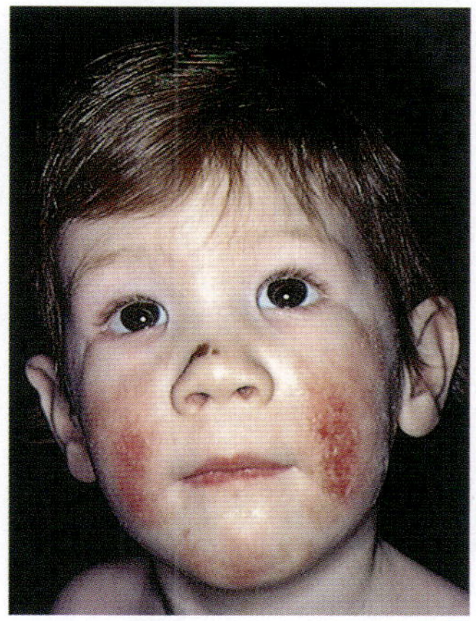

Atopic dermatitis (eczema)

Erythematous papules and vesicles, with weeping, oozing and crusts. Lesions usually on the scalp, forehead, cheeks, forearms, wrists, elbows and backs of knees. Paroxysmal and severe pruritus. Family history of allergies.

Continued

TABLE 22.12 Common skin lesions in children cont'd

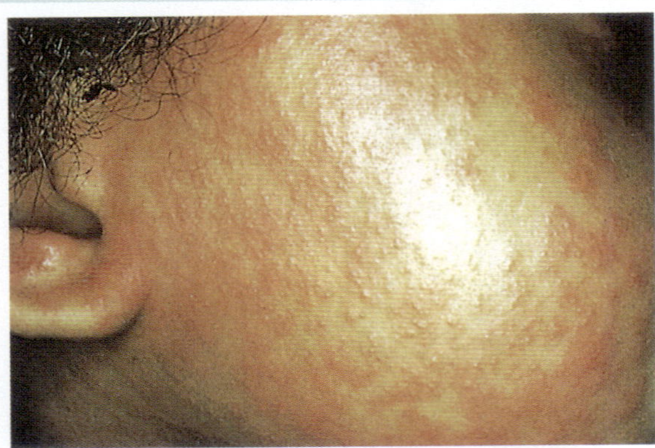

Measles (rubeola) in dark skin

Red-purple maculopapular blotchy rash in dark skin (above) and in light skin (below) appears on the third or fourth day of illness. Rash appears first behind the ears and spreads over the face, then over the neck, trunk, arms and legs; looks 'coppery' and does not blanch. Also characterised by Koplik's spots in the mouth—bluish white, red-based elevations of 1 to 3 mm.

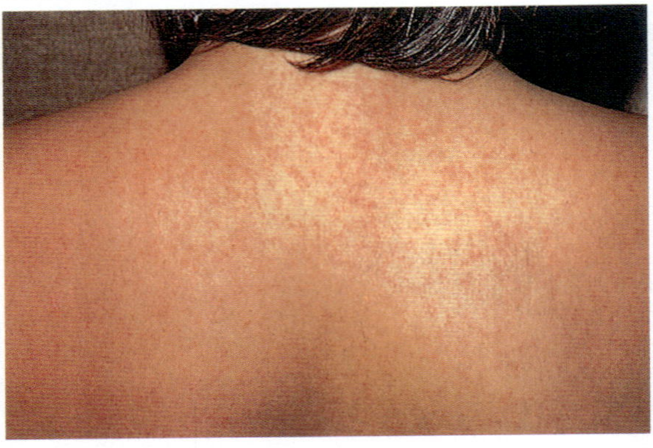

Measles (rubella)

Pink papular rash (similar to rubeola but paler) first appears on the face, then spreads. Distinguished from rubeola by the presence of neck lymphadenopathy and the absence of Koplik's spots.

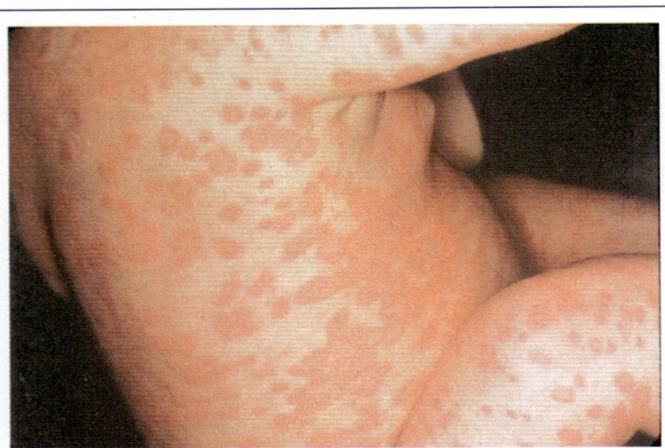

Measles (rubeola) in light skin

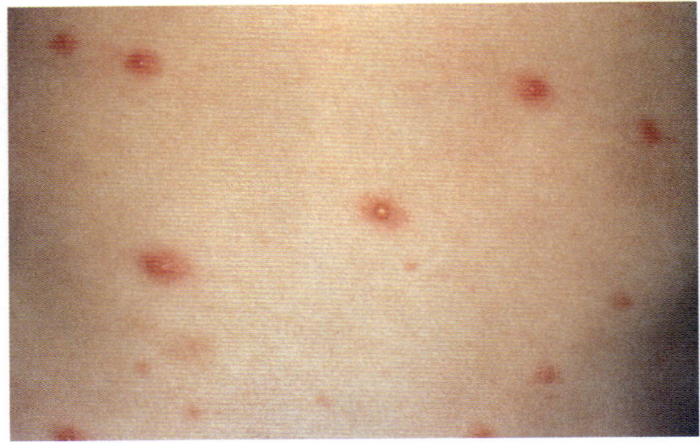

Chickenpox (varicella)

Small tight vesicles first appear on the trunk, then spread to the face, arms and legs (not palms or soles). Shiny vesicles on an erythematous base are commonly described as the 'dewdrop on a rose petal'. Vesicles erupt in succeeding crops over several days and then become pustules, then crusts. Intensely pruritic.

TABLE 22.13 Lesions caused by trauma or abuse

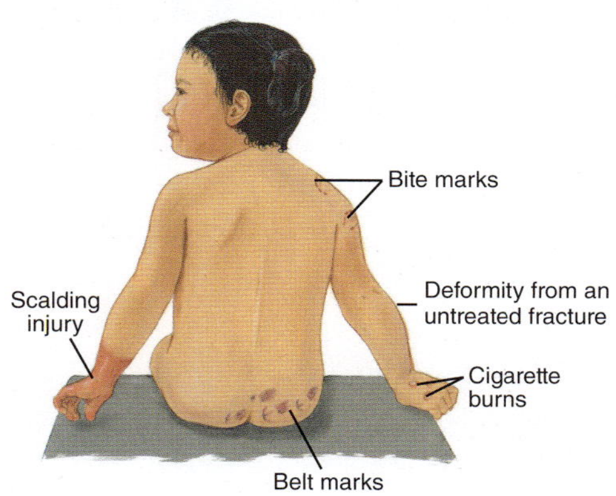

Pattern injury

Pattern injury is a bruise or wound whose shape suggests the instrument or weapon that caused it (e.g. belt buckle, broomstick, burning cigarette, pinch marks, bite marks or scalding hot liquid). Inflicted scalding-water immersion burns usually have a clear border, like a glove or sock, indicating that the body part was held under water intentionally. Deformity results from an untreated fracture because the bone heals out of alignment. These physical signs suggest child abuse, together with a history that does not match the severity or type of injury and indicates an impaired or dysfunctional parent–child relationship.

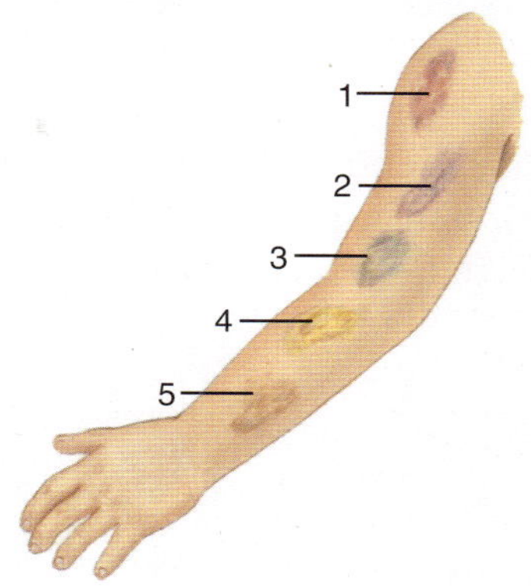

Contusion (bruise)

A large patch of capillary bleeding into tissues. Colour in light-skinned people is usually first 1—red-blue or purple immediately after or within 24 hours of trauma and generally progresses to 2—blue to purple; 3—blue-green; 4—yellow; 5—brown to disappearing. A recent bruise in dark-skinned people is a deep, dark purple. Note that it is not possible to date the age of a bruise from its colour. Pressure on a bruise will not cause it to blanch. A bruise usually occurs from trauma; also from bleeding disorders and liver dysfunction.

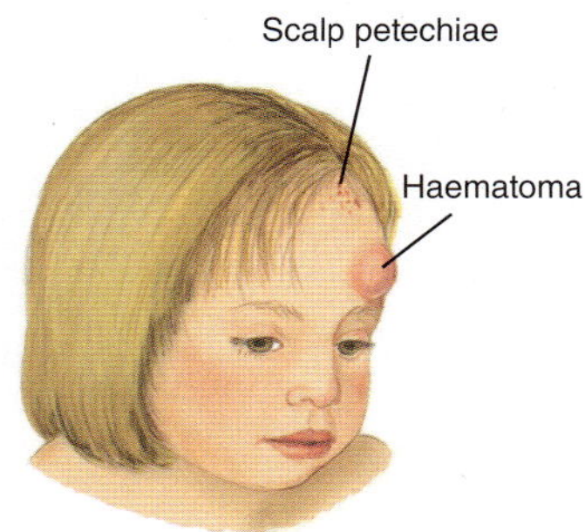

Haematoma

A haematoma is a bruise you can feel. It elevates the skin and is seen as swelling. Multiple petechiae and purpura may occur on the face when prolonged vigorous crying or coughing raises venous pressure.

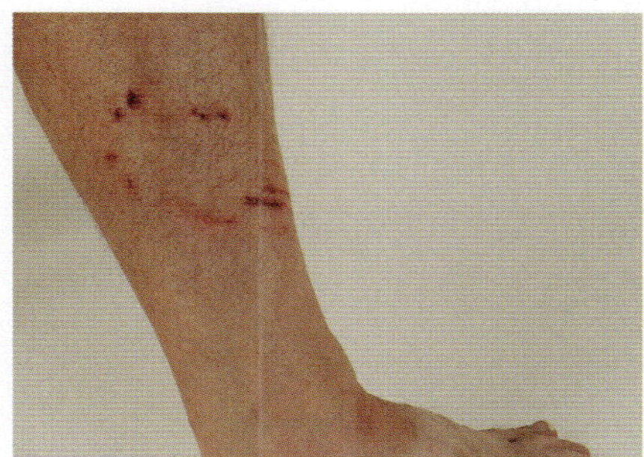

Dog, cat and human bite wounds

The dog bite shown here is a crushing injury with puncture wounds and lacerations. Dog bites on adults occur on the arms or legs; on children they are more often on the face or scalp. Assess for cosmetic repair and risk of infection. An x-ray image shows bone penetration or tooth fragment left in the wound. Cat bites involve deeply punctured tissue, and over half result in infection. Human bites are even more serious because of abundant microorganisms in human saliva. All are treated with appropriate antibiotics.

Advanced practice—additional data

Nurses working in a skin cancer clinic adopt a systematic, detailed and comprehensive approach to skin assessment. In addition to the objective data described previously, nurses working in such a role or midwives caring for pregnant women and newborn babies will need to have advanced inspection and palpation skills to assess these clients.

PROCEDURES AND NORMAL FINDINGS	ABNORMAL FINDINGS AND CLINICAL ALERTS
Additional objective data for infants and children	
Inspect the skin	
Skin colour—general pigmentation. Light-skinned newborns have pink, well-perfused intact skin. Dark-skinned newborns initially have lighter toned skin than their parents because of a pigment function that is not yet in full production. Their full melanotic colour is evident in the nail beds and scrotal folds. The **Mongolian spot** is a common variation of hyperpigmentation in infants of South-East Asian, Pacific Islander and African descent (Figure 22.19). It is a blue-black to purple macular area at the sacrum or buttocks, but sometimes it occurs on the abdomen, thighs, shoulders or arms. It is due to deep dermal melanocytes. It gradually fades during the first year. By adulthood these spots are lighter but are frequently still visible. 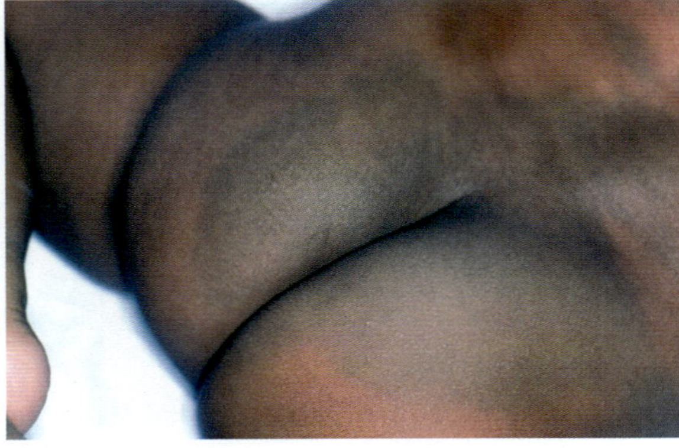 **FIGURE 22.19** Mongolian spot	If you are unfamiliar with **Mongolian spots**, be careful not to confuse them with bruises. Recognition of this normal variation is particularly important when dealing with children who might be erroneously identified as experiencing abuse. **Bruising** is a common soft tissue injury that follows a rapid, traumatic or breech birth.
A **café au lait spot** is a large round or oval patch of light-brown pigmentation (hence, the name 'coffee with milk'), which is usually present at birth (Figure 22.20). Most often these patches are normal.	Six or more café au lait macules, each larger than 1.5 cm in diameter, are diagnostic of neurofibromatosis, an inherited neurocutaneous disease.

PROCEDURES AND NORMAL FINDINGS

ABNORMAL FINDINGS AND CLINICAL ALERTS

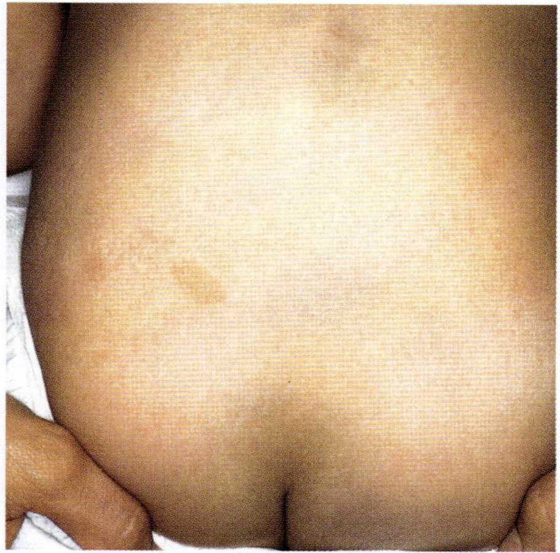

FIGURE 22.20 Café au lait

Moisture
The vernix caseosa is the moist, white, cream cheese-like substance that covers part of the skin in all newborns. Perspiration is present after 1 month of age.

Green-tinged vernix occurs with meconium staining.

In children, excessive sweating may accompany hypoglycaemia, heart disease or hyperthyroidism.

Texture
A common variation occurring in infants is **milia** (Figure 22.21). Milia are tiny white papules on the cheeks, forehead and across the nose and chin caused by sebum that occludes the opening of the follicles. Tell parents not to squeeze the lesions; milia resolve spontaneously within a few weeks.

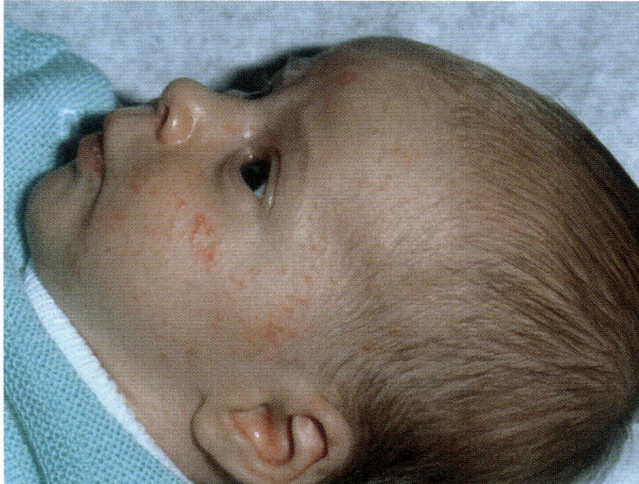

FIGURE 22.21 Milia

PROCEDURES AND NORMAL FINDINGS	ABNORMAL FINDINGS AND CLINICAL ALERTS
Thickness In neonates, the epidermis is normally thin, but you will also note well-defined areas of subcutaneous fat. A baby's skin dimples over joints, but there is no break in the skin. Check for any defect or break in the skin, especially over the length of the spine.	Lack of subcutaneous fat occurs in prematurity and malnutrition.
Mobility and turgor Test mobility and turgor over the abdomen in infants.	Poor turgor, or 'tenting', indicates dehydration or malnutrition.

Erythematous skin colour changes

Three erythematous states are common variations in neonates:

1. A newborn's skin has a beefy red flush for the first 24 hours because of vasomotor instability; then the colour fades to its normal colour.
2. Another finding, the **harlequin colour change**, occurs when the baby is in a side-lying position. The lower half of the body turns red and the upper half blanches with a distinct demarcation line down the midline. The cause is unknown, and its occurrence is transient.
3. Finally, **erythema toxicum** is a common rash that appears in the first 3 to 4 days of life. Sometimes called the 'flea bite' rash or newborn rash, it consists of tiny, punctate, red macules and papules on the cheeks, trunk, chest, back and buttocks (Figure 22.22). The cause is unknown; no treatment is needed.

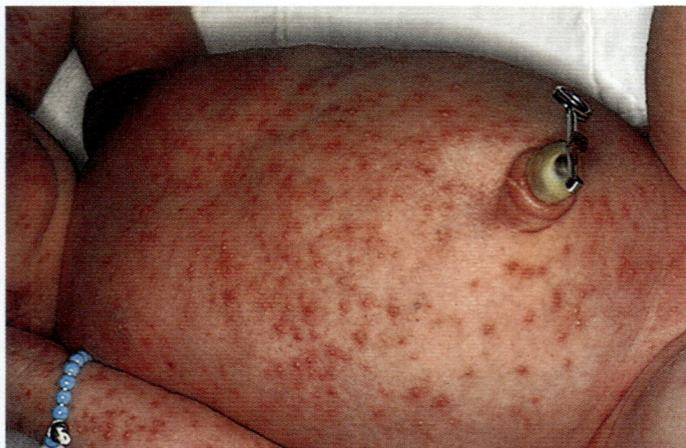

FIGURE 22.22 Erythema toxicum

Cyanotic conditions

PROCEDURES AND NORMAL FINDINGS	ABNORMAL FINDINGS AND CLINICAL ALERTS
A newborn may have **acrocyanosis**, a bluish colour around the lips, hands and fingernails, and feet and toenails. This may last for a few hours and disappear with warming.	Persistent generalised cyanosis indicates distress, such as cyanotic congenital heart disease.

PROCEDURES AND NORMAL FINDINGS

Cutis marmorata is a transient mottling in the trunk and extremities in response to cooler room temperatures (Figure 22.23). It forms a reticulated red or blue pattern over the skin.

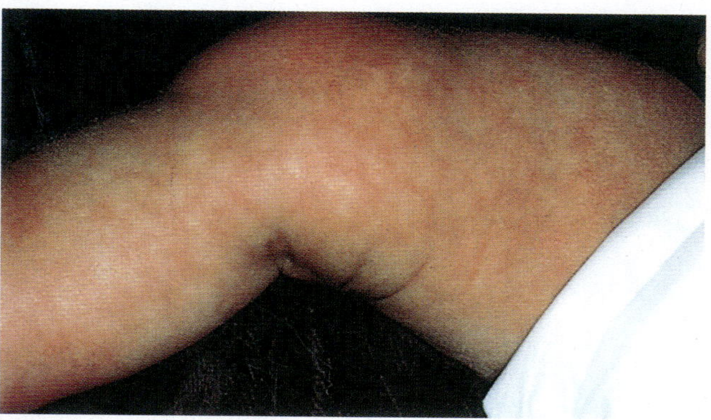

FIGURE 22.23 Cutis marmorata

ABNORMAL FINDINGS AND CLINICAL ALERTS

Persistent or pronounced cutis marmorata occurs with **trisomy 21 (Down syndrome)** or prematurity.

Green-brown discolouration of the skin, nails and cord occurs with passing of meconium in utero, indicating fetal distress.

Other skin colour changes

Physiological jaundice is a common variation in about half of all newborns. A yellowing of the skin, sclera and mucous membranes develops after the third or fourth day of life because of the increased numbers of red blood cells that haemolyse after birth. The haemoglobin in the red blood cells is metabolised by the liver and spleen; its pigment is converted into bilirubin.

Carotenaemia also produces a yellow-orange colour in light-skinned people but no yellowing in the sclera or mucous membranes. It comes from ingesting large amounts of foods containing carotene, a vitamin A precursor. Carotene-rich foods are popular as prepared infant foods, and the absorption of carotene is enhanced by mashing, pureeing and cooking. The colour is best seen on the palms and soles, the forehead, tip of the nose and nasolabial folds, the chin, behind the ears and over the knuckles; it fades to normal colour within 2 to 6 weeks of withdrawing carotene-rich foods from the diet.

Jaundice on the first day of life may indicate haemolytic disease. Jaundice after 2 weeks of age may indicate biliary tract obstruction.

PROCEDURES AND NORMAL FINDINGS

Vascularity or bruising. Some vascular markings are common birthmarks in newborns. A **storkbite** (salmon or strawberry patch) is a flat, irregularly shaped red or pink patch found on the forehead, eyelid or upper lip but most commonly at the back of the neck (nuchal area) (Figure 22.24). It is present at birth and usually fades during the first year.

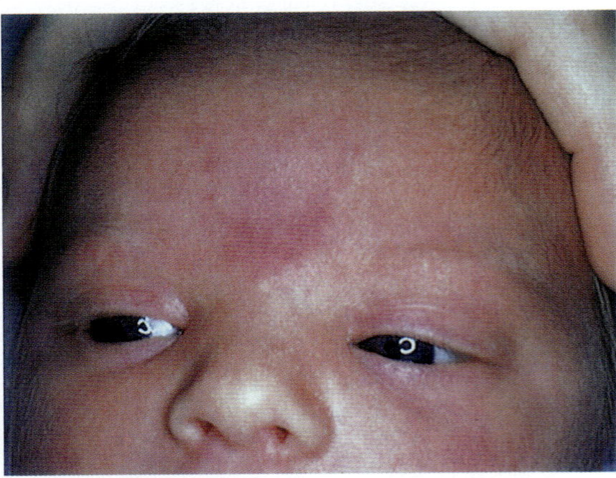

FIGURE 22.24 Storkbite

Inspect the hair and nails

Hair

A newborn's skin is covered with fine downy lanugo (Figure 22.25), especially in a preterm infant. Dark-skinned newborns have more lanugo than lighter skinned newborns. Scalp hair may be lost in the few weeks after birth, especially at the temples and occiput. It grows back slowly.

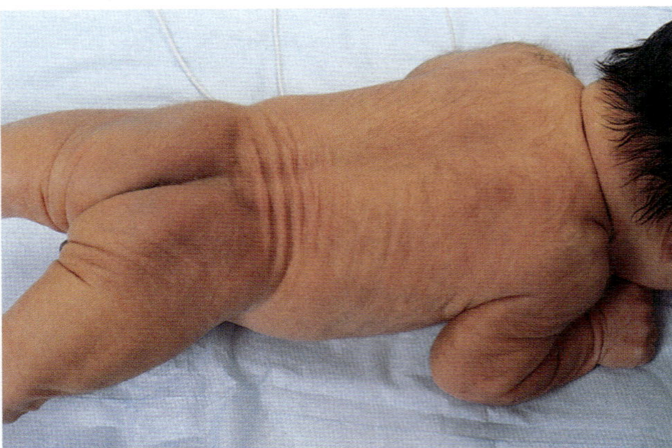

FIGURE 22.25 Lanugo

ABNORMAL FINDINGS AND CLINICAL ALERTS

Port-wine stain, strawberry mark (immature haemangioma), cavernous haemangioma (Table 22.8).

Scaly crusted scalp occurs with seborrhoeic dermatitis (cradle cap) (Table 22.10).

PROCEDURES AND NORMAL FINDINGS	ABNORMAL FINDINGS AND CLINICAL ALERTS
Nails A newborn's nail beds may be blue (cyanotic) for the first few hours of life; then they turn pink.	
Additional objective data for pregnant women	
Striae are jagged linear 'stretch marks' of silver to pink colour that appear during the second trimester on the abdomen, breasts and sometimes thighs. They occur in half of all pregnancies. They fade after delivery but do not disappear. Another skin change on the abdomen is the linea nigra, a brownish black line down the midline (Figure 29.5). **Chloasma** is an irregular brown patch of hyperpigmentation on the face. It may occur with pregnancy or in women taking oral contraceptive pills. Chloasma disappears after delivery or stopping the pill. Vascular spiders occur in two-thirds of pregnancies. These lesions have tiny red centres with radiating branches and occur on the face, neck, upper chest and arms.	

Clinical reasoning and documentation

The following is a continuation of the case study provided at the beginning of this chapter and the initial clinical reasoning process including problem/issue identification and documentation of clinical data. Consult a fundamentals of nursing or medical-surgical nursing text for information about goal setting, nursing interventions and evaluation.

Case study 1 (continued)—Chickenpox

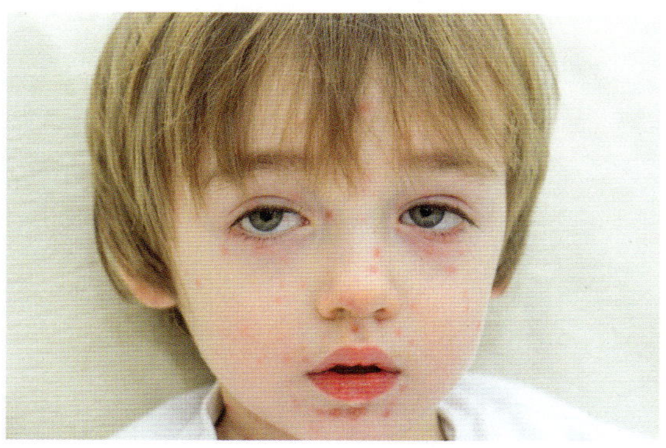

Context

You will recall from the case study described earlier in the chapter that you are a registered nurse working in general practice clinic. One of your roles is to perform an initial health assessment prior to a person consulting with the GP.

Consider the patient's situation

As you will recall, Ethan is aged 3 years old and has been brought to the clinic by his mother. He has had a fever, fatigue and rash for the past 3 days.

Collect cues/information

Your further assessment reveals the following information.

Subjective data

Two weeks ago, Ethan was playing with a child who was subsequently diagnosed as having chickenpox. Ethan's mother reports that Ethan developed a fever 37.7°C to 38.3°C and fatigue and irritability 3 days ago. That evening, Ethan's mother noted 'tiny blisters' on his chest and back.

Yesterday, the blisters on Ethan's chest changed to white with a scab on top. New eruptions of blisters on the shoulders, thighs and face were noted; they caused intense itching and scratching. Ethan's mother confirms that Ethan has not been immunised against chickenpox.

Continued

Clinical reasoning and documentation cont'd

Objective data

Temp 38.0°C, HR 110, R 24.
Skin: Generalised vesiculopustular rash covering the face, trunk, upper arms and thighs. Small vesicles on the face, pustules and red-honey-coloured crusts on the trunk. Otherwise the skin is warm and dry, turgor elastic.
Ears: Tympanic membranes pearl-grey with landmarks visible. No discharge.
Mouth and throat: Mucosa dark pink, no lesions. Tonsils 1+, no exudate. No lymphadenopathy.
Heart: S_1, S_2 heard and regular rhythm.
Lungs: Breath sounds clear.

Process information and identify problems/issues

Collaborative problem

Acute chickenpox (varicella) infection for referral to medical practitioner

Problem statement/nursing diagnoses

Impaired skin integrity related to varicella, infection and scratching
Discomfort related to fever and itchiness

Case study 2 (continued)—Pressure injury

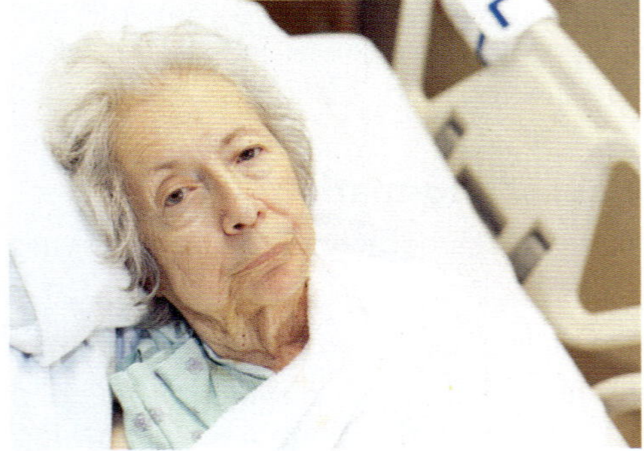

Context

You are a registered nurse in an acute medical ward performing a skin assessment on Mrs Gray at the beginning of your shift.

Consider the patient's situation

Myra Gray is a 79-year-old widow and retired academic, in good health up until recent hospitalisation after a fall. A fractured right hip was diagnosed and followed by hip replacement surgery 2 days ago

Collect cues/information

Subjective data

Mrs Gray reports aching pain in left hip (non-operative side) that she does not normally experience. It is worse after she has been lying in bed for a period of time.

Objective data

Skin on the buttocks, hips and legs generally dry and lacking in moisture. Non-blanching erythema L ischium 2 × 2 cm (Grade 1 pressure injury). Area over L ischium very warm and tender to touch. Needs assistance with repositioning in bed and transfer to chair. Pain rated as 6/10.

Process information and identify problems/issues

Collaborative problems

Pressure injury left hip and pain for referral to medical practitioner to assess and manage pain

Problem statement / nursing diagnoses

Impaired skin integrity left hip related to immobility and pressure
Acute pain related to pressure injury

ADDITIONAL RESOURCES

You can further develop your knowledge and skills relevant to assessment of skin, hair and nails, related pathophysiology, common health issues and nursing interventions by:

- reading chapters of a fundamentals of nursing or medical-surgical nursing textbook
- answering chapter multiple choice questions online. Log onto ClinicalKey Student and search for the text 'Health Assessment, 4th edition'. Choose the section titled 'Teaching material'. In this section you will find question and answer documents for each chapter. Please check instructions on the inside front cover of the book to access online resources
- visiting websites:

  Australasian College of Dermatologists—A to Z of Skin: https://www.dermcoll.edu.au/a-to-z-of-skin/

REFERENCES

1. Cancer Council Australia. 2023. Private ownership and use of solariums in Australia. Available at: https://www.cancer.org.au/about-us/policy-and-advocacy/position-statements/uv/private-solariums
2. Australian Institute of Health and Wellness. Cancer data in Australia: overview of cancer in Australia, 2023. Available at: https://www.aihw.gov.au/reports/cancer/cancer-data-in-australia/contents/overview-of-cancer-in-australia-2023
3. BPac NZ Better Medicine. Reducing the burden of melanoma in New Zealand: prevention and risk assessment 2020. Available at: https://bpac.org.nz/2020/melanoma.aspx
4. Skin Cancer Foundation. 5 Myths of Indoor Tanning, Busted! Available at: https://www.skincancer.org/blog/5-myths-indoor-tanning-busted/
5. Heibel H, Hooey L, Cockerell C. A review of noninvasive techniques for skin cancer detection in dermatology. American Journal of Clinical Dermatology 2020;21:513–524. https://doi.org/10.1007/s40257-020-00517-z
6. Fishbein A, Silverberg J, Wilson E, Ong P. Update on atopic dermatitis: diagnosis, severity assessment, and treatment selection. The Journal of Allergy and Clinical Immunology: In Practice 2020;8(1):91–101. https://doi.org/10.1016/j.jaip.2019.06.044
7. Cancer Council Australia. Position statement—Sun exposure and vitamin D—risks and benefits. 2023. Available at: https://www.cancer.org.au/about-us/policy-and-advocacy/position-statements/sunsmart#jump_3
8. Cancer Council Australia. National Cancer Prevention Policy. 2023. Available at: https://wiki.cancer.org.au/policy/National_Cancer_Control_Policy
9. Napilotano M, Fabbrocini G, Matora F, Genco L, Noto M, Patruno C. Children atopic dermatitis: diagnosis, mimics, overlaps, and therapeutic implication. Dermatologic Therapy 2022;35(12):e15901. https://doi.org/10.1111/dth.15901
10. Jones A, Woods M, Malhotra K. Critical examination of skin care self-management in lymphoedema. British Journal of Community Nursing. 2019 Oct 1;24(Sup10):S6–S10.
11. Delmore BA, Ayello EA. Braden Scales for Pressure Injury Risk Assessment. Advances

in Skin & Wound Care. 2023 Jun 1;36(6): 332–335.
12. Hess CT. Comprehensive patient and wound assessments. Advanced Skin and Wound Care 2019;32(6):287–288.
13. Dhingra G, Ahmad N, Tanwar S, Goyal S, Chaturverdi V, Tanwar K. Nail disorders: an updated review. International Journal of Pharmaceutical Sciences Review and Research 2022;75(2):135–144.
14. Graves S, Stenos J. Tick-borne infectious diseases in Australia. Medical Journal of Australia 2017;206(7):320–324.

UNIT 8

Urinary and bowel function

CHAPTER 23

Abdominal assessment

Written by Carolyn Jarvis
Adapted by Elizabeth Watt

INTRODUCTION

Abdominal assessment is frequently performed in nursing. It forms part of an assessment of nutrition and metabolic function, urinary and bowel function and assessment during pregnancy. Structures relevant to abdominal assessment include all the abdominal organs and the abdominal wall. You will find other relevant anatomy and physiology in Chapters 24 and 25. Information relevant to abdominal examination in pregnancy is detailed in Chapter 29.

Case study

The following case study gives an example of a typical situation involving abdominal assessment and the initial clinical reasoning process. It will help you identify your learning needs.

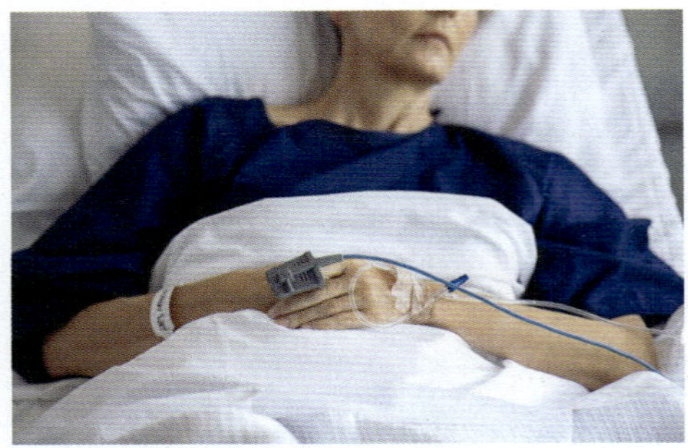

Context

It is 7:30 am and you are on clinical placement in a lower gastrointestinal surgical ward. You go to introduce yourself and perform a primary survey for the patients you will be caring for.

Consider the patient's situation

Ms Samantha Wright is a 55-year-old female who had a laparoscopic anterior bowel resection for adenocarcinoma of the bowel 24 hours ago. She progressed normally in the first 24 hours postoperatively. Her pain was well controlled, and she was tolerating sips of water and able to walk to the toilet with minimal assistance.

This morning she is complaining of abdominal pain and feeling bloated, which has been increasing over several hours. She says she feels nauseated and 'very unwell'.

Questions to further your learning

- What are the possible things that might be going on with Ms Wright?
- What knowledge do you need to be able to predict what might be going on?
- What approach to Ms Wright's health assessment will you take?
- What questions (subjective data) will you ask Ms Wright to extend the health history and why?
- What physical assessment (objective data) will you conduct and why?
- What resources are available to assist in your assessment of Ms Wright?

Assessment plan

Abdominal assessment is commonly performed along with assessing bowel and bladder function and/or nutritional and oral assessment. To be able to perform abdominal assessment, identify problems and plan care, a detailed knowledge of structure and function and developmental and cultural considerations are necessary before you start.

The focus of abdominal assessment outlined in this chapter primarily relates to investigating abdominal pain. You will need to adjust the questioning to fit the purpose of the examination. For example, if the focus of the assessment is about bowel function you would include the questions related to bowel function, but if the abdominal assessment is related to nutrition you would focus on the questions related to that area and expand the questions to include those related to eating, appetite and so on. Through the process of questioning the client or family you may become aware of gaps in the person's knowledge about their health. The opportunity to provide health information is an important part of health assessment.

The main areas for subjective assessment are:

- presenting concern
- food intolerance
- abdominal pain
- nausea/vomiting
- bowel function
- past abdominal history
- health and lifestyle management.

Following subjective data collection, the following sequence is used to collect objective data: **inspection, auscultation, percussion and palpation**. Note that this is a different sequence from other assessments. The main areas for objective assessment are:

- general inspection
- identify abdominal landmarks
- inspection
- auscultation—bowel sounds
- percussion—general tympany
- palpation—surface and light.

Resources available

You will find additional resources and the reference list at the end of this chapter. This chapter also has a video available demonstrating objective data collection related to abdominal assessment. You will find a QR code in the objective data section to enable you to access the video easily on your preferred device.

Structure and function

Surface landmarks

The **abdomen** is a large oval cavity extending from the diaphragm down to the brim of the pelvis. It is bordered at its back by the vertebral column and paravertebral muscles and at the sides and front by the lower rib cage and abdominal muscles (Figure 23.1). Four layers of large, flat muscles form the ventral (anterior) abdominal wall. These are joined at the midline by a tendinous seam, the **linea alba**. One set, the **rectus abdominis**, forms a strip extending the length of the midline, and its edge is often palpable. The muscles protect and hold the organs in place, and they help flex the vertebral column.

Internal anatomy

Internal to the abdominal musculature lies the **peritoneum**, a double envelope of serous membrane that lines the abdominal wall (parietal peritoneum) and covers the surface of most abdominal organs (visceral peritoneum). **The mesentery** consists of double layers of parietal peritoneum which extends from the abdominal wall as pathways for blood vessels, nerves and lymphatics. The mesentery also serves as a supporting network to suspend and stabilise the abdominal organs, called **viscera** (Figure 23.2). The **greater omentum** is a specialised fatty mesentery that overlies the ventral abdomen. Because of the overlying skin, subcutaneous layer, muscles and omentum, you need to be able to visualise each organ that you listen to or palpate through the abdominal wall.

The **solid viscera** are those that maintain a characteristic shape (liver, pancreas, spleen, adrenal glands, kidneys, ovaries and uterus) (Figure 23.2). The liver fills most of the right upper quadrant and extends over to the left midclavicular line. The lower edge of the

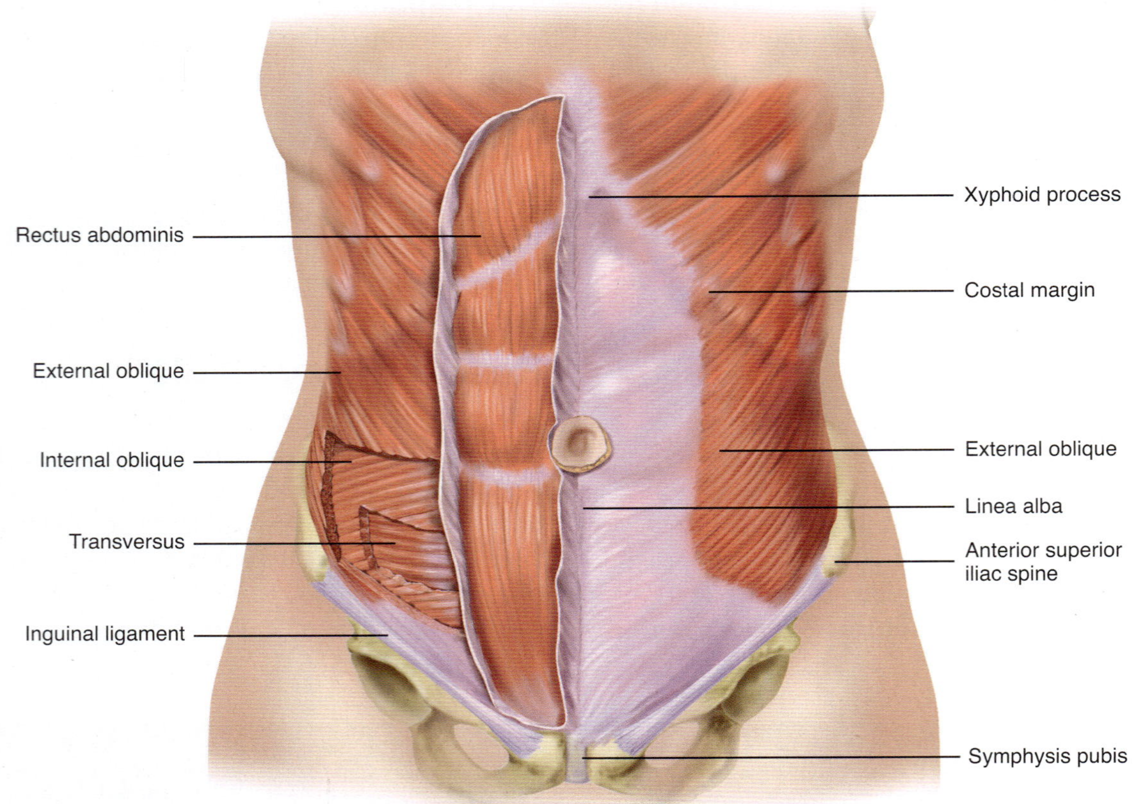

FIGURE 23.1 Abdominal musculature

liver and the right kidney may normally be palpable. The ovaries normally are palpable only on bimanual examination during the pelvic examination.

The shapes of the **hollow viscera** (stomach, gall bladder, small intestine, colon and bladder) depend on the contents. They usually are not palpable, although you may feel a colon distended with faeces or a bladder distended with urine. The stomach is just below the diaphragm, between the liver and spleen. The gall bladder rests under the posterior surface of the liver, just lateral to the right midclavicular line. Note that the small intestine is located in all four quadrants. It extends from the stomach's pyloric valve to the ileocaecal valve in the right lower quadrant, where it joins the colon. The small intestine is divided into three regions: the duodenum (about 25 cm long), the jejunum (about 1 m long) and the ileum (about 2 m long). The small intestine joins the large intestine at the ileocaecal valve. The large intestine is about 1.5 m long and extends from the ileum to the anus. It is divided into four major areas: caecum, colon, rectum and anal canal. The colon is divided according to its position in the abdomen: the ascending colon, the transverse colon, the descending colon and the sigmoid colon. See Chapter 25 for detail about the anatomy of the anus and rectum.

The **spleen** is a soft mass of lymphatic tissue on the posterolateral wall of the abdominal cavity, immediately under the diaphragm (Figure 23.3). It lies obliquely with its long axis behind and parallel to the 10th rib, lateral to the midaxillary line. Its

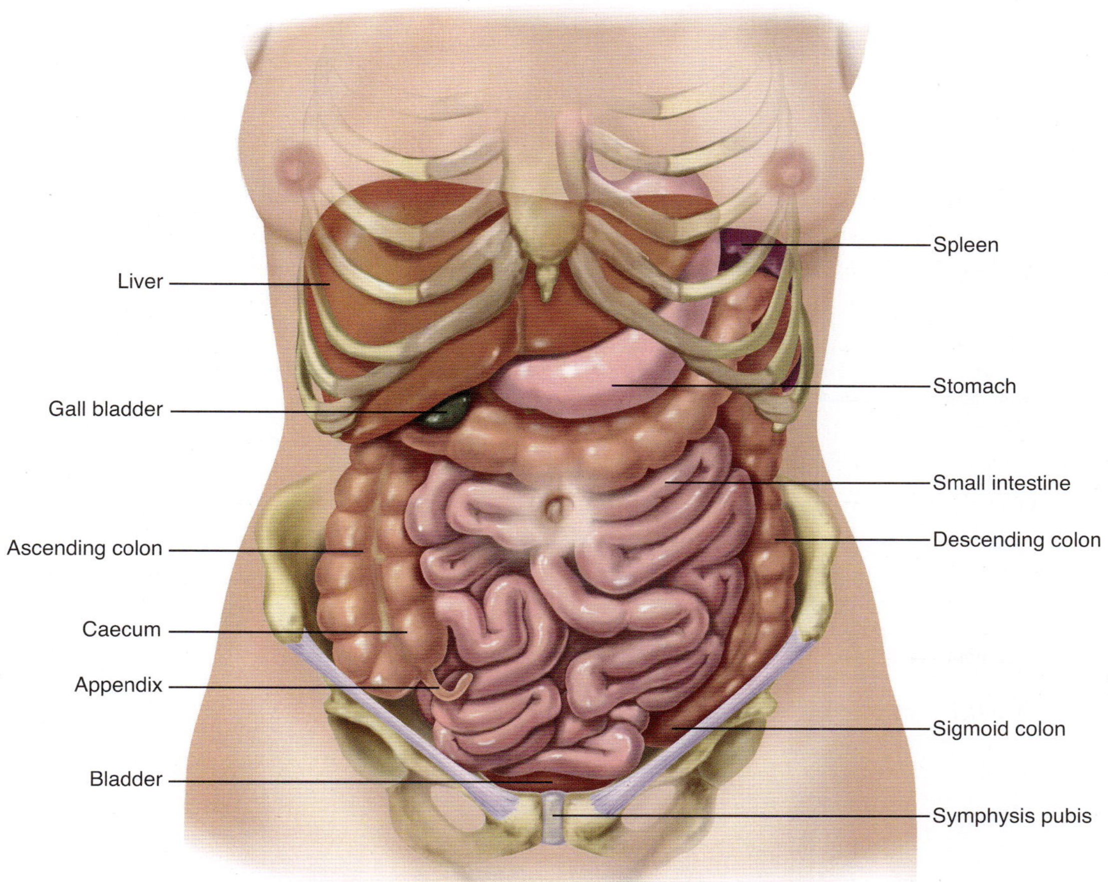

FIGURE 23.2 Abdominal organ location

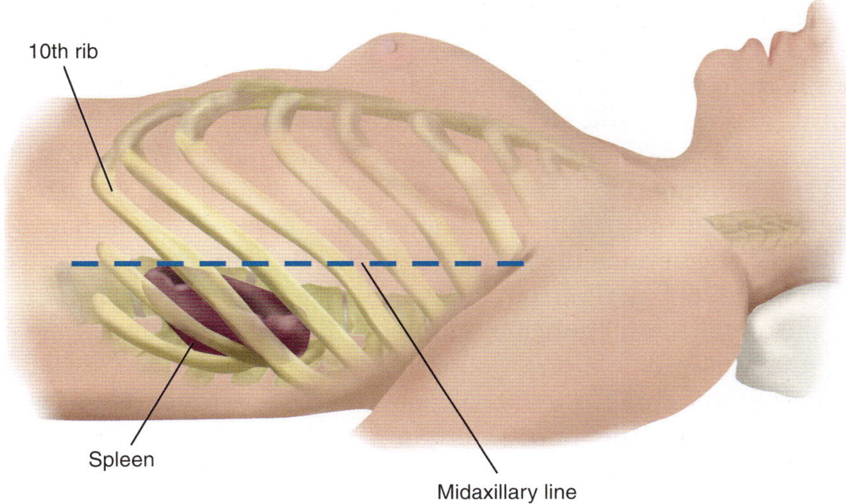

FIGURE 23.3 Position of spleen laterally

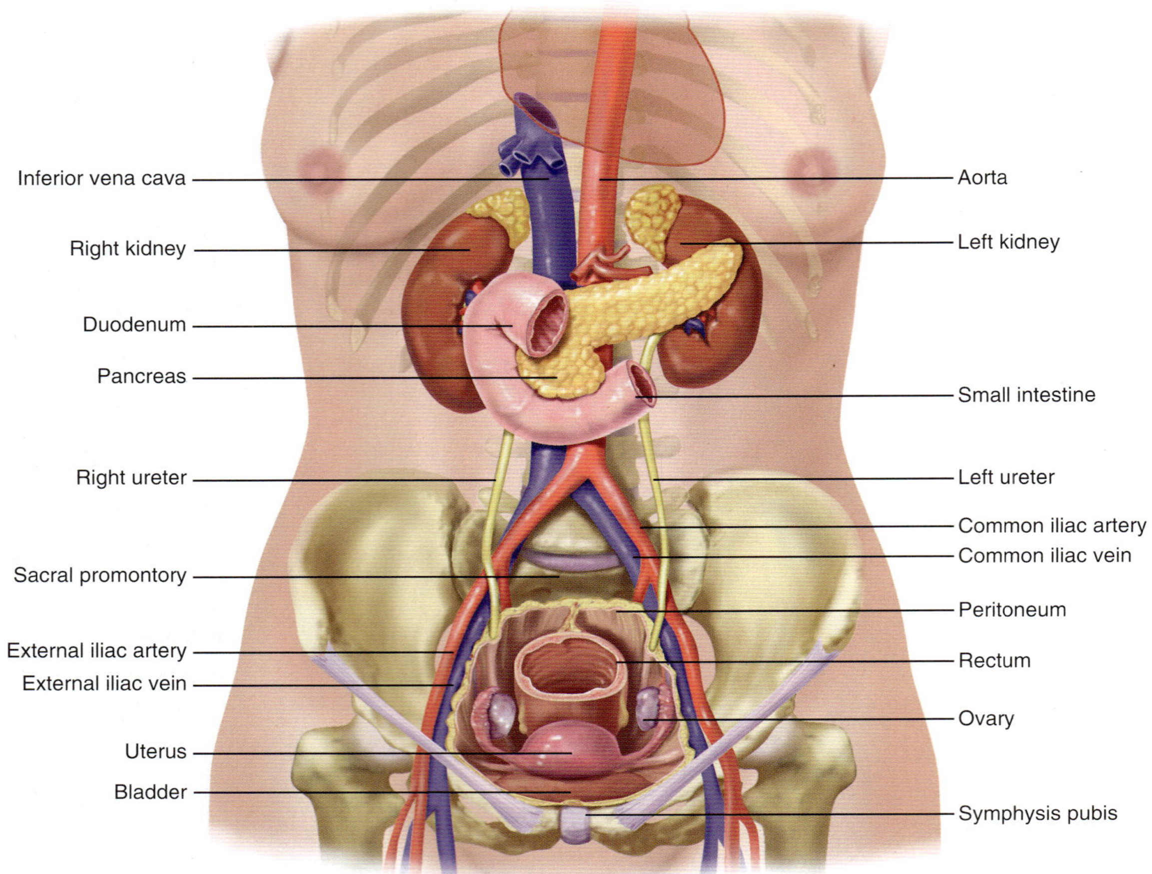

FIGURE 23.4 Major abdominal blood vessels in relation to abdominal organs

width extends from the 9th to the 11th rib, about 7 cm. It is not palpable. If it becomes enlarged, its lower pole moves downwards and towards the midline.

The **aorta** is just to the left of midline in the upper part of the abdomen (Figure 23.4). It descends behind the peritoneum and, at 2 cm below the umbilicus, it bifurcates into the right and left common iliac arteries opposite the fourth lumbar vertebra. You can palpate the aortic pulsations in the upper anterior abdominal wall. The right and left iliac arteries become the femoral arteries in the groin area. Their pulsations are easily palpated at a point halfway between the anterior superior iliac spine and the symphysis pubis.

The **pancreas** is a soft, lobulated gland located behind the stomach. It stretches obliquely across the posterior abdominal wall to the left upper quadrant.

The bean-shaped **kidneys** are retroperitoneal, or posterior to the abdominal contents (Figure 23.5). They are well protected by the posterior ribs and musculature. The 12th rib forms an angle with the vertebral column, the **costovertebral angle**. The left kidney lies here at the 11th and 12th ribs. Because of the placement of the liver, the right kidney rests 1 to 2 cm lower than the left kidney and may sometimes be palpable. The adrenal glands appear as caps on the upper pole of each kidney; they are crucial endocrine glands.

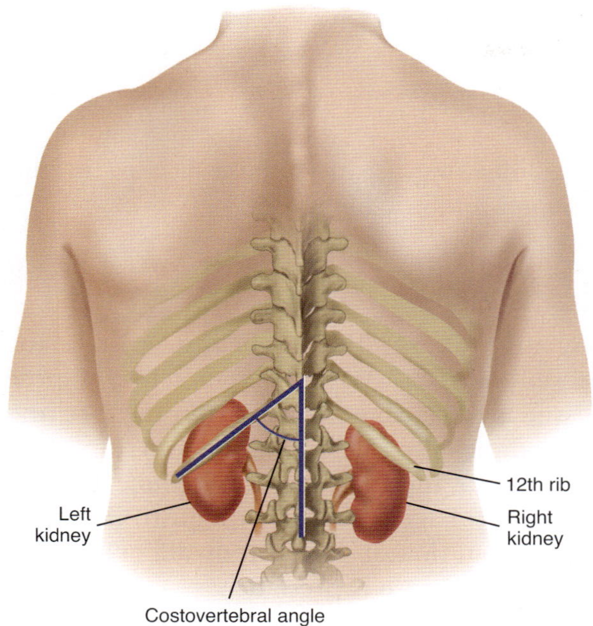

FIGURE 23.5 Position of kidneys posteriorly

You may notice in some people's health records that the abdomen may have been divided into **nine quadrants** (Figure 23.6A). Although this system is not generally used, some regional names persist, such as **epigastric** for the area between the costal margins, umbilical for the area around the **umbilicus** and **hypogastric** or **suprapubic** for the area above the pubic bone. A more common and less complicated description is when the abdomen is divided into four quadrants by a vertial and a horizontal line bisecting the umbilicus (Figure 23.6B).

The anatomical location of the organ by quadrants is:

Right upper quadrant	**Left upper quadrant**
Liver	Stomach
Gall bladder	Spleen
Duodenum	Left lobe of liver
Head of pancreas	Body of pancreas
Right kidney and adrenal gland	Left kidney and adrenal gland
Hepatic flexure of colon	Splenic flexure of colon
Part of ascending and transverse colon	Part of transverse colon and descending colon
Right lower quadrant	**Left lower quadrant**
Caecum	Part of descending colon
Appendix	Sigmoid colon
Right ovary and fallopian tube	Left ovary and fallopian tube
Right ureter	Left ureter
Right spermatic cord	Left spermatic cord
	Midline
	Aorta
	Uterus (if enlarged)
	Bladder (if distended)

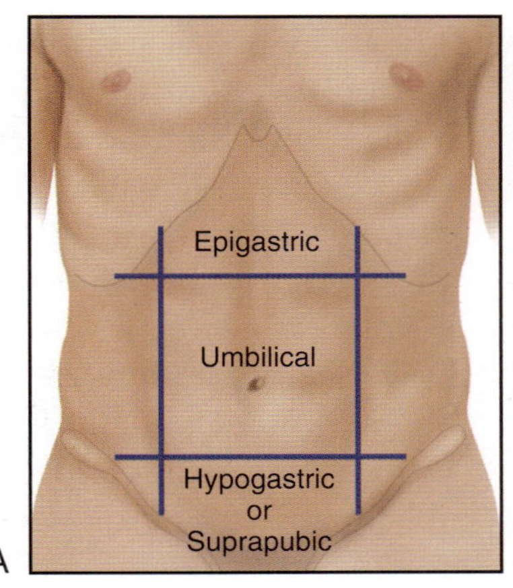

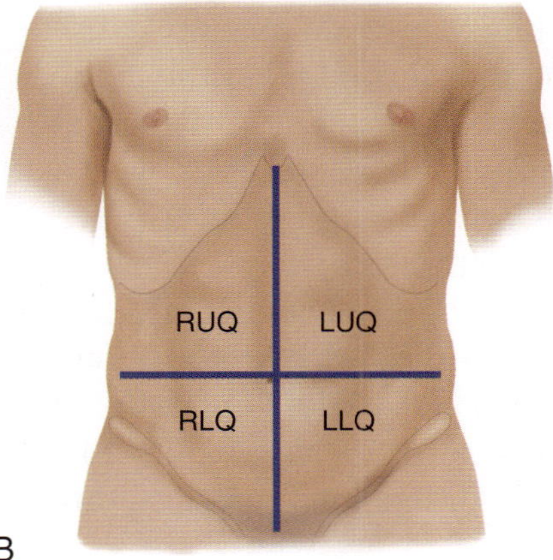

FIGURE 23.6 A Divisions of the abdomen into nine sections, B The abdomen divided into four quadrants

Developmental considerations

Infants and children

In newborns, the umbilical cord shows prominently on the abdomen. It contains two arteries and one vein. The liver takes up proportionately more space in the abdomen at birth than in later life. In healthy term neonates, the lower edge may be palpated 0.5 to 2.5 cm below the right costal margin. Age-related values of expected liver span are listed in the objective data section of the chapter. The urinary bladder is located higher in the abdomen than in the adult. It lies between the symphysis pubis and the umbilicus. Also, during early childhood, the abdominal wall is less muscular, so the appearance is rounded, and the organs may be easier to palpate.

Pregnant women

Nausea and vomiting, or 'morning sickness', is an early sign of pregnancy for many pregnant women, starting between the first and second missed menstrual periods. The cause is unknown but may be due to hormone changes such as the production of human chorionic gonadotrophin. Another symptom is 'acid indigestion' or heartburn (pyrosis) caused by oesophageal reflux. Gastrointestinal motility decreases, which prolongs gastric emptying time. The decreased motility causes more water to be reabsorbed from the colon, which may lead to constipation. Persistent straining to eliminate hard stool, as well as increased venous pressure in the lower pelvis, may lead to haemorrhoids.

The enlarging uterus displaces the intestines upwards and posteriorly and therefore bowel sounds are diminished. The appendix is displaced upwards and to the right. Skin changes on the abdomen, such as striae and the linea nigra, are discussed later in this chapter and in Chapter 29.

Late adulthood (65+ years)

Ageing alters the appearance of the abdominal wall. With further ageing, adipose tissue is redistributed away from the face and extremities to the abdomen and hips; the abdominal musculature may reduce in tone. Changes of ageing occur in the gastrointestinal system but do not significantly affect function when no disease is present.

- Salivation may decrease, causing a dry mouth and a decreased sense of taste. Further changes are discussed in Chapter 21.
- Oesophageal emptying remains normal when there is no disease present until late older age (85 years and older). If oesophageal peristalsis is delayed, this may result in a feeling of fullness after eating, dysphagia and gastro-oesophageal reflux disorder.
- Gastric acid secretion decreases with ageing. This may cause gastric ulceration, pernicious anaemia (because it interferes with vitamin B12 absorption), iron deficiency anaemia and malabsorption of calcium.
- The incidence of gallstones increases with age, occurring in 10 to 20% of adults and being more common in females.[1]
- Liver size and hepatic blood flow decrease with age, particularly after 80 years, although most liver function remains normal. However, several mechanisms of liver metabolism that are responsible for the enzymatic oxidation, reduction and hydrolysis of drugs, especially opioids are affected by age.[2] Prolonged liver

metabolism, in conjunction with decreased renal excretion and age-related changes to absorption and distribution of drugs, can cause increased side effects of many commonly used medications.[3]

- Older people frequently report constipation. However, while there are changes to the enteric nervous system with ageing, gut transit time and colonic motility do not alter significantly with age.[4] The causes of constipation in any age group are multifactorial and include: reduced physical activity; current or recent hospitalisation; low self-reported health; ignoring or delaying the urge to defecate; pelvic organ prolapse (in women); the side effect of some medications; neurological, sensory, mental health, developmental and cognitive disorders; frailty; mobility issues; and underlying bowel disorders.[5]

HEALTH EDUCATION

Promoting liver health

The liver is the largest organ in the body. It has an immense capacity to heal and regenerate, but that capacity is not infinite. Unfortunately, signs of severe liver damage or disease usually do not become apparent until the liver has been significantly harmed. The best protection for the liver is prevention.

Nurse's role

The following points can be emphasised by nurses to encourage people to protect their liver.

Diet and weight control

Obesity, which can lead to metabolic syndrome, can cause a chronic condition called nonalcoholic fatty liver disease, which can progress to liver fibrosis and cirrhosis.[6]

Moderate alcohol consumption

The current Australian Guidelines to Reduce Health Risks from Drinking Alcohol[7] recommend that healthy men and women drink no more than two standard drinks on any day to reduce the lifetime risk of harm from alcohol-related disease or injury.

Use medications wisely

Use prescription and over-the-counter medications only when needed. Be sure to take only the recommended doses. While drug-induced liver injury is rare in the general population, it is more common in hospitalised patients. Several commonly used medications such as amoxicillin/clavulanate can cause drug-induced liver injury.[8] Paracetamol overdose is a significant cause of acute liver failure worldwide, especially in adolescents and young adults.[9] Also, herbal/dietary supplements and illicit drugs can also form toxic compounds that can cause liver damage.[10] Make sure all medications, including over-the-counter medications, complementary therapies and illicit drugs, are reviewed as part of any health history.

Make sure vaccinations are up to date

A vaccine is available for both hepatitis A and hepatitis B (as well as a combination vaccine).

Be aware of the risks for hepatitis

The three leading causes of hepatitis are hepatitis A, hepatitis B and hepatitis C infection. **Hepatitis A** is primarily spread through food or water contaminated by faeces from an infected person. Hepatitis A is not common in Australia and Aotearoa New Zealand. Hepatitis A is more common among specific groups of people including:

- injecting drug users
- men who have sex with men.
- travellers to regions where hepatitis A is common (e.g. countries where there is poor access to clean water or sanitation)
- people who are homeless or people living in extreme poverty.

Hepatitis B is a potentially life-threatening health problem and one of the most common infectious diseases in the world, but the vaccine is safe and gives good protection. Some people infected with hepatitis B will have

HEALTH EDUCATION cont'd

an acute infection and then recover; others will develop a chronic infection which can cause liver damage over time. Hepatitis B is primarily spread through contact with infected blood or body fluids (including saliva, semen, vaginal secretions and breast milk). The most common ways that hepatitis is spread include:

- having vaginal, anal or oral sex without a condom
- tattooing or body piercing with unclean equipment
- medical or dental procedures with unsterile equipment
- sharing and re-use of needles or other injecting equipment
- needlestick injury in the healthcare setting
- mother-to-child transmission at birth
- sharing personal items such as razors and toothbrushes
- having cuts or sores that are uncovered.

Hepatitis C can be acute or chronic and can range from a mild short-term illness to a serious life-long illness. A significant number of people who have chronic infection (15–30%) will develop liver cirrhosis with 20 years, and many will develop primary hepatocellular carcinoma.[11] It is primarily spread through sharing needles, syringes or other injecting equipment by illicit drug users. Other ways in which hepatitis C can be spread include:

- tattooing or body piercing with unclean equipment
- medical or dental procedures with unsterile equipment
- sharing personal items such as razors and toothbrushes.

There are now effective treatments that can cure hepatitis C using direct-acting antiviral medications for 8 to 12 weeks. However, many people have no symptoms until they have had the virus for a long time; therefore, it is important to encourage people who are at risk of infection to have a screening test so they can get started on treatment before they develop liver damage.

More information about liver health and hepatitis is available from the following websites:

- Liver Foundation: www.liver.org.au
- Hepatitis Australia: https://www.hepatitisaustralia.com/
- Hepatitis Foundation of New Zealand: https://www.hepatitisfoundation.org.nz/
- World Health Organization: https://www.who.int/health-topics/hepatitis#tab=tab_1.

Subjective data

Practice note

Before you start the assessment, introduce yourself to the person, confirm the person's identity, discuss the purpose and scope of the assessment, clarify any questions the person may have and obtain verbal consent from the person to perform the assessment.

ASSESSMENT GUIDELINES	CLINICAL SIGNIFICANCE AND CLINICAL ALERTS
Presenting concern	
It is important to ascertain the person's perception of their presenting health concern: *Are you experiencing any abdominal problems?* If they do perceive a problem, ask: *How does this affect your quality of life?*	

ASSESSMENT GUIDELINES	CLINICAL SIGNIFICANCE AND CLINICAL ALERTS
Food intolerance	
• *Are there any foods you cannot eat? What happens if you do eat them: allergic reaction, heartburn, belching, abdominal pain, bloating, indigestion, diarrhoea?* • *Have you sought any assistance from a health professional (medical practitioner, registered nurse, dietitian, pharmacist, natural therapist) for these symptoms?* • *Do you use antacids or any other medication or therapy for these symptoms? Which substance? How often? Does it reduce your symptoms?*	**Food intolerance** such as lactase deficiency (lactose intolerance) resulting in bloating or excessive gas after taking milk products[12] or FODMAP's (fermentable oligosaccharides, disaccharides, monosaccharides and polyols) are types of sugars that are not well digested in the small intestine in people who have irritable bowel syndrome and can cause pain, excess wind and bloating.[13]
Abdominal pain	
Review pain assessment strategies and tools from Chapter 13. Use a pain assessment tool as appropriate to the person's age, context and capacity to communicate. In general, you need to ask the person to describe the following:[14] **Character** • *How would you describe the pain you are experiencing: cramping* (colic type), *burning in pit of stomach, dull, stabbing, aching?* **Onset:** duration, variation • *How did it start? How long have you had it?* **Location** • *Where is the pain? Please point to it* (you could use a body diagram to report these findings). *Is the pain in one spot or does it move around?* **Duration** • *Is the pain constant or does it come and go? Does it occur before or after meals? Does it peak? When?* **Severity** • *How intense is the pain, rated from 1 to 10?* **Pattern** • *What makes the pain worse? Food, position, stress, medication, activity?* • *What have you tried to relieve pain? Rest, heating pad, change in position, medication?* **Associated factors** • *Is the pain associated with any other symptoms? Menstrual period or irregularities, stress, eating too much, fatigue, nausea and vomiting, gas, fever, rectal bleeding, frequent urination, vaginal or penile discharge?*	**Abdominal pain** may be visceral from an internal organ (dull, general, poorly localised), parietal from inflammation of overlying peritoneum (sharp, precisely localised, aggravated by movement) or referred from a disorder in another site. ***Clinical alert:*** Acute abdominal pain can be a sign of serious underlying health issue and requires urgent assessment by a medical practitioner.
Nausea/vomiting	
• *Do you have any nausea or vomiting? How often? How much comes up? What is the colour? Is there an odour?*	**Nausea/vomiting** is a common side effect of many medications, with gastrointestinal disease, early pregnancy.

ASSESSMENT GUIDELINES	CLINICAL SIGNIFICANCE AND CLINICAL ALERTS
• *Is it blood-stained?*	This could be bright red or dark brown coloured (digested blood commonly termed '**coffee-ground**'). **Haematemesis**—vomiting blood- or blood-stained vomit—occurs with gastric or duodenal ulcers, oesophageal varices and upper abdominal trauma.
• *Is the nausea and vomiting associated with any other symptoms such as colicky pain, diarrhoea, fever, chills?*	
• *What foods did you eat in the last 24 hours? Where? At home, school, restaurant? Is there anyone else in the family with same symptoms in last 24 hours?*	Consider **food poisoning** (Chapter 21).
Bowel function	
• *How often do you have a bowel movement?* • *What is the colour? Consistency?* (use Bristol stool chart described in Chapter 25) • *Any diarrhoea or constipation? How long?* • *Any recent change in bowel habits?*	Detailed assessment of bowel function is covered in Chapter 25. Black stools may be tarry due to occult blood **(melaena)** from gastrointestinal bleeding or non-tarry from iron medications. Grey or very pale coloured stools occur with **hepatitis.** Red blood in stools occurs with gastrointestinal bleeding or localised bleeding around the anus.
Past history	
• *Have you had any history of gastrointestinal problems—gastric ulcer or* Helicobacter pylori *infection, gall bladder disease, hepatitis/jaundice, appendicitis, colitis, diverticulitis, Crohn's disease, constipation, hernia?* If so, describe. • *Do you have any history of urinary tract infections, kidney problems, ovarian or menstrual problems?* If so, describe.	***Helicobacter pylori*** a spiral-shaped Gram-negative bacterium. It is one of the most common causes of serious chronic bacterial infections worldwide. *Helicobacter pylori* infection is associated with chronic gastritis, peptic ulcers, gastric mucosa-associated lymphoid tissue lymphoma and gastric adenocarcinoma.[15]
• *Have you ever had any surgery in the abdomen?* Please describe.	Past surgery to the abdomen can predispose the person to **abdominal adhesions** (bands of scar-like tissue), which can cause bowel obstruction (Table 23.2).

ASSESSMENT GUIDELINES	CLINICAL SIGNIFICANCE AND CLINICAL ALERTS
Have you any problems with your abdomen after surgery (if relevant)? Ongoing nausea, vomiting, abdominal pain, food intolerance?	
Health and lifestyle management	
• *What prescribed medications are you currently taking?* • *Are you taking any over-the-counter, complementary or natural therapies?* • *How about alcohol—how much would you say you drink* (estimate in mL or standard drinks) *each day? Each week? What type? When was your last alcoholic drink?* • *How about cigarettes—do you smoke or vape with nicotine included? How many packs/vapes per day? For how long?*	**Gastric ulcer disease** can occur with frequent use of non-steroidal anti-inflammatory drugs, alcohol, smoking and *Helicobacter pylori* infection.
Additional subjective data for infants and children (questions for parents or guardian)	
• *Does the child have abdominal pain?* Please describe what you have noticed and when it started. If the child is able to respond address the question to them: *Do you have any pain? Can you point to where the pain is?* Use a paediatric pain chart to assess the significance of the pain to the child (refer to Chapter 13 for details). Refer also to nutritional assessment and assessment of urinary and bowel function (Chapters 21, 24 and 25).	This symptom is hard to assess with young children. Many conditions of unrelated organ systems are associated with vague abdominal pain (e.g. otitis media). Children may not be able to articulate specific symptoms and often focus on 'the tummy'. Abdominal pain accompanies inflammation of the bowel, constipation, urinary tract infection and anxiety.

Objective data

Preparation

Outline the process for abdominal assessment for the person and ask their consent for you to continue. On some occasions, it may be necessary to have a support person (usually another nurse) present during the examination.

Ensure privacy by closing the door or pulling the screens. Adequate lighting is essential. Expose the abdomen so that it is fully visible by removing or loosening clothing above the costal margin and below the symphysis pubis. Drape (using a clean towel, small sheet or light blanket) below the suprapubic area and across the female breasts.

The following measures will enhance abdominal wall relaxation:

- The person should have emptied the bladder, saving a urine specimen if needed.
- The room should be warm to avoid chilling and tensing of muscles.
- Position the person supine, with the head on a pillow, the knees bent or on a pillow

and the arms at the sides or across the chest. (Note: Discourage the person from placing their arms over the head because this tenses abdominal musculature.)

- Warm the stethoscope endpiece and your hands to avoid abdominal tensing. Your fingernails should be short.
- Enquire about any painful areas. Examine these areas last to avoid any muscle guarding.
- Finally, learn to use distraction: enhance muscle relaxation. For example, encourage slow breathing; use emotive imagery; use a low, soothing voice; and ask the person to relate their abdominal history while you palpate.

Equipment needed

Secondary light source if needed
Stethoscope
Disinfectant wipes (to clean stethoscope endpiece)
One pillow under the person's head
Hand hygiene solution

PROCEDURES AND NORMAL FINDINGS	CLINICAL SIGNIFICANCE AND CLINICAL ALERTS
 A skills video (Abdominal assessment) is available to assist you in your skill development. Scan the QR code to access the video (instructions on the inside front cover of the book to access multimedia resources).	
General inspection	
While collecting subjective data, you will have noticed the colour and moisture of the person's skin and mucous membranes, ease of movement, presence of pain or nausea, hygiene and grooming and height-to-weight ratio. All these factors provide clues to gastrointestinal function and the potential for abdominal health issues. A comfortable person is relaxed quietly on the bed or examining table and has a relaxed facial expression and slow, even respirations.	Restlessness and constant turning to find comfort occur with the colicky pain of gastroenteritis or intestinal (bowel) obstruction (Table 23.1). Absolute stillness, resisting any movement, occurs with the pain of peritonitis. Knees flexed up, facial grimacing and shallow rapid, uneven respirations also indicate pain.
Identify abdominal landmarks	
Identify the following abdominal landmarks: costal margins, symphysis pubis, xiphoid process, inferior-superior illiac spines, umbilicus. Draw an imaginary line with your finger to identify the four abdominal quadrants: right upper quadrant, right lower quadrant, left upper quadrant, left lower quadrant. These quadrants will provide a structure for you to document your findings accurately. See Figure 23.6B.	Refer also to Figures 23.1, 23.2 and 23.6, earlier.

PROCEDURES AND NORMAL FINDINGS	CLINICAL SIGNIFICANCE AND CLINICAL ALERTS

FIGURE 23.6B The abdomen divided into four quadrants

Inspect the abdomen

Umbilicus

Normally, the umbilicus is midline and inverted, with no sign of discolouration, inflammation or hernia. It becomes everted and pushed upwards with pregnancy.

The umbilicus is a common site for skin piercings. The site should not be red or crusted.

Everted with **ascites** (an abnormal buildup of fluid in the peritoneal cavity. Cases include liver disease, abdominal cancers, severe heart or renal failure) (Table 23.2).

Underlying mass

Deeply sunken with obesity.

Enlarged and everted with umbilical hernia.

Bluish periumbilical colour occurs with intraabdominal bleeding (Cullen's sign).

Contour

Stand on the person's side and look down on the abdomen. Then stoop or sit to gaze across the abdomen. Your head should be slightly higher than the abdomen. Determine the profile from the rib margin to the pubic bone. The contour is related to the nutritional and fitness state of the person and normally ranges from flat to rounded (Figure 23.7). A rounded abdomen is a normal finding in a woman who has been pregnant.

Scaphoid abdomen, protuberant abdomen, abdominal distension (see also Table 23.2).

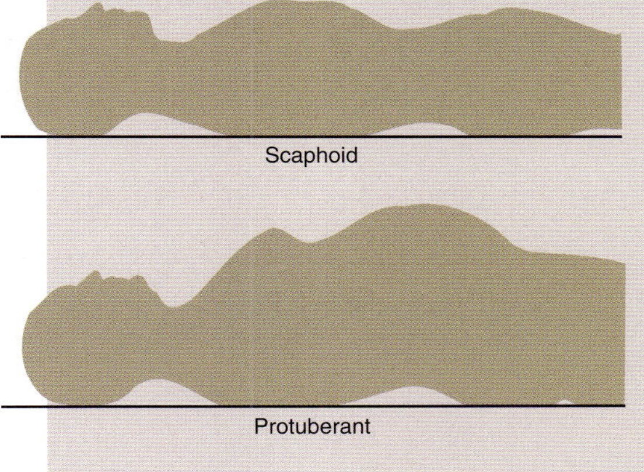

FIGURE 23.7 Common contours of the abdomen

PROCEDURES AND NORMAL FINDINGS	CLINICAL SIGNIFICANCE AND CLINICAL ALERTS
Symmetry	
The abdomen should be symmetrical bilaterally (Figure 23.8). Note any localised bulging, visible mass or asymmetric shape. Even small bulges will be highlighted by shadow. 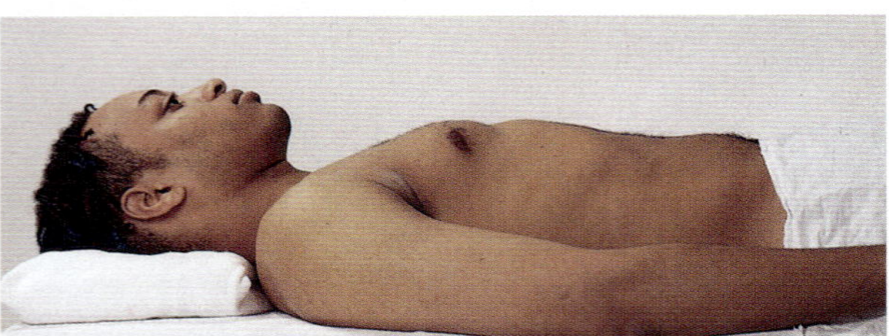 **FIGURE 23.8** Flat abdominal contour	Bulges, **masses**. **Hernia**—protrusion of abdominal viscera through abnormal opening in muscle wall (Table 23.4).
Move to the end of the bed and inspect the person's exposed abdomen for symmetry. Ask the person to take a deep breath to further highlight any change. Ask the person to place their chin on their chest and raise their head off the pillow. The abdomen should stay smooth and symmetrical.	Note any localised bulging. **Umbilical hernia**, enlarged liver or spleen may show. **Diastasis recti**, or a midline longitudinal ridge, is a separation of the abdominal rectus muscles (Table 23.4).
Skin	
The surface is smooth and even, with homogeneous colour. This is a good area to judge skin colour because it is often protected from sun.	Redness with localised inflammation. **Jaundice—**yellow colouration of the skin, sclera of the eye and mucous membranes caused by a buildup of bilirubin in the blood (shows best in natural daylight). Skin glistening and taut occurs with **ascites**.
One common pigment change is **striae** (lineae albicantes), silvery white, linear, jagged marks about 1 to 6 cm long (Figure 23.9). They occur when elastic fibres in the reticular layer of the skin are broken after rapid or prolonged stretching, as in pregnancy or excessive weight gain. Recent striae are pink or blue; then they turn silvery white.	

PROCEDURES AND NORMAL FINDINGS	CLINICAL SIGNIFICANCE AND CLINICAL ALERTS
FIGURE 23.9 Striae	
Pigmented naevi (moles), circumscribed brown macular or papular areas, are common on the abdomen.	Unusual colour or change in shape of mole (Chapter 22). **Petechiae**—small spots of blood under the skin caused by leaking of capillaries. Associated with excessive straining, some medicines such as anticoagulants, infections (such as meningococcal and rubella) and medical conditions. Needs referral to a medical practitioner.
Normally, no lesions are present, although you may note well-healed surgical scars. If a scar is present, draw its location in the person's medical record, indicating the length in centimetres (Figure 23.10). (**Note:** A person may forget a past operation while providing the history. If you note a scar now, ask about it.)	**Cutaneous angiomas** (spider naevi) occur with portal hypertension or liver disease. Lesions, rashes (Chapter 22). A surgical scar alerts you to the possible presence of underlying **adhesions** and excess fibrous tissue.

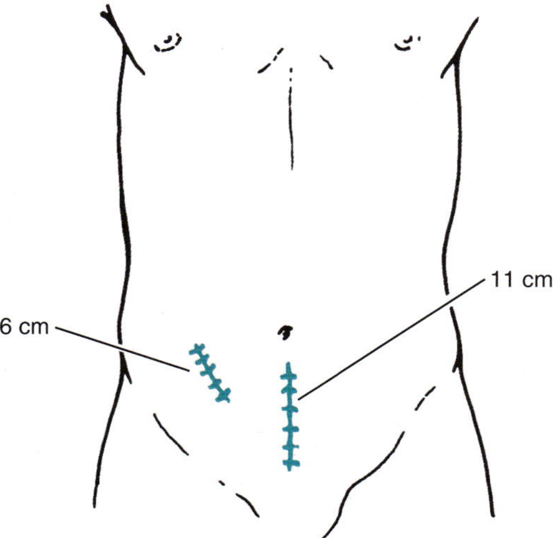

FIGURE 23.10 Diagram of position of scars on the abdomen

PROCEDURES AND NORMAL FINDINGS	CLINICAL SIGNIFICANCE AND CLINICAL ALERTS
Veins are not usually seen, but a fine venous network may be visible in thin people.	Prominent, dilated veins occur with **portal hypertension, cirrhosis,** ascites, or vena caval obstruction. Veins are more visible with malnutrition because of thinned adipose tissue.
Good skin turgor reflects healthy nutrition and hydration. Gently pinch up a fold of skin; then release. Note how long it takes the skin to return to its original position.	Slow return to the original position, referred to as 'poor turgor', occurs with dehydration, which often accompanies gastrointestinal disease.
Pulsation or movement	
Normally, you may see the pulsations from the aorta beneath the skin in the epigastric area, particularly in thin people. Respiratory movement also shows in the abdomen, particularly in males. Finally, waves of peristalsis may be visible in very thin people. These ripple slowly and obliquely across the abdomen.	Marked pulsation of aorta occurs with widened pulse pressure (e.g. hypertension, aortic insufficiency, thyrotoxicosis) and with **aortic aneurysm** (a balloon-like bulge in the aorta). ! ***Clinical alert:*** If you observe marked central abdominal pulsation proceed with caution in performing further examination as this could be caused by an aortic aneurysm (particularly in older adults), which can dissect (the walls of the artery split and become weaker) or rupture. Marked visible peristalsis, together with a distended abdomen, indicates **intestinal or bowel obstruction** (Table 23.1).
Auscultation—bowel sounds	
• Depart from the usual examination sequence and auscultate the abdomen next. This is done because percussion and palpation can increase peristalsis, which would give a false interpretation of bowel sounds. • Use the diaphragm endpiece because bowel sounds are relatively high pitched. • Hold the stethoscope lightly against the skin; pushing too hard may stimulate more bowel sounds (Figure 23.11). • It is usual practice to begin in the right lower quadrant at the ileocaecal valve area because bowel sounds are normally always present here. If bowel sounds are heard in one area it is likely that they will be present throughout the abdomen.[16]	

PROCEDURES AND NORMAL FINDINGS	CLINICAL SIGNIFICANCE AND CLINICAL ALERTS

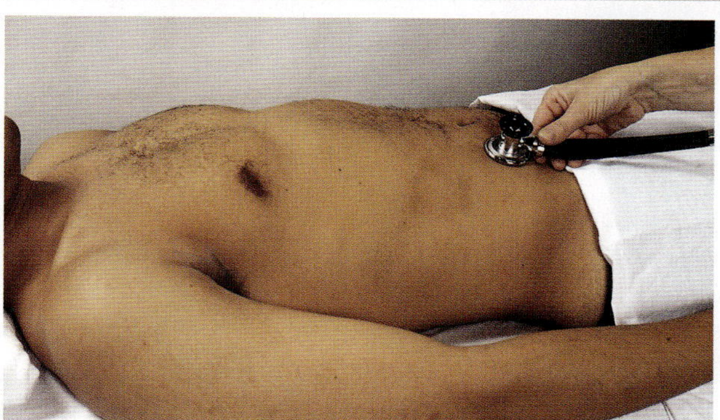

FIGURE 23.11 Placement of the stethoscope for auscultation of the abdomen

Bowel sounds—present or absent

There is no accepted time period that you should listen for bowel sounds—just listen until you hear them. Bowel sounds originate from the movement of air and fluid through the small intestine. Depending on the time elapsed since eating, a wide range of normal sounds can occur.[16]

Bowel sounds are normally high pitched, gurgling, cascading sounds, occurring irregularly anywhere from 5 to 30 times per minute. You don't need to count them—just record if they are present or absent.

A perfectly 'silent abdomen' is uncommon. Listen for at least 4 minutes if bowel sounds are not heard initially.[16]

Two distinct patterns of abnormal bowel sounds may occur:

Hypoactive or absent sounds follow abdominal surgery or with inflammation of the peritoneum.

Hyperactive sounds are loud, high-pitched, rushing, tinkling sounds that signal increased motility (Table 23.5).

Clinical alert: The finding of absent bowel sounds *may* indicate the development of a **paralytic ileus** (intestinal obstruction)—lack of or reduction in the peristaltic movement in the bowel causing a functional obstruction to normal passage of food or fluids—and the person should be referred to a medical practitioner for further assessment if this is a new finding or the person has other symptoms such as abdominal pain, abdominal distension, nausea or vomiting (Table 23.1).

PROCEDURES AND NORMAL FINDINGS	CLINICAL SIGNIFICANCE AND CLINICAL ALERTS
Percussion—general tympany	
Percussion can be used to identify the presence and extent of faecal loading or a distended bladder, especially if there is no access to a bladder ultrasound machine. Percussion is a skill that takes time to master and takes experience to interpret the various sounds. Percussion is rarely used by registered nurses to assess the relative density of abdominal contents, to locate organs or to screen for abnormal fluid or masses (see section titled 'Advanced practice—additional data').	
First, percuss lightly in all four quadrants to determine the prevailing amount of tympany and dullness (Figure 23.12). Move clockwise. **Tympany** should predominate because air in the intestines rises to the surface when the person is supine.	**Dullness** occurs over a distended bladder, faecal loading, adipose tissue, fluid or a mass. **Hyperresonance** is present with gaseous distension (Table 23.5).

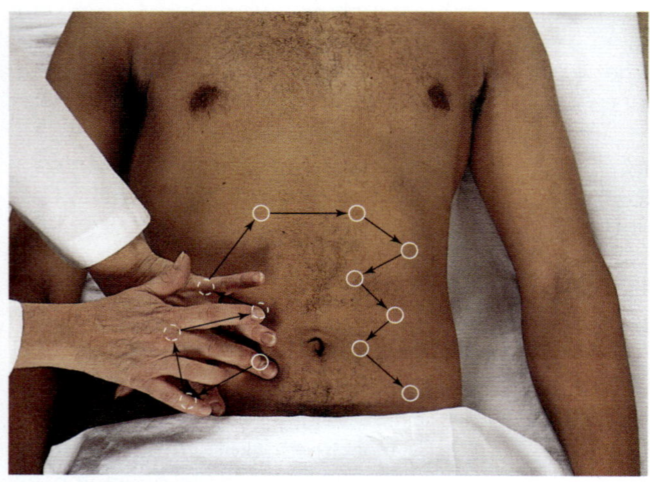

FIGURE 23.12 Position sequence for abdominal percussion

PROCEDURES AND NORMAL FINDINGS	CLINICAL SIGNIFICANCE AND CLINICAL ALERTS
Palpation—surface and light	
Perform palpation to judge the **size, location and consistency of an abnormal mass or tenderness**. Review comfort measures at the beginning of this section. Because most people are naturally inclined to protect the abdomen, use additional measures to enhance complete muscle relaxation.	
• Ask the person to bend their knees.	
• Hold your palpating hand low and parallel to the abdomen. Use the finger pads, not the tips.	Holding the hand high and pointing down could make the person tense up.
• Instruct the person to breathe slowly (in through the nose and out through the mouth).	
• Keep your own voice low and soothing. Conversation may relax the person.	
• Try 'emotive imagery'. For example, you might say, 'Now I want you to imagine you are dozing on the beach, with the sun warming your muscles and the sound of the waves lulling you to sleep. Let yourself relax.'	
Surface palpation	
Begin with **surface palpation**. With the first four fingers close together, depress the skin about 1 cm (Figure 23.13). Make a gentle rotary motion, sliding the fingers and skin together. Then lift the fingers (do not drag them) and move clockwise to the next location around the abdomen. The objective here is not to search for masses but to form an overall impression of the skin surface and superficial musculature. Save the examination of any identified tender areas until last. This method avoids pain and the resulting muscle rigidity that would obscure deeper palpation later in the examination. 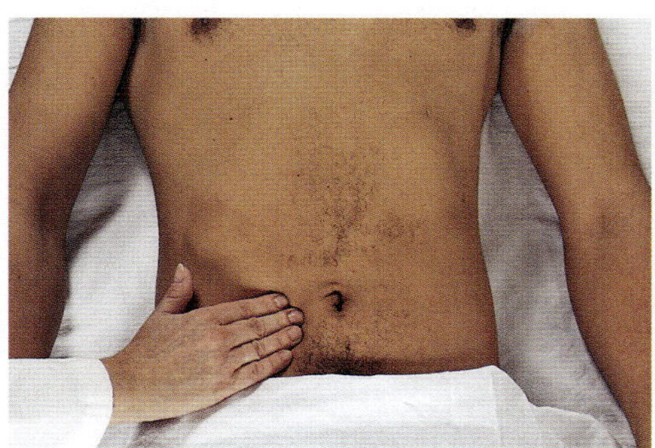 **FIGURE 23.13** Surface palpation	**Muscle guarding—**an involuntary tightening of the muscles (in this case the abdominal muscles) often due to pain on palpation. **Abdominal rigidity—**continuous rigidity of the muscles which can be felt on palpation. It is a protective mechanism accompanying acute inflammation of the peritoneum. Large masses. Tenderness or pain.[12]  ***Clinical alert:*** If the person experiences any significant abdominal tenderness, stop the examination and refer the person to a medical practitioner for further assessment.

PROCEDURES AND NORMAL FINDINGS	CLINICAL SIGNIFICANCE AND CLINICAL ALERTS
As you circle the abdomen, discriminate between voluntary muscle guarding and involuntary rigidity. **Voluntary guarding** occurs when the person is cold, tense or ticklish. It is bilateral, and you will feel the muscles relax slightly during exhalation. Use the relaxation measures to try to eliminate this type of guarding, or it will interfere with deep palpation. If the rigidity persists, it is probably involuntary.	Abdominal rigidity

Light palpation

Now perform **light palpation** using the technique described in surface palpation but push down 5 to 8 cm depending on the amount of abdominal fat (Figure 23.14). Moving clockwise, explore the entire abdomen. The objective of light palpation is to identify masses (location, shape and size).

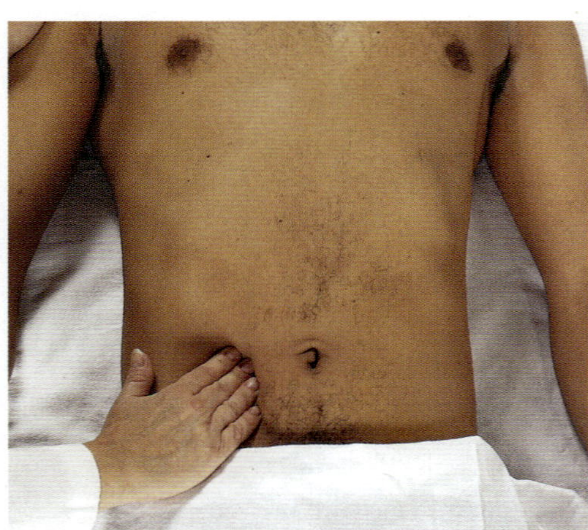

FIGURE 23.14 Light palpation

To overcome the resistance of a very large or obese abdomen, you may need to use a two-handed technique. Place your two hands on top of each other (Figure 23.15). The top hand does the pushing; the bottom hand is relaxed and can be free to focus on the sense of palpation.

With either technique, note the **location, size, consistency and mobility** of masses.

Making sense of what you are feeling is more difficult than it looks. It helps to memorise the anatomy and visualise what is under each quadrant as you palpate. Refer to Figures 23.2 and 23.4.

PROCEDURES AND NORMAL FINDINGS	CLINICAL SIGNIFICANCE AND CLINICAL ALERTS

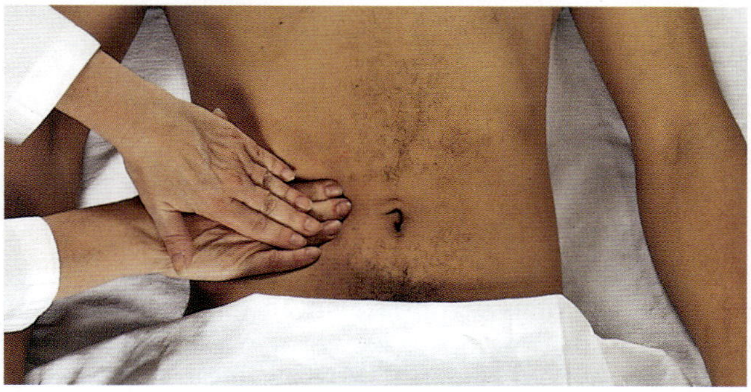

FIGURE 23.15 Two-handed light palpation

Mild tenderness is normally present when palpating the sigmoid colon. Any other tenderness should be investigated.

Tenderness occurs with local inflammation, with inflammation of the peritoneum or underlying organ and with an enlarged organ whose capsule is stretched. **Rebound tenderness** is present when the person experiences a sudden sharp pain on removal of the palpating hand from the abdominal surface.[16]

If you identify a mass, note the following:

- location (quadrant)
- size (measured) and shape
- consistency (soft, firm, hard)
- surface (smooth, nodular)
- mobility (including movement with respirations)
- pulsatility (you can feel a pulse in the mass)
- tenderness.

Clinical alert: If you palpate a pulsatile mass, especially if there is also abdominal tenderness, stop the examination and refer the person to a medical practitioner for further assessment. A pulsatile abdominal mass may indicate the presence of an abdominal aortic aneurysm.

Additional objective data for infants

Inspection

The contour of the abdomen is **protuberant** because of the immature abdominal musculature. The skin contains a fine, superficial venous pattern. This may be visible in lightly pigmented children up to the age of puberty.

A scaphoid shape occurs with dehydration.

Dilated veins may indicate underlying abdominal pathology such as liver enlargement.

Inspect the umbilical cord throughout the neonatal period. At birth, it is white and contains two umbilical arteries and one vein surrounded by mucoid connective tissue, called Wharton's jelly. The umbilical stump dries within a week, hardens and falls off by 10 to 14 days. Skin covers the area by 3 or 4 weeks.

Inflammation.

Discharge or redness after cord falls off.

PROCEDURES AND NORMAL FINDINGS	CLINICAL SIGNIFICANCE AND CLINICAL ALERTS
The abdomen should be symmetrical, although two bulges are common. You may note an **umbilical hernia**. It appears at 2 to 3 weeks and is especially prominent when the infant cries. The hernia reaches maximum size at 1 month (up to 2.5 cm) and usually disappears by 1 year. Another common variation is **diastasis recti**, a separation of the rectus muscles with a visible bulge along the midline.	Refer infants with an umbilical hernia larger than 2.5 cm (Table 23.4) continuing to grow after 1 month to a medical practitioner.
The abdomen shows respiratory movement. The only other abdominal movement you should note is occasional peristalsis, which may be visible because of the thin musculature.	**Marked peristalsis**, together with projectile vomiting in a newborn, suggests pyloric stenosis, an obstruction of the stomach's pyloric valve. Pyloric stenosis is a congenital defect and appears in the second or third week. After feeding, pronounced peristaltic waves cross from left to right, leading to projectile vomiting. Requires referral to a medical practitioner.
Auscultation Auscultation for the presence or absence of bowel sounds. **Percussion** Percussion elicits tympany over the stomach (the infant swallows some air with feeding). Percussing the spleen is not done. The abdomen sounds tympanitic, although it is normal to percuss dullness over the bladder. This dullness may extend up to the umbilicus. **Palpation** Aid palpation by flexing the baby's knees with one hand while palpating with the other (Figure 23.16). Alternatively, you may hold the upper back and flex the neck slightly with one hand.	

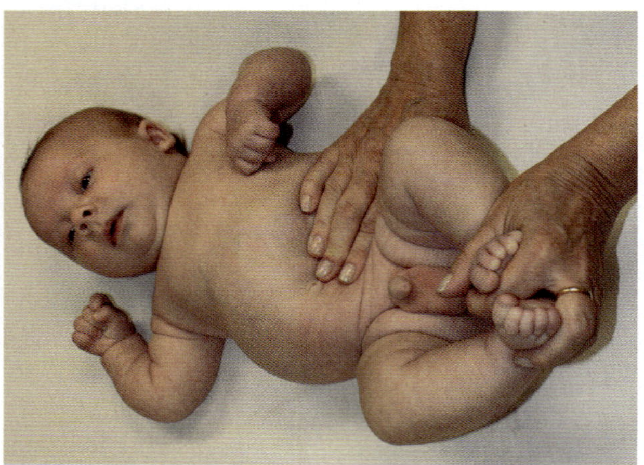

FIGURE 23.16 Abdominal palpation in an infant

PROCEDURES AND NORMAL FINDINGS	CLINICAL SIGNIFICANCE AND CLINICAL ALERTS

Additional objective data for children

Under age 4 years, the abdomen looks protuberant when the child is both supine and standing. After age 4 years, the potbelly remains when standing because of lumbar lordosis, but the abdomen looks flat when supine. Normal movement on the abdomen includes respirations, which remain abdominal until 7 years of age.

A **scaphoid abdomen** is associated with dehydration or malnutrition.

Under 7 years of age, the absence of abdominal respirations occurs with inflammation of the peritoneum.

To **palpate the abdomen**, position the young child on the parent's lap as you sit knee-to-knee with the parent (Figure 23.17). Flex the child's knees up and elevate the head slightly. Hold your entire palm flat on the abdominal surface for a moment before starting palpation. This accustoms the child to being touched. If the child is very ticklish, hold their hand under your own as you palpate or apply the stethoscope and palpate around it.

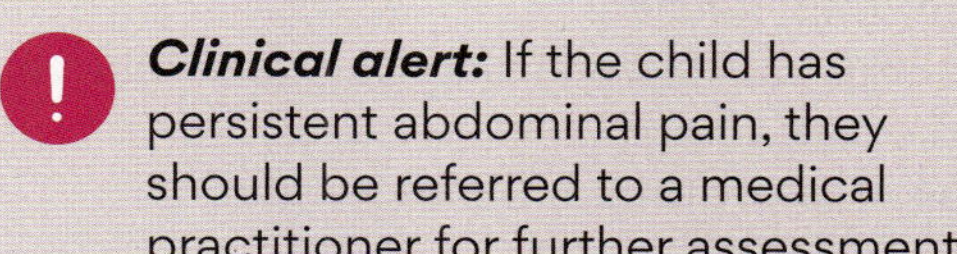

Clinical alert: If the child has persistent abdominal pain, they should be referred to a medical practitioner for further assessment.

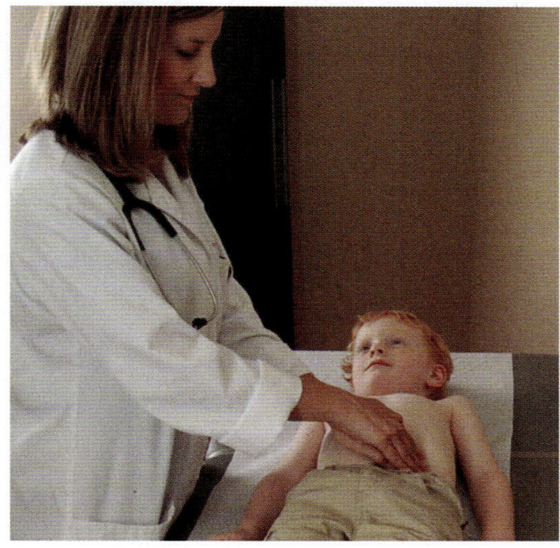

FIGURE 23.17 Light abdominal palpation in a child

Additional objective data for adults over 65 years

As a person ages, on inspection, you may note increased deposits of subcutaneous fat on the abdomen and hips because it is redistributed away from the extremities. The abdominal musculature is often thinner and has less tone than that of the younger adult, so in the absence of obesity you may note peristalsis.

Because of the thinner, softer abdominal wall, the organs may be easier to palpate (in the absence of obesity).

Abdominal rigidity with acute abdominal conditions is less common in older people.

With an **acute abdomen**, the older person often complains of less pain than a younger person would.

Abnormal findings

TABLE 23.1 Clinical portrait of intestinal obstruction

Subjective data

History of previous abdominal surgery with adhesions
Vomiting, nausea
Colicky pain from strong peristalsis above the obstruction
Absence of stool or passage of flatus

Objective data

Restless, ill-appearing person
Distended abdomen
Hyperactive bowel sounds in early obstruction; hypoactive or silent in late obstruction
Tenderness on palpation
Hypovolaemic shock due to dehydration and sepsis may occur (increased pulse, decreased blood pressure, cool skin, dry mucous membranes)

Diagnostic tests

Laboratory: Evidence of dehydration, electrolyte imbalance and possibly sepsis
X-ray: accumulation of fluid and gas in bowel proximal (above) to obstruction

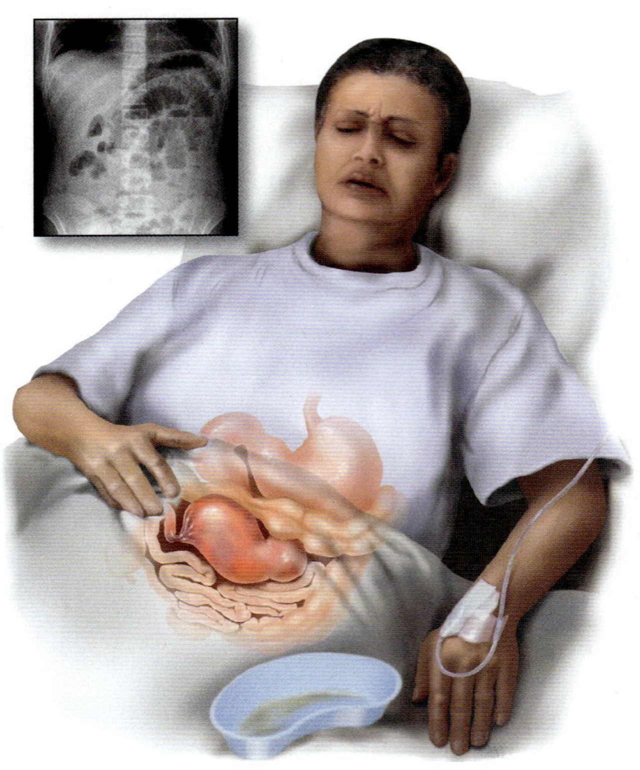

TABLE 23.2 Common causes of abdominal distension

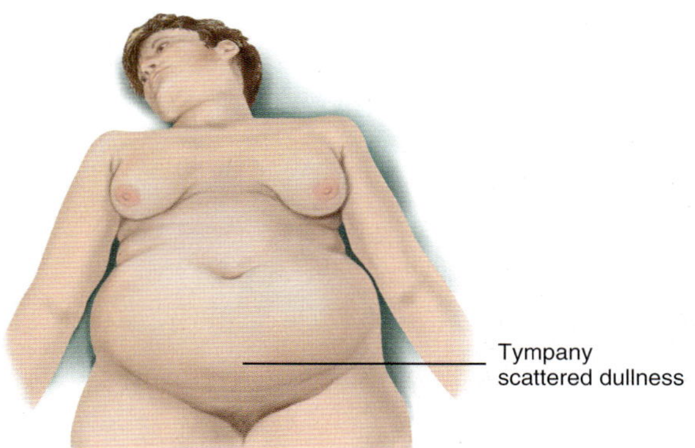

Obesity

Inspection: Uniformly rounded. Umbilicus sunken (it adheres to peritoneum, and layers of fat are superficial to it).
Auscultation: Bowel sounds heard in all four quadrants.
Percussion: Tympany. Scattered dullness over adipose tissue.
Palpation: Soft. May be hard to palpate through thick abdominal wall.

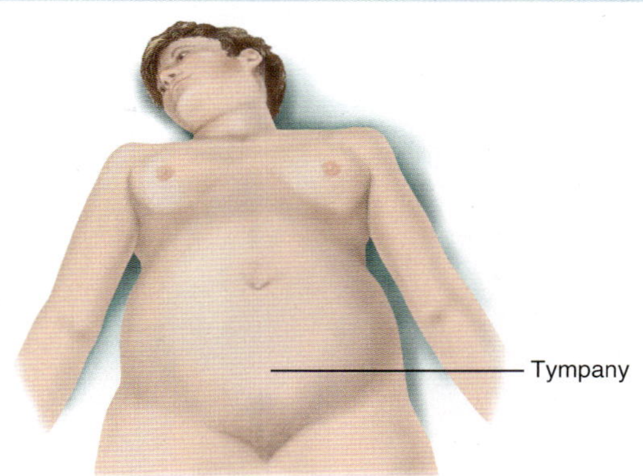

Faecal mass

Inspection: Localised distension.
Auscultation: Bowel sounds heard in all four quadrants.
Percussion: Tympany predominates. Scattered dullness over faecal mass.
Palpation: Firm rope-like mass with faeces in intestines (likely to be in descending colon and sometimes transverse colon).

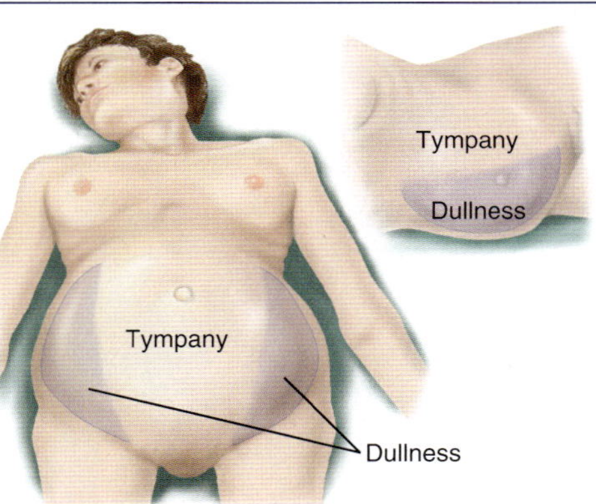

Air or gas

Inspection: Single round curve.
Auscultation: Depends on cause of gas (e.g. decreased or absent bowel sounds with ileus); hyperactive with early intestinal obstruction.
Percussion: Tympany over large area.
Palpation: May have muscle spasm of abdominal wall.

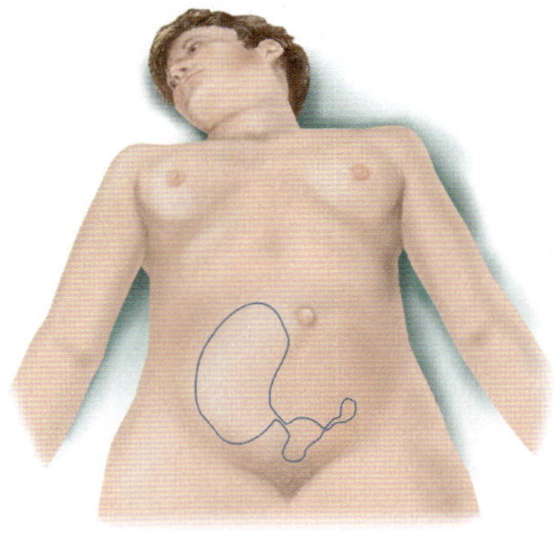

Ovarian cyst (large)

Inspection: Curve in lower half of abdomen, midline. Everted umbilicus.
Auscultation: Bowel sounds heard in all four quadrants.
Percussion—advanced practice: Top dull over fluid. Intestines pushed superiorly. Large cyst produces fluid wave and shifting dullness.
Palpation—advanced practice: Transmits aortic pulsation while ascites does not.

Continued

TABLE 23.2 Common causes of abdominal distension cont'd

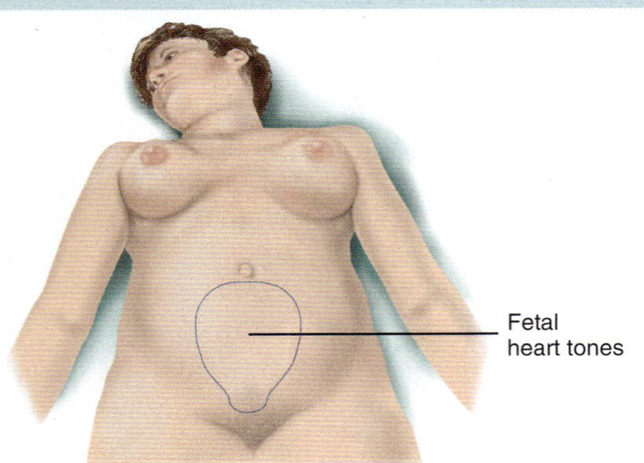

Pregnancy

Obviously a normal finding, pregnancy is included for comparison of conditions causing abdominal distension.

Inspection: Single curve. Umbilicus protruding. Breasts engorged.
Auscultation: Fetal heart tones. Bowel sounds diminished.
Percussion: Tympany over intestines. Dull over enlarging uterus.
Palpation: Fetal parts. Fetal movements.

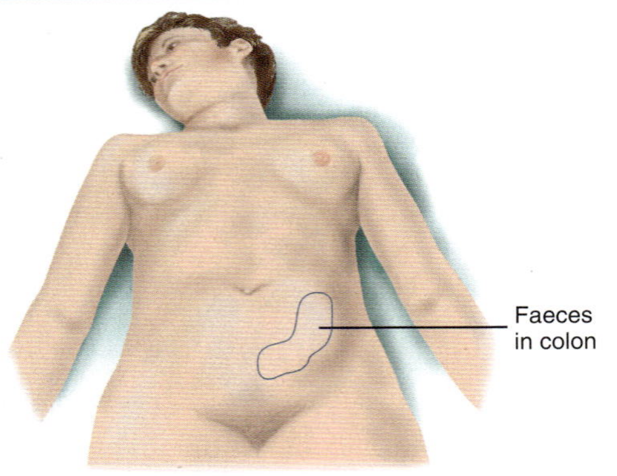

Abdominal mass/tumour

Inspection: Localised distension.
Auscultation: Bowel sounds heard in all four quadrants.
Percussion—advanced practice: Dull over mass if reaches up to skin surface.
Palpation—advanced practice: Define borders. Distinguish from enlarged organ or normally palpable structure.

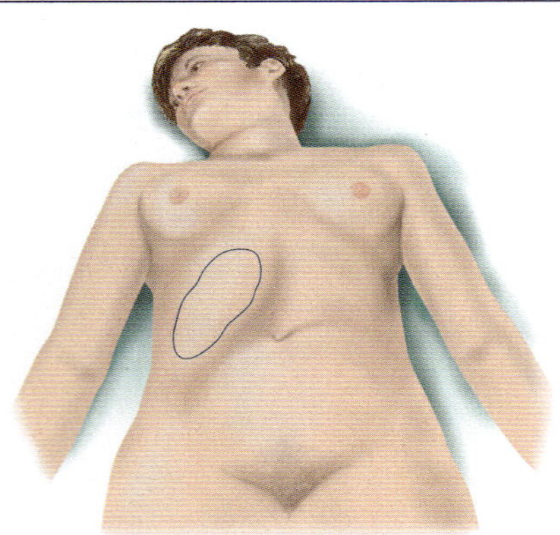

Ascites

Inspection: Single curve. Everted umbilicus. Bulging flanks when supine. Taut glistening skin, recent weight gain, increase in abdominal girth.
Auscultation: Bowel sounds heard in all four quadrants. Diminished over ascitic fluid.
Percussion: Tympany at top where intestines float. Dull over fluid. Produces fluid wave and shifting dullness.
Palpation: Taut skin and increased intraabdominal pressure limit palpation.

TABLE 23.3 Common sites of referred abdominal pain

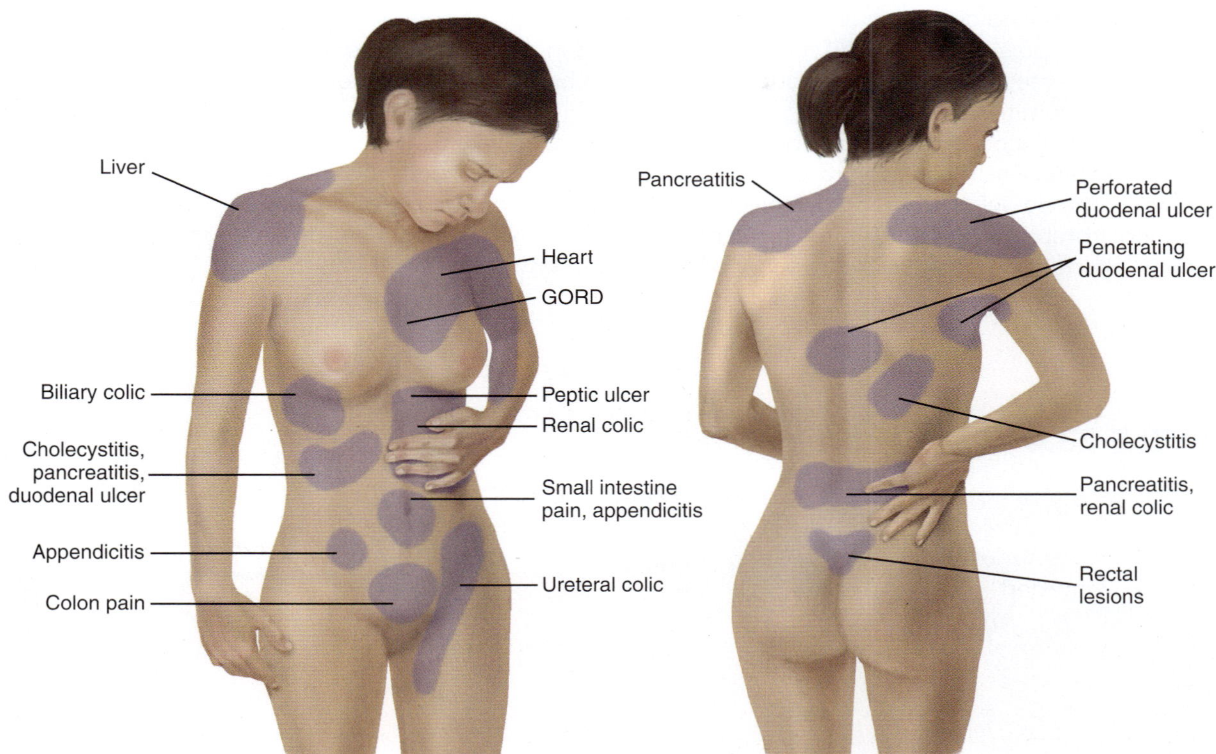

When a person shares a history of abdominal pain, the pain's location may not necessarily be directly over the involved organ. That is because the human brain has no felt image for internal organs. Rather, pain is referred to a site where the organ was in fetal development. Although the organ migrates during fetal development, its nerves persist in referring sensations from the former location. The following are examples, not a complete list.

Liver: Hepatitis may have mild to moderate, dull pain in right upper quadrant or epigastrium, along with anorexia, nausea, malaise, low-grade fever.

Oesophagus: Gastro-oesophageal reflux disease is a complex of symptoms of oesophagitis, including burning pain in midepigastrium or behind lower sternum that radiates upwards, or 'heartburn'. Occurs 30 to 60 minutes after eating; aggravated by lying down or bending over.

Gall bladder: Cholecystitis is biliary colic, sudden pain in right upper quadrant that may radiate to right or left scapula, and which builds over time, lasting 2 to 4 hours after ingesting fatty foods, alcohol or caffeine. Associated with nausea and vomiting and positive Murphy's sign or sudden stop in inspiration with right upper quadrant palpation.

Pancreas: Pancreatitis has acute, boring midepigastric pain radiating to the back and sometimes to the left scapula or flank, severe nausea and vomiting.

Duodenum: Duodenal ulcer typically has dull, aching, gnawing pain, does not radiate, may be relieved by food and may awaken the person from sleep.

Stomach: Gastric ulcer pain is dull, aching, gnawing epigastric pain, usually brought on by food, radiates to back or substernal area. Pain of perforated ulcer is burning epigastric pain of sudden onset that refers to one or both shoulders.

Continued

TABLE 23.3 Common sites of referred abdominal pain cont'd

Appendix: Appendicitis typically starts as dull, diffuse pain in periumbilical region that later shifts to severe, sharp, persistent pain and tenderness localised in the right lower quadrant (McBurney's point). Pain is aggravated by movement, coughing and deep breathing; associated with anorexia, then nausea and vomiting, fever.
Kidney: Kidney stones prompt a sudden onset of severe, colicky flank or lower abdominal pain.
Small intestine: Gastroenteritis presents with diffused, generalised abdominal pain, with nausea, diarrhoea.
Colon: Large bowel obstruction has moderate, colicky pain of gradual onset in lower abdomen, bloating. Irritable bowel syndrome has sharp or burning, cramping pain over a wide area; does not radiate. Brought on by meals, relieved by bowel movement.

TABLE 23.4 Abnormalities on inspection

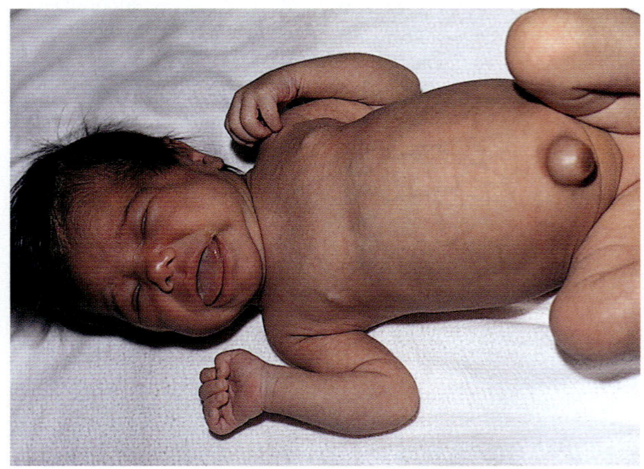

Umbilical hernia

Umbilical hernia is a soft, skin-covered mass that is the protrusion of the omentum or intestine through a weakness or incomplete closure in the umbilical ring. It is accentuated by increased intraabdominal pressure as with crying, coughing, vomiting or straining, but the bowel rarely incarcerates or strangulates. Most umbilical hernias resolve spontaneously by 1 year. In an adult, it can occur with pregnancy, chronic ascites or from chronic intrathoracic pressure (e.g. asthma, chronic bronchitis) and weak abdominal muscles.

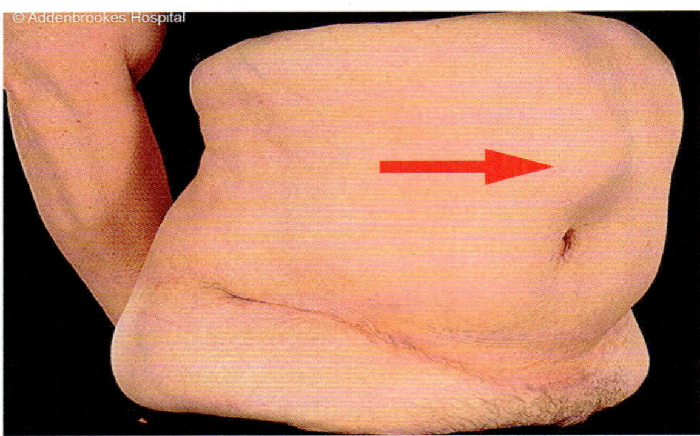

Incisional hernia

A bulge near an old operative scar that may not show when person is supine but is apparent when the person increases intraabdominal pressure by a sit-up, stand or Valsalva manoeuvre.

TABLE 23.4 Abnormalities on inspection cont'd

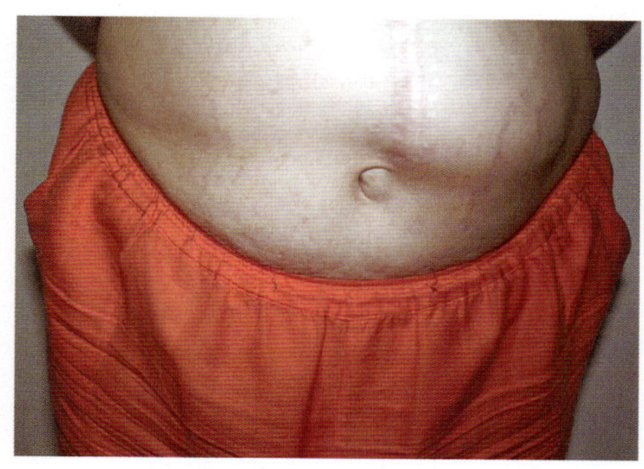

Epigastric hernia

A small protrusion at epigastrium in midline, through the linea alba. Usually, the examiner can feel it rather than observe it. May be palpable only when standing.

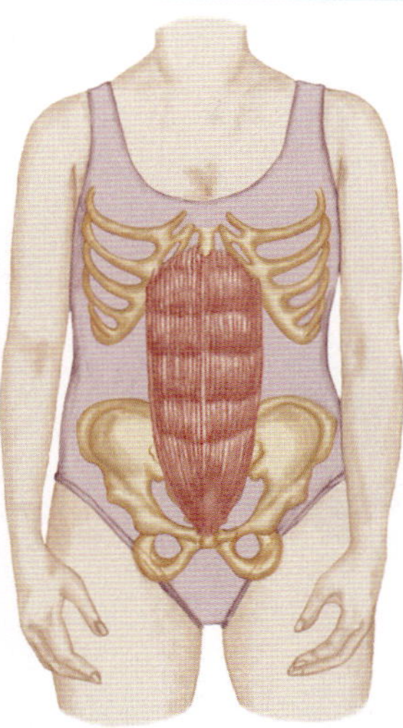

Normal location of rectus muscles of the abdomen

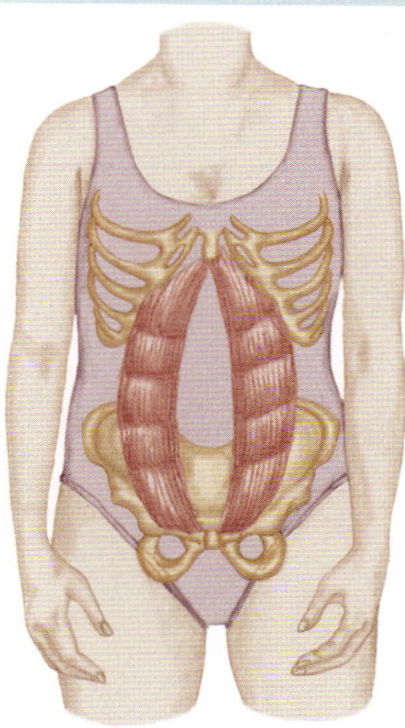

Diastasis recti: separation of the rectus muscles

Diastasis recti

Diastasis recti, or a midline longitudinal ridge, is a separation of the abdominal rectus muscles. Ridge is revealed when intra-abdominal pressure is increased by raising head while supine. Can occur congenitally, during or postpartum, weak abdominal muscles or marked obesity in which prolonged distension or a decrease in muscle tone has occurred. An individualised abdominal muscle exercise program can reduce the separation of the rectus muscles.

TABLE 23.5 Abnormal bowel sounds

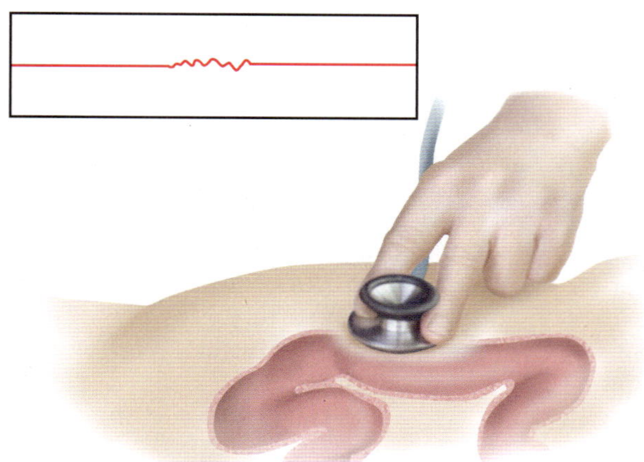

Hypoactive bowel sounds

Diminished or absent bowel sounds signal decreased motility because of inflammation as seen with peritonitis, from paralytic ileus following abdominal surgery or from late bowel obstruction.

Continued

TABLE 23.5 Abnormal bowel sounds cont'd

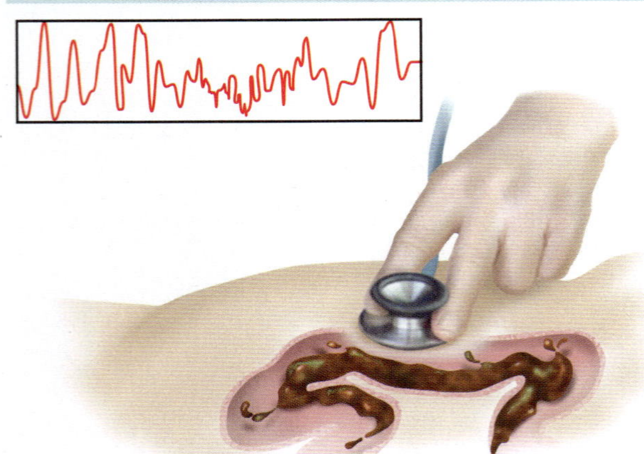

Hyperactive bowel sounds

Loud, gurgling sounds, 'borborygmi', signal increased motility. They occur with early mechanical bowel obstruction (high pitched), gastroenteritis, brisk diarrhoea, laxative use and subsiding paralytic ileus.

Advanced practice—additional data

In addition to the subjective and objective data described previously, the assessments that are described in the following sections require advanced skill and scope of practice. Nurses working in specialist settings and some community nurses would need to develop these skills.

Preparation

Same preparation as previously described.

Equipment needed

Small centimetre ruler
Skin-marking pen
Hand hygiene solution

PROCEDURES AND NORMAL FINDINGS	CLINICAL SIGNIFICANCE AND CLINICAL ALERTS
Auscultate vascular sounds	
As you listen to the abdomen for bowel sounds, note the presence of any **vascular sounds** or **bruits**. Using firmer pressure, listen over the aorta, renal arteries, iliac and femoral arteries, especially in people with hypertension (Figure 23.18). Note location, pitch and timing of a vascular sound. There should be no bruits present.	A **systolic bruit** is a pulsatile blowing sound and occurs with stenosis or occlusion of an artery. **Venous hum and peritoneal friction rub** are rare (Table 23.6).

PROCEDURES AND NORMAL FINDINGS	CLINICAL SIGNIFICANCE AND CLINICAL ALERTS

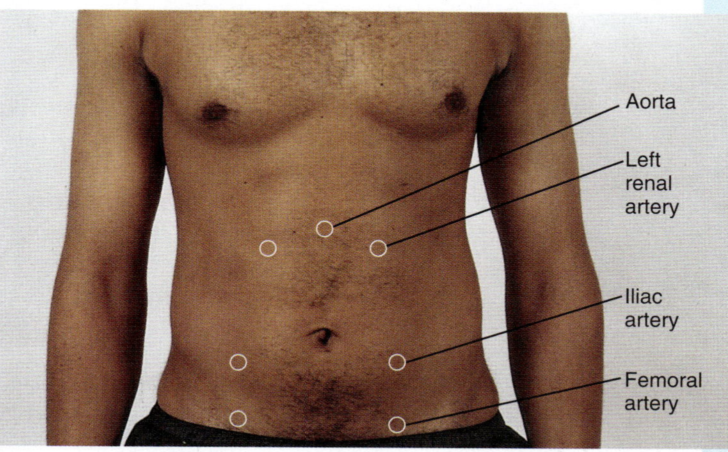

FIGURE 23.18 Sequence for auscultation of vascular sounds in the abdomen

Percussion

Percuss to assess the relative density of abdominal contents, to locate organs and to screen for abnormal fluid or masses.

General tympany

First, percuss lightly in all four quadrants to determine the prevailing amount of tympany and dullness (Figure 23.12). Move clockwise. Tympany should predominate because air in the intestines rises to the surface when the person is supine.

Dullness occurs over a distended bladder, faecal loading, adipose tissue, fluid or a mass.

Hyperresonance is present with gaseous distension.

Liver span

Next, percuss to map out the boundaries of certain organs. Measure the height of the liver in the right midclavicular line. (For a consistent placement of the midclavicular line landmark, remember to palpate the acromioclavicular and the sternoclavicular joints and judge the line at a point midway between the two.)

Begin in the area of lung resonance and percuss down the midclavicular line and the interspaces of the ribs until the sound changes to a dull quality (Figure 23.19). Mark the spot, usually in the fifth intercostal space. Then find abdominal tympany and percuss up the midclavicular line. Mark where the sound changes from tympany to a dull sound, normally at the right costal margin.

PROCEDURES AND NORMAL FINDINGS	CLINICAL SIGNIFICANCE AND CLINICAL ALERTS

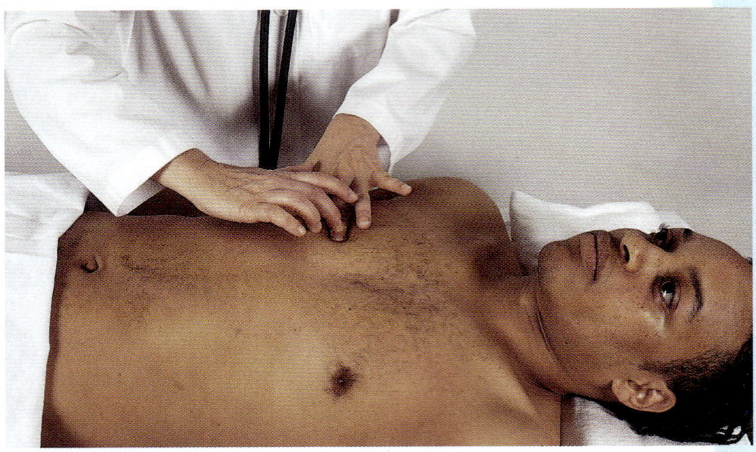

FIGURE 23.19 Percussion to determine liver span

Measure the distance between the two marks; the normal liver span in the adult ranges from 6 to 12 cm (Figure 23.20). The height of the liver span correlates with the height of the person; taller people have longer livers. Also, males have a larger liver span than females of the same height. Overall, the mean liver span is 10.5 cm for males and 7 cm for females.

An enlarged liver span indicates liver enlargement or **hepatomegaly**.

Accurate detection of liver borders is confused by dullness above the fifth intercostal space, which occurs with lung disease (e.g. pleural effusion or lung consolidation). Accurate detection at the lower border is confused when dullness is pushed up with ascites or pregnancy or with gas distension in the colon, which obscures the lower border.

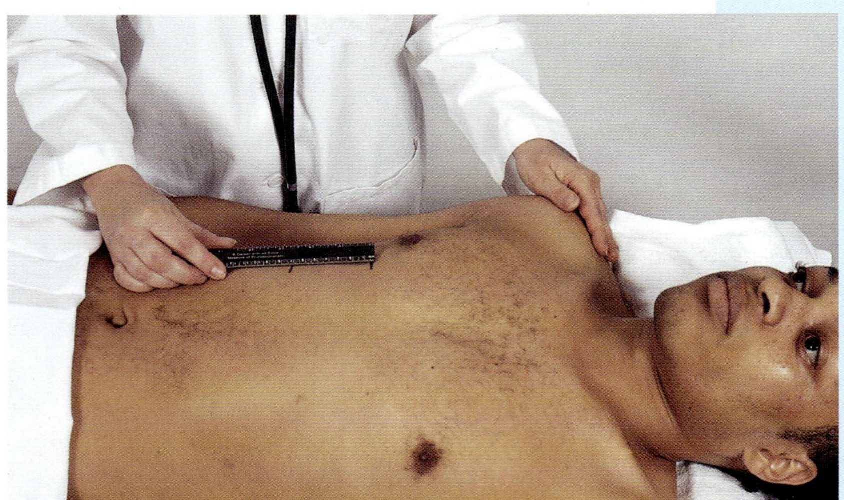

FIGURE 23.20 Measuring liver span

PROCEDURES AND NORMAL FINDINGS	CLINICAL SIGNIFICANCE AND CLINICAL ALERTS
One variation occurs in people with chronic emphysema, in which the liver is displaced downwards by the hyperinflated lungs. Although you hear a dull percussion note well below the right costal margin, the overall span is still within normal limits. Clinical estimation of liver span is important to screen for hepatomegaly and to monitor changes in liver size. However, this measurement is a gross estimate; the liver span may be underestimated because of inaccurate detection of the upper border and/or the lower border is too high.	
Spleen	
Often the spleen is obscured by stomach contents, but you may locate it by percussing for a dull note from the ninth to 11th intercostal space just behind the left midaxillary line (Figure 23.21). The area of **splenic dullness** is normally not wider than 7 cm in adults and should not encroach on the normal tympany over the gastric air bubble.	A dull note forward of the midaxillary line indicates enlargement of the spleen, as occurs with mononucleosis, trauma and infection.

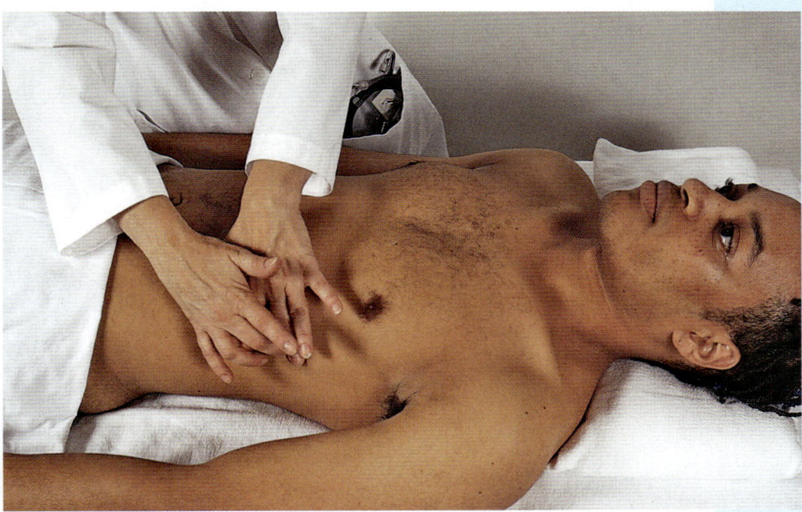

FIGURE 23.21 Percussion of the spleen to determine size

Now percuss in the lowest interspace in the left **anterior axillary line**. Tympany should result. Ask the person to take a deep breath and then percuss. Normally, tympany remains through full inspiration.	At the anterior axillary line, a change in percussion from tympany to a dull sound with full inspiration is a positive spleen percussion sign, indicating splenomegaly. This method will detect mild to moderate splenomegaly before the spleen becomes palpable, as in mononucleosis, malaria or hepatic cirrhosis.

PROCEDURES AND NORMAL FINDINGS	CLINICAL SIGNIFICANCE AND CLINICAL ALERTS
Costovertebral angle tenderness	
Indirect fist percussion causes the tissues to vibrate instead of producing a sound. To assess the kidney, place one hand over the 12th rib at the costovertebral angle on the back (Figure 23.22). Thump that hand with the ulnar edge of your other fist. The person normally feels a thud but no pain. (Although this step is explained here with percussion techniques, its usual sequence in a complete examination is with thoracic assessment, when the person is sitting up and you are standing behind.) 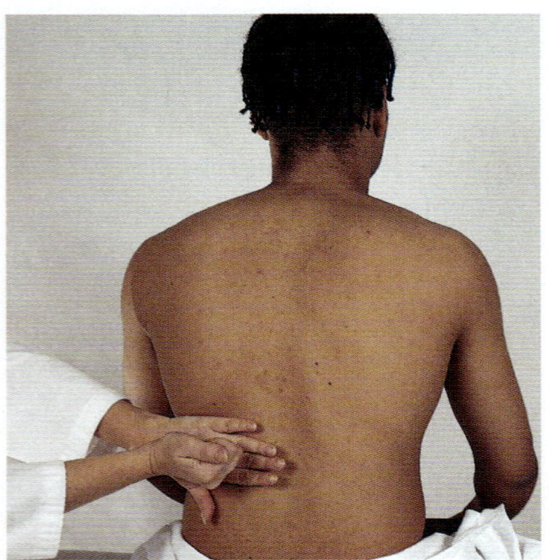 **FIGURE 23.22** Indirect percussion to determine costovertebral tenderness	Sharp pain occurs with inflammation of the kidney or paranephric area.
Palpation of deeper abdominal areas	
Perform palpation to judge the size, location and consistency of certain organs and to screen for an abnormal mass or tenderness. Review comfort measures at beginning of this section. Because most people are naturally inclined to protect the abdomen, use other measures to enhance complete muscle relaxation. Use the techniques described above to perform surface and light palpation.	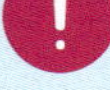 ***Clinical alert:*** If the person experiences any significant abdominal tenderness stop the examination and refer the person to a medical practitioner for further assessment.
Liver	
Next, palpate for specific organs, beginning with the liver in the right upper quadrant (Figure 23.23). Place your left hand under the person's back parallel to the 11th and 12th ribs and lift up to support the abdominal contents. Place your right hand on the right upper quadrant, with fingers parallel to the midline. Push deeply down and under the right costal margin. Ask the person to take a deep breath. It is normal to feel the edge of the liver bump your fingertips as the diaphragm pushes it down during inhalation. It feels like a firm regular ridge. Often, the liver is not palpable and you feel nothing firm.	Except with a depressed diaphragm, a liver palpated more than 1 or 2 cm below the right costal margin is enlarged. Record the number of centimetres it descends and note its consistency (hard, nodular) and tenderness (Table 23.7).

PROCEDURES AND NORMAL FINDINGS	CLINICAL SIGNIFICANCE AND CLINICAL ALERTS

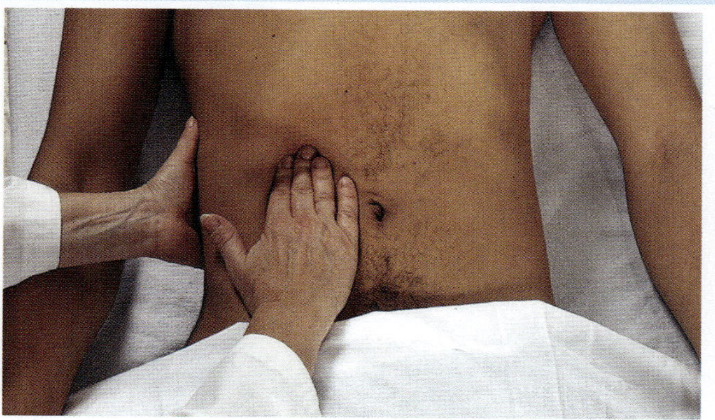

FIGURE 23.23 Palpation of the liver to determine size

Hooking technique. An alternative method of palpating the liver is to stand up at the person's shoulder and swivel your body to the right so that you face the person's feet (Figure 23.24). Hook your fingers over the costal margin from above. Ask the person to take a deep breath. Try to feel the liver edge bump your fingertips.

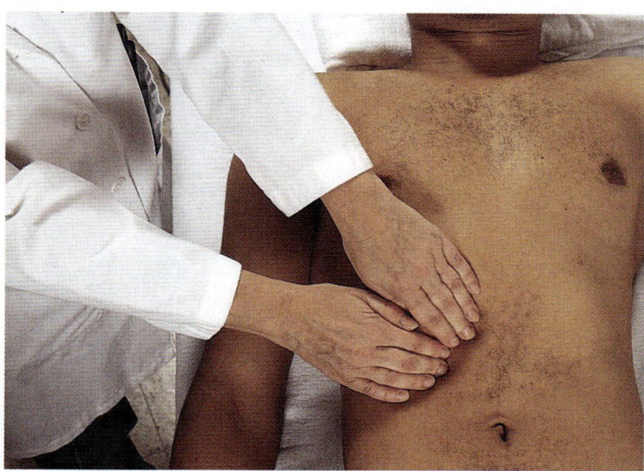

FIGURE 23.24 Palpation of the liver using hooking technique

Spleen

The spleen is not normally palpable and must be enlarged three times its normal size to be felt.

To search for it, reach your left hand over the abdomen and behind the left side at the 11th and 12th ribs (Figure 23.25A). Lift up for support. Place your right hand obliquely on the left upper quadrant with the fingers pointing towards the left axilla and just inferior to the rib margin. Push your hand deeply down and under the left costal margin and ask the person to take a deep breath. You should feel nothing firm.

The spleen enlarges with mononucleosis and trauma (Table 23.7).

! ***Clinical alert:*** If you feel an enlarged spleen refer the person to a medical practitioner; do not proceed with the palpation.

! ***Clinical alert:*** An enlarged spleen is friable and can rupture easily with overpalpation.

Describe the number of centimetres it extends below the left costal margin.

PROCEDURES AND NORMAL FINDINGS	CLINICAL SIGNIFICANCE AND CLINICAL ALERTS

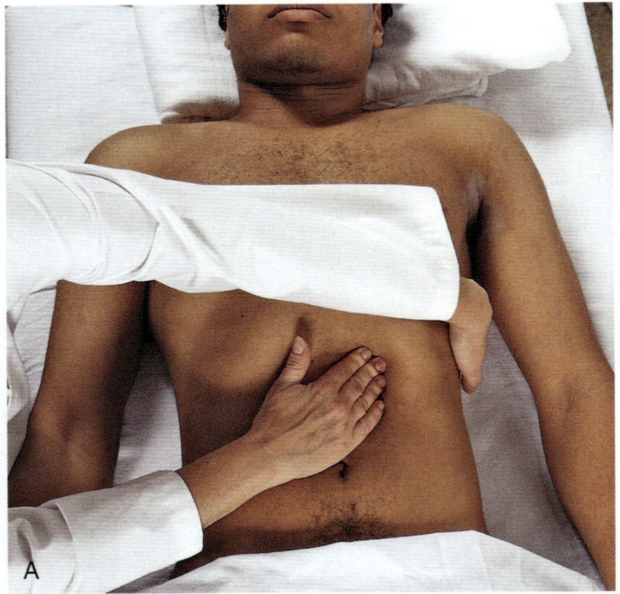

FIGURE 23.25A Palpation of the spleen (if enlarged)

When enlarged, the spleen slides out and bumps your fingertips. It can grow so large that it extends into the lower quadrants. When this condition is suspected, start low so you will not miss it. An alternative position is to roll the person onto their right side to displace the spleen more forwards and downwards (Figure 23.25B). Then palpate as described earlier.

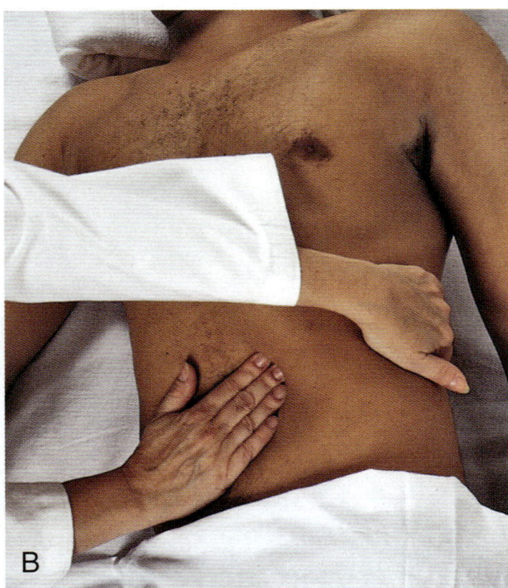

FIGURE 23.25B Palpation of the spleen with person tipped onto their right side

PROCEDURES AND NORMAL FINDINGS	CLINICAL SIGNIFICANCE AND CLINICAL ALERTS
Kidneys	
Search for the right kidney by placing your hands together in a 'duck-bill' position at the person's right flank (Figure 23.26A). Press your two hands together firmly (you need deeper palpation than that used with the liver or spleen) and ask the person to take a deep breath. In most people, you will feel no change. Occasionally, you may feel the lower pole of the right kidney as a round, smooth mass slide between your fingers. Either condition is normal.	Enlarged kidney. Kidney mass.

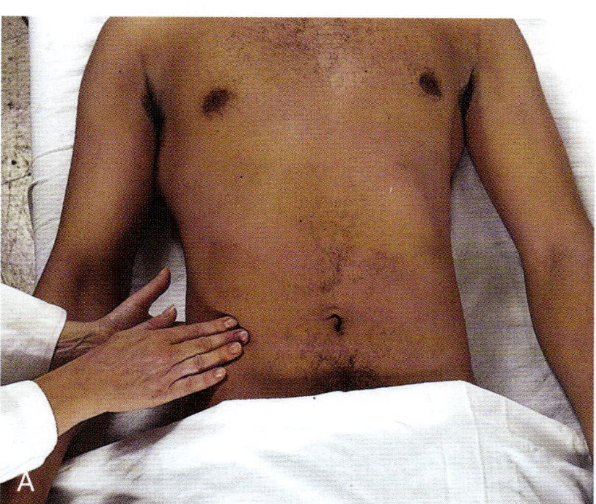

FIGURE 23.26A Duckbill hands palpation of the kidney

The left kidney sits 1 cm higher than the right kidney and is not palpable normally. Search for it by reaching your left hand across the abdomen and behind the left flank for support (Fig. 23.26B). Push your right hand deep into the abdomen and ask the person to breathe deeply. You should feel no change with the inhalation.

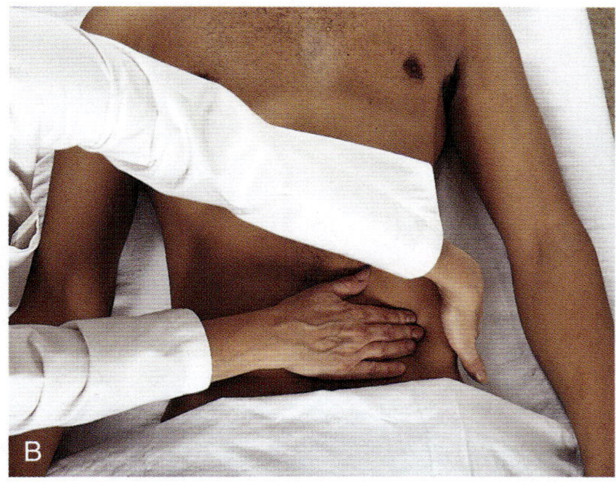

FIGURE 23.26B Bimanual palpation of the kidney

PROCEDURES AND NORMAL FINDINGS	CLINICAL SIGNIFICANCE AND CLINICAL ALERTS

Aorta

Using your opposing thumb and fingers, palpate the aortic pulsation in the upper abdomen slightly to the left of midline (Figure 23.27). Normally, it is 2.5 to 4 cm wide in adults and pulsates in an anterior direction.

Widened with **aneurysm** (Tables 23.6 and 23.7).

Prominent lateral pulsation with aortic aneurysm.

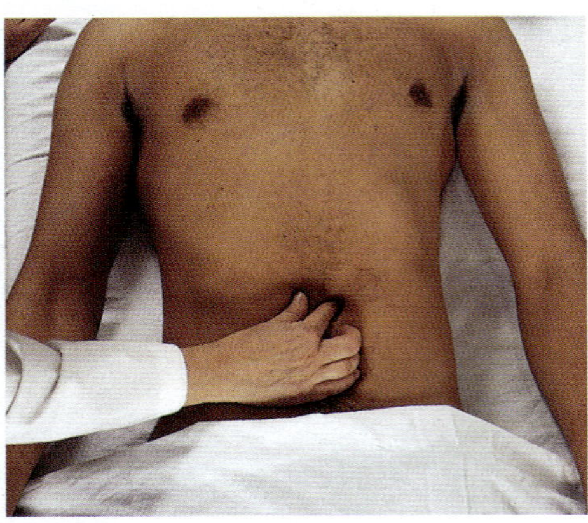

FIGURE 23.27 Palpation of the width of the aortic pulsation

Other deep palpation procedures for advanced practice nurses

Rebound tenderness

Assess rebound tenderness when the person reports abdominal pain or when you elicit tenderness during palpation. Choose a site away from the painful area. Hold your hand at 90 degrees, or perpendicular, to the abdomen. Push down slowly and deeply; then lift your fingers off *quickly* (Figures 23.28A and B). This makes structures that are indented by palpation rebound suddenly. A normal, or negative, response is no pain on release of pressure. Perform this test at the end of the examination because it can cause severe pain and muscle rigidity.

Pain on release of pressure confirms rebound tenderness, which is a reliable sign of peritoneal inflammation. **Peritoneal inflammation** accompanies appendicitis.

Clinical alert: Rebound tenderness in the right lower quadrant when pressure is applied **(Blumberg's sign)** may indicate appendicitis. Refer the person to a medical practitioner for further assessment.

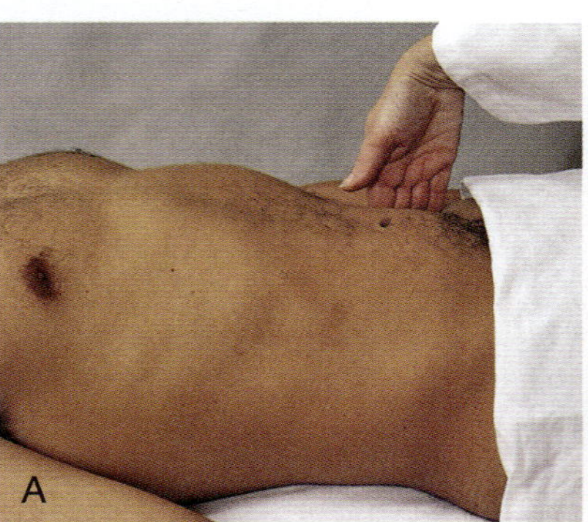

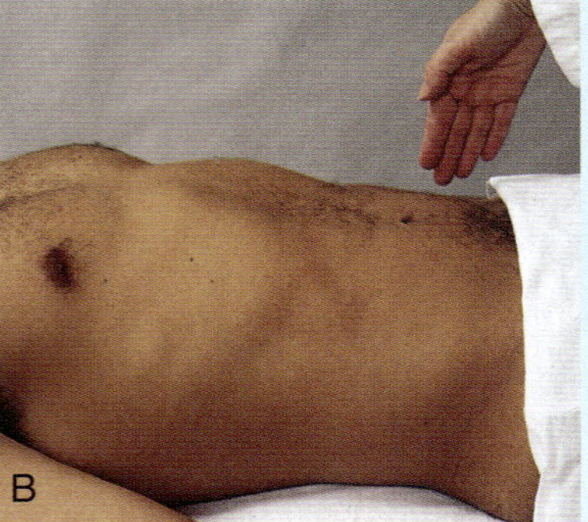

FIGURE 23.28 Rebound tenderness

PROCEDURES AND NORMAL FINDINGS

Murphy's sign
Normally, palpating the liver causes no pain. In a person with inflammation of the gall bladder, or cholecystitis, pain occurs. Hold your fingers under the liver border. Ask the person to take a deep breath. A normal response is to complete the deep breath without pain.

Iliopsoas muscle test
Perform the iliopsoas muscle test when the acute abdominal pain of appendicitis is suspected. With the person supine, lift the right leg straight up, flexing at the hip (Figure 23.29); then push down over the lower part of the right thigh as the person tries to hold the leg up. When the test is negative, the person feels no change.

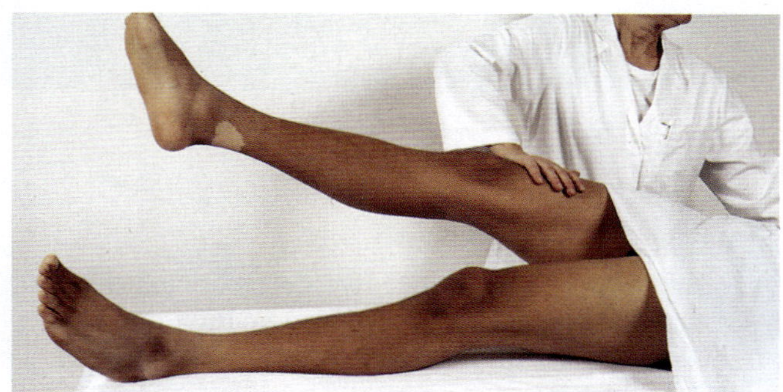

FIGURE 23.29 Iliopsoas muscle test

CLINICAL SIGNIFICANCE AND CLINICAL ALERTS

When the test is positive, as the descending liver pushes the inflamed gall bladder onto the examining hand, the person feels sharp pain and abruptly stops inspiration midway. This sign is less accurate in people older than 60 years—they may not exhibit abdominal tenderness.

When the iliopsoas muscle is inflamed (which occurs with an inflamed or perforated appendix), pain is felt in the right lower quadrant.

Additional objective data for infants

The liver fills the right upper quadrant. It is normal to feel the liver edge at the right costal margin or 1 to 2 cm below. Normally, you may palpate the spleen tip and both kidneys and the bladder. Also easily palpated are the caecum in the right lower quadrant and the sigmoid colon, which feels like a sausage in the left inguinal area.

Make note of the newborn's first stool, a sticky, greenish-black meconium stool within 24 hours of birth. By the fourth day, stools of breast-fed babies are golden-yellow, pasty and smell like sour milk, whereas those of formula-fed babies are brown, yellow, firmer and more faecal smelling.

Additional objective data for children

The liver remains easily palpable 1 to 2 cm below the right costal margin (this is not a sign of hepatomegaly). The edge is soft and sharp and moves easily. On the left, the spleen is also easily palpable with a soft, sharp, movable edge. Usually you can feel 1 to 2 cm of the right kidney and the tip of the left kidney. Percussion of the liver span measures about 3.5 cm at age 2 years, 5 cm at age 6 years and 6 to 7 cm during adolescence.

PROCEDURES AND NORMAL FINDINGS	CLINICAL SIGNIFICANCE AND CLINICAL ALERTS
In assessing abdominal tenderness, remember that young children often answer this question affirmatively no matter how the abdomen feels. Use objective signs to aid assessment, such as a cry changing in pitch as you palpate, facial grimacing, moving away from you and guarding. School-age children have a slim abdominal shape as they lose the potbelly. This slimming trend continues into adolescence. Adolescents may be embarrassed with exposing their abdomen, and adequate draping is necessary. The physical findings are the same as those listed for adults.	 ***Clinical alert:*** If the child experiences any significant abdominal tenderness, stop the examination, and refer the child to a medical practitioner for further assessment.

Abnormal findings for advanced practice

TABLE 23.6 Abdominal friction rubs and vascular sounds

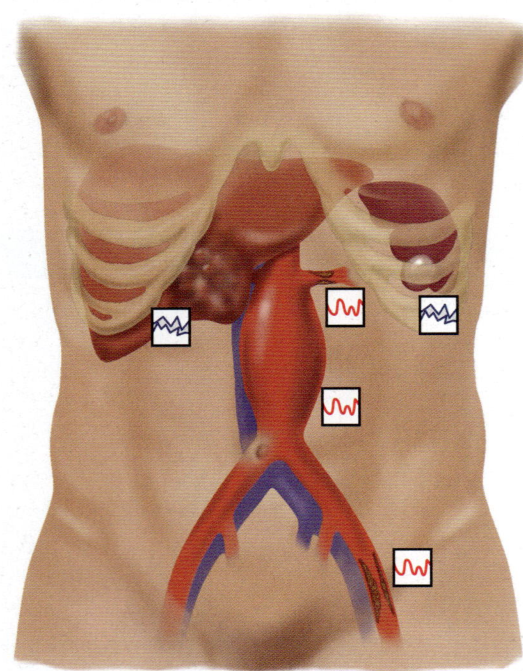

Peritoneal friction rub

A rough, grating sound, like two pieces of leather rubbed together, indicates peritoneal inflammation. Occurs rarely. Usually occurs over organs with a large surface area in contact with the peritoneum.
Liver—friction rub over lower right rib cage, from abscess or metastatic tumour.
Spleen—friction rub over lower left rib cage in left anterior axillary line, from abscess, infection or tumour.

Vascular sounds

Arterial—a **bruit** indicates turbulent blood flow, as found in constricted, abnormally dilated or tortuous vessels. Listen with the bell. Occurs with the following three conditions:
Aortic aneurysm—murmur is harsh, systolic or continuous and accentuated with systole. Note in a person with hypertension.
Renal artery stenosis—murmur is midline or towards flank, soft, low-to-medium pitch.
Partial occlusion of femoral arteries
Venous hum—occurs rarely. Heard in the periumbilical region. Originates from the inferior vena cava. Medium pitch, continuous sound, pressure on bell may obliterate it. May have palpable thrill. Occurs with portal hypertension and cirrhotic liver.

TABLE 23.7 Abnormalities on palpation of enlarged organs

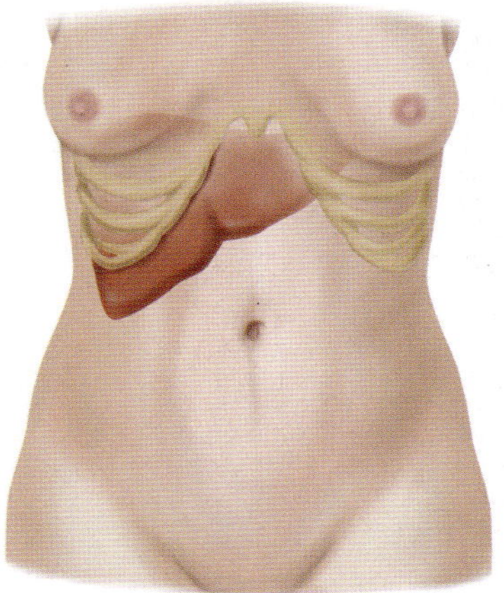

Enlarged liver

An enlarged, smooth and nontender liver occurs with fatty infiltration, portal obstruction or cirrhosis, high obstruction of inferior vena cava and lymphocytic leukaemia.
The liver feels enlarged and smooth but is tender to palpation with early heart failure, acute hepatitis or hepatic abscess.

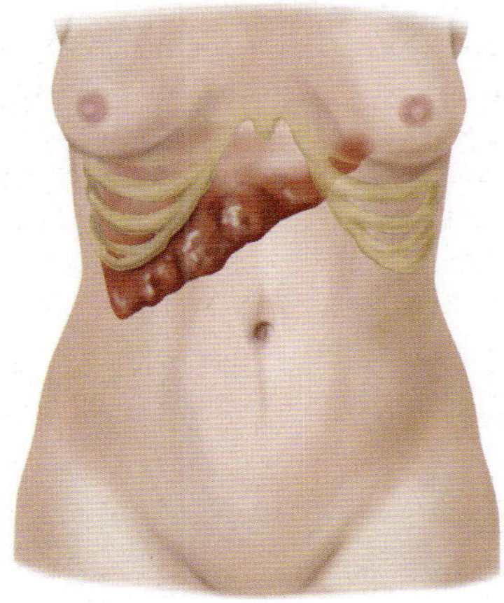

Enlarged nodular liver

An enlarged and nodular liver occurs with late portal cirrhosis, metastatic cancer or tertiary syphilis.

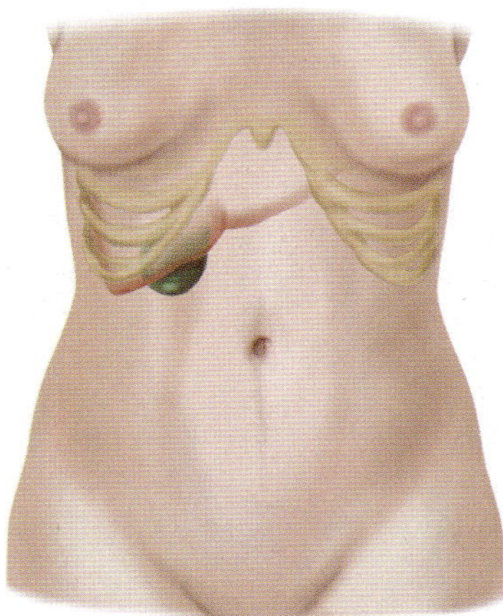

Enlarged gall bladder

An enlarged, tender gall bladder suggests acute cholecystitis. Feel it behind the liver border as a smooth and firm mass like a sausage, although it may be difficult to palpate because of involuntary rigidity of abdominal muscles. The area is exquisitely painful to fist percussion and inspiratory arrest (Murphy's sign) is present.
An enlarged, nontender gall bladder also feels like a smooth, sausage-like mass. It occurs when the gall bladder is filled with stones, as with common bile duct obstruction.

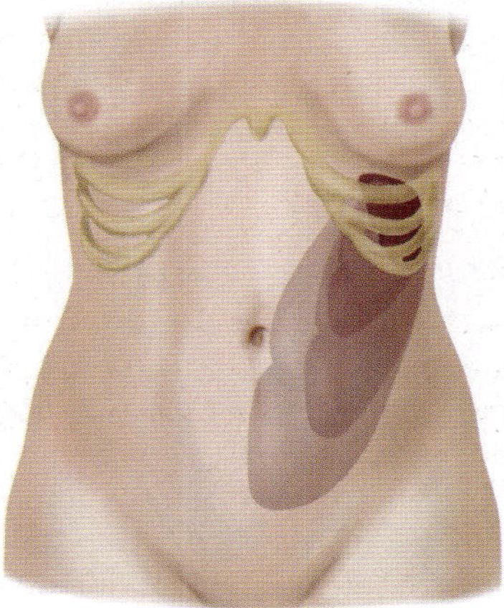

Enlarged kidney

Enlarged with hydronephrosis, cyst or neoplasm. May be difficult to distinguish an enlarged kidney from an enlarged spleen because they have a similar shape. Both extend forwards and down. However, the spleen may have a sharp edge, whereas the kidney never does. The spleen retains the splenic notch, whereas the kidney has no palpable notch. Percussion over the spleen is dull, whereas over the kidney it is tympanitic because of the overriding bowel.

Continued

TABLE 23.7 Abnormalities on palpation of enlarged organs cont'd

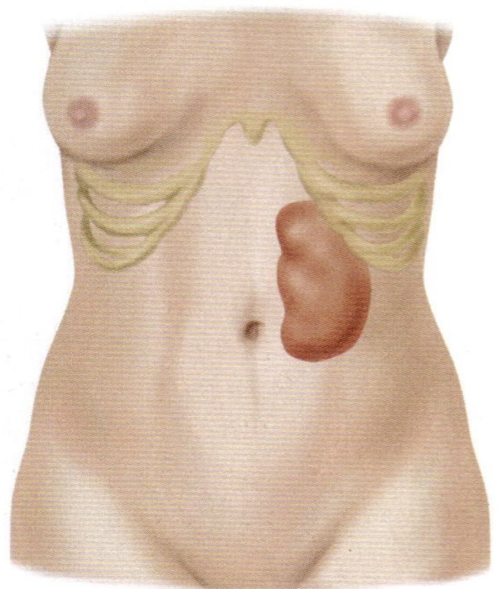

Enlarged spleen

Because any enlargement superiorly is stopped by the diaphragm, the spleen enlarges down and to the midline. When extreme, it can extend down to the left pelvis. It retains the splenic notch on the medial edge. When splenomegaly occurs with acute infections (mononucleosis), it is moderately enlarged and soft, with rounded edges. When the result of a chronic cause, the enlargement is firm or hard, with sharp edges. An enlarged spleen is usually not tender to palpation; it is tender only if the peritoneum is also inflamed.

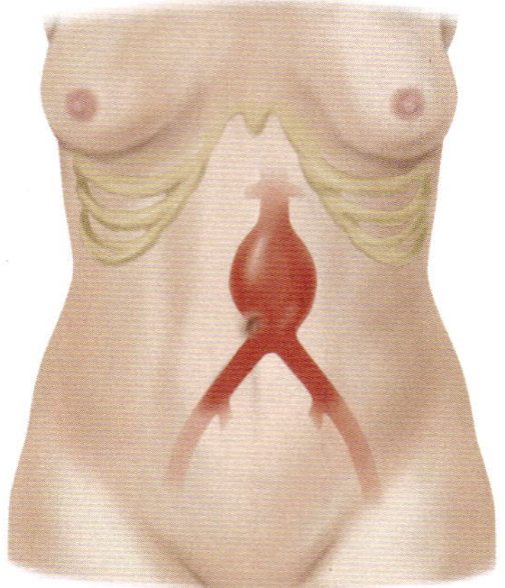

Aortic aneurysm

Most aortic aneurysms (more than 95%) are located below the renal arteries and extend to the umbilicus. About 80% of these are palpable during routine physical examination and feel like a pulsating mass in the upper abdomen just to the left of midline. You will hear a bruit. Femoral pulses are present but decreased.
More information on abdominal aneurysm is provided in Table 23.6.

Clinical reasoning and documentation

The following case studies give examples of typical situations involving abdominal assessment and the clinical reasoning process including problem/issue identification. Consult a fundamentals of nursing or medical-surgical nursing text for information about goal setting, nursing interventions and evaluation.

Case study 1 (continued)—Postoperative nausea and abdominal pain

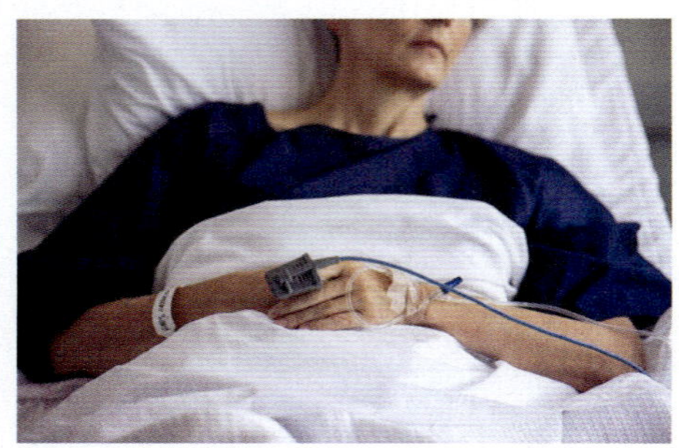

Context

You will recall from the case study described earlier in the chapter that you are on clinical placement in a lower gastrointestinal surgical ward.

Consider the patient's situation

Ms Samantha Wright is a 55-year-old female who had a laparoscopic anterior bowel resection for adenocarcinoma of the bowel 24 hours ago. She progressed normally in the first 24 hours postoperatively. Her pain was well controlled; she was tolerating sips of water and was able to walk to the toilet with minimal assistance.

Collect cues/information

Your further assessment reveals the following information.

Clinical reasoning and documentation cont'd

Subjective data

In the last hour she has complained of abdominal pain and feeling bloated, which had been increasing over several hours. She says she feels nauseated and 'very unwell'. She hasn't been able to drink or eat any breakfast due to nausea. Last drink was at 1:00 am (about 100 mL). Does not feel up to having a shower. She says she has not been passing wind or had any abdominal gurgling.

Objective data

Temp 36.5°C, BP 120/70, HR 94, RR 16

Oral mucous membranes and lips are dry. Peripheral IV remains on 8hrly rate.

Resting in bed, appears pale, and she is taking in deep breaths, which she says reduces her nausea. The abdomen appears rounded and tense (a change from 24 hours ago). No bowel sounds present on auscultation. Laparoscopy wounds are clean and occlusive dressings are intact.

On palpation, abdominal wall is tense. She expresses discomfort on light palpation—no further assessment undertaken until medical consultation.

Process information and identify problems/issues

Collaborative problem

Possible bowel obstruction—nausea, abdominal bloating and lack of bowel sounds post abdominal surgery—requires medical assessment

Problem statements/nursing diagnoses

Nausea related to possible acute bowel obstruction

Abdominal pain related to possible bowel obstruction

Potential for anxiety related to change in health state and need for further assessment

Case study 2—Acute abdominal pain

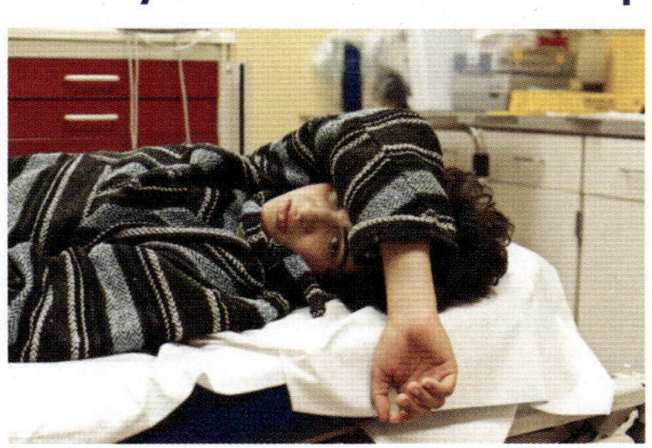

Context

You are a registered nurse working in triage in an emergency department. An initial assessment is conducted to assess the urgency of the person's need for medical care.

Consider the patient's situation

Dan Groves is a 17-year-old male high school student who presents at the emergency department with abdominal pain. He is accompanied by his parents (Jo and Peter).

Collect cues/information

Subjective data

Two days ago, Dan noted general abdominal pain in the umbilical region. Now the pain is sharp and severe, and Dan points to a location in the right lower quadrant. His pain score is 9/10 at rest. No bowel movement for 2 days. Nausea and vomiting off and on for 1 day. He says that no one else in his household has these symptoms and that he has only eaten home-prepared meals in the past few days.

Objective data

Temp 38°C, BP 112/70, HR 116, RR 18

Lying on side, with knees drawn up under chin. Resists any movement. Face tight and occasionally grimacing. Cries out with any sudden movement.

No bowel sounds present on auscultation.

On palpation, abdominal wall is rigid and board-like. Extreme tenderness to light palpation in the right lower quadrant—no further assessment undertaken until medical consultation.

Process information and identify problems/issues

Collaborative problem

Acute abdominal pain in the right lower quadrant (? appendicitis)—requires urgent medical assessment

Problem statements/nursing diagnoses

Nausea related to possible acute appendicitis

Abdominal pain related to possible acute appendicitis

Potential for anxiety related to uncertain diagnosis and need for further assessment

ADDITIONAL RESOURCES

You can further develop your knowledge and skills relevant to abdominal assessment, related pathophysiology, common health issues and nursing interventions by:

- reading chapters of a fundamentals of nursing or medical-surgical textbook.
- Answering chapter multiple choice questions online. Log into ClinicalKey Student and search for the text 'Health Assessment, 4th edition. Choose the section titled 'Teaching material'. In this section you will find question and answer documents for each chapter. Please check instructions on the inside front cover of the book to access online resources
- visiting websites:

  Radiology masterclass—Abdominal x-ray: https://www.radiologymasterclass.co.uk/tutorials/abdo/abdomen_x-ray/anatomy_introduction.

REFERENCES

1. Sun H, Warren J, Yip J, Ji Y, Hao S, Han W, et al. Factors influencing gallstone formation: a review of the literature. Biomolecules. 2022 Apr 6;12(4):550.
2. Drenth-van Maanen AC, Wilting I, Jansen PA. Prescribing medicines to older people: how to consider the impact of ageing on human organ and body functions. British Journal of Clinical Pharmacology. 2020 Oct;86(10):1921–1930.
3. Knights K, Darroch S, Rowland A, Bushell M. Pharmacology for health professionals. 6th ed. Chatswood, NSW: Elsevier; 2022.
4. Marieb EM, Keller SM. Essentials of human anatomy & physiology. 13th Global ed. UK: Pearson; 2022.
5. Werth BL, Christopher SA. Potential risk factors for constipation in the community. World Journal of Gastroenterology. 2021 Jun 6;27(21):2795.
6. Pouwels S, Sakran N, Graham Y, Leal A, Pintar T, Yang W, et al. Non-alcoholic fatty liver disease (NAFLD): a review of pathophysiology, clinical management and effects of weight loss. BMC Endocrine Disorders. 2022 Dec;22(1):1–9.
7. National Health and Medical Research Council: Australian guidelines to reduce health risks from drinking alcohol. Canberra: Commonwealth of Australia; 2020. Available at: https://www.nhmrc.gov.au/about-us/publications/australian-guidelines-reduce-health-risks-drinking-alcohol
8. Li X, Tang J, Mao Y. Incidence and risk factors of drug-induced liver injury. Liver International. 2022 Aug;42(9):1999–2014.
9. Fathelrahman A. Ten challenges associated with management of paracetamol overdose: an update on current practice and relevant evidence from epidemiological and clinical studies. Journal of Clinical and Diagnostic Research. 2021 Mar 1;15:FE01–FE06.
10. Nash E, Sabih AH, Chetwood J, Wood G, Pandya K, Yip T, et al. Drug-induced liver injury in Australia, 2009–2020: the increasing proportion of non-paracetamol cases linked with herbal and dietary supplements. Medical Journal of Australia. 2021 Sep 20;215(6):261–268.
11. World Health Organization (WHO). Hepatitis. 2023. Available at https://www.who.int/health-topics/hepatitis#tab=tab_1
12. Li A, Zheng J, Han X, Jiang Z, Yang B, Yang S, et al. Health implication of lactose intolerance and updates on its dietary management. International Dairy Journal. 2023 Feb 3:105608.
13. Monash University, The low FODMAP diet, 2023. Available at: https://www.monashfodmap.com/
14. Dunlap JJ, Patterson S. Assessing abdominal pain. Gastroenterology Nursing. 2020 May 1;43(3):267–270.
15. Aumpan N, Mahachai V, Vilaichone RK. Management of *Helicobacter pylori* infection. JGH Open. 2023 Jan;7(1):3–15.
16. Talley NJ, O'Connor S. Clinical examination: a systematic guide to physical diagnosis. 9th ed. Chatswood: Elsevier; 2021.

CHAPTER 24

Assessing urinary function

Written by Carolyn Jarvis
Adapted by Elizabeth Watt

INTRODUCTION

Assessment of urinary tract function is a frequent assessment area for nurses in a variety of healthcare settings. However, many people with urinary problems, in particular urinary incontinence, will be reluctant to discuss their specific problem, so you need to approach this assessment with tact and empathy.

Structures relevant to assessment of urinary tract function include the kidneys, ureters, bladder and urethra. The upper urinary tract consists of the kidneys and ureters. The lower urinary tract consists of the bladder and urethra. The male prostate gland, while not related to the urinary tract in terms of urine production, drainage of urine, storage and elimination of urine (voiding), is an important structure to consider in this chapter as any enlargement of the prostate can lead to obstructed urine flow through the urethra. The structure and function of the prostate gland is described in Chapter 27. Likewise, the pelvic floor muscles play an important role in the maintenance of continence (Chapter 26).

Case study

The following case study gives an example of a typical situation involving assessment of urinary function and the initial clinical reasoning process. It will help you to identify your learning needs.

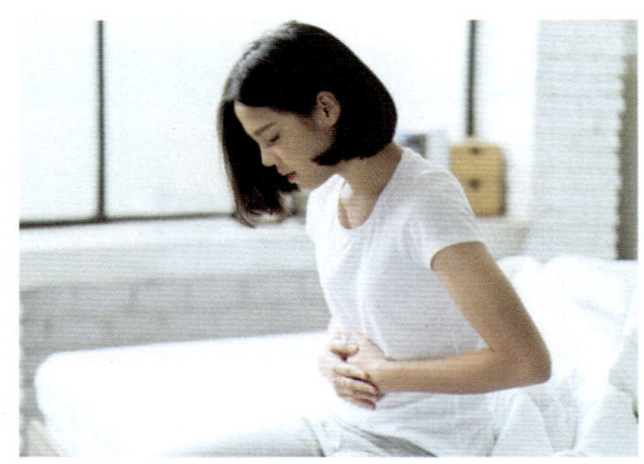

Context

You are a registered nurse working as a practice nurse in a busy community multidisciplinary health clinic. The role includes screening assessments for people who have not attended the clinic previously.

Consider the patient's situation

Ms Chee Wan Ching is a 26-year-old woman attending the clinic following sudden onset today of dysuria, urinary frequency and urgency.

Questions to further your learning

- What are the possible things that might be going on with Ms Chee?
- What knowledge do you need to be able to predict what might be going on?
- What approach to Ms Chee's health assessment will you take?
- What questions (subjective data) will you ask Ms Chee to extend the health history and why?
- What physical examination (objective data) will you conduct and why?
- What resources are available to assist in your assessment of Ms Chee?

Assessment plan

The extent of the questioning and examination will depend on the person's main health concern. You need to keep in mind the intimate and private nature of many aspects of this assessment; therefore, it is important to ensure the privacy and comfort of the environment and be mindful of the need for some people to have a health professional of the same gender performing the assessment. You also need to keep in mind that bladder problems often coincide with bowel problems, especially constipation and, in men, erectile dysfunction, so you may need to assess these areas as well (Chapters 23, 25 and 27). There are common terms that the general public uses to describe urine and the process of voiding—for example, 'wee' and 'pee' and 'having a leak'. While the correct terms are used in the assessment guidelines below, you may need to adjust your language when you are collecting the subjective information.

There are also many assessment tools available to help collect subjective data, specifically for the presence and severity of urinary symptoms, including incontinence, and the impact of these symptoms on the quality of life. These validated assessment tools are used in clinical practice and research.[1] For example:

- assessment of incontinence and lower urinary tract symptoms in men (ICIQ—MLUTS Male lower urinary tract symptoms questionnaire)
- assessment of incontinence and lower urinary tract symptoms in women (ICIQ—FLUTS Female lower urinary tract symptoms questionnaire)
- assessment of lower urinary tract symptoms in men (I-PSS—International Prostate Symptom Score)
- impact of lower urinary tract symptoms on quality of life (ICIQ—LUTSqol).

Through the process of questioning the person or family you may become aware of gaps in the person's knowledge about living a healthy lifestyle. The opportunity to provide health information is an important part of health assessment. The main areas for subjective assessment are:

- presenting concern
- usual urinary pattern
- fluid intake (type and amount)
- pain
- lower urinary tract symptoms
- other symptoms (including fever, weight gain/loss, fatigue)
- past history (including obstetric history)
- health and lifestyle management
- environmental issues related to bladder function.

Objective data collection focuses on further explanation related to the person's symptoms that have been revealed in the history taking. Some of the areas for objective assessment required for assessing urinary tract function are described in other chapters and will only be mentioned briefly in this chapter. Other relevant areas for assessment could include bowel function (Chapters 23 and 25), nutrition (Chapter 21), mobility (Chapter 20) and neurological function (Chapter 12). The main areas for objective assessment are:

- general inspection
- vital signs
- abdominal examination
- inspection of genitalia
- post-void residual urine volume
- examination of urine
- fluid balance chart or voiding diary.

Resources available

You will find additional resources and the reference list at the end of this chapter.

Structure and function

The urinary system has several important functions including the regulation of blood volume and composition; assisting in the regulation of blood pressure; production of hormones (calcitriol and erythropoietin); regulation of blood glucose levels; excretion of wastes in the urine; passing urine from the kidney to the bladder via the ureters; storage of urine in the bladder; emptying the stored urine from the bladder via the urethra.[2]

Kidneys

The bean-shaped **kidneys** are retroperitoneal, or posterior, to the abdominal contents (Figure 24.1). They are well protected by the posterior ribs and musculature. The 12th rib forms an angle with the vertebral column, the **costovertebral angle** (Figure 24.2). The left kidney lies here at the 11th and 12th ribs. An average-sized adult kidney is 10 to 12 cm long and 5 to 7 cm wide and weighs 130 to 150 g.[2] Each kidney is covered by three layers of tissue: the renal capsule, adipose capsule and renal fascia, which all help to maintain the position of the kidney and protect it from trauma. Near the centre of each kidney is a narrowing (the renal hilum) through which the ureter, renal artery and renal vein, lymphatic vessels and nerves enter and exit. A longitudinal section through the kidney (Figure 24.3) reveals two distinct regions; the outer layer (renal cortex) and the inner layer (the medulla). The medulla consists of several pyramid-shaped structures (the renal pyramids) that narrow, forming the renal papillae. The renal cortex contains the functional unit of the kidney, the nephron. There are more than 1 million nephrons in each healthy kidney. Each

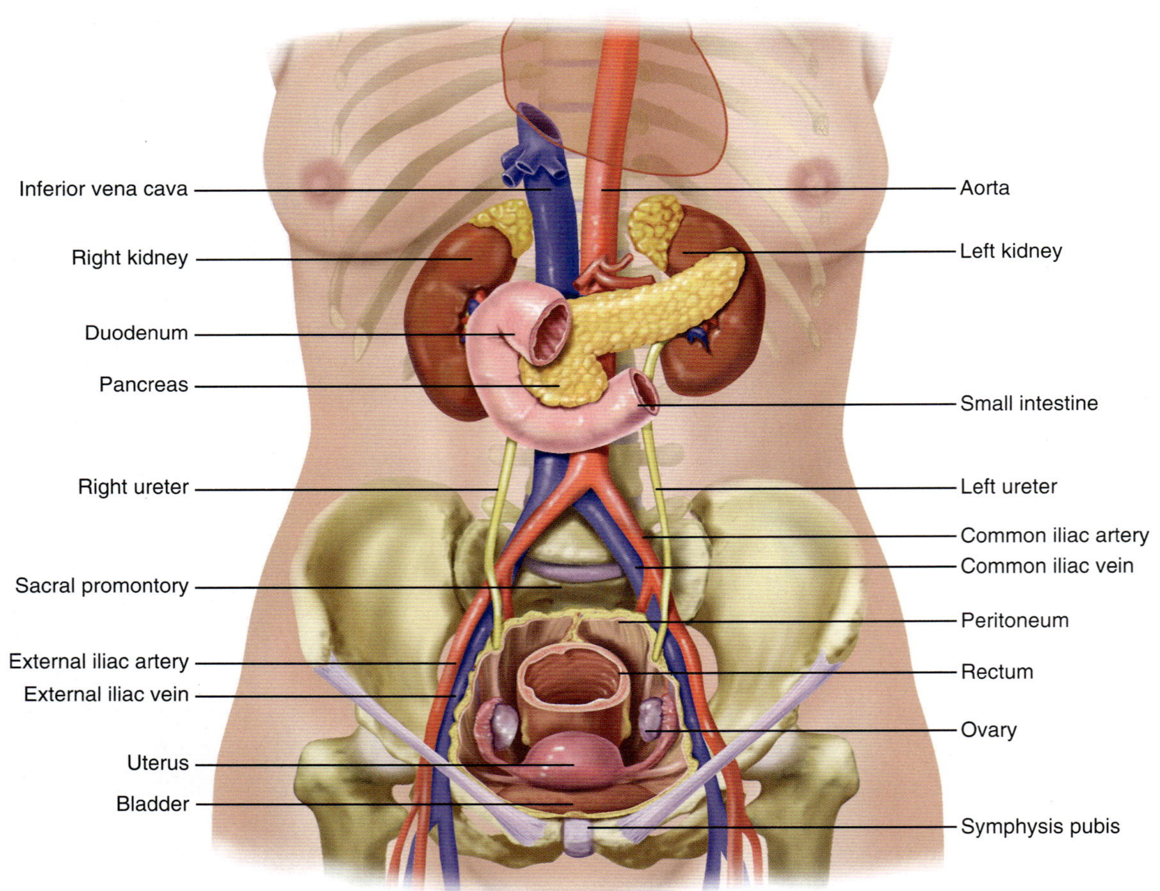

FIGURE 24.1 Location of major blood vessels and organs

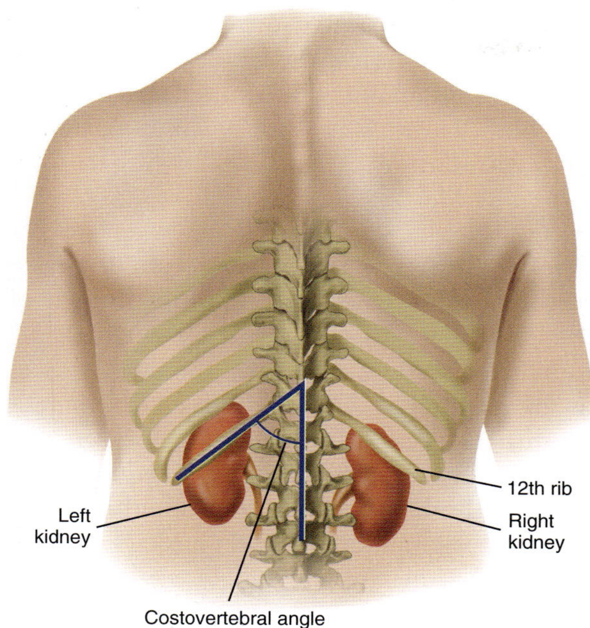

FIGURE 24.2 Location of kidneys—posterior view

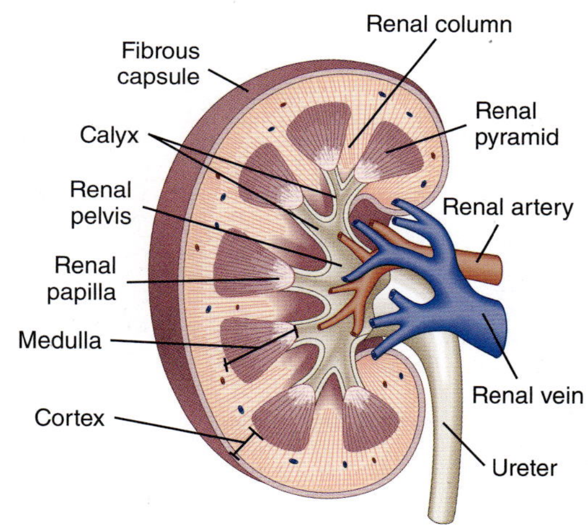

FIGURE 24.3 Structures of the kidney

nephron is a complex system comprising a glomerulus, Bowman's capsule and tubular system (proximal convoluted tubule, the loop of Henle and the distal convoluted tubule). Several nephrons merge into a collecting duct that empties via the papillae to the minor calyx, the renal pelvis, eventually draining into the ureters. The two kidneys receive 25% of the resting cardiac output into the renal arteries. In adults, renal blood flow is about 1,200 mL per minute. The amount of filtrate formed in the renal corpuscle (a Bowman's capsule and a glomerulus) of both kidneys each minute is known as the glomerular filtration rate. The urine output does depend on intake of fluids, but the normal adult output of urine is 1,500 to 1,600 mL every 24 hours.

Ureters

The two ureters extend in a continuous tube from the renal pelvis (pelvoureteric junction) to the trigone of the bladder (vesicoureteric junction) and carry urine from the kidney. Peristaltic contractions of the muscle walls of the ureters help move urine down each ureter into the bladder. Each ureter is 25 to 30 cm long and has a diameter of 3 to 4 mm.[3] Three layers of muscle form the ureters (the mucosa, the lamina propria and the muscularis). The inner layer (the mucosa) is composed of transitional epithelium which can stretch to accommodate a varying volume of fluid. The distal end of the ureter enters the bladder on an angle at the vesicoureteric junction. The muscle of bladder and ureter in combination with the angle of entry of the ureter into the bladder acts as a valve-like mechanism to prevent reflux of urine back up into the ureter from the bladder during micturition.

Bladder

The urinary bladder is a hollow, distensible, muscular organ designed to store and expel urine. It lies in the pelvic cavity posterior to the symphysis pubis. In men, the bladder lies directly anterior to the rectum, and in women it is anterior to the vagina and inferior to the uterus.[2] The size and shape of the bladder changes to comply with the amount of urine it contains. At the base of the bladder there is a triangular area called the trigone. The two upper corners of the trigone contain the two ureteral openings and the lower corner is where the urethral orifice is located.

The bladder is constructed of four layers of tissue. The inner surface of the bladder is lined with transitional cell epithelium that prevents reabsorption of urine. The muscle of the bladder consists of three layers of smooth muscle (the detrusor muscle). The outermost layer (the adventitia) is composed of fibroelastic connective tissue. The serosa, a layer of the visceral peritoneum, lies over the superior surface of the bladder. Parasympathetic nerve fibres stimulate the detrusor muscle during urination. In males, the bladder neck forms the internal urinary sphincter. In females, the bladder neck is a far weaker structure than in men.[3]

Urethra

The urethra is a small tube from the base of the bladder (bladder neck) to the outside of the body. In women, the urethra is 3.5 to 5.5 cm in length and leaves the bladder neck at an angle. The entire length of the female urethra acts as a sphincter mechanism and contributes to continence during bladder filling. The urethral orifice lies between the clitoris and the vaginal opening (Figure 24.4). The relative shortness of the female urethra and its

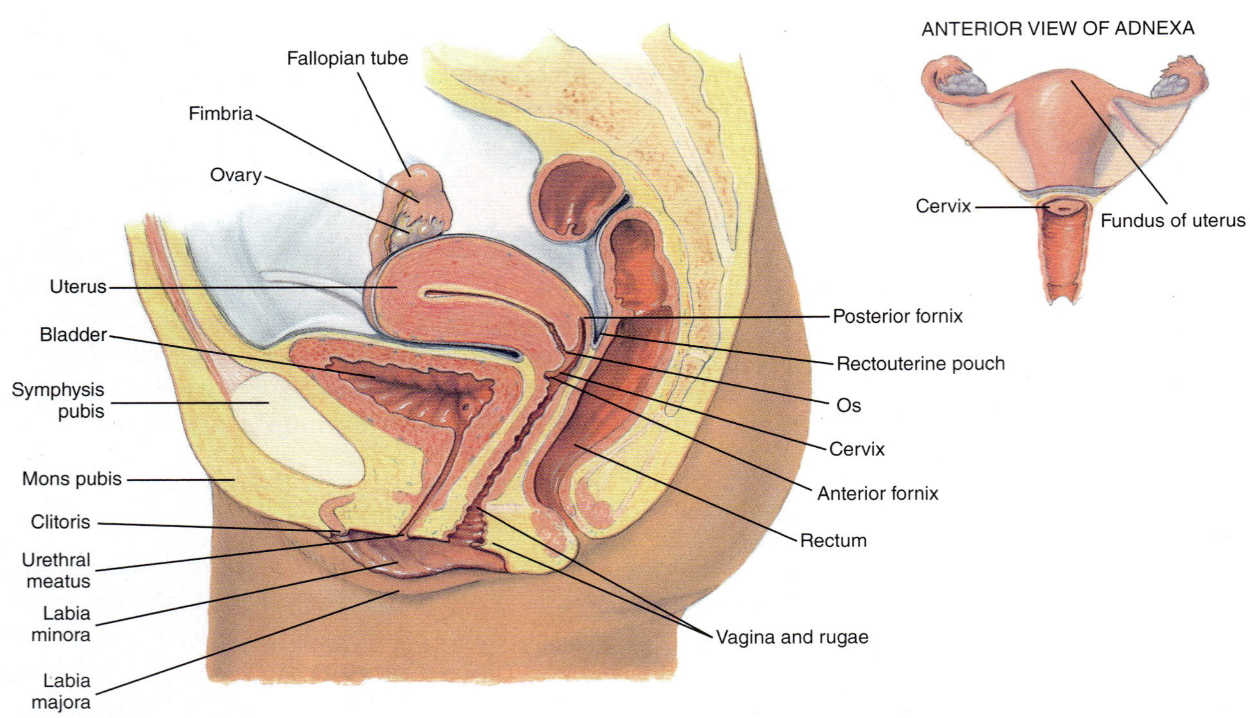

FIGURE 24.4 Female pelvic organs

position close to the vagina and anus predisposes women to urinary tract infection from ascending movement of bacteria up the urethra into the bladder. In females, the urinary meatus is located between the labia minora, anterior to the vagina and posterior to the clitoris.

In males, the urethra is 18 to 23 cm long and is divided into three sections: the prostatic urethra, the membranous urethra and the spongy (or penile) urethra[4] (Figure 24.5). The prostatic urethra originates at the bladder neck and travels through the prostate gland. The membranous urethra passes through the deep muscle of the perineum. These two sections form the sphincter mechanism in males. The spongy urethra consists of four parts: the bulbous urethra, pendulous urethra, fossa navicularis and the meatus. The male urethra transverses the corpus spongiosum and its meatus forms a slit at the glans tip. The urethra consists of a mucosa and muscularis with circular smooth muscle fibres continuous with the wall of the bladder.

Prostate gland

In men, the **prostate gland** lies in front of the anterior wall of the rectum and 2 cm behind the symphysis pubis. It surrounds the bladder neck and the urethra and secretes a milky, slightly acidic fluid which contributes to sperm motility, viability and volume of semen[5] (see also Chapter 27).

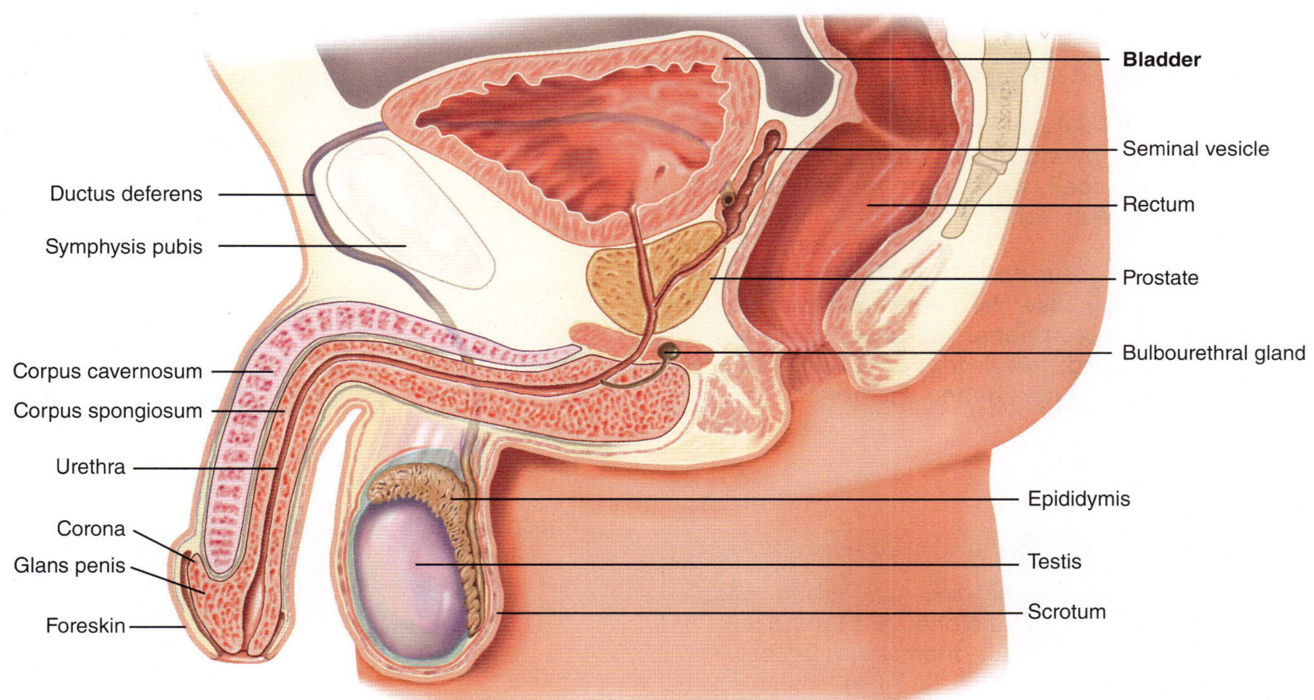

FIGURE 24.5 Male pelvic organs

Developmental considerations

Infants and children

At birth, the kidneys occupy a large portion of the abdominal cavity. Urine formation occurs at the third month of fetal development and contributes to the volume of amniotic fluid. At birth, the bladder is in the abdomen and, as the child grows, it becomes a pelvic structure. In infants and children, micturition is an involuntary act occurring about 20 times per day. As children develop, the frequency of voiding decreases and mean voiding volume increases. At 2 or 3 years of age children become aware of bladder filling and begin to inhibit voiding by contracting the pelvic floor muscles. As the central nervous system develops, children learn to inhibit the detrusor muscle activity, which enables them to achieve continence.

Adults and late adulthood (65+ years)

Kidney and bladder function change as people age. The kidneys decrease in size and weight, as does the glomerular filtration rate. Under normal circumstances, these changes do not cause any problems with maintaining homeostasis. However, the decrease in function puts older people more at risk for health problems with rapid changes to blood volume or other insults.

Physiological changes related to ageing occur in the bladder and urethra. For example, changes to the female bladder, urethra, vagina and pelvic floor due to decreasing estrogen following menopause can cause these structures to become less vascular, thinner and less elastic.

The muscles that surround the urethra and support the bladder can lose strength, causing changes to the anatomical positioning of these structures. As people age, they may experience increasing episodes of nocturia (the need to urinate at night). The bladder reduces in muscle tone and capacity to hold urine, which can result in increased urinary frequency.

In most men, the prostate gland gradually enlarges as they age. This enlargement is termed benign prostatic hypertrophy. It does not raise a man's risk for prostate cancer, but benign enlargement of the prostate can cause significant and bothersome lower urinary tract symptoms including urinary urgency, frequency, poor stream, hesitancy, post-micturition dribble and acute or chronic urinary retention, which can impact significantly on a man's quality of life. Treatment can include ongoing monitoring of symptoms, medications and surgical interventions.[6]

Cultural and social considerations

Chronic kidney disease is a major health problem in the Australian and Aotearoa New Zealand community, causing a significant and ongoing health burden on the person, their family and the healthcare system. Diseases that cause irreversible damage to the glomerulus or tubules result in permanent alterations in renal function. Chronic kidney disease (CKD) or end-stage kidney disease (ESKD) are the terms used to describe the resulting decline in kidney function from these processes. CKD is damage to the kidneys or reduced renal function lasting more than 3 months.[7]

It is estimated that 11% of Australians over the age of 18 years have biomedical signs of CKD, and most are over 65 years of age.[8] Aboriginal and Torres Strait Islander people, especially those living in remote communities, have about twice the risk of developing CKD than non-Indigenous Australians.[8] The incidence of CKD in the overall Aotearoa New Zealand population has not been estimated, but a study in Auckland found the overall prevalence to be 13%, with a higher incidence in Pacific Islanders (particularly Samoans) and Māori.[9]

A major risk factor for CKD is diabetes mellitus. Other risk factors include hypertension, having existing heart failure or history of myocardial infarction or stroke, family history of CKD, obesity, having smoked or being a current smoker, being over 60 years of age and having a history of acute kidney injury.[10]

Urinary incontinence is another health problem that causes significant effects on the person's health and wellbeing. Urinary incontinence is defined as the complaint of any involuntary loss of urine.[11] Urinary incontinence is not considered a normal part of ageing. Its causes are multifactorial and include pregnancy, childbirth, obesity, chronic constipation, change in cognitive state and problems with mobility and dexterity.[12]

Around one in four Australians over the age of 15 years experience bladder or bowel control problems. Most (80%) are women.[13] In Aotearoa New Zealand, 25 to 34% of adult women and 5 to 22% of adult men have experienced urinary incontinence.[14]

Urinary incontinence can significantly affect the person's perception of their general health, their daily activities, sexuality, social function, mental health and vitality.[15,16] To try to reduce symptoms, people may reduce their fluid intake, increase the frequency of voiding and avoiding social contact.[17] Many people who experience bladder symptoms or incontinence are reluctant to seek help because of embarrassment; therefore, it is important to include continence-related questions in any assessment of urinary tract function.

HEALTH EDUCATION

Promoting healthy bladder habits

People need information about normal bladder and bowel functioning and the typical risk factors for continence problems. Healthy bowel and bladder habits form an important part of a healthy lifestyle.

Nurse's role

The Continence Foundation of Australia[18] recommends five important steps aimed at promoting good bowel and bladder habits that should form part of your health education for all people. These include the following:

- **Practising good toilet habits.** It is normal for people to void between four and eight times per day and no more than once at night. Good toileting habits include not going to the toilet 'just in case' as this may result in a smaller functional bladder capacity over time. People should be encouraged to relax when voiding to empty the bladder fully and to go to the toilet only when their bladder is full and they have the need to void (except before going to bed at night, which most people do routinely).
- **Looking after the pelvic floor muscles.** Most people should be doing regular pelvic floor exercises as part of their general fitness program. For pregnant women pelvic floor exercises help the body

HEALTH EDUCATION cont't

to cope with the increasing weight of the baby and aid in recovery after birth. A health education program should include information about the location of the pelvic floor muscles, which muscles need to be contracted, the pattern of contractions and how often they need to be contracted.

- **Maintaining good bowel habits.** Avoid constipation because this can put pressure on the bladder and the pelvic floor, weakening these muscles. It is also important to encourage people to eat a healthy diet that is high in fibre with plenty of fresh fruit and vegetables and with only small amounts of highly processed foods. It is also important to keep active because this will reduce the risk of constipation.
- **Drinking plenty of fluids.** Aim for 1 to 1.5 litres of fluid per day, mostly water. This will need to be adjusted according to the level of activity and the ambient temperature. People should drink enough fluid to keep the urine a pale yellow colour and to limit their intake of caffeine (including cola and sports drinks) and alcohol—these are irritants to the bladder.
- **Seeking help when symptoms persist.** Our role is to provide information for people so they can make informed choices about the health care that will best suit their needs. This means we must be informed about the services that are available. The Continence Foundation of Australia or Continence New Zealand is a good place to refer people for information about bladder, bowel and pelvic floor health and local continence services:
  - **Continence Foundation of Australia:** https://www.continence.org.au
  - **Continence New Zealand**: https://www.continence.org.nz

Subjective data

Practice note

Before you start the assessment, introduce yourself to the person, confirm the person's identity, discuss the purpose and scope of the assessment, clarify any questions the person may have and obtain verbal consent from the person to perform the assessment.

ASSESSMENT GUIDELINES	CLINICAL SIGNIFICANCE AND CLINICAL ALERTS
Presenting concern	
• *Are you experiencing any problems with your bladder (e.g. passing urine or being able to control the flow of urine) that you are worried about>?* It is important to ascertain the person's perception of their urinary tract function. If they do perceive a problem, ask: *How does this affect your quality of life?*	

ASSESSMENT GUIDELINES	CLINICAL SIGNIFICANCE AND CLINICAL ALERTS
Usual urinary pattern	
• *How often do you empty your bladder (pass urine) during the day?* • *How often do you get up to empty your bladder overnight?* • *Have you noticed any changes in your usual voiding patterns? Can you describe this change for me?* • *How long has this been happening?* • *What have you been doing about this?* There will be detailed questions in the following sections that will help you detail the signs/symptoms the person may be experiencing.	There is a usual pattern to voiding over a 24-hour period, although there is variation between people. It is normal for an adult to void 3- to 5-hourly during the daytime and not need to void overnight. The adult bladder capacity is normally about 500 mL.[3] **Oliguria**—diminished quantity, < 400 mL/24 hours. **Polyuria**—excessive quantity. **Anuria**—no urine production. This should not be confused with **urinary retention**, where urine is formed in the kidney and stored in the bladder but the person is unable to void or unable to completely empty their bladder.
Characteristics of the urine	
• *What colour is your urine?* • *Does it have an unpleasant odour? (If so, describe.) Is the urine clear, cloudy or blood-stained? Does it contain mucus?*	Urine should normally be clear, light-yellow coloured and have a non-offensive odour. **Cloudy**—urinary tract infection (or significant protein in the urine). **Haematuria**—blood in the urine, which can be **microscopic** or **macroscopic**. May indicate urinary tract infection, bladder or renal cancer, urinary calculi and chronic inflammation of the bladder. ! ***Clinical alert:*** When there is blood in urine, or a colour change lasting more than a day, the person should seek medical advice. Some colour changes are temporary or harmless. They can be the result of some medications, foods, **vitamin supplements** and dyes. These can include blue-, orange- and tea-coloured urine.

ASSESSMENT GUIDELINES	CLINICAL SIGNIFICANCE AND CLINICAL ALERTS
Assessment of '**fluid balance**' is often conducted for hospitalised patients using a fluid balance chart to record intake and output over a 24-hour period. It is often difficult for people to accurately estimate the amount of fluid they consume in a day. In community and primary care settings, accurate assessment of fluid intake and output is also important for those people with renal and urinary tract health problems, and others—for example, with heart failure. The person (or their carer) should be asked to keep a written record usually over three 24-hour periods. See further information in the voiding diary section below.	It is important to ascertain the types of fluids consumed over the day and night because some types of fluids are known to irritate the bladder in certain people such as caffeine-containing fluids such as coffee and cola drinks. Alcohol is a diuretic and can cause exacerbation of urinary symptoms, especially frequency and urgency.
Pain	
Review pain assessment strategies and tools from Chapter 13. Use a pain assessment tool as appropriate to the person's age, context and capacity to communicate. In general, ask the person to describe the following: **Character** • *How would you describe the pain you are experiencing: dull, stabbing, aching, burning?* **Onset:** Duration, variation • *How did it start? How long have you had it?* **Location** • *Where is the pain? Please point to it* (you could use a body diagram to report these findings). • *Is the pain in one spot or does it move around?* **Duration** • *Is the pain constant or does it come and go? Does it peak?* (for example, when urinating, after urinating) **Severity** • *How intense is the pain—rate from 1 to 10.* **Pattern** • *What makes the pain worse: voiding or having bowels opened, sexual intercourse?* **Associated factors** • *Is the pain associated with any other symptoms*? Possibilities include menstrual period or irregularities, stress, fatigue, nausea and vomiting, frequent urination (see also the next point, lower urinary tract symptoms, below), vaginal or penile discharge. • *What have you tried to relieve pain: rest, heating pad, fluids, medication?*	There are several sites for pain associated with upper and/or lower urinary tract dysfunction. Keep in mind that pain may be referred from another organ or site and may be associated with general symptoms such as fever or nausea. **Flank pain** (costovertebral angle) is usually associated with a disorder of the renal pelvis or kidney, especially when it is unilateral. A continuous dull ache is associated with chronic obstruction or infection. An acute pain in the flank region may be the result of acute obstruction of the renal pelvis or proximal (upper) ureter and is commonly termed '**renal colic**'. Pain may also radiate to upper lateral aspect of the abdomen. It is often described as moderate to severe in intensity and will cause the person to seek help. The pain tends to occur in waves during which the pain intensifies for periods of time as the pressure in the ureter and renal pelvis increases in response to the peristaltic waves. If the obstruction is in the lower ureter the pain may also radiate to the inguinal area and/or groin and upper thigh. A person with this type of pain should also be questioned about **haematuria**, fever and other urinary tract symptoms that might indicate infection (e.g. cloudy, foul-smelling urine, dysuria, frequency).[19] See also Table 24.1.

ASSESSMENT GUIDELINES	CLINICAL SIGNIFICANCE AND CLINICAL ALERTS
	Lower urinary tract and pelvic pain—most commonly caused by urinary tract infection (including prostatitis in the male). **Dysuria** (painful urination) is a common symptom related to urinary tract dysfunction. Typically, the person complains of burning on urination, which is associated with lower urinary tract infection and, less commonly, prostatitis in men.  ***Clinical alert:*** People with pain indicating renal colic and signs and symptoms of infection need urgent medical referral for further assessment and intervention to prevent septicaemia.
Lower urinary tract symptoms	
Storage symptoms	
Daytime voiding frequency (see questions related to usual urinary pattern above).	**Increased daytime frequency**—voiding more than eight times per day. It is important to consider the volume of urine per void and fluid intake when assessing urinary frequency (see objective assessment—fluid balance assessment/voiding diary). The increased urinary frequency could be the result of an unusually high fluid intake or an underlying problem with such as a urinary tract infection or a problem with renal function.

ASSESSMENT GUIDELINES	CLINICAL SIGNIFICANCE AND CLINICAL ALERTS
Urgency • *Do you feel that you can delay going to the toilet?* • *Do you ever feel you can't get to the toilet in time?* • *Do you ever lose urine on the way to the toilet?*	**Urinary urgency** is the complaint of sudden, compelling desire to pass urine that is difficult to defer.[11] It can lead to urge urinary incontinence if the person is unable to quickly respond to the desire to void. Urinary urgency can be a debilitating symptom that significantly affects activities of daily living and decreases a person's quality of life.[20,21] Urgency often accompanies urinary frequency.
Nocturia • *Do you need to get up at night to pass urine? How often?* • *How long has this been occurring?* • *Has it increased over this time?*	**Nocturia** is the number of times urine is passed during the main sleep period. Having woken to pass urine for the first time, each urination must be followed by sleep or the intention to sleep. This should be quantified using a bladder diary.[11] Normally, an adult should not wake more than once overnight to void. Nocturia is commonly associated with benign prostatic enlargement in men over the age of 50 years and can be severe. Some men must void more than six times per night; this results in sleep disturbance, relationship tensions and a general decrease in health and wellbeing.[22] Other causes are heart failure, urinary tract infection, hyperglycaemia and diuretic medication.

ASSESSMENT GUIDELINES	CLINICAL SIGNIFICANCE AND CLINICAL ALERTS
Urinary incontinence • *Do you ever leak urine when you don't want to?* Keep in mind that the person may not have disclosed their urinary incontinence previously, even to a close family member. You need to approach the questions with tact and have a supportive approach. People will frequently underestimate their urinary symptoms, especially if they have urinary incontinence. Often, if asked directly about urinary incontinence, they will answer 'no'. However, if you ask about whether they use pads so their clothes don't get wet they may answer 'yes'. This happens because people are embarrassed; and some may have had the problem for a long time and now consider it 'normal'.	**Urinary incontinence** is the complaint of involuntary loss of urine.[11] A comprehensive assessment of urinary incontinence takes time and expertise to determine the exact type of urinary incontinence. The person may need referral to a continence nurse specialist or other continence health professional for further assessment and advice. The International Continence Society[11] classifies the varying types of urinary incontinence according to the typical symptoms.
• *When does the leakage occur: changing position, coughing, sneezing, laughing or no provocation?* • *How much urine is lost?* (estimate in terms of dampness to clothing) • *How often does this happen?*	**Stress urinary incontinence** is the complaint of involuntary loss of urine on effort or physical exertion including sporting activities, or on sneezing or coughing.[11] This type of incontinence is often caused by weakness of the pelvic floor muscles. Usually, small amounts of urine are leaked.
• *Do you ever lose urine because you cannot get to the toilet in time?*	**Overactive bladder (OAB)** is the term used to describe urinary urgency, usually accompanied by increased daytime frequency and/or nocturia, with urinary incontinence (OAB-wet) or without (OAB-dry), in the absence of urinary tract infection or other detectable disease.[11] **Urgency urinary incontinence** is the involuntary loss of urine associated with urgency.[11] The person may not be able to inhibit the urge, and this can result in the entire bladder contents being leaked. Urge incontinence can be caused by several factors including neurological conditions such as stroke and multiple sclerosis and local causes such as **urinary tract infection**, **bladder pain syndrome**, **bladder stones** or **prostatic enlargement.**[23]

ASSESSMENT GUIDELINES	CLINICAL SIGNIFICANCE AND CLINICAL ALERTS
	Mixed urinary incontinence includes the complaints of both stress and urgency urinary incontinence—that is, involuntary loss of urine associated with urgency and with effort or physical exertion including sporting activities or on sneezing or coughing.[11]
• *Do you ever lose urine at night when you are asleep?*	**Nocturnal enuresis** is the complaint of involuntary voiding that occurs at night during the main sleep period (i.e. bedwetting).[11] It most commonly occurs in children but can also occur in adults. Loss of urine at night can also occur in people who have acute or chronic urinary retention (see below).
• *Does urine leak regardless of what you are doing?* • *Do you feel that you completely empty your bladder after you have been to the toilet?*	**Continuous urinary leakage** is the complaint of continuous involuntary loss of urine. It can be a sign of anatomical abnormality—for example, a fistula formation from bladder to vagina, or continuous overflow of urine where there is an acute or chronic obstruction causing **urinary retention** with some overflow of urine (**retention with overflow**). **Urinary retention** is the complaint of the inability to empty the bladder completely.[1] The most common cause of urinary retention is enlargement of the prostate gland in men.
• *Do you have trouble getting to the toilet: walking, rising from a chair to standing, walking to the toilet, opening doors, sitting/standing to toilet?* • *Are you able to undress/redress for toileting unassisted?* See also below on environmental factors.	**Functional incontinence** is urinary leakage associated with impairment of the person's mobility, dexterity or cognitive function.[24] This type of incontinence is a significant problem for frail older people and people with a disability. The person's or their carer's answers to these questions may lead to the need for a more in-depth assessment of the home environment and referral to an occupational therapist.

ASSESSMENT GUIDELINES	CLINICAL SIGNIFICANCE AND CLINICAL ALERTS
Voiding symptoms	
Urinary stream • *Do you feel that the force at which you pass urine has decreased?* For men • *Do you ever find that you need to stand closer to the toilet or urinal? If so, how long has this been happening?* • *Do you find it difficult to start passing urine?*	**Slow urinary stream** is the perception of a slower than previous urinary stream or in comparison with others.[11] If the person has a severe slowing of the urinary stream, they may describe it as a dribble or trickle. Sometimes described as a weak stream. **Intermittency/interrupted stream** is starting and stopping the urinary stream during one episode of voiding.[11] **Hesitancy** is the complaint of a delay in initiating voiding (when the person is ready to pass urine).[11] All these symptoms can be associated with poor detrusor (bladder) contraction and bladder outlet obstruction.
Straining • *Do you ever have to strain (bear down) to start or continue urinating?* • *Do you ever have to strain to completely empty your bladder?*	**Straining** is using intensive muscular effort to initiate, maintain or improve the urinary stream.[11] This is abnormal and may indicate an underlying dysfunction of the detrusor or bladder outlet obstruction.
Post-micturition symptoms • *Do you ever dribble urine after going to the toilet? How often does this happen? Does the leakage stop after a small loss of urine?* • *Do you feel that you empty your bladder completely when you have gone to the toilet? If no: How long have you had this feeling?*	**Post-micturition leakage (dribble)** is a symptom most commonly affecting men where there is a further small loss of urine after urination is completed.[11] **Feeling of incomplete emptying** is the perception that the bladder is not fully emptied following voiding.[11] This may or may not indicate that the person has a raised **post-void residual (PVR)**—the volume of urine left in the bladder at the completion of voiding.[11] See more detail below.

ASSESSMENT GUIDELINES	CLINICAL SIGNIFICANCE AND CLINICAL ALERTS
Difficulty or complete inability to void • *Do you feel that you need to pass urine but can't?*	The three most likely causes of significant difficulty with voiding are urinary retention (acute or chronic) and oliguria or anuria. People experiencing severe pain or who have undergone surgery (especially with epidural anaesthesia) can experience transient difficulty in voiding and may require urinary catheterisation until their general health improves. Acute and chronic retention of urine is most often associated with enlargement of the prostate in men. **Acute urinary retention** can cause significant lower abdominal pain and restlessness. **Chronic urinary retention** can result in renal damage due to increased pressures and/or infection in the urinary tract.
Lack of sensation of the need to void • *Do you have any sensation to pass urine?* • *Do you lose urine but have no sensation of this happening?*	Lack of sensation to void is associated with neurogenic dysfunction of the bladder which can be caused by disease or injury of the central or peripheral nervous system (e.g. multiple sclerosis, spinal cord injury, spina bifida, diabetes mellitus). For some people the bladder contracts without the sensation of the need to void, causing urinary incontinence. For others, the bladder may fail to contract (atonic bladder) resulting in retention of urine.[23] The bladder can retain large amounts of urine which can cause further damage to the detrusor muscle and increased pressures in the urinary tract resulting in renal damage.

ASSESSMENT GUIDELINES	CLINICAL SIGNIFICANCE AND CLINICAL ALERTS
Other symptoms (including fever, weight gain/loss, fatigue)	
Fever • *Have you experienced fever now or recently?* **Nausea and vomiting** • *Have you experienced nausea and/or vomiting now or recently? Anorexia?* **Weight gain/loss and peripheral oedema** • *Have you had a weight increase/loss now or recently?* • *Do you have any swelling in your lower legs?* • *Are you experiencing excessive thirst?* **Fatigue/lethargy** • *Have you experienced fatigue now or recently?* **For men** Questions related to erectile dysfunction (see Chapter 27). **Any other symptoms** • *Have you experienced any other symptoms such as headaches or itchy skin?*	Fever is associated with infection of the urinary tract and may be accompanied by other symptoms. The presence of a high body temperature with other symptoms such as flank pain, nausea and chills usually indicate the need for urgent referral to a medical practitioner. Nausea and vomiting can accompany pain and fever or can be a sign of increased creatinine levels indicating renal failure. Weight gain/loss in a person with a renal disorder is an indicator of general fluid balance. Fatigue and lethargy can be associated with chronic urinary tract disorders including renal failure.
Past history (including obstetric history)	
• *Do you or your family have any past history of renal or urinary tract health problems (infection, urinary stones, cancer)?* • *Do you or your family have any past history of neurological disorders?* • *Do you have diabetes? For how long? Current treatment?* • *Have you had any problem with your bowel function, including constipation?* • *History of mental health problems?* **For men** • *Any history of prostate cancer in your family?* **For women**—obstetric history • *How many births?* • *Were forceps used for any of these?* • *Did you have an episiotomy?* • *What were the babies' birthweights?* • *Did you have any bladder control issues after the births?* • *Menopausal symptoms?* **Surgical history** • *Have you had any surgery such as gynaecological, spinal or bowel?*	**Diabetes mellitus** is a major risk factor for renal failure and bladder dysfunction. **Constipation** is a risk factor for urinary incontinence and voiding dysfunction. There is a higher incidence of prostate cancer in men who have a first-degree relative with the disease. Pregnancy and childbirth are risk factors for developing urinary incontinence. **Obesity** is a risk factor for developing urinary incontinence. Older people may experience **acute confusion** rather than the more typical symptoms of urinary tract infection (e.g. frequency, urgency and dysuria).

ASSESSMENT GUIDELINES	CLINICAL SIGNIFICANCE AND CLINICAL ALERTS
Health and lifestyle management	
Activity and exercise • *What regular exercise do you take?* • *Are you able to manage your personal hygiene and toileting?* **Smoking/vaping** • *How much? For how long?* **Continence aids and appliances** • *Do you use any continence aids to assist you with toileting or incontinence (commodes, urinals, toilet seats, grab bars and rails)? If so, which ones? For how long? How effective are they?* **Incontinence products** • *Do you use any incontinence products to assist you with bladder leakage (pads, pants, condom (sheath) drainage catheters, sometimes referred to as external catheters)? If so, which ones? For how long? How effective are they?* **Medications** • *What medications are you currently taking (both over the counter and prescribed)?* **Screening** (for men over 50 years) • *Do you discuss prostate cancer screening with your GP?*	Some exercise activities can contribute to bladder symptoms and pelvic floor dysfunction, especially high-impact activities or those that cause increased intra-abdominal pressure. Smoking is a known risk factor for bladder and renal cancer and can contribute to urinary dysfunction. It is common for a person with urinary incontinence to self-manage their problem. You may need to assess the effectiveness of these aids and appliances and the person's knowledge of matters such as skin care, fluid intake and voiding position. They may need referral to a continence nurse specialist for further assessment and advice. Many medications affect bladder function, in particular anticholinergics, antidepressants and sedatives. Polypharmacy is a major contributor to the risk of incontinence in older people.
Environmental issues related to bladder function	
Mobility and dexterity issues • *Do you have any mobility and dexterity issues related to getting to and from the toilet and/or dressing/undressing?* • *Do you have any vision problems?* **Home environment** • *Is your toilet easy to get to? Do you have enough room in your toilet* (especially if the person uses walking aids)*?* **Work environment** • *Do you have easy access to the toilet at work?* • *Are there any restrictions related going to the toilet at work?* • *Do you have access to water whenever you need it?*	All these factors may contribute to urinary incontinence or other voiding dysfunction and can significantly affect the person's ability to cope with the problem.
Additional subjective data for infants and children (questions for parents or guardian)	
• *Does your child have any problem urinating?* • *Do they have any pain with urinating, crying or holding the genitals?* • *Any other symptoms or signs—for example, not feeding normally?* • *Do you think that your child has a urinary tract infection?* • *What makes you think that? What are the signs and symptoms you have noticed?*	

ASSESSMENT GUIDELINES	CLINICAL SIGNIFICANCE AND CLINICAL ALERTS
Toilet training (if child older than 2 to 2½ years of age.) • *Has toilet training started? How is it progressing?*	
Bed wetting (if child 5 years or older) • *Does the child wet the bed at night?* • *How often? Nightly?* • *Is this a problem for child or for you (parents)?* • *What have you done about this?* • *How does the child feel about it?* • *Any daytime wetting?*	Nocturnal enuresis

Objective data

Preparation

The positioning of the person depends on the area being assessed.

Equipment needed

You may need:

- urine jug or jar to collect a clean specimen
- urine testing equipment (dipsticks)
- non-sterile gloves
- portable bladder scanner and ultrasound transmission gel
- paper towel or tissues to remove ultrasound gel
- disinfectant wipes (to clean ultrasound transducer)
- hand hygiene solution (use before and after the physical examination).

PROCEDURES AND NORMAL FINDINGS	ABNORMAL FINDINGS AND CLINICAL ALERTS
General inspection	
While collecting subjective data, you will have noticed the person's height-to-weight ratio, body shape, ability to move around with ease, presence of persistent cough, level of hygiene and grooming, any obvious body odour and the person's general demeanour. All these factors provide clues to the person's urinary tract function and potential risk factors for dysfunction.	
Vital signs	
Temperature and blood pressure—see Chapter 10.	It is important to assess for the presence of fever, which may be related to infection and could indicate the need for urgent assessment by a medical practitioner. One of the consequences of renal impairment or renal failure is hypertension.

PROCEDURES AND NORMAL FINDINGS	ABNORMAL FINDINGS AND CLINICAL ALERTS
Abdominal examination	
Inspection, percussion and palpation of the lower abdomen to determine bladder distension (Chapter 23). Normally the bladder would not be palpable above the symphysis pubis after voiding.	Lower abdominal pain on palpation may accompany **urinary retention** or **urinary tract infection.**
Inspection of the genitalia (if indicated)	
Inspect for urethral discharge and excoriation. See Chapters 26 and 27 for details.	**Urethral discharge** is abnormal. See Table 24.1 for an image of urethral discharge.
Post-void residual (urine volume)	
The portable bladder scanner is commonly used by nurses in hospitals and in the community to assess post-void residual (PVR) urine volume. The use of this specialised piece of equipment has reduced the need for intermittent urethral catheterisation to assess residual volume. There are various scanning devices available. Most will have an integrated digital screen, a transducer that is placed on the lower abdomen and a printer for displaying the bladder volume measurements. You need to read the instructions for the scanner that you are using, but the following are general guidelines: • Explain the procedure to the person. • Have the person void into the collection jug or jar as usual—the volume of this void should be measured. Save the sample for dipstick testing after the scan is completed. (The scan should be performed as soon as possible after the person has voided to obtain accurate results.) • Ask the person to lie down (use one pillow if tolerated) and remove clothing on the lower abdomen down to the level of the symphysis pubis. • Have the scanning device placed on a trolley beside the person. • Wipe the transducer head with a disposable disinfectant wipe and allow to dry. • Turn the device on—male or female setting (male setting for a woman who has had a hysterectomy). • Apply transmission gel to the transducer head. • Place the transducer head onto the abdomen about 2.5 cm above the symphysis pubis and pointing down towards the bladder. Move the transducer head around until you have the bladder positioned centrally on the scanner screen, then avoid moving the transducer during scanning process.	An increased **PVR** is not necessarily a clinical problem, but in situations where there is high pressure in the bladder, an increased PVR can lead to infection, **hydronephrosis** and **renal insufficiency.**[23] Multiple ultrasounds may be needed to identify a trend. In a healthy person the PVR should normally be no more than 50 mL. A PVR over 250 mL is significant (incomplete bladder emptying) and over 350 mL increases the risk for upper urinary tract dilation and renal damage.[25] However, an acceptable PVR is very patient-specific, and you should always check with the attending medical officer as to what is considered acceptable for a particular person. Keep in mind that the amount of PVR must be interpreted considering the volume of urine the person had in their bladder in the first place. For example, if the person voided 100 mL and had a PVR of 100 mL, the finding is significant. Whereas a person who has voided 300 mL and has a PVR of 100 mL on one occasion may not be significant.

PROCEDURES AND NORMAL FINDINGS	ABNORMAL FINDINGS AND CLINICAL ALERTS

- The scanning device will signal when the scanning is complete.
- Remove the transducer head from the abdomen and clean. Offer the person tissues to wipe their abdomen and assist them, if necessary, to redress.
- Label the printed results with the date and time, the volume voided before the bladder scan and the person's name and date of birth. The printed results should be fixed into the person's medical history/progress notes. (Note: some scanners use thermal printing that fades over time. In this case photocopy the results.)

In the normal adult bladder there should be less than 50 mL of urine left in the bladder after voiding.[25]

Examination of urine

Collect a clean specimen of urine

- You should always collect a clean specimen for urinalysis, either freshly voided or taken aseptically from an access/ sample port in the tubing of a catheter drainage bag.
- Ask the person to void into a clean container (urinal, bed pan or clean urine measuring jug).
- The specimen should be tested as soon as possible after collection.
- For a person with a urethral or suprapubic catheter, the drainage bag tubing should be positioned so there are loops at the level of the bladder (so the urine collects in the tubing rather than dripping into the urine drainage bag). When the urine has collected in the tubing, aseptically draw about 10 mL of the urine from the access/sample port in the tubing.

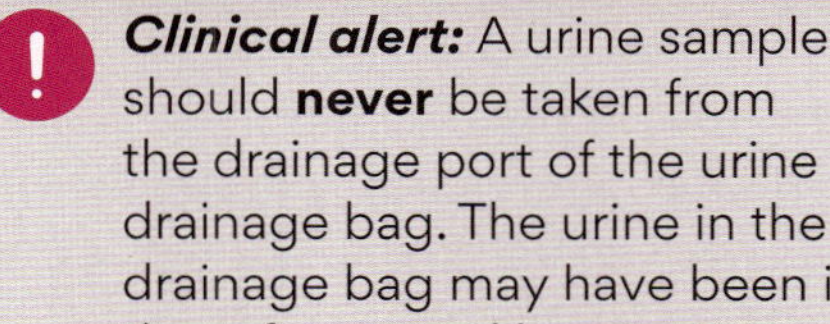

Clinical alert: A urine sample should **never** be taken from the drainage port of the urine drainage bag. The urine in the drainage bag may have been in there for several hours—it is not a fresh specimen.

Never disconnect the tubing from the catheter to take a urine specimen: this breaks the closed system and increases the risk of urinary tract infection.

Characteristics

- Volume of void, colour, clarity and odour.
- Urine should normally be clear, light-yellow coloured and have a non-offensive odour.

Urinalysis

- Urinalysis (Figure 24.6) can produce quick and useful information on the person's health status and bladder and kidney function. It may indicate the need for further investigations such as midstream urine for microscopy and culture. There are various brands of reagent strips that test for a variety of urine characteristics and abnormalities. These need to be stored and used in keeping with the manufacturer's instructions. The following are general guidelines:
    - Wear non-sterile gloves.
    - Open the reagent strip container and remove a reagent strip. Avoid touching the reagent test pads on the stick.

PROCEDURES AND NORMAL FINDINGS	ABNORMAL FINDINGS AND CLINICAL ALERTS
• Dip the stick into the urine specimen making sure that all of the reagent test pads are moistened. Remove the stick, making sure you don't flick the stick causing spray. Start timing the test. Let the stick drain above the urine container to reduce dripping of urine. • Some test pads can be read immediately; others require a specific time for the result to be finalised. Follow the instructions on the container for the time requirements (Figure 24.6). • After the required time frame, compare the colour of the reagent test pad to the chart for the specific test located on the reagent strip container. Avoid touching the urine-soaked reagent strip on the container chart. Discard the test strip and then your gloves into the waste bin. • Perform hand hygiene. • Record the results.	
• Normal urine dip stick (reagent strip) test results: • pH—4.5–8.0 (average 5.0–6.0) • bilirubin—none or trace • urobilinogen—none or trace • protein—none • blood—none • glucose—none • ketones—none • specific gravity—1.005–1.030 • leucocyte esterase—none • nitrite—none	! ***Clinical alert:*** A person should be referred to a medical or nurse practitioner where there is a positive finding for blood, protein, nitrates or leucocytes.

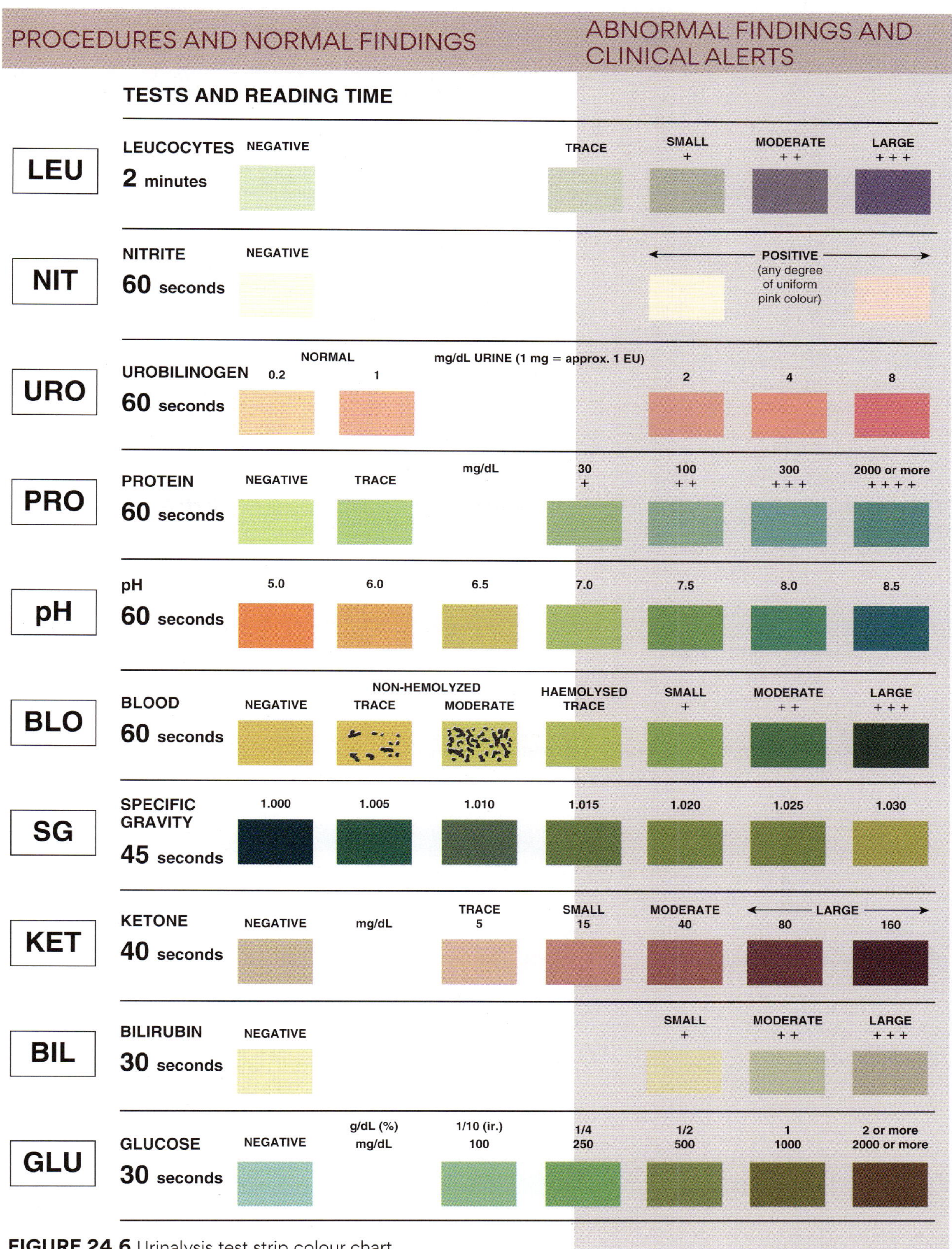

FIGURE 24.6 Urinalysis test strip colour chart

PROCEDURES AND NORMAL FINDINGS	ABNORMAL FINDINGS AND CLINICAL ALERTS
Fluid balance chart or voiding diary	
In hospitalised people, a **'fluid balance'** chart is commonly issued to record intake and output as well as type and amount of fluid intake and any accompanying voiding symptoms. In situations where estimation of fluid balance is vital to the overall health of the person, urinary catheterisation may be required so accurate, frequent urine volumes may be obtained. **A voiding diary** (sometimes called a bladder chart, bladder diary or frequency/volume chart) can be used to record a person's voiding and incontinence pattern over a period of time. The form used will depend on the information to be elicited such as information on intake and types of fluids, volume voided, accompanying symptoms such as urgency, dysuria, incontinence and precipitating factors, use of continence pads. This data is sometimes combined with a bowel chart/diary. It is common practice to collect at least 3 full (24-hour) days of charting to establish if a voiding pattern exists. During this time the person or their carer should make no attempt to alter their usual patterns, as the purpose of the chart is to establish the person's usual voiding patterns. You need to review and interpret the following data from the voiding diary: **Pattern of urinary elimination** • Voiding frequency during the daytime • Presence and severity of nocturia (each void is preceded by sleep) • Proportion of urine formed overnight (voided volume after going to bed to sleep including the first void of the morning) • 24-hour frequency • Maximum voided volume • Average voided volume (sum of volumes voided divided by the number of voids) • 24-hour total voided volume **Patterns of urinary leakage**[25] • Frequency of incontinence episodes and relationship to voiding and precipitating events (e.g. coughing, sneezing) • Volume of leakage **Fluid consumption** • Intake compared with output • Patterns of intake • Types of fluids • Relationship of intake and voiding or incontinence	Output should be roughly similar to intake. In an adult the amount of urine produced per hour is 0.5 mL/kg/hr or 30 to 40 mL per hour in an average-sized adult. Proportion of urine voided overnight. Up to one-third of daily urine production overnight is considered normal.

PROCEDURES AND NORMAL FINDINGS	ABNORMAL FINDINGS AND CLINICAL ALERTS
Additional objective data for infants and children	
It may be difficult to get an accurate measurement of urine volume in infants and young children. Observing the number of wet nappies and the colour and concentration of urine can give an indication of urine output. In sick children, urinary catheterisation may be required to accurately measure urine output.	The expected urine output for infants and young children is 1 mL/kg/h.

Abnormal findings

TABLE 24.1 Urinary tract–related problems

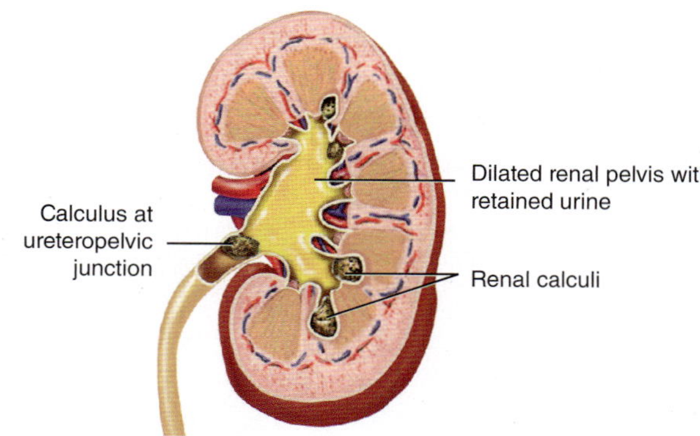

Renal calculi (stones)

Renal stones (crystals of calcium oxalate or uric acid) form in kidney tubules and then migrate and become urgent when they pass into ureter, become lodged and obstruct urine flow, causing hydronephrosis. They cause abrupt severe flank pain with radiation to the groin or abdomen, nausea and vomiting, restlessness, gross or microscopic haematuria.

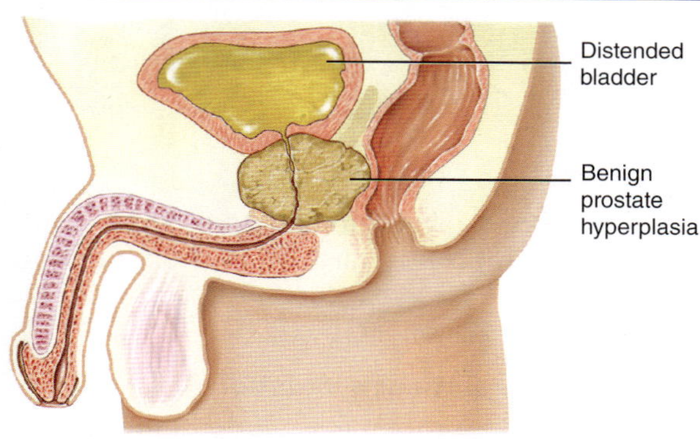

Acute urinary retention

Inability to pass urine with bladder distension and lower abdominal pain. Common in older men due to bladder outlet obstruction from benign prostatic hypertrophy (Chapter 26).

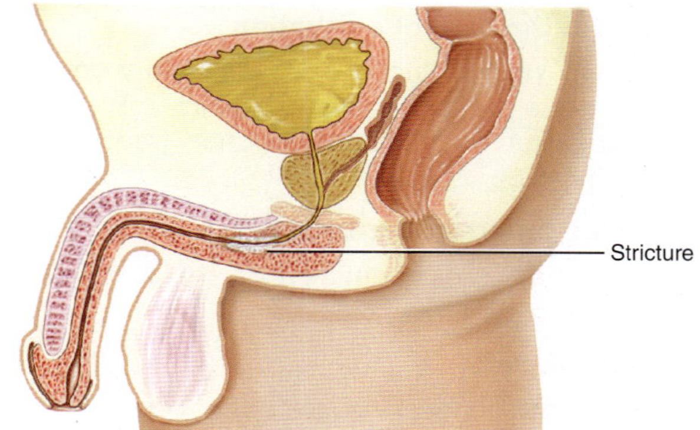

Urethral stricture

Pinpoint, constricted opening at meatus or inside along urethra. Occurs congenitally or secondary to urethral injury. Gradual decrease in force and calibre of urine stream is most common symptom. Shaft feels indurated along ventral aspect at site of stricture.

Clinical reasoning and documentation

The following is a continuation of the case study provided at the beginning of this chapter and the clinical reasoning process including problem/issue identification. Consult a fundamentals of nursing or medical-surgical nursing text for information about goal setting, nursing interventions and evaluation.

Case study 1 (continued)—Lower urinary tract symptoms

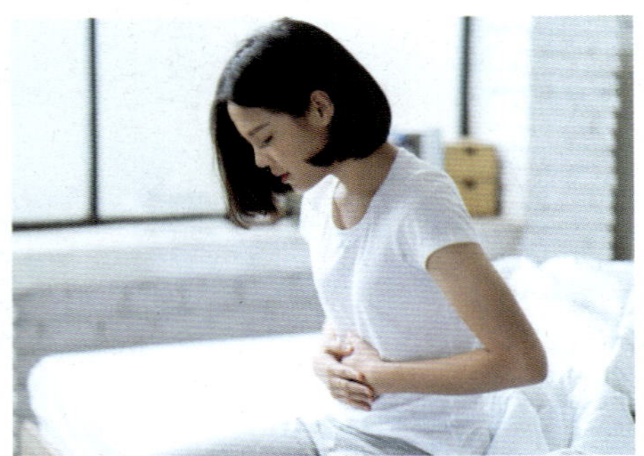

Context

You will recall from the case study described earlier in the chapter that you are a registered nurse working as a practice nurse in a busy community multidisciplinary health clinic. The role includes screening assessments for people who have not attended the clinic previously.

Consider the patient's situation

Ms Chee Wan Ching is a 26-year-old woman attending a general practice clinic following sudden onset today of dysuria, urinary frequency and urgency.

Collect cues/information

Your further assessment reveals the following information.

Subjective data

Ms Chee has no fever, nausea or flank pain but is complaining of suprapubic pain and discomfort. She has never had a urinary tract infection and has no past medical health problems or surgery. She has recently started a sexual relationship with her boyfriend of 3 months. She takes the oral contraceptive pill but no other medications. Her last sexual health check and cervical screening test was 1 year ago.

Objective data

Vital signs: Temp 37°C, HR 72/min, RR 14/min, BP 110/70

Suprapubic tenderness on palpation. No other areas of tenderness noted. Urine—cloudy and foul smelling. Dipstick test: pH 7.0, protein nil, leucocytes +++, nitrites +++, blood (microscopic) +.

Process information and identify problems/issues

Collaborative problem

Probable urinary tract infection - refer to medical practitioner

Problem statements/nursing diagnoses

Pain—dysuria related to probable UTI

Knowledge deficit about UTI prevention and management (including antibiotic therapy and follow-up)

Case study 2—Urinary incontinence

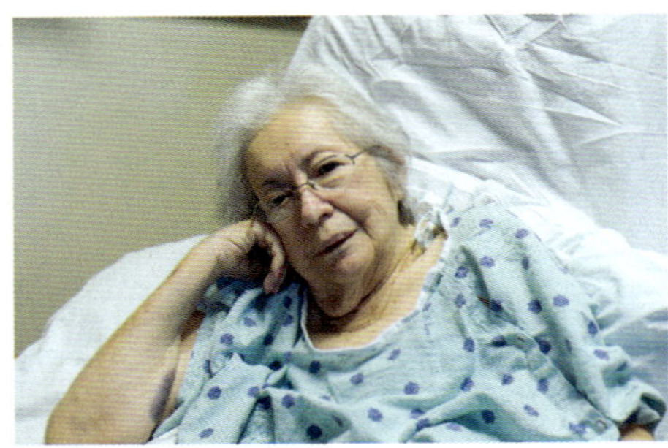

Context

You are on a clinical placement in an acute respiratory medical ward on a morning shift. You introduce yourself to one of your allocated patients, Mrs Jennifer Guyatt.

Consider the patient's situation

Mrs Guyatt, aged 84 years, was admitted to the ward 3 days ago with pneumonia. As you assist her to get ready for breakfast you notice that her bed is very wet with urine.

Collect cues/information

Subjective data

Mrs Guyatt says she is very concerned because she did not realise that she had wet herself so

Clinical reasoning and documentation cont't

much. She says that she normally doesn't have any problem with incontinence but has noticed she is leaking urine when she coughs, and it has been getting worse since the chest infection started. She is very embarrassed about wetting the bed.

She says that she is only aware of urine leaking when she coughs. She has a productive cough that is difficult to control, and it comes without warning. She has been changing her underwear frequently to deal with it and sometimes has put a towel under her bottom when she is in bed to try to keep the sheets dry. She says she hasn't mentioned it to the nursing staff previously. She has been trying not to drink too much so she doesn't wet herself. She says her cough is still troublesome, but she feels it is improving.

Mrs Guyatt has opened her bowels each day of her admission.

She had three normal vaginal deliveries many years ago and has not had any gynaecological problems. She says she occasionally gets a urinary tract infection, which is successfully treated by her GP with oral antibiotics. She doesn't think she has had an infection for the past 3 years.

Objective data

Bed sheets and clothing obviously wet with urine. Odour non-offensive.

Inspection of skin—perineal and upper thighs—skin pink and intact. No evidence of skin irritation.

Bowels opened each day—last was Bristol 3.

Previous 24-hour intake—approximately 1,000 mL of fluid intake and 900 mL urine output.

Small urine sample obtained—urine clear but dark yellow, dipstick test: pH 6, SG 1.025, no other abnormalities detected.

Vital signs within normal limits—afebrile.

Process information and identify problems/issues

Collaborative problem

Stress urinary incontinence related to persistent coughing/weakened pelvic floor muscles—needs referral to the continence service when discharged

Problem statements/nursing diagnoses

Risk of fluid volume deficit related to reduced fluid intake

Risk of skin breakdown (incontinence associated dermatitis) in genital area and upper thighs related to persistent urine loss and damp clothing

Knowledge deficit about stress urinary incontinence, cough and the need to drink enough fluids

ADDITIONAL RESOURCES

You can further develop your knowledge and skills relevant to assessment of urinary function, related pathophysiology, common health issues and nursing interventions by:

- reading chapters of a fundamentals of nursing or medical-surgical nursing textbook
- answering chapter multiple choice questions online. Log onto ClinicalKey Student and search for the text 'Health Assessment, 4th edition'. Choose the section titled 'Teaching material'. In this section you will find question and answer documents for each chapter. Please check instructions on the inside front cover of the book to access online resources
- visiting websites

  Caregiving, dementia and incontinence—Free online learning short course: https://www.futurelearn.com/courses/caregiving-dementia-incontinence/3

ADDITIONAL RESOURCES cont't

Continence Foundation of Australia: www.continence.org.au

Continence New Zealand: www.continence.org.nz

International Continence Society: www.ics.org

Kidney Health Australia: www.kidney.org.au

Chronic kidney disease management handbook https://kidney.org.au/health-professionals/ckd-management-handbook

Kidney Health Australia, First Nations Resources https://kidney.org.au/health-professionals/health-professional-resources/hp-resources-first-nations-australians

Medical Journal of Australia—Recommendations for culturally safe clinical kidney care for First Nations Australians: a guideline summary: https://www.mja.com.au/journal/2023/219/8/recommendations-culturally-safe-clinical-kidney-care-first-nations-australians

Kidney Health New Zealand: www.kidneys.co.nz

Prostate Cancer Foundation of Australia: www.prostate.org.au

Prostate Cancer Foundation New Zealand: www.prostate.org.nz

REFERENCES

1. The International Consultation on Incontinence Group, Bristol Urological Institute. 2023. Available at: https://iciq.net/
2. Tortora GJ, Derrickson B, Burkett B, Cooke J, DiPietro F. Principles of anatomy and physiology. 2022. Milton, Qld.: John Wiley & Sons.
3. Marieb EM, Keller SM. Essentials of human anatomy & physiology. 13th Global ed. UK: Pearson; 2022.
4. Montayre J, Macdiarmid R, McDonald EM, Saravanakumar P. Urinary system. In: Tompkins, Z. editor, Applied anatomy and physiology: An interdisciplinary approach, Chatswood: Elsevier; 2020. pp. 361–382.
5. Grodensky M. Male genital and reproductive function. Banasik J (editor). Pathophysiology. 7th ed. St Louis, Elsevier. 2022. pp. 636–650.
6. Devlin CM, Simms MS, Maitland NJ. Benign prostatic hyperplasia—what do we know? BJU International. 2021. Apr;127(4):389–399.
7. Australian Institute of Health and Welfare. Chronic kidney disease: Australian facts—summary. Canberra: Australian Institute of Health and Welfare, 2023. Available at: https://www.aihw.gov.au/reports/chronic-kidney-disease/chronic-kidney-disease/contents/summary
8. Australian Institute of Health and Welfare. How many people are living with chronic kidney disease in Australia? Canberra: Australian Institute of Health and Welfare, 2023. Available at: https://www.aihw.gov.au/reports/chronic-kidney-disease/chronic-kidney-disease/contents/how-many-people-are-living-with-ckd
9. Tafuna'i M, Turner RM, Richards R, Sopoaga FA, Walker R. The prevalence of chronic kidney disease in Samoans living in Auckland, New Zealand. Nephrology. 2022. Mar;27(3):248–259.
10. Kidney Health Australia. Statistics—Risk factors of kidney disease. Available at: https://

kidney.org.au/your-kidneys/know-your-kidneys/know-the-risk-factors
11. International Continence Society. Glossary. 2023. Available at: https://www.ics.org/glossary
12. Ermer-Seltun JM, Engberg S. Continence care Nursing: an overview. In Ermer-Seltun JM, Engberg S. (eds) Core curriculum: Continence Management. 2nd ed. Wound, Ostomy and Continence Nursing Society. Wolters Kluwer: Philadelphia 2022. pp. 32–43.
13. Continence Foundation of Australia. Understanding incontinence. 2023. Available at: https://www.continence.org.au/incontinence/understanding-incontinence
14. Continence New Zealand. Epidemiology—statistics. 2023. Available at: https://www.continence.org.nz/pages/Epidemiology-Statistics/102/
15. Pizzol D, Demurtas J, Celotto S, Maggi S, Smith L, Angiolelli G, et al. Urinary incontinence and quality of life: a systematic review and meta-analysis. Aging Clinical and Experimental Research. 2021 Jan;33:25–35.
16. Veronese N, Smith L, Pizzol D, Soysal P, Maggi S, Ilie PC, et al. Urinary incontinence and quality of life: a longitudinal analysis from the English Longitudinal Study of Ageing. Maturitas. 2022. Jun 1;160:11–15.
17. Aydin Avci İ, Öz Yildirim Ö, Yildirim E, Bulgak M. Non-medication coping strategies for urinary incontinence in older adults: factors associated with frequency of use. International Urogynecology Journal. 2022 May;33(5):1259
18. Continence Foundation of Australia. Good bladder habits for everyone. 2023. Available at: https://www.continence.org.au/information-incontinence-english/good-bladder-habits-for-everyone
19. Talley NJ, O'Connor S. Clinical examination: a systematic guide to physical diagnosis. 9th ed. Chatswood: Elsevier; 2021.
20. Kant P, Inbaraj LR, Franklyn NN, Norman G. Prevalence, risk factors and quality of life of lower urinary tract symptoms (LUTS) among men attending primary care slum clinics in Bangalore: a cross-sectional study. Journal of Family Medicine and Primary Care. 2021 Jun;10(6):2241.
21. Mehr AA, Kreder KJ, Lutgendorf SK, Ten Eyck P, Greimann ES, Bradley CS. Daily symptom associations for urinary urgency and anxiety, depression and stress in women with overactive bladder. International Urogynecology Journal. 2022 Apr;33(4):841–850.
22. Aucar N, Fagalde I, Zanella A, Capalbo O, Aroca-Martinez G, Favre G, et al. Nocturia: its characteristics, diagnostic algorithm and treatment. International Urology and Nephrology. 2023 Jan;55(1):107–114.
23. Cobley J, Wyndaele M, Hashim H. Pathophysiology of urinary incontinence. Surgery. 2023 Mar 21. https://doi.org/10.1016/j.mpsur.2023.02.010
24. Shaw C, Wagg A. Urinary and faecal incontinence in older adults. Medicine. 2021 Jan 1;49(1):44–50.
25. Nelles K. Primary assessment of patients with urinary incontinence and voiding dysfunction. In Ermer-Seltun JM, Engberg S. editors. Core curriculum: Continence Management. 2nd ed. Wound, Ostomy and Continence Nursing Society. Wolters Kluwer: Philadelphia. 2022. pp. 44–66.

CHAPTER 25

Assessing bowel function

Written by Carolyn Jarvis
Adapted by Elizabeth Watt

INTRODUCTION

Many people have a primary problem concerned with bowel elimination or can develop a bowel health issue secondary to illness, hospitalisation, medical treatments or change of lifestyle. Because so many body systems are involved, as you progress through this chapter you also need to consider the structure and function related to eating (mouth, teeth and throat) and nutrition (Chapter 21) and the small and large bowel (Chapter 23), as well as the anus and rectum described in this chapter.

Case study

The following case study will help you identify your learning needs.

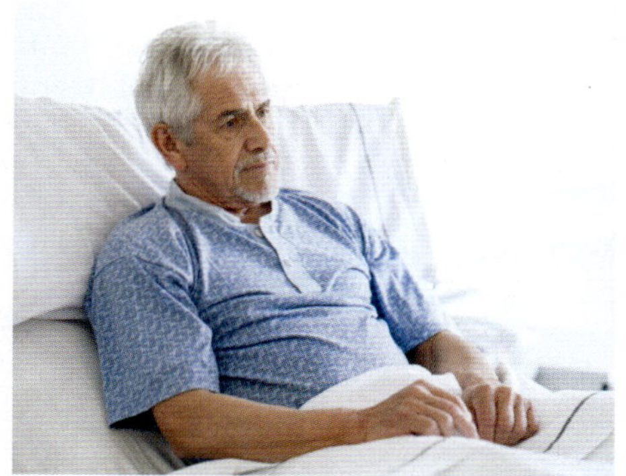

Context

You are a registered nurse working on an orthopaedic surgical ward. The assessment was performed as part of a general survey on meeting the patient at the start of a shift.

Consider the patient's situation

Mr Jerry Wishart is a 78-year-old man who had a left total knee replacement 2 days ago. He was previously well with no major health problems other than severe osteoarthritis in the left knee and milder osteoarthritis in the right knee. The surgical procedure went well, with no complications. Today Mr Wishart is due to be discharged to a rehabilitation hospital and tells you he has not his opened his bowels for 3 days and he is feeling bloated and uncomfortable.

Questions to further your learning

- What are the possible things that might be going on with Mr Wishart?
- What knowledge do you need to be able to predict what might be going on?
- What approach to Mr Wishart's health assessment will you take?
- What questions (subjective data) will you ask Mr Wishart to extend the health history and why?
- What physical examination (objective data) will you conduct and why?
- What resources are available to assist in your assessment of Mr Wishart?

Assessment plan

Assessment of bowel function is a frequent assessment area for nurses in a variety of healthcare settings. The extent of the questioning and examination will depend on the person's main health concern. Some people will focus on their bowel function and have strong beliefs about what they consider normal. It is also an area of health that people will frequently self-manage. You need to screen hospitalised, frail or immobilised people for risk of constipation and put interventions in place to prevent constipation developing. Many people with bowel problems, in particular faecal incontinence, will be reluctant to discuss their problem, so approach these questions with tact and empathy.

Through the process of questioning the client or family you may become aware of gaps in the person's knowledge about living a healthy lifestyle. The opportunity to provide health information is an important part of health assessment. The main areas for subjective assessment are:

- presenting concern
- usual bowel pattern
- history of change or disturbance in bowel function
- bowel symptoms
- anal symptoms
- medications
- past history
- health and lifestyle management
- environmental issues related to bowel function
- bowel diary.

People who have bowel problems frequently have skin excoriation and/or anal abnormalities. The findings of subjective data collection will guide you in deciding the extent of the physical examination. In most cases, assessment of bowel function is done in conjunction with an abdominal examination (Chapter 23). In addition, many people who have bowel problems also have mobility issues, altered nutrition, skin problems and urinary problems. See Chapters 20, 21 and 24 for details of these assessments.

The main areas for objective assessment are:

- general inspection
- abdominal examination
- inspection of the skin and perianal area
- specimen screening—inspection of stool.

Resources available

You will find additional resources and the bibliography at the end of this chapter.

Structure and function

Anus and rectum

The **anal canal** is the outlet of the gastrointestinal tract and is about 3.8 cm long in adults. It is lined with modified skin (having no hair or sebaceous glands) that merges with rectal mucosa at the anorectal junction.

The anal canal is surrounded by two concentric layers of muscle, the **sphincters** (Figure 25.1). The internal sphincter is under involuntary control by the autonomic nervous system. The external sphincter surrounds the internal sphincter but also has a small section overriding the tip of the internal sphincter at the opening. It is under voluntary control. Faecal continence is achieved by a combination of a competent, closed anal sphincter, normal anorectal sensation and reflexes, adequate rectal capacity and compliance, conscious control, as well as other factors such as stool consistency.[1] The pelvic floor also plays an important role in maintaining faecal continence and successful defecation.[2] Except for the passing of faeces and gas, the sphincters keep the anal canal tightly closed. The **intersphincteric groove** separates the internal and external sphincters and is palpable.

The **anal columns** (or columns of Morgagni) are folds of mucosa. These extend vertically down from the rectum and end in the **anorectal junction** (also called the mucocutaneous junction, pectinate or dentate line). This junction is not palpable, but it is visible on proctoscopy. Each anal column contains an artery and a vein. Under

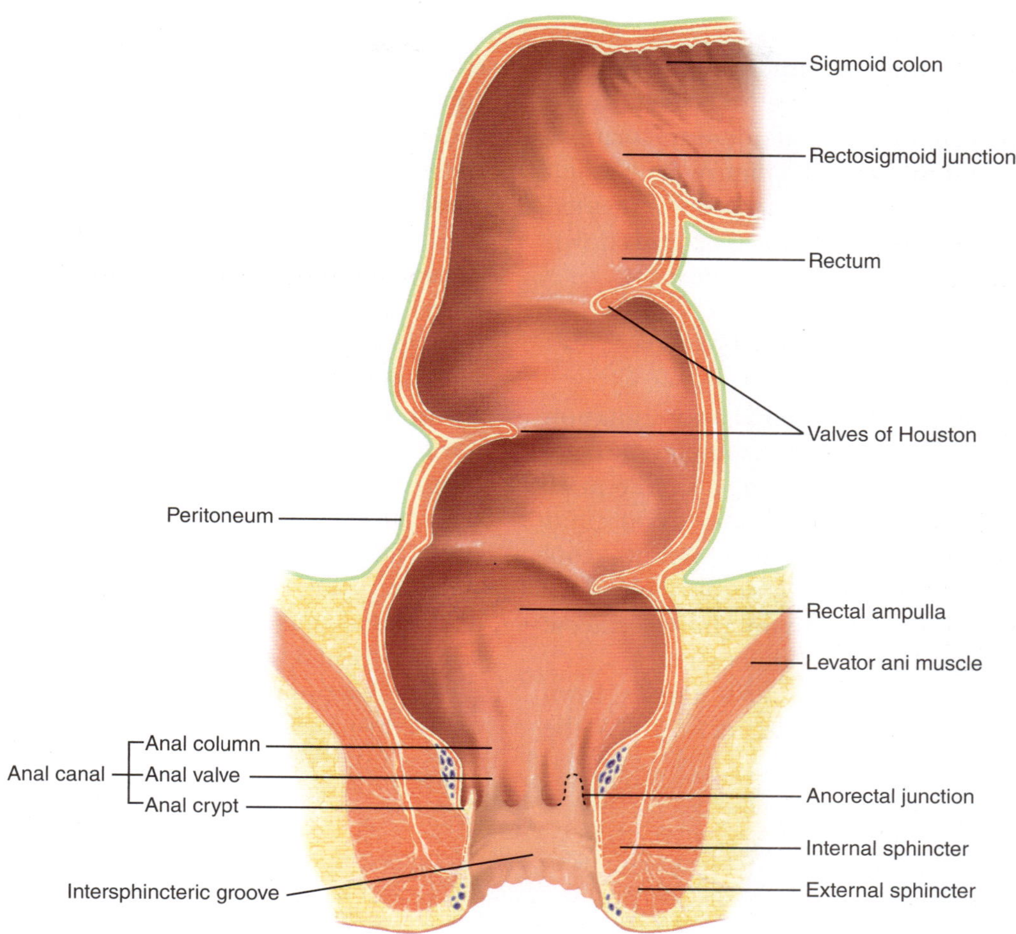

FIGURE 25.1 Anatomy of the lower bowel, rectum and anus

conditions of chronic increased venous pressure, the vein may enlarge, forming a haemorrhoid. At the lower end of each column is a small crescent fold of mucous membrane, the **anal valve**. The space above the anal valve (between the columns) is a small recess, the **anal crypt**.

The canal slants forwards towards the umbilicus, forming a distinct right angle with the rectum, which rests back in the hollow of the sacrum. Although the rectum contains only autonomic nerves, numerous somatic sensory nerves are present in the anal canal and external skin, so a person feels sharp pain from any trauma to the anal area.

The **rectum**, which is approximately 12 cm long, is the distal portion of the large intestine. It extends from the sigmoid colon, at the level of the third sacral vertebra and ends at the anal canal. Just above the anal canal, the rectum dilates and turns posteriorly, forming the rectal ampulla. The rectal interior has three semilunar transverse folds called the **valves of Houston**. These folds cover half the circumference of the rectal lumen. Their function is unclear, but they may serve to hold faeces as the flatus passes. The lowest is within reach of palpation, usually on the person's left side and must not be mistaken for an intrarectal mass.

The **peritoneum** covers only the upper two-thirds of the rectum. In males, the anterior part of the peritoneum reflects down to within 7.5 cm of the anal opening, forming the **rectovesical pouch** (Figure 25.2) then covers the bladder. In females, this is termed the **recto-uterine pouch** and extends down to within 5.5 cm of the anal opening.

Defecation

Faecal continence is achieved by a combination of a competent, closed anal sphincter, normal anorectal sensation and reflexes, adequate rectal capacity and compliance, conscious control as well as other factors such as stool consistency.[1] The pelvic floor also plays an important role in maintaining faecal continence and successful defecation.[2]

Peristaltic movements push faeces from the sigmoid colon into the rectum. As the rectal walls distend, the defecation reflex is stimulated via nerve impulses and the sacral spinal cord, resulting in contraction of the rectal muscles, an increase in pressure within the rectum and relaxation of the **internal anal sphincter**.[1] The internal sphincter is a smooth muscle innervated by the autonomic nervous system. As the rectum distends, more faeces enter the rectum. At the same time, impulses travel to the brain to create conscious awareness of the need to defecate. The **external sphincter** is voluntarily controlled. Voluntary constriction of the levator ani muscles will close the anus and defecation can be delayed for a period. At the time of defecation, the external sphincter relaxes.[2] A voluntary contraction of abdominal muscles during forced expiration with a closed glottis (Valsalva manoeuvre) causes a rise in intraabdominal pressure to be exerted to assist in expelling faeces.

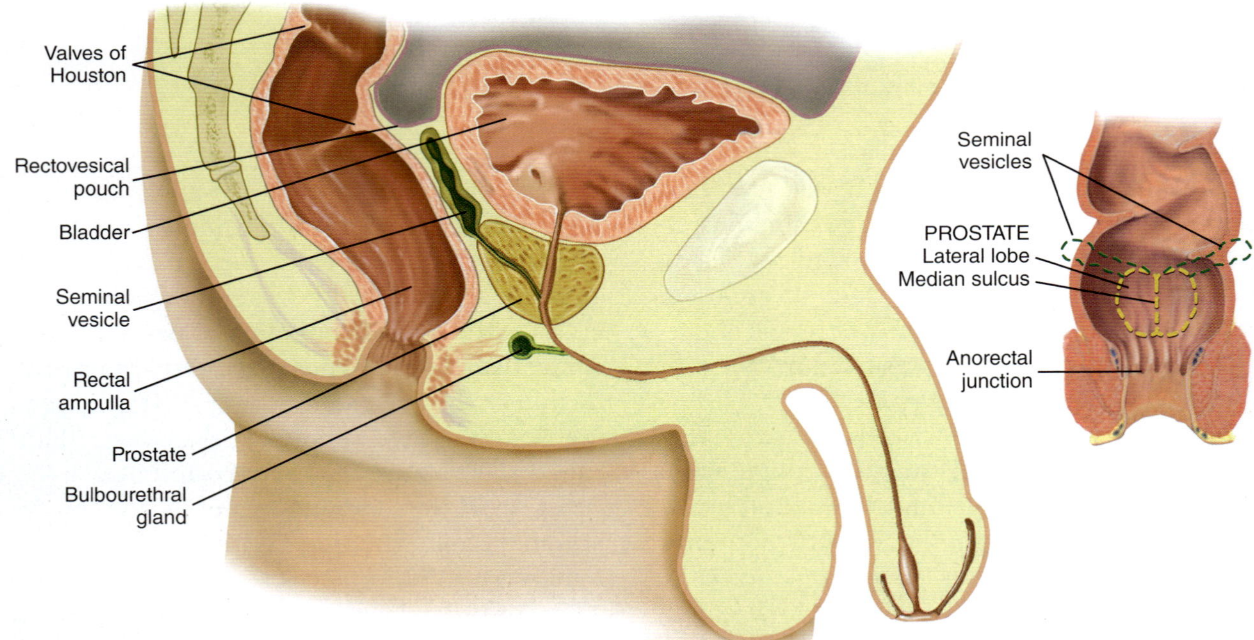

FIGURE 25.2 Anatomy of the male pelvis and related structures

Regional structures

In females, the uterine cervix lies in front of the anterior rectal wall and may be palpated through it (Chapter 26). In males, the prostate gland lies in front of the anterior wall and 2 cm behind the symphysis pubis (Chapter 27).

The combined length of the anal canal and the rectum is about 16 cm in adults. The average length of the examining finger is from 6 to 10 cm, bringing many rectal structures within reach.

The sigmoid colon is named from its S-shaped course in the pelvic cavity. It extends from the iliac flexure of the descending colon and ends at the rectum. It is 40 cm long and is accessible to examination only through the colonoscope. The flexible fibreoptic endoscope provides a view of the entire mucosal surface of the sigmoid, as well as the colon.

Developmental considerations

Infants

The first stool passed by a newborn is dark green meconium and occurs within 24 to 48 hours of birth, indicating anal patency. From that time on, the infant usually has a stool after each feeding. This response to eating is a wave of peristalsis called the gastrocolic reflex, which continues throughout life, although children and adults usually produce no more than one or two stools per day.

The infant passes stools by reflex. Voluntary control of the external anal sphincter cannot occur until the nerves supplying the area have become fully myelinated, usually around 1½ to 2 years of age. Toilet training usually starts after age 2 years.

Late adulthood (65+ years)

There is a widely accepted belief that people are more likely to develop health problems related to bowel function as they age. While there is degeneration of the enteric nervous system with age, gut transit time and colonic motility tend to be consistent throughout life,[2] and most older people maintain the same frequency of bowel movements that they had in their younger years. Known changes that occur with ageing that can affect defecation include a decrease in the resting anal sphincter pressure and impaired rectal sensation.[3] However, bowel function is more likely to be influenced by other factors such as chronic disease, immobility and the various treatments for these health problems. There is evidence that the composition of the gut microbiota changes with age, which may lead to greater susceptibility to disease, altered inflammatory and immune response, decreased insulin sensitivity and increased risk of frailty.[4]

Cultural and social considerations

Colorectal cancer is the fourth most common cancer in Australian men and women.[5] There is an increase in the incidence of colorectal cancer with ageing, rising sharply after the age of 50 years. The lifetime risk of developing colorectal cancer for Australians to age 85 years is one in 19.[5] While the incidence of colorectal cancer in older Australians has decreased over time, the incidence in colorectal cancer in people aged up to 39 years has more than doubled over a 20-year period.[5] The same trend is occurring internationally. While the reasons for the increased incidence in the younger age group have not been identified, it is likely to be related to lifestyle factors such as obesity, lack of physical activity and poor diet.[6]

In non-Indigenous Australians, there is a 69.8% 5-year survival rate for men and a 71.0% 5-year relative survival rate for women.[5] Colorectal cancer is the third most common cancer in Aotearoa New Zealand. The incidence of colorectal cancer for non-Indigenous New Zealanders has reduced over time, but the incidence has increased in Māori people and is now like non-Indigenous New Zealanders.[7] The survival rate from colorectal cancer (and other cancers) in Māori people is lower than non-Māori in Aotearoa New Zealand due to socioeconomic disparities, comorbidity, access to cancer screening and treatment and follow-up when a cancer diagnosis is made.[8] There are also higher colorectal cancer incidence and mortality rates for Indigenous Australians.[5] For more information about colorectal cancer and screening programs see 'Health education' below.

Like urinary incontinence, faecal incontinence has a significant impact on the person. Faecal incontinence is defined as the complaint of involuntary loss of faeces (may be solid and/or liquid).[9] It is estimated that faecal incontinence affects more than 7% of adults[10] and up to 50% in people living in residential care.[11] Risk factors for faecal incontinence include abnormal anal sphincter or pelvic floor function; congenital anorectal malformations; secondary to degenerative neurological disease; obstruction and impaction with overflow; environmental factors such as poor toilet facilities; and inadequate care. In addition, advanced age, dementia or cognitive impairment, frailty, reduced mobility, urinary incontinence and any condition that creates frequent, loose, large-volume, watery stools also predispose a person to incontinence—for example, inflammatory bowel disease.[11]

HEALTH EDUCATION

National Bowel Cancer Screening Program

The incidence of colorectal cancer in Australia and Aotearoa New Zealand has been described above. Risk factors for colorectal cancer include obesity, unhealthy diet (high in fat, high red meat consumption, high salt intake, low fruit and vegetable intake), low physical activity, active and passive smoking, low socioeconomic status and low educational levels.[12] Also, colorectal cancer is more common in people over 50 years of age and in those who have a positive family history of colorectal cancer, especially at a younger age. The signs and symptoms that have been associated with colorectal cancer include rectal bleeding, persistent change in bowel habits, unexplained weight loss, unexplained anaemia and raised blood inflammatory markers.[13]

Colorectal cancer screening with an immunochemical faecal occult blood test (iFOBT) has been shown to significantly reduce the morbidity and mortality from bowel cancer.[14] Screening aims to detect colorectal cancer before any obvious signs and symptoms, improving long-term survival. People with a family history of bowel cancer or other risk factors need more intensive screening with regular colonoscopy and other diagnostic tests.

In Australia, the federal government funds the National Bowel Cancer Screening Program.[15] When people turn 50 years of age, they receive an invitation through the mail to complete an iFOBT in their own home, free of charge. They receive a kit with instructions and all the equipment needed to collect two faecal specimens quickly and cleanly. When they have collected the specimens, they return them

HEALTH EDUCATION cont'd

by mail to a pathology laboratory for analysis. Of those invited, 43.8% returned a completed kit for analysis.[14] The New Zealand Ministry of Health has funded a similar program for non-Indigenous New Zealanders aged 60 to 74 years of age and from 50 years of age for Māori and Pacific Islander people.[16]

Nurse's role

Take the opportunity to encourage people to collect and return their iFOBT—it may just save their life!

People with a positive iFOBT result will be advised to discuss the result with their medical practitioner, who will generally refer them for further investigations, usually a colonoscopy.

For more information visit the following websites:

- National (Australian) Bowel Cancer Screening Program: https://www.health.gov.au/our-work/national-bowel-cancer-screening-program
- National (Australian) Indigenous Bowel Cancer Screening Program: https://www.health.gov.au/our-work/national-bowel-cancer-screening-program/indigenous
- Ministry of Health (New Zealand) National Bowel Cancer Program: https://www.health.govt.nz/our-work/preventative-health-wellness/screening/national-bowel-screening-programme.

Subjective data

Practice note

Before you start the assessment, introduce yourself to the person, confirm the person's identity, discuss the purpose and scope of the assessment, clarify any questions the person may have and obtain verbal consent from the person to perform the assessment.

ASSESSMENT GUIDELINES	CLINICAL SIGNIFICANCE AND CLINICAL ALERTS
Presenting concern	
• *Are you experiencing any problems with your bowel function?* It is important to ascertain the person's perception of their bowel function. If they do perceive that they have a bowel problem, ask: *How does this affect your quality of life?*	
Usual bowel pattern	
• *Do you have a regular bowel movement? How often?* • *Do you have any pain while passing a bowel movement?* • *Is this relieved when you have finished?*	The **frequency** of bowel movements varies from person to person. Appearance and consistency of the stool is more relevant than frequency of bowel movements. **Pain** may be due to a local condition such as **haemorrhoids** (varicose veins in the rectum or anus), **anal fissures** (a small split in the anal mucosa), **constipation** or pathology within the colon.

ASSESSMENT GUIDELINES	CLINICAL SIGNIFICANCE AND CLINICAL ALERTS
History of change or disturbance in bowel pattern	
• *Have you noticed any change in usual bowel habits? Can you describe this change?* See questions related to constipation below. • *Do you have loose stools or diarrhoea? When did this start?* • *Is the diarrhoea associated with nausea and vomiting, abdominal pain, something you ate recently? What have you done about it? Did this help?*	**Diarrhoea** (three or more loose stools in a day) can occur with **gastroenteritis, ulcerative colitis, Crohn's disease and irritable bowel syndrome.** ***Clinical alert:*** Any recent persistent change in bowel pattern could indicate an underlying disease or malignancy; therefore, the person should be referred to a medical practitioner for further assessment.
Have you eaten take away food or at a restaurant recently? Does anyone else in your group or family have the same symptoms?	Consider food poisoning.
• *Have you travelled overseas or to a remote or rural area during the past 6 months?* • *Do you live with a pet or farm animals? If so, are they up to date with their immunisations and/or worming treatments?*	Consider parasitic infection or water borne infection.
• *Have you noticed that it is difficult to have a bowel movement (constipation)?* • *Do your stools have a hard consistency? How often does this occur?* • *How often do you have a bowel movement?* • *Do you have to strain to have a bowel movement? When did this start? How often does this occur?* • *Do you feel that you have completely emptied your bowel when you have been to the toilet? How often does this occur?* • *Do you feel that there is a blockage or obstruction when you empty your bowel? How often does this occur?* • *Do you need to support your perineum or in any way assist having a bowel movement? How often does this occur?* • *What have you done about it? Did this help?*	**Functional constipation** is characterised by two or more of the following criteria for at least 3 months (Rome IV criteria[17]): • straining during more than 25% of defecations • sensation of incomplete evacuation with more than 25% of defecations • sensation of anorectal obstruction/blockage more than 25% of defecations • use of manual manoeuvres to facilitate more than 25% of defecations (e.g. support of pelvic floor, digital evacuation) • fewer than three spontaneous bowel movements per week • there is insufficient criteria for irritable bowel syndrome. **Opioid constipation** involves most of above symptoms when initiating, changing or increasing opioid therapy. Some people may have functional constipation exacerbated by opioid use.[17]

ASSESSMENT GUIDELINES	CLINICAL SIGNIFICANCE AND CLINICAL ALERTS
Bowel symptoms	
Rectal bleeding Blood in the stool: • *Have you ever had black-coloured or bloody stools?* • *When did you first notice blood in the stools?* • *What is the colour? Bright red or dark red to black?* • *How much blood? Is it spotting on the toilet paper or outright passing of blood with the stool?* • *Do the bloody stools have a particular smell?*	Black stools may be tarry due to occult blood (**melaena**) from gastrointestinal bleeding or non-tarry from ingestion of iron medications. Bright red blood can be from a bleeding haemorrhoid or anal fissure or can be an indicator of a tumor in the bowel. ! ***Clinical alert:*** Bright red blood in stools occurs with intestinal bleeding or localised bleeding around the anus and with colon and rectal cancer. If the person is reporting black-coloured stools when not taking iron replacement therapy, this could indicate upper gastrointestinal bleeding. In either case the person should be referred to a medical practitioner for further assessment.
• *Have you ever experienced clay-coloured stools?*	**Clay** colour (pale grey) indicates absent bile pigment. This is associated with disease of the liver and/or gall bladder.
• *Have you ever experienced frothy stool?*	**Steatorrhoea** is excessive fat in the stool as in malabsorption of fat.
Flatus • *Can you control wind?* Passage of flatus is a normal finding. • *Do you feel that you have excessive wind? Are you able to distinguish between flatus and stool?*	The amount of flatus can be affected by diet and underlying intestinal pathology such as food sensitivities. Inability to control the passage of flatus can indicate anal sphincter dysfunction.
Urgency • *Do you have any difficulty making it to the toilet in time? How often? What happens? How long can you hang on?* With normal bowel control the person can usually defer for a long period after the first urge to defecate.	Consider **faecal incontinence** (also see the questions in the next section). If the person is unable to defer defecation even when the stool consistency is normal, they are likely to have poor external anal sphincter function. In this situation the person should be referred to a nurse continence nurse specialist, medical practitioner or continence physiotherapist for further assessment.

ASSESSMENT GUIDELINES	CLINICAL SIGNIFICANCE AND CLINICAL ALERTS
Faecal incontinence	**Faecal incontinence** is the complaint of involuntary loss of faeces (may be solid and/or liquid).[9]

ASSESSMENT GUIDELINES

Faecal incontinence

- *Do you ever experience any leakage from the bowel? Were you aware of this happening? Was it liquid or solid stool? How often does this happen? Does it happen only after you have used your bowels?*

If leakage (stool and faecal leakage or faecal leakage without stool) is a problem, note the day of the week, date and time of this occurrence.

- *Can you describe the amount of faecal leakage or stool (small, medium or large)?*[18]

Description of stool

Ask the person to describe their bowel movement using the Bristol stool chart (Figure 25.3). The Bristol stool chart is a validated tool for describing stool appearance, its consistency and form. It is a seven-point scale. Types 3 and 4 are the most usual or 'normal' consistency.

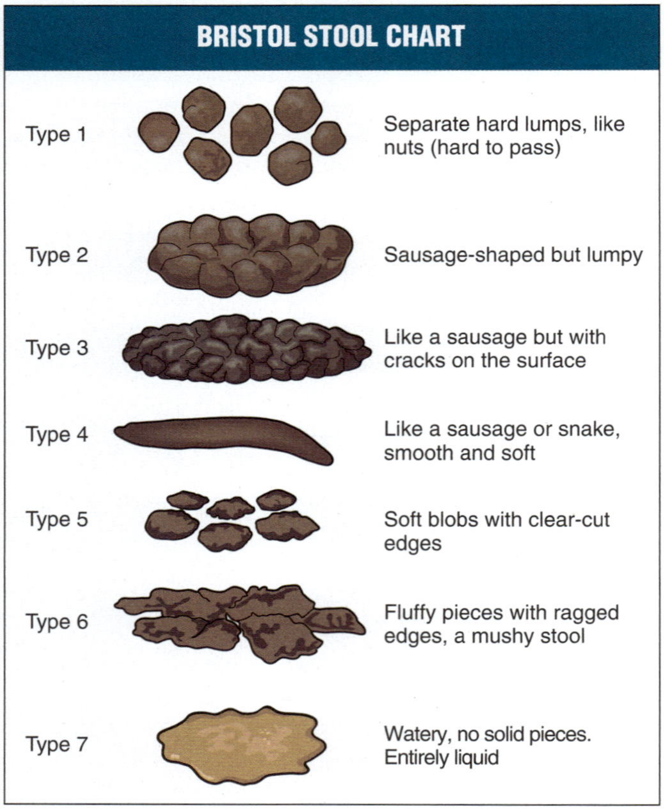

BRISTOL STOOL CHART

Type 1	Separate hard lumps, like nuts (hard to pass)
Type 2	Sausage-shaped but lumpy
Type 3	Like a sausage but with cracks on the surface
Type 4	Like a sausage or snake, smooth and soft
Type 5	Soft blobs with clear-cut edges
Type 6	Fluffy pieces with ragged edges, a mushy stool
Type 7	Watery, no solid pieces. Entirely liquid

FIGURE 25.3 Bristol stool chart

CLINICAL SIGNIFICANCE AND CLINICAL ALERTS

Faecal incontinence is the complaint of involuntary loss of faeces (may be solid and/or liquid).[9]

ASSESSMENT GUIDELINES	CLINICAL SIGNIFICANCE AND CLINICAL ALERTS
Anal symptoms	
• *Have you experienced any problems in anal area: itching, pain or burning, haemorrhoids? How do you treat these?* • *Do you use any haemorrhoid preparations?* • *Have you ever had an anal fissure or anal fistula? When did this occur? How was this treated?*	**Pruritus** is itching.
Medications	
• *What* medications *do you take—prescription, over-the-counter, traditional and complementary therapies?* • *Do you use laxatives or stool softeners? Which ones? How often do you use them?* • *Do you take iron replacement therapy?* • *Do you ever use suppositories or enemas to move your bowels? How often?* If the person has experienced faecal leakage, *Have you used any medications to prevent or lessen the leakage?*	Many prescription medications can cause bowel problems (e.g. opioid medications, iron supplements, some antidepressants). It is important to note what laxatives a person takes regularly. If these are stopped abruptly for any reason this could result in sudden and severe constipation, especially if the laxatives have been taken over many years.
Past history	
• *Do you have any family history: polyps in the bowel or cancer in the colon or rectum, inflammatory bowel disease, haemorrhoids?* • *Have you had any surgery or have you experienced any medical condition that may have contributed to disturbed bowel function?* (e.g. gynaecological surgery, abdominal surgery, neurological disease) • *Do you have a bowel stoma?* **For women**—obstetric history: • *How many pregnancies and births have you had?* • *Did you have a long second stage of labour? Were forceps used for any deliveries?* • *Did you have an episiotomy? What were the babies' birthweights?* • *Did you have any bowel control issues after the births?*	A strong family history of **bowel polyps** or colorectal cancer is a risk factor for the person. A **bowel stoma** is a small opening in the abdomen which is used to remove faeces into a collection bag. It can be permanent or temporary (used to enable the bowel to heal after surgery). The type of stoma depends on its position in the bowel. Common bowel stomas are an **ileostomy** or a **colostomy**. Pregnancy, labour and delivery, especially prolonged labour and instrumental delivery, can damage the anal sphincter, which can predispose the woman to faecal incontinence.[19]

ASSESSMENT GUIDELINES	CLINICAL SIGNIFICANCE AND CLINICAL ALERTS
Health and lifestyle management	
Diet and fluids • *What is the usual amount of high-fibre foods in your daily diet? These include cereals/grains, apples, pears or other fruits, vegetables, legumes and wholegrain breads.* • *Do you take fibre supplements? Which ones? How often?* • *Do you eat spicy foods? Does this affect your digestion?* • *How many glasses of water do you drink each day?*	High-fibre foods of the soluble type (beans, prunes, barley, carrots, broccoli, cabbage) lower cholesterol, while insoluble fibre foods (cereals, wheatgerm) reduce the risk of constipation and colorectal cancer. Also, fibre foods stabilise blood sugar and help certain gastrointestinal disorders. Inadequate fluid intake is significantly related to developing constipation. If you find significant risk factors in this area, you may need to complete a more detailed nutritional assessment (Chapter 21).
Activity and exercise • *What regular exercise do you undertake?* • *Describe your usual day in terms of exercise and activity.* If the person has a very sedentary lifestyle, ask: *What do you feel is stopping you being more active?*	Lack of activity and exercise are significantly related to developing constipation. Lack of activity may be related to another health problem such as chronic obstructive pulmonary disease, which can cause significant breathlessness on exertion.
Smoking/vaping • *How many packs per day (or vapes)? For how long?*	Smoking can affect bowel function and is a risk factor for colorectal cancer.
Screening • If they are aged 50 years or older, ask about the date of their last bowel cancer screening or colonoscopy.	Early detection for cancer. See 'Health education' above.
Incontinence pads or pants When people disclose bowel control issues ask them: • *Do you ever need to wear a pad to protect your clothes?* • *What type of pad do you use? How often do you use a pad?* This may give you an indication of the severity of the problem.	
Environmental issues related to bowel function	
Make a judgement about whether the following questions are relevant to the person's situation: • *Do you need assistance to get to the toilet?* Ask the person to describe the level of assistance required. • *Do you need assistance with toileting?* (e.g. undressing, getting onto the toilet, wiping/cleaning, getting off the toilet, redressing, handwashing etc.). Ask the person to describe the level of assistance required.	Some people will have difficulties getting to the toilet or with activities associated with toileting that may cause them to be incontinent. These need to be investigated so appropriate interventions can be put in place to improve the situation.

ASSESSMENT GUIDELINES	CLINICAL SIGNIFICANCE AND CLINICAL ALERTS
• *Do you find it difficult to get to the toilet?* (e.g. stairs, distance from living area or bedroom). Ask the person to describe the difficulty. • *Do you use toileting aids?* (e.g. commode chairs, raised toilet seats, support rails)	
Bowel diary	
If the person is experiencing bowel dysfunction, more detailed information can be obtained by asking them to complete a bowel diary. A bowel diary is used to collect information about the frequency, amount and consistency of bowel movements over a period, preferably at least 1 week. The person is asked to complete a simple chart that details the date and time, description (using the Bristol stool chart, Figure 25.3) and adding in notes about bowel-related symptoms (see previous questions). The data from the chart provides useful information about the severity of symptoms (including incontinence episodes) and the person's actual bowel elimination patterns.	
Additional subjective data for infants and children (questions for parents or guardian)	
Anal irritation • *Have you ever noticed any irritation in your child's anal area: redness, raised skin, frequent itching?*	In children, pinworms are a common cause of intense itching and irritated anal skin.
Bowel movements • *Are you able to describe your child's bowel movements? What is the frequency? Do they experience any problems with their bowels? Any pain or straining with bowel movements?* If the child is over 4 years of age, ask: *Are there any issues with soiling or inability to control bowel movements?*	Assess usual elimination pattern. **Faecal incontinence in children** older than age 4 years (an age at which bowel continence would be expected) can be primary—the child has never attained bowel continence; or secondary—when the soiling occurs after a period of continence.[20]

Objective data

The findings of subjective data collection will guide you in the extent of the examination required. You may also need to perform an abdominal examination (Chapter 23). Many people who have bowel problems may also have urinary problems, immobility or nutritional issues. See Chapters 21, 23 and 24 for details of these assessments.

Preparation

If a perianal skin examination is needed, the person will need to remove their pants/trousers/shorts, as well as underwear and/or stockings. Ask the person to move into the left (or right) lateral position on a bed or examination couch. Use a sheet, blanket or towel to cover the person.

Make sure the room is warm and that privacy is maintained.

Equipment needed

Penlight
Non-sterile gloves
Hand hygiene solution

PROCEDURES AND NORMAL FINDINGS	ABNORMAL FINDINGS AND CLINICAL ALERTS
General inspection	
While collecting subjective data, you will have noticed the person's height-to-weight ratio, body shape, ability to move around with ease, level of hygiene and grooming, any obvious body odour and the person's general demeanour. All these factors provide clues to the person's bowel function and risk factors for dysfunction.	
Abdominal examination	
An abdominal examination should be conducted to identify any factors that can indicate bowel dysfunction. See Chapter 23 for details.	A bloated or rigid abdomen. The absence of bowel sounds or hyperactive bowel sounds. Dullness on percussion, especially over the left lower quadrant—may indicate faecal mass. Tenderness or mass on palpation.
Inspection of the skin and perianal area	
Wear non-sterile gloves. Spread the buttocks wide apart and observe the perianal region. The anus normally looks moist and hairless, with coarse folded skin that is more pigmented than the perianal skin. The anal opening is tightly closed. No lesions are present. Skin is clean.	Inflammation. Lesions or scars. Linear split—**fissure**. Flabby skin sac—haemorrhoid. Shiny blue skin sac—thrombosed haemorrhoid. Small round opening in anal area—**fistula** (Table 25.1). Perineal soiling may indicate loss of anal sphincter tone and/or poor hygiene practices.

PROCEDURES AND NORMAL FINDINGS	ABNORMAL FINDINGS AND CLINICAL ALERTS
Inspect the sacrococcygeal area. Normally, it appears smooth and even.	Inflammation or tenderness, swelling, tuft of hair or dimple at tip of coccyx may indicate a **pilonidal cyst** (Table 25.1).
Instruct the person to breathe in, hold the breath and bear down by performing a **Valsalva manoeuvre**. No break in skin integrity or protrusion through the anal opening should be present. Describe any abnormality in clock-face terms, with 12 o'clock as the anterior point towards the symphysis pubis and 6 o'clock towards the coccyx.	Appearance of fissure or **haemorrhoids**. Circular red doughnut of tissue—rectal prolapse.
Specimen screening—inspection of stool	
Inspect the faecal specimen. Normally, the **colour** is light to dark brown (depends on diet) and the consistency is soft. Use the **Bristol stool chart** (Figure 25.3) to determine consistency. Estimate the **amount** of faeces in cups. See 'Health education' above for information about the National Bowel Screening Program.	Jelly-like mucus shreds mixed in stool may indicate inflammation. Bright red blood on the stool surface indicates rectal bleeding. Bright red blood mixed with faeces indicates possible colonic bleeding. Black tarry stool with distinct malodour (**melaena**) indicates upper gastrointestinal bleeding with blood partially digested. (Must lose more than 50 mL from upper gastrointestinal tract to be considered melaena.) **Black stool**—also occurs with ingesting iron supplements. **Pale grey (clay coloured) stool**—absent bile pigment such as in obstructive jaundice. **Pale yellow, greasy stool**—increased fat content (steatorrhoea), as occurs with malabsorption syndrome.
Additional objective data for infants and children	
For newborns, hold the feet with one hand and flex the knees up onto the abdomen. Note the presence of the anus. Confirm a patent rectum and anus by noting the first meconium stool passed within 24 to 48 hours of birth. To assess sphincter tone, check the **anal reflex**. Gently stroke the anal area and note a quick contraction of the sphincter.	**Imperforate anus**—a congenital anal malformation where the normal anal opening has not been formed.
Note that the buttocks are firm and rounded with no masses or lesions. The **mongolian spot** is a common variation of hyperpigmentation in newborns (Chapter 22).	**Meningocele** (sac containing meninges that protrude through a defect in the bony spine).

PROCEDURES AND NORMAL FINDINGS	ABNORMAL FINDINGS AND CLINICAL ALERTS
The **perianal skin** is free of lesions. However, nappy rash is common in children younger than 1 year of age and is exhibited as a generalised reddened area with papules or vesicles.	Pustules or reddened skin may indicate secondary infection of nappy rash. Signs of physical or sexual abuse such as anal abrasions or perianal tears (Chapter 5). Fissure is a common cause of constipation or rectal bleeding in children (painful, so the child does not defecate). Inspect the **perianal region** of a school-age child or adolescent while examining the genitalia.

Abnormal findings

TABLE 25.1 Abnormalities of the anus and perianal region

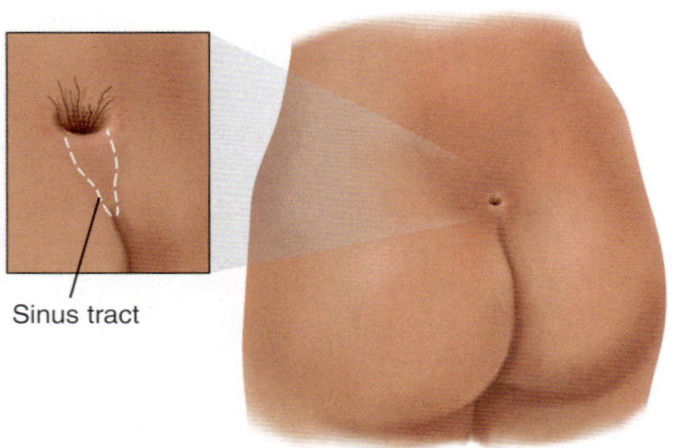

Pilonidal cyst or sinus

A hair-containing cyst or sinus located in the midline over the coccyx or lower sacrum. Often opens as a dimple with visible tuft of hair and, possibly, an erythematous halo. Or may appear as a palpable cyst. When advanced, has a palpable sinus tract. Although it is a congenital disorder, the lesion is first diagnosed between the ages of 15 and 30 years.

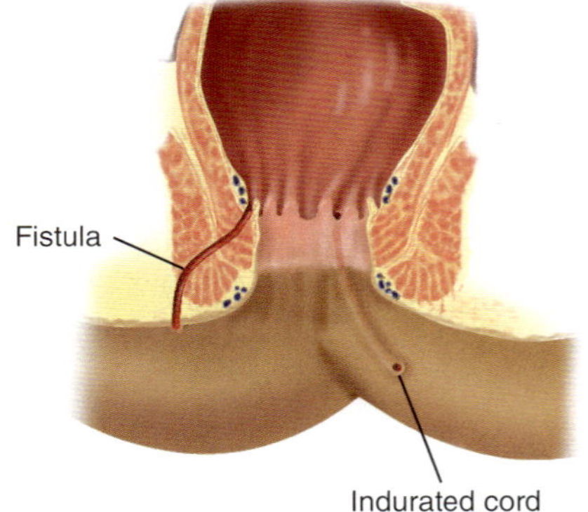

Anorectal fistula

A chronically inflamed gastrointestinal tract creates an abnormal passage from the inner anus or rectum out to the skin surrounding the anus. May result from a local abscess. The red, raised tract opening may drain serosanguinous or purulent matter when pressure is applied.

TABLE 25.1 Abnormalities of the anus and perianal region cont'd

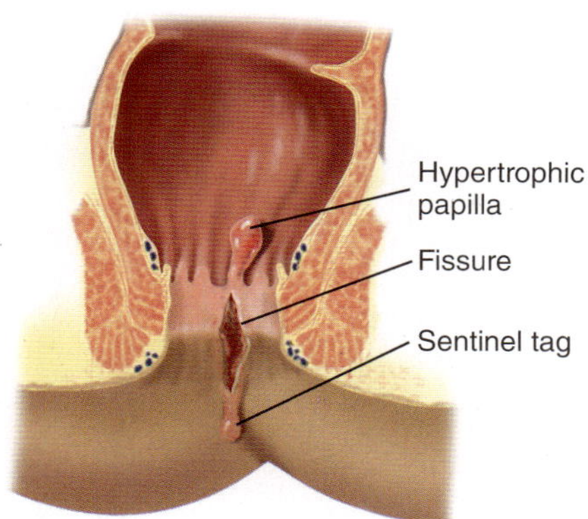

Anal fissure

A painful longitudinal tear in the superficial mucosa at the anal margin. Most fissures (> 90%) occur in the posterior midline area. They are frequently accompanied by a papule of hyperplastic skin (called a sentinel tag) on the anal margin below. Fissures often result from trauma such as passing a large, hard stool or from irritant diarrhoeal stools. The person has itching, bright bleeding (may be noticed on the toilet paper or on the stool) and significant pain on defecation. As resulting spasm in the sphincters makes the area painful to examine, local anaesthesia may be indicated.

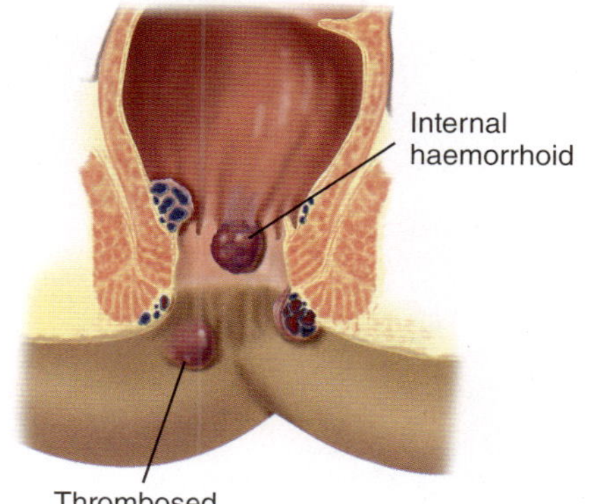

Haemorrhoids

These painless, flabby papules are due to a varicose vein of the haemorrhoidal plexus. An external haemorrhoid originates below the anorectal junction and is covered by anal skin. When thrombosed, it contains clotted blood and becomes a painful, swollen, shiny blue mass that itches and bleeds with defecation. When it resolves, it leaves a painless, flabby skin sac around the anal orifice. An internal haemorrhoid originates above the anorectal junction and is covered by mucous membrane. When the person performs a Valsalva manoeuvre, it may appear as a red mucosal mass. It is not palpable. All haemorrhoids result from increased portal venous pressure, as occurs with straining at stool, chronic constipation, pregnancy, obesity, chronic liver disease or the low-fibre diet common in Western society.

Continued

TABLE 25.1 Abnormalities of the anus and perianal region cont'd

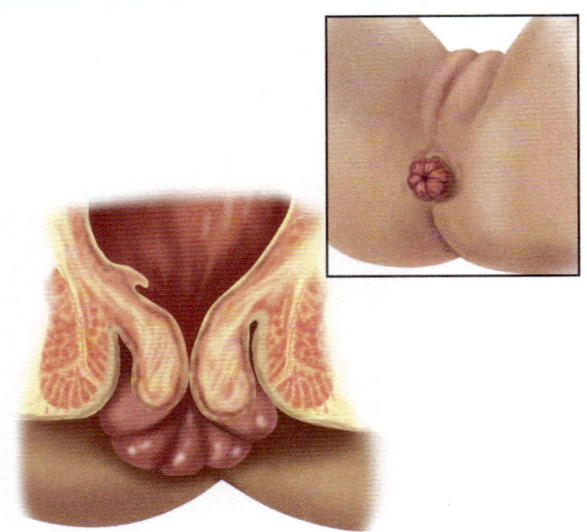

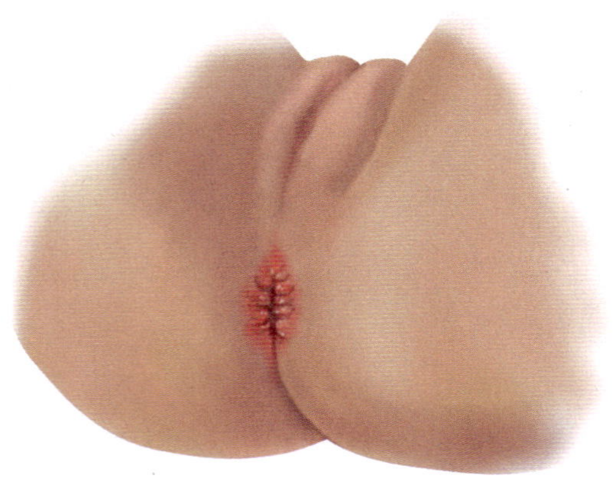

Rectal prolapse

The rectal mucous membrane protrudes through the anus, appearing as a moist red doughnut with radiating lines. When prolapse is incomplete, only the mucosa bulges. When complete, it includes the anal sphincters. Occurs following a Valsalva manoeuvre, such as straining at stool or with exercise.

Pruritus ani

Intense perianal itching is manifested by red, raised, thickened, excoriated skin around the anus. Common causes are pinworms in children and anal fissures, dermatitis, chronic diarrhoea, fungal infections in adults. The area is swollen and moist, and with a fungal infection it appears dull greyish pink. The skin is dry and brittle and itchy.

Advanced practice—additional data

Nurses working in the acute care setting rarely perform a screening rectal examination, but they may need to perform a rectal examination as part of assessing a person with severe constipation before deciding on the most appropriate treatment. You need to make a clinical judgement about the need to perform a rectal examination. In addition to the objective assessment described previously, nurse continence specialists and other advanced practice nurses may perform this assessment as part of an advanced assessment of constipation and faecal incontinence.

Fully explain the procedure to be performed and get the person's consent. Make sure the room is warm and privacy is maintained.

Preparation

As described in the objective data section.

Equipment needed

Lubricant gel
Non-sterile gloves
Hand hygiene solution

PROCEDURES AND NORMAL FINDINGS	ABNORMAL FINDINGS AND CLINICAL ALERTS

Palpate the anus and rectum

Drop lubricating gel onto your gloved index finger. Instruct the person that palpation is not painful but may feel like needing to move the bowels. Place the pad of your index finger gently against the anal verge (Figure 25.4). You will feel the sphincter tighten, then relax. As it relaxes, flex the tip of your finger, and slowly insert it into the anal canal in a direction towards the umbilicus.

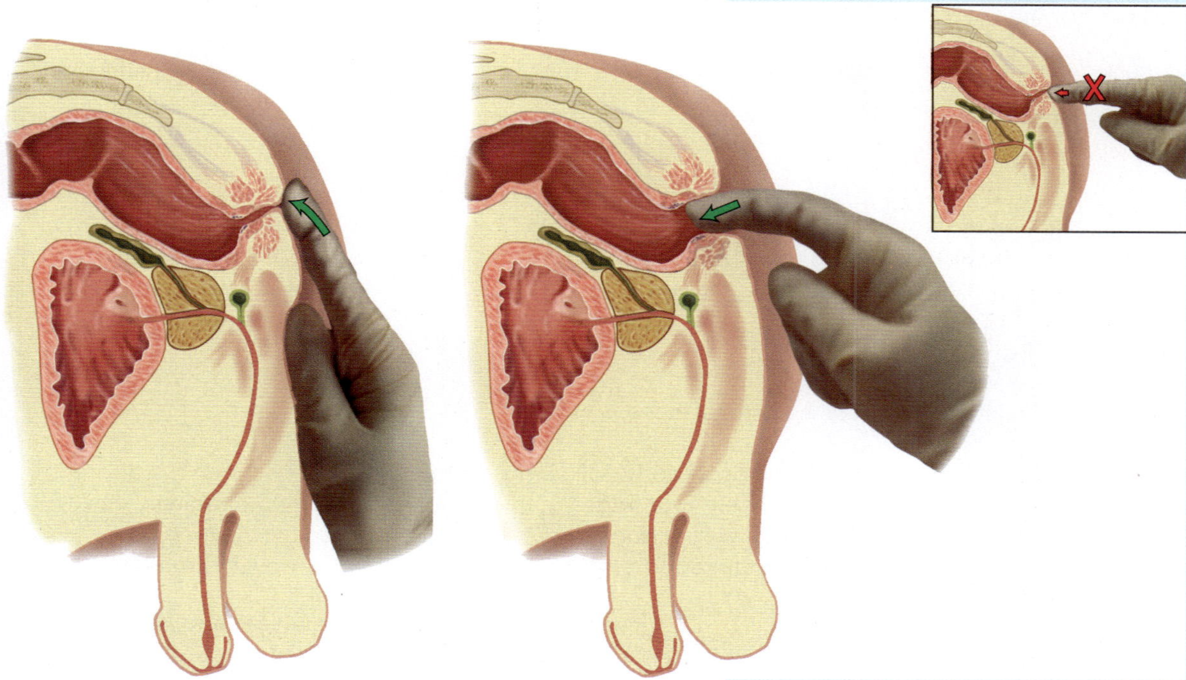

FIGURE 25.4 Palpating the anus and rectum

Rotate your examining finger to palpate the entire muscular ring. The canal should feel smooth and even. Note the intersphincteric groove circling the canal wall. To assess tone, ask the person to tighten the muscle. The sphincter should tighten evenly around your finger with no pain to the person.

Use a bidigital palpation with your thumb against the perianal tissue (Figure 25.5). Press your examining finger towards it. This manoeuvre highlights any swelling or tenderness and helps assess the bulbourethral glands.

Decreased tone.
Increased tone occurs with inflammation and anxiety.
Tenderness.

PROCEDURES AND NORMAL FINDINGS	ABNORMAL FINDINGS AND CLINICAL ALERTS

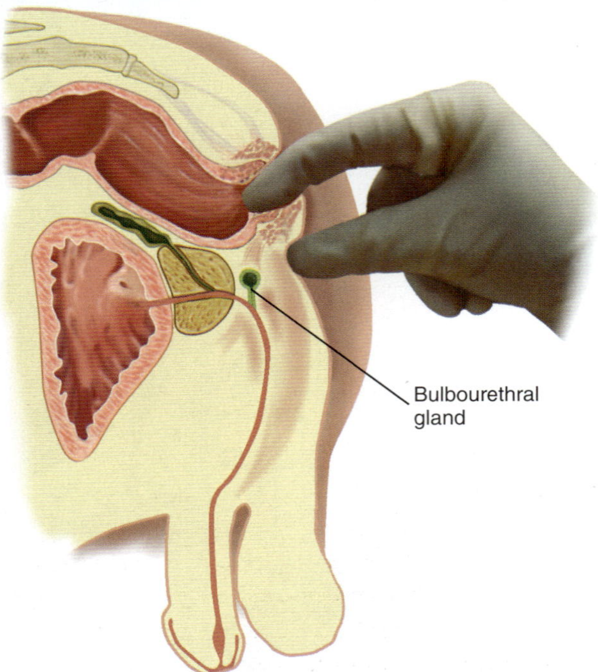

FIGURE 25.5 Bidigital palpation of the perianal tissue

Above the anal canal, the rectum turns posteriorly, following the curve of the coccyx and sacrum. Insert your finger further and explore all around the rectal wall. It normally feels smooth with no nodularity. Promptly report any mass you discover for further examination.

Internal haemorrhoid above anorectal junction is not palpable unless thrombosed.

A soft, slightly movable mass may be a polyp.

A firm or hard mass with irregular shape or rolled edges may signify carcinoma (Table 25.2).

Palpate any stool in the rectum and assess consistency. Stool should be soft.

Presence of hard stool in the rectum in addition to a history that indicates **constipation** is significant and requires further assessment. You may also need to perform an abdominal palpation to determine the extent of the faecal loading before prescribing treatment for constipation.

Withdraw your examining finger; normally, no bright red blood or mucus is on the glove. To complete the examination, offer the person tissues to remove the lubricant and help the person to a more comfortable position.

Abnormal findings for advanced practice

TABLE 25.2 Abnormalities of the rectum

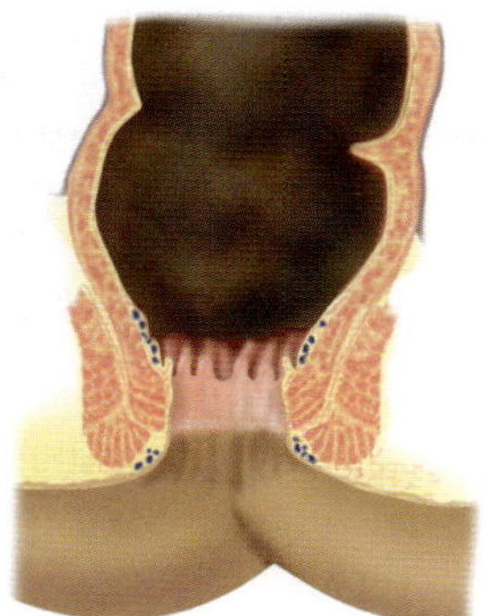

Faecal impaction

A collection of hard, desiccated, immovable faeces in the rectum. The obstruction often results from decreased bowel motility, in which more water is reabsorbed from the stool. For example, in people who have spinal cord injuries, poor diet, lack of exercise, opiate use or cognitive impairment. The person may complain of constipation or of diarrhoea and/or faecal incontinence as a faecal stream passes around the impaction.

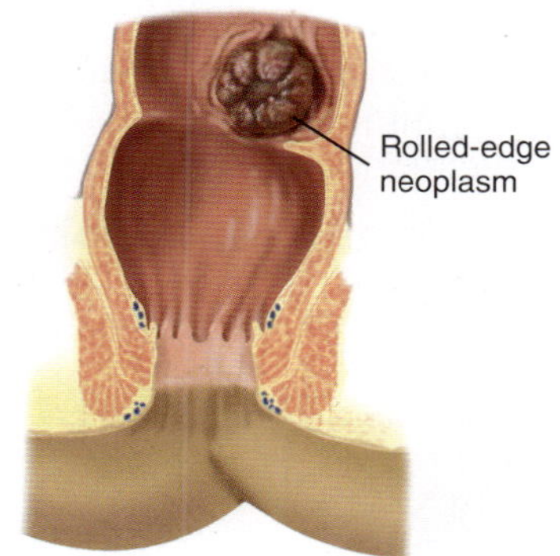

Carcinoma

A malignant neoplasm in the rectum is asymptomatic, thus the importance of routine bowel cancer screening. An early lesion may be a single firm nodule, which may bleed. As the lesion grows, it has an irregular cauliflower shape and is fixed and stone hard.

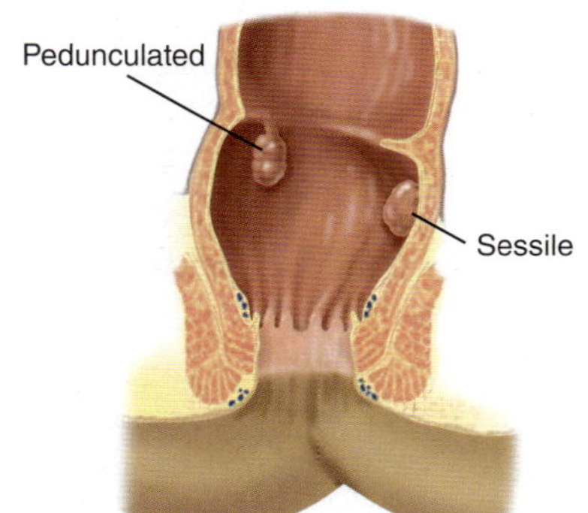

Rectal polyp

A protruding growth from the rectal mucous membrane that is common. The polyp may be *pedunculated* (on a stalk) or *sessile* (a mound on the surface, close to the mucosal wall). The soft nodule is difficult to palpate. Colonoscopy is needed as well as biopsy to screen for a malignant growth.

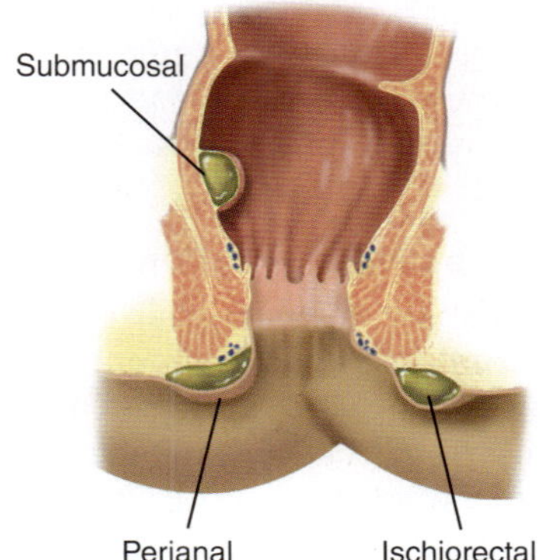

Abscess

A localised cavity of pus from infection in a pararectal space. Infection usually extends from an anal crypt. Characterised by persistent throbbing rectal pain. Termed by the space it occupies such as a perianal abscess is superficial around the anal skin and appears red, hot, swollen, indurated and tender. An ischiorectal abscess is deep and tender to bidigital palpation. It occurs laterally between the anus and ischial tuberosity and is uncommon.

Clinical reasoning and documentation

The following case studies give examples of typical situations involving bowel assessment and the clinical reasoning process including problem/issue identification. Consult a fundamentals of nursing or medical-surgical nursing text for information about goal setting, nursing interventions and evaluation.

Case study 1 (continued)—Postoperative constipation

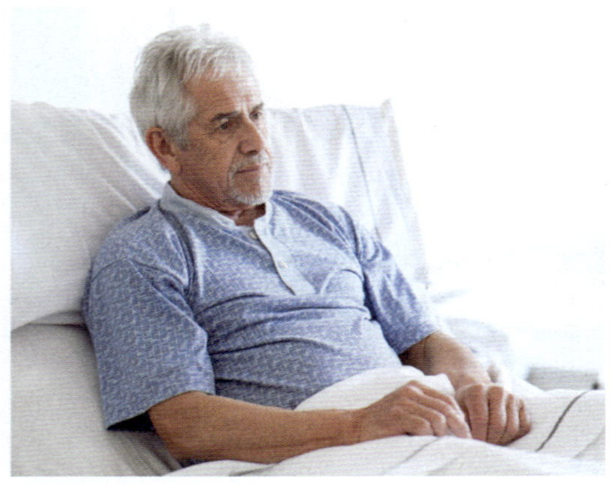

Context

You will recall from the case study described earlier in the chapter that you are a registered nurse working on an orthopaedic surgical ward. Your assessment was performed as part of a general survey on meeting the patient at the start of a shift.

Consider the patient's situation

Mr Jerry Wishart is a 78-year-old man who had a left total knee replacement 2 days ago. He was previously well with no major health problems other than severe osteoarthritis in the left knee and milder osteoarthritis in the right knee. The surgical procedure went well with no complications.

Collect cues/information

Your further assessment reveals the following information.

Subjective data

Mr Wishart expressed concern that he has not opened his bowels for 3 days and he is feeling bloated and uncomfortable. Normally he has a bowel movement every day and has a soft formed stool, which he estimates is Bristol score 3 or 4 using the Bristol stool chart.

He has been eating small amounts of food but feels that his appetite is not good. He normally makes his own breakfast muesli, which contains raw oats and oat bran as well as dried fruit and nuts. While in hospital he has been eating buttered toast for breakfast with a cup of tea. He normally eats several pieces of fresh fruit per day but has not been ordering fruit from the menu.

He is drinking tea when offered but not drinking much water because he says it tastes bad.

He took Panadol Osteo for joint pain relief before surgery.

Objective data

Sitting out of bed for most of the day and walking a short distance several times per shift with a gutter frame and assistance. Requiring regular pain medication—oxycodone and paracetamol, which has good effect.

Slightly rounded abdomen. Bowel sounds present on auscultation. Abdomen soft on palpation, firm mass in left lower quadrant with mild tenderness—consistent with a faecal mass.

Rectal examination not performed.

Process information and identify problems/issues

Collaborative problems

Constipation related to recent surgery, narcotic pain medication, reduced mobility and change of diet.

Problem statement / nursing diagnoses

Constipation related to decreased bowel motility secondary to recent surgery, narcotic pain medication, reduced mobility and change of diet.

Clinical reasoning and documentation cont'd

Case study 2—Acute diarrhoea

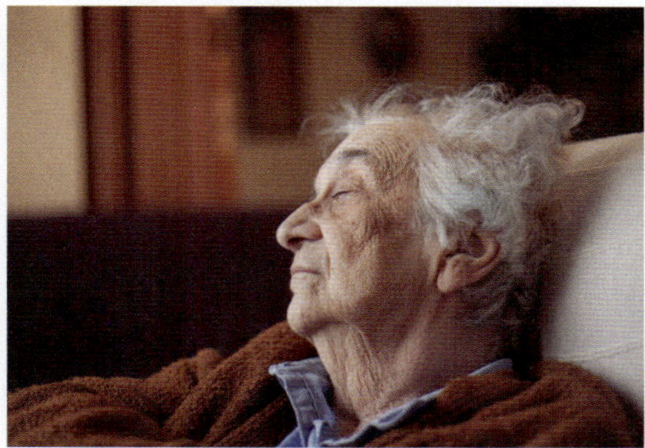

Context

You are a registered nurse working in a residential aged care facility.

Consider the patient's situation

On the afternoon shift, an aged care worker informs you that one of the residents has had several episodes of very loose bowel actions. Mrs Edna Grey is a 94-year-old woman who has lived in the aged care facility for 18 months. She was admitted to the facility following surgery for a left fractured neck of femur. She needs assistance with most activities of daily living; she has no cognitive impairment.

Collect cues/information

Subjective data

Mrs Grey says that she started to feel unwell earlier in the day with gripey abdominal pain, slight nausea and has since had three or four episodes of very loose and watery bowel actions. She says that she has eaten very little today and doesn't feel like drinking. She is concerned about getting assistance to get to the toilet quickly because she feels she needs to go urgently.

She normally has one bowel movement per day, which is easy to pass. She has only eaten food provided to her from the nursing home in the past few days.

She says she had a lot of visitors over the weekend, including several of her great grandchildren (aged 3 and 5).

Objective data

Appears pale. Afebrile. Vital signs within normal limits.

Mouth and oral mucous membranes dry. Tongue coated white. Water jug ¾ full (was changed early in the day).

Slightly rounded abdomen. Hyper resonant bowel sounds present on auscultation. Abdomen soft on palpation.

Rectal examination not performed. Perineal skin intact and not red.

Aged care worker reported that she had seen a bowel action in the toilet—Bristol 6 to 7.

Process information and identify problems/issues

Collaborative problems

Acute diarrhoea related to unknown cause—potentially an infection or food poisoning – for referral to a medical practitioner

Potential for infection outbreak related to acute diarrhoea

Problem statement/nursing diagnoses

Potential for fluid volume deficit related to acute diarrhoea

Potential for electrolyte imbalance related to acute diarrhoea

Potential for skin breakdown related to frequent bowel actions, wiping and cleansing

Potential for faecal incontinence related to faecal urgency and very loose stools

ADDITIONAL RESOURCES

You can further develop your knowledge and skills relevant to assessment of bowel function, related pathophysiology, common health issues and nursing interventions by:

- reading chapters of a fundamentals of nursing or medical-surgical nursing textbook
- answering chapter multiple choice questions online. Log onto ClinicalKey Student and search for the text 'Health Assessment, 4th edition'. Choose the section titled 'Teaching material'. In this section you will find question and answer documents for each chapter. Please check instructions on the inside front cover of the book to access online resources
- visiting websites

  Continence Foundation of Australia: https://www.continence.org.au

  Australian Association of Stomal Therapy Nurses: https://stomaltherapy.au

REFERENCES

1. On WH, Lim, WH, Yap K. Gastrointestinal system. In Tompkins, Z. editor, Applied anatomy and physiology: An interdisciplinary approach, Chatswood: Elsevier; 2020.
2. Marieb EM, Keller SM. Essentials of human anatomy and physiology. 13th Global ed. New York: Pearson; 2022.
3. Camilleri M (2022). The aging gastrointestinal tract: digestive and motility problems. In: Wang TC, Camilleri M, Lebwohl B, Wang KK, Lok AS (editors). Yamada's Textbook of Gastroenterology (pp. 505–511).
4. Ghosh TS, Shanahan F, O'Toole PW. The gut microbiome as a modulator of healthy ageing. Nature Reviews Gastroenterology & Hepatology. 2022 Sep;19(9):565–584.
5. Australian Institute of Health and Welfare (AIHW). Cancer in Australia 2021. Cancer series no.133. Cat. no. CAN 144. Canberra: AIHW; 2021. Available at: https://www.aihw.gov.au/reports/cancer/cancer-in-australia-2021/related-material
6. di Martino E, Smith L, Bradley SH, Hemphill S, Wright J, Renzi C, et al. Incidence trends for twelve cancers in younger adults: a rapid review. British Journal of Cancer. 2022 Jun 1;126(10): 1374–1386.
7. Te Aho o Te Kahu, Cancer Control Agency. He Pūrongo Mate Pukupuku o Aotearoa 2020, The State of Cancer in New Zealand 2020. Wellington: Te Aho o Te Kahu, Cancer Control Agency. 2021. Available at: https://www.tewhatuora.govt.nz/our-health-system/data-and-statistics/new-cancer-registrations-2020/
8. Gurney J, Stanley J, McLeod M, Koea J, Jackson C, Sarfati D. Disparities in Cancer-specific survival between Māori and non-Māori New Zealanders, 2007–2016. JCO Global Oncology. 2020 Jun;6:766–774.
9. International Continence Society (ICS). Glossary. 2023. Available at: https://www.ics.org/glossary
10. Bharucha AE, Knowles CH, Mack I, Malcolm A, Oblizajek N, Rao S, et al. Faecal incontinence in adults. Nature Reviews Disease Primers. 2022 Aug 10;8(1):53.
11. Musa MK, Saga S, Blekken LE, Harris R, Goodman C, Norton C. The prevalence, incidence, and correlates of fecal incontinence among older people residing in care homes: a systematic review. Journal of the American Medical Directors Association. 2019 Aug 1;20(8):956–962.
12. Lewandowska A, Rudzki G, Lewandowski T, Stryjkowska-Góra A, Rudzki S. Risk factors

for the diagnosis of colorectal cancer. Cancer Control. 2022 Jan 6;29:10732748211056692

13. Moullet M, Funston G, Mounce LT, Abel GA, de Wit N, Walter FM, et al. Pre-diagnostic clinical features and blood tests in patients with colorectal cancer: a retrospective linked-data study. British Journal of General Practice. 2022 Aug 1;72(721):e556–e563.
14. Australian Institute of Health and Welfare (AIHW). National Bowel Cancer Screening Program: monitoring report 2022. Cat. no. CAN 148. Canberra: AIHW; 2022. Available at: https://www.aihw.gov.au/reports/cancer-screening/nbcsp-monitoring-2022/summary
15. Australian Government, Department of Health and Aged Care. National Bowel Screening Program. 2023. Available at: https://www.health.gov.au/our-work/national-bowel-cancer-screening-program
16. Ministry of Health New Zealand. National Bowel Screening Program. 2023. Available at: https://www.health.govt.nz/our-work/preventative-health-wellness/screening/national-bowel-screening-programme
17. Rome Foundation. Rome IV criteria for functional gastrointestinal disorders. 2021. Available at: https://theromefoundation.org/rome-iv/rome-iv-criteria/
18. Bliss DZ, Igualada-Martinez P, Engberg S, Herbert JH, Gurvich OV, Igbedioh C, et al. Standard questions for a bowel diary to assess fecal incontinence in adults: a consensus project of the International Continence Society. Continence. 2023. 6:100588. https://doi.org/10.1016/j.cont.2023.100588
19. Gallo G, Realis Luc A, Trompetto M. Epidemiology, anorectal anatomy, physiology and pathophysiology of continence. In: Docimo L, Brusciano L (eds). Anal Incontinence: Clinical Management and Surgical Techniques. 2023 (pp. 9–17). Cham: Springer International Publishing.
20. Garza JM. Fecal Incontinence in Children. In: Faure C, Thapar N, Di Lorenzo C (eds). Pediatric Neurogastroenterology: Gastrointestinal Motility Disorders and Disorders of Gut Brain Interaction in Children 2023 Jan 1 (pp. 545–552). Cham: Springer International Publishing.

CHAPTER 26

UNIT 9

Assessing sexuality and reproductive function

Female sexual and reproductive assessment

Written by Carolyn Jarvis
Adapted by David Lee

INTRODUCTION

Many health issues and their treatments can have an adverse effect on a person's sexuality and sexual functioning. In some settings, a sexual or reproductive health issue will be the primary reason for the person seeking health care. It is an area of practice that many health professionals are reluctant to address due to embarrassment, perceived lack of time or other priorities and the feeling that they don't have the skills.[1] However, sexual and reproductive health is important to a person's general health and wellbeing. Health professionals should not wait for the person to bring up the issue; it should be part of a general health assessment.

Assessing female reproductive function is closely linked to assessing bladder and bowel function and breast health (refer to Chapters 23, 24, 25 and 28). In this chapter we will explore communicating effectively about sexual and reproductive health, which is also relevant to the following chapter related to male reproductive health.

It should be noted that while this chapter focuses on female reproductive health, we emphasise the importance of not making assumptions about a person's sexual orientation and gender identity. This important point needs to be considered when devising an assessment plan.

Case study

The following case study will help you identify your learning needs.

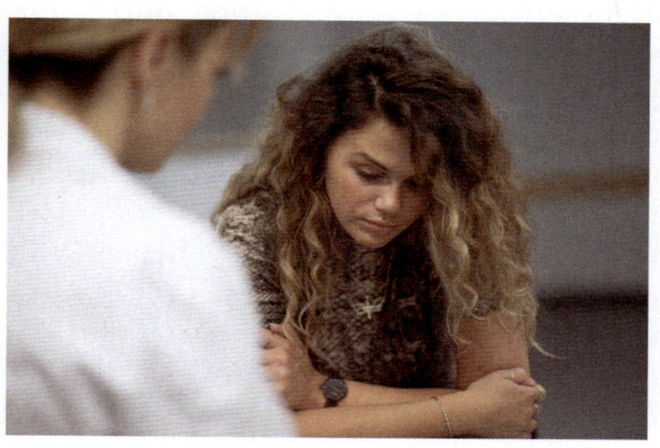

Context

You are a registered nurse working in a women's health clinic.

Consider the patient's situation

Ms Jacinta Knight, a 27-year-old woman, presents at the clinic with urinary burning, vaginal itch and discharge for 4 days.

Questions to further your learning

- What are the possible things that might be going on with Ms Knight?
- What knowledge do you need to be able to predict what might be going on?
- What approach to Ms Knight's health assessment will you take?
- What questions (subjective data) will you ask Ms Knight to extend the health history and why?
- What physical examination (objective data) will you conduct and why?
- What resources are available to assist in your assessment of Ms Knight?

Assessment plan

To assess sexual and reproductive function, identify potential or actual problems and plan care, a detailed knowledge of structure and function, developmental and cultural and social considerations are necessary before you start. You also need to consider your approach to communication and use of language around gender and gender identity. Detailed questions and physical examination techniques related to urinary and bowel functions are covered in Chapters 23, 24 and 25.

The person's responses to the opening questions suggested in the subjective data section will guide the sequence of the rest of the health interview. In most cases, it will be a relief for the person to raise their concerns with a health professional, even if they need referral to a nurse or medical practitioner for further specialised health assessment. Through the process of questioning the client or family you may become aware of gaps in the person's knowledge about living a healthy lifestyle. The opportunity to provide health information is an important part of health assessment.

The main areas for subjective assessment are:

- presenting concern
- general health history
- sexual health history
- reproductive health history
- health and lifestyle management.

Following subjective data collection, you will get a sense of the areas needed to be examined for objective assessment. Only the relevant areas should be examined.

The main areas for physical examination are:

- general inspection
- inspection of external genitalia.

Resources available

You will find additional resources and the reference list at the end of this chapter.

Structure and function

External genitalia

The external genitalia are called the **vulva** or pudendum (Figure 26.1). The **mons pubis** is a round, firm pad of adipose tissue covering the symphysis pubis. After puberty, it is covered with hair in the pattern of an inverted triangle. The **labia majora** are two rounded folds of adipose tissue extending from the mons pubis down and around to the perineum. After puberty, hair covers the outer surfaces of the labia, whereas the inner folds are smooth and moist and contain sebaceous follicles.

Inside the labia majora are two smaller, darker folds of skin, the **labia minora**. These are joined anteriorly at the clitoris where they form a hood or prepuce. The labia minora are joined posteriorly by a transverse fold, the **frenulum** or fourchette. The **clitoris** is a small, pea-shaped erectile body, homologous with the male penis and highly sensitive to tactile stimulation.

The labial structures encircle a boat-shaped space or cleft, termed the **vestibule**. Within it are numerous openings. The **urethral meatus** appears as a dimple 2.5 cm posterior to the clitoris. Surrounding the urethral meatus are the tiny, multiple **paraurethral (Skene's) glands**. Their ducts are not visible but open posterior to the urethra at the 5 and 7 o'clock positions.

The **vaginal orifice** is posterior to the urethral meatus. It appears either as a thin median slit or as a large opening with irregular edges, depending on the presentation of the membranous **hymen**. The hymen is a thin, circular or crescent-shaped fold that may cover part of the vaginal orifice or may be absent completely. On either side, and posterior to the vaginal orifice, are two **vestibular (Bartholin's) glands**, which secrete a clear lubricating mucus during intercourse. Their ducts are not visible but open in the groove between the labia minora and the hymen.

Pelvic floor muscles and perineum

The bony pelvis forms the solid structure for the muscles and ligaments of the anterior, posterior and lateral pelvic walls and pelvic

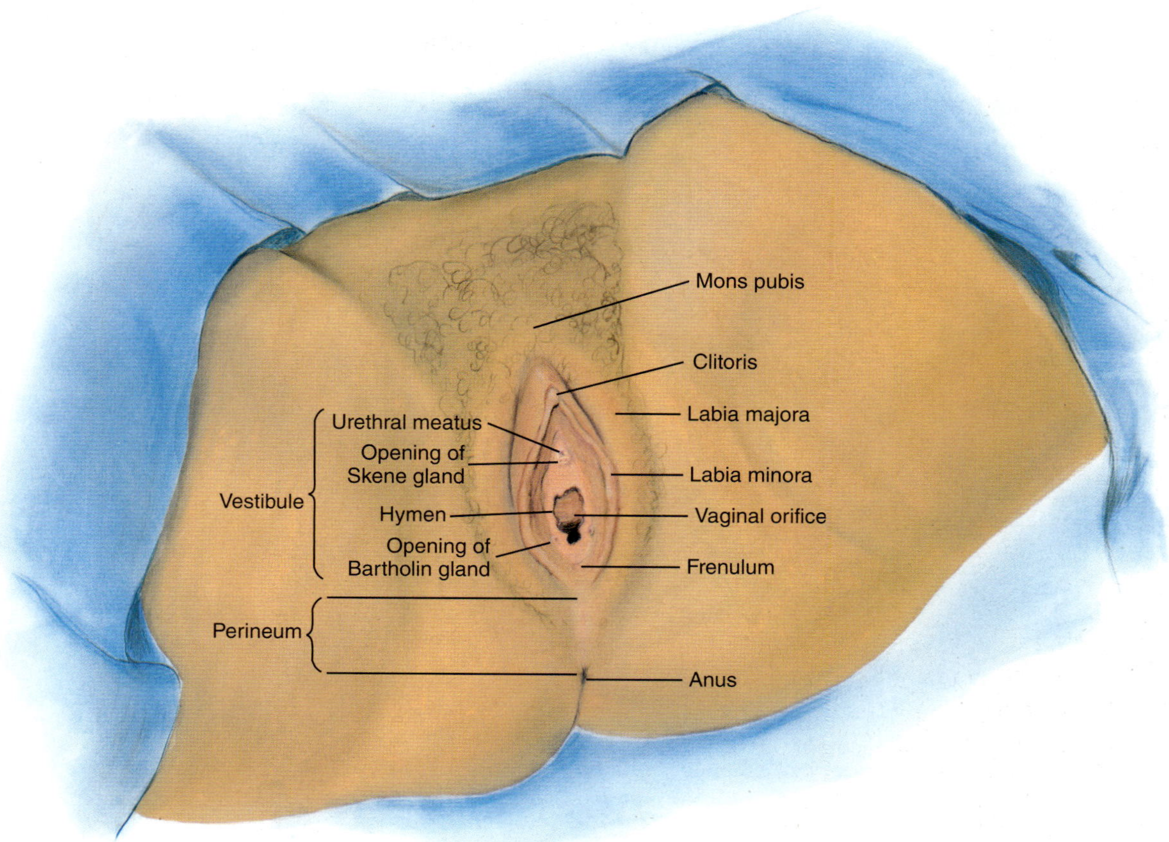

FIGURE 26.1 External female genitalia

floor, which play such an important role in supporting the position of the pelvic organs. The pelvic floor muscles include the coccygeus muscle and the levator ani and are referred to as the pelvic diaphragm, which stretches from the pubic bone anteriorly to the coccyx posteriorly and from the right and left lateral pelvic walls. The anal canal, urethra and vagina pass through the pelvic diaphragm. The levator ani muscles support the pelvic organs and functions as a sphincter for the anal canal and urethra.[2]

The perineum is located inferior to the pelvic diaphragm. The perineum extends from the symphysis pubis anteriorly to the coccyx posteriorly and the ischial tuberosities laterally. The muscles of the perineum are in two layers, superficial and deep. The superficial layer includes the superficial transverse perineal, bulbospongiosus and the ischiocavernosus muscles, which help to maintain erection of the clitoris. The deep layer of the perineum includes the deep transverse perineal muscle, the external urethral sphincter and external anal sphincter, which assist in maintaining urinary and faecal continence.[2]

Internal genitalia

The internal genitalia include the **vagina**, a flattened, tubular canal extending from the orifice up and backwards into the pelvis (Figure 26.2). It is 9 cm long and sits between the rectum posteriorly and the bladder and urethra anteriorly. Its walls are in thick

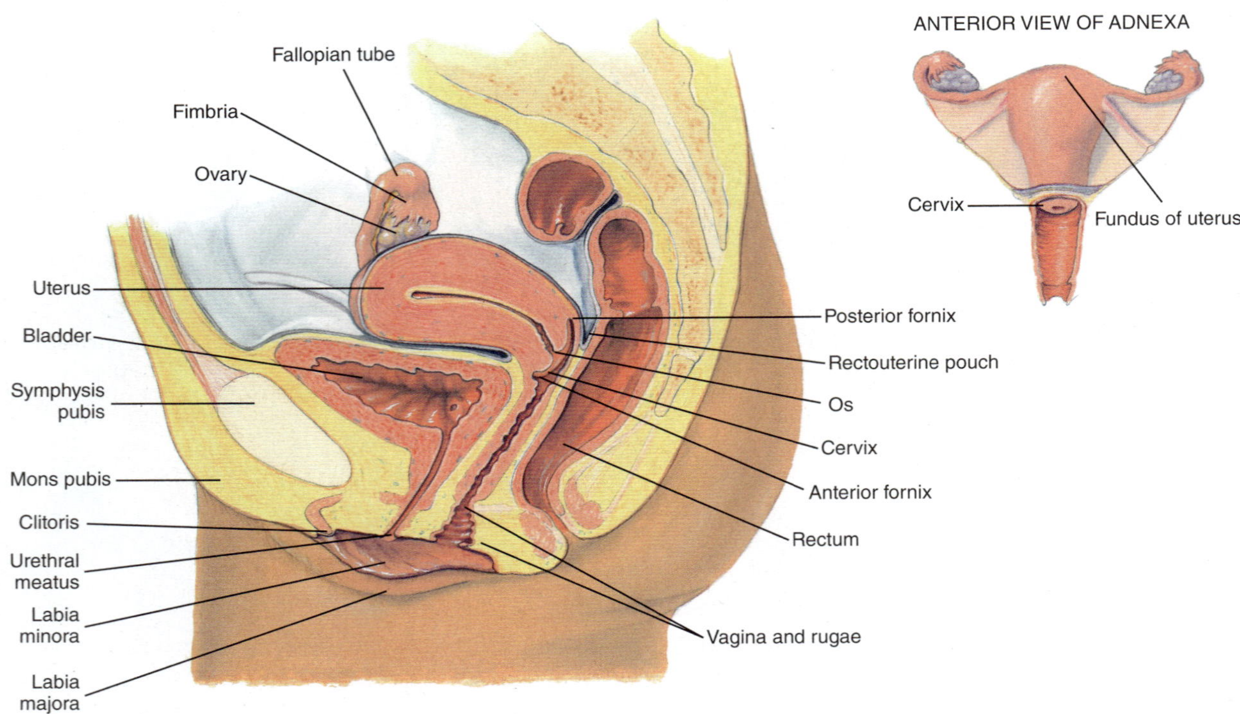

FIGURE 26.2 Female pelvic anatomy

transverse folds, or **rugae**, enabling the vagina to dilate widely during childbirth.

At the end of the canal, the uterine **cervix** projects into the vagina. In the nulliparous female, the cervix appears as a smooth doughnut-shaped area with a small circular hole, or **os**. After childbirth, the os is slightly enlarged and irregular. The cervical epithelium is of two distinct types. The vagina and cervix are covered with smooth, pink, stratified squamous epithelium. Inside the os, the endocervical canal is lined with columnar epithelium that looks red and rough. The point where these two tissues meet is the **squamocolumnar junction** and is not visible.

A continuous recess is present around the cervix, termed the **anterior fornix** in front and the **posterior fornix** at the back. Behind the posterior fornix, another deep recess is formed by the peritoneum. It dips down between the rectum and cervix to form the **rectouterine pouch** or **cul-de-sac of Douglas**.

The **uterus** is a pear-shaped, thick-walled, muscular organ. It is flattened anteroposteriorly, measuring 5.5 to 8 cm long by 3.5 to 4 cm wide and 2 to 2.5 cm thick. It is freely movable, not fixed and usually tilts forwards and superior to the bladder (a position labelled as anteverted and anteflexed; see Figure 26.21, later).

The **fallopian tubes** are two pliable, trumpet-shaped tubes, 10 cm in length, extending from the uterine fundus laterally to the brim of the pelvis. There they curve posteriorly, their fimbriated ends located near the **ovaries**. The two ovaries are located one on each side of the uterus at the level of the anterior superior iliac spine. Each is oval shaped, 3 cm long by 2 cm wide by 1 cm thick and serves to develop ova (eggs) and the female hormones.

HEALTH EDUCATION

Human papilloma virus vaccine

In Australia and Aotearoa New Zealand vaccination to prevent human papillomavirus (HPV) infection is part of the National Immunisation Program Schedule. HPV consists of a group of viruses that can cause skin and genital warts and some cancers, including cervical cancer. The vaccine targets HPV, the virus responsible for most cases of cervical cancer. It is recommended for girls and boys (usually 12–13 years of age) *before* they become sexually active because it is not effective if the person is already infected with HPV. There are a few formulations of the HPV vaccine—there is a bivalent, quadrivalent and 9-valent HPV vaccine (9vHPV). The 9vHPV vaccine requires a single dose only in immunocompetent people and is protective of cervical intraepithelial cancer (CIN) but also other cancers derived from HPV (anal cancer in men which is rare and oral cancer).[3]

HPV is a very common sexually transmitted virus. Most people who have had sex have been infected at some point in their lives. Most people never even know they have HPV because the virus usually does not cause any symptoms. However, sometimes the virus lingers in a woman's cervix and can cause changes that may eventually lead to cervical cancer. Other than the vaccine, the only way to prevent HPV is to abstain from all sexual activity. With the introduction of HPV immunisation, it is estimated that in countries with high uptake of the vaccination, cervical cancer will be nearly eliminated.[4]

Nurse's role

It is important to remind women that being immunised against HPV does not mean that women can forget about routine cervical screening tests (CST). The vaccine will protect against the major types of HPV that cause cervical cancer, but not all types. CST are recommended for women (people who have a cervix) from 25 years old. In Australia, this diagnostic test screens for HPV subtypes through a nucleic acid amplification test (DNA testing). Women are advised to screen every 5 years if normal until the age of 69 years old.[5] Abnormal CST has a robust follow-up algorithm, so reassure the woman that she will be contacted if there is an abnormal result.

In Aotearoa New Zealand, the CST changed to HPV primary screening in September 2023.[6]

Visit the following websites for more information:

- National (Australian) Cervical Cancer Screening Program: https://www.health.gov.au/our-work/national-cervical-screening-program
- Health New Zealand Government Understanding HPV Primary Screening: https://www.tewhatuora.govt.nz/for-the-health-sector/ncsp-hpv-screening/understand-hpv-primary-screening/.

Developmental considerations

Infants and adolescents

At birth, the external genitalia are engorged because of the presence of maternal estrogen. The structures recede in a few weeks, remaining small until puberty. The ovaries are in the abdomen during childhood. The uterus is small with a straight axis and no anteflexion.

At puberty, estrogens stimulate the growth of cells in the reproductive tract and the development of secondary sex characteristics. The first signs of puberty are breast and pubic hair development, beginning between the ages of 8½ and 13 years. Menarche occurs during the latter half of this sequence, just after the peak of growth velocity.

TABLE 26.1 Sex maturity ratings in girls

Stage 1: Preadolescent. No pubic hair. Mons and labia covered with fine vellus hair as on the abdomen.

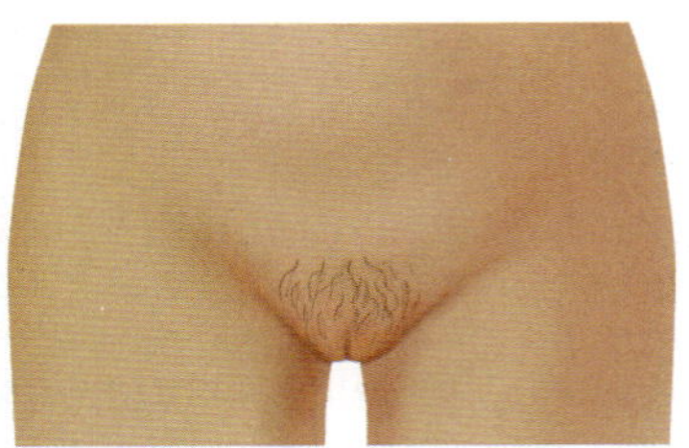

Stage 2: Growth sparse and mostly on the labia. Long, downy hair, slightly pigmented, straight or only slightly curly.

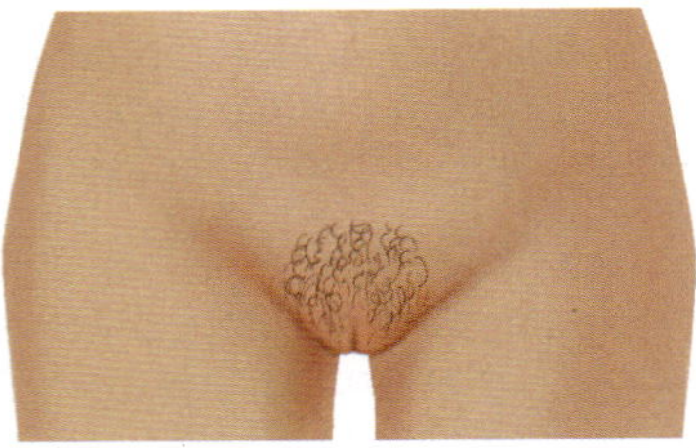

Stage 3: Growth sparse and spreading over the mons pubis. Hair is darker, coarser and curlier.

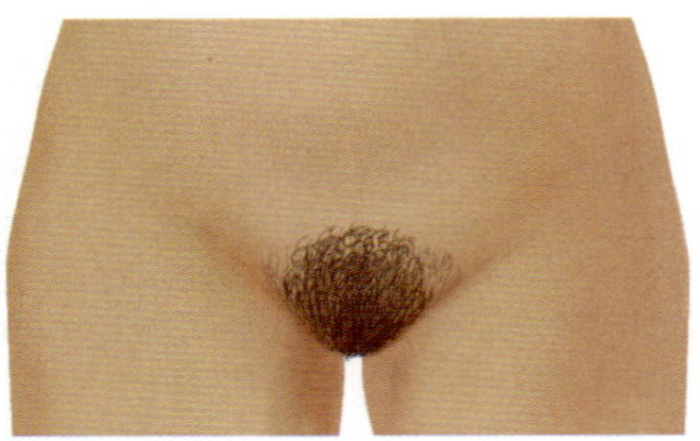

Stage 4: Hair is adult in type but over a smaller area; none on the medial thigh.

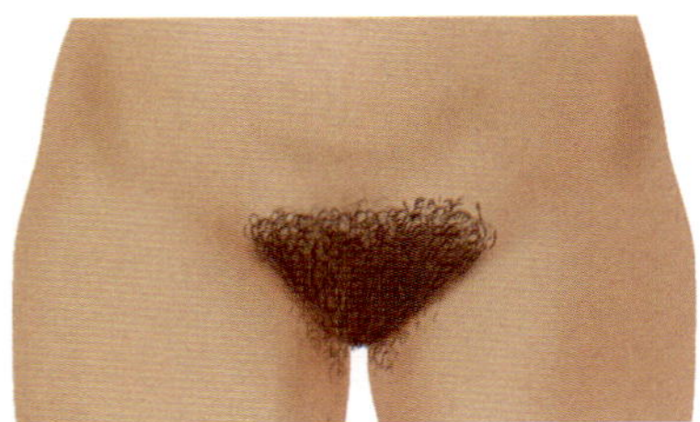

Stage 5: Adult in type and pattern; inverse triangle. Also on the medial thigh surface.

Adapted from Tanner 1962[7]

Irregularity of the menstrual cycle is common during adolescence because of the girl's occasional failure to ovulate. With menarche, the uterine body flexes on the cervix. The ovaries are now in the pelvic cavity.

Tanner's table on the five stages of pubic hair development (sex maturity ratings) is helpful in teaching girls the expected sequence of sexual development (Table 26.1). These data may not necessarily generalise to all people because there are wide individual variations in development.

Adult women

A woman will experience an average of 450 to 500 menstrual bleeds (or 'periods') throughout her lifetime. The menstrual cycle start is counted from the first day of a period and ends on the first day of bleeding of the next cycle. The menstrual cycle varies for each person and averages between 21 and 42 days. Periods (bleeding) tends to last between 4 and 8 days and loses 40 to 150 mL of menstrual fluid, which ranges from bright red to brownish in colour.[2]

The ovulatory phase of the period (mid-cycle) occurs before day 14 (of a 28-day cycle) when there is a surge of luteinising hormone, which stimulates mature follicles in an ovary to release an egg (ovulation). This is the time when fertility is high and pregnancy is most likely to occur.[2] Some women may experience this phase of their cycle when she experiences 'period pain' (mittelschmerz) unilaterally localised on either side of the abdomen and may be described as 'a twinge' to 'severe abdominal pain' lasting a few minutes to a few hours.[2]

The menstrual cycle is a conjoint of hormonal hypothalamus control and hormonal release from the ovaries and aims to prepare the body for pregnancy. The resultant of a non-pregnant state will result in a period. This complex hormonal relationship ends up with ovulation (release of eggs from the ovaries) and thickens the lining of the endometrium (proliferative phase) (Figure 26.3). Further to preparing the woman for pregnancy, the menstrual cycle has no other known physiological features.

The vaginal microbiome (or environment) has an important role in sexual and reproductive health and provides a protective physical and immunological barrier to invasive organisms. The vaginal microbiome protects pathogens from bypassing the cervix through metabolism of glycogen, which produces lactic acid and acidifies the vaginal environment. The optimal vaginal microbiota is dominated by beneficial *Lactobacillus* species (e.g. *L. crispatus*, *L. iners*). A healthy vaginal pH is typically less than 4.5, in which *Lactobacillus* can survive but is too acidic for several other types of bacteria.[8] Changes in the microbiome may be caused hormonally, neurologically, physiologically or by medical treatments such as antibiotic use. These factors can cause a change in the pH towards a less acidic environment and enable other vaginal bacteria or *Candida* species to overgrow, causing infection.[8]

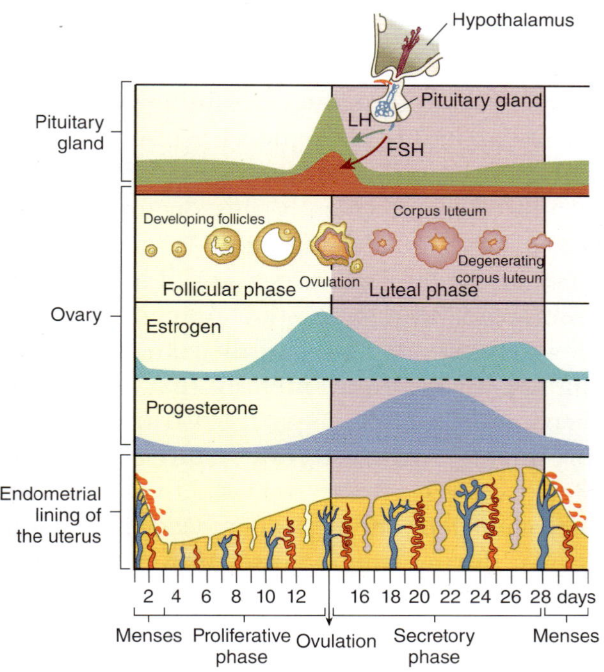

FIGURE 26.3 Events of the menstrual cycle

Fertility, infertility and pregnancy choices

Society places demands, and perhaps high expectations and pressure, on women to be fertile. Perhaps one of the most important scientific breakthroughs has been the oral contraceptive pill, and more recently long-acting reversible contraception, which has provided women with a choice of planning their personal life journey. Two-thirds of Australian women are on a form of contraception.[9]

Women who choose not to go down the medical contraceptive pathway also have a choice in accessing an emergency contraceptive pill (morning-after pill) as soon as possible after unprotected sex (can be taken up to 120 hours or 5 days after unprotected sex depending on the type of drug).[10] The morning-after pill is available 'over the counter' from local pharmacies, without the need for a medical prescription.

Unplanned pregnancies remain an issue in Australia, although there is no accurate data on the rates of unintended pregnancies. However, it is estimated that one in four pregnancies in Australia are unplanned.[11] The incidence of unintended pregnancy is similar in Aotearoa New Zealand (183 per 1,000 pregnancies).[12] In an Australian study, 25 to 33% of women who had an unintended pregnancy opted for a termination of pregnancy (TOP).[11]

There are safe and effective options for women who choose a termination. This can be a medical choice (using mifepristone and misoprostol) or a surgical termination. Surgical TOP (STOP) is usually done up to 12 weeks' gestation and medical TOP (MTOP) up to 9 weeks' gestation.[13] The cost of these procedures may not be fully covered by the Australian public health insurance, Medicare (there may be a 'gap cost' in addition to the Medicare rebate). The access to MTOP became more accessible with the Australian Pharmaceutical Benefits Scheme allowing medical practitioners and GPs to prescribe the medicines. In the past, this was restricted to specially licensed medical practitioners.

In Aotearoa New Zealand, 18.6% of known pregnancies ended in an abortion in 2020. Termination of pregnancy was decriminalised in 2020.[14] Legislative changes in the Aotearoa New Zealand Parliament in 2021 means that doctors, midwives, nurse practitioners and registered nurses can provide abortions (subject to scopes of practice and training), a person seeking an abortion no longer needs a referral from a doctor to access abortion services, and counselling is not mandatory but must be offered.

The shift of women planning pregnancy past 30 years of age has increased since the 1970s. Unfortunately, this also means an increase in 'infertility' because the fertile period appears to decline in women after 30 years of age. Assisted reproductive techniques, such as in-vitro fertilisation, has improved vastly since the 1980s and has successfully assisted many women towards healthy family planning.

Pregnant women

A complete discussion of pregnancy assessment is presented in Chapter 29. In summary, shortly after the first missed menstrual period, the genitalia show signs of the growing fetus. The cervix softens (Goodell's sign) at 4 to 6 weeks and the vaginal mucosa and cervix look cyanotic (Chadwick's sign) at 8 to 12 weeks. These changes occur because of increased vascularity and oedema of the cervix and hypertrophy and hyperplasia of the cervical glands. The isthmus of the uterus softens (Hegar's sign) at 6 to 8 weeks.

The greatest change is in the uterus itself. It increases in capacity by 500 to 1,000 times its non-pregnant state, at first because of hormone stimulation and then because of the increasing size of its contents.[2] A non-pregnant uterus has a flattened pear shape. Its early growth encroaches on the space occupied by the bladder, producing the symptom of urinary frequency. By 10 to 12 weeks' gestation, the uterus becomes globular in shape and is too large to stay in the pelvis. At 20 to 24 weeks, the uterus has an oval shape. It rises almost to the liver, displacing the intestines superiorly and laterally.

Women over 65 years

In contrast to the slowly declining hormones in ageing males, a female's hormonal milieu decreases rapidly. **Menopause** is cessation of the menses. Usually this occurs around 48 to 53 years, although a wide variation of ages from 35 to 60 years exists. The stage of menopause includes the preceding 1 to 2 years of decline in ovarian function, shown by irregular menses that gradually become further apart. Ovaries stop producing progesterone and estrogen. Because cells in the reproductive tract are estrogen-dependent, decreased estrogen levels during menopause bring dramatic physical changes.

The uterus reduces in size because of decreased myometrium. The ovaries atrophy to 1 to 2 cm and are not palpable after menopause. Ovulation still may occur sporadically after menopause. The sacral ligaments relax and the pelvic musculature weakens, predisposing the woman to pelvic organ prolapse, particularly in women who have had vaginal births. The cervix decreases in size and looks paler with a thick, glistening epithelium.

The vagina becomes shorter, narrower and less elastic because of increased connective tissue. The vaginal epithelium atrophies, becoming thinner and drier. This results in a fragile mucosal surface that is at risk for bleeding and vaginitis. Decreased vaginal secretions leave the vagina dry and at risk for irritation and pain with intercourse (dyspareunia). The vaginal pH becomes more alkaline and decreased glycogen content occurs from the decreased estrogen. These factors also increase the risk of vaginitis (infection or inflammation of the vagina) because they create a suitable medium for pathogens.

In late older age, externally, the mons pubis looks smaller because the fat pad atrophies. The labia and clitoris gradually decrease in size. Pubic hair becomes thin and sparse. However, sexual desire and sexuality do not diminish with age.

Cultural and social considerations

There are varying cultural considerations to do with assessing sexual and reproductive function in women, including for some woman the requirement to be examined only by a female healthcare practitioner. Ascertain the woman's requirements before beginning the examination.

Family relationships and violence

You will have read Chapter 5—family violence—for guidance on assessment in this area. Family violence also includes socio-cultural issues such as female-genital mutilation, forced marriage and arranged child-marriage from birth. Questions about family violence in history taking should be offered routinely and questions asked with respect, courteously and in a way that values ethical principles of autonomy, beneficence, non-maleficence, justice and informed consent in a safe and private environment.

Communicating effectively with people about sexuality and sexual function

Our perceptions of our sexuality affect the way we view ourselves as humans. The World Health Organization[15] has a definition of human sexuality that is useful to consider:

> *[Sexuality is]... a central aspect of being human throughout life and encompasses sex, gender identities and roles, sexual orientation, eroticism, pleasure, intimacy and reproduction. Sexuality is experienced and expressed in thoughts, fantasies, desires, beliefs, attitudes, values, behaviours, practices, roles and relationships. While sexuality can include all of these dimensions, not all of them are always experienced or expressed. Sexuality is influenced by the interaction of biological, psychological, social, economic, political, cultural, ethical, legal, historical, religious and spiritual factors.*

It is clear to see from this definition that sexuality is an important aspect of human existence and therefore should not be ignored by nurses and other healthcare clinicians. These definitions also remind us that sexuality is much broader than just 'sexual function'.

Part of the difficulty in addressing a sexual health problem is in overcoming the embarrassment of the person and the health professional. There is evidence that people want to discuss their sexual problems with health professionals, but they find that health professionals are often unwilling or reluctant to do so.[16,17] Several studies have found that registered nurses rarely discuss sexuality and sexual function because they feel fear and embarrassment in raising or discussing the issues.[16–18] Communicating with the person about their sexuality and sexual function is clearly an important skill for nurses and other health professionals. Health concerns in this area are likely to cause significant distress for the person, and therefore you need to approach the assessment in a tactful and empathic way. Privacy is of upmost importance, along with the need to establish a trusting relationship with the person. See Chapter 7 for more information about communication skills in health assessment.

Another aspect of communicating effectively in healthcare settings is not making assumptions. In the context of sexuality and sexual health, this includes not making assumptions about a person's sexual orientation and gender identity. Specifically, this means assuming that the person identifies as heterosexual, lesbian, gay, bisexual or a particular gender. Language is important in conveying acceptance of the person and respect for their self-worth and inherent dignity.[19] Therefore, it is important to understand commonly used terminology related to gender identity and sexuality. The following terms are a general guide; each person has their own preferred language describing their sexuality and terms evolve and change over time (adapted from):[19,20]

- **Biological sex** (*What sex were you assigned at birth?*)—an anatomical descriptor of the person's genitals, chromosomes, hormones and other physical and reproductive traits.
- **Gender or gender identity** (*What is your current gender identity?*)—the way in which a person identifies or expresses their masculine or feminine characteristics (male, female or other identity). A person's gender identity or gender expression is not always exclusively male or female and may change over time. The gender identity of the person may be reflected in the pronouns they use to describe themselves (for example, he/him/she/her/they/their). *What pronouns do you use?*
- **Cisgender**—people who identify their gender in the same way that was legally assigned to them at birth.
- **Heterosexual**—a person who is sexually and/or romantically attracted to the opposite gender.
- **Sexual orientation**—a person's romantic and/or sexual attraction towards another person including (but not confined to) heterosexual, gay, lesbian, bisexual, pansexual, asexual or same-sex attracted.
- **Asexual**—a sexual orientation that reflects little to no sexual attraction, either within or outside relationships. People who identify as asexual can still experience romantic attraction across the sexuality continuum. While asexual people do not experience sexual attraction, this does not necessarily imply a lack of libido or sex drive.
- **LGBTIQ+**—acronym for lesbian, gay, bisexual, transgender, intersex/intersex and queer/questioning people collectively.

- **Lesbian**—refers to women whose sexual and/or romantic attraction is towards other people who identify as women.
- **Gay**—a person whose primary sexual and/or romantic attraction is towards other people who identify as men. The term is most used to refer to men, although some women use it.
- **Bisexual**—a person whose sexual and/or romantic attraction is to people of the same sex or gender as well as people of other genders.
- **Non-binary**—a person who does not identify exclusively as male or female. A non-binary person might identify as gender fluid, trans masculine, trans feminine or could be agender (without a feeling of having any gender or having neutral feelings about gender).
- **Pansexual**—a person whose sexual and/or romantic attraction to others is not restricted by gender, regardless of their gender identity.
- **Queer**—an umbrella term covering a range of sexual orientations and gender identities. Some LGBTIQ+ people may still perceive 'queer' to be an insult.
- **Gender dysphoria**—defined in DSM-5[21] as the 'distress caused and experiences as a result of the sex and gender they were assigned at birth'. The removal of the word 'disorder' from previous DSM editions sought to destigmatise and reduce societal discrimination against gender-diverse people. These clinical criteria are used to access gender affirmation treatments hormonally or surgically.
- **Transgender**—or 'transgender and gender diverse' are terms for people whose gender identity is different than that legally assigned to them at birth. These people may also refer to themselves as 'trans', 'transsexual' or 'transgender'. Being transgender is not related to the person's sexual orientation; a transgender person may be heterosexual, gay, lesbian, bisexual or another sexual orientation. Trans and gender diverse people may take steps to live in their nominated sex with or without medical treatment (see 'Transition') and they should be referred to as their preferred gender regardless of whether or not they have used medical or surgical treatment.
- **Transition**—transition may involve social, medical and/or legal processes to affirm a person's gender identity.
- **Intersex**—refers to people who are born with physical, hormonal or genetic characteristics that do not conform to biological norms for male or female bodies. Intersex people have a diversity of bodies and identities.
- **Brotherboy**—a culturally specific term to describe Aboriginal and Torres Strait Islander transgender men.
- **Sistergirl**—a culturally specific term to describe Aboriginal and Torres Strait Islander transgender women.
- **Takatāpui**—a Māori term, meaning 'intimate companion of the same sex'. It is culturally specific and not easily translated into English. Māori and Pacific Islander peoples have their own terms for gender identity (see 'Takatāpui—a resource hub' in the 'Additional resources' section).

Be cautious about recording information about sexual orientation, gender identity or intersex condition in a person's medical or health record. You should seek consent from the person and inform them about why the information is needed and to whom it will be made available. There is no legal requirement to disclose or to document a disclosure.[22,23] There are many excellent resources available to health professionals to assist them in communicating and engaging with people from diverse backgrounds, and some of these are referred to in the 'Additional resources' section at the end of this chapter.

Subjective data

Practice note

Before you start the assessment, introduce yourself to the person, confirm the person's identity, discuss the purpose and scope of the assessment, clarify any questions the person may have and obtain verbal consent from the person to perform the assessment.

As you approach the health assessment interview it is important that you:

- don't make assumptions about the person's gender identity and sexual orientation based on appearance
- use open and inclusive questions that are gender neutral and inclusive
- encourage the person to discuss their sexual orientation, gender identity and relationship status
- respect a person's choice not to disclose their sexual or gender identity
- respond positively when the person is prepared to be open about their sexual orientation, gender identity or intersex condition
- ask how they would like to be addressed and what pronouns they use if you are unsure of how to address the person
- begin with open-ended questions to assess individual needs
- be flexible with the structure of this part of the health assessment to ensure you follow up with the issues that are important to the person first, and then complete the other relevant areas.

ASSESSMENT GUIDELINES	CLINICAL SIGNIFICANCE AND CLINICAL ALERTS
Presenting concern	
It is important to ascertain the person's perception of their sexual and/or reproductive health. From the presenting concern, the person would be able to provide you with some insight into their symptoms and perhaps other health issues. If they do perceive a problem, ask: *How does this affect your quality of life?* The responses to these questions will guide the sequence of the rest of the subjective data collection. Take the cues from the person. If the person is unable to articulate their health concern, use questions below to assist them to verbalise their health situation. A suggested approach: • *I would like to ask you some questions to find out more about how I can help you today. Some of the questions might appear intrusive and personal but will assist me in identifying your healthcare needs. Is it OK with you if I ask these questions?*	

ASSESSMENT GUIDELINES	CLINICAL SIGNIFICANCE AND CLINICAL ALERTS
• *What brings you here today? What concerns do you have about your sexual and reproductive health?*	
General health history	
Recent illness • *Have you experienced any recent illness?*	
Personal health history • *Have you had any surgery?* • *Do you have any medical conditions?* • *Do you have any allergies?* • *Do you have any health difficulties such as with mobility, pain or disability?*	
Family history • *Do you or any significant family member have a history of diabetes, epilepsy, clotting disorders, hypertension or cardiovascular disease or reproductive cancer?*	
Current and past cigarette smoking/vaping • *How many cigarettes do you smoke per day? How many vapes? How long have you been smoking/vaping?*	**Oral contraceptives**, together with cigarette smoking, increase the risk of cardiovascular health issues.
Current and past alcohol and illicit substance use • *How much alcohol do you drink (glasses, bottles, cans etc.)? How often do you drink alcohol (every day, every week etc.)? How long have you been drinking that amount of alcohol?* • *Have you used illicit or prescription drugs not prescribed for you? What drugs? How much? How often (including injecting drug use)?*	Personal health risks as well as putting the person at risk of unsafe sex or sexual violence.
Current medication • *Are you taking any prescribed medications, complementary and traditional therapies or over-the-counter medications?*	Oral contraceptives increase glycogen content of vaginal epithelium, providing fertile medium for some organisms which cause **vaginitis**. Broad-spectrum antibiotics alter balance of normal flora, which can predispose to **candida vaginal infection.**
Social history (see also Chapter 8) • *What is your highest educational achievement? High school, TAFE or university?* • *What are your living arrangements?* • *Do you have contact and support from family members? Friends?* • *Do you have any hobbies and/or regular activities?*	

ASSESSMENT GUIDELINES	CLINICAL SIGNIFICANCE AND CLINICAL ALERTS
Sexual health history	
Start with a general statement and question such as: '*When I conduct a health assessment, I ask people about their sexual health. Is it alright with you if I ask questions about your sexual health?*' This may help you open the discussion with the person. Only ask questions that are relevant to the situation.	
Genital signs and symptoms If a woman presents with symptoms, then concentrate on a symptom history—length of time, precipitating factors, pain, improvement and experience. Ask about current or past symptoms related to urethral, vaginal or anal discharge (amount, odour, colour and character). Questions may include: • *Have you experienced any abnormal vaginal or rectal bleeding, genital rashes, lumps or sores?* 'If yes, ask the person to describe the sign or symptom: • *When did it start?* • *What have you done about it, and did this reduce the symptom?* Normal vaginal discharge is small, clear or cloudy and always non-irritating.	Abnormal vaginal discharge may be described as white, yellow-green, grey, curd-like and/or foul smelling. Suggests **vaginal infection**; character of discharge often suggests causative organism. May be acute or chronic.
• If the person has an abnormal vaginal discharge, ask: *Is this associated with vaginal itching, rash or pain with intercourse?*	Occurs because of irritation from discharge. **Dyspareunia** (pain with sexual intercourse) occurs with **vaginitis** of any cause.
• *Do you ever experience a feeling of fullness or dragging in the vagina, perineum or rectum?* If yes, ask the person to describe the sign or symptom: • *When did it start?* • *What have you done about it? Did it help?*	These symptoms (and sometimes urinary and/or bowel symptoms) may indicate **pelvic organ prolapse**. **Cystocele**—anterior vaginal wall defect causing the bladder to prolapse posteriorly into the vagina. **Rectocele**—posterior vaginal wall defect causing the rectum to prolapse anteriorly into the vagina. These symptoms require further assessment by a medical or nurse practitioner.
Urinary or bowel symptoms or lower abdominal pain • *Have you experienced any problem with your bladder or bowel or experienced any abdominal pain?* (Ask about urinary symptoms such as urgency, slow stream, feeling of incomplete emptying or incontinence; typical bowel symptoms such as constipation, difficulty in defecation or feeling of incomplete emptying.) If yes, ask the person to describe the sign or symptom: • *When did it start?* • *What have you done about it? Did it help?*	**Urinary or faecal incontinence** or bothersome lower urinary tract symptoms can significantly affect a person's sexuality and sexual function and requires further assessment. For details about assessment of urinary function, see Chapter 24; bowel function, see Chapter 25; and assessment of abdominal pain, see Chapter 23.

ASSESSMENT GUIDELINES	CLINICAL SIGNIFICANCE AND CLINICAL ALERTS
Breast symptoms • *Have you experienced any pain or other abnormal symptoms in your breasts?* If yes, ask the person to describe the sign or symptom: • *When did it start?* • *What have you done about it? Did it help?*	Breast symptoms are often associated with hormonal changes. Any unusual change in the breast should be further assessed and/or referred to a medical practitioner. For details about breast assessment see Chapter 28.
Sexual activity (if relevant) • *Are you currently sexually active?* • *At what age did you have your first sexual contact?* • *When was the last time that you had sex?* • *Do you have a regular or casual sexual partner? How long have you been with this person?* • *What type of sexual contact do you have—oral, vaginal, anal?* • *How many sexual partners have you had in the past 12 months?* • *Have you had sex that you can't remember because of alcohol or substance use?* • *Any history with a partner from overseas?* **Contraception** (if relevant) • *Are you currently using contraception to avoid pregnancy? What specifically?* • If on the combined oral contraceptive pill, ask about adherence: *Have you missed any pills in the past two packs?* • If on the progestogen only pill, ask about adherence; *Have you taken the pill at the same time daily in the past two packets?* • If using long active reversible contraception, some women will have amenorrhoea and others will have a 'breakthrough bleed'. • If using an intrauterine device: *Have you had any side effects?* • *Do you use condoms?* • *Do you use the morning-after pill? When? Any side effects?*	Determining the person's sexual practices will enable you to identify areas for health education or the need for further questioning to identify risk factors for sexually transmitted infections (STIs), personal safety and/or the need for specific physical examination and other investigations.
Assess knowledge of effects, precautions and side effects of contraceptive. • *Are you happy with this form of contraception?* • *Have you experienced any side effects? If so, what? How have you managed this?*	This information will give direction to possible areas for further discussion and health information or the need for referral to family planning or sexual health services.

ASSESSMENT GUIDELINES	CLINICAL SIGNIFICANCE AND CLINICAL ALERTS
Sexually transmitted infection (STI) • *Do you have any symptoms today?* Ask about an abnormal vaginal discharge, pain passing urine or any abnormal bleeding. • *Have you or your partner ever been diagnosed with a STI (e.g. chlamydia)?* • *If so, what symptoms did you experience? How long ago? How was it treated?* • *Have you ever had a test for HIV or hepatitis B or C?* Screen for knowledge of prevention of STIs including use of condoms.	An **STI** includes all conditions that can be transmitted during intercourse or intimate sexual contact with an infected partner.
Sexual function and satisfaction (if relevant) • *Are you satisfied with the sexual relationship you have with your partner(s)?* • *Are you satisfied with the way you and your partner(s) communicate about sex?* • *Are you satisfied with your ability to respond sexually?*	There are validated sexual health/satisfaction assessment tools available (e.g. the female sexual function questionnaire).
• *Have you experienced any sexual difficulties or dysfunction?* Ask about: • low sexual desire or sexual arousal • vaginal dryness (lack of lubrication, 'wetness', on arousal or during sexual activity) • difficulty in achieving an orgasm, lack of sexual satisfaction • pain during intercourse • other sexual issues. If they are experiencing any difficulties, ask: *How much does this bother you?* (scale of 1–5; 1 is not bothered at all, 5 is extremely bothered).	**Dyspareunia** is pain with sexual intercourse that can be deep or superficial. **Vaginismus** is an involuntary spasm or contraction of the pelvic floor muscles making penetration painful or impossible causing personal and/or relationship distress. Women who are concerned about their sexual health should be referred to a medical or nurse practitioner or sexual health clinic for further assessment.
Family violence, sexual abuse, assault or unwanted sexual experiences (if relevant) See questions and approach to assessment described in Chapter 5 for detail on assessment related to screening for family violence and abuse.	May prompt need for follow-up and referral for counselling. See Chapter 5.
Reproductive health history	
Menstrual history • *What was the date of your last normal menstrual period?*	**LMP**—last menstrual period.
• *At what age did you have your first period?*	**Menarche**—mean age at onset at 12 or 13 years; delayed onset suggests endocrine or underweight problem. **Primary amenorrhoea**—failure to start menstruating by 17 years of age.[24]

ASSESSMENT GUIDELINES	CLINICAL SIGNIFICANCE AND CLINICAL ALERTS
• *How often are your periods?* Cycle—normally every 18 to 45 days.	**Amenorrhoea** is absence of menses. **Secondary amenorrhoea** is the cessation of menstruation for 6 months or more.[24] **Polycystic ovary syndrome** is a complex hormonal condition associated with irregular menstrual periods, excessive facial and body hair, acne, weight gain, cysts on the ovaries, reduced fertility and an increased risk of insulin insensitivity and therefore type 2 diabetes.
• *How many days does your period last?* Duration—average 3 to 7 days.	
• *Usual amount of flow: light, medium, heavy?* • *How many pads or tampons do you use each day or hour?* If relevant—*How often do you change the menstrual cup?*	**Menorrhagia** is heavy menses. **Endometriosis** is a condition that affects 10% of adult women. Symptoms include menorrhagia, pelvic pain, bloating, nausea, infertility and fatigue. Women with these symptoms need prompt referral to a specialist for diagnosis and management.
• *Have you noticed any clotting?*	Clotting indicates heavy flow or vaginal pooling.
• *Do you experience any pain or cramps before or during period? How do you treat it? Does it interfere with your day-to-day activities?* • *Do you experience any other associated symptoms: bloating, breast tenderness, moodiness?* • *Do you have any spotting between periods?*	**Dysmenorrhoea** is the experience of painful periods.
• *Do you experience any abnormal vaginal bleeding (post-coital, bleeding between periods)?* • *If so, what have you done about it?* • *Do you take medication to regulate your menstrual cycle (contraceptive pill or other hormonal medication)?*	Bleeding between periods can be an indication of hormonal imbalance or a side effect of hormonal contraception. Abnormal vaginal bleeding can also be present with infection or changes in the cervix and uterus that require further assessment by a medical practitioner.
Menopause • *Have your periods slowed down or stopped?*	**Menopause** is the cessation of menstruation, usually considered to be after 12 months of menstruation stopping.
• *Do you experience any associated symptoms of menopause (e.g. hot flushes, numbness and tingling, headache, palpitations, drenching sweats, mood swings, vaginal dryness, itching)? What have you done about these symptoms if any?*	**Perimenopausal period** from 40 to 55 years has hormone shifts, resulting in vasomotor instability.

ASSESSMENT GUIDELINES	CLINICAL SIGNIFICANCE AND CLINICAL ALERTS
If using menopausal hormone therapy (MHT), ask: • *What is the dosage? How effective is the medication in reducing the menopausal side effects? Any unwanted effects of the medication? How long have you been using hormone replacement therapy?* • *Are you using any other therapies to help relieve menopausal symptoms?* Ask about herbs and other complementary therapies, exercise and yoga.	Side effects of **menopausal hormone therapy** include fluid retention, breast pain or enlargement and vaginal bleeding.
• *Has menopause affected your quality of life and sense of wellbeing?* • *If yes, in what ways?*	Although this is a normal life stage, reaction varies from acceptance to feelings of loss.
Obstetric history • *Have you ever been pregnant?*	
• *How many times have you been pregnant?*	**Gravida** is the number of pregnancies.
• *How many births have you had?*	**Para** is the number of births (over 20 weeks' gestation—live or stillborn).
• *Have you had any miscarriages (spontaneous abortion) or a termination of pregnancy (induced abortion)?* The woman may not want to share this information. Be aware that partners and other family members may not be aware of this history, therefore it is important to try to consult with a woman by herself in the first instance. For each pregnancy describe: duration, any complication, labour and birth, baby's sex, birth weight, condition. • *Are you planning a pregnancy? Do you think you may be pregnant now? What symptoms have you noticed?*	**Abortion** is interrupted pregnancy, including elective termination of pregnancy (medical or surgical) and spontaneous miscarriage.
• *Have you ever had any problems becoming pregnant?*	**Infertility** is considered present after 1 year of engaging in unprotected sexual intercourse without becoming pregnant.
Health and lifestyle management	
Cervical screening test • *Have you had a CST (previously known as the Pap test)?* • *When was your last CST?* • *Have you had any previously abnormal CST (or Pap test) result?* Take the opportunity to reinforce the need for regular CST.	**Cervical screening tests** should be conducted at 25 years of age and every 5 years up to 69 years of age unless abnormality detected. If any abnormality detected, there will be recommendations about diagnostic tests. The CST has become easier in that women do not require an invasive speculum examination. In fact, most screening can be done by a self-collected high vaginal swab (see 'Additional resources' section for links to information about self-collection).

ASSESSMENT GUIDELINES	CLINICAL SIGNIFICANCE AND CLINICAL ALERTS
Immunisation • *Have you been immunised against human papillomavirus (HPV)?* A single dose of a 9vHPV vaccine is enough to protect against cervical cancer. For more information about HPV vaccination see the 'Health education' section of this chapter.	**HPV** can cause cancers of the penis, anus, cervix, vulva, vagina and throat. The virus causes genital warts. Warts that are visible are caused by a subtype of HPV that is benign and is self-limiting. Warts cause a lot of angst but are self-limiting as they will resolve spontaneously with time. Treatments of genital warts are cosmetic. For more information about HPV vaccination, see the section titled 'Health education' earlier in the chapter.
• *Have you been immunised against hepatitis B?* Hepatitis B vaccination is part of the immunisation schedule in Australia and Aotearoa New Zealand. Most Australians under the age of 30 would have been given the vaccine and the herd immunity is high (>80%), but there are subpopulations that may not have been vaccinated. These include migrants, those whose parents are vaccine conscientious objectors and those who missed out at school.	**Hepatitis B** is a sexually transmissible infection and vertical transmission from mother to baby continues to be the main way of acquiring hepatitis B with long-term sequelae that include hepatocellular carcinoma.
• *Have you been immunised against measles, mumps and rubella (MMR)?* While this is not sexually transmitted, an unvaccinated pregnant woman may vertically transmit the infections to their unborn baby and cause significant morbidity and mortality. It is therefore important to ascertain that women of child-bearing age have had the MMR vaccine before they start family planning.	
Breast health Ask questions about breast health awareness. • *Have you ever had a mammogram or breast ultrasound?*	For more information on assessment of breast health, see Chapter 28.
Safer sex practices See points in the sexual health history above.	
Activity and exercise Ask about usual activity and exercise patterns. See Chapters 17, 19 and 20.	Part of a general health history. May provide an opportunity to provide more information about the importance of exercise to general health and wellbeing.
Additional subjective data for infants and children (questions for parent or guardian)	
• *Does your child have any problem urinating?* • *Have you noticed any evidence of pain with urinating such as crying or holding their genitals?* • *Has your child had a previous urinary tract infection?*	For more information on assessing urinary function, see Chapter 24.

ASSESSMENT GUIDELINES	CLINICAL SIGNIFICANCE AND CLINICAL ALERTS
• *Has your child experienced any problems in the genital area such as itching, rash, vaginal or anal discharge?*	Occurs with poor perineal hygiene or insertion of foreign body in vagina/rectum.
Questions related to suspected child abuse Read the important information about the Australian legal requirements about mandatory reporting. See Chapter 5 for details and a specific approach to screening.	For more information about signs and symptoms related to child abuse, see Chapter 5.
Additional subjective data for preadolescents and adolescents	
Use the following questions, as appropriate, to assess sexual growth and development and sexual behaviour. Use the same principles as discussed at the beginning of the health history section related to the approach to gender identity and sexual orientation outlined in the sexual health history. Ask questions that seem appropriate for a girl's age, but be aware that norms vary widely. Around age 9 or 10, girls start to develop breasts and pubic hair. • *Have you ever seen charts and pictures of normal growth patterns for girls? Let us go over these now.*	
• *Have your periods started? How did you feel? Were you prepared or surprised?*	Assess the attitude of the girl and parents. Note inadequate preparation or attitude of distaste.
• *Who in your family do you talk to about your body changes and about sex information? How do these talks go? Do you think you get enough information?* • *What about sex education classes at school? Is there a teacher, a nurse, doctor or counsellor to whom you can talk?*	
• *Often girls your age have questions about having sex. Do you have questions?* If appropriate in the situation, ask further questions about sexual activity (use similar questions to that of adults outlined in the previous section including questions about STI protection and prevention of unplanned pregnancy if relevant).	Determining the young person's sexual practices will enable you to identify areas for health education or the need for further questioning to identify risk factors for STIs and/or the need for specific physical examination and other investigations.
Questions related to suspected child abuse Read the important information about the Australian legal requirements about mandatory reporting of suspected child abuse. See Chapter 5 for details and a specific approach to screening.	For more information about signs and symptoms related to child abuse, see Chapter 5.

ASSESSMENT GUIDELINES	CLINICAL SIGNIFICANCE AND CLINICAL ALERTS
Additional subjective data for women over 65 years	
• *Have you experienced any vaginal itching, discharge or pain with sexual activity?*	Associated with **atrophic vaginitis**—inflammation, thinning and dryness of the vaginal tissue and labia due to a reduction in estrogen following menopause. Can also cause urinary symptoms such as urgency, dysuria and incontinence.

Objective data

The techniques and extent of the objective data collection in this area will depend on the presenting signs and symptoms. Nurses working in sexual health clinics and some urological settings may need to develop skill in a more advanced assessment of female sexual and reproductive function. For most nurses, asking questions about the woman's reproductive health will be sufficient for a nursing assessment.

Practice note

Physical examination, including inspection of the genitalia, is only performed when there is a valid reason to do so.

In the case of a child or adolescent, the parent or guardian normally provides informed consent for assessment and treatment. Young people have the legal right to confidential health care unless they cannot be considered a mature minor and/or there is a significant concern or risk—for example, harm to self or physical or sexual abuse. It is generally accepted that most young people over the age of 16 years can give informed consent. Those under 16 years may sometimes be considered mature minors where it is legally permissible for a mature adolescent to consent to assessment and treatment.[25] The mature minor (Gillick principle) is confirmed in Australian common law.[26] However, it is always advisable to obtain verbal consent from a child or adolescent before an examination and this should be documented in the health history.

Preparation

Before you start, explain what you are going to assess and why; answer any questions the woman may have; and gain her consent to be examined.

- Ask if she would like a partner, family member or friend to be present.
- Ask her to empty her bladder before the examination.
- Allow the woman to undress in privacy.
- Explain each step in the examination before you do it.
- Assure the woman that she can stop the examination at any point if she feels any discomfort.
- Communicate throughout the examination. Maintain a dialogue to share information.

If an examination of the external genitalia is necessary, the woman should be assisted to lie down in the supine position with one or two pillows under her head. Ensure privacy before exposing the genital area and cover as much bare skin as possible. Have the woman place her ankles together and let her knees drop to the side exposing the perineal area. If the woman has a partner, friend or family member present, ask them to stand at the top (head) of the bed or examination couch to support the woman.

Equipment needed

Non-sterile gloves
Appropriate lighting (examination light)
Hand hygiene solution

PROCEDURES AND NORMAL FINDINGS	ABNORMAL FINDINGS AND CLINICAL ALERTS
General inspection	
While collecting subjective data you will have noticed the condition of the person's skin, hair, posture, height-to-weight ratio, body shape, level of hygiene and grooming and general demeanour. All these factors provide clues to the woman's sexual and reproductive health.	
Inspection of external genitalia	
Skin colour (Figure 26.4) 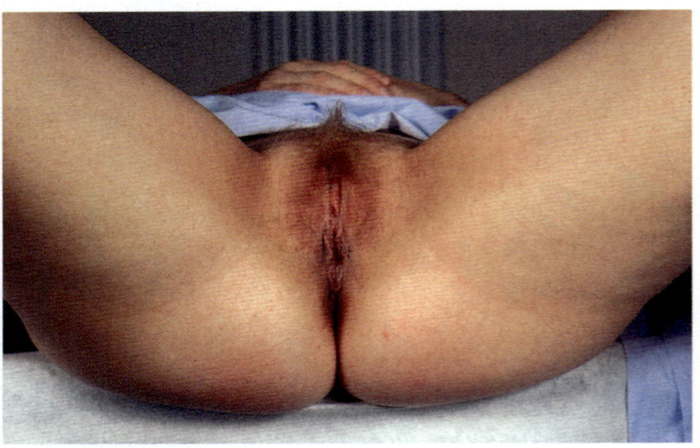 **FIGURE 26.4** Normal female genital skin colour	
Hair distribution is in the usual female pattern of inverted triangle, although it normally may trail up the abdomen towards the umbilicus. However, it is not uncommon for women to remove some or all the pubic hair.	Consider delayed puberty if no pubic hair or breast development has occurred by age 13 years. Nits or lice at the base of pubic hair.
Labia majora normally are symmetrical, plump and well formed. In the nulliparous (woman who has never had a baby) woman, labia meet in the midline; after a vaginal birth, the labia are usually gaping and slightly shrivelled.	Swelling.

PROCEDURES AND NORMAL FINDINGS	ABNORMAL FINDINGS AND CLINICAL ALERTS
No lesions should be present, except for occasional sebaceous cysts. These are yellowish, 1-centimetre nodules that are firm, non-tender and often multiple.	Be aware that not all lesions are abnormal. There are normal anatomical variants, however.  ***Clinical alert:*** If any suspicious lesion is identified, the woman should be referred to a medical or nurse practitioner for further assessment.
With your gloved hand, separate the labia majora to inspect (Figure 26.5): 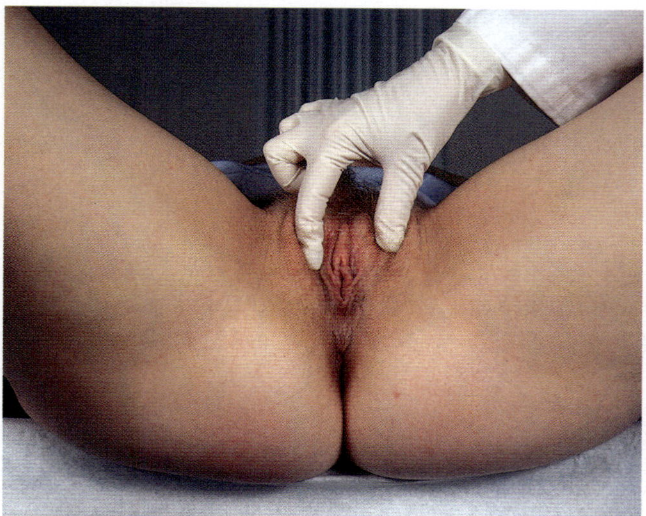 **FIGURE 26.5** Hand position for labial separation	Excoriation, nodules, rash or lesions (Table 26.2).
Clitoris	
Labia minora are dark pink and moist, usually symmetrical.	**Inflammation** or lesions.
Urethral opening appears stellate or slit-like and is midline.	**Polyp.**
Vaginal opening, or introitus, may appear as a narrow vertical slit or as a larger opening.	Foul-smelling, irritating **discharge**.
Perineum is smooth. A well-healed episiotomy scar, midline or mediolateral, may be present after a vaginal birth.	
Anus has coarse skin of increased pigmentation (Chapter 25).	
Additional objective data for infants and children	
Preparation A parent or guardian should be present. • Infant—place them on the examination table. • Toddler/preschooler—place on the parent's lap. Frog-leg position—hips flexed, soles of the feet together and up to the buttocks.	

PROCEDURES AND NORMAL FINDINGS	ABNORMAL FINDINGS AND CLINICAL ALERTS

- School-age girl—place them on the examination table, frog-leg position; drape if appropriate.

During childhood, a routine screening is limited to inspecting the external genitalia to determine:

- the structures are intact
- the vagina is present.

A newborn's genitalia are somewhat engorged. The labia majora are swollen, the labia minora are prominent and protrude beyond the labia majora, the clitoris looks relatively large and the hymen appears thick. Because of transient engorgement, the vaginal opening is more difficult to see now than it will be later. Place your thumbs on the labia majora. Push laterally while pushing the perineum down and try to note the vaginal opening above the hymenal ring. Do not palpate the clitoris because it is very sensitive.

Ambiguous genitalia are rare but are suggested by a markedly enlarged clitoris, fusion of the labia (resembling scrotum) and palpable mass in fused labia (resembling testes).

Clinical alert: Any abnormalities should be referred to a medical practitioner for further assessment.

A sanguineous vaginal discharge or leucorrhoea (mucoid discharge) is normal during the first few weeks because of the maternal estrogen effect. (This also may cause transient breast engorgement and secretion.) During the early weeks, the genital engorgement resolves and the labia minora atrophy and remain small until puberty (Figure 26.6).

Lesions, rash.

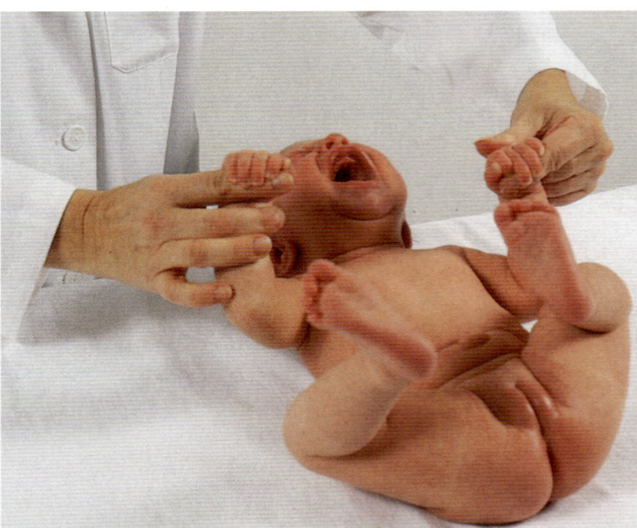

FIGURE 26.6 Newborn female labial engorgement

PROCEDURES AND NORMAL FINDINGS	ABNORMAL FINDINGS AND CLINICAL ALERTS
Between the ages of 2 months and 7 years, the labia majora are flat, the labia minora are thin, the clitoris is relatively small and the hymen is tissue-paper thin. Normally, no irritation or foul-smelling discharge is present.	Poor perineal hygiene. **Excoriations.** During and after toddler age, foul-smelling discharge occurs with lodging of foreign body, pinworms or infection.
In a young school-age girl (7–10 years), the mons pubis thickens, the labia majora thicken and the labia minora become slightly rounded. Pubic hair appears beginning around age 11 years, although sparse pubic hair may occur as early as age 8 years. Normally, the hymen is perforate (Table 26.3). Almost always in these age groups, an external examination will suffice. If needed, an internal pelvic examination is best performed by a paediatric gynaecologist using specialised instruments.	Absence of pubic hair by 13 years indicates delayed puberty. **Amenorrhoea** in adolescents, together with bluish and bulging hymen, indicates imperforate hymen and warrants referral.
Additional objective data for women over 65 years	
Natural vaginal lubrication is decreased; to avoid a painful examination, take care to lubricate the examining hand adequately. Menopause and the resulting decrease in estrogen production cause numerous physical changes. Pubic hair gradually decreases, becoming thin and sparse in later years. The skin is thinner and fat deposits decrease, leaving the mons pubis smaller and the labia flatter. Clitoris size also decreases after age 60 years.	

Abnormal findings

TABLE 26.2 Abnormalities of the external genitalia

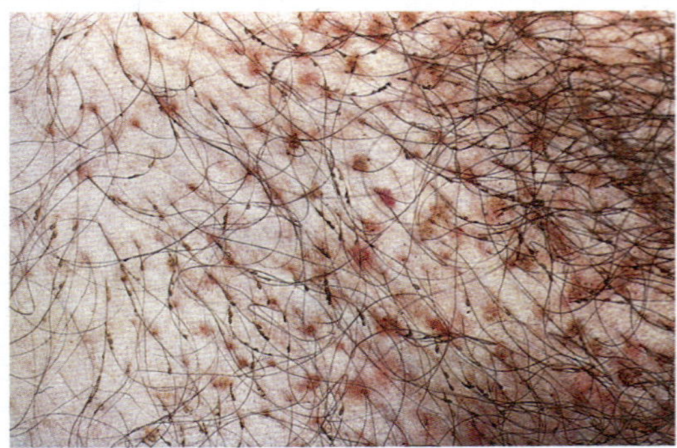

Pediculosis pubis (crab lice)

The person will complain of severe perineal itching. Appears as excoriations and erythematous areas. May see little dark spots (lice are small), nits (eggs) adherent to pubic hair near roots. Usually localised in pubic hair, occasionally in eyebrows or eyelashes.

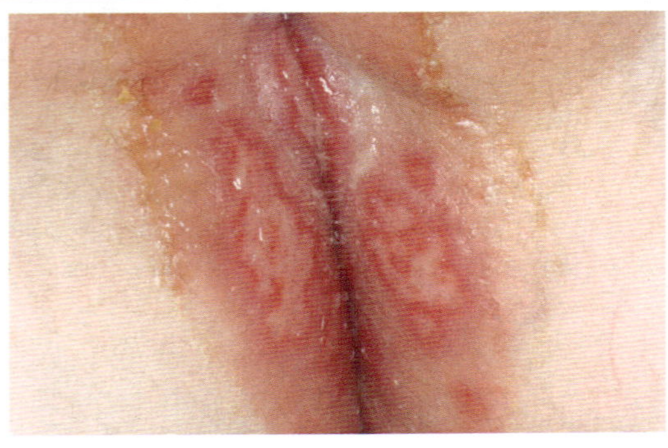

Herpes simplex virus—type 2 (genital herpes)

The person will complain of episodes of local pain, dysuria and fever. Appears as clusters of small, shallow vesicles with surrounding erythema; erupt on genital areas and inner thigh. Also, inguinal adenopathy, oedema. Vesicles on labia rupture in 1 to 3 days, leaving painful ulcers. Initial infection lasts 7 to 10 days. Virus remains dormant indefinitely; recurrent infections last 3 to 10 days with milder symptoms.

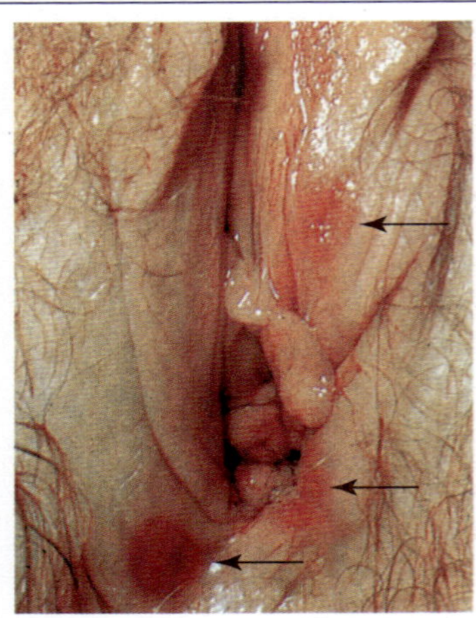

Syphilitic chancre

Begins as a small, solitary silvery papule that erodes to a red, round or oval, superficial ulcer with a yellowish serous discharge. Palpation—nontender indurated base; can be lifted like a button between thumb and finger. Nontender inguinal lymphadenopathy.

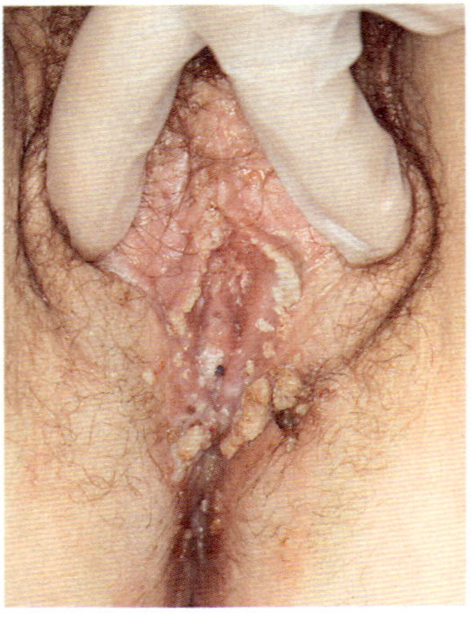

Human papillomavirus (HPV) genital warts

The painless warty growths may be unnoticed by the woman (this image shows an advanced case). They are caused by HPV virus, commonly types 6 and 11. These types are not associated with cervical cancer.

TABLE 26.2 Abnormalities of the external genitalia cont'd

The lesions appear as pink or flesh-coloured, soft, pointed, moist, warty papules. Single or multiple in a cauliflower-like patch. Occur around vulva, introitus, anus, vagina and cervix.
HPV infection is common among sexually active women, especially adolescents, regardless of ethnicity or socioeconomic status. Risk factors include early age at menarche and multiple sexual partners. The long incubation period (6 weeks to 8 months) makes it difficult to establish history of exposure.

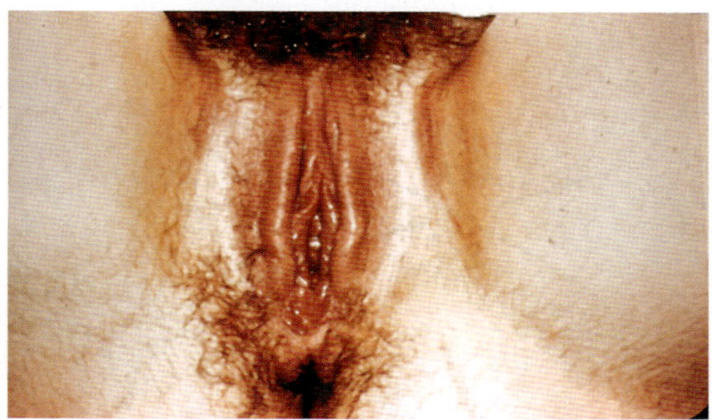

Red rash—contact dermatitis

The person will have a history of skin contact with an allergenic substance in the environment, intense pruritus. The primary lesions appear as red, swollen vesicles. They may have weeping of lesions, crusts, scales, thickening of skin or excoriations from scratching. May result from a reaction to feminine hygiene spray or synthetic underclothing.

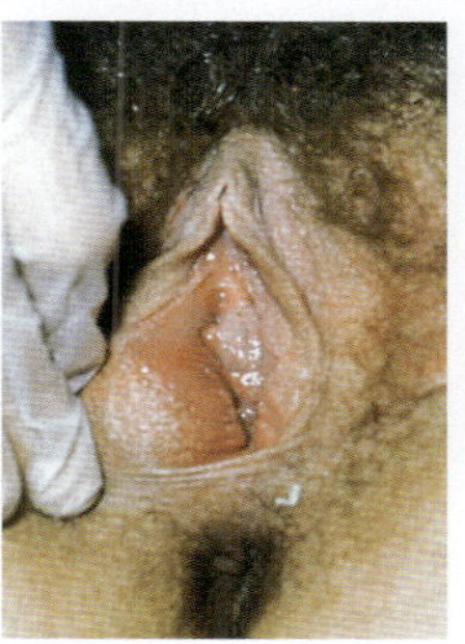

Abscess of Bartholin's gland

The person complains of local pain, which can be severe.
On inspection, the overlying skin is red and hot. The posterior part of the labia is swollen; palpable fluctuant mass and tenderness. Mucosa shows a red spot at the site of the duct opening; can express purulent discharge.

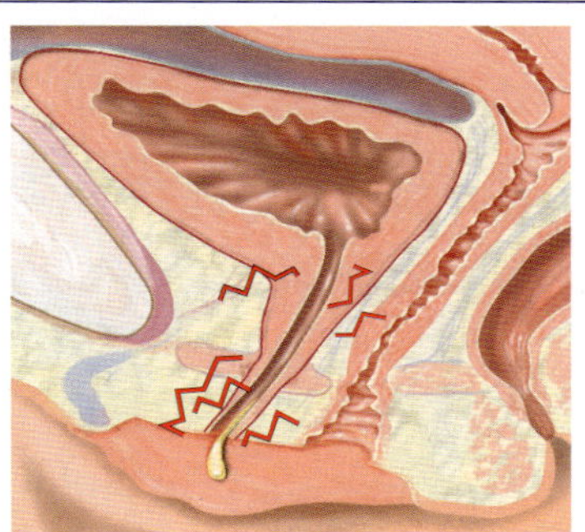

Urethritis

Urethritis

The person complains of dysuria and a burning sensation.
Palpation of anterior vaginal wall shows erythema, tenderness, induration along urethra, purulent discharge from meatus. May be caused by *Neisseria gonorrhoeae*, *Chlamydia* or *Staphylococcus* infection.

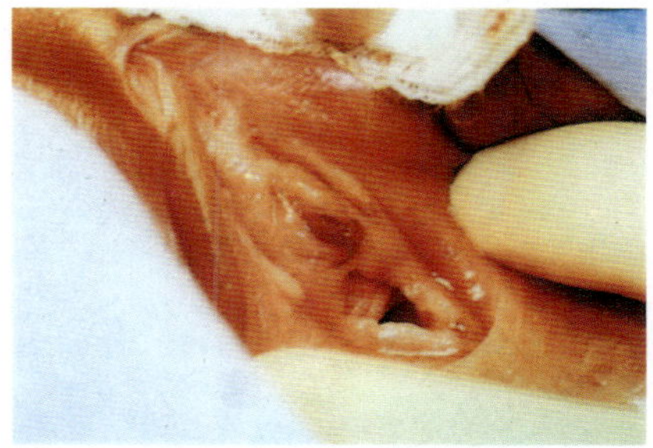

Urethral caruncle

The person complains of tenderness, painful urination, urinary frequency, haematuria, dyspareunia or may be asymptomatic.
The lesion appears as a small, deep red mass protruding from the meatus; usually secondary to urethritis or skenitis; lesion may bleed on contact.

TABLE 26.3 Abnormalities in paediatric genitalia

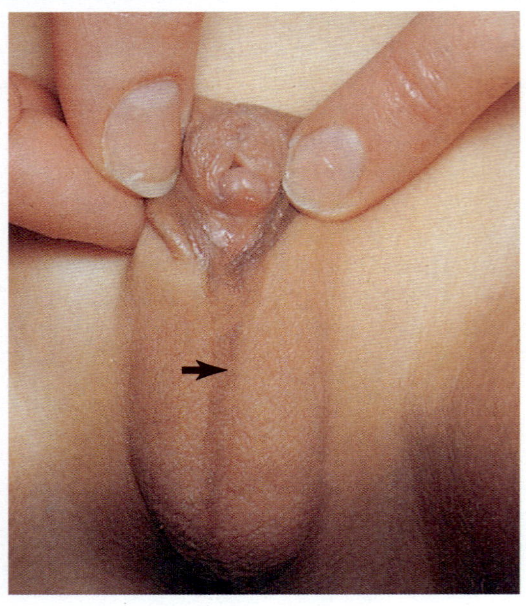

Ambiguous genitalia

Intersex is a congenital condition where the person is born with several sex characteristics including chromosome patterns, genitals and sex organs that, for a variety of reasons, do not fit typical binary male or female development. Ambiguous means the enlarged clitoris may look like a small penis with hypospadias, and the fused labia looks like an incompletely formed scrotum with absent testes. The family must be referred for further assessment and support.

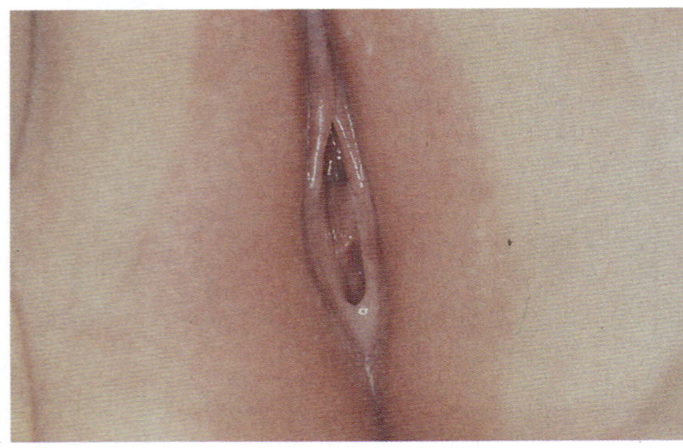

Vulvovaginitis in a child

This is an acute, nonspecific vulvovaginitis in a child. Symptoms include pruritus and burning when urine touches excoriated area. Examination shows red and shiny vulva and surrounding area. Common causes of vulvovaginitis in a prepubertal child include infection from a respiratory or bowel pathogen, *Candida albicans* infection, STI or presence of a foreign body.

Advanced practice—additional objective data

In addition to the objective assessment outlined above, the assessments that are described in the following sections require advanced skill and scope of practice. Nurses working in specialist women's health and sexual health settings and urological and continence nurses need to develop these skills. Advanced assessment for infants and children would be performed by specialist neonatal and paediatric nurses, some midwives and maternal and child health nurses.

Practice note

Physical examination, including vaginal inspection and palpation, are intimate invasive assessments and are only performed when there is a valid reason to do so.

It is critical that clear communication with the person is maintained throughout the procedure to ensure the person fully understands the purpose, nature and extent of the assessment. You will have to make a professional judgement about the need for another health professional (a chaperone) to be present during the examination.

Preparation

See previous comments about positioning of the woman. Internal examination usually follows examination of external structures. Take time to reconfirm consent to be examined internally. Familiarise yourself with the vaginal speculum before the examination. Practise opening and closing the blades, locking them into position and releasing them. Try both metal and plastic types. Note that the plastic speculum locks and unlocks with a resounding click that can be alarming to an uninformed woman.

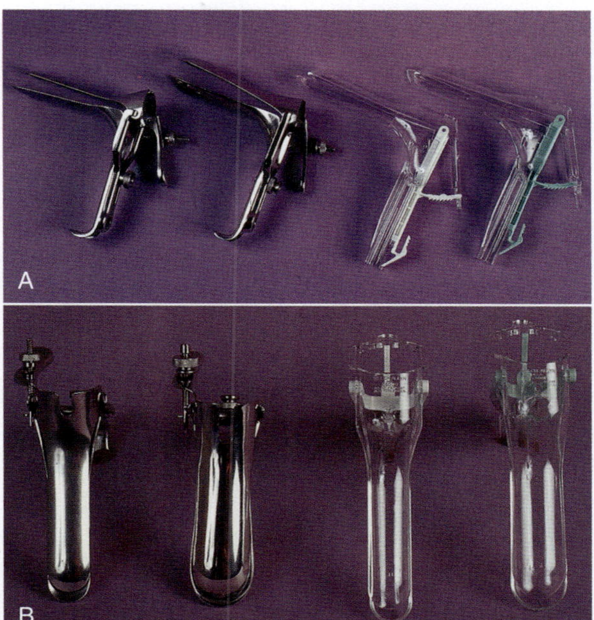

FIGURE 26.7 Vaginal speculum

Equipment needed

In addition to the equipment listed previously you will require:

- vaginal speculum of appropriate size (Figure 26.7)
- materials for cytological study—this depends on the preference of the laboratory; make yourself familiar with the equipment and how to collect, prepare and transport the specimen
- specimen containers for specific STI cultures if needed
- warm water (to lubricate vaginal speculum)
- non-sterile gloves
- water-based lubricant (depending on the purpose and extent of the examination).

PROCEDURES AND NORMAL FINDINGS	ABNORMAL FINDINGS AND CLINICAL ALERTS
Inspection	
In addition to the detailed inspection described previously, you may need to assess for pelvic organ prolapse and stress incontinence. While observing the perineum, ask the woman to cough and note any loss of urine when coughing. Observe for any sign of bulging of the vaginal walls at the introitus and bulging of the urethral meatus. There should be no prolapse of the vaginal walls and no urine loss during coughing.	Loss of urine when coughing is an indicator of **stress incontinence**. Bulging of the anterior vaginal wall is termed a **cystocele** where the pelvic musculature fails to support the bladder and it falls posteriorly into the vagina. This can cause voiding dysfunction and incontinence. Similarly, a bulge in the posterior vaginal wall is termed a **rectocele**. A rectocele can cause defecatory dysfunction and can contribute to constipation.  ***Clinical alert:*** Any degree of pelvic organ prolapse should be referred to a medical practitioner for further assessment.

PROCEDURES AND NORMAL FINDINGS	ABNORMAL FINDINGS AND CLINICAL ALERTS

Palpation

Assess the urethra and Skene's glands

Dip your gloved finger in a bowl of warm water to lubricate. Then insert your index finger into the vagina, and gently milk the urethra by applying pressure up and out. This procedure should produce no pain. If any discharge appears, culture it (Figure 26.8).

Tenderness.
Induration along urethra.
Urethral discharge.

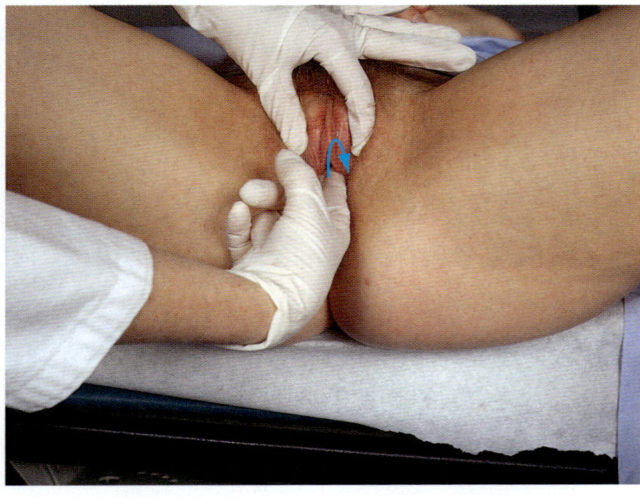

FIGURE 26.8 Palpation of the urethra and Skene's glands

Assess Bartholin's glands

Palpate the posterior parts of the labia majora with your index finger in the vagina and your thumb outside (Figure 26.9). Normally, the labia feel soft and homogeneous.

Swelling (Table 26.2).
Induration.
Pain with palpation.
Erythema around or discharge from duct opening.

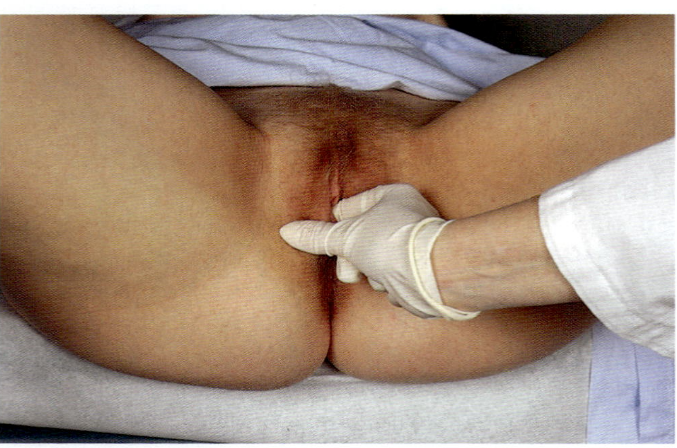

FIGURE 26.9 Palpation of Bartholin's glands

PROCEDURES AND NORMAL FINDINGS	ABNORMAL FINDINGS AND CLINICAL ALERTS
Palpate the perineum	
Normally, it feels thick, smooth and muscular in a nulliparous woman and may be thinner and more rigid in a multiparous woman.	Tenderness. Paper-thin perineum.
Palpate the vagina	
Insert a gloved finger into the vagina and assess for tenderness, descent of the cervix, anterior and posterior vaginal wall. If no specimens are being collected, a water-based lubricant can be applied to your gloved fingers.	Tenderness. Descent of cervix into vagina. **Anterior or posterior prolapse.**
Assessment of pelvic muscle strength	
This is performed to: • establish a baseline of neuromuscular function and contractility of the pelvic floor muscles • assess the woman's ability to identify, isolate, contract and relax the pelvic floor muscles.[28] Good pelvic muscle function is important in maintaining the position of pelvic organs and structures and in maintaining urinary and faecal continence.	Digital palpation of pelvic floor muscle assessment is subjective and hard to quantify reliably, but it does offer a clinically useful way to determine pelvic floor muscle function.[27]
This should be performed in the supine position with hips and knees flexed and relaxed. Depending on the purpose of the assessment (and the findings from the assessment in the supine position), it can be repeated in the standing position. • Begin by inserting one gloved finger (index finger) into the woman's vagina (about 4 cm). If you cannot feel the vaginal walls tightly around one examining finger you may need to use two fingers (index and middle fingers). • If using one finger, ask the woman to 'lift and squeeze' or 'pull up and tighten' the pelvic floor muscles around your finger. If using two examining fingers, spread the fingers laterally in the anterior–posterior position and ask the woman to 'lift and squeeze' or 'pull up and tighten' the pelvic floor muscles around your fingers. You should feel a brisk contraction of the muscles firmly and evenly around your fingers. The **modified Oxford grading system** is used to quantify pelvic floor muscle strength: • 0/5 = nil/none (no discernible peri-vaginal muscle contraction)	Absent or decreased contraction—little sensation of pressure on the examiner's fingers. Inability to maintain the contraction ($<$ 3 seconds). Women with poor pelvic floor muscle strength are likely to experience urinary incontinence and should be referred to a nurse continence specialist or continence physiotherapist for further assessment and development of an individualised pelvic floor muscle-strengthening program.

PROCEDURES AND NORMAL FINDINGS	ABNORMAL FINDINGS AND CLINICAL ALERTS
• 1/5 = flicker (fluttering or quivering of the peri-vaginal muscle contraction) • 2/5 = weak (weak contraction of the peri-vaginal muscles with or without elevation/lifting) • 3/5 = moderate (compressing the examiner's fingers with or without elevation or lifting of the fingers) • 4/5 = good (a firm contraction with good compression of the examiner's fingers causing elevation/lifting of the examiner's fingers) • 5/5 = strong (strong contraction of the peri-vaginal muscles on the examiner's fingers and strong elevation/lifting of the examiner's fingers. • **Assess the duration of the contraction** (in seconds)—normally 3 to 6 seconds. • **Number of contractions** that can be performed before the muscle fatigues. • **Assess how fast the woman can contract the muscles**. Make sure you allow the woman to rest the muscles for a few seconds between contractions. • **Assess extent of muscle movement**. Normally the contraction should lift the examiner's fingers upwards. Note the evenness of the contraction (anterior–posterior, circumferential).[28,29]	
Inspection of internal genitalia	
Select the proper-sized speculum. Warm and lubricate the speculum under warm running water. A good technique is to dedicate one hand to the person and the other hand to picking up equipment in the room. For example, hold the speculum in your left hand (the equipment hand), with the index and the middle fingers surrounding the blades and your thumb under the thumbscrew. This prevents the blades from opening painfully during insertion. With your right index and middle fingers (the patient hand), push the introitus down and open to relax the pubococcygeal muscle (Figure 26.10). Tilt the width of the blades obliquely and insert the speculum past your right fingers, applying any pressure *downwards*. This avoids pressure on the sensitive urethra above it.	

PROCEDURES AND NORMAL FINDINGS

ABNORMAL FINDINGS AND CLINICAL ALERTS

FIGURE 26.10 Position for insertion of a vaginal speculum

Ease insertion by informing the woman of what you are doing. Tell her you are placing the speculum externally. This method relaxes the perineal muscles and opens the introitus. (With experience, you can combine speculum insertion with assessing the support of the vaginal muscles.) As the blades pass your right fingers, withdraw your fingers. Now change the hand holding the speculum to your right hand and turn the width of the blades horizontally. Continue to insert in a 45-degree angle *downwards* towards the small of the woman's back (Figure 26.11). This matches the natural slope of the vagina.

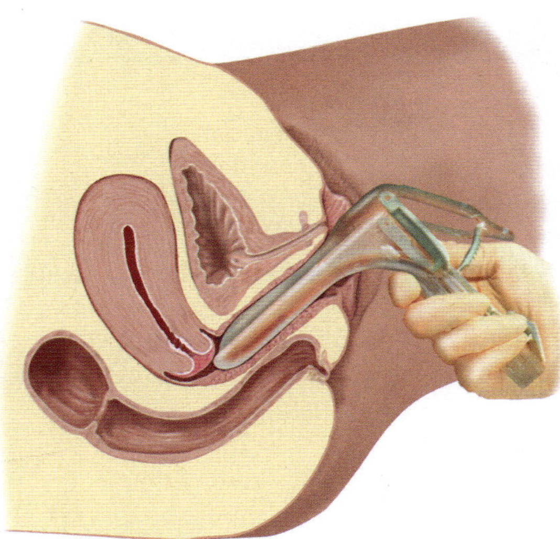

FIGURE 26.11 Longitudinal view of a vaginal speculum in situ

PROCEDURES AND NORMAL FINDINGS	ABNORMAL FINDINGS AND CLINICAL ALERTS
After the blades are fully inserted, open them by squeezing the handles together (Figure 26.12). The cervix should be in full view. Sometimes this does not occur (especially with beginning examiners) because the blades are angled above the location of the cervix. Try closing the blades, withdrawing about halfway and reinserting in a more *downwards* plane. Then slowly sweep upwards. Once you have the cervix in full view, lock the blades open by tightening the thumbscrew.	

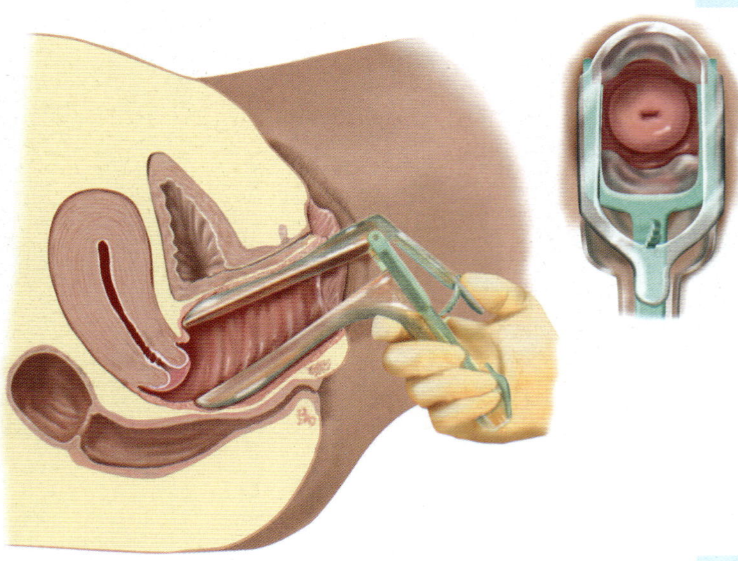

FIGURE 26.12 Longitudinal view of a vaginal speculum with blades opened/View of cervical os

Inspect the cervix and its os

PROCEDURES AND NORMAL FINDINGS	ABNORMAL FINDINGS AND CLINICAL ALERTS
Note:	
Colour Normally the cervical mucosa is pink and even. During the second month of pregnancy it looks blue (Chadwick's sign) and after menopause it is pale.	Redness, inflammation. Pallor with anaemia. Cyanotic other than with pregnancy (Table 26.4).
Position Midline, either anterior or posterior. Projects 1 to 3 cm into the vagina.	Lateral position may be due to adhesion or tumour. Projection of more than 3 cm may be a prolapse.
Size Diameter is 2.5 cm.	Hypertrophy of more than 4 cm occurs with inflammation or tumour.

PROCEDURES AND NORMAL FINDINGS	ABNORMAL FINDINGS AND CLINICAL ALERTS
Os This is small and round in the nulliparous woman. In the parous woman, it is a horizontal irregular slit and may show healed lacerations on the sides (Figure 26.13).	

NORMAL VARIATIONS OF THE CERVIX

Nulliparous

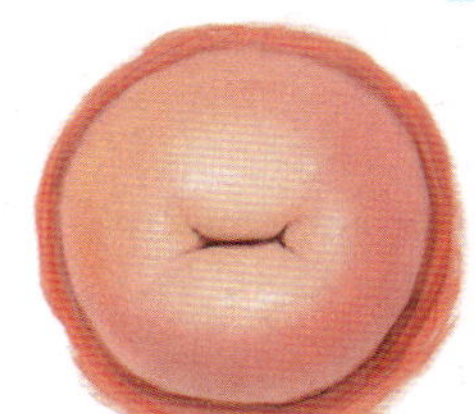

LACERATIONS

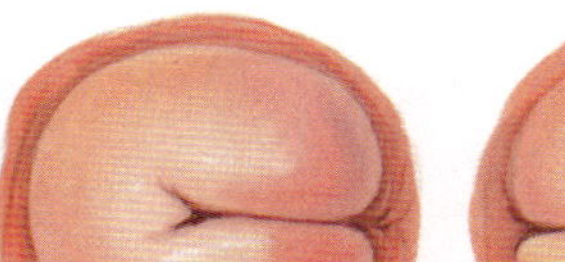

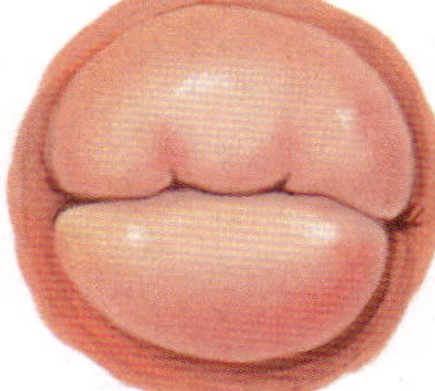

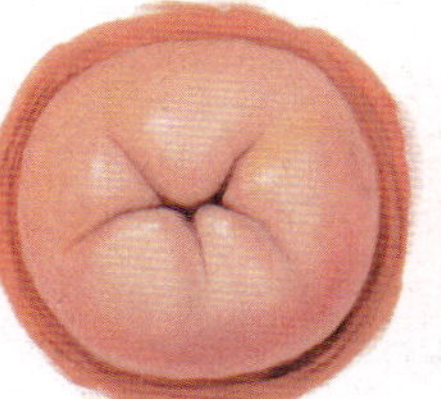

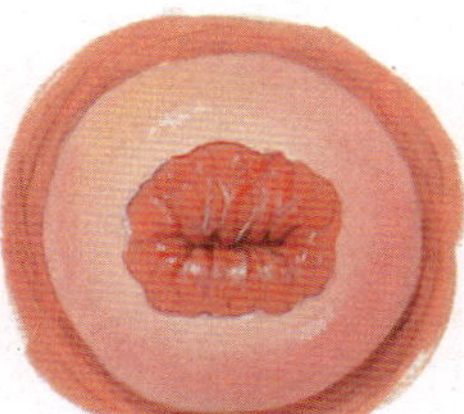

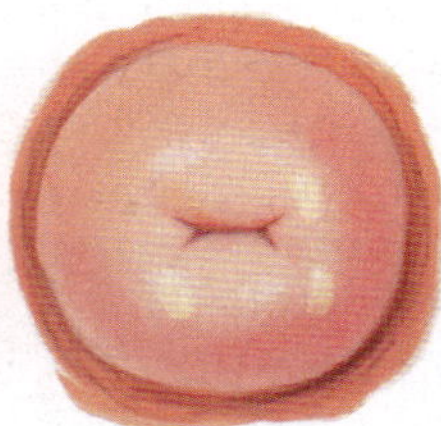

FIGURE 26.13 Normal and abnormal findings on inspection of the cervical os

PROCEDURES AND NORMAL FINDINGS	ABNORMAL FINDINGS AND CLINICAL ALERTS
Surface This is normally smooth, but **cervical eversion**, or ectropion, may occur normally after vaginal deliveries. The endocervical canal is everted or 'rolled out'. It looks like a red, beefy halo inside the pink cervix surrounding the os. It is difficult to distinguish this normal variation from an abnormal condition (e.g. erosion or carcinoma) and biopsy may be needed.	Surface reddened, granular and asymmetrical, particularly around os. **Friable**, bleeds easily. Any lesions: white patch on cervix; strawberry spot. Refer any suspicious red, white or pigmented lesion for biopsy (Table 26.4).
Nabothian cysts are benign growths that commonly appear on the cervix after childbirth. They are small, smooth, yellow nodules that may be single or multiple. Less than 1 cm, they are retention cysts caused by obstruction of cervical glands.	**Cervical polyp**—bright red growth protruding from the os (Table 26.4).
Cervical secretions Depending on the day of the menstrual cycle, secretions may be clear and thin, or thick, opaque and stringy. Always they are odourless and non-irritating. If secretions are copious, swab the area with a thick-tipped swab. This method sponges away secretions and you have a better view of the structures.	Foul-smelling, irritating, with yellow, green, white or grey discharge (Table 26.5).

PROCEDURES AND NORMAL FINDINGS	ABNORMAL FINDINGS AND CLINICAL ALERTS

Obtain cervical smears and cultures

The **CST** screens for HPV subtypes that are precursors to cervical cancers. Do not obtain during the woman's menses or if a heavy infectious discharge is present. Instruct the woman not to douche, have intercourse or put anything into the vagina within 24 hours before collecting the specimens.

Should the CST screening test detect high-risk HPV 16 and/or 18, the laboratory may request further tests that are diagnostic. These tests will vary in method of collection, but it may consist of a liquid based cytology such as a ThinPrep.

Laboratories may vary in method of collection of the CST (see Figure 26.14 for an example of ThinPrep technique). A cervical smear on to a microscopy slide is rarely requested, but the following techniques may be used in collecting extra samples for diagnostic tests.

NATIONAL CERVICAL SCREENING PROGRAM GUIDELINES

CERVIX SAMPLING CARD

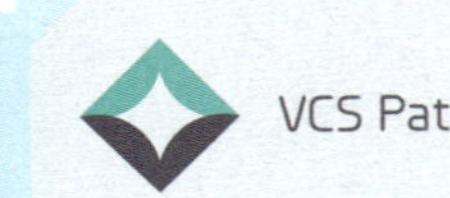

A GUIDE TO TAKING A HIGH-QUALITY CERVICAL SAMPLE

If you would like to watch a video demonstrating the correct technique for taking a high-quality Cervical Screening Test (CST) visit www.vcs.org.au/pathology/for-practitioners/general-resources/

For more information about CST technique, the new National Cervical Screening Program, and testing for HPV, contact VCS Pathology on 03 9250 0300 and ask to speak to a Liaison Physician or email LiaisonTeam@acpcc.org.au

CERVICAL SCREENING: RECOMMENDED TECHNIQUES AND INSTRUMENTS FOR TAKING A CERVICAL SAMPLE

FOR PRE-MENOPAUSAL WOMEN

Cervical sampler broom: rotate 3-5 times

or

Cervex-Brush ® Combi: insert central part of the brush into os and rotate clockwise twice

or

Spatula: rotate once or twice, taking care to keep contact with the ecto-cervix

plus:

Endocervical brush: insert ensuring that you can see the lower row of the bristles and make a quarter rotation

FOR PERI AND POST-MENOPAUSAL WOMEN

Cervical sampler broom: rotate 3-5 times

plus:

Endocervical brush: insert ensuring that you can see the lower row of the bristles and make a quarter rotation

or

Cervix-Brush ® Combi: insert central part of the brush into os and rotate clockwise twice

or

Spatula: rotate once or twice, taking care to keep contact with the ecto-cervix

plus:

Endocervical brush: insert ensuring that you can see the lower row of the bristles and make a quarter rotation.

FOR THINPREP

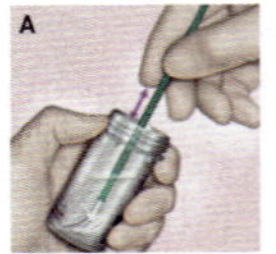

A. Cervical sampler Broom / Cervex-Brush ® Combi: rinse the broom/brush as quickly as possible into the vial by pushing the broom into the bottom of the vial 10 times, forcing the bristles apart. As a final step, swirl the broom vigorously to further release material. Discard the collection device.

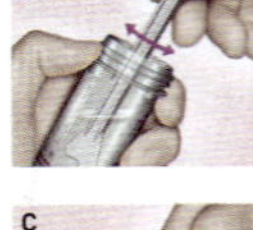

B. Spatula (Plastic): Rinse the spatula as quickly as possible into the vial by swirling the spatula vigorously in the vial 10 times. Discard the spatula.

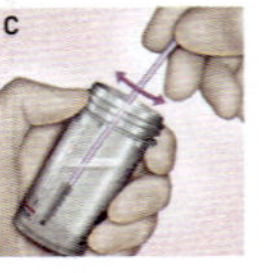

C. Endocervical Brush: Rinse the brush as quickly as possible in the solution by rotating the device in the solution 10 times while pushing against the vial wall. Swirl the brush vigorously to release material. Discard the brush.

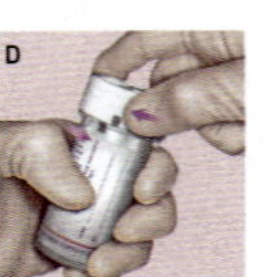

D. Tighten the cap so that the black line on the cap passes the black line on the vial.

Images supplied by Hologic (Australia) Pty Ltd

RECORDING PATIENT DETAILS

Record the patient's surname, first name and date of birth on the vial.

OR

Apply sticker with details.

Record the patient's information and medical history on the request form.

VCS IS ABLE TO PROCESS THINPREP AND SUREPATH

ThinPrep

- Do not leave any part of the sampling device in the fluid.

SurePath

- Instruments should be broken off and left in the fluid

Sampling instrumments

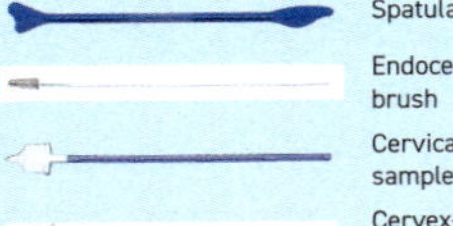

SPECIAL NOTES

Eversion: take care to sample the squamo-columnar junction. This is the junction where the columnar epithelium of the endocervical canal meets the squamous epithelium of the vagina. It is the area where changes occur.

Pregnancy: do not use the endocervical brush or Cervex-Brush ® Combi.

www.acpcc.org.au

FIGURE 26.14 Cervical screening sampling instructions

PROCEDURES AND NORMAL FINDINGS

ABNORMAL FINDINGS AND CLINICAL ALERTS

NATIONAL CERVICAL SCREENING PROGRAM GUIDELINES

CERVIX SAMPLING CARD

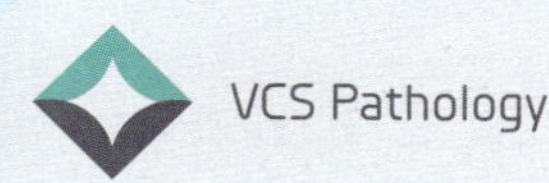

This resource is a guide for practitioners to assist them in identifying visual cervical appearances.

The images shown here are some examples of cervices you may see when taking a cervical sample.

Visual cervical abnormality may need further investigation even if screening tests are negative.

If you are uncertain about the appearance of the cervix, we recommend you seek a second opinion.

Further investigation not required in asymptomatic patients

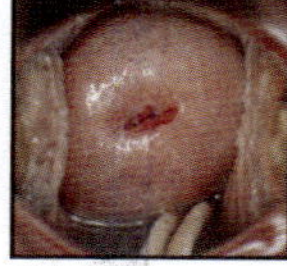
Nulliparous [1]

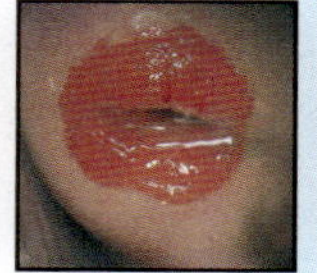
Eversion / ectropion

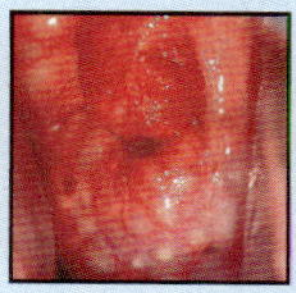
Nabothian follicles

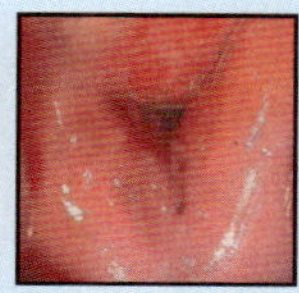
Multiparous

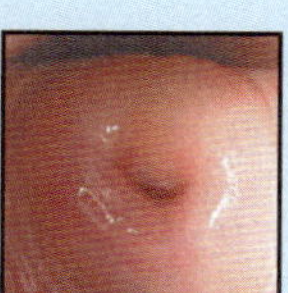
Atrophy

Consider further investigation

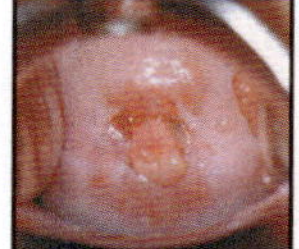
Polyp

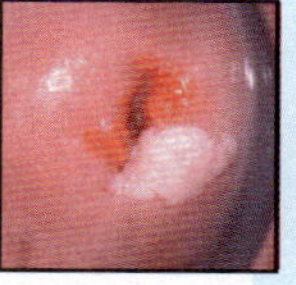
Cervical wart

Should be investigated

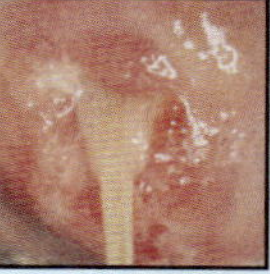
Mucopurulent discharge [3]

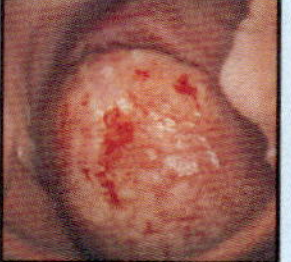
Cancer [2]

Post-intervention - further investigation not required in asymptomatic patients

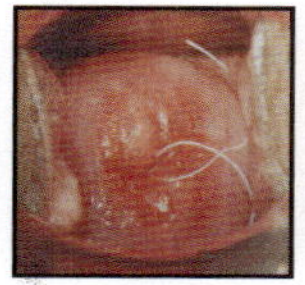
Intra Uterine Device (IUD)

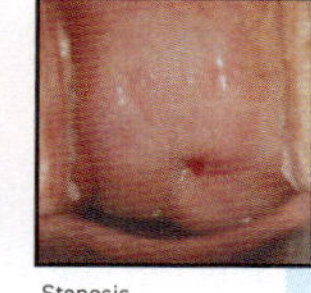
Stenosis

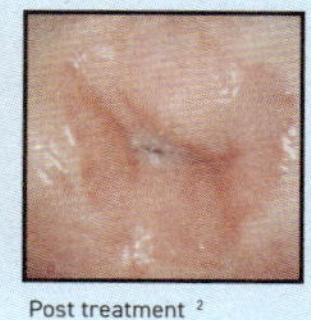
Post treatment [2]

Reproduced with permission from:

1 Wolfendale, Margaret, 1995. Taking Cervical Smears. British Society for Clinical Cytology: page 12.
2 Burghardt, Erich, 1984. Colposcopy Cervical Pathology Textbook and Atlas. Georg Thiem Verlag. Germany: pages 162 & 174.
3 Cartier, René, 1984. Practical Colposcopy. Laboratoire Cartier. Switzerland: page 168.

www.acpcc.org.au

Corp-Mkt-Pub-11 V8

FIGURE 26.14 Cervical screening sampling instructions cont'd

Vaginal pool

Use a cotton-swab and collect a high-vaginal sample that may pool at the end of the speculum. Transfer this on to a pH test. Discard the swab and leave the pH test until you complete the genital exam. Read the pH and document this. Gently rub the blunt end of an Ayre spatula (or cervical brush depending on the equipment required by the particular laboratory) over the vaginal wall under and lateral to the cervix (Figure 26.15).

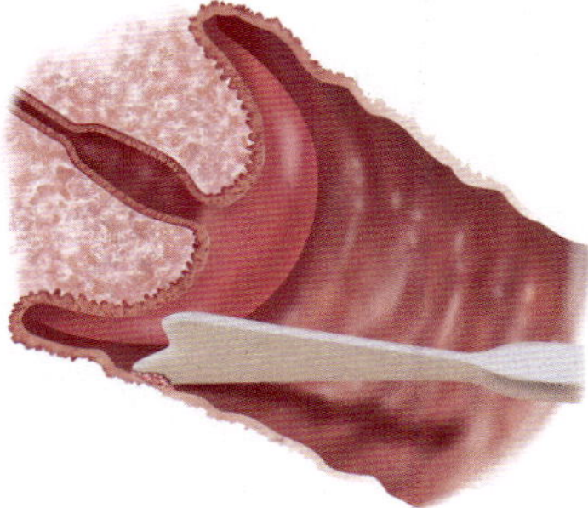

FIGURE 26.15 Position of spatula on the vaginal wall lateral to the cervix

The **vaginal pH** in pre-menopausal women is usually acidic with a pH range between 3.5 and 4.5. The less acidic the environment may cause an overgrowth of normal vaginal flora, leading to symptoms; and also trichomoniasis, which is sexually transmitted.

PROCEDURES AND NORMAL FINDINGS	ABNORMAL FINDINGS AND CLINICAL ALERTS

Collection of a cervical specimen (Figure 26.16)
Insert the bifid end of the Ayre spatula into the vagina with the more pointed bump into the cervical os. Rotate it 360 to 720 degrees, using firm pressure. The rounded cervix fits snugly into the spatula's groove. The spatula scrapes the surface of the squamocolumnar junction and cervix as you turn the instrument. It is important not to screen adolescents and women under 25 years old whose endocervical cells have not yet migrated into the endocervical canal.

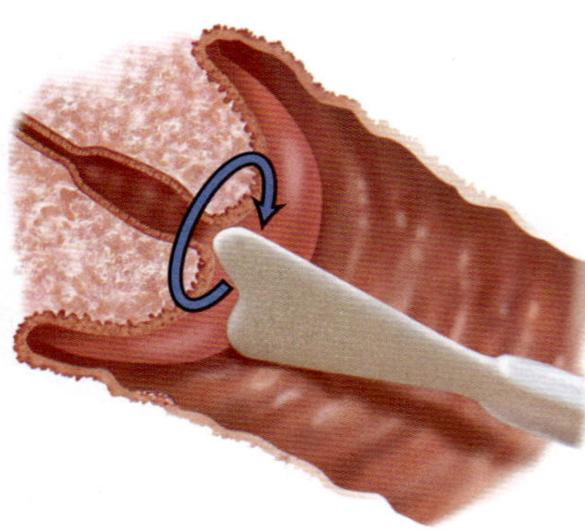

FIGURE 26.16 Position of spatula in the cervical os

Endocervical specimen (Figure 26.17)
Insert a cervical brush (instead of a cotton applicator) into the os. The woman may feel a slight pinch with the brush and scant bleeding may occur.

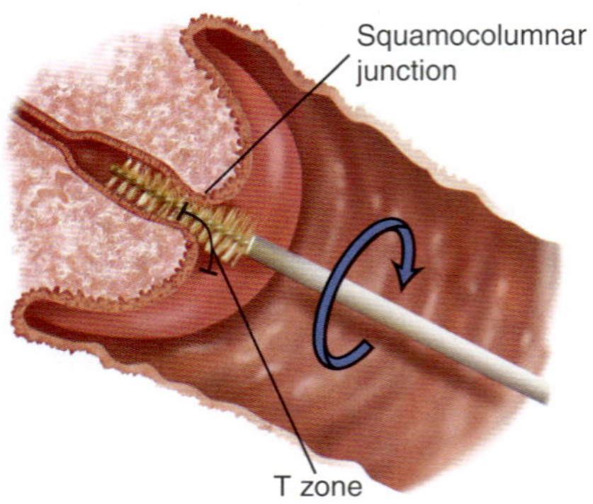

FIGURE 26.17 Endocervical specimen

PROCEDURES AND NORMAL FINDINGS	ABNORMAL FINDINGS AND CLINICAL ALERTS
Rotate the brush 720 degrees in *one* direction in the endocervical canal, either clockwise or counterclockwise. Then rotate the brush gently on a slide to deposit all the cells. Rotate in the opposite direction from the one in which you obtained the specimen. Avoid leaving a thick specimen that would be hard to read under the microscope. Immediately (within 2 seconds) spray the slide with fixative to avoid drying.	
For the woman after hysterectomy whose cervix has been removed, collect a scrape from the end of the vagina and a vaginal pool.	CSTs from a 'vault smear' regardless of whether the hysterectomy was performed because of benign or invasive gynaecological disease. While there is an absence of a cervix, post-surgery, HPV may, albeit less commonly, affect cells of the vagina leading to vaginal intraepithelial neoplasia or recurrence of previously treated cervical or vaginal cancer.
Immediately spray the slides with fixative. The frosted ends of the slides should be labelled with the woman's name. Send these to the laboratory with the following necessary data: • date of specimen • woman's date of birth • date of last menstrual period • any hormone medication • if pregnant, estimated date of delivery • known infections • prior surgery or radiation • prior abnormal cytology • abnormal findings on physical examination.	
These data are important for accurate interpretation; for example, a specimen may be interpreted as positive unless the laboratory technicians know the woman has had prior radiation treatment. Newer methods of cervical screening use a liquid-based thin-layer preparation. Instead of transferring the cervical sample onto a slide, the swab with the sample is deposited into a transportation fluid. The thin uniform layer of suspended cervical cells has improved sensitivity and a lower false-positive rate.	
To screen for STIs, and if you note any abnormal vaginal discharge, obtain a specimen of the discharge. Insert a sterile cotton applicator into the os, rotate it 360 degrees and leave it in place for 10 to 20 seconds for complete saturation. Insert into a labelled specimen container. Follow laboratory guidelines for collection, preparation and transport of specimens for possible STI.	

PROCEDURES AND NORMAL FINDINGS	ABNORMAL FINDINGS AND CLINICAL ALERTS
Inspect the vaginal wall	
Loosen the thumbscrew but continue to hold the speculum blades open. Slowly withdraw the speculum, rotating it as you go, to fully inspect the vaginal wall. Normally, the wall looks pink, deeply rugated, moist and smooth and is free of inflammation or lesions. Normal discharge is thin and clear, or opaque and stringy, but always odourless.	Inflammation or lesions. **Leucoplakia** appears like a spot of dried white paint. Vaginal discharge is thick, white and curd-like with candidiasis; profuse, watery, grey-green and frothy with trichomoniasis; or any grey, green-yellow, white or foul-smelling discharge (Table 26.5).
When the blade ends near the vaginal opening, let them close, but be careful not to pinch the mucosa or catch any hairs. Turn the blades obliquely to avoid stretching the opening. Place the metal speculum in a basin to be cleaned later and soaked in a sterilising and disinfecting solution; discard the plastic variety. Discard your gloves and wash hands.	
Bimanual examination	
Drop lubricant onto the index and middle fingers of your gloved hand (Figure 26.18). With the index and middle fingers extended, the last two flexed onto the palm and the thumb abducted; gently insert your fingers into the vagina, with any pressure directed posteriorly. Wait until the vaginal walls relax, then insert your fingers fully.	

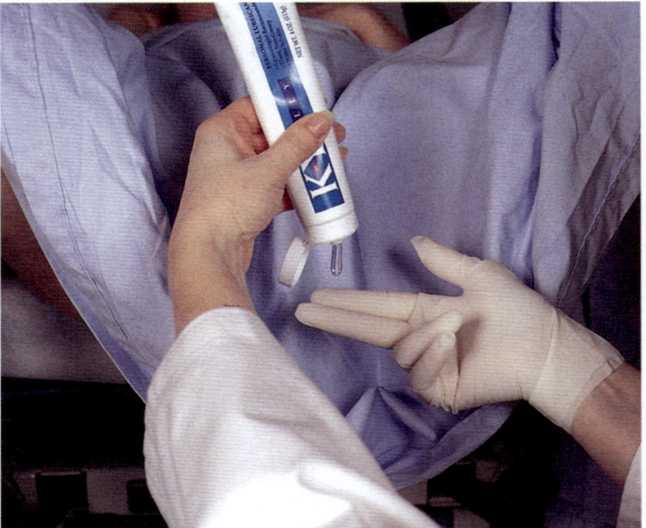

FIGURE 26.18 Lubricant placed on the middle two fingers of a gloved hand

PROCEDURES AND NORMAL FINDINGS	ABNORMAL FINDINGS AND CLINICAL ALERTS
You will use both hands to palpate the internal genitalia to assess their location, size and mobility and to screen for any tenderness or mass. One hand is on the abdomen while the other (often the dominant, more sensitive hand) inserts two fingers into the vagina (Figure 26.19). It does not matter which you choose as the intravaginal hand; try each way and settle on the more comfortable method for you.	
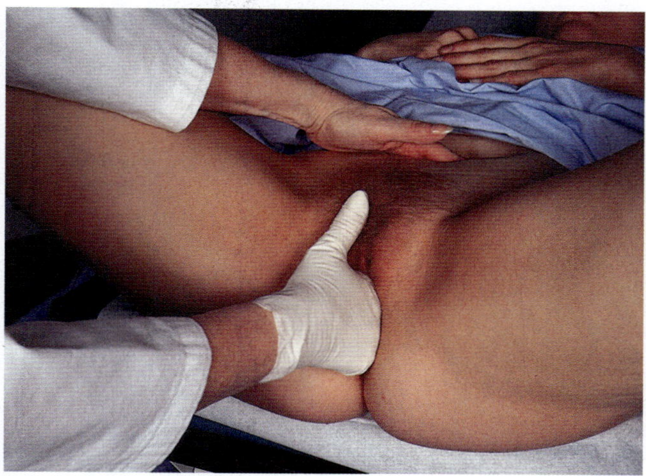 **FIGURE 26.19** Palpation of the vaginal wall	
Palpate the vaginal wall. Normally, it feels smooth and has no area of induration or tenderness.	Nodule. Tenderness.
Cervix Locate the cervix in the midline, often near the anterior vaginal wall. The cervix points in the opposite direction of the fundus of the uterus. Palpate using the palmar surface of the fingers. Note these characteristics of a normal cervix:	
• **Consistency**—feels smooth and firm, has the consistency of the tip of the nose. It softens and feels velvety at 5 to 6 weeks of pregnancy (Goodell's sign).	Hard with malignancy. Nodular.
• **Contour**—evenly rounded.	Irregular.
• **Mobility**—with a finger on either side, move the cervix gently from side to side. Normally, this produces no pain (Figure 26.20).	Immobile with malignancy.

PROCEDURES AND NORMAL FINDINGS	ABNORMAL FINDINGS AND CLINICAL ALERTS

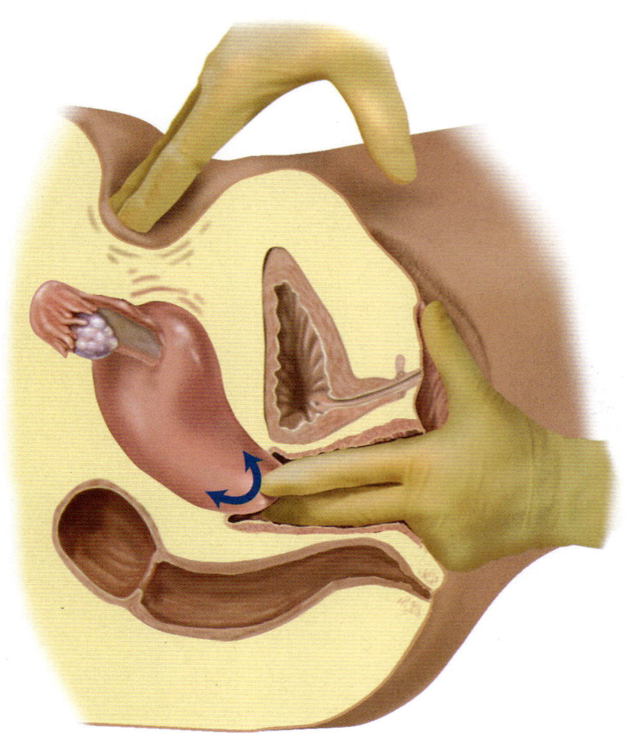

FIGURE 26.20 Female pelvis—palpation of the uterus

Palpate all around the fornices; the wall should feel smooth.

Painful with inflammation or ectopic pregnancy.

Next, use your abdominal hand to push the pelvic organs closer for your intravaginal fingers to palpate. Place your hand midway between the umbilicus and the symphysis; push down in a slow, firm manner, fingers together and slightly flexed. Brace the elbow of your pelvic arm against your hip and keep it horizontal. The woman must be relaxed.

Uterus

With your intravaginal fingers in the anterior fornix, assess the uterus. Determine the position, or *version*, of the uterus (Figure 26.21). This compares the long axis of the uterus with the long axis of the body. In many women, the uterus is anteverted; you palpate it at the level of the pubis with the cervix pointing posteriorly. Two other positions occur normally (midposition and retroverted), as well as two aspects of flexion, where the long axis of the uterus is not straight but is flexed.

PROCEDURES AND NORMAL FINDINGS	ABNORMAL FINDINGS AND CLINICAL ALERTS

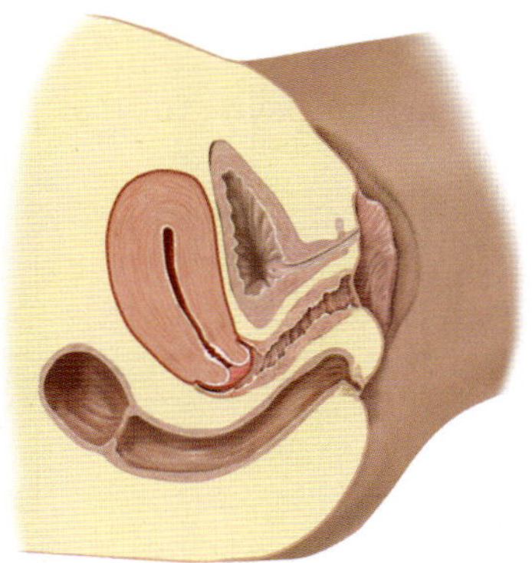

Anteverted

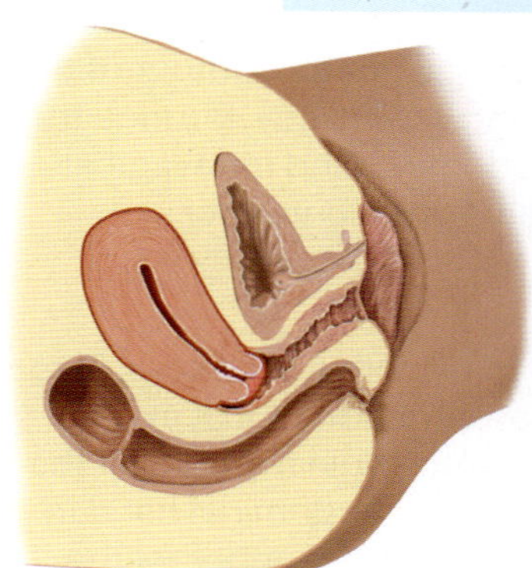

Midposition

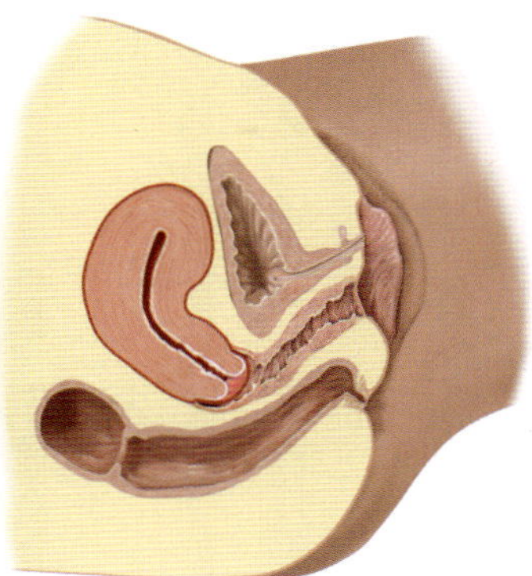

Anteflexed

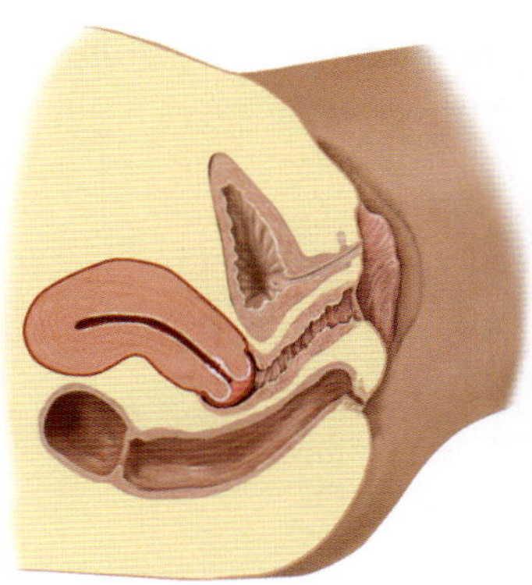

Retroflexed

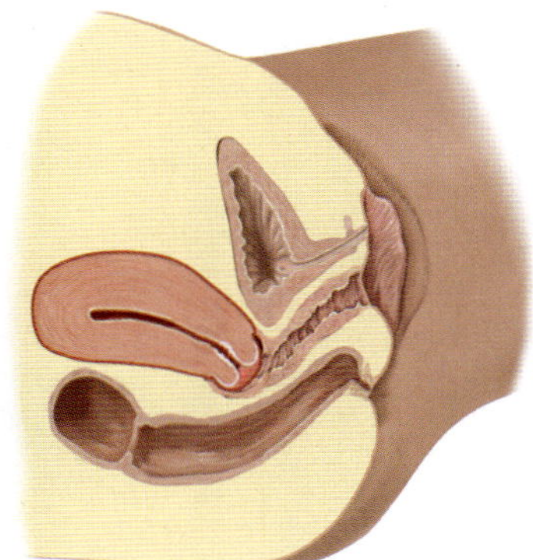

Retroverted

FIGURE 26.21 Position of the uterus in the female pelvis

PROCEDURES AND NORMAL FINDINGS	ABNORMAL FINDINGS AND CLINICAL ALERTS
Palpate the uterine wall with your fingers in the fornices. Normally, it feels firm and smooth, with the contour of the fundus rounded. It softens during pregnancy. Bounce the uterus gently between your abdominal and intravaginal hand. It should be freely movable and nontender.	Enlarged uterus (Table 26.6). Lateral displacement. Nodular mass. Irregular, asymmetrical uterus. Fixed and immobile. Tenderness.
Adnexa Move both hands to the right to explore the adnexa. Place your abdominal hand on the lower quadrant just inside the anterior iliac spine and your intravaginal fingers in the lateral fornix (Figure 26.22). Push the abdominal hand in and try to capture the ovary. Often, you cannot feel the ovary. When you can, it normally feels smooth, firm and almond shaped and is highly movable, sliding through the fingers. It is slightly sensitive but not painful. The fallopian tube is not palpable normally. No other mass or pulsation should be felt.	**Enlarged adnexa.** Nodules or mass in adnexa. Immobile. Markedly tender (Table 26.7). Pulsation or palpable fallopian tube suggests ectopic pregnancy; this warrants immediate referral.

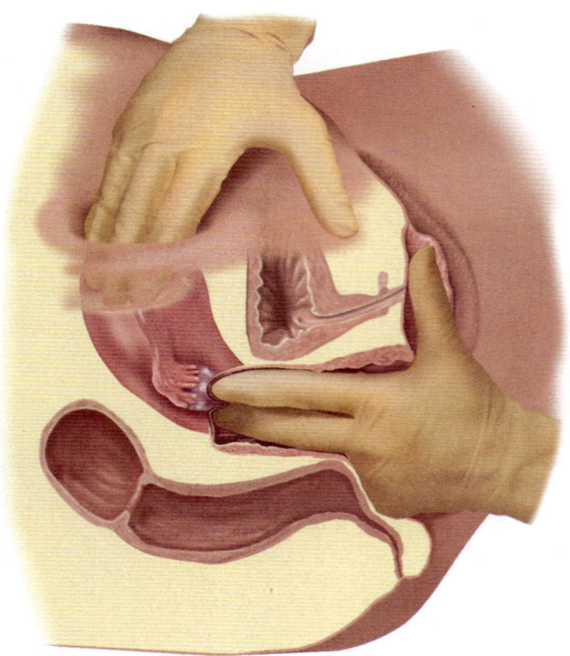

FIGURE 26.22 Female pelvis—palpation of the ovaries

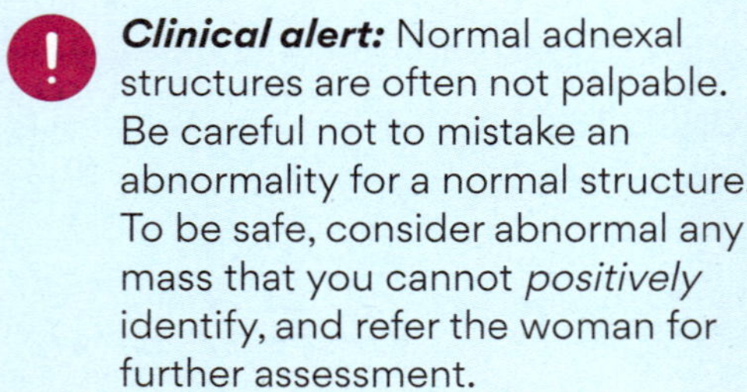

Clinical alert: Normal adnexal structures are often not palpable. Be careful not to mistake an abnormality for a normal structure. To be safe, consider abnormal any mass that you cannot *positively* identify, and refer the woman for further assessment.

PROCEDURES AND NORMAL FINDINGS	ABNORMAL FINDINGS AND CLINICAL ALERTS
Move to the left to palpate the other side. Then, withdraw your hand and check secretions on the fingers before discarding the glove. Normal secretions are clear or cloudy and odourless. Following the examination make sure you give the woman tissues to clean herself and allow time for her to redress before completing the assessment.	
Additional objective data for adolescents	
Adolescent girls have special needs during a genitalia examination. Examine her alone, without a parent present. Assure her of privacy and confidentiality. Allow plenty of time for health education and discussion of pubertal progress. Assess her growth velocity and menstrual history and use the sexual maturity rating charts to teach breast and pubic hair development. Assure her that increased vaginal fluid (physiological **leucorrhoea**) is normal because of the estrogen effect. Perform a pelvic examination when contraception is desired or when the girl's sexual activity includes intercourse. Although the techniques of the examination are listed in the adult section, you will need to provide extra time and psychological support for an adolescent having her first pelvic examination. The experience of the first pelvic examination determines how the adolescent will approach future care. Your accepting attitude and gentle, unhurried approach are important. You have a unique teaching opportunity here. Take the time to teach, using the girl's own body as illustration. Your frank discussion of anatomy and sexual behaviour communicates that these topics are acceptable to discuss and not taboo with healthcare providers. This affirms the girl's self-concept.	
During the bimanual examination, note that the adnexa are not palpable in adolescents.	Pelvic or adnexal mass.
Additional objective data for pregnant women	
Depending on the week of gestation of the pregnancy, inspection shows the enlarging abdomen. The height of the fundus ascends gradually as the fetus grows. At 16 weeks, the fundus is palpable halfway between the symphysis and umbilicus; at 20 weeks, at the lower edge of the umbilicus; at 28 weeks, halfway between the umbilicus and the xiphoid; and at 34 to 36 weeks, almost to the xiphoid. Then, close to term, the fundus drops as the fetal head engages in the pelvis (Chapter 29).	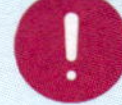 ***Clinical alert:*** Any serious abdominal pain in a woman who could be or is pregnant should be referred to a medical practitioner urgently for further assessment. Serious abdominal pain in very early pregnancy could be an ectopic pregnancy, which can be life-threatening (Table 26.7).

PROCEDURES AND NORMAL FINDINGS	ABNORMAL FINDINGS AND CLINICAL ALERTS
The external genitalia show hyperaemia of the perineum and vulva because of increased vascularity. Varicose veins may be visible in the labia or legs. Haemorrhoids may show around the anus. Both are caused by interruption in venous return from the pressure of the fetus.	
See Chapter 29 for further details of assessment during pregnancy.	
Additional objective data for women over 65 years	
Natural lubrication is decreased; to avoid a painful examination, take care to lubricate instruments and the examining hand adequately. Use the Pedersen speculum (rather than the Graves) because its narrower, flatter blades are more comfortable in women with vaginal stenosis or dryness.	
Internally, the rugae of the vaginal walls decrease, and the walls look pale pink because of the thinned epithelium. The cervix shrinks and looks pale and glistening. It may retract, appearing to be flush with the vaginal wall. In some, it is hard to distinguish the cervix from the surrounding vaginal mucosa. Alternatively, the cervix may protrude into the vagina if the uterus has prolapsed.	Refer any suspicious red, white or pigmented lesion for biopsy. Vaginal atrophy increases the risk of infection and trauma.
With the bimanual examination, you may need to insert only one gloved finger if vaginal stenosis exists. The uterus feels smaller and firmer, and the ovaries are not palpable normally.	Refer any mass for prompt evaluation.
Prior surgery for a hysterectomy does not preclude the need for routine gynaecological care, including cervical screening. Cervical screening can help detect gynaecological malignancies even when the cervix has been removed. Be aware that older women may have special needs and will appreciate the following plans of care: for those with arthritis, taking a mild analgesic or anti-inflammatory before the appointment may ease joint pain in positioning; schedule appointment times when joint pain or stiffness is at its least; allow extra time for positioning and 'un positioning' after the examination; and be careful to maintain dignity and privacy.	

Abnormal findings for advanced practice

TABLE 26.4 Abnormalities of the pelvic musculature—pelvic organ prolapse

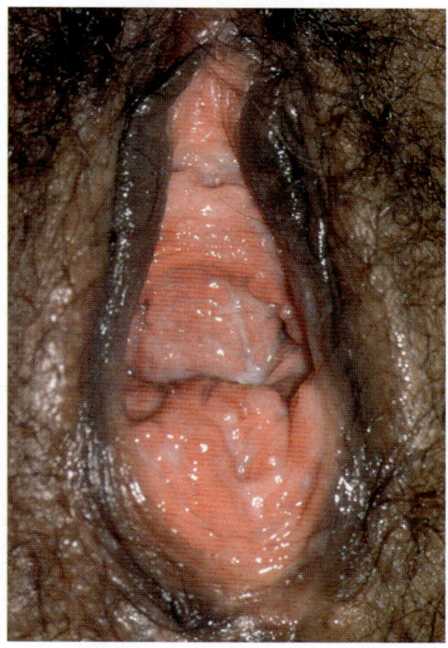

Cystocele

The woman may complain of a feeling of pressure in the vagina or stress incontinence. With straining or standing, note introitus widening and the presence of a soft, round anterior bulge. The bladder, covered by vaginal mucosa, prolapses into vagina.

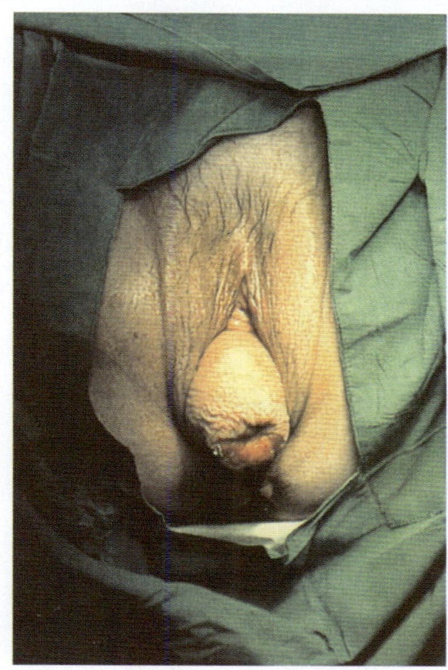

Uterine prolapse

With straining or standing, the uterus protrudes into vagina. Prolapse is graded: 1st degree, cervix appears at introitus with straining; 2nd degree, cervix bulges outside introitus with straining; 3rd degree (in this case), whole uterus protrudes even without straining—essentially, uterus is inside out.

TABLE 26.5 Abnormalities of the cervix

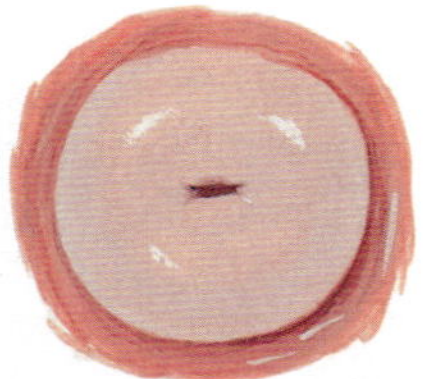

Bluish cervix—cyanosis

Bluish discolouration of the mucosa occurs normally in pregnancy (Chadwick's sign at 6 to 8 weeks' gestation) and with any other condition causing hypoxia or venous congestion (e.g. heart failure, pelvic tumour).

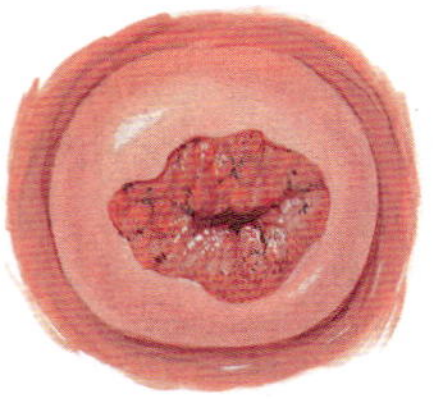

Erosion

Cervical lips inflamed and eroded. Reddened granular surface is superficial inflammation, with no ulceration (loss of tissue). Usually secondary to purulent or mucopurulent cervical discharge. Biopsy needed to distinguish erosion from carcinoma; cannot rely on inspection.

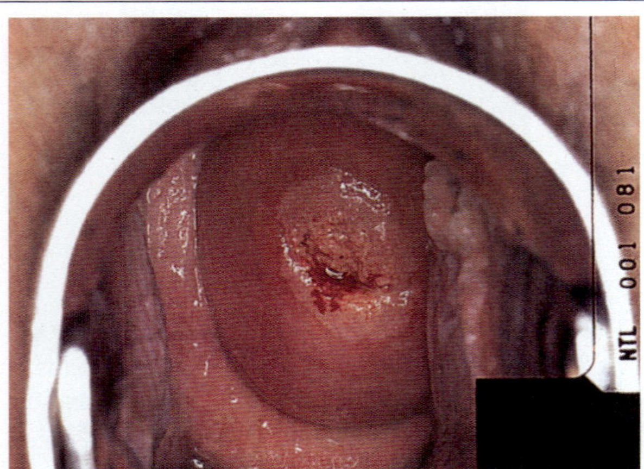

Human papillomavirus (HPV, condylomata)

The virus can appear in various forms when affecting cervical epithelium. Here, warty growth appears as abnormal thickened white epithelium. Visibility of lesion is enhanced by acetic acid (vinegar) wash, which dissolves mucus and temporarily causes intracellular dehydration and coagulation of protein. This must be treated as it can progress to cervical cancer.

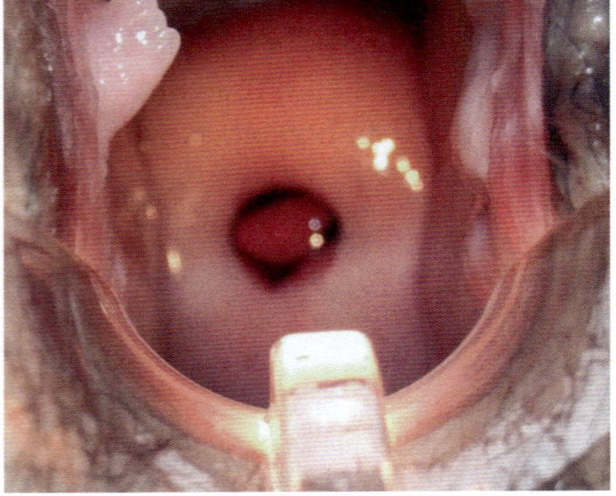

Polyp

The person may have mucoid discharge or bleeding.
The polyp will appear as a bright red, soft, pedunculated growth emerging from os. It is a benign lesion, but this must be determined by biopsy. May be lined with squamous or columnar epithelium.

TABLE 26.5 Abnormalities of the cervix cont'd

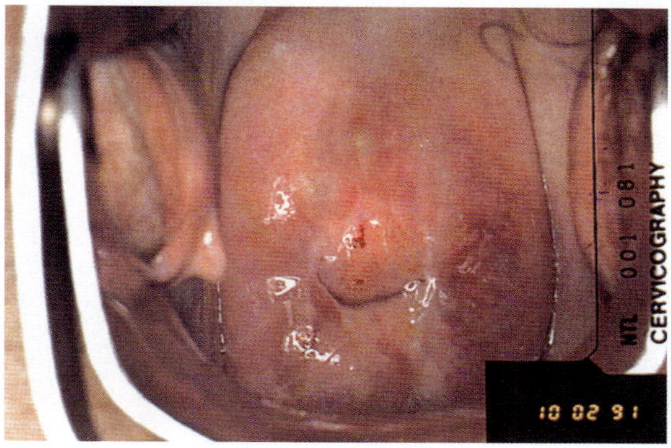

Cervical cancer

The person may complain of bleeding between menstrual periods or after menopause, unusual vaginal discharge.
Chronic ulcer and induration are early signs of carcinoma, although the lesion may or may not show on the exocervix. (Here, lesion is mostly around the external os.) Diagnosed by CST, colposcopy and biopsy.

TABLE 26.6 Vulvovaginal infections

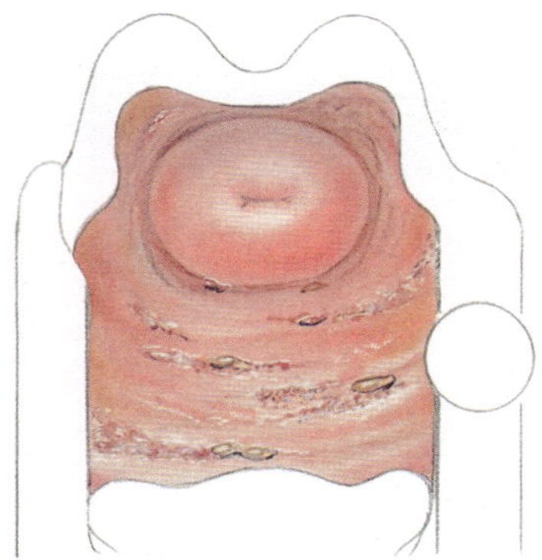

Atrophic vaginitis

Postmenopausal vaginal itching, dryness, burning sensation, dyspareunia, mucoid discharge (may be flecked with blood).
Pale mucosa with abraded areas that bleed easily; may have bloody discharge. Labial mucosa may appear to be thin and fragile, bleeding easily on touch.

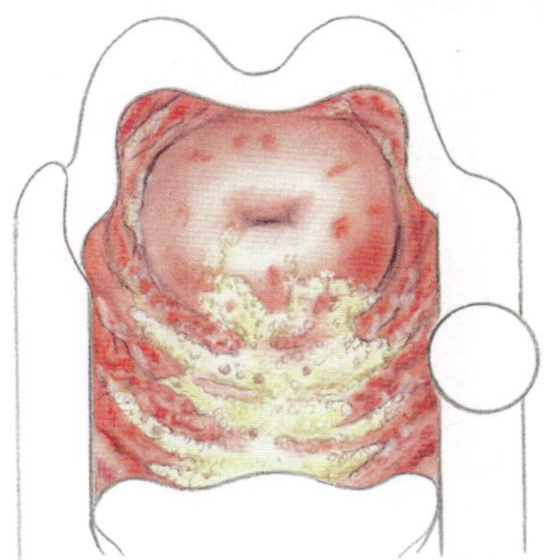

Trichomoniasis

Pruritus, watery and often malodorous vaginal discharge, urinary frequency, terminal dysuria. Symptoms are worse during menstruation when the pH becomes optimal for the organism's growth.
Vulva may be erythematous. Vagina diffusely red, granular, occasionally with red, raised papules and petechiae ('strawberry' appearance). Frothy, yellow-green, foul-smelling discharge. Microscopic examination of saline wet mount specimen shows characteristic flagellated cells.

Continued

TABLE 26.6 Vulvovaginal infections cont'd

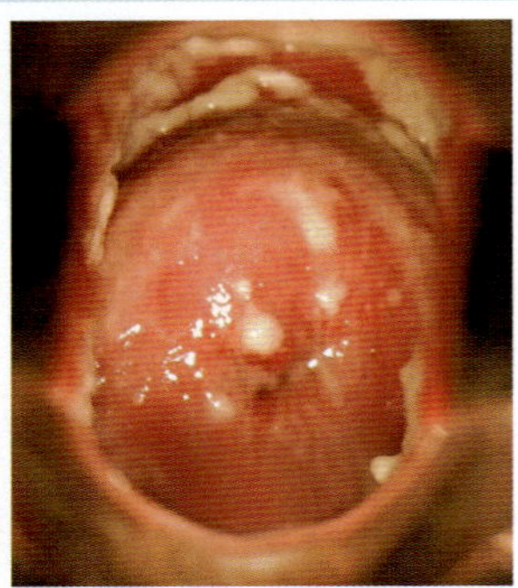

Candidiasis (moniliasis)

Intense pruritus, thick whitish discharge.

Vulva and vagina are erythematous and oedematous. Discharge is usually thick, white and curdy, 'like cottage cheese'. Diagnose by microscopic examination of discharge on potassium hydroxide wet mount.

Predisposing causes—recent use of antibiotics or some oral contraceptives, more alkaline vaginal pH (as with menstrual periods, postpartum, menopause), also pregnancy from increased glycogen and diabetes types 1 and 2.

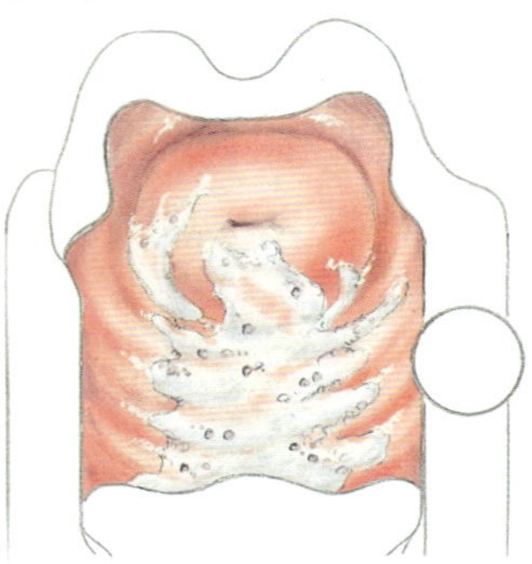

Bacterial vaginosis (*Gardnerella vaginalis, Haemophilus vaginalis* or nonspecific vaginitis)

Profuse discharge, 'constant wetness' with a 'foul, fishy, rotten' odour.

Thin, creamy, grey-white, malodorous discharge. No inflammation on the vaginal wall or cervix because this is a surface parasite. Microscopic view of saline wet mount specimen shows typical 'clue cells'.

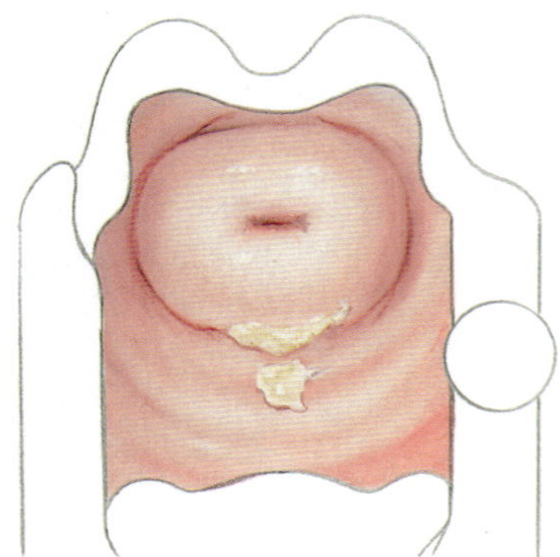

Chlamydia

Minimal symptoms. May have urinary frequency, dysuria or vaginal discharge, postcoital bleeding. May have yellow or green mucopurulent discharge, friable cervix or cervical motion tenderness. Signs are subtle, easily mistaken for gonorrhoea. The two are important to distinguish because antibiotic treatment is different; if the wrong drug is given or if the condition is untreated, chlamydia can ascend the reproductive tract to cause pelvic inflammatory disease and result in infertility.

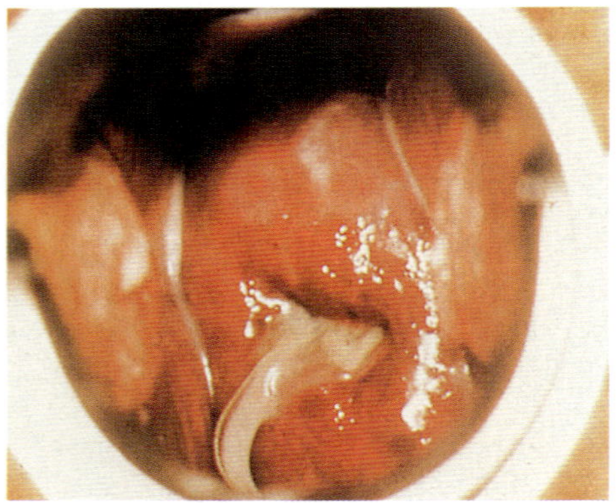

Gonorrhoea

Variable symptoms: vaginal discharge, dysuria, abnormal uterine bleeding, abscess in Bartholin's or Skene's glands; most cases are asymptomatic.

Often no signs are apparent. May have purulent vaginal discharge. Diagnose by positive culture of the organism. If the condition is untreated, it may progress to acute salpingitis or pelvic inflammatory disease.

TABLE 26.7 Uterine enlargement

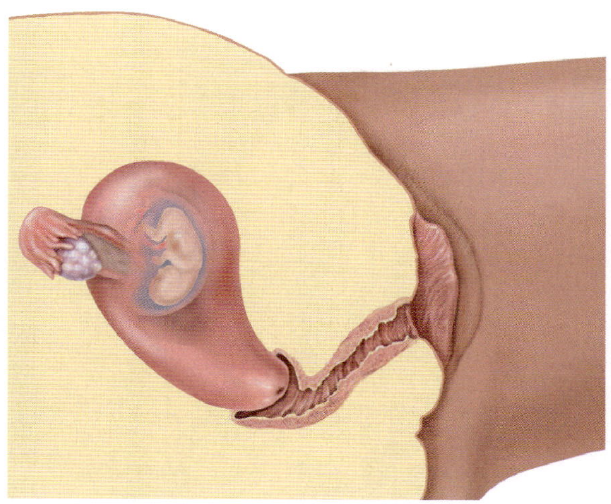

Pregnancy

Obviously a normal condition, pregnancy is included here for comparison.

Amenorrhoea, fatigue, breast engorgement, nausea, changes in food tolerance, weight gain.

Early signs: cyanosis of vaginal mucosa and cervix (Chadwick's sign). Palpation—soft consistency of cervix, enlarging uterus with compressible fundus and isthmus (Hegar's sign at 10 to 12 weeks).

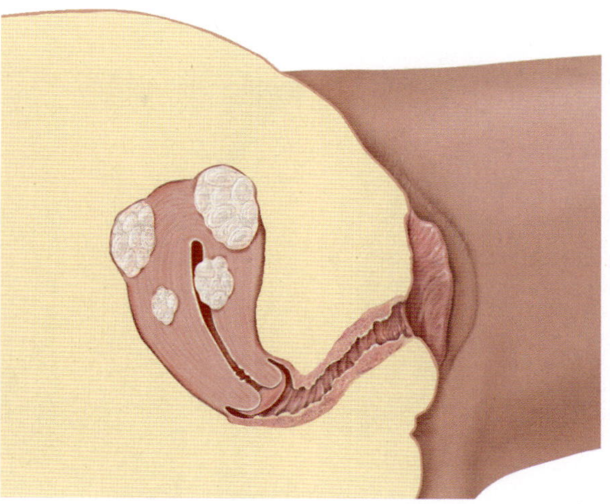

Myomas (leiomyomas, uterine fibroids)

Symptoms vary, depending on size and location. Often no symptoms. When symptoms do occur, include vague discomfort, bloating, heaviness, pelvic pressure, dyspareunia, urinary frequency, backache or hypermenorrhoea if myoma disturbs endometrium. Heavy bleeding produces anaemia.

Uterus irregularly enlarged, firm, mobile and nodular with hard, painless nodules in the uterine wall.

They are usually benign. Myomas are estrogen dependent; after menopause, the lesions usually regress but do not disappear. Surgery may be indicated.

Continued

TABLE 26.7 Uterine enlargement cont'd

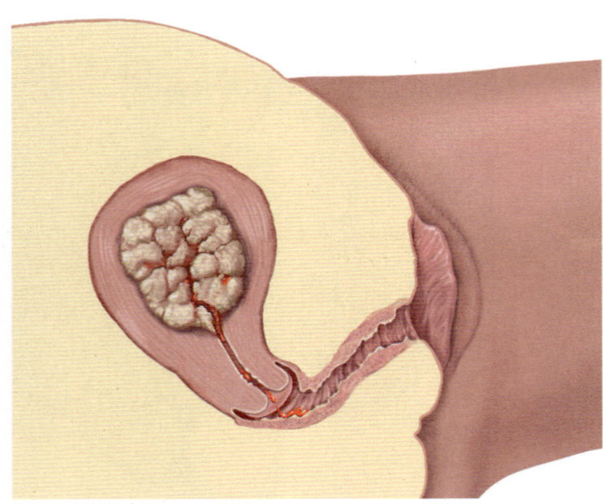

Carcinoma of the endometrium

Abnormal and intermenstrual bleeding before menopause; postmenopausal bleeding or mucosanguineous discharge. Pain and weight loss occur late in the disease.

Uterus may be enlarged.

CSTs are rarely effective in detecting endometrial cancer. Women with abnormal vaginal bleeding or at high risk should have an endometrial tissue sample. Risk factors for endometrial cancer are early menarche, late menopause, history of infertility, failure to ovulate, tamoxifen, unopposed estrogen therapy (which continually stimulates the endometrium, causing hyperplasia) and obesity (which increases endogenous estrogen).

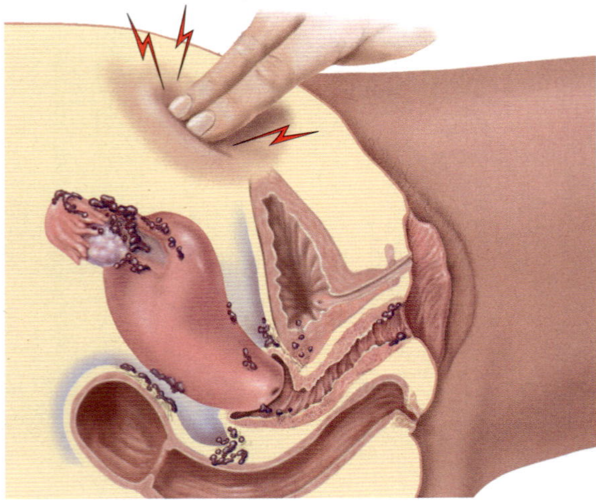

Endometriosis

Symptoms include cyclic or chronic pelvic pain, occurring as dysmenorrhoea or dyspareunia, low backache. Also, may have irregular uterine bleeding or hypermenorrhoea or may be asymptomatic.

Uterus fixed, tender to movement. Small, firm nodular masses tender to palpation on posterior aspect of fundus, uterosacral ligaments, ovaries, sigmoid colon. Ovaries often enlarged.

Masses are aberrant growths of endometrial tissue scattered throughout pelvis as a result of transplantation of tissue by retrograde menstruation. Ectopic tissue responds to hormone stimulation; builds up between periods, sloughs during menstruation. May cause infertility from pelvic adhesions, tubal obstruction, decreased ovarian function.

TABLE 26.8 Adnexal enlargement

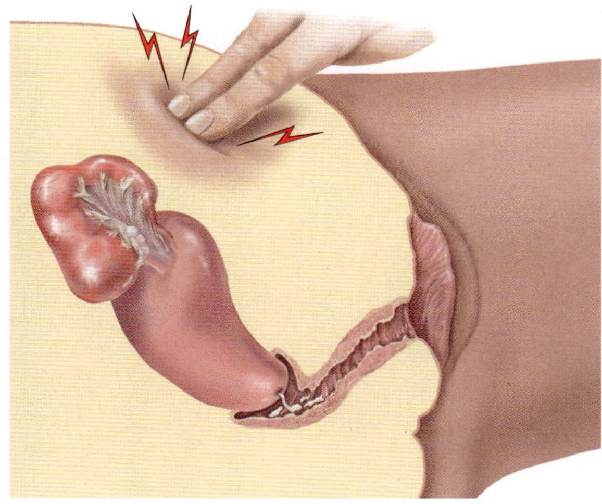

Fallopian tube mass—acute salpingitis (pelvic inflammatory disease)

Sudden fever above 38°C, suprapubic pain, and tenderness.

Acute—rigid board-like lower abdominal musculature. May have purulent discharge from cervix. Movement of uterus and cervix causes intense pain. Pain in lateral fornices and adnexa. Bilateral adnexal masses difficult to palpate because of pain and muscle spasm. Chronic—bilateral, tender, fixed adnexal masses. Complications include ectopic pregnancy, infertility and reinfection. Pelvic inflammatory disease usually caused by *Neisseria gonorrhoeae* or *Chlamydia trachomatis.*

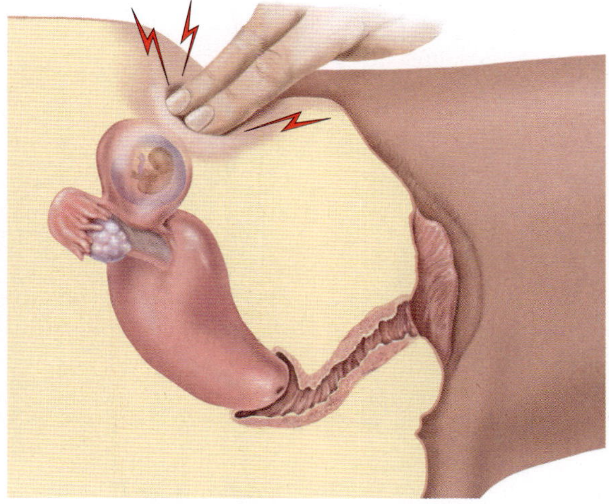

Fallopian tube mass—ectopic pregnancy

Amenorrhoea or irregular vaginal bleeding, pelvic pain.

Softening of cervix and fundus; movement of cervix and uterus causes pain; palpable tender pelvic mass, which is solid, mobile and unilateral. Late signs may indicate rupture: decreased blood pressure, tachycardia, diaphoresis, shock. This is a medical emergency and requires urgent medical referral.

Continued

TABLE 26.8 Adnexal enlargement cont'd

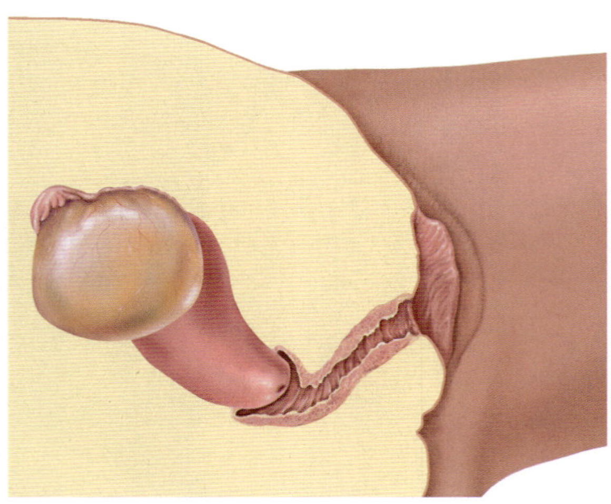

Fluctuant ovarian mass—ovarian cyst

Usually asymptomatic.
Smooth, round, fluctuant, mobile, nontender mass on ovary. Some cysts resolve spontaneously within 60 days but must be followed closely.

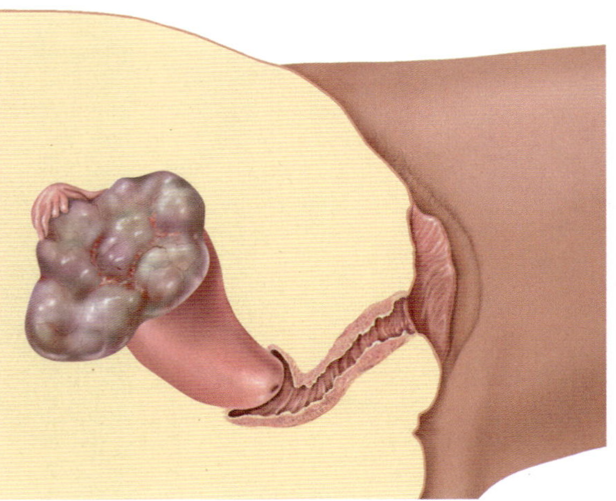

Solid ovarian mass—ovarian cancer

Usually asymptomatic. May have abdominal enlargement from fluid accumulation.
May or may not be able to palpate a solid tumour on the ovary. Heavy, solid, fixed, poorly defined mass suggests malignancy; benign mass may feel mobile and solid.
Biopsy necessary to distinguish the two types of masses. CSTs do not detect ovarian cancer.

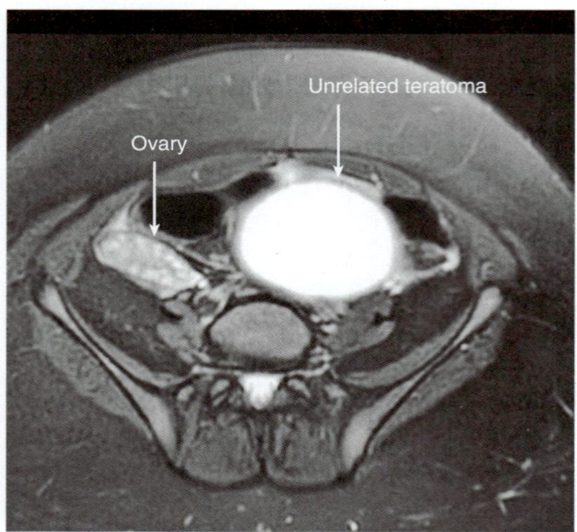

Polycystic ovary syndrome

The woman will usually experience amenorrhoea for 3 months or infrequent periods, infertility, hyperandrogenism (acne, facial hirsutism, hair loss), weight gain. May also have insulin resistance and diabetes.
This MRI image shows a right ovary with multiple cysts.

Clinical reasoning and documentation

The following is a continuation of the case study provided at the beginning of this chapter and the clinical reasoning process including problem/issue identification. Consult a fundamentals of nursing or medical-surgical nursing text for information about goal setting, nursing interventions and evaluation.

Case study (continued)—Genital symptoms

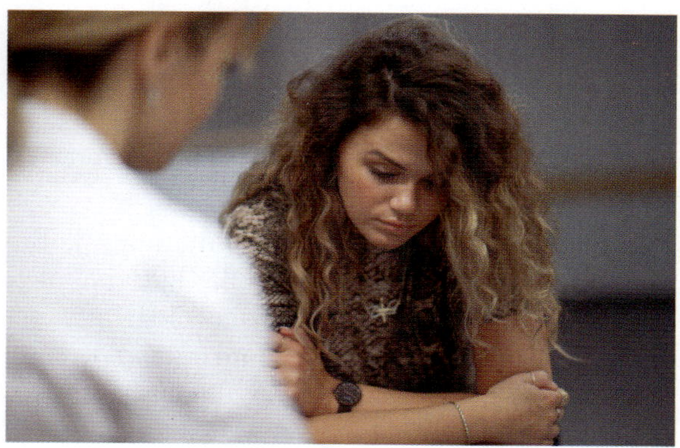

Context

You will recall that you are a registered nurse working at a women's health clinic.

Consider the patient's situation

Ms Jacinta Knight, a 27-year-old woman, presents with urinary burning, vaginal itching and discharge for 4 days.

Collect cues/information

Your further assessment reveals the following information.

Subjective data

3 weeks ago: Ms Knight was treated at a GP clinic for bronchitis with erythromycin, following a respiratory tract virus that progressed to a bacterial infection. No history of asthma, generally healthy but has been very busy at work, working long hours. She says she was very tired before becoming ill. Non-smoker. She says the chest infection improved within 5 days after commencing antibiotics and taking 3 days off work.

She has never been pregnant.

4 to 5 days ago: Noted burning on urination, intense vaginal itching, thick white discharge. Says her husband has no symptoms.

No previous history of vaginal infection, urinary tract infection or pelvic surgery.

Monogamous sexual relationship. Has used combined oral contraceptive pill for 7 years with no side effects. Ms Knight has consented to physical examination of genitalia.

Objective data

On inspection, vulva and vagina erythematous and oedematous. Thick, white, curd-like discharge clinging to vaginal walls and labia.

Process information and identify problems/issues

Collaborative problem

Likely *Candida* vaginitis following antibiotic use and illness

Problem statements/nursing diagnoses

Pain and discomfort related to inflammation and itch

Knowledge deficit related to prevention and treatment of candida (thrush) infection

ADDITIONAL RESOURCES

You can further develop your knowledge and skills relevant to female sexual and reproductive assessment, related pathophysiology, common health issues and nursing interventions by:

- reading chapters of a fundamentals of nursing or medical-surgical nursing textbook
- answering chapter multiple choice questions online. Log onto ClinicalKey Student and search for the text 'Health Assessment, 4th edition'. Choose the section titled 'Teaching material'. In this section you will find question and answer documents for each chapter.

ADDITIONAL RESOURCES cont'd

Please check instructions on the inside front cover of the book to access online resources

- visiting websites

Jean Hailes for Women's Health: http://jeanhailes.org.au

New Zealand Sexual Health Society (Inc.): www.nzshs.org

LGBTIQ+ Health Australia: https://www.lgbtiqhealth.org.au

Community and Public Health (New Zealand): https://www.cph.co.nz/your-health/lgbtqiaplus-health/

Australian Centre for the Prevention of Cervical Cancer—Clinician resources: https://acpcc.org.au/practitioners/resources/.

REFERENCES

1. Kelder I, Sneijder P, Klarenbeek A, Laan E. Communication practices in conversations about sexual health in medical healthcare settings: a systematic review. Patient Education and Counseling. 2022 Apr 1;105(4):858–868.
2. Tortora GJ, Derrickson B, Burkett B, Cooke J, Di Pietro F, Diversi T, et al. Principles of Anatomy and Physiology, 3rd Asia-Pacific Edition. John Wiley & Sons; 2022.
3. Australian Government, Department of Health and Aged Care. National Immunisation Handbook. Australian Government. 2023. Available at: https://immunisationhandbook.health.gov.au/contents/vaccine-preventable-diseases/human-papillomavirus-hpv
4. Rahangdale L, Mungo C, O'Connor S, Chibwesha CJ, Brewer NT. Human papillomavirus vaccination and cervical cancer risk. The BMJ. 2022 Dec 15;379.
5. Australian Government Department of Health. National Cervical Screening Program. 2023. Available at: https://www.health.gov.au/our-work/national-cervical-screening-program
6. Te Whatu Ora—Health New Zealand. The national cervical screening programme (NCSP) HPV primary screening. 2023. Available at: https://www.tewhatuora.govt.nz/for-the-health-sector/ncsp-hpv-screening/
7. Tanner JM: Growth at adolescence. Oxford, 1962, Blackwell Scientific.
8. Champer M, Wong AM, Champer J, Brito IL, Messer PW, Hou JY, et al. The role of the vaginal microbiome in gynaecological cancer. BJOG: An International Journal of Obstetrics & Gynaecology. 2018;125(3):309–315.
9. Family Planning NSW. Contraception in Australia 2005–2018. Ashfield, Sydney: FPNSW; 2020. Available at: https://www.fpnsw.org.au/sites/default/files/assets/Contraception-in-Australia_2005-2018_v20200716.pdf
10. Sexual Health Victoria. Emergency contraceptive pill (morning after pill). 2021. Available at: https://shvic.org.au/for-you/contraception/emergency-contraception/morning-after-pill-emergency-contraception
11. Taft AJ, Shankar M, Black KI, Mazza D, Hussainy S, Lucke JC. Unintended and unwanted pregnancy in Australia: a cross-sectional, national random telephone survey of prevalence and outcomes. Medical Journal of Australia. 2018 Nov 5;209(9):407–408.
12. Ministry of Health. 2022. Abortion Services Aotearoa New Zealand: Annual Report 2022. Wellington: Ministry of Health. Available at: https://www.health.govt.nz/system/files/documents/publications/abortion-services-aotearoa-new-zealand-annual-report-2022-oct22.pdf
13. Sexual Health Victoria. Abortion. 2021. Available at: https://shvic.org.au/for-you/abortion

14. Ministry of Health. 2021. New Zealand Aotearoa Abortion Clinical Guideline. Wellington: Ministry of Health. Available at: https://www.health.govt.nz/system/files/documents/publications/new_zealand_aotearoa_abortion_clinical_guideline.pdf
15. World Health Organization. Defining sexual health. Report of a technical consultation on sexual health. 28–31 January 2002, Geneva. Geneva: WHO; 2006.
16. McGrath M, Low MA, Power E, McCluskey A, Lever S. Addressing sexuality among people living with chronic disease and disability: a systematic mixed methods review of knowledge, attitudes, and practices of health care professionals. Archives of Physical Medicine and Rehabilitation. 2021 May 1;102(5):999–1010.
17. Ollivier R, Aston M, Price S. Let's talk about sex: a feminist poststructural approach to addressing sexual health in the healthcare setting. Journal of Clinical Nursing 2019;28(3–4):695–702.
18. Azar M, Kroll T, Bradbury-Jones C. How do nurses and midwives perceive their role in sexual healthcare? BMC Women's Health. 2022 Dec;22(1):1.
19. Australian Human Rights Commission. Terminology. 2023. Available at: https://humanrights.gov.au/our-work/lgbti/terminology#:~:text=LGBTI%3A%20An%20abbreviation%20which%20is,of%20the%20broader%20LGBTI%20movement
20. Australian Institute of Family Studies. LGBTIQA+ glossary of common terms. Australian Government. 2023. Available at: https://aifs.gov.au/resources/resource-sheets/lgbtiqa-glossary-common-terms#this
21. American Psychiatric Association (APA). Diagnostic and statistical manual of mental disorders. 5th ed. Arlington, VA: American Psychiatric Association; 2013.
22. Victorian Government—Department of Health. Community health pride—LGBTIQ+ inclusive practice resources. 2022. Available at: https://www.health.vic.gov.au/community-health/community-health-pride-lgbtiq-inclusive-practice-resources
23. Victorian Government. LGBTIQ+ inclusive language guide. 2022. Available at: https://www.vic.gov.au/inclusive-language-guide
24. Talley NJ, O'Connor S. Clinical examination: a systematic guide to physical diagnosis. 9th ed. Chatswood, NSW: Elsevier; 2021.
25. Royal Children's Hospital. Engaging with and assessing the adolescent patient. 2019. Available at: https://www.rch.org.au/clinicalguide/guideline_index/Engaging_with_and_assessing_the_adolescent_patient/
26. Australian Law Reform Commission, Australian Government. Capacity and health information. 2010. Available at: https://www.alrc.gov.au/publication/for-your-information-australian-privacy-law-and-practice-alrc-report-108/68-decision-making-by-and-for-individuals-under-the-age-of-18/capacity-and-health-information/
27. Guevara GV, editor. Digital palpation of the pelvic floor muscles. International Continence Society; 2018. Available at: https://www.ics.org/committees/standardisation/terminologydiscussions/digitalpalpationofthepelvicfloormuscles
28. Dickinson T. Advanced assessment of the patient with urinary incontinence and voiding dysfunction. In: Ermer-Seltun JM, Engberg S, editors. Wound, Ostomy and Continence Nurses Society Core Curriculum: Continence Management. 2nd ed. Philadelphia: Wolters Kluwer; 2022.
29. Newman DK, Laycock J. Clinical evaluation of the pelvic floor muscles. In: Baessler K, Schüssler B, Burgio KL, et al., editors. Pelvic floor re-education principles and practice. 2nd ed. London: Springer; 2008. pp. 91–104.

CHAPTER 27

Male sexual and reproductive assessment

Written by Carolyn Jarvis
Adapted by David Lee

INTRODUCTION

You learnt in the previous chapter that sexual and reproductive health is important to a person's general health and wellbeing. Health professionals should not wait for the person to bring up the issue; it should be part of a general health assessment. The male reproductive structures include the penis and scrotum externally and the testes, epididymis and ductus deferens internally. They also include glandular structures accessory to the genital organs (the prostate, seminal vesicles and bulbourethral glands). As the organs, muscles and structures of the urinary tract, abdomen and bowel are relevant to male sexual and reproductive function you should also revise Chapters 23, 24 and 25.

It should be noted that while this chapter focuses on male reproductive health, we emphasise the importance of not making assumptions about a person's sexual orientation and gender identity. This important point needs to be considered when devising an assessment plan.

Case study

The following case study will help you identify your learning needs.

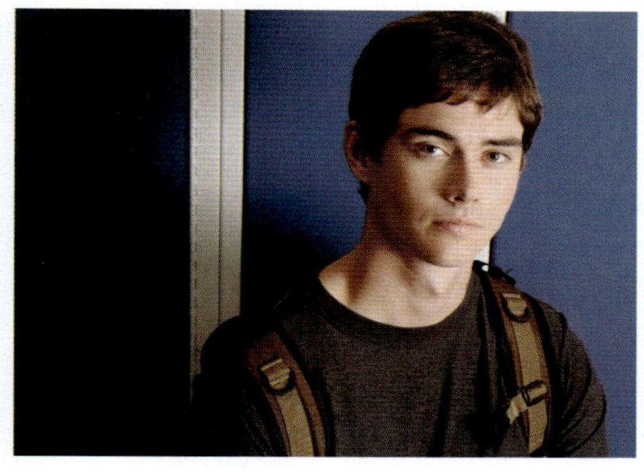

Context

You are a registered nurse working in a university student health centre.

Consider the patient's situation

Mr Ryan Wilson is a 19-year-old student who has experienced acute onset of painful urination, urinary frequency and urgency 2 days ago.

Questions to further your learning

- What are the possible things that might be going on with Mr Wilson?
- What knowledge do you need to be able to predict what might be going on?
- What approach to Mr Wilson's health assessment will you take?
- What questions (subjective data) will you ask Mr Wilson to extend the health history and why?
- What physical examination (objective data) will you conduct and why?
- What resources are available to assist in your assessment of Mr Wilson?

Assessment plan

Assessment of male reproductive function is closely linked to assessing bladder function. Health issues in this area are likely to cause significant distress to the man and his partner and therefore you need to approach the assessment in a tactful and empathic way. Privacy is of upmost importance, and you need to establish a trusting relationship with the person. Detailed questions and physical examination techniques related to urinary and bowel function and the prostate are covered in Chapters 24 and 25. Assessment covers:

- presenting concern
- general health history
- genitourinary/reproductive health history
- sexual health history
- health and lifestyle management.

Following subjective data collection, you will get a sense of the areas needed to be examined for objective data collection. For most nurses asking questions about the man's reproductive health will be enough for a nursing assessment. Physical examination, including inspecting the genitalia, is only performed when there is a valid reason to do so. There needs to be awareness to be mindful that some men may prefer a male clinician and allow for this in your plan. This is particularly so in some cultures and religions including Australia's Indigenous populations where 'men's business' and 'women's business' are separated, and gender-specific health workers are welcomed.

The main areas for physical examination are:

- general inspection
- inspection of external genitalia.

Resources available

You will find additional resources and the reference list at the end of this chapter.

Structure and function

External genitalia

PENIS

The penis is composed of three cylindrical columns of erectile tissue: the two corpora cavernosa on the dorsal side and the corpus spongiosum ventrally (Figure 27.1). At the distal end of the shaft, the corpus spongiosum expands into a cone of erectile tissue, the glans. The shoulder where the glans joins the shaft is the corona. The urethra transverses the corpus spongiosum and its meatus forms a slit at the glans tip (see Chapter 24 for more detail on the structure of the male urethra). Over the glans, the skin folds in and back on itself, forming a hood or flap. This is the foreskin or prepuce. The frenulum is a fold of the foreskin extending from the urethral meatus ventrally.

SCROTUM

The scrotum is a loose protective sac, which is a continuation of the abdominal wall (Figure 27.2). After adolescence, the scrotal skin is deeply pigmented and has large sebaceous follicles. The scrotal wall consists of thin skin lying in folds, or rugae, and the underlying cremaster muscle. The cremaster muscle controls the size of the scrotum by responding to ambient temperature. This is to keep the testes at 3°C below abdominal temperature, the best temperature for producing sperm. When it is cold, the muscle contracts, raising the sac and bringing the testes closer to the body to absorb heat necessary for sperm viability. As a result, the scrotal skin looks corrugated. When it is warmer, the muscle relaxes, the scrotum lowers and the skin looks smoother.

Internal reproductive structures

TESTES

Inside the scrotum a septum separates the sac into two halves. In each scrotal half is a testis, which produces sperm. The testis has a solid oval shape, which is compressed laterally and measures 4 to 5 cm long by 3 cm wide in adults. The testis is suspended vertically by the spermatic cord. The left testis is lower than the right because the left spermatic cord is longer. Each testis is covered by a double-layered membrane, the tunica vaginalis, which separates it from the scrotal wall. The two layers are lubricated by fluid so the testis can

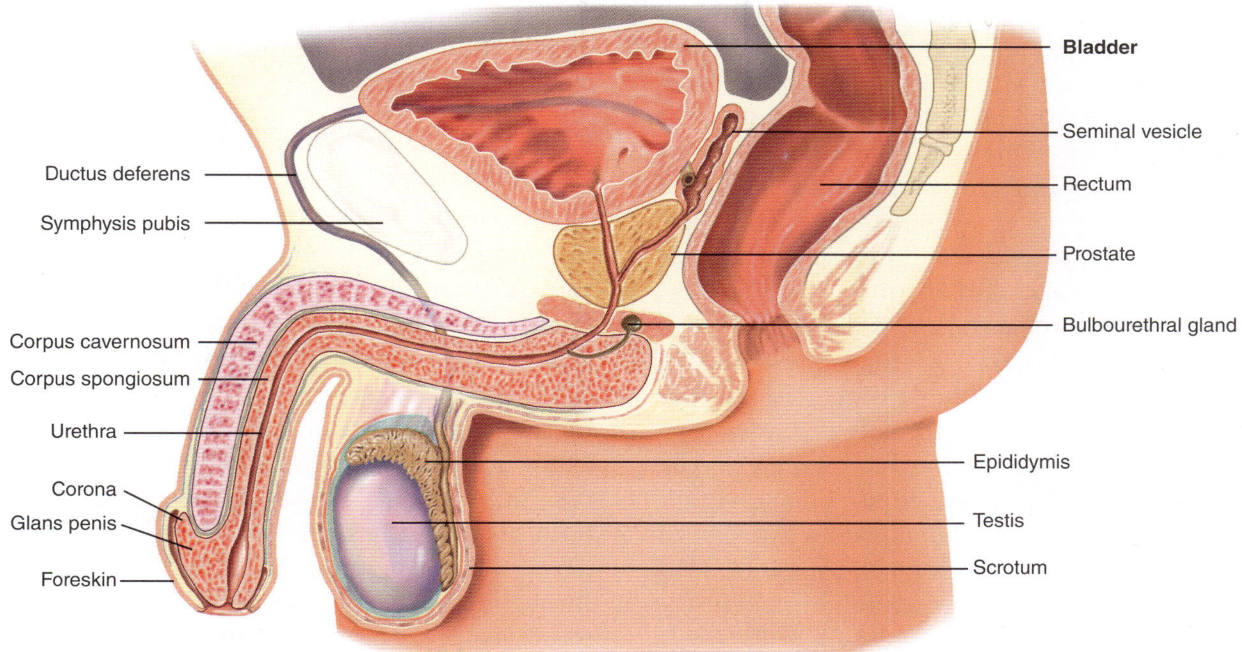

FIGURE 27.1 Male pelvic organs

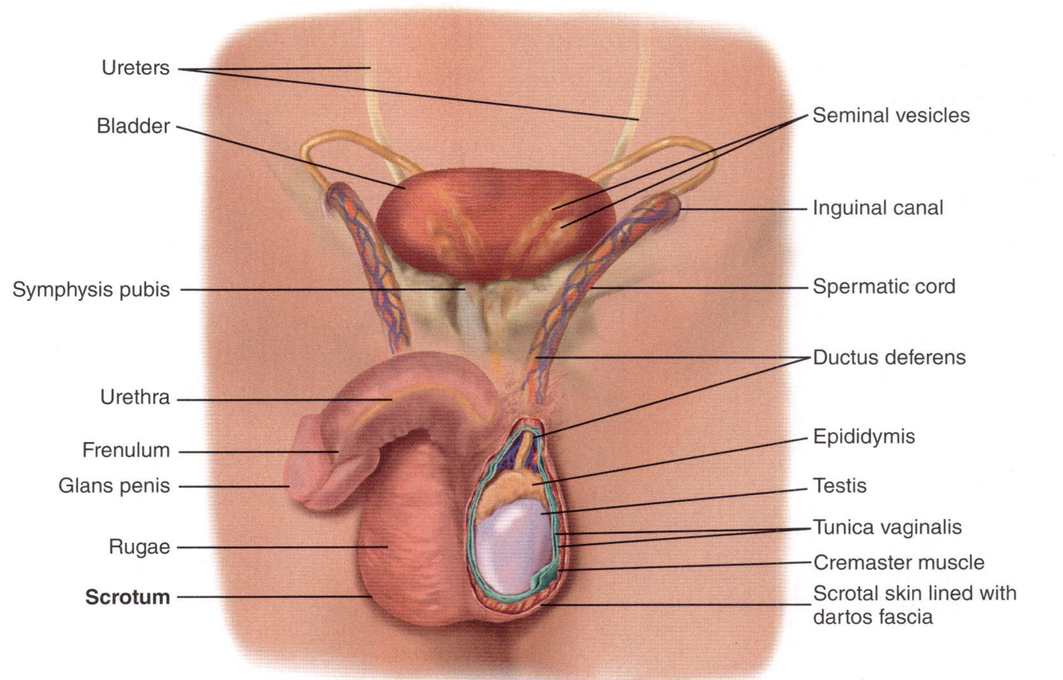

FIGURE 27.2 Male genitourinary anatomy

slide a little within the scrotum; this helps prevent injury.

Sperm are transported along a series of ducts. First, the testis is capped by the **epididymis**, which is a markedly coiled duct system and the main storage site of sperm. It is a comma-shaped structure, curved over the top and the posterior surface of the testis. Occasionally (in 6–7% of males), the epididymis is anterior to the testis.

The lower part of the epididymis is continuous with a muscular duct, the **ductus deferens**. This duct approximates with other vessels (arteries and veins, lymphatics, nerves) to form the **spermatic cord**. The spermatic cord ascends along the posterior border of the testis and runs through the tunnel of the inguinal canal into the abdomen. Here, the ductus deferens continues back and down behind the bladder, where it joins the duct of the seminal vesicle to form the **ejaculatory duct**. This duct empties into the urethra.

The **lymphatics** of the penis and scrotal surface drain into the inguinal lymph nodes, whereas those of the testes drain into the abdomen. Abdominal lymph nodes are not accessible to clinical examination.

PROSTATE GLAND

In males, the **prostate gland** lies in front of the anterior wall of the rectum and 2 cm behind the symphysis pubis. It surrounds the bladder neck and the urethra and has 15 to 30 ducts that open into the urethra. The prostate secretes a thin, milky alkaline fluid that helps sperm viability. It is a bilobed structure with a round or heart shape. It measures 2.5 cm long and 4 cm in diameter. The two lateral lobes are separated by a shallow groove called the **median sulcus**.

The two **seminal vesicles** project like rabbit ears above the prostate. The seminal vesicles secrete a fluid that is rich in fructose, which nourishes the sperm and contains prostaglandins. The two **bulbourethral** (Cowper's) **glands** are each the size of a pea and are located inferior to the prostate on either side of the urethra. They secrete a clear, viscid mucus.

PELVIC FLOOR MUSCLES AND PERINEUM

The bony pelvis forms the solid structure for the muscles and ligaments of the anterior, posterior and lateral pelvic walls and pelvic floor, which play such an important role in supporting the position of the pelvic organs. The pelvic floor muscles include the coccygeus muscle and the levator ani and are referred to as the pelvic diaphragm, which stretches from the pubic bone anteriorly to the coccyx posteriorly and from the right and left lateral pelvic walls. The anal canal and urethra pass through the pelvic diaphragm. The levator ani muscles support the pelvic organs and functions as a sphincter for the anal canal and urethra.[1]

The perineum is located inferior to the pelvic diaphragm. The perineum extends from the symphysis pubis anteriorly to the coccyx posteriorly and the ischial tuberosities laterally. The muscles of the perineum are in two layers, superficial and deep. The superficial layer includes the superficial transverse perineal, bulbospongiosus and the ischiocavernosus muscles, which help to maintain erection of the penis and facilitate ejaculation. The deep layer of the perineum includes the deep transverse perineal muscle, the external urethral sphincter and external anal sphincter, which assist in maintaining urinary and faecal continence as well as ejaculation.[1]

INGUINAL AREA

The **inguinal area**, or groin, is the juncture of the lower abdominal wall and the thigh (Figure 27.3). Its diagonal borders are the anterior superior iliac spine and the symphysis pubis. Between these landmarks lies the **inguinal ligament** (Poupart's ligament). Superior to the ligament lies the **inguinal canal**, a narrow tunnel passing obliquely between layers of abdominal muscle. It is 4 to

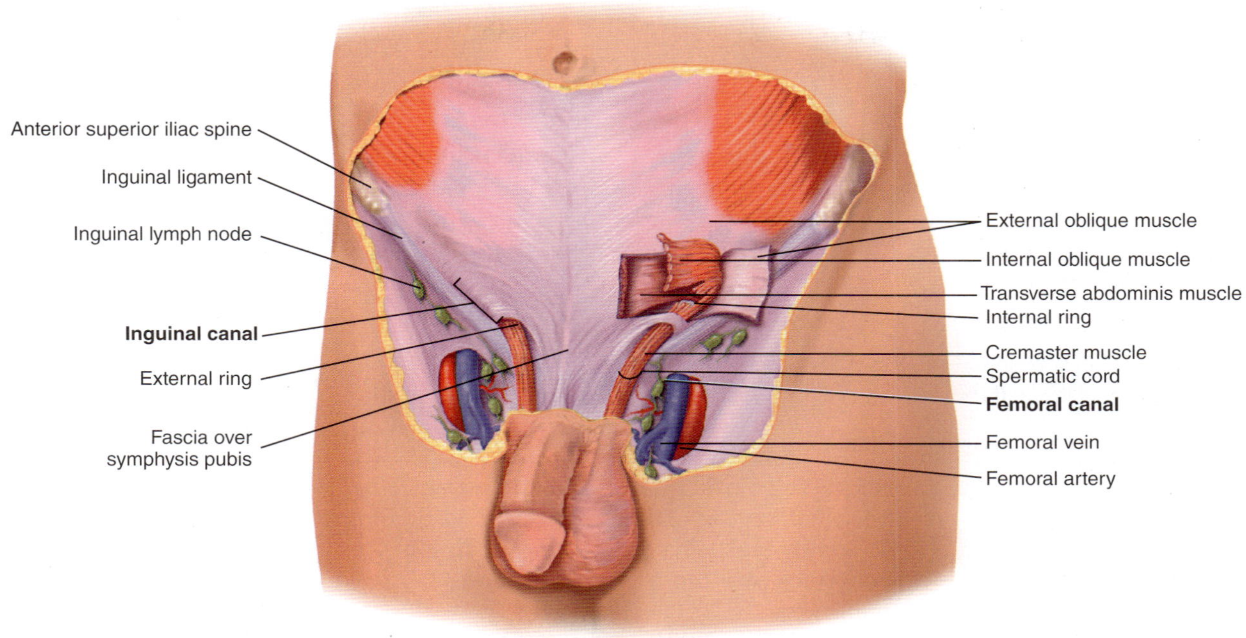

FIGURE 27.3 Structures of the male inguinal area

6 cm long in adults. Its openings are an internal ring, located 1 to 2 cm above the midpoint of the inguinal ligament and an external ring, located just above and lateral to the pubis.

Inferior to the inguinal ligament is the **femoral canal**. It is a potential space located 3 cm medial to and parallel with the femoral artery. You can use the artery as a landmark to find this space. There are superficial and deep lymph nodes around the inguinal canal located in the femoral triangle of Scarpa. Lymph nodes are glands that function to maintain blood fluid balance, filter waste and are a protective defence system from pathogens. These lymph nodes may be palpable in thinner men and are smooth, mobile in consistency and nontender when palpated. The inguinal lymph nodes can become painful and enlarged (lymphadenitis) when there is localised infection. Knowledge of these anatomical areas in the groin is useful because they are potential sites for a hernia, which is a loop of bowel protruding through a weak spot in the musculature.

Developmental considerations

Infants

Prenatally, the testes develop in the abdominal cavity near the kidneys. During the later months of gestation the testes migrate, pushing the abdominal wall in front of them and dragging the ductus deferens, the blood vessels and nerves behind. The testes descend along the inguinal canal into the scrotum before birth. At birth, each testis measures 1½ to 2 cm long and 1 cm wide. Only a slight increase in size occurs during the prepubertal years.

Adolescents

Puberty begins sometime between the ages of 9½ and 13. The first sign is enlargement of the testes. Next, pubic hair appears then penis size increases. The stages of development are documented in Tanner's sexual maturity ratings (Table 27.1). The complete change in development from a preadolescent to an adult takes about 3 years, although the normal range is 2 to 5 years.

The level of sexual development at the end of puberty remains constant through young and middle adulthood, with no further

TABLE 27.1 Sex maturity ratings in boys

Developmental Stage	Pubic hair	Penis	Scrotum
1	No pubic hair. Fine body hair on the abdomen (vellus hair) continues over the pubic area.	Preadolescent, size and proportion the same as during childhood.	Preadolescent, size and proportion the same as during childhood.
2	Few straight slightly darker hairs at base of penis. Hair is long and downy.	Little or no enlargement.	Testes and scrotum begin to enlarge. Scrotal skin reddens and changes in texture.
3	Sparse growth over the entire pubis. Hair darker, coarser and curly.	Penis begins to enlarge, especially in length.	Further enlarged.
4	Thick growth over the pubic area but not on the thighs. Hair coarse and curly as in adults.	Penis grows in length and diameter, with development of glans.	Testes almost fully grown; scrotum darker.

TABLE 27.1 Sex maturity ratings in boys cont'd

5 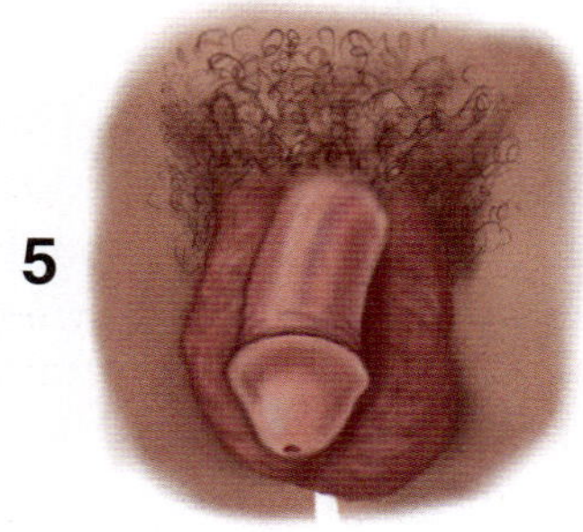	Growth spread over medial thighs, although not yet up towards umbilicus. After puberty, pubic hair growth continues until the mid-20s, extending up the abdomen towards the umbilicus.	Adult size and shape.	Adult size and shape.

genital growth and no change in circulating sex hormone. The male does not experience a definite end to fertility as the female does. Around age 40 years, the production of sperm begins to decrease, although it continues into the 80s and 90s.

Testosterone (or androgen) and estrogen are important hormones in both men and women. When blood levels are depleted or elevated, physiological, physical, emotional and psychological concerns may arise. Men have higher levels of testosterone than women and lower levels of estrogen. Testosterone maintains sex drive, production of sperm, muscle strength and bone mass and plays a role in overall wellbeing and energy levels. Low levels of testosterone (hypogonadism) may lead to mood changes, poor concentration, lethargy, low libido or sex drive, hot flushes and sweats, reduced body hair growth, reduced muscle strength and breast enlargement (gynaecomastia).[2] The misuse of steroids and other performance and image enhancing drugs have significant and detrimental impact on physiology, neurological function and mental health.[3]

Adults—men over 65 years

At male puberty, the prostate gland undergoes a very rapid increase to more than twice its prepubertal size. During young adulthood its size remains fairly constant. The prostate gland commonly starts to enlarge during the middle adult years. This **benign prostatic hypertrophy** is a common condition affecting more than 20% of men by 60 years of age and 40% of men over 70 years of age.[4] It is thought that hypertrophy is caused by hormonal imbalance that leads to the proliferation of benign adenomas. These gradually impede voiding because they obstruct the urethra.

Prostate cancer is the most common cancer that occurs in men and the second leading cause of cancer deaths in men. The crude prostate cancer incidence rate in Australia estimated 189 cases per 100,000 men in 2022. This rate is expected to rise, due to longer lifespan and more men over the age of 70 years by 2033. The lifetime risk of developing prostate cancer is one in five for Australian men.[5] In Aotearoa New Zealand males, the incidence of prostate cancer is estimated to be one in 13 to age 75.[6]

Prostate cancer is essentially a disease of older men, with 63% diagnosed after 65 years of age; it is rare before the age of 40 and its incidence rises rapidly after age 60.[7,8]

The cause of prostate cancer is unknown. Apart from advancing age and being male, the strongest established risk factor is a family history of the disease; the risk depends on the number of relatives affected. Genetic mutations (BRCA gene) as well as genetic conditions such as Lynch syndrome may lead to a higher risk of prostate cancer.[9] People from an African ethnicity appear to have a higher risk in developing prostate cancer.[10]

In the early stages of prostate cancer, the man is likely to be asymptomatic, making early detection difficult. Men who request a prostate-specific antigen serology test should be given information about the benefits and harms of testing.[9] Men with a family history of prostate cancer or other risk factors should be offered prostate-specific antigen testing every 2 years from age 40–45 to 69 years old.[11]

In ageing males, the amount of pubic hair decreases, and the remaining hair turns grey. Penis size decreases. Due to decreased tone of the dartos muscle, the scrotal contents hang lower, the rugae decrease and the scrotum looks pendulous. The testes decrease in size and are less firm to palpation. Increased connective tissue is present in the tubules, so these become thickened and produce less sperm. As men age their testosterone levels decline slowly, from about the age of 40 years. Some older men will develop very low testosterone levels (androgen deficiency), which will cause symptoms like the female menopause such as fatigue, hot flushes, decreased sexual drive and osteoporosis.[12]

Although a wide range of differences can occur, older males may find that an erection takes longer to develop and that it is less full or firm. Once obtained, the erection may be maintained for longer periods without ejaculation. Ejaculation is shorter and less forceful, and the volume of seminal fluid is less than when the man was younger. After ejaculation, rapid detumescence (return to the flaccid state) occurs, especially after 60 years of age. This occurs in a few seconds as compared with minutes or hours in younger males. Erectile dysfunction has been defined as the persistent inability to achieve or maintain an erection sufficient for satisfactory sexual intercourse.[13] The incidence of erectile dysfunction increases with age, occurring in up to 50% of men aged 40 to 70 years.[14] Apart from advancing age, risk factors include smoking/vaping, alcohol abuse, obesity and metabolic syndrome, lack of physical activity, diabetes, cardiovascular disease, neurological conditions, some medications and psychological factors.[13]

Cultural and social considerations

There is a marked inequality in Australian men's health—men have a shorter life expectancy than women and die more often than women from preventable diseases. While men are seeking out health care more frequently than in previous years, they often present when a condition or illness is advanced and are unlikely to seek help for mental ill-health.[15] There is a higher rate of risk-taking behaviour, suicide, accidents and poorer mental health outcomes including violence, anger, substance and alcohol misuse.[16] There is a similar situation for men in Aotearoa New Zealand.[17] To address the specific needs of men's health, the Australian Government has developed a focused health strategy to promote men's health with the goal of 'every man and boy in Australia is supported to live a long, fulfilling and healthy life'.[15] The five priority areas of the strategy are mental health, chronic conditions, sexual and reproductive health and conditions where men are over-represented (such as injuries and risk taking) and healthy ageing.

As has been discussed in previous chapters, a range of determinants influence health including individual factors, social, economic, environmental, cultural and political contexts.[15] You will also appreciate that there are some population groups that are more at risk than others. In Australia, the National Men's Health Strategy 2020–2030 focuses on Aboriginal and Torres Strait Islander males, males from socioeconomically disadvantaged backgrounds, males living in rural and remote areas, males with disability including mental illness, males from culturally and linguistically diverse backgrounds, members of the LGBTIQ+ community, male veterans, socially isolated males and men in the criminal justice system.[15]

Gender identity and sexuality

Gender has been thought of throughout history as binary—female or male. In the recent past, it has been recognised that not all people fall comfortably into this binary. Globally, the legal frameworks have not caught up with correcting gender preference politics such as in birth certificates, marriage certificates or passports, although this is gradually being discussed by governments and organisations. In Australia it is estimated that approximately 3.5% of the adult population identify as LGBTIQ+.[18] In Aotearoa New Zealand, 4.4% of the adult population identifies as LGBTIQ+, 0.5% of the population identify as transgender or non-binary.[19] For a list of relevant terminology relevant to gender diversity, see Chapter 26.

However, despite the acceptance of LGBTIQ+ as a norm in sexuality, at least in developed nations, there are still significant barriers to health and wellbeing in this group. In Australia, LGBTIQ+ people continue to experience high levels of discrimination in many aspects of their lives. There remains high rates of suicide and suicide attempts, depression and anxiety, especially in trans and gender diverse people who have lower self-reported health than the general population.[20] The point has been made previously in this text (Chapter 9) that many trans and gender diverse people have had previous experience of discrimination, misgendering and disrespectful communication, often avoiding contact with health care professionals and missing important health screening.[20,21] Your approach to the person is critical in gaining their trust, including asking the person if there are any terms they use for their body parts, ensure they understand what is going to happen and why and continuously reconfirming consent to touch them in a new location.[22]

Treatment as prevention, pre- and post-exposure HIV prophylaxis

In Australia, there were 552 diagnosed cases of human immunodeficiency virus (HIV) in 2021, a 48% reduction since 2012 and 39% decrease since 2019.[23] Male-to-male sex is the major HIV risk exposure in Australia, accounting for 68% of notifications in 2021, followed by heterosexual sex (27%) and injecting drug use. In 2022 in Aotearoa New Zealand, 135 people (109 men and 20 women) were notified with HIV. Of the 135 people, 80 involved men who had sex with men, 27 people acquired HIV through heterosexual contact and one through perinatal transmission.[24]

Highly affective antiretroviral drug therapy has reduced the morbidity of acquired immunodeficiency syndrome (AIDS) related diseases and significantly reduced the risk of acquiring AIDS. Evidence has shown that a person living with HIV on combined antiretroviral treatment who adheres to the medication regimen will have a close to zero viral load and have a zero risk of transmitting HIV.[25]

The use of a two-drug combined antiretroviral therapy as HIV *post-exposure* prophylaxis lacks research evidence and is likely to be ineffective.[26] On the other hand, HIV *pre-exposure* prophylaxis (PrEP) has an efficacy of 99% if taken every day.[26,27] However, men need to be reminded that these drugs do not prevent other sexually transmitted infections (STI), so condoms should always be used. These drugs are potent, safe, with few side effects and convenient with one-pill, once-daily dosing. However, adherence is critical for long-term efficacy. Men using PrEP need regular monitoring for drug side effects and HIV screening.[26]

Infant male circumcision

Circumcision is an elective surgical procedure involving removal of the male foreskin. It is a procedure that has been performed for thousands of years for cultural and religious reasons. There are high rates of male circumcision still practised in some countries, but in Australia and Aotearoa New Zealand, male circumcision remains a controversial procedure and is not routinely performed. It is estimated that worldwide 37 to 39% of men are circumcised, with approximately 13% of newborn Australians being circumcised each year.[28]

A foreskin is usually fully retractile by up to age 10 years, but this is variable. Genital hygiene needs to be taught in early childhood to help prevent penile problems like balanitis, phimosis and paraphimosis. Genital hygiene includes retracting back and gently stretching the foreskin as well as using soap alternatives for genital skin care.[28]

Communicating effectively with people about sexuality and sexual function

Discussing sexuality is an important part of health assessment, although many nurses do not feel comfortable in discussing these issues. Read the section titled 'Communicating effectively with people about sexuality and sexual function' in Chapter 26 before you continue to work through this chapter.

HEALTH EDUCATION

Testicular self-examination/ testicular awareness

Testicular cancer accounts for 1.2% of all male cancers. The lifetime risk of developing testicular cancer is one in 193 for Australian men.[29] And although the prognosis is very good, testicular cancer has the potential to significantly impact on the man's quality of life. In Aotearoa New Zealand, there has been a trend for increasing rates of testicular cancer, especially in Māori men.[30] It is primarily a disease of young males, with incidence being most frequent in males aged between 15 and 44 years.

Although the pathogenesis of testicular cancer is unclear, several risk factors have been identified including having undescended testis as an infant (cryptorchidism), family history (father, brother) of testicular cancer, infertility, HIV and AIDS, history of congenital hypospadias (abnormality of the penis and urethra), previous testicular cancer and intersex variations.[31] If identified early almost all testicular cancers are curable.

HEALTH EDUCATION cont'd

Men are advised to become aware of the normal size and consistency of their testicles so they can recognise any changes that may occur. Healthy Male recommends that men regularly perform testicular self-examination so they develop a sense of what is normal for them. It only takes a few minutes to perform.

Nurse's role

Points to include for health teaching are:

- Testicular self-examination involves feeling the testes, one at a time, using the fingers and thumb.
- It is usually easier after a warm shower or bath (warm water relaxes the scrotal sac).
- Advise the man to use the palm of one hand to support the scrotum, then gently roll one testis between the thumb and fingers to feel for any lumps or swelling in or on the surface of the testis (or any changes from the last testicular self-examination).
- Normally a testis has a smooth surface and feels firm. It is normal for one testis to feel slightly bigger than the other.
- Using the thumb and fingers continue along the back of the testis to feel the epididymis (a soft coiled tube that carries the sperm from the testis to the ductus deferens).
- If there are any changes to how the testes feel normally, or if the man is concerned, advise him to see his local doctor (GP) as soon as possible.

For more information see the following websites:

- Healthy Male (Australia): https://www.healthymale.org.au/mens-health/testicular-cancer
- Healthy Male video—testicular self-examination https://youtu.be/DwPhOLKfVYY?si=j9Px3TosK6ElJLw0
- Testicular Cancer NZ: https://testicular.org.nz.

Subjective data

Practice note

Before you start the assessment, introduce yourself to the person, confirm the person's identity, discuss the purpose and scope of the assessment, clarify any questions the person may have and obtain verbal consent from the person to perform the assessment. As you approach the health assessment interview it is important that you:

- don't make assumptions about the person's gender identity and sexual orientation based on appearance
- use open and inclusive questions that are gender neutral and inclusive
- encourage the person to discuss their sexual orientation, gender identity and relationship status
- respect their choice to not disclose their sexual or gender identity
- respond positively when the person is prepared to be open about their sexual orientation, gender identity or intersex condition
- ask how they would like to be addressed (he/she/they) if you are unsure
- begin with open-ended questions to assess individual needs
- be cautious about recording information about sexual orientation, gender identity or intersex condition in a person's health record. Seek consent from the person and inform them about why the information is needed and to whom it will be made available.

ASSESSMENT GUIDELINES	CLINICAL SIGNIFICANCE AND CLINICAL ALERTS
Presenting concern	
It is important to ascertain the person's perception of their sexual and/or reproductive health. From the presenting concern, the person would be able to provide you with some insight into their symptoms and perhaps other health issues. If they do perceive a problem, ask: *How does this affect your quality of life?* The responses to these questions will guide the sequence of the rest of the subjective data collection. Take the cues from the person. If the person cannot articulate their health concern, use the questions below to assist them to verbalise their health situation. A suggested approach: • *I would like to ask you some questions to find out more about how I can help you today. Some of the questions might appear intrusive and personal but will assist me in identifying your healthcare needs. Is it OK with you if I ask these questions?* • *What brings you here today? Do you have any issues with your sexual and reproductive health?*	
General health history	
Recent illness • *Have you experienced any recent illness?*	
Personal health history • *Have you had any surgery, medical conditions, allergies or other health difficulties related to mobility, pain or disability?* Ask specifically about genital, prostate, bladder or bowel surgery (Chapters 23, 24 and 25).	Chronic illness and treatments can contribute to sexual dysfunction.
Family history Ask about significant family history of diabetes, epilepsy, clotting disorders, hypertension or cardiovascular disease, prostate and testicular cancers, etc.	There is an increased incidence of prostate cancer in men with a first-degree relative who has/had prostate cancer.
Current and past cigarette smoking/vaping • *How many cigarettes/vapes do you smoke per day? For how long have you been smoking?*	Smoking causes cardiovascular disease, which can reduce fertility and cause erectile dysfunction.
Current and past alcohol and illicit substance use Ask the person to be specific about how much alcohol, how often and for how long. • *Which drugs do you use? How much and how often (including injecting drug use)?*	Personal health risks as well as putting the person at risk of unsafe sex or sexual violence.
Current medication Ask about use of prescribed medications, complementary and traditional therapies and over-the-counter medications.	Broad-spectrum antibiotics alter balance of normal flora, which can predispose to *Candida* genital skin infection.

ASSESSMENT GUIDELINES	CLINICAL SIGNIFICANCE AND CLINICAL ALERTS
Psychosocial history (see also Chapter 8 and Chapter 11) • *What is your highest educational achievement? High school, TAFE or university?* • *Living arrangements?* • *Contact and support from family members? Friends?* • *Are you involved in any hobbies and activities?*	
Genitourinary/reproductive health history	
Urinary symptoms or lower abdominal pain • *Have you experienced any problem with your bladder or voiding?* (urinary symptoms such as urgency, slow stream, feeling of incomplete emptying or incontinence) • *Have you experienced any problems with bowel function?* • *Have you experienced any abdominal pain?* If the symptom is present, ask the person to describe the sign or symptom: • *When did it start?* • *What have you done about it? Did the treatment help?*	**Urinary or faecal incontinence** or **lower urinary tract symptoms** can significantly affect a person's sexuality and sexual function and requires further assessment. It is rare for men under the age of 60 years to suffer from a **urinary tract infection.** Unlike in women, the anatomical sites of the male genitalia has no direct contact with the anorectal region. Should an individual present with mild symptoms of urethritis, no high sexual risk, but also urinary frequency including nocturnal frequency, consider a mid-stream urine for testing for bacteriuria. For details about assessment of urinary function, see Chapter 24; bowel function, see Chapter 25; and assessment of abdominal pain, see Chapter 23.
Genital signs and symptoms • *Have you experienced any problem with your penis—foreskin, pain, lesions, itch, redness?*	
Urethral discharge • *How much (scant, a lot)? Has that increased or decreased?* • *Can you describe the colour? Any odour?* • *Is there any discharge associated with pain or with urination?*	**Urethral discharge** occurs with infection. Some penile infections will be sexually transmitted. STIs can cause pain on voiding and lower abdominal pain. People with a suspected STI should be referred to a medical or nurse practitioner or sexual health clinic for diagnosis and treatment.
Scrotum and testicles • *Have you noticed any difference with your scrotum? Any pain?*	**Epididymitis** is an inflammation of the epididymis and caused by pathogens, some of which may be sexually transmitted. **Hydrocoele** is collection of serous fluid in the tunica vaginalis, surrounding the testis. A **varicocoele** is dilated, tortuous varicose veins in the spermatic cord due to incompetent valves within the vein, which permit reflux of blood.

ASSESSMENT GUIDELINES	CLINICAL SIGNIFICANCE AND CLINICAL ALERTS
	Hydrocoeles and varicocoeles may cause scrotal enlargement; an ultrasound will confirm whether these lumps might be cancerous.
• *Have you noticed any bulge or swelling in the scrotum? For how long?* • *Have you ever been told you have a hernia?* • *Have you ever experienced any dragging, heavy feeling in scrotum?*	Possible **scrotal hernia**. A **hernia** is a loop of bowel protruding through a weak spot in the musculature and the section of the bowel moves down the inguinal canal and into the scrotal sac.
• *Have you noticed any lump or swelling on testes?*	**Testicular cancer**—see 'Health education' section. **Testicular torsion**—a sudden twisting of spermatic cord, can occur at any age but most commonly in men between the onset of puberty and the mid-20s. The blood supply to the testes is occluded due to twisting of the spermatic cord and can lead to scrotal necrosis. ! ***Clinical alert:*** Any report of severe pain in the testes or scrotum should be referred to a medical practitioner. It is considered a medical emergency.
Breast symptoms • *Have you experienced any pain or other abnormal symptoms in your breasts?* If present, ask the person to describe the sign or symptom: • *When did it start?* • *What have they done about it, and did this reduce the symptom?*	**Breast cancer** is rare in men; the lifetime risk of being diagnosed with breast cancer is 1 in 672. The median age at diagnosis was 70.5 years.[32] Age and a known *BRAC1* or *BRAC2* gene mutation are known risk factors. ! ***Clinical alert:*** Any unusual change in the breasts should be further assessed and/or referred to a medical practitioner. For details about breast assessment, see Chapter 28.
Sexual health history	
Start with a general statement and a question such as: '*When I conduct a health assessment, I ask people about their sexual health. Is it alright with you if I ask questions about your sexual health?*' This may help you open up the discussion with the person. Only ask the questions that are relevant to the situation.	

ASSESSMENT GUIDELINES	CLINICAL SIGNIFICANCE AND CLINICAL ALERTS
Sexual history • *Are you currently sexually active?* • *At what age was your first sexual contact?* • *When was the last time you had sex?* • *Do you have a regular or casual sexual partner? How long have you been with this person?* • *What type of sexual contact do you have—oral, vaginal, anal?* • *How many sexual partners have you had in the past 12 months?* • *Have you had sex that you can't remember because of alcohol or substance use?* • *Any history with partners from overseas?*	Determining the person's sexual practices will enable you to identify areas for health education or the need for further questioning to identify risk factors for STI and/or the need for specific physical examination and other investigations.
Contraception (if relevant) • *What do you do to protect your partner from unplanned pregnancy?*	
History of sexually transmitted infection (STI) • *Have you (or your partner) had any current symptoms or past history of STI?* Ask about gonorrhoea, chlamydia, genital warts (HPV) and syphilis. • *If so, what symptoms did you experience? How long ago? How was it treated?* • *Have you ever had a test for HIV or hepatitis B or C?* Screen for knowledge of prevention of STIs and use of condoms. See 'Additional resources' section.	An **STI** includes all conditions that can be transmitted during intercourse or intimate sexual contact with an infected partner.
Sexual function and satisfaction (if relevant) • *Are you satisfied with the sexual relationship you have with your partner(s)?* • *Are you satisfied with the way that you and your partner communicate about sex?* • *Are you satisfied with your ability to respond sexually?* **Sexual difficulties or dysfunction** Ask relevant questions—for example: • *Have you experienced low sexual desire or sexual arousal?* • *Have you experienced erectile dysfunction (ability to get an erection, hardness, staying hard)?* • *Have you ever had trouble in achieving an orgasm, lack of sexual satisfaction (able to ejaculate (cum), pain or discomfort on ejaculation)?* • *Have you experienced loss of urine during sexual activity?* • *Have you experienced any other sexual issue?* • *If you are experiencing any difficulties, how much does this bother you?* (scale of 1–5; 1 is not bothered at all/5 is extremely bothered)	There are validated sexual health/satisfaction and erectile function assessment tools available (e.g. the Male Sexual Health Questionnaire). Men who are concerned about their sexual function should be referred to a medical or nurse practitioner or sexual health clinic for further assessment. Erectile dysfunction has been defined as the persistent inability to achieve or maintain an erection sufficient for satisfactory sexual intercourse.[33] ! ***Clinical alert:*** While it is normal that male erectile function decreases with ageing, the man should be screened for cardiovascular disease risk factors because these are also associated with erectile dysfunction.[13]

ASSESSMENT GUIDELINES	CLINICAL SIGNIFICANCE AND CLINICAL ALERTS
Family violence, sexual abuse, assault or unwanted sexual experiences (if relevant) See questions and approach to assessment described in Chapter 5 for detail on assessment related to screening for family violence and abuse	May prompt need for follow-up and counselling. See also Chapter 5 for detail on assessment.
Health and lifestyle management	
Prostate For men over 50 years of age or men with a family history of prostate cancer, ask: *Have you had a discussion with a health professional about prostate health?*	See 'Developmental considerations' earlier in the chapter.
Testicular self-examination • *Do you perform testicular self-examination?* See the 'Health education' section in teaching testicular awareness.	
Immunisation • *Have you been immunised against human papillomavirus (HPV)?*	**HPV** can cause cancers of the penis, anus and genital warts. Men can be asymptomatic carriers of the virus and pass it on to sexual partners. For more information about HPV vaccination see the section titled 'Health education' in Chapter 26.
• *Have you been immunised against hepatitis B?* Hepatitis B vaccination is part of the Immunisation Schedule in Australia and Aotearoa New Zealand. Most Australians under the age of 30 would have been given the vaccine and the herd immunity is high, more than 80%, but there are subpopulations that may not have been vaccinated. These include migrants, those whose parents are vaccine conscientious objectors and those who missed out at school (Chapter 3).	**Hepatitis B** is an STI and vertical transmission from mother to baby continues to be the main way of acquiring hepatitis B with long-term sequelae that include hepatocellular carcinoma.
Safer sex practices See points in sexual health history above.	
Activity and exercise Ask about usual activity and exercise patterns. See Chapters 17, 19 and 20.	Part of a general health history. May provide an opportunity to provide more information about the importance of exercise to general health and wellbeing.
Additional subjective data for infants and children (questions for parent or guardian)	
• *Does your child have any problem urinating? Does his urine stream look straight?* • *Have you noticed any evidence of pain with urinating such as crying or holding the genitals?* • *Has your child had a previous urinary tract infection?*	If the infant/child has any voiding issues refer to Chapter 24 for specific areas for assessment.

ASSESSMENT GUIDELINES	CLINICAL SIGNIFICANCE AND CLINICAL ALERTS
• *Has your child experienced any problems with genital area: itching, rash, anal discharge?*	Occurs with poor perineal hygiene or insertion of foreign body in the rectum.
• *Any problem with the child's penis or scrotum: sores, swelling, discolouration?*	
• *Are you aware if his testes are descended?*	
• *Has he ever had an inguinal hernia or hydrocoele?*	**Hydrocoele** is the collection of serous fluid in tunica vaginalis, surrounding testis. **Inguinal hernia** is a bulging of the contents of the abdomen through a weak area in the lower abdominal wall.
• *Have you ever noticed any swelling in his scrotum during crying or coughing?*	**Scrotal hernia.**
Questions related to suspected child abuse Read the important information about the Australian legal requirements about mandatory reporting of suspected child abuse. See Chapter 5 for details and a specific approach to screening.	For more information about signs and symptoms related to child abuse refer to Chapter 5.
Additional subjective data for preadolescents and adolescents	
Use the following questions regarding sexual growth and development and sexual behaviour. Use the same principles as discussed in the previous sections related to approach to gender identity and sexual orientation outlined in the sexual health history. Ask questions that seem appropriate for the boy's age, but be aware that norms vary widely. Do not be concerned if a boy will not discuss sexuality with you or respond to offers for information. He may not wish to let on that he needs or wants more information. You do well to 'open the door'. The adolescent may come back at a future time. At about age 12 to 13 years, but sometimes earlier, boys start to change and grow hair around the penis and scrotum. • *What changes have you noticed?* • *Have you ever seen charts and pictures of normal growth patterns for boys? Let us go over these now.* • *Who in your family do you talk to about your body changes and about sex information? How do these talks go? Do you think you get enough information?* • *What about sex education classes at school? Is there a teacher, a nurse, a doctor or a counsellor to whom you can talk?*	

ASSESSMENT GUIDELINES	CLINICAL SIGNIFICANCE AND CLINICAL ALERTS
• *Boys around age 12 to 13 years have a normal experience of fluid coming out of the penis at night, called nocturnal emissions or 'wet dreams'. Has this happened to you?*	Occasionally a boy confuses this with a sign of STI or feels guilty.
• *Often boys your age have questions about having sex. Do you have questions?* If appropriate in the situation, ask further questions about sexual activity (use similar questions to that of adults outlined in the previous section including questions about STI protection and preventing unplanned pregnancy if relevant).	Determining the young person's sexual practices will enable you to identify areas for health education or the need for further questioning to identify risk factors for STI and/or the need for specific physical examination and other investigations.
Questions related to suspected child abuse Read the important information about the Australian legal requirements about mandatory reporting of suspected child abuse. See Chapter 5 for details and a specific approach to screening.	For more information about signs and symptoms related to child abuse refer to Chapter 5.

Objective data

Preparation

Men's concerns are similar to those experienced by females during examinations of the genitalia: modesty, fear of pain, cold hands, negative judgement or memory of previously uncomfortable examinations. Also, he may fear comparison to others or fear having an erection during the examination and that this would be misinterpreted by the examiner.

During physical examination your demeanour should be confident and relaxed. Use a firm deliberate touch, not a soft, stroking one. If an erection does occur, do not stop the examination or leave the room. This only focuses more attention on the erection and increases embarrassment. Reassure the male that this is a normal physiological response to touch (it is healthy), just as when the pupil constricts in response to bright light. Proceed with the rest of the examination if the man consents. It is preferable not to have a family member or friend present during sexual health history taking and examinations. However, another health professional of the appropriate gender may be present at the person's request.

In the case of a child or adolescent, the parent or guardian normally provides informed consent for assessment and treatment. Young people have the legal right to confidential health care unless they cannot be considered a mature minor and/or there is a significant concern or risk—for example, harm to self or physical or sexual abuse. It is generally accepted that most young people over the age of 16 years can give informed consent. Those under 16 years may sometimes be considered mature minors where it is legally permissible for a mature adolescent to consent to assessment and treatment.[34] The mature minor (Gillick principle) is confirmed in Australian common law.[35] However, it is always advisable to obtain verbal consent from a child or adolescent before an examination, and this should be documented in the health history.

In addition:

- The bladder should *not* be emptied before a genital examination when the person has symptoms. Urinating before an examination will flush any discharge and signs on examination. Testing for STI requires a urine specimen for laboratory testing (first-void urine—that is, the urine is voided straight into a sterile urine collection container).
- Allow him to undress in privacy.

For the examination of the external genitalia the man should be assisted to lie down in the supine position with one or two pillows under his head. Ensure privacy before exposing the genital area and cover as much bare skin as possible.

If the man has a chaperone present, ask them to stand at the top (head) of the bed or examination couch to support the man.

- Explain each step in the examination before you do it.
- Assure the man he can stop the examination at any point if he feels any discomfort.
- Communicate throughout the examination. Maintain a dialogue to share information.

Equipment needed

Non-sterile gloves
Appropriate lighting (good examination lighting)
Hand hygiene solution

PROCEDURES AND NORMAL FINDINGS	CLINICAL SIGNIFICANCE AND CLINICAL ALERTS
General inspection	
While collecting subjective data you will have noticed the condition of the person's skin, hair, posture, height-to-weight ratio, body shape, level of hygiene and grooming and general demeanour. All these factors provide clues to the man's sexual and reproductive health.	
Inspection of external genitalia	
Penis	
Ask the man to retract the prepuce (foreskin). It should move easily. Inspect the dorsal and the ventral aspect, noting skin colour, erythema, lesions, ulcers or blisters. The glans looks smooth and without lesions. Some cheesy smegma may have collected under the foreskin (this is normal). After inspection, ask the man to slide the foreskin back to the original position. The skin normally looks wrinkled, hairless and without lesions. The dorsal vein may be apparent (Figure 27.4).	**Inflammation.** **Lesions**—nodules, solitary ulcer (chancre), grouped vesicles or superficial ulcers, wart-like papules (Table 27.2). **Inflammation**—Lesions on glans or corona. Discharge (Table 27.3). **Phimosis**—unable to retract the foreskin. **Paraphimosis**—unable to return foreskin to original position.

PROCEDURES AND NORMAL FINDINGS	CLINICAL SIGNIFICANCE AND CLINICAL ALERTS
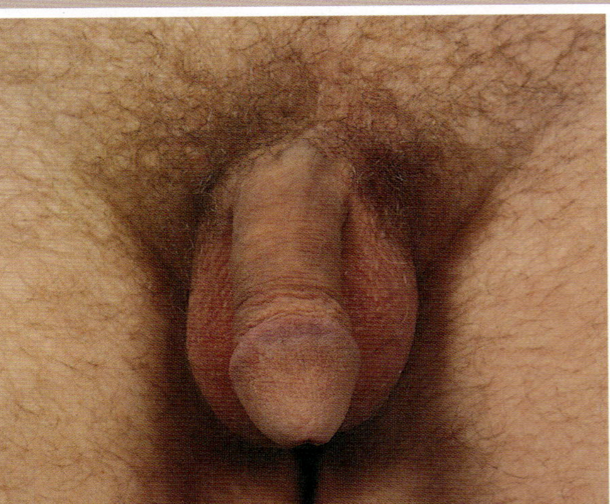 FIGURE 27.4 Penis and scrotum	
The urethral meatus is positioned just about centrally.	**Hypospadias**—ventral location of meatus. **Epispadias**—dorsal location of meatus (Table 27.4).
At the base of the penis, pubic hair distribution is consistent with age. Hair is without lice.	**Pubic lice** or nits can be seen with the unaided eye. Excoriated skin usually accompanies.
Scrotum	
Inspect the scrotum skin as the male holds the penis out of the way. Alternatively, you hold the penis out of the way with the back of your hand (Figure 27.5). Scrotal size varies with ambient room temperature. Asymmetry is normal, with the left scrotal half usually lower than the right.	**Scrotal swelling** (oedema) may be taut and pitting. This occurs with heart failure, renal failure or local inflammation.
Inspect the skin of the inner thighs for redness or lesions.	Lesions.
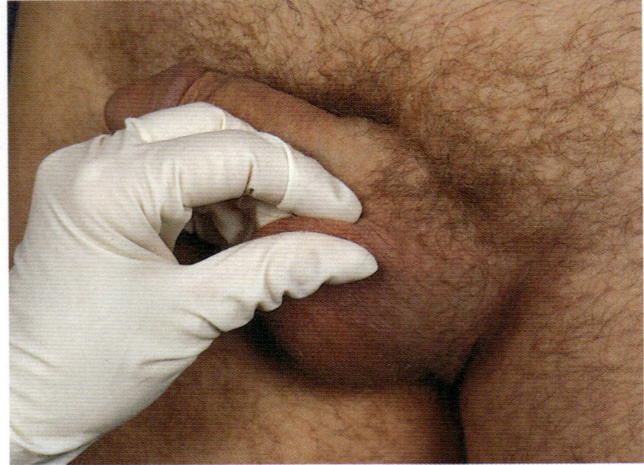 FIGURE 27.5 Hand position for inspection of the scrotum and perineum	

PROCEDURES AND NORMAL FINDINGS	CLINICAL SIGNIFICANCE AND CLINICAL ALERTS
Additional objective data for infants and children	
A parent or guardian should be present. For an infant or toddler, perform this procedure straight after the abdominal examination (Chapter 23). In a preschool-age to young school-age boy (3 to 8 years of age), leave their underpants on until just before the examination. In an older school-age boy or adolescent, offer an extra drape, as with adults. Reassure the child and parents of normal findings.	
Inspect the penis and scrotum Penis size is usually small in infants (2–3 cm) (Figure 27.6) and in young boys until puberty. In obese boys, the penis looks even smaller because of folds of skin covering the base.	Rarely, what appears to be a very small penis may be an enlarged clitoris in a genetically female infant. Enlarged penis—precocious puberty. Redness, swelling, lesions.
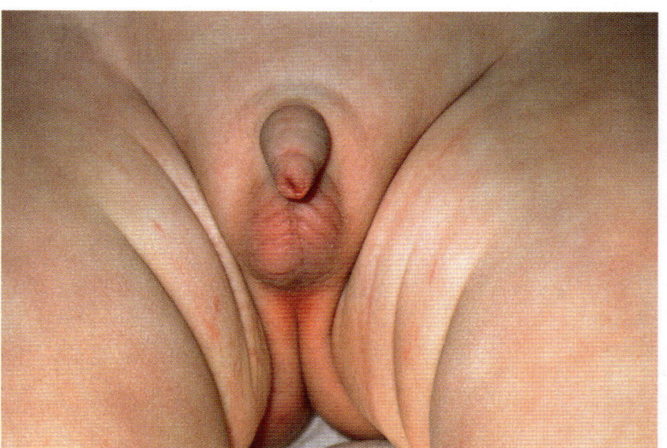 **FIGURE 27.6** Infant penis and scrotum	
The **urethral meatus** should be located centrally in the tip of the penis.	Discharge (Table 27.3). **Hypospadias**, **epispadias** (Table 27.4).
The **foreskin** is normally tight during the first 3 months and should not be retracted because of the risk of tearing the membrane attaching the foreskin to the shaft. This leads to scarring and, possibly, to adhesions later in life. In infants older than 3 months of age, retract the foreskin gently to check the glans and meatus. It should return to its original position easily.	**Phimosis**—unable to retract the foreskin. **Paraphimosis**—the foreskin cannot be slipped forward once it is retracted. Dirt and smegma collecting under foreskin.
Scrotal rugae are well formed in full-term infants. Size varies with ambient temperature, but overall, an infant's scrotum looks large in relation to the penis. No bulges, either constant or intermittent, are present.	

PROCEDURES AND NORMAL FINDINGS	CLINICAL SIGNIFICANCE AND CLINICAL ALERTS
Additional objective data for adolescents	
Adolescents show wide variation in normal development of the genitals. Using the sex maturity charts (Table 27.1), note: • enlargement of the testes and scrotum (Table 27.5) • pubic hair growth • darkening of scrotal colour • roughening of scrotal skin • increase in penis length and width • axillary hair growth.	
Additional objective data for adults over 65 years	
In older males, you may note thinner, greying pubic hair and the decreased size of the penis. The size of the testes may be decreased and may feel less firm. The scrotal sac is pendulous with fewer rugae.	

Abnormal findings

TABLE 27.2 Male genital lesions

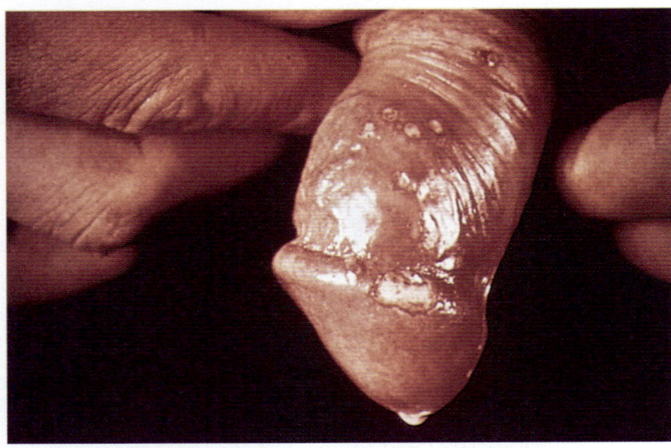

Genital herpes—HSV-2 infection

Clusters of small vesicles with surrounding erythema, which are often painful, erupt on the glans or foreskin. These rupture to form superficial ulcers. An STI, the initial infection lasts 7 to 10 days. The virus remains dormant indefinitely; recurrent infections last 3 to 10 days with milder symptoms.

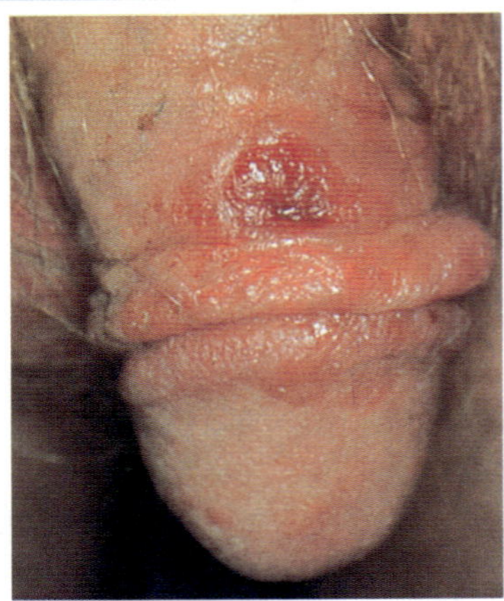

Syphilitic chancre

Begins within 2 to 4 weeks of infection as a small, solitary, silvery papule that erodes to a red, round or oval, superficial ulcer with a yellowish serous discharge. Palpation reveals a nontender indurated base that can be lifted like a button between the thumb and the finger. Lymph nodes enlarge early but are nontender. This is an STI.

TABLE 27.2 Male genital lesions cont'd

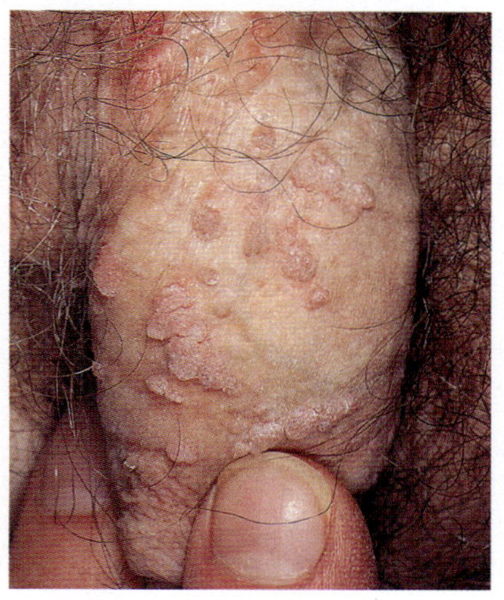

Genital warts

Soft, pointed, moist, fleshy, painless papules may be single or multiple in a cauliflower-like patch. They occur on the shaft of the penis, behind the corona or around the anus where they may grow into large grape-like clusters.
These are caused by HPV and are one of the most common STIs. The HPV infection is correlated with early onset of sexual activity, infrequent use of condoms and multiple sexual partners.

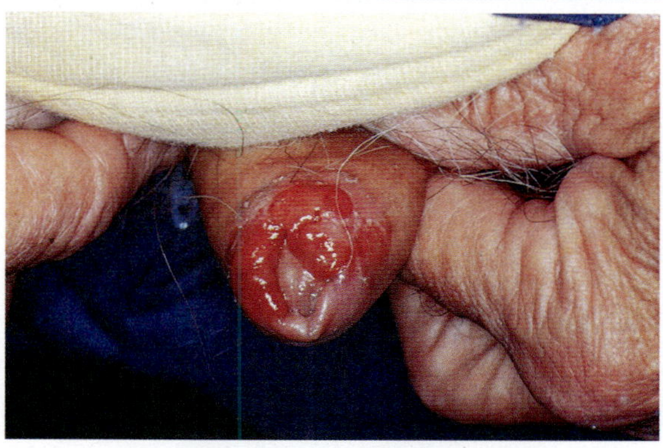

Carcinoma

Begins as red, raised warty growth or as an ulcer, with watery discharge. As it grows, may necrose and slough. Usually painless. Almost always on glans or inner lip of foreskin and following chronic inflammation. Enlarged lymph nodes are common.

Mpox (previously known as 'monkey pox')

Mpox is a rare virus of the Poxviridae family, (*Orthopoxvirus* strain) with close links to smallpox, cow pox and variola. The virus remained endemic in central, east and west Africa after eradication of smallpox in the 1980s. In the Northern hemisphere's summer of 2022, there was a global outbreak of mpox that affected GBMSM populations (mpox Clade IIB). Typically, the virus is passed on through close skin-to-skin contact and causes very painful mucosal blisters, with men presenting with severe proctitis, urethritis and systemic illness 1 to 21 days after close contact. The initial symptoms usually begin with a sore throat. Preventive measures include a non-replicating MVA-BN vaccine, which was available with very short supplies at the start of the outbreak. Men at risk (gay, bisexual and men who have sex with men) were recommended to have two doses of the vaccine 4 weeks apart, if they had not had a smallpox vaccine previously.

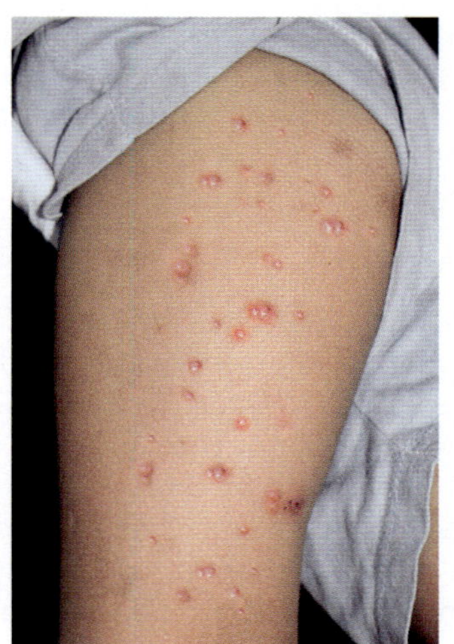

TABLE 27.3 Urethritis and proctitis—sexually transmitted infections

Non-specific urethritis or non-gonococcal urethritis

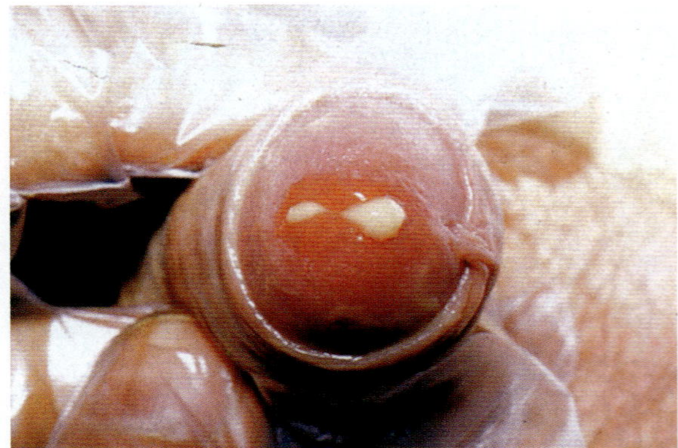

The history of the presenting complaint will include mild non-specific penile symptoms to acute painful symptoms. Penile inflammation caused by a bacteria includes urethral itch and discomfort, burning or tingling passing urine and meatal redness. There may also be a urethral discharge and if any discharge, the patient may complain of the underpants being stained. Symptoms are usually present from 7 to 60 days after sex.

Forty to fifty per cent of all non-gonococcal urethritis will end up with no aetiological agent identified. Of the common STIs, 30% will test positive for *Chlamydia trachomatis* and 30% *Mycoplasma genitalium* and 1% will test positive for *Neisseria gonorrhoea.*

Gonococcal urethritis

Gonococcal urethritis presents with acute obvious urethral symptoms that includes moderate to copious yellowish greenish pus-like discharge. This is associated with pain—moderate to extreme—burning to razor sharp pain, passing urine. This usually occurs 24 hours to 7 days after a sexual encounter.

The physical examination will identify gonococcal urethritis because of its prominent signs. A specimen collected by swab of the discharge (not the meatal or urethral skin) for a Gram stain identifying Gram-negative diplococci intracellularly and extracellularly will confirm the diagnosis. However, if there are no facilities for microscopy, a first-void urine is sufficient for a nucleic acid amplification test diagnosis and treatment is symptomatic.

Viral urethritis

The presenting complaint will include severe pain passing urine, associated with an erythematous meatus. There is usually an absence of discharge. There may be some systemic illness with mild fevers and complaints of generalised aches and pains. The examination reveals a rather erythematous meatus. The most common aetiological agent is adenovirus. Herpes virus (HSV1 and/or HSV2) will also cause typical symptoms and examination may reveal blisters or lesions on the meatus and adjacent skin. HSV, however, has a shorter natural history than adenovirus. Treatment is conservative measures with push fluids and local anaesthetic cream or gel.

Proctitis/proctocolitis

The presenting complaint will include mild to severe anorectal pain, pruritus ani and an observed mucous discharge on toilet paper. There may be spasms/pain (tenesmus) with passing motion. The symptoms may appear 24 hours to 3 weeks after an anal sexual encounter. The aetiological agents most related to proctitis include *Neisseria gonorrhoea*, *Chlamydia trachomatis*, *Mycoplasma genitalium* and herpes simplex virus. Anoscopy may be performed by a clinician who is trained in the procedure, and this will yield any abnormal discharge or lesions inferior of the anorectal dentate line. Other causes of anorectal discomfort include haemorrhoids, where blood on the toilet paper after defecating is a common complaint (haematochezia).

TABLE 27.4 Abnormalities of the penis

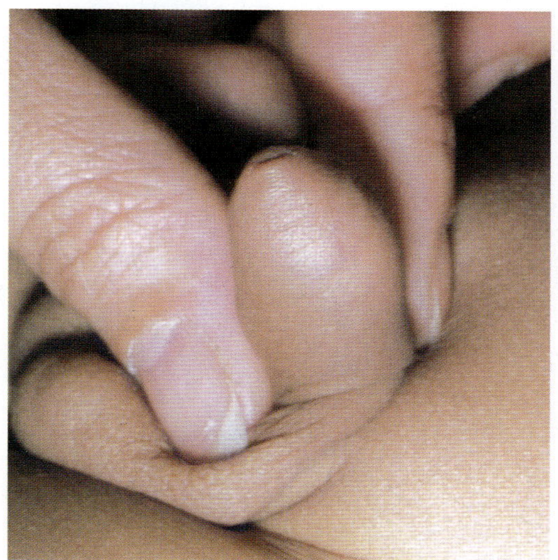

Phimosis

Foreskin is advanced and fixed so tight it is impossible to retract over glans. May be congenital or acquired from adhesions secondary to infection. Poor hygiene leads to retained dirt and smegma, which increases risk of inflammation or calculus formation.

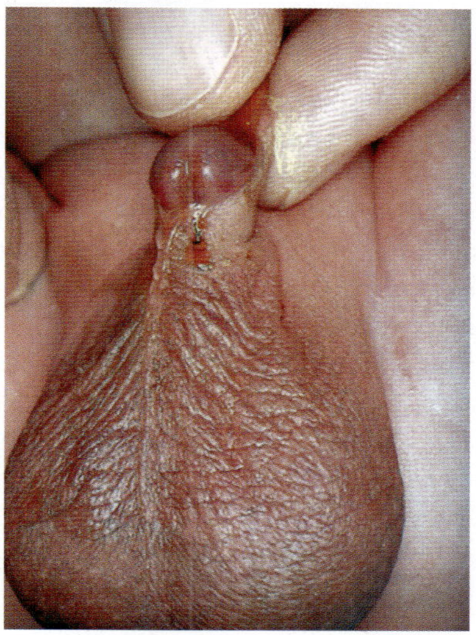

Hypospadias

Urethral meatus opens on the ventral (under) side of glans, shaft or at the penoscrotal junction. A groove extends from the meatus to the normal location at the tip. This is a congenital defect that is important to recognise at birth. Newborns should not be circumcised because surgical correction may use foreskin tissue to extend urethral length.

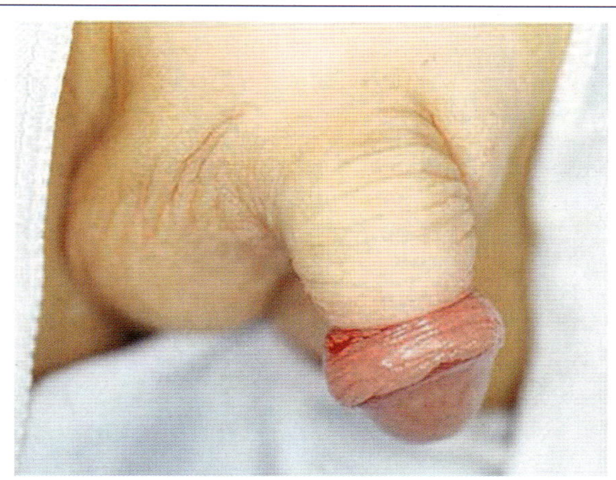

Paraphimosis

Foreskin is retracted and fixed. Once retracted behind glans, a tight or inflamed foreskin cannot return to its original position. Constriction impedes circulation, so glans swells. If untreated, it may compromise arterial circulation. It is important to make sure the foreskin is placed back to its normal position after urinary catheterisation.

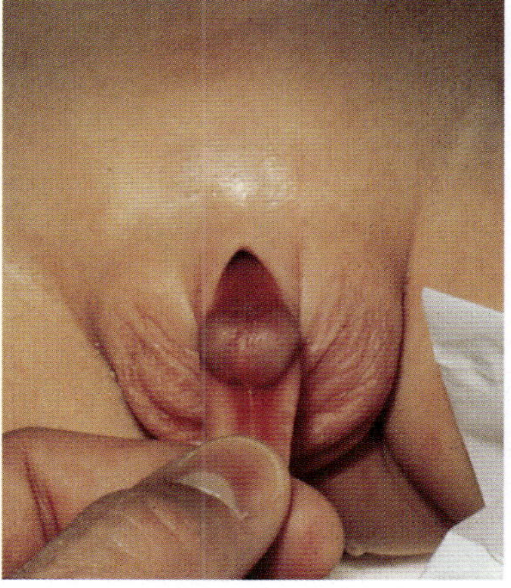

Epispadias

Meatus opens on the dorsal (upper) side of glans or shaft above a broad, spade-like penis. Rare; less common than hypospadias but more disabling because of associated urinary incontinence and separation of pubic bones.

TABLE 27.4 Abnormalities of the penis cont'd

Peyronie's disease

Hard, nontender, subcutaneous plaques palpated on dorsal or lateral surface of penis. May be single or multiple and asymmetrical. They are associated with painful bending of the penis during erection. Plaques are fibrosis of covering of corpora cavernosa. Usually occurs after 45 years. Its cause is trauma to the erect penis such as an unexpected change in angle during intercourse. More common in men with diabetes, gout and Dupuytren's contracture of the palm.

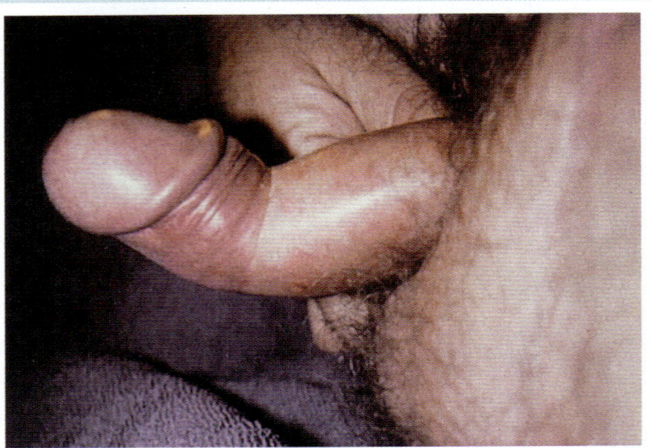

TABLE 27.5 Abnormalities in the scrotum

DISORDER	CLINICAL FINDINGS	DISCUSSION
Absent testis cryptorchidism 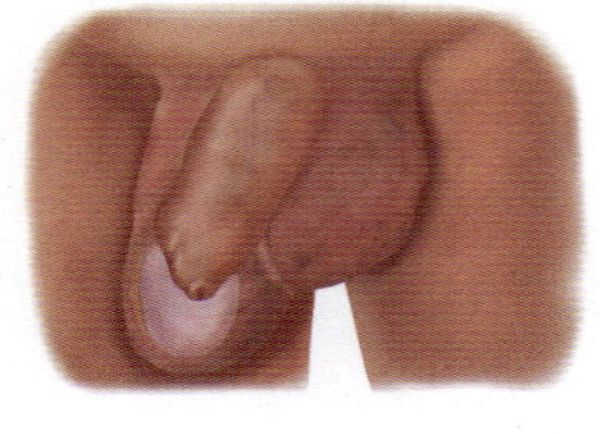	Empty scrotal half. Inspection—in true maldescent, atrophic scrotum on affected side. Palpation—no testis.	True cryptorchidism—testes that have never descended. Incidence at birth is 3 to 4%; half of these descend in first month. Incidence with premature infants is 30%; in adults 0.7 to 0.8%. True undescended testes have a histological change by 6 years, causing decreased spermatogenesis and infertility.
Small testis 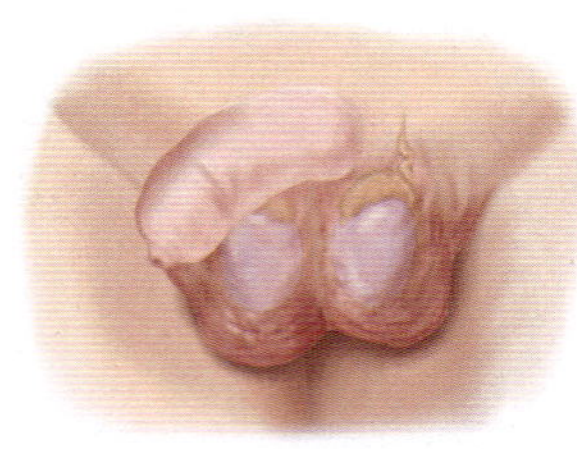	Palpation—small and soft (rarely may be firm). Small testis.	Small and soft (< 3.5 cm) indicates atrophy as with cirrhosis, hypopituitarism, following estrogen therapy or as a sequela of orchitis. Small and firm (< 2 cm) occurs with Klinefelter's syndrome (hypogonadism).

Continued

TABLE 27.5 Abnormalities in the scrotum cont'd

DISORDER	CLINICAL FINDINGS	DISCUSSION
Testicular torsion 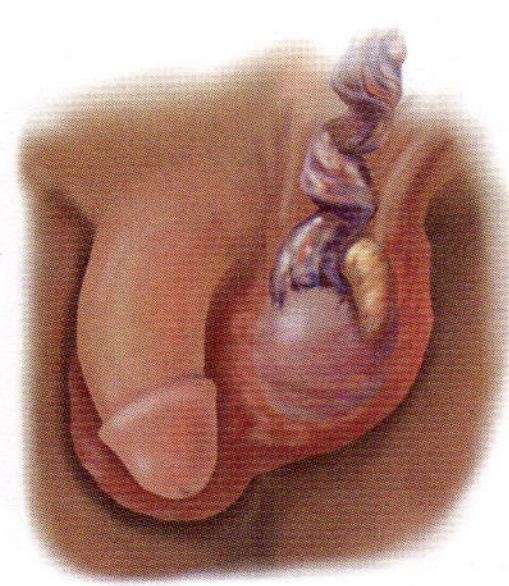	Excruciating pain in the testicle of sudden onset, often during sleep or following trauma. May also have lower abdominal pain, nausea and vomiting, no fever. Inspection—red, swollen scrotum, one testis (usually left) higher owing to rotation and shortening. Palpation—cord feels thick, swollen, tender, epididymis may be anterior, cremasteric reflex is absent on side of torsion.	! ***Clinical alert:*** Sudden twisting of the spermatic cord. Occurs in late childhood, early adolescence, into the mid-20s. Torsion occurs usually on the left side. Faulty anchoring of testis on wall of scrotum allows testis to rotate. The anterior part of the testis rotates medially towards the other testis. Blood supply is cut off, resulting in ischaemia and engorgement. This is an emergency requiring surgery; testis can become gangrenous in a few hours.
Epididymitis 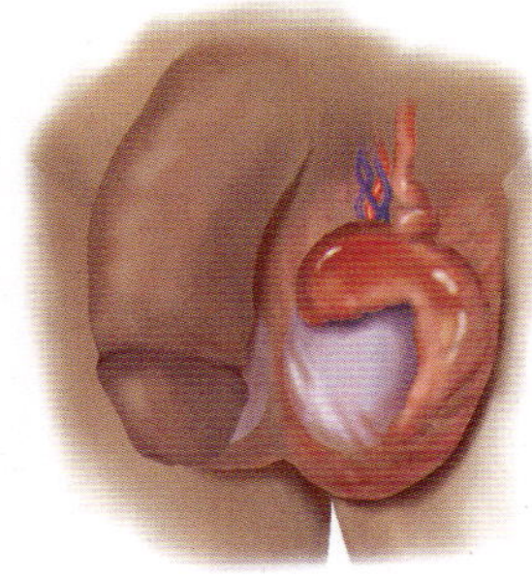	Severe pain of sudden onset in the scrotum, somewhat relieved by elevation (a positive Phren's sign); also rapid swelling, fever. Inspection—enlarged scrotum; reddened. Palpation—exquisitely tender; epididymis enlarged, indurated; may be hard to distinguish from testis. Overlying scrotal skin may be thick and oedematous. Laboratory—white blood cells and bacteria in urine.	Acute infection of epididymis commonly caused by prostatitis, after prostatectomy because of trauma of urethral instrumentation or due to chlamydia, gonorrhoea or another bacterial infection. Often difficult to distinguish between epididymitis and testicular torsion.
Spermatic cord varicocoele 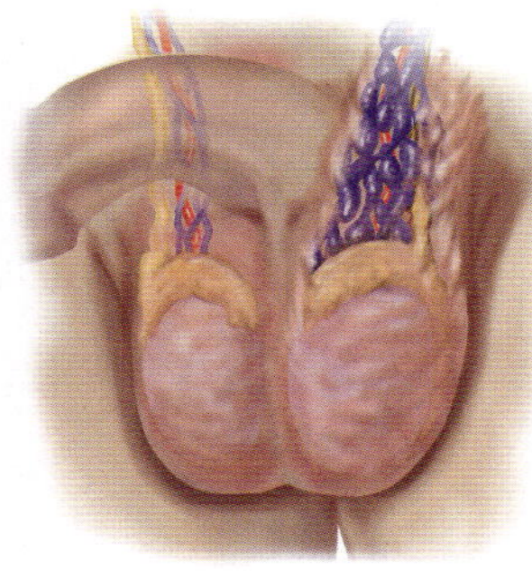	Dull pain; constant pulling or dragging feeling; or may be asymptomatic. Inspection—usually no sign. May show bluish colour through light scrotal skin. Palpation—when standing, feel soft, irregular mass posterior to and above testis; collapses when supine, refills when upright. Feels distinctive, like a 'bag of worms'. The testis on the side of the varicocoele may be smaller owing to impaired circulation.	A varicocoele is dilated, tortuous varicose veins in the spermatic cord due to incompetent valves within the vein, which permit reflux of blood. Most often on left side, perhaps because left spermatic vein is longer and inserts at a right angle into left renal vein. Common in young males. Screen at early adolescence; early treatment is important to prevent potential infertility when an adult.

TABLE 27.5 Abnormalities in the scrotum cont'd

DISORDER	CLINICAL FINDINGS	DISCUSSION
Spermatocoele 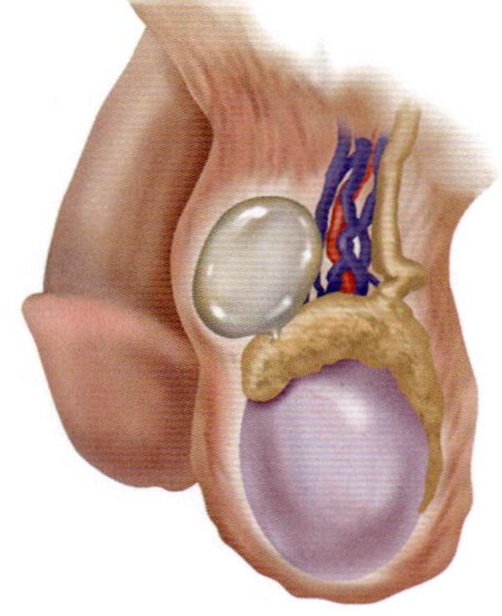	Painless, usually found on examination. Palpation—round, freely movable mass lying above and behind testis. If large, feels like a third testis.	Retention cyst in epididymis. Cause unclear but may be obstruction of tubules. Filled with a thin, milky fluid that contains sperm. Most spermatocoeles are small (< 1 cm); occasionally, they may be larger and then mistaken for hydrocoele.
Early testicular tumour 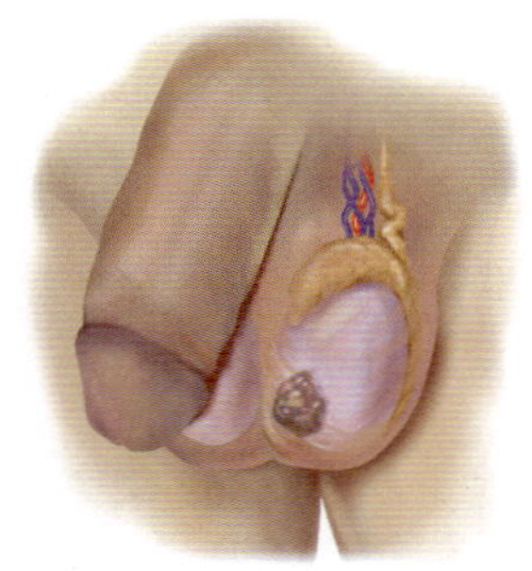	Painless, found on examination. Palpation—firm nodule or harder than normal section of testicle.	Most testicular tumours occur between the ages of 18 and 35. Practically all are malignant. Must biopsy to confirm. The most important risk factor is undescended testis, even those surgically corrected. Early detection is important in prognosis, but practice of testicular self-examination is currently low.
Diffuse tumour 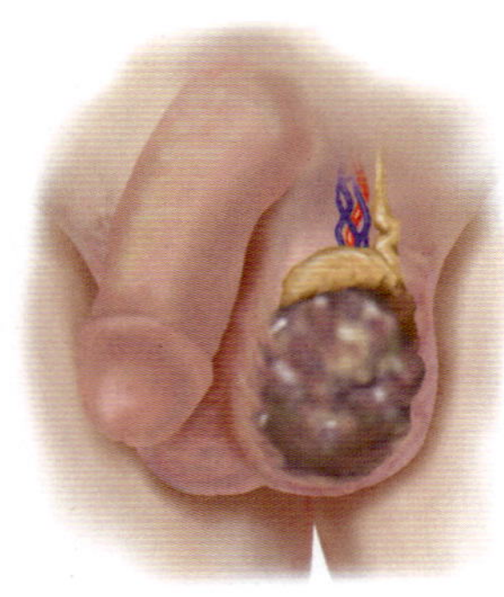	Enlarging testis (most common symptom). When enlarges, has feel of increased weight. Inspection—enlarged. Palpation—enlarged, smooth, ovoid, firm. Important—firm palpation does not cause usual sickening discomfort as with normal testis.	Diffuse tumour maintains shape of testis.

Continued

TABLE 27.5 Abnormalities in the scrotum cont'd

DISORDER	CLINICAL FINDINGS	DISCUSSION
Hydrocoele 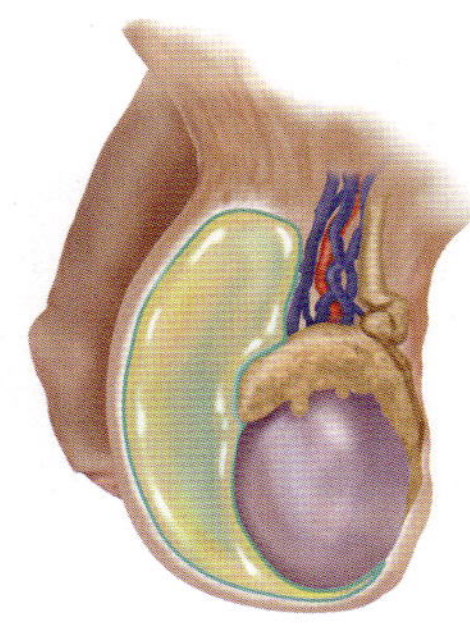	Painless swelling, although the person may complain of weight and bulk in scrotum. Inspection—enlarged scrotum. Palpation—nontender mass, able to get fingers above the mass (in contrast to scrotal hernia).	Cystic. Circumscribed collection of serous fluid in tunica vaginalis, surrounding testis. May occur following epididymitis, trauma, hernia, tumour of testis or spontaneously in newborns.
Scrotal hernia 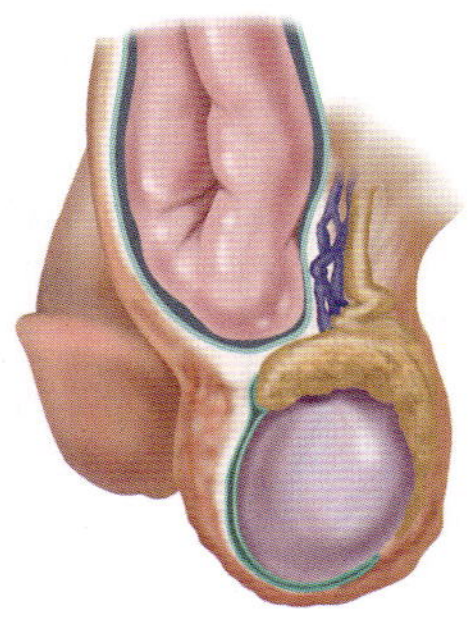	Swelling, may have pain with straining. Inspection—enlarged, may reduce when supine. Palpation—soft mushy mass, palpating fingers cannot get above the mass. Mass is distinct from the testicle that is normal.	Scrotal hernia usually due to indirect inguinal hernia.
Orchitis 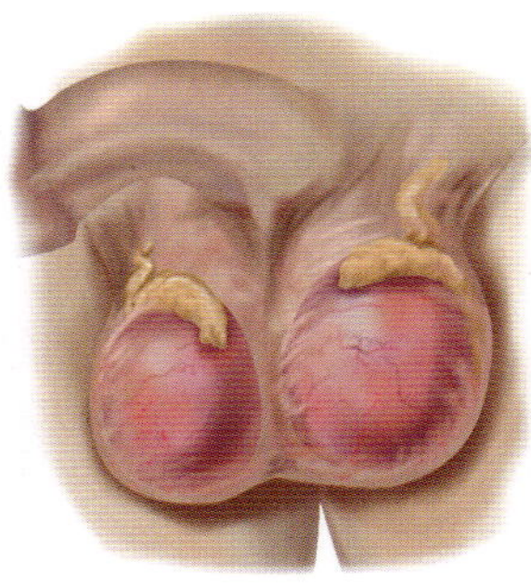	Acute or moderate pain of sudden onset, swollen testis, feeling of weight, fever. Inspection—enlarged, oedematous, reddened. Palpation—swollen, congested, tense and tender; hard to distinguish testis from epididymis.	Acute inflammation of testis. Most common cause is mumps; can occur with any infectious disease. May have associated hydrocoele that does transilluminate.
Scrotal oedema 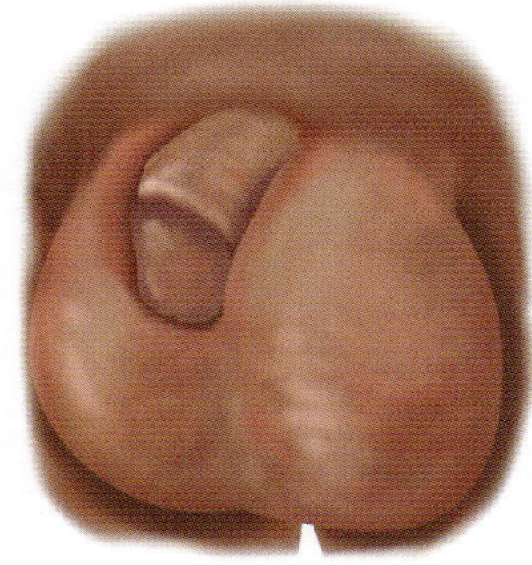	Tenderness. Inspection—enlarged, may be reddened (with local irritation). Palpation—taut with pitting. Probably unable to feel scrotal contents.	Accompanies marked oedema in the lower half of the body such as congestive heart failure, renal failure and portal vein obstruction. Occurs with local inflammation: epididymitis, torsion of spermatic cord. Also obstruction of inguinal lymphatics produces lymphoedema of scrotum.

Advanced practice—additional data

In addition to the objective data described previously, the assessments described in the following section require advanced skill and scope of practice. Nurse practitioners and nurses working in specialist men's health and sexual health settings, as well as urological and continence nurses, need to develop these skills. Advanced assessment for infants and children is performed by specialist neonatal and paediatric nurses, some midwives and maternal and child health nurses.

Physical examination of male genitals and rectum are intimate, invasive assessments and are only performed when there is a valid reason to do so. It is critical that clear communication with the person is maintained throughout the procedure to ensure the person fully understands the purpose, nature and extent of the assessment. You will have to make a professional judgement about the need for another health professional (a chaperone) to be present during the examination.

Preparation

Position the person supine for most of the examination. Cover them with sheet or blanket when possible. In addition to the equipment listed previously you will require the following.

Equipment needed

Sterile specimen for specific STI cultures if needed
Penlight torch
Magnifying glass (when the person presents with lesion, warts and skin changes)
Non-sterile gloves and lubricating gel
Hand hygiene solution

PROCEDURES AND NORMAL FINDINGS	CLINICAL SIGNIFICANCE AND CLINICAL ALERTS
Inspection and palpation of external genitalia	
Penis	
With gloved hands, compress the glans anteroposteriorly between your thumb and forefinger (Figure 27.7). The meatus edge should appear pink, smooth and without discharge.	**Stricture**—narrowed opening. Edges that are red, everted, oedematous, along with purulent discharge, suggest **urethritis** (Table 27.3).

PROCEDURES AND NORMAL FINDINGS	CLINICAL SIGNIFICANCE AND CLINICAL ALERTS
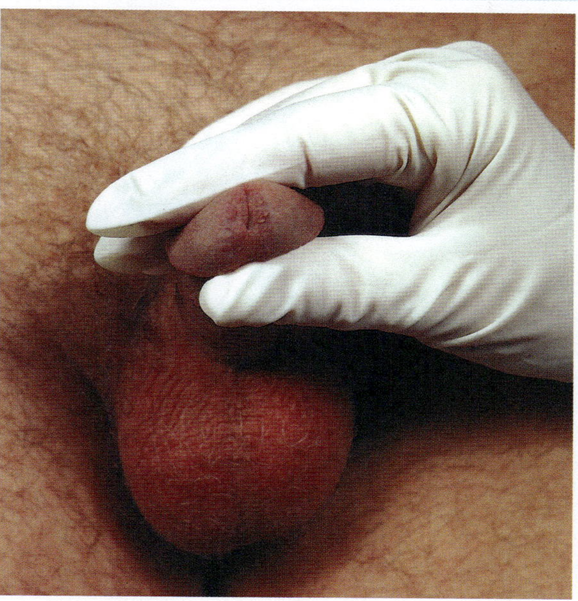 **FIGURE 27.7** Position of the hands to inspect the penile meatus	
If you note urethral discharge, collect a smear for microscopic examination and culture. If no discharge shows but the man gives a history of it, ask him to milk the shaft of the penis. This should produce a drop of discharge.	***Clinical alert:*** For men who have sex with men, STIs may be asymptomatic. It is important to collect specimens from appropriate sites to test for STIs. In sexually active men who have sex with men, for those with more than one partner, a screen is recommended at least twice a year. For those with more than five partners, 4- to 6-monthly screening is recommended. Specimens should include oropharyngeal swabs, first void urine and an anorectal swab (which can be collected by the person) for gonorrhoea and chlamydia. Blood tests are done to detect HIV and syphilis.
Palpate the shaft of the penis between your thumb and first two fingers. Normally, the penis feels smooth, semi-firm and nontender.	**Nodule or induration.** **Tenderness.**

PROCEDURES AND NORMAL FINDINGS	CLINICAL SIGNIFICANCE AND CLINICAL ALERTS
Scrotum and testes	
Spread rugae out between your fingers. Lift the sac to inspect the posterior surface. Normally, no scrotal lesions are present, except for the commonly found sebaceous cysts. These are yellowish, 1-centimetre nodules and are firm, nontender and often multiple.	**Inflammation.**
Palpate gently each scrotal half between your thumb and first two fingers (Figure 27.8). The scrotal contents should slide easily. Testes normally feel oval, firm and rubbery, smooth and equal bilaterally and are freely movable and slightly tender to moderate pressure. Each epididymis normally feels discrete, softer than the testis, smooth and nontender. 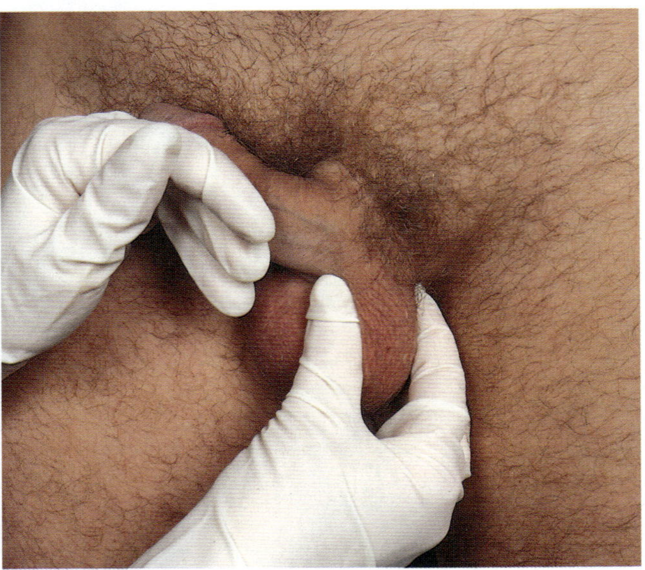 **FIGURE 27.8** Position of hands to palpate the scrotum and testes	**Absent testis**—may be a temporary migration or true cryptorchidism (Table 27.5). **Atrophied testes**—small and soft. **Fixed testes.** **Nodules** on testes or epididymis. Marked **tenderness**. An indurated, swollen and tender epididymis indicates **epididymitis**. ***Clinical alert:*** Any abnormality of the testis needs referral to a medical practitioner.
Palpate each spermatic cord between your thumb and forefinger, along its length from the epididymis up to the external inguinal ring (Figure 27.9). You should feel a smooth, nontender cord.	Thickened cord. Soft, swollen and tortuous cord—see the discussion of varicocoele, Table 27.5.

PROCEDURES AND NORMAL FINDINGS	CLINICAL SIGNIFICANCE AND CLINICAL ALERTS

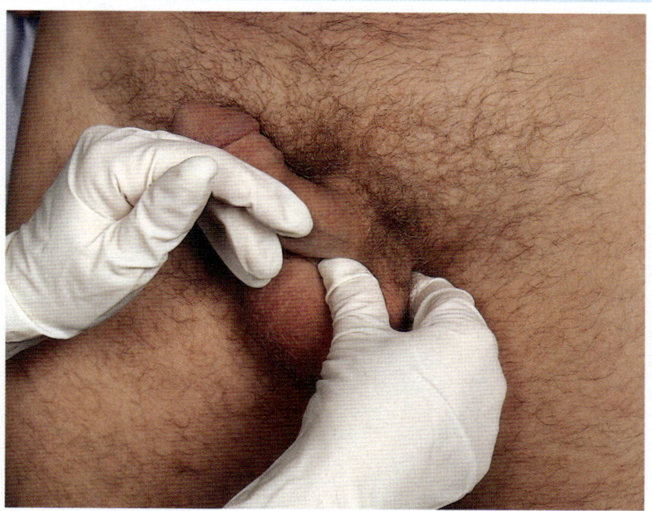

FIGURE 27.9 Palpation of the epididymis

Normally, no other scrotal contents are present. If you do find a mass, note:

- any tenderness
- if the mass is distal or proximal to the testis
- if you can place your fingers over it
- if it reduces when the person lies down
- if you can auscultate bowel sounds over it.

Abnormalities in the scrotum: hernia, tumour, orchitis, epididymitis, hydrocoele, spermatocoele, varicocoele (Table 27.5).

Clinical alert: Any scrotal mass needs referral to a medical practitioner.

Inspect and palpate for hernia

With the man in a standing position, inspect the inguinal region for a bulge as he strains down. Normally, none is present.

Bulge at the external inguinal ring or at the femoral canal. (A hernia may be present but easily reduced and may appear only intermittently with an increase in intra-abdominal pressure.)

Palpate the inguinal canal (Figure 27.10). For the right side, ask the male to shift his weight onto the left (unexamined) leg. Place your right index finger low on the right scrotal half. Palpate up the length of the spermatic cord, invaginating the scrotal skin as you go, to the external inguinal ring. It feels like a triangular slit-like opening, and it may or may not admit your finger. If it will admit your finger, gently insert it into the canal and ask the person to 'bear down'. Normally, you feel no change. Repeat the procedure on the left side.

A palpable herniating mass bumps your fingertip or pushes against the side of your finger.

PROCEDURES AND NORMAL FINDINGS	CLINICAL SIGNIFICANCE AND CLINICAL ALERTS

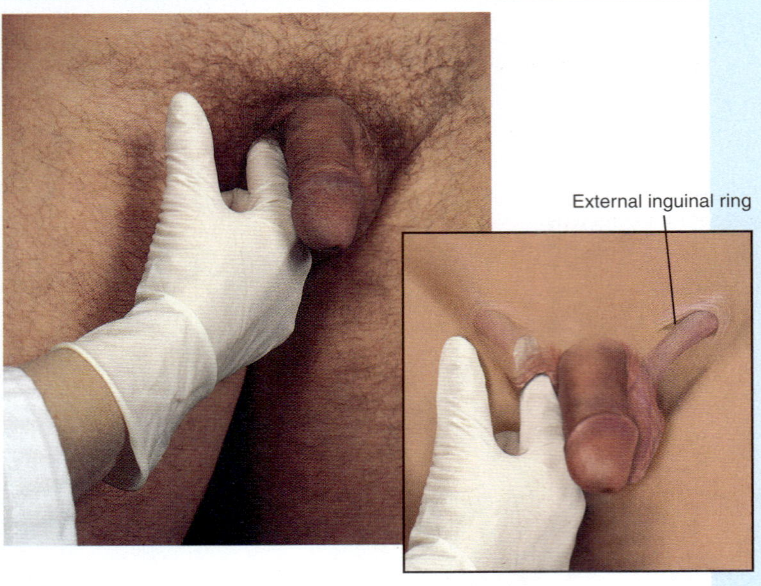

FIGURE 27.10 Palpation of the inguinal canal

Palpate the femoral area for a bulge. Normally you feel none.

Palpate inguinal lymph nodes

Palpate the horizontal chain along the groin inferior to the inguinal ligament and the vertical chain along the upper inner thigh.

It is normal to palpate an isolated node on occasion; it then feels small (less than 1 cm), soft, discrete and movable (Figure 27.11).

Clinical significance: Enlarged, hard, matted, fixed nodes.

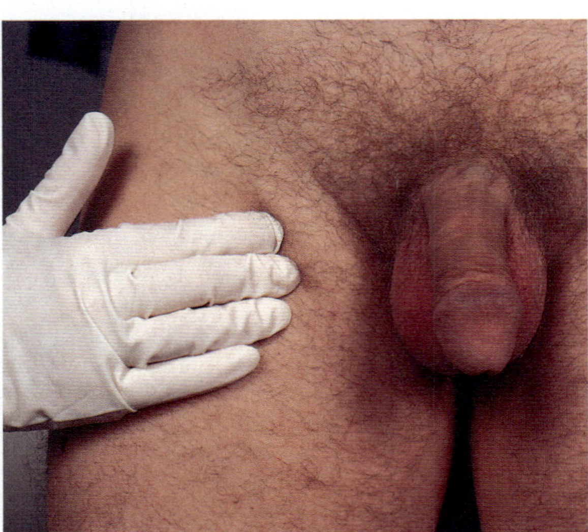

FIGURE 27.11 Palpation of the inguinal lymph nodes

PROCEDURES AND NORMAL FINDINGS	CLINICAL SIGNIFICANCE AND CLINICAL ALERTS

Palpate the prostate gland via the rectum

Drop lubricating gel onto your gloved index finger. Instruct the person that palpation is not painful but may feel like needing to move the bowels. Place the pad of your index finger gently against the anal verge (Figure 27.12). You will feel the sphincter tighten, then relax. As it relaxes, flex the tip of your finger and slowly insert it into the anal canal in a direction towards the umbilicus. *Never* approach the anus at right angles with your index finger extended. Such a jabbing motion does not promote sphincter relaxation and is painful.

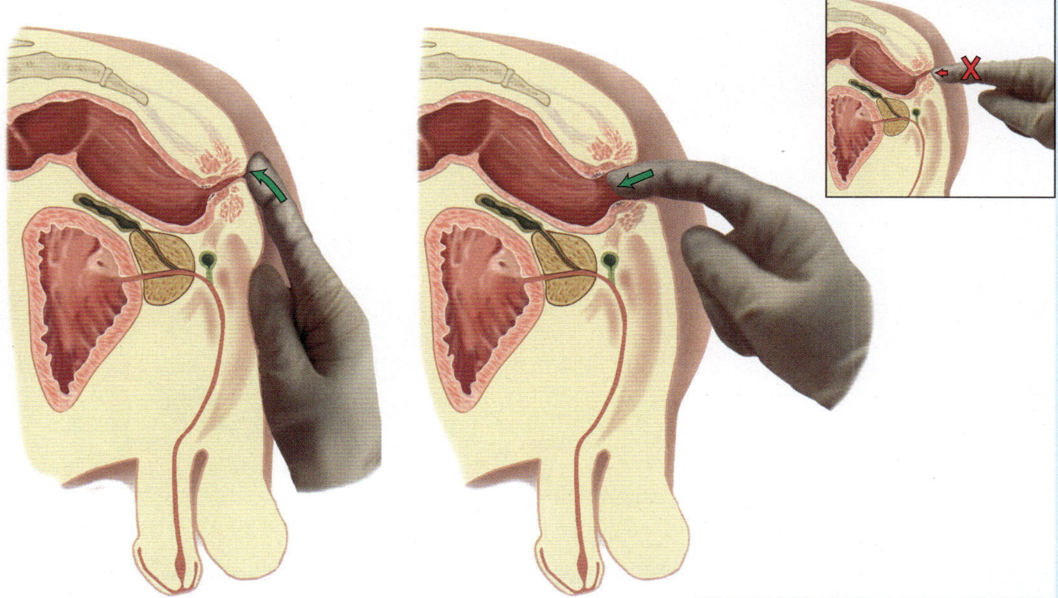

FIGURE 27.12 Position of index finger for insertion into rectum

PROCEDURES AND NORMAL FINDINGS	CLINICAL SIGNIFICANCE AND CLINICAL ALERTS
Prostate gland On the anterior wall in the male, note the elastic, bulging prostate gland (Figure 27.13). Palpate the entire prostate in a systematic way, but note that only the superior and part of the lateral surfaces are accessible to examination. Press into the gland at each location, because when a nodule occurs, it will not project *into* the rectal lumen. The surface should feel smooth and muscular; search for any distinct nodule or diffuse firmness. Note these characteristics: • **size**—2.5 cm long by 4 cm wide; should not protrude more than 1 cm into the rectum • **shape**—heart shape, with palpable central groove • **surface**—smooth • **consistency**—elastic, rubbery • **mobility**—slightly movable • **sensitivity**—nontender to palpation.	Occasionally, digital examination of the prostate can cause a feeling of warmth, flushing and on occasion a vagal response. Enlarged or atrophied gland. Flat with no groove. Nodular. Hard; or boggy, soft, fluctuant. Fixed. Tender. Enlarged, firm smooth gland with central groove obliterated suggests benign prostatic hypertrophy. Swollen, exquisitely tender gland accompanies prostatitis. Any stone-hard, irregular, fixed nodule indicates carcinoma—needs referral to a medical practitioner (Table 27.6).

PROCEDURES AND NORMAL FINDINGS	CLINICAL SIGNIFICANCE AND CLINICAL ALERTS

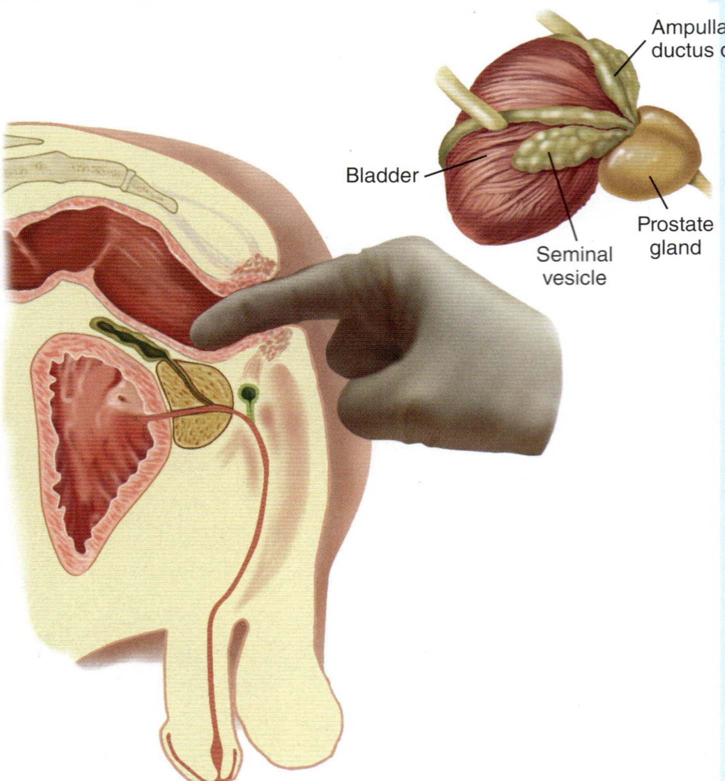

FIGURE 27.13 Position of the index finger for palpation of the prostate gland

Additional objective data for infants and children

Palpate the scrotum and testes

The **cremasteric reflex** is strong in infants, pulling the testes up into the inguinal canal and abdomen from exposure to cold, touch, exercise or emotion. Take care not to elicit the reflex:

- Keep your hands warm and palpate from the external inguinal ring down
- Block the inguinal canals with the thumb and forefinger of your other hand to prevent the testes from retracting (Figure 27.14).

PROCEDURES AND NORMAL FINDINGS

FIGURE 27.14 Palpation of the infant scrotum and testes

Normally, the testes are descended and are equal in size bilaterally (1.5–z2 cm until puberty). It is important to document that you have palpated the testes. Once palpated, they are considered descended, even if they have retracted momentarily at the next visit.

If the scrotal half feels empty, search for the testes along the inguinal canal and try to milk them down. Ask the toddler or child to squat with the knees flexed up; this pressure may force the testes down. Or, have a young child sit cross-legged to relax the reflex (Figure 27.15).

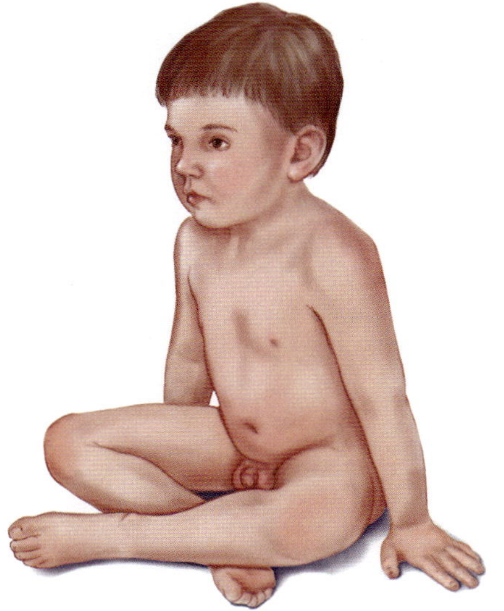

FIGURE 27.15 Position for a young child to relax their scrotum for palpation of the testes

CLINICAL SIGNIFICANCE AND CLINICAL ALERTS

Cryptorchidism is undescended testes (those that have never descended). Undescended testes are common in premature infants. They occur in 3 to 4% of term infants, although most have descended by 3 months of age. The age at which a child should be referred differs among physicians (Table 27.5).

PROCEDURES AND NORMAL FINDINGS	CLINICAL SIGNIFICANCE AND CLINICAL ALERTS
Migratory testes (physiological cryptorchidism) are common because of the strength of the cremasteric reflex and the small mass of the prepubertal testes. Note that the affected side has a normally developed scrotum (with true cryptorchidism, the scrotum is atrophic) and that the testis can be milked down. These testes descend at puberty and are normal.	
Palpate the epididymis and spermatic cord as described in the adult section. A common scrotal finding in a boy under 2 years of age is a **hydrocoele**, or fluid in the scrotum. It appears as a large scrotum and usually disappears spontaneously.	A **hydrocoele** is a cystic collection of serous fluid in the tunica vaginalis, surrounding the testis (Table 27.5).
Inspect the inguinal area for a bulge. If you do not see a bulge but the parent gives a positive history of one, try to elicit it by increasing intra-abdominal pressure. Ask the boy to hold his breath and strain down or have him blow up a balloon.	
If a hernia is suspected (Table 27.7), palpate the inguinal area. Use your little finger to reach the external inguinal ring.	

Abnormal findings for advanced practice

TABLE 27.6 Abnormalities of the prostate gland

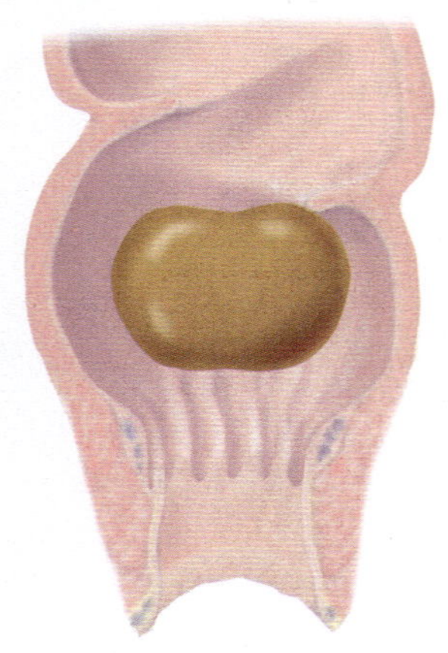

Benign prostatic hypertrophy

Urinary frequency, urgency, hesitancy, straining to urinate, weak stream, intermittent stream, sensation of incomplete emptying, nocturia. A symmetrical nontender enlargement, commonly occurs in males beginning in the middle years. The prostate surface feels smooth, rubbery or firm (like the consistency of the nose), with the median sulcus obliterated.

Continued

TABLE 27.6 Abnormalities of the prostate gland cont'd

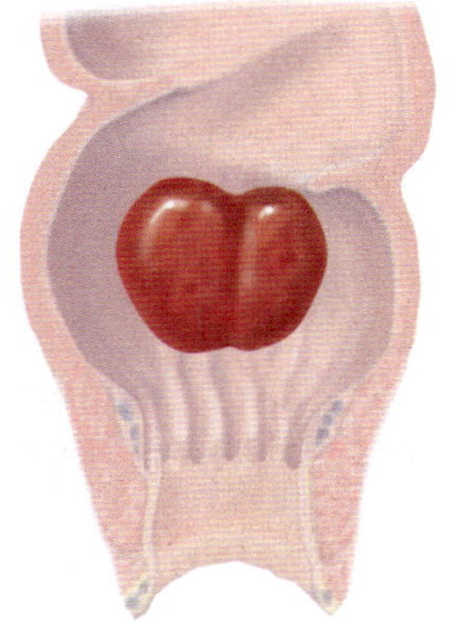

Prostatitis

Fever, chills, malaise, urinary frequency and urgency, dysuria, urethral discharge, dull, aching pain in perineal and rectal area.
An exquisitely tender enlargement is *acute* inflammation of the prostate gland yielding a swollen, slightly asymmetrical gland that is quite tender to palpation.
With a chronic inflammation, the signs can vary from tender enlargement with a boggy feel to isolated firm areas due to fibrosis. Or the gland may feel normal.

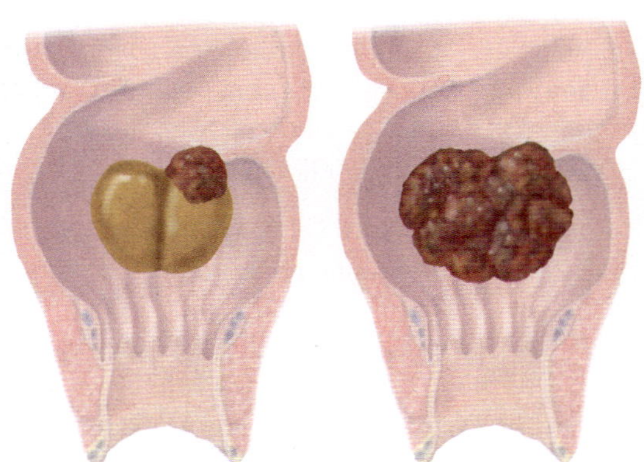

Carcinoma

Asymptomatic until advanced. Frequency, nocturia, haematuria, weak stream, hesitancy, pain or burning on urination, continuous pain in the lower back, pelvis and thighs.
A malignant neoplasm often starts as a single hard nodule on the posterior surface, producing asymmetry and a change in consistency. As it invades normal tissue, multiple hard nodules appear or the entire gland feels stone-hard and fixed. The median sulcus is obliterated.

TABLE 27.7 Inguinal and femoral hernias

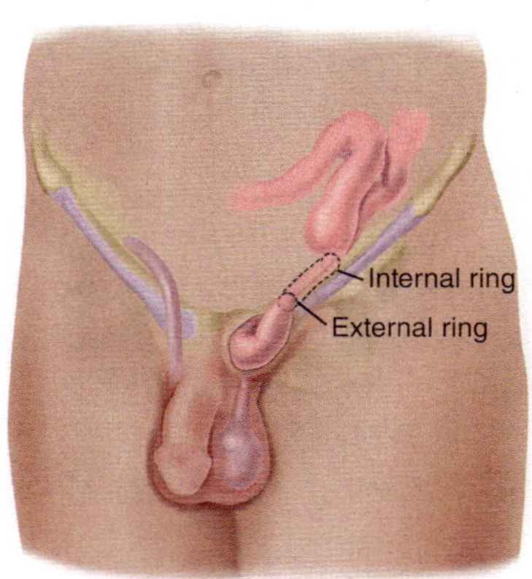

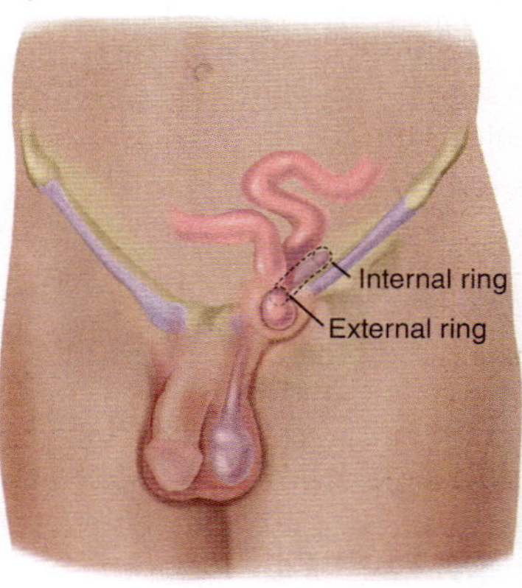

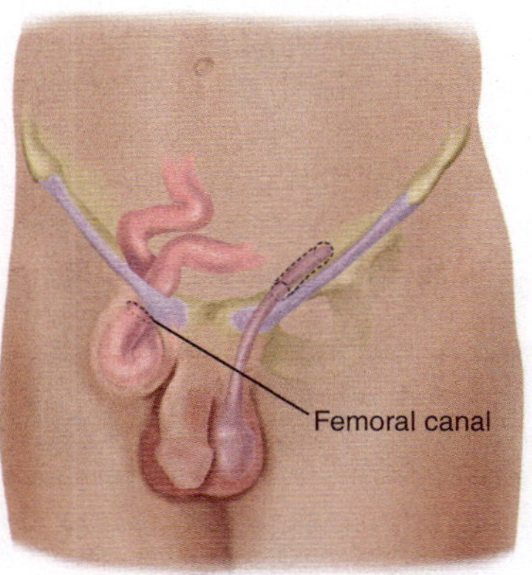

	Indirect Inguinal	Direct Inguinal	Femoral
Course	The sac herniates through the internal inguinal ring; can remain in the canal or pass into the scrotum.	Directly behind and through the external inguinal ring, above the inguinal ligament; rarely enters the scrotum.	Through the femoral ring and canal, below the inguinal ligament, more often on the right side.

TABLE 27.7 Inguinal and femoral hernias cont'd

Clinical symptoms and signs	Pain with straining; soft swelling that increases with increased intra-abdominal pressure; may decrease when lying down.	Usually painless; round swelling close to the pubis in the area of the internal inguinal ring; easily reduced when supine.	Pain may be severe, and may become strangulated.
Frequency	Most common; 60% of all hernias. More common in infants under 1 year and in males 16 to 20 years of age.	Less common; occurs most often in men over 40; rare in women.	Least common; 4% of all hernias; more common in women.
Cause	Congenital or acquired.	Acquired weakness; brought on by heavy lifting, muscle atrophy, obesity, chronic cough or ascites.	Acquired; due to increased abdominal pressure, muscle weakness or frequent stooping.

Notes:
Reducible—the contents will return to the abdominal cavity by lying down or with gentle pressure.
Incarcerated—a herniated bowel cannot be returned to the abdominal cavity.
Strangulated—the blood supply to the hernia is shut off. Accompanied by nausea, vomiting and tenderness.

Clinical reasoning and documentation

The following is a continuation of the case study provided at the beginning of this chapter and the clinical reasoning process including problem/issue identification. Consult a fundamentals of nursing or medical-surgical nursing text for information about goal setting, nursing interventions and evaluation.

Case study (continued)—STI symptoms

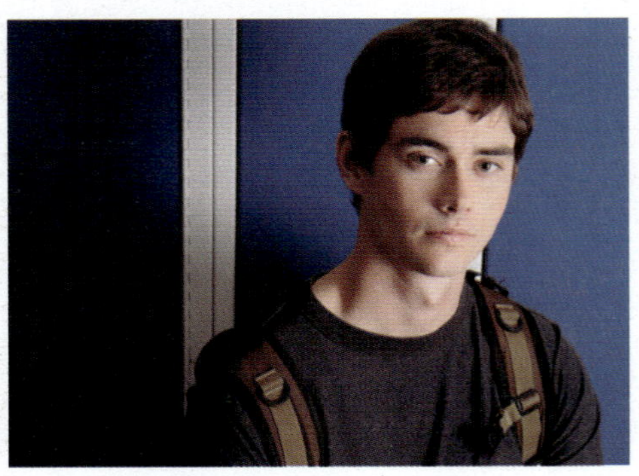

Context

You will recall from earlier in the chapter that you are a registered nurse working in a university student health centre.

Consider the patient's situation

Mr Ryan Wilson is a 19-year-old student who has experienced acute onset of painful urination, urinary frequency and urgency for 2 days.

Collect cues/information

Your further assessment reveals the following information.

Subjective data

Mr Wilson is concerned he has an STI because of an episode of unprotected intercourse with a new female partner 6 days ago. Has no known allergies or any significant medical or surgical history. He did not use a condom and

Clinical reasoning and documentation cont'd

says he tends not to use condoms. He is in contact with the sexual partner, who says she has no symptoms.

Noted some thick penile discharge. He states he has no flank pain, no abdominal pain, no fever or genital skin rash.

Objective data

Temp 37°C; HR 72/min; RR 16/min. No lesions or inflammation around penis or scrotum. Urethral meatus has mild oedema with purulent urethral discharge.

Urine slightly cloudy, light yellow in appearance. Urine dipstick—pH6, blood—trace, leucocytes small, no other abnormalities detected.

Process information and identify problems/issues

Collaborative problem

Urethral discharge—possible STI

Needs full STI screen and first void urine specimen collected

Problem statement/nursing diagnosis

Knowledge deficit about STI and pregnancy prevention

Dysuria/pain related to urethral inflammation

ADDITIONAL RESOURCES

You can further develop your knowledge and skills relevant to male sexual and reproductive health assessment, related pathophysiology, common health issues and nursing interventions by:

- reading chapters of a fundamentals of nursing or medical-surgical nursing textbook
- answering chapter multiple choice questions online. Log onto ClinicalKey Student and search for the text 'Health Assessment, 4th edition'. Choose the section titled 'Teaching material'. In this section you will find question and answer documents for each chapter. Please check instructions on the inside front cover of the book to access online resources.
- visiting websites

  Andrology Australia: www.andrologyaustralia.org

  Healthy Male: www.healthymale.org.au

  New Zealand Sexual Health Society (Inc.): www.nzshs.org

  LGBTIQ+ Health Australia: https://www.lgbtiqhealth.org.au

  Rainbow Health Australia: https://rainbowhealthaustralia.org.au

  TransHub (see information for clinicians): https://www.transhub.org.au

  Community and Public Health (NZ): https://www.cph.co.nz/your-health/lgbtqiaplus-health/

  Rainbow Youth (NZ): https://ry.org.nz.

REFERENCES

1. Tortora GJ, Derrickson B, Burkett B, Cooke J, Di Pietro F, Diversi T, et al. Principles of Anatomy and Physiology, 3rd Asia-Pacific Edition. John Wiley & Sons; 2022.
2. Healthy Male. Clinical summary guide—androgen deficiency. Melbourne: Andrology Australia; 2022. Available at: https://www.healthymale.org.au/files/inline-files/4_Androgen%20Deficiency_CSG_Healthy%20Male%202022.pdf
3. Sharma A, Grant B, Islam H, Kapoor A, Pradeep A, Jayasena CN. Common symptoms associated with usage and cessation of anabolic androgenic steroids in men. Best Practice & Research Clinical Endocrinology & Metabolism. 2022 Aug 12:101691.
4. Patel RM, Bariol S. National trends in surgical therapy for benign prostatic hyperplasia in Australia. ANZ Journal of Surgery 2019;89(4):345–349.
5. Australian Institute of Health and Welfare. Cancer data in Australia—cancer risk data visualisation—prostate cancer. Canberra: AIHW; 2023. Available at: https://www.aihw.gov.au/reports/cancer/cancer-data-in-australia/contents/cancer-risk-data-visualisation
6. Prostate Cancer Foundation New Zealand. Prostate cancer now New Zealand's most diagnosed cancer. 2022. Available at: https://prostate.org.nz/2022/08/prostate-cancer-now-new-zealands-most-diagnosed-cancer/
7. Cancer Council. Types of cancer—prostate cancer. 2023. Available at: https://www.cancer.org.au/cancer-information/types-of-cancer/prostate-cancer
8. Prostate Cancer Foundation New Zealand. Prostate cancer. 2023. Available at: https://prostate.org.nz/prostate-cancer/
9. Cancer Council Victoria and Department of Health Victoria. Optimal care pathway for men with prostate cancer, 2nd edn, Cancer Council Victoria, Melbourne. 2021. Available at: https://www.cancer.org.au/assets/pdf/prostate-cancer-2nd-edition
10. National Institute of Health and Care Excellence. Prostate cancer: diagnosis and management. UK NICE guideline [NG131]. 2021. Available at: https://www.nice.org.uk/guidance/ng131/chapter/Context
11. Rashid P, Zargar-Shoshtari K, Ranasinghe W. Prostate-specific antigen testing for prostate cancer: Time to reconsider the approach to screening. Australian Journal of General Practice. 2023 Mar 1;52(3):91–95.
12. Hackett G, Kirby M, Rees RW, Jones TH, Muneer A, Livingston M, et al. The British Society for Sexual Medicine guidelines on male adult testosterone deficiency, with statements for practice. The World Journal of Men's Health. 2023 Jan 1;41.
13. Lowy M, Ramanathan V. Erectile dysfunction: causes, assessment and management options. Australian Prescriber. 2022 Oct;45(5):159.
14. Colson MH, Cuzin B, Faix A, Grellet L, Huyghes E. Current epidemiology of erectile dysfunction, an update. Sexologies 2018; 27(1):e7–e13.
15. Australian Government Department of Health. National Men's Health Strategy 2020–2030. 2019. Available at https://www.health.gov.au/resources/publications/national-mens-health-strategy-2020-2030?language=en
16. Australian Institute of Health and Welfare. The health of Australia's males. Canberra: Australian Institute of Health and Welfare, 2023. Available from: https://www.aihw.gov.au/reports/men-women/male-health
17. Ministry of Health. New Zealand Health Strategy. Wellington: Ministry of Health. 2023. Available at: https://www.health.govt.nz/system/files/documents/publications/new-zealand-health-strategy-jul23.pdf
18. Wilson T, Temple J, Lyons A, Shalley F. What is the size of Australia's sexual minority population? BMC Research Notes. 2020 Dec;13:1–6.
19. Stats New Zealand. LGBT+ population of Aotearoa: Year ended June 2021. New Zealand Government. 2022. Available at: https://www.stats.govt.nz/information-releases/lgbt-plus-population-of-aotearoa-year-ended-june-2021/#:~:text=4.4%20percent%20of%20the%20Aotearoa,the%20year%20ended%20June%202021
20. Hill AO, Bourne A, McNair R, Carman M, Lyons A. Private lives 3: The health and wellbeing of LTGBTIQ people in Australia. ARCSHS Monograph Series No. 122.

Melbourne, Australia: Australian Research Centre in Sex, Health and Society, La Trobe University. 2020. Available at: https://www.latrobe.edu.au/__data/assets/pdf_file/0009/1185885/Private-Lives-3.pdf
21. Haire BG, Brook E, Stoddart R, Simpson P. Trans and gender diverse people's experiences of healthcare access in Australia: A qualitative study in people with complex needs. PloS ONE. 2021 Jan 28;16(1):e0245889.
22. Vermeir E, Jackson LA, Marshall EG. Improving healthcare providers' interactions with trans patients: recommendations to promote cultural competence. Healthcare Policy. 2018 Aug;14(1):11.
23. King J, McManus H, Kwon A, Gray R, McGregor S 2022. HIV, viral hepatitis and sexually transmissible infections in Australia: annual surveillance report 2022, The Kirby Institute, UNSW Sydney, Sydney, Australia. http://doi.org/10.26190/sx44-5366. Available at: https://www.kirby.unsw.edu.au/research/reports/asr2022
24. University of Otago, AIDS epidemiology group. Epidemiological surveillance newsletter. Issue 83—May 2023. 2023. Available at: https://www.otago.ac.nz/__data/assets/pdf_file/0018/307233/aids-new-zealand-newsletter-issue-82-may-2023-0244567.pdf
25. World Health Organization. The role of HIV viral suppression in improving individual health and reducing transmission: policy brief. Geneva: World Health Organization; 2023. Available at: https://www.who.int/publications/i/item/9789240055179
26. Australasian Society for HIV Viral Hepatitis and Sexual Health Medicine (ASHM). National Prep Clinical Guidelines. ASHM. 2023. Available at: https://hivmanagement.ashm.org.au
27. Centers for Disease Control and Prevention (CDC). Pre-Exposure Prophylaxis (PrEP). US Department of Health and Human Services. 2022. Available at: https://www.cdc.gov/hiv/risk/prep/index.html#:~:text=Pre%2Dexposure%20prophylaxis%20(or%20PrEP,use%20by%20at%20least%2074%25.
28. Prabhakaran S, Ljuhar D, Coleman R, Nataraja RM. Circumcision in the paediatric patient: a review of indications, technique and complications. Journal of Paediatrics and Child Health 2018;54(12):1299–1307.
29. Australian Institute of Health and Welfare. Cancer data in Australia—cancer risk data visualisation—testicular cancer. Canberra: AIHW; 2023. Available at: https://www.aihw.gov.au/reports/cancer/cancer-data-in-australia/contents/cancer-risk-data-visualisation
30. Gurney JK. The puzzling incidence of testicular cancer in New Zealand: what can we learn? Andrology 2019;7(4):394–401.
31. Cancer Council. Testicular Cancer. 2023. Available at: https://www.cancer.org.au/cancer-information/types-of-cancer/testicular-cancer
32. Australian Institute of Health and Welfare. Cancer data in Australia—cancer risk data visualisation—male breast cancer. Canberra: AIHW; 2023. Available at: https://www.aihw.gov.au/reports/cancer/cancer-data-in-australia/contents/cancer-risk-data-visualisation
33. Argiolas A, Argiolas FM, Argiolas G, Melis MR. Erectile dysfunction: treatments, advances and new therapeutic strategies. Brain Sciences. 2023 May 15;13(5):802.
34. Royal Children's Hospital. Engaging with and assessing the adolescent patient. 2019. Available at: https://www.rch.org.au/clinicalguide/guideline_index/Engaging_with_and_assessing_the_adolescent_patient/
35. Australian Law Reform Commission, Australian Government. Capacity and health information. 2010. Available at: https://www.alrc.gov.au/publication/for-your-information-australian-privacy-law-and-practice-alrc-report-108/68-decision-making-by-and-for-individuals-under-the-age-of-18/capacity-and-health-information/

CHAPTER 28

Breasts assessment

Written by Carolyn Jarvis
Adapted by Elizabeth Pascoe

INTRODUCTION

The breasts, or mammary glands, are present in both females and males, although in males they are rudimentary throughout life. The female breasts are accessory reproductive organs whose function is to produce milk for nourishing newborns. However, in most Western cultures, female breasts signify more than their primary purpose of lactation. Women are surrounded by messages that feminine norms of beauty and desirability are enhanced by, and dependent on, the size of the breasts and their appearance. More recently, women leaders have tried to refocus this attitude, stressing women's self-worth as individual human beings, not as stereotyped sexual objects. The intense cultural emphasis is gradually changing, yet the breasts are still crucial to a woman's self-concept and her perception of her femininity.

Case study

The following case study provides an example of a typical situation involving assessing the female breast and the initial clinical reasoning process. It will help you to identify your learning needs.

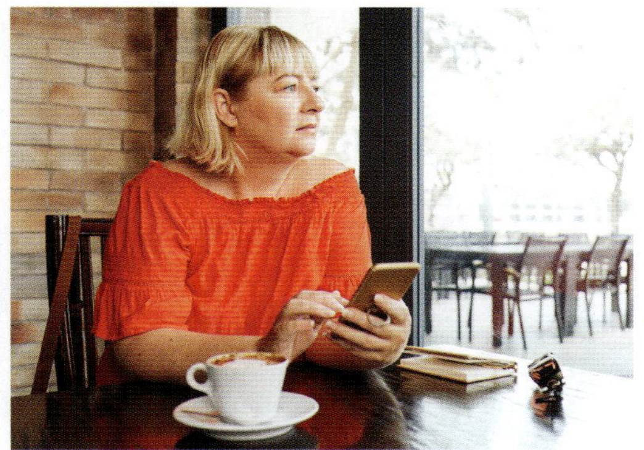

Context

You are a registered nurse working in a hospital emergency department.

Consider the patient's situation

Ms Justine Klein, a 48-year-old woman, was admitted to the emergency department following a minor traffic accident having sustained a mild concussion. Neurological assessment is being conducted at half-hourly intervals, and the discharge plan is to continue assessment for 4 hours. After medical reassessment she will be discharged home with GP review in 24 hours. During her admission, Ms Klein informed you that she had noticed a lump in her right breast 2 weeks ago.

Questions to further your learning

- What are the possible things that might be going on with Ms Klein?
- What knowledge do you need to be able to predict what might be going on?
- What approach to Ms Klein's health assessment will you take?
- What questions (subjective data) will you ask Ms Klein to extend the health history and why?
- What physical examination (objective data) will you conduct and why?
- What resources are available to assist in your assessment of Ms Klein?

Assessment plan

Matters of the breast affect a woman's body image and generate deep emotional responses that may be observed as you discuss the woman's history. One woman may be acutely embarrassed talking about her breasts, as evidenced by lack of eye contact, minimal response, nervous gestures or inappropriate humour. Another woman may talk wryly and disparagingly about the size or development of her breasts.

Young adolescents are acutely aware of their own development in relation to their peers. Or a woman who has found a breast lump may come to you with fear, high anxiety and even panic. Although many breast lumps are benign, women often assume the worst possible outcome—cancer, disfigurement and death. While you are collecting the subjective data, tune in to cues for these behaviours. While rare, men can also have breast signs or symptoms. These will be addressed in the subjective and objective data collection sections of this chapter.

Subjective assessment enables you to get information directly from the person about signs and symptoms they are experiencing. For the breasts, the main areas for subjective assessment are:

- presenting concern
- pain
- lump
- discharge
- rash
- swelling
- trauma
- history of breast disease
- surgery
- health and lifestyle management.

For the axillae:

- tenderness, a lump or swelling
- rash.

After collecting subjective data, you will get a sense of the areas needed to be examined. The main areas for physical examination are:

- general inspection
- inspecting the breasts
- palpating the breasts
- male breasts.

Resources available

You will find additional resources and the reference list at the end of this chapter.

Structure and function

Surface anatomy

The **breasts** lie anterior to the pectoralis major and serratus anterior muscles (Figure 28.1). The breasts are located between the second and sixth ribs, extending from the side of the sternum to the midaxillary line. The superior lateral corner of breast tissue, called the axillary **tail of Spence**, projects up and laterally into the axilla.

The **nipple** is just below the centre of the breast. It is rough, round and usually protuberant; its surface looks wrinkled and indented with tiny milk duct openings. The **areola** surrounds the nipple for a 1- to 2-centimetre radius. In the areola are small elevated sebaceous glands, called the Montgomery glands. These secrete a protective lipid material during lactation. The areola also has smooth muscle fibres that cause nipple erection when stimulated. Both the nipple and the areola are more darkly pigmented than the rest of the breast surface; the colour varies from pink to brown depending on the person's skin colour and parity.

Internal anatomy

The breast is composed of (1) glandular tissue, (2) fibrous tissue including the suspensory ligaments and (3) adipose tissue (Figure 28.2). The **glandular tissue** contains 15 to 20 lobes radiating from the nipple, and these are composed of lobules. Within each lobule are clusters of alveoli that produce milk. Each lobe empties into a lactiferous duct. The 15 to 20 lactiferous ducts form a collecting duct system converging towards the nipple. There, the ducts form ampullae, or lactiferous sinuses, behind the nipple, which are reservoirs for storing milk. The suspensory ligaments, or **Cooper's ligaments**, are fibrous bands extending

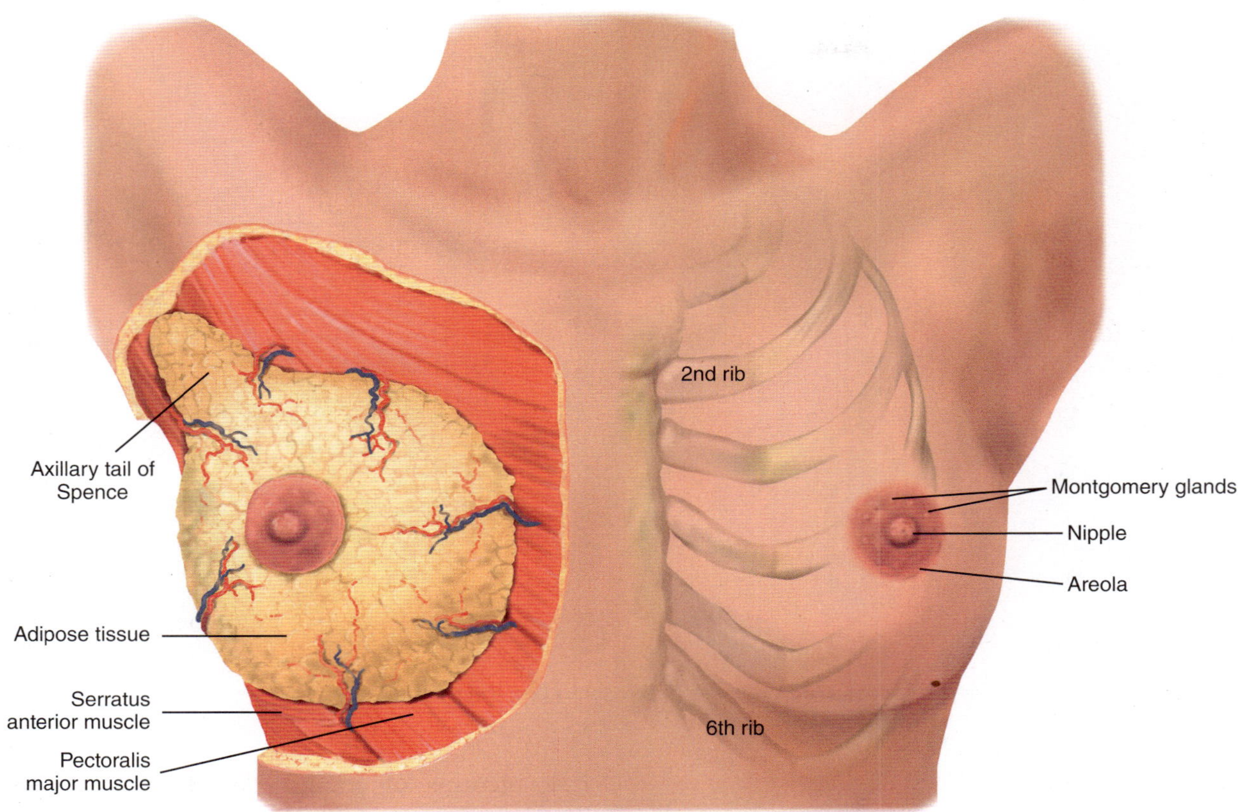

FIGURE 28.1 Anterior chest wall and breast anatomy

vertically from the surface to attach on chest wall muscles. These support the breast tissue. They become contracted in cancer of the breast, producing pits or dimples in the overlying skin.

The lobes are embedded in **adipose tissue**. These layers of subcutaneous and retromammary fat provide most of the bulk of the breast. The relative proportion of glandular, fibrous and fatty tissue varies depending on age, menstrual cycle, pregnancy, lactation and general nutritional state.

The breast may be divided into four quadrants by imaginary horizontal and vertical lines intersecting at the nipple (Figure 28.3). This makes a convenient map to describe clinical findings. In the upper outer quadrant, note the axillary **tail of Spence**, the cone-shaped breast tissue that projects up into the axilla, close to the pectoral group of axillary lymph nodes. The upper outer quadrant is the site of most breast tumours.

Lymphatics

The breast has extensive lymphatic drainage. Most of the lymph, more than 75%, drains into the ipsilateral (same side) axillary nodes.

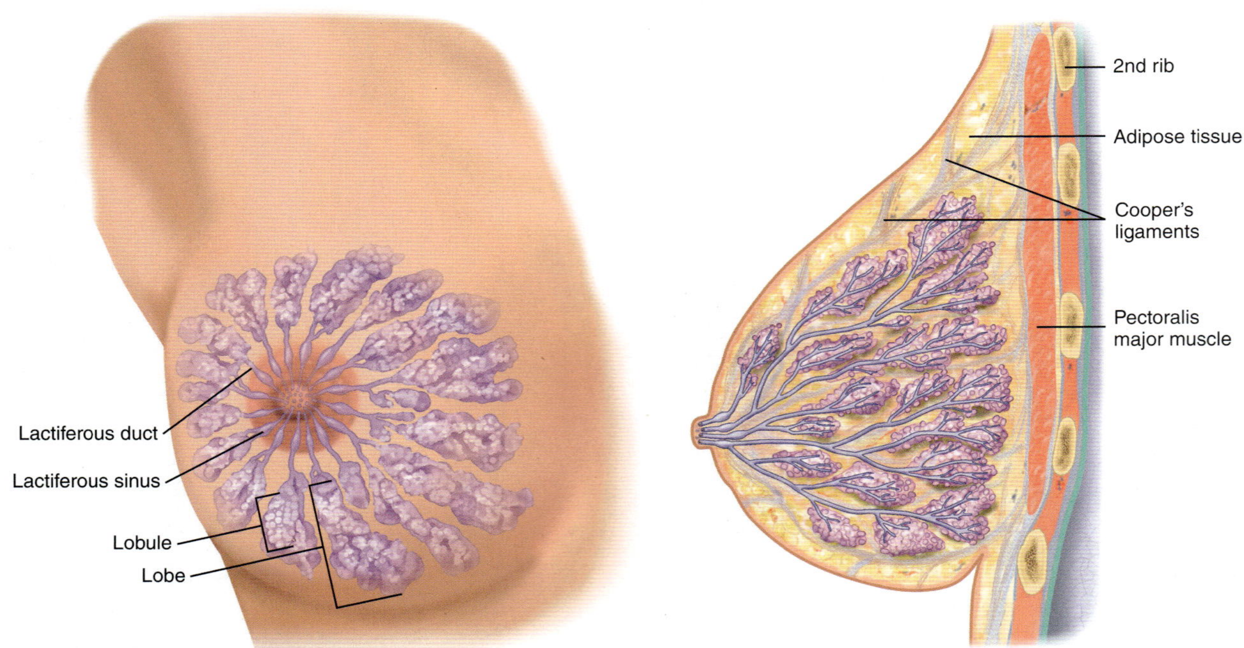

FIGURE 28.2 Anterior and lateral view of breast structure including the duct system

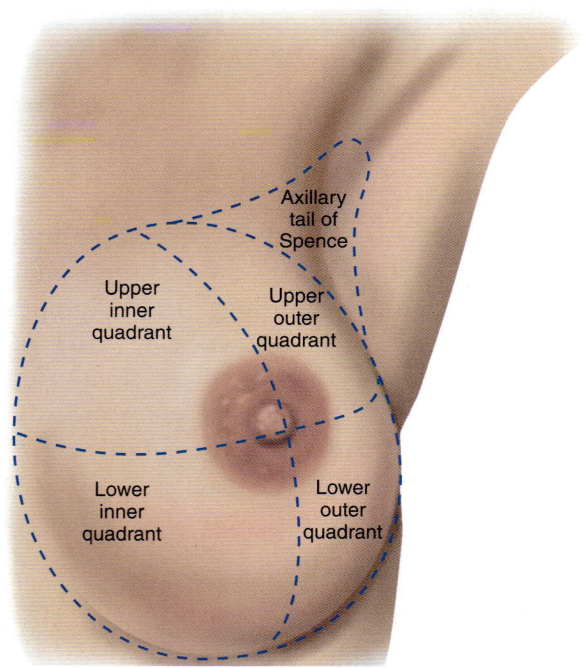

FIGURE 28.3 Anatomical mapping of breast areas for documenting breast examination findings

Four groups of axillary nodes are present (Figure 28.4):

- **central axillary nodes**—high up in the middle of the axilla, over the ribs and serratus anterior muscle. These receive lymph from the other three groups of nodes
- **pectoral** (anterior)—along the lateral edge of the pectoralis major muscle, just inside the anterior axillary fold
- **subscapular** (posterior)—along the lateral edge of the scapula, deep in the posterior axillary fold
- **lateral**—along the humerus, inside the upper arm.

From the central axillary nodes, drainage flows up to the infraclavicular and supraclavicular nodes.

A smaller amount of lymphatic drainage does not take these channels but flows directly up to the infraclavicular group, deep into the chest or into the abdomen or directly across to the opposite breast.

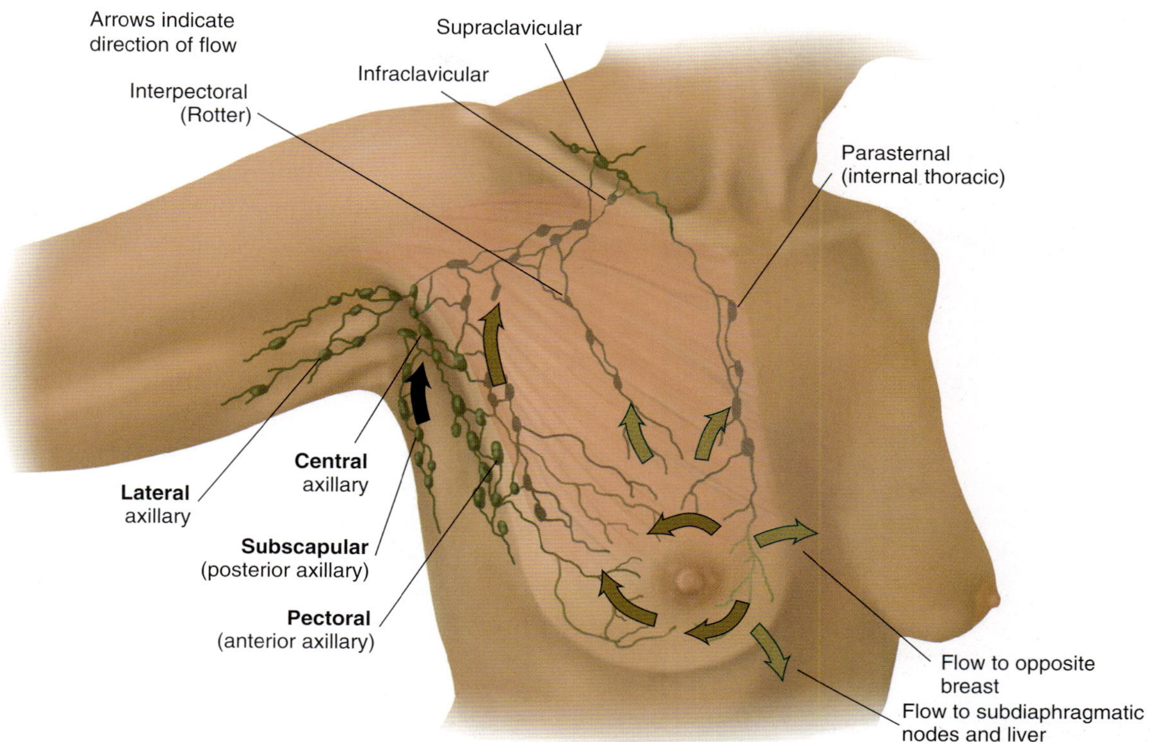

FIGURE 28.4 Location of lymph glands and lymph drainage system of the breast, anterior chest wall and axilla

Developmental considerations

During embryonic life, ventral epidermal ridges, or 'milk lines', are present; these curve down from the axilla to the groin bilaterally (Figure 28.5). The breast develops along the ridge over the thorax and the rest of the ridge usually atrophies. Occasionally a **supernumerary nipple** (i.e. an extra nipple) persists and is visible somewhere along the track of the mammary ridge (Figure 28.6).

At birth, the only breast structures present are the lactiferous ducts within the nipple. No alveoli have developed. Little change occurs until puberty. However, at birth, some infants appear to have breast tissue. This is a normal response to maternal hormones and disappear within the first week of life.

Adolescents

At puberty, the estrogen hormones stimulate breast changes. The breasts enlarge, mostly because of extensive fat deposition. The duct system also grows and branches and masses of small, solid cells develop at the duct endings. These are potential alveoli.

Knowledge about the factors that influence the timing of onset of puberty is still being studied. What is known is that the process is complex and multifactorial. Physiological factors include endocrine events involving the hypothalamus–pituitary–gonadal axis and changes to cellular networks controlling gonadotrophin-releasing hormone. These mechanisms are likely to be influenced

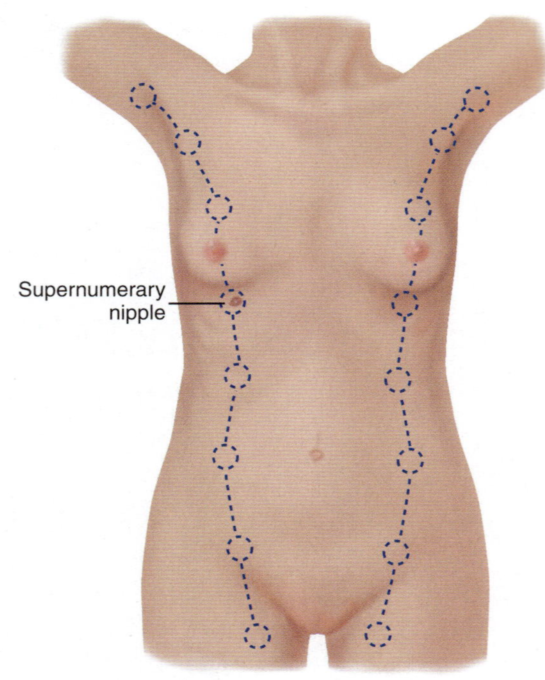

FIGURE 28.5 Potential location of a supernumerary nipple

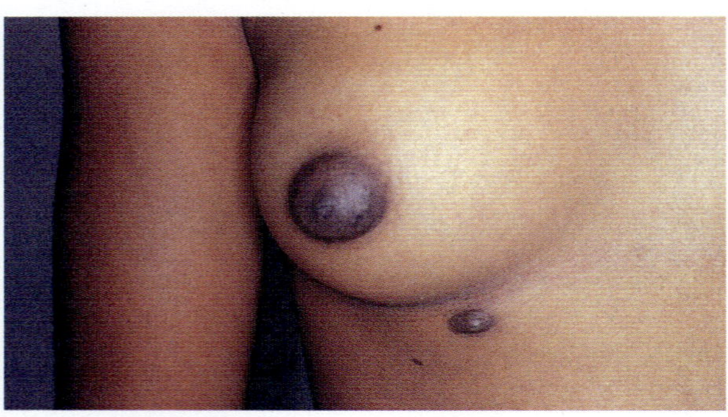

FIGURE 28.6 Supernumerary nipple and areolar complex

by regulatory gene networks, epigenetic changes, exposure to endocrine disrupting chemicals, maternal and childhood obesity, physical inactivity, social factors and low birthweight.[1–3] While the relative risk of each of the factors associated with the timing of onset of puberty is not specifically determined, level of BMI is increasingly cited as an important influencing factor.[1–3] While the specific mechanisms for this remain unclear, it is hypothesised that increased fat deposition might facilitate the production of higher levels of estrogen.[2]

Occasionally, one breast may grow faster than the other, producing a temporary asymmetry. This may cause some distress; reassurance is necessary. Tenderness is also common due to the influence of reproductive hormones, particularly estrogen. Although the age of onset varies widely, the five stages of breast development follow this classic description of sexual maturity rating, or **Tanner staging** (Table 28.1).

Full breast development from stage 2 to stage 5 takes an average of 3 years, although the range is 1.5 to 6 years. The beginning of breast development precedes menarche (beginning of menstruation) by about 2 years. Menarche occurs in breast development stage 3 or 4, usually just after the peak of the adolescent growth spurt around age 12 years. This aids in assessing the development of adolescent girls and increases their knowledge about their own development.

The breasts of a non-pregnant woman change with the ebb and flow of hormones during the monthly menstrual cycle. Nodularity increases from midcycle up to menstruation. During the 3 to 4 days before menstruation, the breasts feel full, tight, heavy and occasionally sore. The breast volume is smallest on days 4 to 7 of the menstrual cycle.

Pregnant women

During pregnancy, breast changes start during the second month and are an early sign of pregnancy for most women. Pregnancy stimulates the expansion of the ductal system and supporting fatty tissue as well as development of the true secretory alveoli. Thus, the breasts enlarge and feel more nodular. The nipples are larger, darker and

TABLE 28.1 Sexual maturity rating in girls

STAGE		
Preadolescent: Only a small, elevated nipple	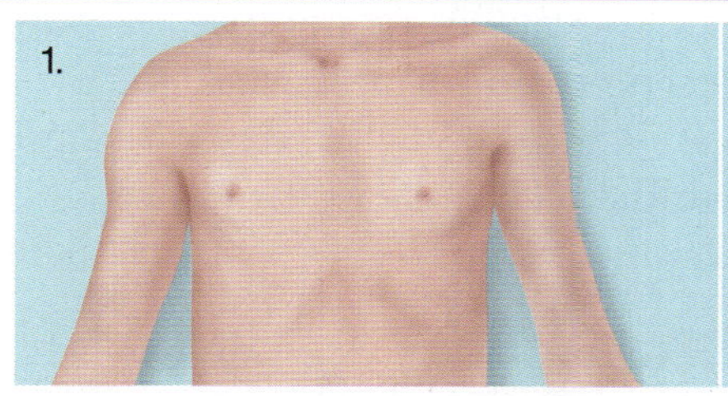	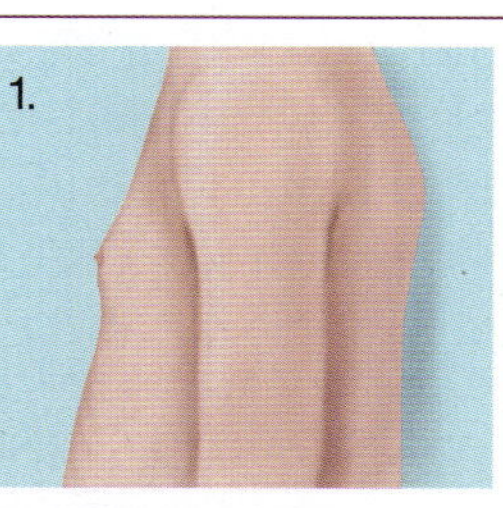
Breast bud stage: A small mound of breast and nipple develops; the areola widens	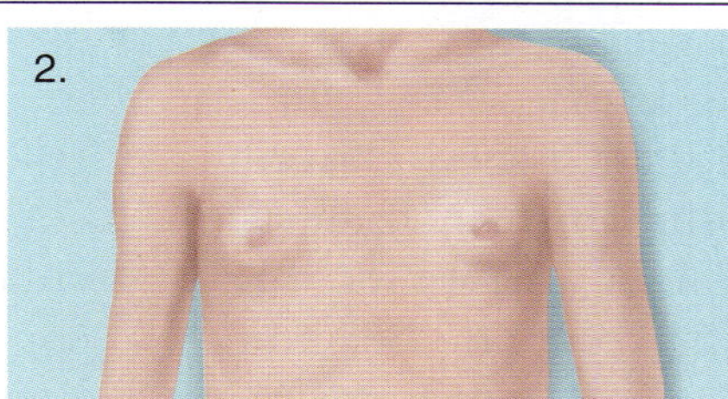	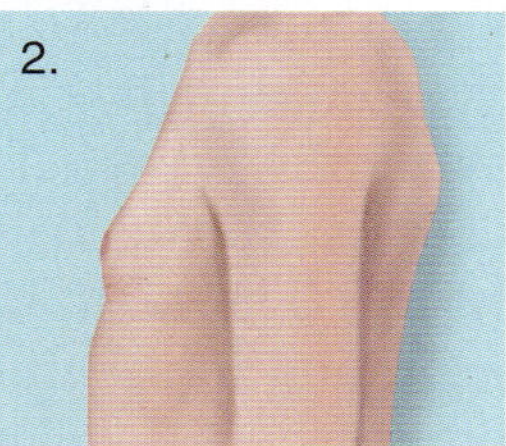
The breast and areola enlarge; the nipple is flush with the breast surface	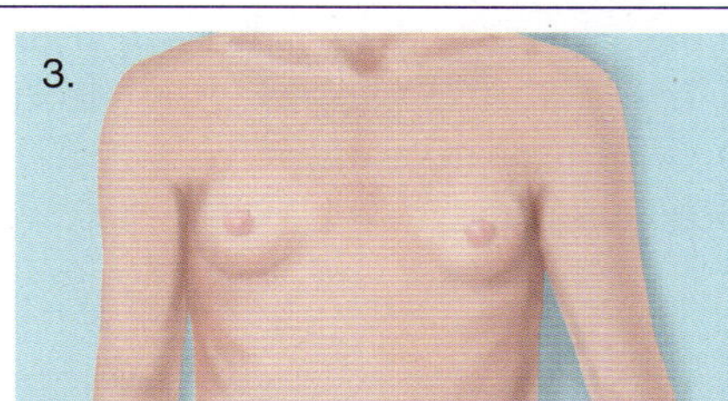	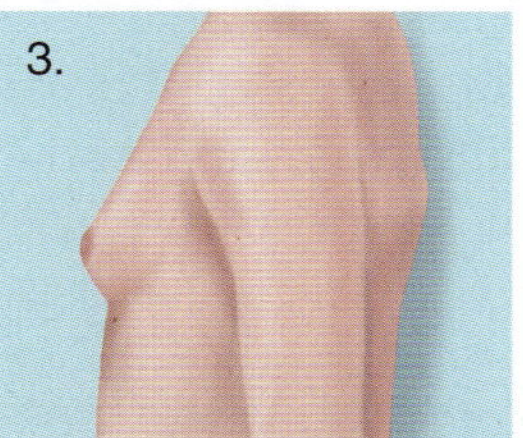
The areola and nipple form a secondary mound over the breast	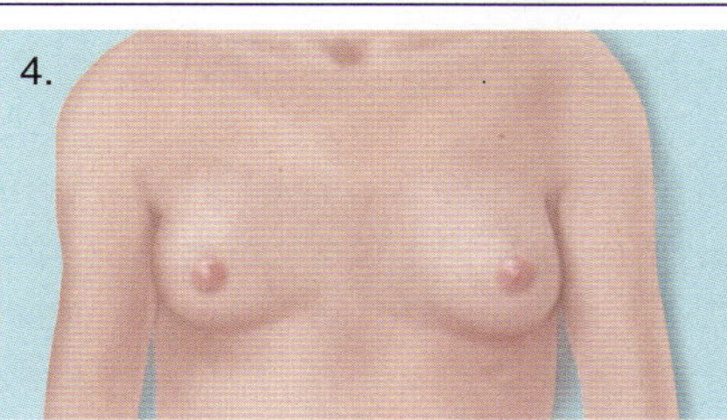	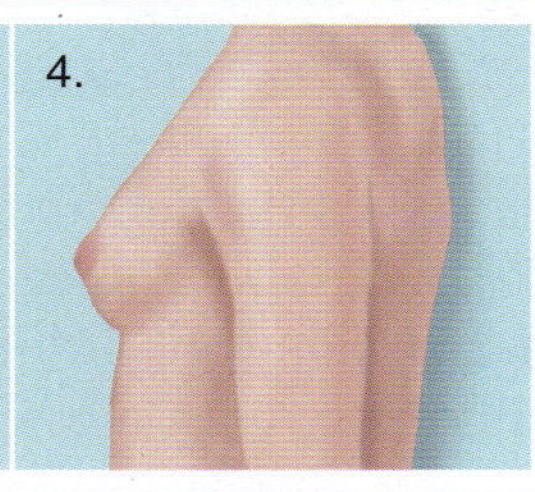
Mature breast: Only the nipple protrudes; the areola is flush with the breast contour (the areola may continue as a secondary mound in some normal women)	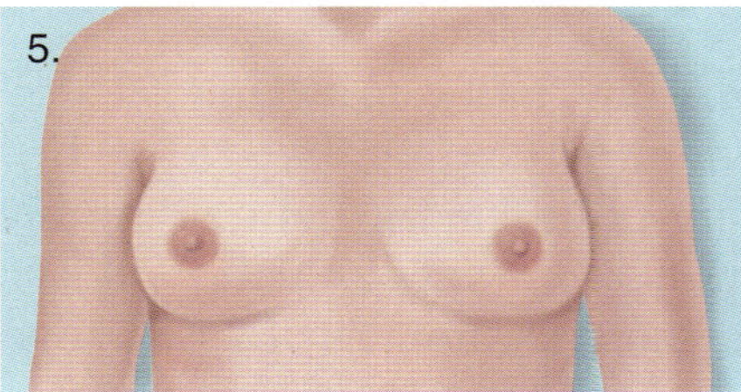	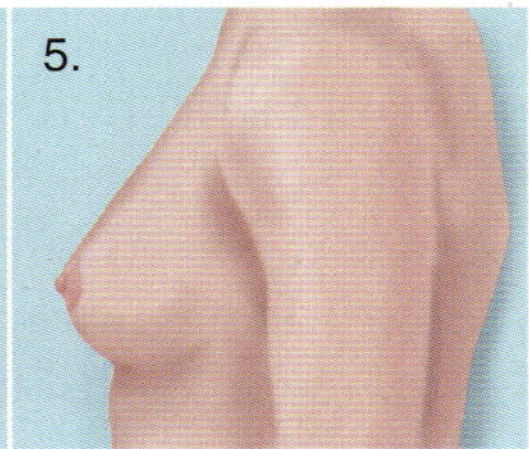

more erectile. The areolae become larger and grow a darker brown as pregnancy progresses and the tubercles become more prominent. The brown colour fades after lactation, but the areolae never return to the original colour. A venous pattern is prominent over the skin surface (Figure 28.4).

After the fourth month, **colostrum** may be expressed. This thick yellow fluid is the precursor for milk, containing the same amount of protein and lactose but practically no fat. The breasts produce colostrum for the first few days after birth. It is rich with antibodies that protect the newborn against infection, so breastfeeding is important. Milk production (lactation) begins 1 to 3 days postpartum. The whitish colour is from emulsified fat and calcium caseinate.

Women over 65 years

After menopause, ovarian secretion of estrogen and progesterone decreases, which causes the breast glandular tissue to atrophy. This is replaced with fibrous connective tissue. The fat envelope atrophies also, beginning in the middle years and becoming marked in the eighth and ninth decades. These changes decrease breast size and elasticity so the breasts droop and sag, looking flattened and flabby. Drooping is accentuated by kyphosis in some older women.

The decreased breast size makes inner structures more prominent. Around the nipple the lactiferous ducts are more palpable and feel firm and stringy because of fibrosis and calcification. The axillary hair decreases.

Male breasts

The male breast is a rudimentary structure consisting of a thin disc of undeveloped tissue underlying the nipple. The areola is well developed, although the nipple is relatively small. During adolescence, it is common for the breast tissue to temporarily enlarge, producing **gynaecomastia**. This condition is usually unilateral and temporary. Reassurance is necessary for adolescent males, whose attention may be focused on his body image. Gynaecomastia may reappear in males over 65 years and may be due to testosterone deficiency.

Cultural and social considerations

The age at which menarche occurs is reported to be variable across countries and races. The mean age of onset of menarche is also changing, with a lowering of the age of first menstruation reported. Non-Indigenous Australian women experience their first menstrual period (menarche) between 12 and 14 years of age, which is comparable to findings reported in Europe and in the United States.[4,5] Data from Aotearoa New Zealand reports age of first menstruation is 13.2 years.[6] Nevertheless, the authors further clarify that a school-by-school analysis indicates that nearly 50% of Aotearoa New Zealand girls start menstruation during years 7 and 8 and late primary-school age. The lowering of age on onset of menarche is reported in countries such as South Korea, where the mean age has dropped from 12.3 years to 12.0 years.[1] To date, there is no specific data on age of onset of menarche in Indigenous Australian women.

Breast cancer

Breast cancer is the most common cancer that occurs in Australian and Aotearoa New Zealand women. The risk of developing breast cancer to age 85 years is one in eight for Australian women and one in 668 for Australian men.[7] There are similar rates of breast cancer in Aotearoa New Zealand.[8]

The incidence of breast cancer varies with different cultural groups. Although the incidence of breast cancer is significantly lower in Indigenous Australian women than in non-Indigenous women, Indigenous women have significantly lower 5-year crude survival rates (85% and 91% crude survival, respectively).[9] In Aotearoa New Zealand, breast cancer registration among Māori women is approximately 30% higher than non-Māori women.[8] Further, Māori women are 1.5 times more likely to die from the disease than non-Māori, mainly because they tend to present with late-stage breast cancer at the time of diagnosis.[10]

In Australia, non-Indigenous women are significantly more likely to have had a mammogram through the BreastScreen Australia Program than are Indigenous women. In 2018–19, the age-standardised participation rate for non-Indigenous women aged 50 to 74 years was 55% compared with 38% for Indigenous Australian women in the same age range.[11] Although there is no single main factor influencing Indigenous women's decisions to use the BreastScreen Australia Program service, in addition to lack of easy access to services, there are historical and culturally related influences. Indigenous distrust of non-Indigenous institutions and beliefs about cancer and Western medical treatments (e.g. institutionalised racism, lack of cultural sensitivity, use of medical jargon and perceived lack of confidentiality in services because of kinship relations) are contributing factors.[12] Similarly, there are a range of cultural and social reasons why Māori and Pacific Islander women tend not to have regular screening mammograms.[13]

Cultural and social issues associated with diet and exercise are gaining attention. Mounting interest in the role that lifestyle factors such as diet, exercise, body weight and consumption of alcohol have on breast cancer incidence and survival and/or comorbidity and mortality has led researchers to evaluate the effects of these factors on the disease. Maintaining a healthy weight (especially after menopause), eating a healthy, balanced diet and cutting down on alcohol consumption are mainstay modifiable risk-factor recommendations to reduce the risk of developing breast cancer.[14]

Physical activity currently provides the strongest evidence for improving physical function and improving quality of life across multiple general health and cancer-specific domains.[15] At least 150 minutes of moderate-intensity or 75 minutes of vigorous-intensity aerobic exercise (e.g. walking, jogging, cycling, swimming) each week and two to three resistance exercise (i.e. lifting weights) sessions each week that target the major muscle groups are recommended.[15]

Despite the potential therapeutic effects of lifestyle factors on breast cancer prevention, they are not as significant when compared with non-modifiable factors. Familial history, inherited or acquired genetic mutations, age, gender (being a woman), breast density and having previous breast issues are the most significant risk factors. Nevertheless, in women with a high genetic risk, the absolute risk can be reduced by changing modifiable risk factors.[16]

HEALTH EDUCATION

Teaching breast awareness

When completing a breast assessment or other relevant health assessment, take the opportunity to discuss breast awareness strategies. Remember to reinforce that there are no right or wrong breast awareness techniques.

If the woman is unsure what she should do, suggest she adopt behaviours that are comfortable to do from time to time. For example, view her breasts in the mirror when dressing or undressing, or to feel her breasts while in the shower or bath, lying down or while dressing. Stress that breast awareness will familiarise her with her own breasts and

HEALTH EDUCATION cont'd

their normal variation. Emphasise the absence of lumps, not the presence of them. However, do encourage her to report any unusual finding promptly to her GP.

Focus on the positive aspects of breast awareness. Women know their own breast shape, size and feel, so small changes can be detected early.

- **Knowledge of risk factors and breast awareness** techniques should increase confidence in detecting changes and seeking further assessment from a health professional. Cancer Australia now provides dedicated information on breast cancer for men—Men can get breast cancer too: https://breastcancerinmen.canceraustralia.gov.au.
- **Educational materials are helpful reinforcements.** Cancer Australia provides a simple video on breast changes: https://www.youtube.com/watch?v=iCvFMTJgD1I.
- **Culturally sensitive information on breast awareness** for Australian Aboriginal and Torres Strait Islander women is available via the Cancer Australia website: Looking after your breasts, find breast cancer early and survive: https://www.canceraustralia.gov.au/key-initiatives/aboriginal-and-torres-strait-islander-health/looking-after-your-breasts%2C-find-breast-cancer-early-and-survive.
- In Aotearoa New Zealand, the Breast Cancer Foundation has information on breast awareness: https://www.breastcancerfoundation.org.nz/breast-awareness.

Assessing breast cancer risk—breast cancer screening tool

During a clinical breast examination, in addition to breast awareness, there is also an opportunity to assess the woman's breast cancer risk, including family history.

Using breast cancer risk assessment tools in the clinical setting has the potential to improve health substantially by reducing breast cancer incidence through cancer prevention and by more effective early detection programs for high-risk people.

- For clinicians, internationally, breast cancer risk assessment tools such as the Gail Model[17] has been validated among Australian women to effectively stratify a screened population aged 50 to 69 years according to the risk of future invasive breast cancer.[18]
- In Australia, eviQ[19] provides breast cancer genetic referral guidelines to health practitioners.
- For women, iPrevent, a web-based tool developed by the Peter MacCallum Cancer Centre, helps Australian women to understand their personal breast cancer risk and act upon it. The tool is available at: https://www.petermac.org/iprevent.

Subjective data

Practice note

Before you start the assessment, introduce yourself to the person, confirm the person's identity, discuss the purpose and scope of the assessment, clarify any questions the person may have and get verbal consent from the person to perform the assessment.

ASSESSMENT GUIDELINES	CLINICAL SIGNIFICANCE AND CLINICAL ALERTS
Presenting concern	
• *Do you think that you have any problems with your breasts?* It is important to ascertain the person's perception of their presenting health concern. If they do perceive a problem, ask: *How does this affect your quality of life and sexuality?*	
Pain	
• *Do you have any pain or tenderness in your breasts? When did you first notice it?* • *Where is the pain? Localised or all over? Is the painful spot sore to touch? Do you feel a burning or pulling sensation?*	! ***Clinical alert:*** **Mastalgia** (pain in the breast) may occur with trauma, inflammation, infection and benign breast disease. Seek medical advice.
• *Is the pain cyclic? Any relation to your menstrual period?* • *Is the pain related to a specific cause? Is the pain brought on by strenuous activity, especially involving one arm, a change in activity, touch during sex, from an underwire bra or exercise?*	Cyclic pain is common with normal breasts (commonly associated with the menstrual cycle) and benign breast (fibrocystic) disease. Oral contraceptives can also cause breast tenderness.
Lump	
• *Have you ever noticed a lump or thickening in the breast? Where?* • *When did you first notice it? Has it changed at all since then?* • *Does the lump have any relation to your menstrual period?* • *Have you noticed any change in the overlying skin: redness, warmth, dimpling or swelling?*	Carefully explore the presence of any lump. A lump present for many years and exhibiting no change may not be serious but still should be explored. Approach any recent change or new lump with suspicion.
Discharge	
• *Have you noticed any discharge from the nipple?* • *When did you first notice this?* • *What colour is the discharge?* • *Consistency—thick or runny?* • *Any odour?*	**Galactorrhoea** (lactation not associated with childbirth). Note medications that may cause clear nipple discharge: oral contraceptives, phenothiazines, diuretics, digitalis, steroids, methyldopa, calcium channel blockers. **Bloody or blood-tinged** discharge is always significant. Any discharge with a lump is significant. ! ***Clinical alert:*** If any discharge is noted, the person should be referred to a medical practitioner for further assessment.

ASSESSMENT GUIDELINES	CLINICAL SIGNIFICANCE AND CLINICAL ALERTS
Rash	
• *Have you noticed any rash on either breast?* • *When did you first notice this?* • *Where did it start? On the nipple, areola or the surrounding skin?*	**Paget's disease of the nipple.** Inflammatory malignant neoplasm of the nipple and areola that is usually associated with carcinoma in deeper breast tissue. Paget's disease starts with a small crust on the nipple apex, then spreads to the areola. Eczema (superficial dermatitis) or other dermatitis rarely starts at the nipple unless it is due to breastfeeding. It usually starts on the areola or surrounding skin and then spreads to the nipple. ***Clinical alert:*** If any rash on the breast is noted, the person should be referred to a medical practitioner for further assessment.
Swelling	
• *Have you noticed any swelling in the breasts? In one spot or all over?* • *Is it related to your menstrual period, pregnancy or breastfeeding? If relevant, when was your last menstrual period? Do you usually have any associated breast symptoms with your menstrual cycle?* • *Any change in bra size?*	
Trauma	
• *Have you experienced any trauma or injury to the breasts?* • *Did it result in any swelling, lump or break in the skin?*	A lump from an injury is due to local haematoma or oedema and should resolve shortly. Or trauma may cause a woman to feel the breast and find a lump that was actually there before.
History of breast disease	
• *Do you have any history of breast disease yourself?* • *What type? How was this diagnosed?* • *When did this occur?* • *How is it being treated?*	Past breast cancer increases the risk of recurrent cancer (Table 28.2). The presence of benign breast disease makes the breasts more difficult to examine; the general lumpiness may conceal a new lump.

ASSESSMENT GUIDELINES	CLINICAL SIGNIFICANCE AND CLINICAL ALERTS
• *Is there a history of any breast cancer in your family? Who? Sister, mother, maternal grandmother, maternal aunts, daughter?* • *At what age did this relative have breast cancer?*	Breast cancer occurring in certain family members increases the risk (Table 28.2).
Surgery	
• *Have you ever had surgery on the breasts?* (choose whichever is relevant) • *Was this a biopsy? What were the biopsy results?* • *Mastectomy—prophylactic or for treatment of the breast cancer?* • *Breast reconstruction?* • *Mammoplasty—augmentation or reduction?*	
Health and lifestyle management	
• *Do you take oral contraceptives? For how long?* • *For post-menopausal women—are you taking menopausal hormone therapy? Type? For how long?* • *Are you taking any other medications?*	**Oral contraceptives** may control symptoms of benign (fibrocystic) breast disease. Combined **menopausal hormone therapy** can increase the risk of breast cancer in some women. There is variation in the risk with other variables such as race/ethnicity, body mass index and breast density.
• *Do you routinely inspect and feel your breasts?* • *Are you aware of what you should be looking for?* • *Do you know when to seek medical advice?* Breast awareness and mammograms are complementary screening measures. Cancer Australia and the Breast Cancer Foundation NZ advocate a 'Breast Aware' approach to encourage women to report unusual breast changes. This approach involves the woman being aware of how her breasts normally look and feel so she may be better able to recognise any changes.[20,21] (See 'Health education' earlier in the chapter.)	A suggested **breast awareness** approach is offered by Cancer Australia (see 'Health education' earlier in the chapter). ***Clinical alert:*** Inform the woman that if she notices any of the following changes in either of her breasts when performing regular breast awareness, she should contact her GP without delay: • a new lump or lumpiness, especially if it is in one breast • nipple discharge • a change in the size or shape of the breast or nipple • a change in the skin over the breast such as redness or dimpling • an unusual, persistent pain, especially if it is in one breast.[21] See the 'Additional resources' section at the end of the chapter for links to resources for health teaching related to breast awareness.

ASSESSMENT GUIDELINES	CLINICAL SIGNIFICANCE AND CLINICAL ALERTS
• *Have you ever had mammography, a screening x-ray examination of the breasts? When was the last x-ray?*	**Screening mammograms** are an effective way of detecting early signs of breast cancer in older women, but they are not effective in young women. Younger women's breasts are very dense and appear like white cotton wool on a mammogram. Free screening mammograms are offered to all women over 40 years of age living in Australia. As women become older, their breasts become less dense and so screening mammogram becomes an effective means of revealing cancers too small to be detected by the woman or by the most experienced examiner. In Australia, women aged 50 to 74 years are recommended to have a free screening mammogram every 2 years. In Aotearoa New Zealand, free screening[22] is offered biannually to women aged 45 to 69 years. In Australia, women aged 75 years and older are also offered free screening mammogram every 2 years.[11] It is important for women to continue with breast awareness practices because lumps may become palpable between mammograms.
Axilla	
Tenderness, lump or swelling • *Have you experienced any tenderness or lump in the underarm area?* • *Where? When did you first notice this?* **Rash** • *Any axillary rash? Please describe it.* • *Does it seem to be a reaction to deodorant?*	Breast tissue extends up into the axilla. Also, the axilla contains many lymph nodes.
Additional subjective data for preadolescents	
• *Have you noticed your breasts changing? How long has this been happening?* • *Many girls notice other changes in their bodies that come with growing up. What have you noticed?* • *What do you think about all this?*	Developing breasts are the most obvious sign of puberty and the focus of attention for most girls, especially in comparison with peers. Assess each girl's perception of her own development and provide teaching and reassurance as indicated.

ASSESSMENT GUIDELINES	CLINICAL SIGNIFICANCE AND CLINICAL ALERTS
Additional subjective data for pregnant women	
• *Have you noticed any enlargement or fullness in the breasts?* • *Is there any tenderness or tingling?* • *Do you have a history of inverted nipples?* • *Are you planning to breastfeed your baby? See Chapter 29.*	Breast changes are expected and normal during pregnancy. Assess the woman's knowledge and provide reassurance. Inverted nipples may need special care in preparation for breastfeeding. Breastfeeding exclusively for the first 6 months provides the perfect food and antibodies for the baby, decreases the risk of ear infections, promotes bonding and provides relaxation. It is also protective against breast cancer.
Additional subjective data for menopausal women	
• *Have you noticed any change in the breast contour, size or firmness?* **Note:** Change may not be as apparent to obese women or to women whose earlier pregnancies have already produced breast changes.	Decreased estrogen level causes decreased firmness. A rapid decrease in estrogen level causes actual shrinkage.
Risk factor profile for breast cancer	
Breast cancer is the second most common cause of cancer-related death for Australian women.[11] However, early detection and improved treatment have increased survival rates. The outcomes for women diagnosed with breast cancer have improved significantly for both Indigenous and non-Indigenous women aged 50 to 74 years who took part in the screening program, with a similar mortality rate reported for this age group.[11] Note the risk factors listed in Table 28.2.	The best way to detect a person's risk for breast cancer is by asking the right history questions. Table 28.2 highlights risk factors for breast cancer, and from these you can fashion your questions. Be aware that most breast cancers occur in women with risk factors classified as nonmodifiable. Just because a woman does not report the cited risk factors does not mean you or she should fail to consider breast cancer seriously.

TABLE 28.2 Breast cancer risk factors

Modifiable and nonmodifiable factors that may increase risk of breast cancer

	Risk factor	Relative risk
Nonmodifiable	Gender (female greater than male)	High
	Increasing age (higher risk after age 65)	High
	Genetic profile—Several genes have been identified that substantially influence risk of breast cancer (so-called rare, high-penetrant genes) including BRCA1, BRCA2, TP53, PTEN, CD1 and STK11.[23]	
	Family history (two or more first-degree relatives, younger than age 50 at diagnosis)	High
	Breast density (including persistent density after menopause)	High
	Abnormal breast biopsy (atypia or lobular carcinoma in situ)	High
	Geographic location (exposure to chemical or ionising radiation)	Moderate (depending on exposure)
	History of chest radiation	Moderate
	Personal history of breast cancer	Moderate
	Endogenous hormone levels (high levels of estrogen or testosterone)	Moderate
	Diethylstilboestrol exposure (secondary to mother's use)	Low
	Personal history of other cancers (endometrium, ovary or colon)	Low
May be modifiable	Personal history of increase bone density (signifies increased endogenous estrogen)	Low
Modifiable	Exogenous hormone use (e.g. estrogen, progesterone or testosterone)	Low
	Birth control pills (recent and long-term use)	Low
	Age at first full-term pregnancy (after 30 years of age)	Low
	Occupational exposure	Low (depending on specific chemicals)
	Lifestyle risks (alcohol, diet, weight, exercise, smoking)	Low
	High socioeconomic status	Low
	Absence of breastfeeding	Low
	Absence of full-term pregnancy	Low

Adapted from Table 47-1 in Lester 2018[16]

Objective data

Irrespective of whether the person has had a clinical breast examination performed for the first time or many times, sensitivity to body image, privacy when performing the examination and awareness of cultural norms and practices should be acknowledged and provided. Remember to ensure the room in which you perform the examination is warm and well lit. Also, warm your hands before you begin.

Preparation

Ask the woman to sit up and face you. Use a short gown, open at the back and lift it up to the woman's shoulders during inspection. During palpation when the woman is supine, cover one breast with the gown while examining the other. Be aware that many women are embarrassed to have their breasts examined; use a sensitive but matter-of-fact approach. After your examination, be prepared to discuss breast awareness techniques.

Equipment needed

Small pillow
Hand hygiene solution

PROCEDURES AND NORMAL FINDINGS	CLINICAL SIGNIFICANCE AND CLINICAL ALERTS
General inspection	
While collecting subjective data, you will have noticed the condition of the person's skin, hair, posture, height-to-weight ratio, body shape, level of hygiene and grooming and general demeanour. All these factors provide clues to the woman's overall health.	
Inspecting the breasts	
Symmetry size and shape	
Note symmetry of size and shape (Figure 28.7). It is common to have a slight asymmetry in size; often the left breast is slightly larger than the right. 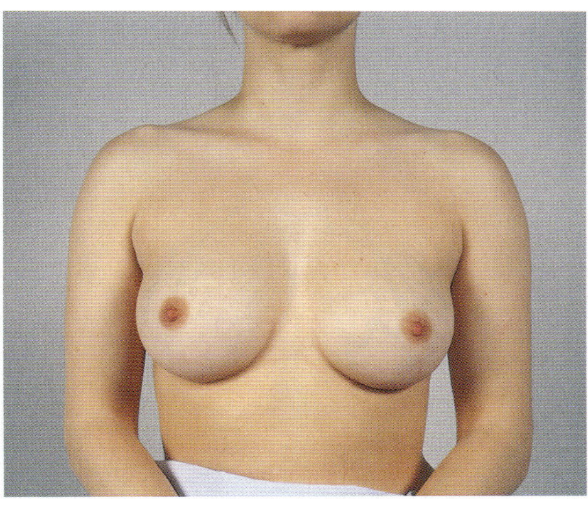 **FIGURE 28.7** Position to assess the symmetry and size of the breasts	A sudden increase in the size of one breast may signify inflammation or new growth.

PROCEDURES AND NORMAL FINDINGS	CLINICAL SIGNIFICANCE AND CLINICAL ALERTS
Skin	
The skin is normally smooth and of even colour. Note any localised areas of redness, bulging or dimpling. Also, note any skin lesions or focal vascular pattern. A fine blue vascular network is visible normally during pregnancy. Pale linear striae, or stretch marks, often follow pregnancy.	**Hyperpigmentation** (darkening of the skin). Redness and heat with inflammation. Unilateral dilated superficial veins in a non-pregnant woman. **Oedema** (Table 28.3). Normally no oedema is present. Oedema exaggerates the hair follicles, giving an 'orange-peel' look (also called *peau d'orange*).
Lymphatic drainage areas	
Observe the axillary and supraclavicular regions. Note any bulging, discolouration or oedema.	
Nipples	
The nipples should be symmetrically placed on the same plane on the two breasts. Nipples usually protrude, although some are flat and some are inverted. They tend to stay in their original condition. Distinguish a recently retracted nipple from one that has been inverted for many years or since puberty. Normal nipple inversion may be unilateral or bilateral and usually can be pulled out (i.e. it is not fixed).	Deviation in pointing (Table 28.3). Recent nipple retraction signifies acquired disease (Table 28.3).
Note any dry scaling, any fissure or ulceration and bleeding or other discharge.	Explore any discharge, especially in the presence of a breast mass.
A **supernumerary nipple** is a normal and common variation (Figure 28.6). An extra nipple along the embryonic 'milk line' on the thorax or abdomen is a congenital finding. Usually, it is 5 to 6 cm below the breast near the midline and has no associated glandular tissue. It looks like a mole, although a close look reveals a tiny nipple and areola. It is not significant; merely distinguish it from a mole.	Rarely, additional glandular tissue, called a supernumerary breast, is present.
Screening for skin retraction	
Direct the woman to change position while you check the breasts for skin retraction signs. First ask her to lift the arms slowly over the head. Both breasts should move up symmetrically (Figure 28.8).	**Retraction** signs are due to fibrosis in the breast tissue, usually caused by growing neoplasms. The fibrosis shortens with time, causing contrasting signs with the normally loose breast tissue. Note a lag in movement of one breast.

PROCEDURES AND NORMAL FINDINGS	CLINICAL SIGNIFICANCE AND CLINICAL ALERTS

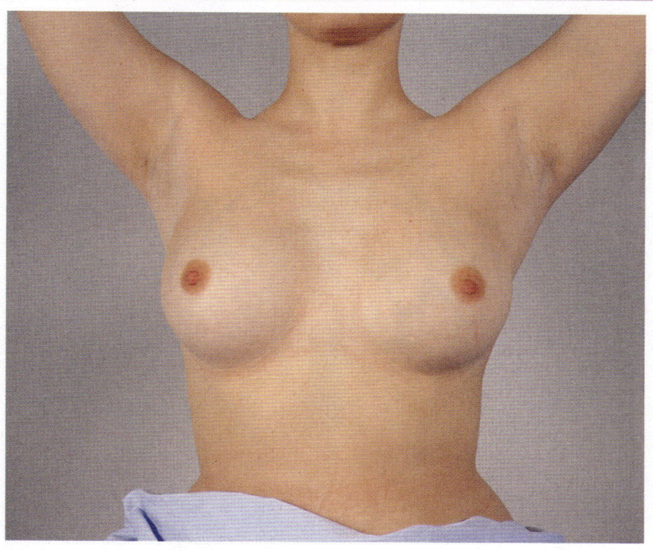

FIGURE 28.8 Retraction manoeuvre (arms up)

Next ask her to push her hands onto her hips (Figure 28.9) and to push her two palms together (Figure 28.10). These manoeuvres contract the pectoralis major muscle. A slight lifting of both breasts will occur.

Note a **dimpling** or a pucker, which indicates skin retraction (Table 28.3).

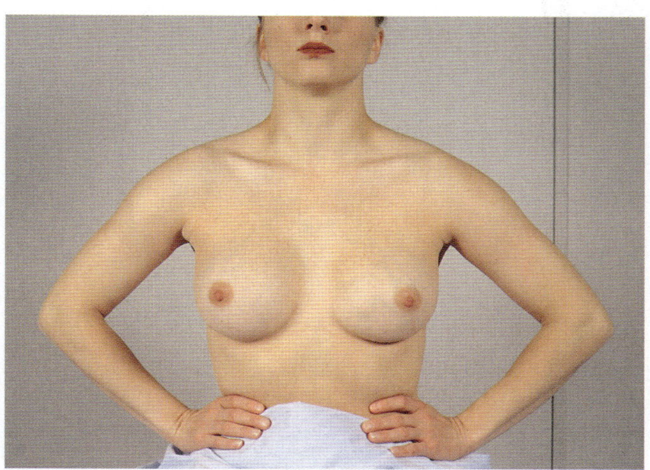

FIGURE 28.9 Retraction manoeuvre (hands pressing at the hips)

PROCEDURES AND NORMAL FINDINGS	CLINICAL SIGNIFICANCE AND CLINICAL ALERTS
FIGURE 28.10 Retraction manoeuvre (hands pressing together)	
Ask women with large pendulous breasts to lean forward while you support her forearms. Note the symmetrical free-forward movement of both breasts (Figure 28.11).	Note fixation to the chest wall or skin retraction (Table 28.3).

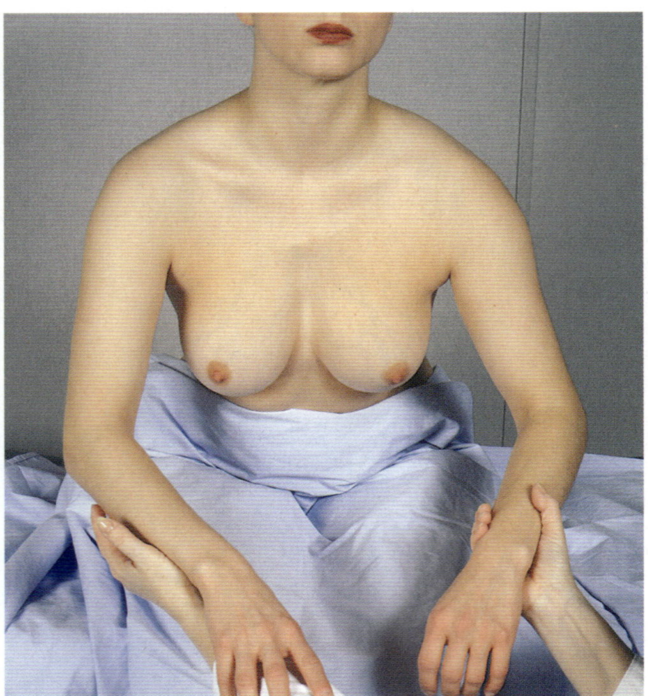

FIGURE 28.11 Leaning forward movement

PROCEDURES AND NORMAL FINDINGS	CLINICAL SIGNIFICANCE AND CLINICAL ALERTS

Palpating the breasts

Help the woman to a supine position. Tuck a small pad under the side to be palpated and raise her arm over her head. These manoeuvres will flatten the breast tissue and displace it medially. Any significant lumps will then feel more distinct (Figure 28.12).

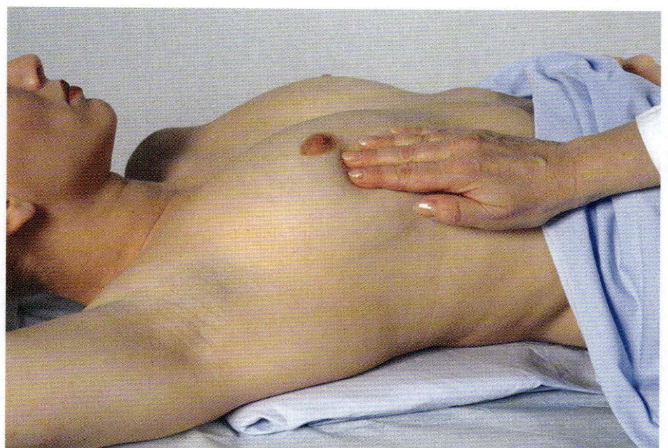

FIGURE 28.12 Light palpation of the breast

Use the pads of your first three fingers and make a gentle rotary motion on the breast. Vary your pressure so you are palpating light, medium and deep tissue in each location.

Start high in the axilla and palpate down just lateral to the breast. Proceed in overlapping vertical lines ending at the sternal edge. In every pattern, take care to palpate every square inch of the breast and to examine the tail of Spence high into the axilla. Be consistent and thorough in your approach to each woman.

In nulliparous women, normal breast tissue feels firm, smooth and elastic. After pregnancy, the tissue feels softer and looser. Premenstrual engorgement is normal from increasing progesterone. This consists of a slight enlargement, a tenderness to palpation and a generalised nodularity; the lobes feel prominent and their margins more distinct.

Heat, redness and swelling in non-lactating and non-postpartum breasts may indicate inflammation.

Also, normally you may feel a firm transverse ridge of compressed tissue in the lower quadrants. This is the inframammary ridge and it is especially noticeable in large breasts. Do not confuse it with an abnormal lump.

PROCEDURES AND NORMAL FINDINGS	CLINICAL SIGNIFICANCE AND CLINICAL ALERTS
After palpating over the four breast quadrants, palpate the nipple (Figure 28.13). Note any induration or subareolar mass. With your thumb and forefinger, gently depress the nipple tissue into the well behind the areola. The tissue should move inwards easily. If the woman reports spontaneous nipple discharge, press the areola inwards with your index finger—repeat from a few different directions. If any discharge appears, note its colour and consistency.	Except in pregnancy and lactation, discharge is abnormal (Table 28.4). Note the number of discharge droplets and the quadrant(s) producing them. Blot the discharge on a white gauze pad to ascertain its colour. Document and report any discharge to a medical practitioner.

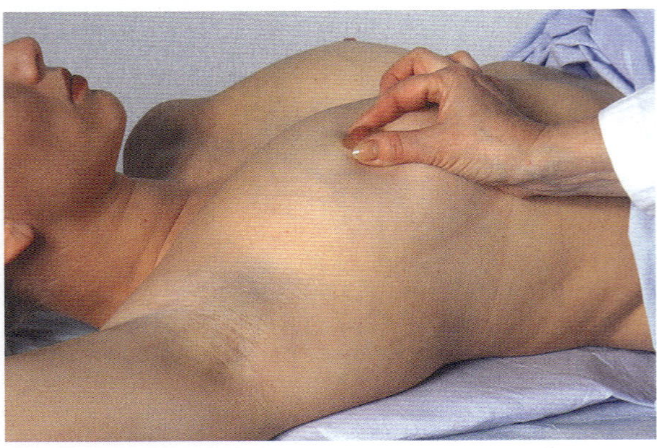

FIGURE 28.13 Palpation of the nipple and areola

For women with large pendulous breasts, you may palpate by using a bimanual technique (Figure 28.14). The woman is in a sitting position, leaning forwards. Support the inferior part of the breast with one hand. Use your other hand to palpate the breast tissue against your supporting hand.

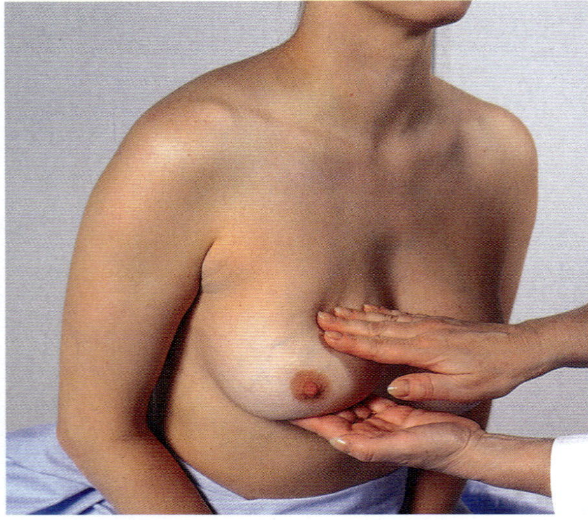

FIGURE 28.14 Bimanual palpation for a woman with larger breasts

PROCEDURES AND NORMAL FINDINGS	CLINICAL SIGNIFICANCE AND CLINICAL ALERTS

If the woman mentions a breast lump that she has discovered herself, examine the unaffected breast first to learn a baseline of normal consistency for this woman.

If you do feel a lump or mass, note the following characteristics (Figure 28.15).

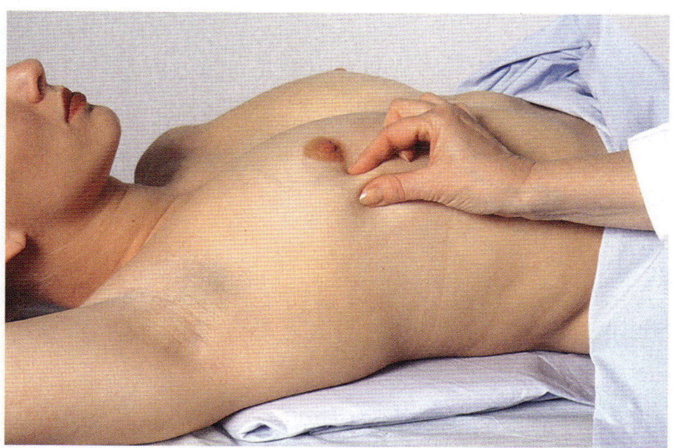

FIGURE 28.15 Palpation of a breast mass

If you detect a lump or change in breast tissue, record as follows:

- **Location**—using the breast as a clock face, describe the distance in centimetres from the nipple (e.g. '7:00, 2 cm from the nipple'). Or diagram the breast in the woman's record and mark in the location of the lump.
- **Size**—judge in centimetres in three dimensions: width × length × thickness.
- **Shape**—state whether the lump is oval, round, lobulated or indistinct.
- **Consistency**—state whether the lump is soft, firm or hard.
- **Movable**—is the lump freely movable, or is it fixed when you try to slide it over the chest wall?
- **Distinctness**—is the lump solitary or multiple?
- **Nipple**—is it displaced or retracted?
- **Note the skin over the lump**—is it erythematous, dimpled or retracted?
- **Tenderness**—is the lump tender to palpation?
- **Lymphadenopathy**—are any regional lymph nodes palpable?

See Tables 28.5 and 28.6 for descriptions of common breast lumps with these characteristics.

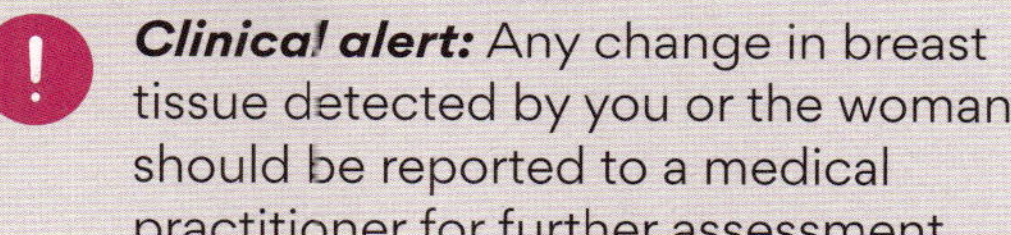

Clinical alert: Any change in breast tissue detected by you or the woman should be reported to a medical practitioner for further assessment.

PROCEDURES AND NORMAL FINDINGS	CLINICAL SIGNIFICANCE AND CLINICAL ALERTS

Male breasts

Your examination of the male breast can be much more abbreviated, but do not omit it. Combine a breast check technique with that of the anterior thorax. Inspect the chest wall, noting the skin surface and any lumps or swelling. Palpate the nipple area for any lump or tissue enlargement (Figure 28.16). It should feel even, with no nodules. Palpate the axillary lymph nodes.

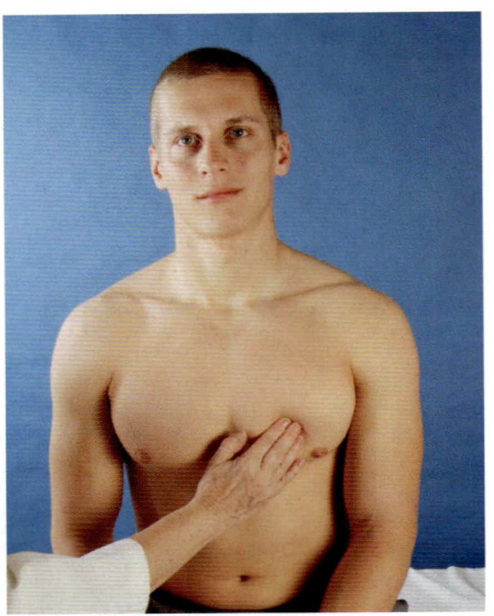

FIGURE 28.16 Light palpation of the male breast

A normal male breast has a flat disc of undeveloped breast tissue beneath the nipple. Adolescents are acutely aware of his body image. Reassure him that this change is normal, common and temporary. In contrast, obese males have an increase of fatty, not glandular, tissue.

Gynaecomastia is an enlargement of this breast tissue, making it clinically distinguishable from the other tissues in the chest wall (Figure 28.17). It feels like a smooth, firm, movable disc. This occurs normally during puberty. It usually affects only one breast and is temporary.

Gynaecomastia also occurs with use of anabolic steroids, some medications and some disease states.

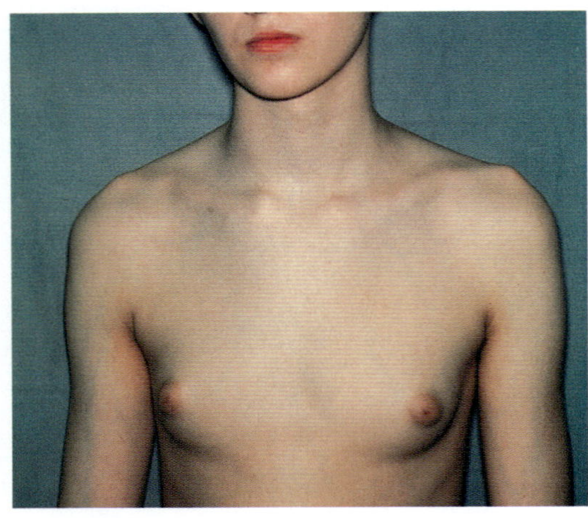

FIGURE 28.17 Adolescent gynaecomastia

PROCEDURES AND NORMAL FINDINGS	CLINICAL SIGNIFICANCE AND CLINICAL ALERTS
Additional objective data for infants and children	
In neonates, the breasts may be enlarged and visible due to maternal estrogen crossing the placenta. They may secrete a clear or white fluid called 'witch's milk'. These signs are not significant and are resolved within a few days to a few weeks.	
Note the position of the nipples on the prepubertal child. They should be symmetrical, just lateral to the midclavicular line, between the fourth and fifth ribs. The nipple is flat and the areola is darker pigmented.	**Premature thelarche** is early breast development with no other hormone-dependent signs (pubic hair, menses).
Additional objective data for adolescents	
Adolescent breast development usually begins between 8 and 10 years of age. Expect some asymmetry during growth. (Distinguish breast development from extra adipose tissue present in obese children.) Record the stage of development using Tanner's staging described in Table 28.1. Use the chart to teach adolescents about normal developmental stages and to assure them of their own normal progress. Consider BMI when evaluating breast budding before 8 years of age because it may be difficult to distinguish breast budding from adipose tissue. With maturing adolescents, palpate the breasts as you would with adults. The breasts normally feel firm and uniform. Note any mass. Discuss breast awareness techniques that young women can routinely practise. If required, demonstrate how to use finger pads and flats of fingers to feel near the surface and deeper in the breast tissue and under the arm.	Note **precocious development**, occurring before age 8 years. It is usually normal but also occurs with thyroid dysfunction, stilboestrol ingestion or ovarian or adrenal tumour. Note delayed development, occurring with hormonal failure or anorexia nervosa beginning before puberty or with severe malnutrition. At this age, a mass is almost always a **benign fibroadenoma** or a cyst (Table 28.4).
Additional objective data for pregnant women	
A delicate blue vascular pattern is visible over the breasts. The breasts increase in size, as do the nipples. Jagged linear stretch marks, or striae, may develop if the breasts have a large increase. The nipples also become darker and more erectile. The areolae widen, grow darker and contain the small, scattered, elevated Montgomery glands. On palpation, the breasts feel more nodular and thick yellow colostrum can be expressed after the first trimester.	
Additional objective data for lactating women	
Colostrum changes to milk production around the third postpartum day. At this time, the breasts may become engorged, appearing enlarged, reddened and shiny and feeling warm and hard. Frequent feeding helps drain the ducts and sinuses and stimulate milk production.	One section of the breast surface appearing red and tender indicates a blocked duct. ! ***Clinical alert:*** A lactating woman who is experiencing nipple soreness or pain should be referred to a midwife or maternal and child health nurse for advice.

PROCEDURES AND NORMAL FINDINGS	CLINICAL SIGNIFICANCE AND CLINICAL ALERTS
Additional objective data for women over 65 years	
On inspection, the breasts may look pendulous, flattened and sagging. Nipples may be retracted but can be pulled outwards. On palpation, the breasts feel more granular and the terminal ducts around the nipple feel more prominent and stringier. Thickening of the inframammary ridge at the lower breast is normal, and it feels more prominent with age. Reinforce the value of breast awareness. Women over 50 years old have an increased risk of breast cancer.	Because atrophy causes shrinkage of normal glandular tissue, cancer detection is somewhat easier. Any palpable lump should be referred.

Abnormal findings

TABLE 28.3 Signs of retraction and inflammation in the breasts

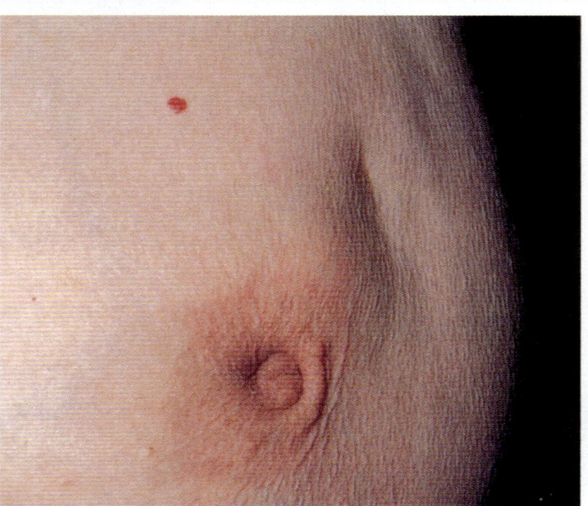

Dimpling

The shallow dimple (also called a skin tether) shown here is a sign of skin retraction. Cancer causes fibrosis, which contracts the suspensory ligaments. The dimple may be apparent at rest, with compression or with lifting of the arms. Also note the distortion of the areola here as the fibrosis pulls the nipple towards it.

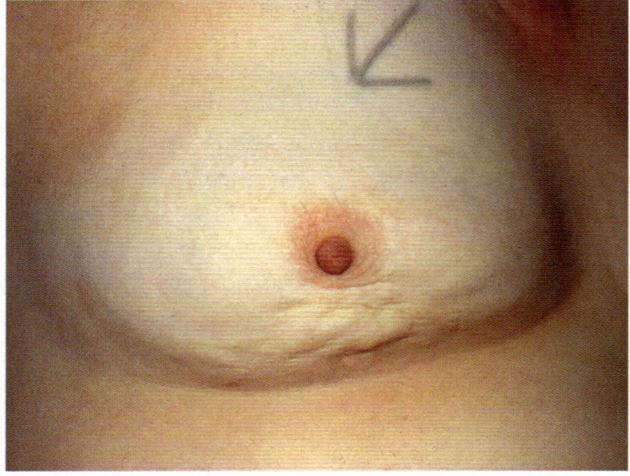

Oedema (peau d'orange)

Lymphatic obstruction produces oedema. This thickens the skin and exaggerates the hair follicles, giving a pig-skin or orange-peel look. This condition suggests cancer. Oedema usually begins in the skin around and beneath the areola, the most dependent area of the breast. Also note nipple infiltration here.

Continued

TABLE 28.3 Signs of retraction and inflammation in the breasts cont'd

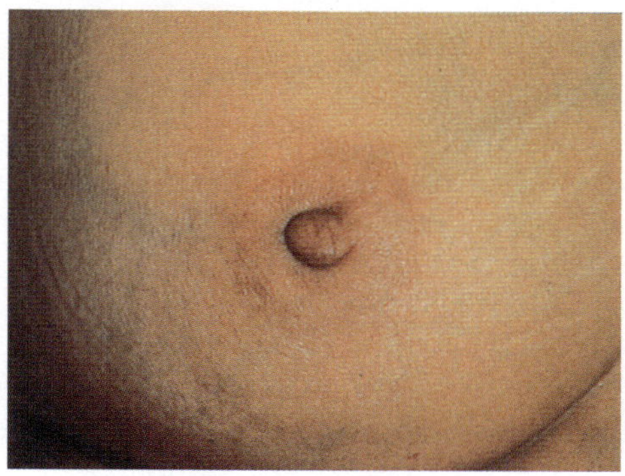

Deviation in nipple pointing

An underlying cancer causes fibrosis in the mammary ducts, which pulls the nipple angle towards it. Here, note the swelling behind the right nipple and that the nipple tilts laterally.

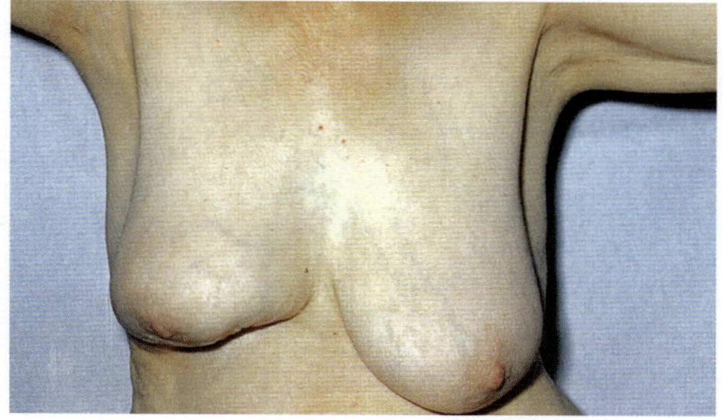

Fixation

Asymmetry, distortion or decreased mobility with the elevated arm manoeuvre. As cancer becomes invasive, the fibrosis fixes the breast to the underlying pectoral muscles. Here, note the right breast is held against the chest wall.

TABLE 28.4 Breast lumps

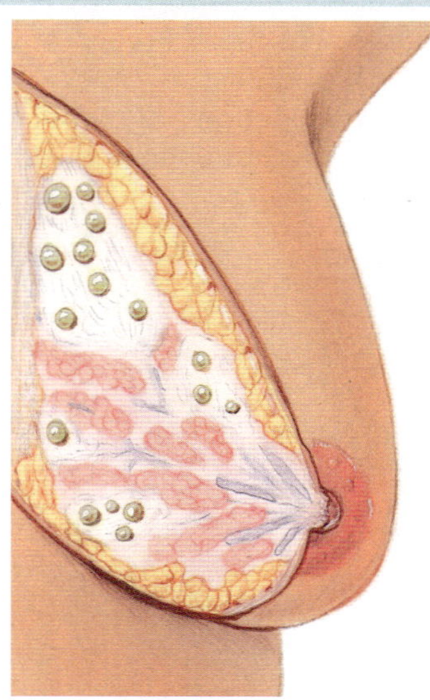

Benign breast disease (formerly fibrocystic breast disease)

Multiple tender masses. 'Fibrocystic disease' is a meaningless term because it covers too many entities. Six diagnostic categories exist, based on symptoms and physical findings:

- swelling and tenderness (cyclic discomfort)
- mastalgia (severe pain, both cyclic and noncyclic)
- nodularity (significant lumpiness, both cyclic and noncyclic)
- dominant lumps (including cysts and fibroadenomas)
- nipple discharge (including intraductal papilloma and duct ectasia)
- infections and inflammations (including subareolar abscess, lactational mastitis, breast abscess and Mondor's disease).

About 50% of all women have some form of benign breast disease. Nodularity occurs bilaterally; regular, firm nodules that are mobile, well demarcated and feel rubbery, like small water balloons. Pain may be dull, heavy and cyclic or just before menses as nodules enlarge. Some women have nodularity but no pain and vice versa. Cysts are discrete, fluid-filled sacs. Dominant lumps and nipple discharge must be investigated carefully and may need a biopsy to rule out cancer. Nodularity itself is not premalignant but may produce difficulty in detecting other cancerous lumps.

Continued

TABLE 28.4 Breast lumps cont'd

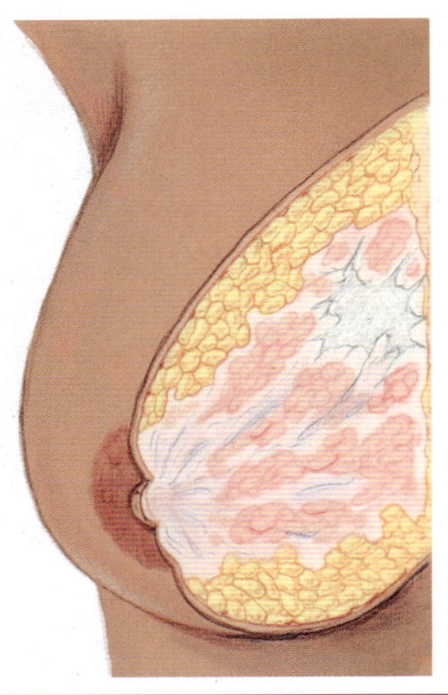

Cancer

Solitary unilateral nontender mass. Single focus in one area, although it may be interspersed with other nodules. Solid, hard, dense and fixed to underlying tissues or skin as cancer becomes invasive. Borders are irregular and poorly delineated. Grows constantly. Often painless, although the person may have pain. Most common in upper outer quadrant. Usually found in women 30 to 80 years of age; increased risk in ages 40 to 44 years and in women older than 50 years. As cancer advances, signs include firm or hard irregular axillary nodes; skin dimpling; nipple retraction, elevation and discharge.

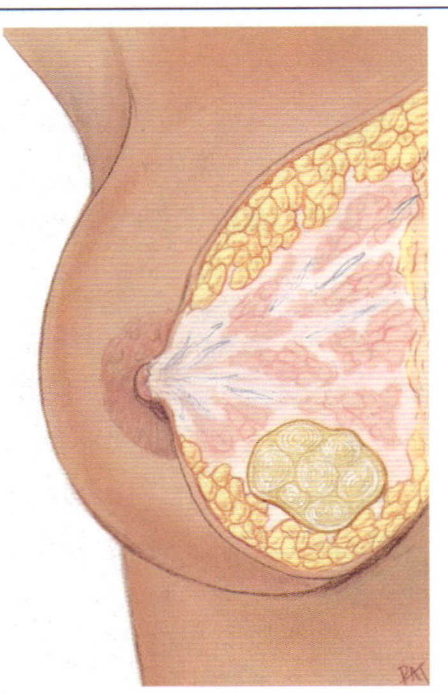

Fibroadenoma

Solitary nontender mass. A category of benign breast disease that deserves mention because of its frequency and characteristic appearance. Solid, firm, rubbery and elastic. Round, oval or lobulated; 1 to 5 cm. Freely movable, slippery; fingers slide it easily through tissue. Most common between 15 and 30 years of age but can occur up to 55 years. Grows quickly and constantly. Benign, although it must be diagnosed by biopsy.

TABLE 28.5 Differentiating breast lumps

	Fibroadenoma	Benign Breast Disease	Cancer
Likely age	15 to 30 years, can occur up to 55 years	30 to 55 years, decreases after menopause	30 to 80 years, risk increases after 50 years
Shape	Round lobular	Round, lobular	Irregular, star-shaped
Consistency	Usually firm, rubbery	Firm to soft, rubbery	Firm to stony hard

TABLE 28.5 Differentiating breast lumps cont'd

	Fibroadenoma	Benign Breast Disease	Cancer
Demarcation	Well demarcated, clear margins	Well demarcated	Poorly defined
Number	Usually single	Usually multiple, may be single	Single
Mobility	Very mobile, slippery	Mobile	Fixed
Tenderness	Usually none	Tender, usually increases before menses, may be noncyclic	Usually none, can be tender
Skin retraction	None	None	Usually
Pattern of growth	Grows quickly and constantly	Size may increase or decrease rapidly	Grows constantly
Risk to health	None; they are benign—must diagnose by biopsy	Benign, although general lumpiness may mask other cancerous lump	Serious, needs early treatment

Advanced practice—additional data

In addition to previous objective assessment, nurses working in specialist women's health and breast care settings may need to develop these advanced skills. Preparation and communication continue to be important parts of practice to support women undergoing this assessment. No additional equipment is required.

PROCEDURES AND NORMAL FINDINGS	CLINICAL SIGNIFICANCE AND CLINICAL ALERTS
Inspect and palpate axillary lymph nodes	
Examine the axillae while the woman is sitting. Inspect the skin, noting any rash or infection. Lift the woman's arm and support it yourself so her muscles are loose and relaxed. Use your right hand to palpate the left axilla (Figure 28.18). Reach your fingers high into the axilla. Move them firmly down in four directions: (1) down the chest wall in a line from the middle of the axilla, (2) along the anterior border of the axilla, (3) along the posterior border and (4) along the inner aspect of the upper arm. Move the woman's arm through range-of-motion to increase the surface area you can reach.	

PROCEDURES AND NORMAL FINDINGS	CLINICAL SIGNIFICANCE AND CLINICAL ALERTS
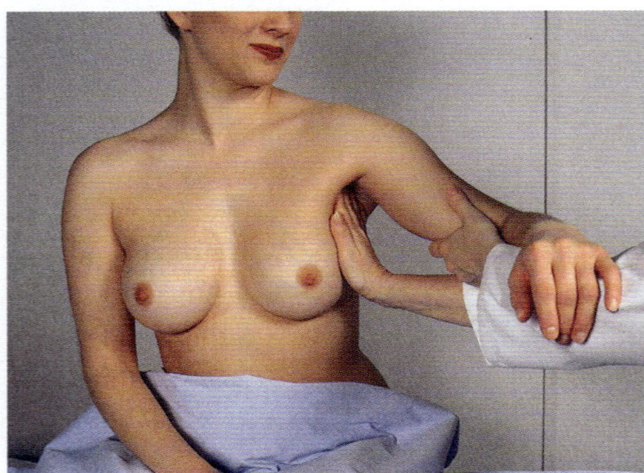 FIGURE 28.18 Palpation of the axilla	
Usually nodes are not palpable, although you may feel a small, soft, nontender node in the central group. Expect some tenderness when palpating high in the axilla. Note any enlarged and tender lymph nodes.	Nodes may enlarge with any local infection of the breast, arm or hand and with breast cancer metastases.

Abnormal findings for advanced practice

TABLE 28.6 Abnormal nipple discharge

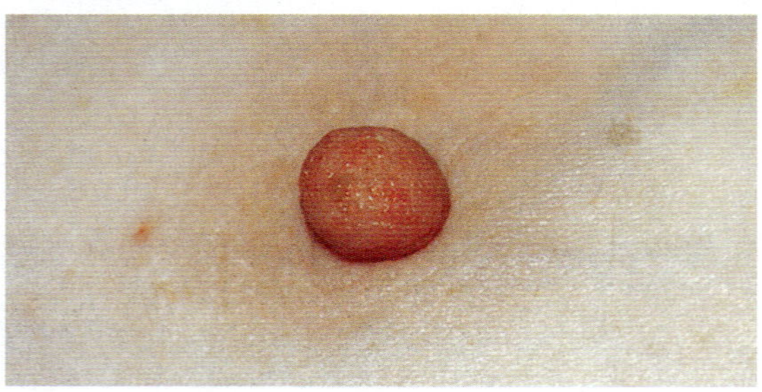

Mammary duct ectasia

Paste-like matter in subareolar ducts produces sticky, purulent discharge that may be white, grey, brown, green or bloody. A light green, single duct discharge is shown here. Caused by stagnation of cellular debris and secretions in the ducts, leading to obstruction, inflammation and infection. Occurs in women who have lactated; usually occurs in perimenopause. Itching, burning or drawing pain occurs around the nipple. May have subareolar redness and swelling. Ducts are palpable as rubbery, twisted tubules under areola. May have a palpable mass, soft or firm, poorly delineated. Not malignant but needs biopsy.

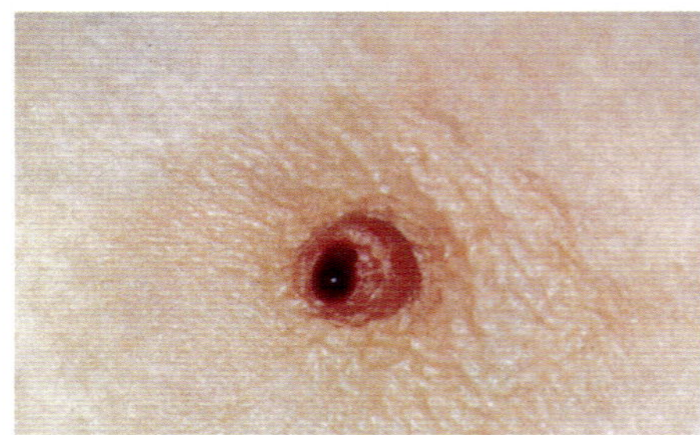

Carcinoma

Bloody nipple discharge that is unilateral and from a single duct requires further investigation. Although there was no palpable lump associated with the discharge shown here, mammography revealed a 1-centimetre, centrally located, ill-defined mass.

TABLE 28.6 Abnormal nipple discharge cont'd

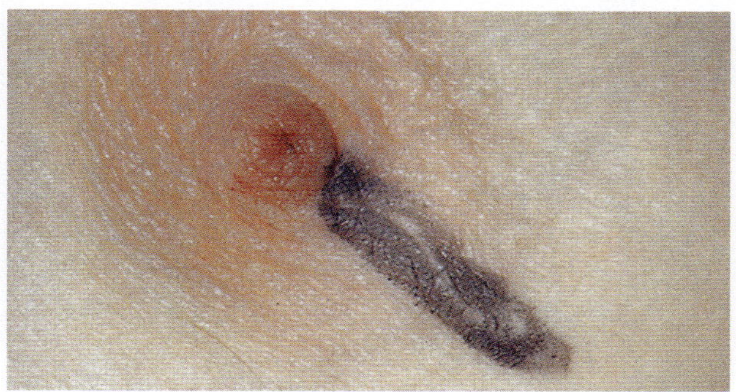

Intraductal papilloma

Serous or serosanguineous discharge, which is spontaneous, unilateral or from a single duct. Lesion consists of tiny tumours, 2 to 3 mm. Often there is a palpable nodule in the underlying duct (highlighted here). Papillomas affect women 40 to 60 years of age; most are benign. Refer any bloody discharge for careful evaluation, including biopsy, to rule out cancer.

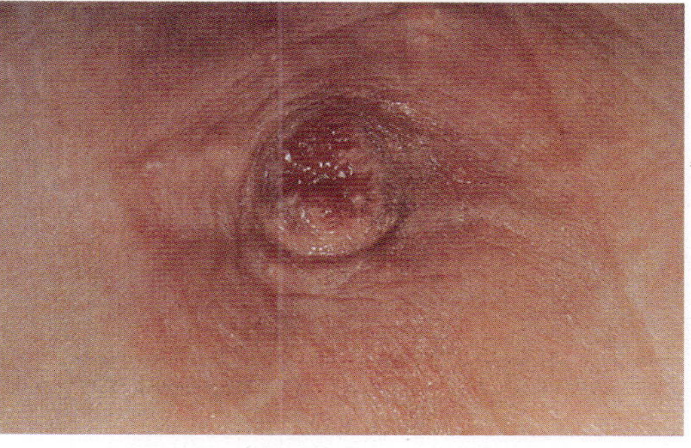

Paget's disease (intraductal carcinoma)

Early lesion has unilateral, clear, yellow discharge and dry, scaling crusts, friable at nipple apex. Spreads outwards to areola with erythematous halo on areola and crusted, eczematous, retracted nipple. Later lesion shows nipple reddened, excoriated, ulcerated, with bloody discharge when surface is eroded and an erythematous plaque surrounding the nipple. Symptoms include tingling, burning and itching.

Except for the redness and occasional cracking from initial breastfeeding, any dermatitis of the nipple area must be carefully explored and referred immediately.

TABLE 28.7 Disorders occurring during lactation

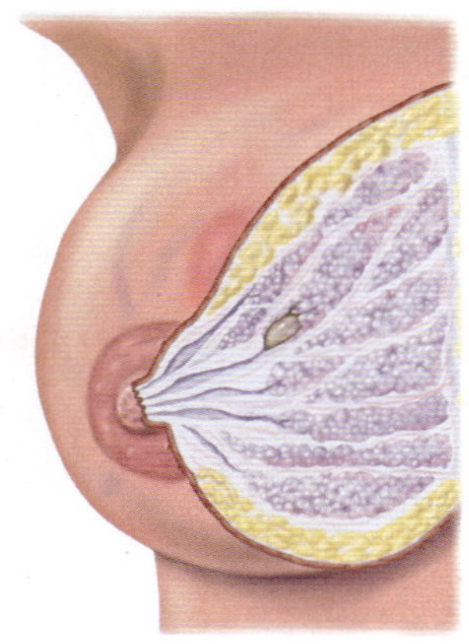

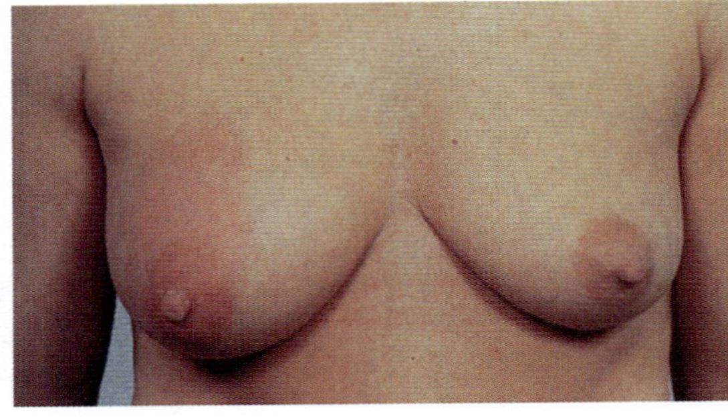

Plugged duct

A common and not serious condition. One milk duct is clogged. One section of the breast is tender; may be reddened. No infection. It is important to keep the breast as empty as possible and milk flowing. The woman should nurse her baby frequently, on the affected side first to ensure complete emptying and manually express any remaining milk. A plugged duct usually resolves in less than a day.

Mastitis

An inflammatory mass before abscess formation. Usually occurs in a single quadrant. The area is red, swollen, tender, very hot and hard, here forming outwards from areola upper edge, in the right breast. Also, the woman has a headache, malaise, fever, chills and sweating, increased pulse and flu-like symptoms. May occur during the first 4 months of lactation from infection or from stasis from plugged duct. Treat with rest, local heat to the area, antibiotics and frequent nursing to keep the breast as empty as possible. Must not wean now or the breast will become engorged and the pain will increase. The mother's antibiotics are not harmful to the infant. Usually resolves in 2 to 3 days.

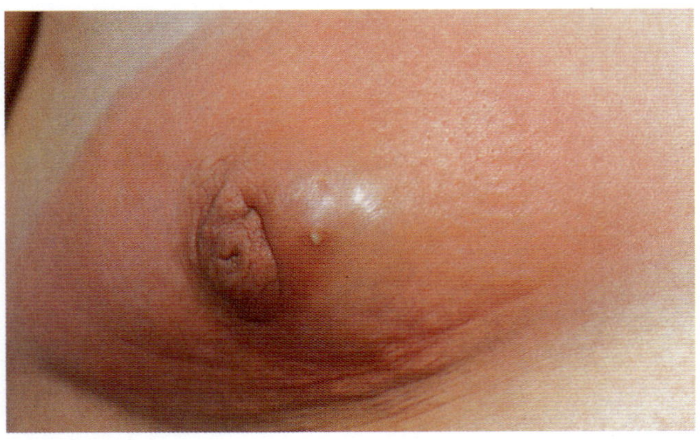

Breast abscess

A rare complication of generalised infection (e.g. mastitis) if untreated. A pocket of pus accumulates in one local area. Here, extensive nipple oedema and an abscess is 'pointing' at 3:00 on areolar margin. Must temporarily discontinue nursing on the affected breast; manually express milk and discard. Continue to nurse on the unaffected side. Treat with antibiotics, surgical incision and drainage.

TABLE 28.8 Abnormalities in the male breast

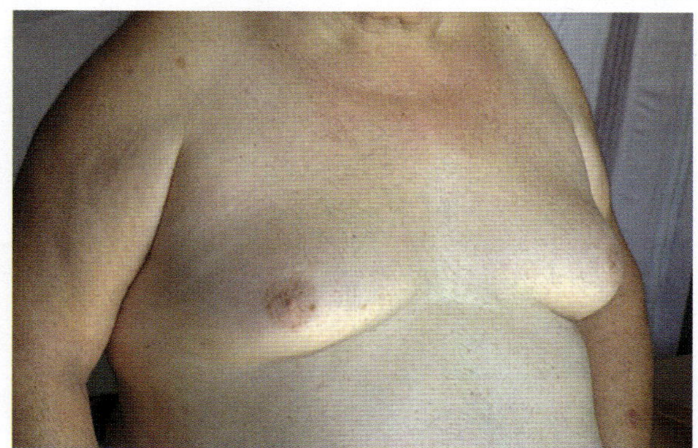

Gynaecomastia

Non-inflammatory enlargement of male breast tissue. This is physiological at puberty, unilateral, usually mild and transient. Gynaecomastia occurs commonly in males over 65 years because of changing hormone levels. It is bilateral and may be tender.

It also occurs bilaterally from hormone stimulation (e.g. on estrogen for cancer of the prostate); Cushing's syndrome; cirrhosis of liver as unable to metabolise estrogen completely; leukaemia occasionally; and sometimes with medication—digitalis, isoniazid, spironolactone and phenothiazines; testicular tumour, lung cancer; adrenal disease; and thyrotoxicosis.

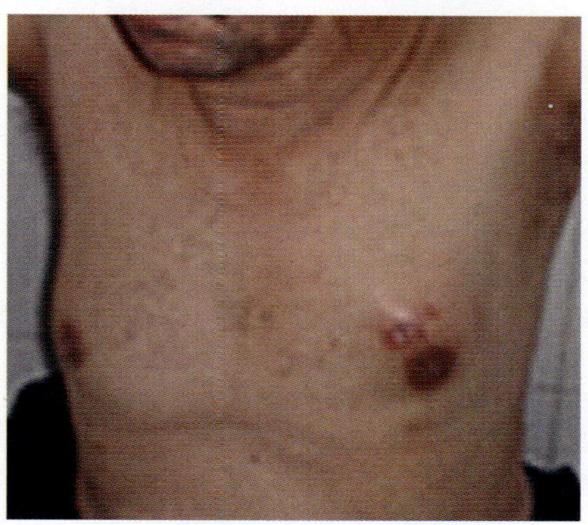

Carcinoma

Fewer than 1% of all breast cancer occurs in men. The lesion is a hard, irregular, nontender mass, most often directly under the areola, fixed to the area and may have nipple retraction. Mass is noticeable early because of minimal breast tissue. There is also early spread to axillary lymph nodes due to minimal breast tissue.

Clinical reasoning and documentation

The following is a continuation of the case study provided at the beginning of this chapter and the clinical reasoning process including problem/issue identification. Consult a fundamentals of nursing or medical-surgical nursing text for information about goal setting, nursing interventions and evaluation.

Case study (continued)—A breast lump

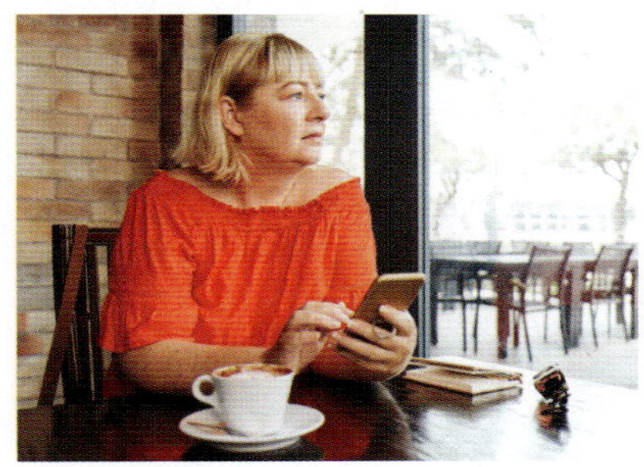

Context

You will recall from the case study described earlier in the chapter that you are a registered nurse working in an emergency department.

Consider the patient's situation

Ms Justine Klein, a 48-year-old woman, was admitted to the emergency department following a minor traffic accident having sustained a mild concussion. Neurological assessment is being conducted at half-hourly intervals and the discharge plan is to continue assessment for 4 hours. After medical reassessment she will be discharged home with GP review in 24 hours. During her admission, Ms Klein informed you that she had noticed a lump in her right breast 2 weeks ago.

Clinical reasoning and documentation cont'd

Collect cues/information

Your further assessment reveals the following information.

Subjective data

Ms Klein works fulltime as a secondary school teacher. She is married, with two children (aged 12 and 15 years).

She described the breast lump as a firm, non-movable area 'the size of a pea' in the upper outer quadrant of the breast, tender on touch only. She has not noticed any skin changes or nipple discharge. Ms Klein is not currently taking any medications.

Her last menstrual period was 20 days ago. Her cycle is on average every 28 days and regular.

There is no history of breast disease in self or family. She states that she has been feeling very anxious for the past 2 days and has not been able to sleep well or concentrate at work. '*I just know it's cancer.*' Ms Klein reports that her lack of sleep may have contributed to the road traffic accident. No complaints of headache.

Objective data

Voice trembling and visibly anxious during history. Sitting posture stiff and rigid. Her neurological assessment has been within normal limits. She is oriented to time, name and place. Pupils are equal and reacting briskly to light.

Vital signs: Temp 37°C, BP 148/78, HR 92/min, RR 16/min

Breasts symmetrical, nipples everted. No skin lesions, no dimpling, no retraction, no fixation. On palpation: Left breast firm, no mass, no tenderness, no discharge. Right breast firm, with 1 cm × 1 cm mass at 10 o'clock position, 5 cm from the nipple. The right breast lump is firm, oval, with smooth discrete borders, non-movable, tender to palpation. No other mass. No nipple discharge.

Process information and identify problems/issues

Collaborative problem

Breast mass requiring further assessment (referral to medical practitioner)

Problem statement/nursing diagnosis

Anxiety related to unknown diagnosis

ADDITIONAL RESOURCES

You can further develop your knowledge and skills relevant to breasts assessment of the breasts, related pathophysiology, common health issues and nursing interventions by:

- reading chapters of a fundamentals of nursing or medical-surgical nursing textbook
- answering chapter multiple choice questions online. Log onto ClinicalKey Student and search for the text 'Health Assessment, 4th edition'. Choose the section titled 'Teaching material'. In this section you will find question and answer documents for each chapter. Please check instructions on the inside front cover of the book to access online resources.
- visiting websites

  Cancer Australia—Looking after your breasts, find breast cancer early and survive—resources for Aboriginal and Torres Strait Islander women: https://www.canceraustralia.gov.au/key-initiatives/aboriginal-and-torres-strait-islander-health/looking-after-your-breasts%2C-find-breast-cancer-early-and-survive

ADDITIONAL RESOURCES cont'd

The Breast Cancer Foundation NZ—provide targeted information on breast awareness to the LGBTIQ+ community: https://www.breastcancerfoundation.org.nz/breast-cancer/types-of-breast-cancer/breast-cancer-in-the-lgbtiq-community

The Breast Cancer Foundation NZ—Māori and Pacific Islander women: https://www.breastcancerfoundation.org.nz/what-we-do/awareness-and-education/awareness-campaigns.

REFERENCES

1. Cho H, Han J-W. Obesity-related factors in older women with early menarche. Healthcare 2023; 11:557. Available at: https://doi.org/10.3390/healthcare 11040557
2. Idris MI, Wolday SJ, Habteselassie F, Ghebremichael L, Andemariam M, Azmera R, et al. Factors associated with early age at menarche among female secondary school students in Asmara: a cross-sectional study. Global Reproductive Health 2020; 6(2):e51. Available at: http://dx.doi.org/10.1097?GRH.000000000000051.
3. Worthman CM, Dockray S, Marceau K. Puberty and the evolution of developmental science. Journal of Research on Adolescence 2019;29(1):9–31.
4. Biro FM, Pajak A, Wolff MS, Pinney SM, Windham GC, Galvez MP, et al. Age of menarche in a longitudinal US cohort. Journal of Pediatric and Adolescent Gynecology 2018;31(4):339–345. Available at: https://doi.org/10.1016/j.pag.2018.05.002
5. Markevych I, Astell-Burt T, Altag H, Triebner K, Standl M, Flexeder C, et al. Residential green space and age at menarche in German and Australian adolescent girls: a longitudinal study. International Journal of Hygiene and Environmental Health 2022; 240:113917. Available at: https://doi.org/10.1016/j.ijheh.2021.113917
6. Donovan S, Telfar-Barnard L. Age of first menstruation in New Zealand: findings from first ever national-level data and implications for age-appropriate education and support. The New Zealand Medical Journal 2019:132(1500):100–102. Available at http://www.nzma.org.nz/journal.
7. Australian Government Cancer Australia. Breast cancer in Australia statistics. 2023. Available at: https://www.canceraustralia.gov.au/cancer-types/breast-cancer/statistics
8. Health New Zealand. Cancer web tool. New Zealand Government. 2023. Available at: https://www.tewhatuora.govt.nz/our-health-system/data-and-statistics/nz-health-statistics/health-statistics-and-data-sets/cancer-data-and-statistics/cancer-web-tool/
9. Australian Institute of Health and Welfare (AIHW) Cancer in Australia 2021. Cancer series no. 133. Cat.no. CAN 144. Canberra: AIHW; 2021. Available at: https://www.aihw.gov.au/reports/cancer/cancer-in-australia-2021/summary
10. Kim DH, Clepulis L, Keenan R, Lao C, Hodgson F, Bullen C, et al. Prevalence of invasive cancer in a large general practice population in New Zealand. Journal of Primary Health Care 2020;12 (3): 215–224. Available at: https://doi.org/10.1071/HC19113
11. Australian Institute of Health and Welfare (AIHW). BreastScreen Australia monitoring report 2021. Cat no. CAN 140. Canberra: AIHW; 2021. Available at: https://www.aihw.gov.au/reports/cancer-screening/breastscreen-australia-monitoring-report-2021/summary
12. Davies A, Gurney J, Garvey G, Diaz A, Segelov E. Cancer care disparities among Australian

and Aotearoa New Zealand indigenous peoples. Current Opinion in Supportive and Palliative Care 2021;15 (3):162–168. Available at: https://doi.org/10.1097/SPC0000000000000558
13. Lawrenson R, Lao C, Jacobson G, Seneviratne S, Scott N, Sarfati D, et al. Outcomes in different ethnic groups of New Zealand patients with screen-detected vs non-screen detected breast cancer. Journal of Medical Screening 2019; 26(4):197–203. Available at https://doi.org.10.1177/0969141319844801
14. Cancer Research UK 2023. Reducing your risk of breast cancer. Available at: http://www.cancerresearchuk.org
15. Clinical Oncology Society of Australia. COSA position statement on exercise in cancer care. Version 3. 2020. Clinical Oncology Society of Australia. Available at: https://www.cosa.org.au/advocacy/position-statements/exercise-in-cancer-care/
16. Lester J. Chapter 47: Early-stage breast cancer. In: Henke-Yarbro C, Frogge D, Holmes-Gobel B, editors. Cancer nursing: principles and practice. 8th edition. Burlington MA: Jones and Bartlett Learning LLC; 2018, pp. 1279–1334.
17. National Cancer Institute [NCI]. Breast cancer risk assessment tool. 2019. Available at: https://bcrisktool.cancer.gov/
18. Nickson C, Procopio P, Velentzis LS, Carr S, Devereux L, Mann GB, et al. Prospective validation of the NCI breast cancer risk assessment tool (Gail Model) on 40,000 Australian women. Breast Cancer Research 2018;20:155. Available at: http://doi.org.10.1186/s13058-018-1084-x
19. Cancer Institute NSW. NSW Government eviQ 2023. Breast cancer—referring to genetics. Available at: https://www.eviq.org.au/cancer-genetics/referral-guidelines/1620-breast-cancer-referring-to-genetics
20. Breast Cancer Foundation NZ. 2023. Breast awareness. Breast Cancer in NZ. Available at https://www.breastcancerfoundation.org.nz/breast-awareness
21. Cancer Australia. Breast cancer awareness. 2023. Available at: https://www.canceraustralia.gov.au/cancer-types/breast-cancer/awareness/breast-cancer-awareness
22. National Screening Unit (NSU). Breast Screening. BreastScreen Aotearoa. 2023. Available at: https://www.timetoscreen.nz/breast-screening/
23. Wendt C, Margolin S. Identifying breast cancer susceptibility genes: a review of the genetic background in familial breast cancer. Acta Oncologica 2019;58(2):135–146. Available at: http://doi.org.10.1080/0284186X.2018.1529428

CHAPTER 29

Assessing pregnant women

Written by Carolyn Jarvis
Adapted by Nicki Hartney

INTRODUCTION

Pregnancy and childbirth result in significant physiological changes in women. These changes include the growth of the fetus, placenta and uterus, as well as complex endocrine and circulatory changes. Most women experience good health during pregnancy. For many, their care can be managed by a midwife or a medical practitioner or by using a shared model combining the two. The elements of woman-centred care include choice, control and continuity of care; women are encouraged to be an active participant in their own care. Midwives are required to practise according to the Midwife Standards of Practice and engage in referral and collaboration with other healthcare providers when either maternal or fetal health issues are recognised.[1,2]

This chapter gives a brief overview of the changes to structure and function that occur during normal pregnancy and the approach to routine antenatal assessment. For a detailed description of labour and puerperium you are advised to consult a midwifery textbook. In the context of this chapter, 'woman' describes a pregnant person. Keep in mind that pregnant people may identify as gender diverse, non-binary or transgender. Fundamental to person-centred care is tailoring non-judgemental and respectful care to the person to ensure their experience of care aligns with their identify, values and beliefs.

Case study

The following case study gives an example of a typical situation involving pregnancy assessment and the clinical reasoning process including problem/issue identification. Consult a midwifery textbook for information about pregnancy care.

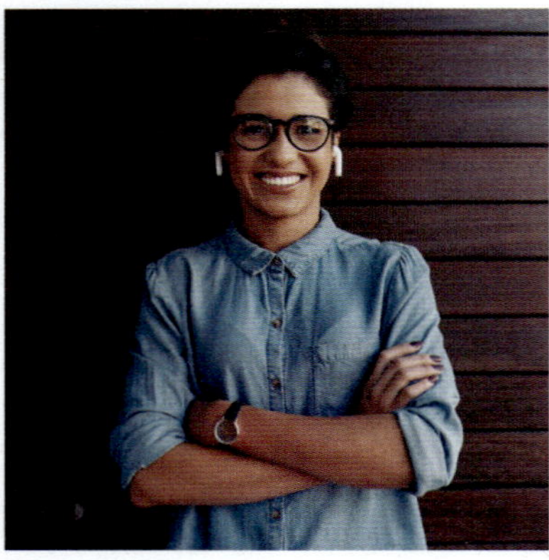

Context

You are a registered nurse working as a practice nurse in a general practice clinic.

Consider the patient's situation

Ms Imani Otieno, a 29-year-old woman, presents at the clinical reporting that she feels unwell and has missed her period.

Questions to further your learning

- What are the possible things that might be going on with Ms Otieno?
- What knowledge do you need to be able to predict what might be going on?
- What approach to Ms Otieno's health assessment will you take?
- What questions (subjective data) will you ask Ms Otieno to extend the health history and why?
- What physical examination (objective data) will you conduct and why?
- What resources are available to assist in your assessment of Ms Otieno?

Assessment plan

Pregnancy assessment is most commonly conducted by midwives, but registered nurses may also need to conduct a health assessment if the woman is seeking health care to confirm a pregnancy or for non–pregnancy related health issues. During pregnancy an extensive health history is obtained at the first antenatal visit. This provides a comprehensive database for establishing an appropriate model of care and for monitoring the progress of both the woman's health and that of her fetus throughout the pregnancy. This approach also provides the opportunity for considerable insight into the woman's needs and concerns that can be addressed through personalised health promotion and education.

The main areas for subjective assessment are:

- menstrual history
- gynaecological history
- obstetric history
- current pregnancy
- medical history
- family history
- general health history
- nutritional history
- environment/hazards.

Following subjective data collection, you will get a sense of the areas needed to be examined for objective data. Only the relevant areas should be examined. The main areas for physical examination are:

- general inspection
- measuring blood pressure
- inspecting and palpating the skin, mouth and breasts
- peripheral vascular assessment
- auscultating heart and lung sounds
- abdominal examination
- auscultating the fetal heart
- screening for maternal and fetal health.

Resources available

You will find additional resources and the reference list at the end of this chapter.

Structure and function

Fertilisation, embryology and placental development

The first day of the menses is day 1 of the menstrual cycle, which is generally referred to as being of 28 days' duration. There is, however, acknowledgement that there are cycle lengths ranging from 15 to 45 days, with length variations primarily occurring in the follicular phase of the menstrual cycle.[3] During the secretory phase of the menstrual cycle, the corpus luteum secretes a large amount of progesterone to act on the estrogen-prepared endometrium to convert it into a secretory tissue to prepare for implantation, which occurs 7 days after ovulation. Implantation is completed at 14 days after ovulation when the next menstrual cycle would be due.[3]

At the beginning of the menstrual cycle, 15 to 20 primary follicles are stimulated by the follicle-stimulating hormone but only 6 to 12 enlarge and eventually one follicle becomes dominant and begins to function independently of the follicle-stimulating hormone. Ovulation is triggered by the mid-cycle action of luteinising hormone, occurring in response to sustained high levels of estrogen released from the developing follicle. Progesterone production rises immediately after the luteinising hormone surge and this pre-ovulatory increase may be important in follicular rupture. Fertilisation occurs in the ampulla of the fallopian tube and viability of the sperm is thought to be about 5 days.[4]

Although one sperm penetrates the ovum, many more are required to support the passage of the spermatozoa through the corona radiata of the oocyte. The acrosome (head of the sperm) reaction with release of enzymes through the acrosomal membrane must occur for successful penetration of the corona radiata and zona pellucida by the sperm. After sperm entry, the sperm–ovum interaction binds the sperm to a glycoprotein. Once this has occurred enzyme release changes the zona pellucida making the oocyte impenetrable to any other sperm. After entering the cytoplasm of the oocyte, the sperm undergoes rapid morphological changes including sex determination, which is dependent on whether the sperm entering the oocyte has an X or a Y chromosome. The nuclei of the male and female pronuclei fuse and chromatin strands intermingle resulting in the diploid number (46) of chromosomes, causing the formation of the **zygote**.[3]

The zygote remains in the ampulla for the first 24 hours and is then propelled by ciliary action down the fallopian tube for the next few days while undergoing simultaneous rapid cell division. At the 12 to 16 cell stage (about 3 days after fertilisation), the zygote becomes a solid cluster of cells referred to as the **morula** and by days 3 to 4 reaches the uterine cavity. The series of rapid mitotic cell divisions of the zygote results in the formation of the **blastocyst**, which organises into two layers: the inner cell mass (to form the embryo) and the trophoblast (which will become the placenta).[3]

Approximately 5 to 6 days after fertilisation (7 to 9 days after ovulation), the blastocyst adheres to the endometrium (implantation).[3] During the secretory phase of the menstrual cycle, the endometrium and, under the control of ovarian steroids, biochemical, physiological and morphological changes have occurred to prepare for implantation. Once implantation has occurred, the blastocyst absorbs nourishment from the decidua and secretes human chorionic gonadotrophin (hCG) to stimulate growth and secretory activity of the corpus luteum to produce steroid hormones for its continued growth as well as that of the decidua. The levels of hCG steadily increase and can first be detected in maternal serum and urine approximately 7 days after ovulation or around the time of implantation. The major function of hCG is to maintain the corpus luteum during early pregnancy to ensure secretion of progesterone and other substances until placental production is adequate by approximately 10 to 12 weeks' gestation.[4]

Pre-embryonic development occurs from the time of fertilisation and zygote formation until 2 weeks' gestation. The embryonic period lasts from 2 weeks after fertilisation until the end of the eighth week, the period of organogenesis, which is a critical time for human development. As they develop, organ systems are susceptible to external influences which may lead to serious congenital abnormalities.

By the end of the eighth week, the embryo, identified as a 'fetus', has already developed a distinct human appearance.[4] During the fetal period, the fetus grows rapidly; tissues and organs differentiate and mature. Calculation of the estimated date of birth using Nägele's rule (presented later in this chapter) assists in this calculation.

The placenta and chorion (outer membrane) develop from the trophoblast layer of the blastocyst cells. Other extraembryonic tissues that develop from the inner cell mass include the amnion (inner membrane), the yolk sac, allantois (part of the yolk sac during the embryonic period) and extra-embryonic mesoderm from which the umbilical cord and blood vessels of the placenta are derived.[4] Placental function commences at the end of the third week and by about 10 to 12 weeks of the pregnancy its function is well established.[3]

The placenta has four major activities including metabolic (nutrient supply), immunological (fetal protection against maternal rejection), transport (i.e. gas exchange, nutrients, waste) and endocrine. Placental endocrine activities are important in maintaining a pregnancy including metabolic adaptations in the mother and fetus. Four major hormones synthesised by the placenta include hCG, human placental lactogen, steroid hormones (including estrogens and progesterone) and mediators such as proteins and growth factors. Maternal and fetal circulations are separated by layers of tissue referred to as the placental membrane or placental barrier.[3]

A woman who is pregnant for the first time is referred to as a **primigravida**, and after birth she is called a **primipara**. A **multigravida** is a woman who has previously carried a fetus to the point of viability. The woman is referred to as a **multipara** after birth.

Physiological changes during pregnancy

FIRST TRIMESTER (THE FIRST 12 WEEKS)

The first missed menstrual cycle is a probable sign of pregnancy and is highly suggestive when the second one is also missed. The woman may be led to believe that she has had a cycle but has instead experienced an implantation bleed occurring about the time of the expected menstrual cycle. Increased breast tenderness and tingling around the nipple often occur from about 4 to 6 weeks; nipples become more erect; and increased breast size and vascularity are usually evident by the end of the second month. In addition, there is enlargement of the sebaceous glands around the nipples (Montgomery's glands), due to hormonal changes. During the first trimester, the ductal system of the woman's breast proliferates under the influence of the hormone estrogen whereas the lobular formation is enhanced by progesterone. Milk secretion is inhibited by high levels of placental hormones including progesterone.[3]

Uterine hyperplasia begins after implantation and is driven by estrogen and growth factors. The three layers of the myometrium become more clearly defined as the uterine muscle undergoes hyperplasia and subsequent hypertrophy (increase in length and thickness of existing muscle fibres). Uterine quiescence is mediated by progesterone, relaxin, nitric oxide and prostacyclin.[4] By 12 weeks, the uterine fundus can be located at the brim of the maternal pelvis (Figure 29.1).

Maternal cardiovascular changes begin to occur, with stroke volume and cardiac output

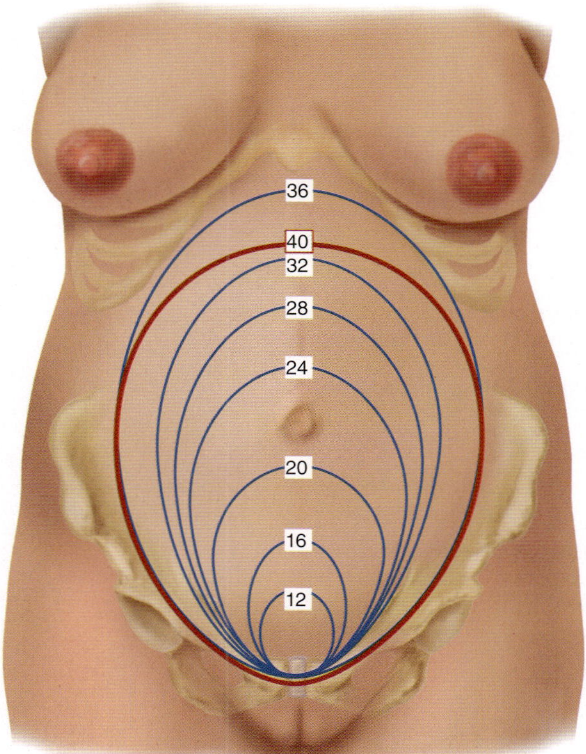

FIGURE 29.1 Height of fundus at weeks of gestation

increasing and systemic vascular resistance decreasing, thereby contributing to increased renal plasma flow and glomerular filtration.[3] Even though there is increased cardiac output and blood volume, a healthy woman's blood pressure, especially the diastolic pressure, can decrease slightly in the second trimester.[3]

There is a range of symptoms that can be experienced in the first trimester of pregnancy (Figure 29.2). A woman can experience nausea with or without vomiting occurring at any time during the day or night, starting about 6 weeks after the onset of the last normal menstrual period and continuing for 6 to 12 weeks or even longer for some. The exact cause and function of the nausea and vomiting is unknown, and the most common hormonal theories are related to rapidly increasing and high levels of estrogen, hCG and possibly thyroxine[4] and can be managed through frequent small low-fat content meals. This condition is usually self-limiting and not associated with adverse fetal outcomes. The woman requires ongoing supportive care to manage her symptoms including consideration of pharmacological treatment if symptoms are severe. A few women develop hyperemesis gravidarum, which occurs when there is nausea and excessive vomiting. If this condition is not managed it can result in dehydration and metabolic imbalance and can be life threatening for the woman.[3]

There can be an increase in frequency of urination (due to pressure of the growing uterus in the pelvis) and excessive fatigue that could be related not only to the hormonal

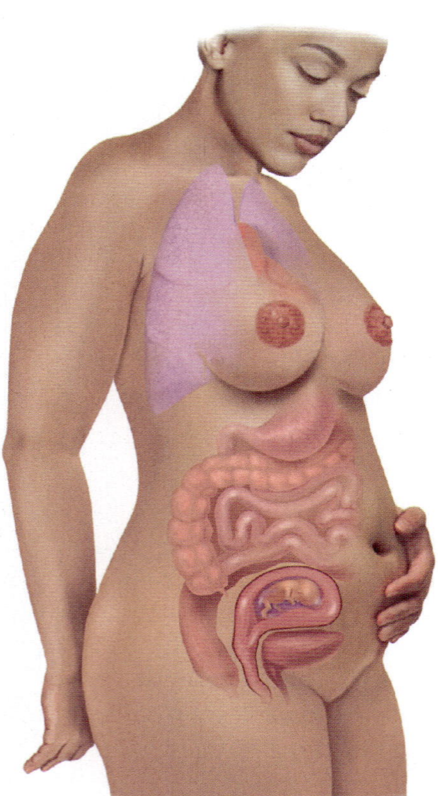

FIGURE 29.2 First trimester physiological changes

shifts due to pregnancy but also to the impact of nausea or nausea and vomiting. Minor disorders such as reflux oesophagitis (heartburn) and constipation occur because of maternal physiological adaptations to pregnancy and, in particular, in response to the effect of the hormone progesterone on smooth muscle and connective tissue.[4]

Positive signs of pregnancy include fetal heart sounds, fetal movements and palpation of fetal body parts confirmed through ultrasound.[5] By 8 to 10 weeks, a fetal heart rate using, for example, Doppler ultrasonography can be heard and movements identified in a real-time ultrasound even earlier.[3]

SECOND TRIMESTER (WEEKS 13 TO 27)

By weeks 12 to 16, the nausea, vomiting, fatigue and urinary frequency of the first trimester improve (due to changes in hormone levels). Protein and carbohydrate needs increase, thereby contributing to weight gain.

By the end of the second trimester, the woman can experience heartburn due to the smooth muscle relaxant influence of the hormone progesterone that also can cause constipation. There is a need to prevent or care for existing haemorrhoids. Increased estrogen and progesterone levels can result in increased blood flow causing soft, swollen gums, which lead to bleeding gums. Further, there is increased risk of urinary tract infection due to decreased bladder and ureter tone.[3] The maternal blood volume rises and the haemoglobin level begins to fall due to haemodilution; the blood pressure decreases slightly whereas the heart rate increases by 10 to 20 beats per minute and most women develop a systolic murmur during this trimester. Cardiac output usually peaks at 20 to 32 weeks.[5]

There is increased skin pigmentation including darkening over the forehead and cheeks—called **chloasma gravidarum**—and a darkened line from the maternal umbilicus to the symphysis pubis referred to as the **linea nigra**. Other cutaneous changes include, for example, the appearance of spider naevi and capillary haemangiomas and the breakdown of connective tissue over the abdomen, breasts or thighs referred to as stretch marks. The fresh tissue breakdown appears as reddish irregular marks[3] and older ones are faded and silver in appearance.

During the second trimester of pregnancy, there is further lobular growth with formation of new alveoli and ducts and dilation of the lumens of the breast. The breasts become more nodular, the nipples larger and more deeply pigmented and the areolae broadened. Prolactin stimulates production of colostrum, which is produced as early as 16 weeks.

The uterus moves into the abdominal cavity to displace the intestines, becoming more ovoid in shape. The woman will experience tension and stretching of the broad ligament that could be painful for her. Uterine contractions, referred to as Braxton Hicks, are irregular, usually painless and assist in the circulation of blood to the placenta.[4] The woman recognises fetal movement ('quickening') at approximately 16 to 20 weeks (the multigravida earlier). By 20 weeks of pregnancy the uterus is expected to be at the level of the maternal umbilicus.[3]

There is increasing vascularity of the vagina, pelvic viscera and perineal structures and increased vascularity and vasocongestion of the perineal body. There can be increases in vaginal discharge that is thick, white and acidotic to contribute to the inhibition of pathogenic colonisation of the vagina.[3]

THIRD TRIMESTER (WEEK 28 TO BIRTH)

During the third trimester of pregnancy, the woman is likely to experience fatigue and dyspnoea on exertion due to the increased weight and pressure exerted by the enlarged uterus. Urinary frequency is increased due to the pressure of the fetal presenting part on the bladder, which is pulled up and out of the true pelvis because of the enlarging uterus. This enlargement also displaces the intestines and stomach and a hiatal hernia may develop with associated heartburn and decreased stomach capacity. Haemorrhoids (varicosities of the rectum) are worsened by constipation and the relaxation impact of the hormone progesterone on the large bowel.

The woman's heart is slightly displaced to the left as a consequence of the enlarged uterus. The diastolic pressure reaches its lowest point by mid-pregnancy and then gradually returns to non-pregnant baseline values by term of pregnancy. This is thought to be related to a lag in compensation for changes in peripheral resistance. The maternal blood volume peaks at 32 to 34 weeks' gestation and oedema frequently occurs; blood return from the lower extremities is reduced.[3]

As pregnancy advances, the fetal placental unit grows and the level of placental hormones, antagonistic to insulin increase, leads to decreased sensitivity or resistance to insulin. This means that insulin is less effective at stimulating glucose uptake. The dominant effect in the second and third trimesters is related to the high levels of human placental lactogen (hPL), but human placental growth hormone, prolactin, cortisol and progesterone are also involved. Levels of hPL increase markedly after 20 weeks. hPL is a powerful insulin antagonist and consequently there are decreased peripheral tissue responses to insulin with increased levels of circulating glucose and amino acids also available to the fetus.[4]

The woman can experience backache and contributing factors might include postural changes resulting in lumbar lordosis with overstretched abdominal muscles, strained back muscles and broad ligament pain (Figure 29.3). The increased elasticity of connective and collagen tissue leads to relaxation and hypermobility of the pelvic joints; separation of the symphysis pubis results in instability of the sacroiliac joint and the centre of gravity shifts due to increased cervicodorsal curvature resulting in difficulty in walking.[3] The woman may experience numbness of the arms and hands due to fluid retention of pregnancy, compressing the median nerve; this is commonly referred to as 'carpal tunnel syndrome' and for most women will resolve spontaneously after the pregnancy.[3]

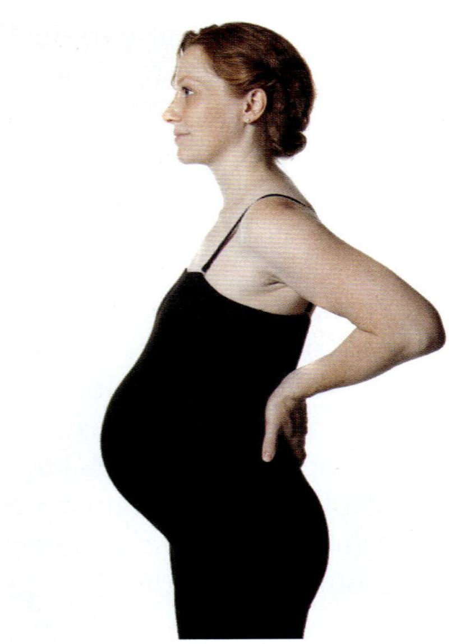

FIGURE 29.3 Postural changes

On abdominal examination the fetus can usually be easily palpated and movements observed; the growth of the fundus of the uterus continues to rise until 36 weeks when it reaches the level of the maternal xiphisternum. The uterus remains at this level until engagement of the fetal presenting part occurs. Approximately 2 weeks before going into labour, the primigravida woman experiences 'lightening' when the presenting part, normally the fetal head, moves down into the pelvis. Symptoms include a lower-appearing fundus, urinary frequency, increased vaginal secretions from increased pelvic congestion and increased lung capacity. In a multigravida woman, engagement of the presenting part may occur at any time in late pregnancy or not until labour. The haemodynamic effect of maternal position in late pregnancy can have an impact when the woman is in a supine position and the enlarged uterus may compress the vena cava to reduce venous return to the heart. In turn, this can lead to a decrease in the cardiac output, maternal blood pressure and uterine perfusion.[6]

The cervix, in preparation for labour, begins to thin (efface) and open (dilate). A thick **mucus plug (operculum)**, formed in the cervix as a mechanical barrier during pregnancy, is expelled at variable times before or during labour. Braxton Hicks contractions are irregular and painless but increase as pregnancy advances. When labour commences, uterine contractions are painful and increase in frequency, intensity and duration to achieve progressive effacement and dilatation of the cervix. Normal labour typically occurs between 37 and 42 weeks and pregnancy is considered to be post term after 42 weeks.[5]

Determining weeks of gestation

If fertilisation occurs, according to Nägele's rule,[5] the average length of a human gestation is 280 days (40 weeks), measured from the first day of the last normal menstrual period, equal to 10 lunar months or just over 9 calendar months (this rule is based on a 28-day cycle; if a longer cycle—for example, a 31-day cycle—10 days are added to the due date). Estimation of the date of birth or estimation of the due date can be achieved by counting forwards 9 months and adding

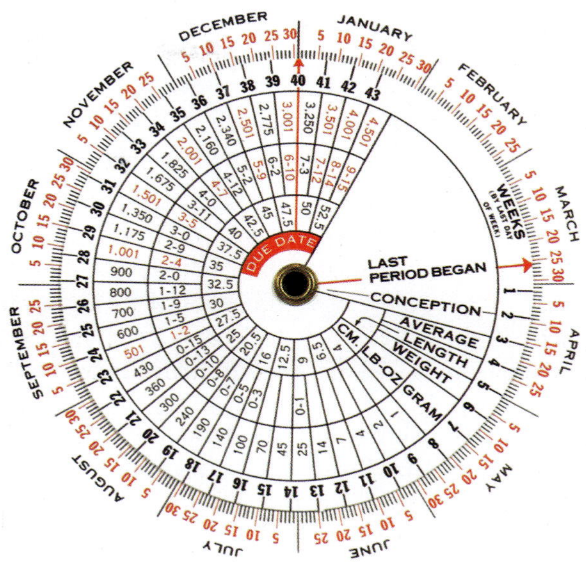

FIGURE 29.4 Pregnancy wheel

7 days from the first day of the last normal menstrual period.[5] A pregnancy wheel can be used to assist in determining the estimation of the due date and weeks of a gestation (Figure 29.4).

Weight gain in pregnancy

Weight gain during pregnancy reflects increased maternal stores as well as those of the developing fetus and placenta. Approximately 62% of the gain is water, 30% fat and 8% protein. About 25% of the total weight gain is related to the fetus, 11% to the placenta and amniotic fluid and the remainder to the mother. Optimal weight gain during pregnancy varies with maternal pre-pregnancy weight; greater weight gain is generally recommended for underweight women and a lower weight gain for those who are overweight. Body mass index (BMI) and energy expenditure must also be considered.[3] Woman with a BMI either below or above the healthy range is most likely to require extra care during pregnancy.

Underweight women can have a BMI lower than 18.5 and are at risk of a preterm birth and a low-birthweight infant, whereas women with a BMI greater than 25 have increased risk of gestational diabetes, fetal macrosomia, congenital heart defects, preterm birth and stillbirth. Woman with a normal pre-pregnancy BMI are expected to gain approximately 11.5 to 16 kg.[7]

Developmental considerations

In industrialised countries, risks for pregnant adolescents are largely psychosocial. Young women are at risk for the downward cycle of poverty beginning with an incomplete education, failure to limit family size and continuing with failure to establish a vocation and become independent. She may be unprepared emotionally to be a mother. Her social situation may be stressful. She may not have the support of her family, her partner or their family. Medical risks for a pregnant adolescent are generally related to poverty, inadequate nutrition, substance abuse and sometimes sexually transmitted infections (STIs), poor health before pregnancy and emotional and physical abuse from her partner. The proportion of women who gave birth and were teenagers in 2018 varied by place of residence, ranging from a low of 1.1% in the Australian Capital Territory to 6.0% in the Northern Territory. The proportion of Australian teenage mothers (younger than 20) has steadily declined since 2002 (4.9%) to a rate of 2.0% in 2018.[8] In Aotearoa New Zealand, the teenage fertility rate is approximately 3.9% for women aged under 20 years. This is a significant decrease from previous statistics.[9]

While evidence suggests that adolescents are at risk for pregnancy-induced hypertension, preterm birth and perinatal mortality,[5] it is unclear whether these risks are associated with physiological change or social factors. For social reasons, the adolescent often seeks health care later, and early antenatal care has been shown to provide optimal management. In 2018, 11.9% of Aboriginal and Torres Strait Islander mothers were teenagers, compared with 1.5% of non-Indigenous mothers.[8] Proportionately more Aboriginal and Torres Strait Islander mothers have their babies at a younger age than non-Indigenous mothers.[8] Similarly, in Aotearoa New Zealand, Māori and Pacific Islander birth rates are higher in lower socioeconomic communities.[10]

Since the advent of assisted conception, more women older than 40 years of age are now becoming pregnant. In Australia, the proportion of mothers aged 40 or older made up 4.4% of women giving birth in 2018 compared with 3.4% in 2006.[8]

Women of 'later maternal age' (over 35 years) are often more prepared emotionally and financially to parent, but they are more at risk for infertility and age-related anomalies. With reproductive ageing the primary changes occur in the ovary and follicles and particularly the oocytes. Oocytes of the woman over 35 years have been found to have abnormal chromosomes due to meiotic nondisjunction.[3] Once conception has occurred, the woman is at increased risk of having a child with congenital abnormalities, particularly trisomy 21, commonly known as Down syndrome. Further issues include a decline in fertility, due in part to: a decrease in the number and health of eggs to be ovulated; a decrease in ovulation; and other gynaecological conditions such as endometriosis and early onset of menopause.

Women of later maternal age are also at risk of spontaneous abortions, in part because of the increase in genetically abnormal embryos.[11] Since the incidence of chronic medical conditions such as diabetes type 2 and hypertension increase with age, a pregnant woman over the age of 35 years is considered to be at risk of complications related to these diseases.[6] The increased incidence of hypertension places the woman at risk of placental abruption and pre-eclampsia that, in turn, increases the risk of intrauterine growth restriction. There are still wide variances in maternal deaths between developed and developing countries. In Australia women aged under 20 and over 40, with higher parity, of Aboriginal and Torres Strait Islander origin or with remote or very remote usual residence were among those at increased risk of maternal death.[12] Maternal deaths worldwide are due to severe bleeding (mostly postpartum), infection (soon after birth), hypertensive disorders of pregnancy and obstructed labour.[13]

In Australia, the current recommendation is for all women to be offered first trimester screening for fetal genetic abnormality.[7] This screening involves an ultrasound between 11 and 13 weeks' gestation measuring the fetal nuchal translucency thickness, combined with a maternal blood test that analyses pregnancy-associated placental protein-A (PAPP-A) and beta-human chorionic gonadotrophin (B-hCG). In addition to this, a noninvasive prenatal test (NIPT) is also available from 10 weeks' gestation. This test analyses maternal blood for cell-free deoxyribonucleic acid, with a greater than expected number of relevant chromosome fragments present in genetic fetal abnormality such as trisomy 21 (Down syndrome). The NIPT test may be offered as a first-line test, combined with first trimester screening or in addition to first trimester screening where intermediate risk has been identified.[7] Women who present later in pregnancy (14–20 weeks) are offered second trimester maternal serum screening for fetal chromosomal anomaly. All of these tests are gestation specific, so a known accurate gestation is required and can be determined by early ultrasound, prior to 13 weeks' gestation.

Women who return a high-risk result are offered genetic counselling and diagnostic testing such as **chorionic villus sampling** where a small sample of **chorionic villi** is removed, either abdominally or transvaginally, between 11 and 14 weeks or amniocentesis, in which a small amount of amniotic fluid is removed, is performed after 15 weeks under ultrasound guidance.[7]

Cultural and social considerations

In Australia, women are encouraged to make their own decisions about their pregnancy and birth experience supported by a woman-centred approach to maternity care. Key issues include having a safe birth, feeling in control within the birth environment, developing supportive relationships with their carer or carers and being treated with dignity and respect. The concept of woman-centred care is intended to place the focus on the woman's individual unique needs, expectations and aspirations, rather than the needs of institutions or maternity service professionals. The application of this care is to recognise the woman's right to self-determination in terms of choice, control and continuity of care.[7]

In Australia, 44% of pregnancy care models have a midwife as the lead maternity carer. Models of care range from caseload, where a known midwife provides care across the continuum, to a known midwife for some aspects of care—for example, pregnancy care only, through to fragmented care where the woman is cared for by a variety of midwives across her pregnancy, birth and postnatal period.[14] In Aotearoa New Zealand, midwives work in partnership with women, providing continuity of midwifery care throughout the woman's experience. Primary maternity care is provided by lead maternity carers, selected by women to provide their care. Lead maternity carers can be either midwives, GPs with a diploma in obstetrics or obstetricians. Lead maternity carers take responsibility for the care provided to women throughout pregnancy and up to 6 weeks following, including managing labour and birth.[15] In both countries midwives work collaboratively with other health professionals when necessary to meet any additional medical, health or social needs of mothers and their babies.

In promoting woman-centred care there is an increase in the range of maternity care models available to Australian women of diverse cultural and social backgrounds to support improved birth outcomes. Considering cultural traditions could include, for example, the traditions of Aboriginal and Torres Strait Islander women, in which the risk of not birthing on Country and potentially away from family can result in distress and increase in clinical and medical risk.[7] In Aotearoa New Zealand, midwifery practice is guided by 'Tūranga Kaupapa', which are statements that express the cultural values related to childbirth of Māori. These statements describe the wāhine Māori and their whānau values and philosophies and provide guidance for healthcare providers.[16]

Women living in rural and remote regions of Australia frequently need to travel to access maternity care due to the centralisation of health services. This issue can be exacerbated by the need for ongoing care throughout the pregnancy, particularly for higher risk pregnancies, and the requirement for hospitalisation before and after the birth. Even in a low-risk pregnancy where a woman has local access to a healthcare provider, she may still have to travel a considerable distance in anticipation of the birth or for some aspects of her antenatal and/or postnatal care. Women of childbearing age living in rural and remote regions of Australia need access to an appropriately skilled workforce and associated infrastructure, not all of which can be provided in every community. While outreach and telehealth services have provided some improvement in care access, there is still a requirement for a woman who experiences health issues during pregnancy to separate from her family and community, with likely psychosocial and financial hardship.[17]

Pregnancy is a life event with profound psychological and social meaning for the woman and for her family and community. Pregnancy is a unique period in a woman's life that is surrounded by customs, traditions, beliefs and spiritual practices. Adopting a partnership approach to care, respecting beliefs, sharing knowledge and supporting informed decision-making positions midwives to tailor care to a woman's individual needs. Creating a safe and trusting relationship is fundamental to building rapport and provides an environment in which the woman feels in control, respected and heard.[16]

Some complications of pregnancy occur more frequently in certain groups. Women who live in developing countries may not have the advantages of a skilled attendant for pregnancy and birth, let alone technology. Every day 800 women die from preventable pregnancy or childbirth causes, with 95% of these deaths occurring in low and lower middle-income communities. Common causes of these maternal deaths include haemorrhage, infection, hypertension, complications during delivery and unsafe abortion.[13]

Australian demographic data for 2018 show that 291,712 women gave birth to 295,976 babies. This was a 4% decrease in mothers compared with 2015. The mean age of Aboriginal and Torres Strait Islander women who gave birth in 2018 was 26.2 years, compared with 30.9 years for non-Indigenous mothers. In contrast, 7.9% of Aboriginal and Torres Strait Islander mothers were aged 35 or older, compared with 20.4% of non-Indigenous mothers.[8]

From 2011 to 2020 in Australia, there were 194 maternal deaths that occurred during pregnancy or within 42 days of the end of pregnancy. The maternal mortality ratio was relatively stable between 2011 and 2020, with the maternal mortality ratio ranging between 5.0 and 8.4 per 100,000 women who gave birth. These data should be interpreted with caution due to the rarity of maternal deaths in Australia and associated volatility of small numbers. Aboriginal and Torres Strait Islander women were three times more likely to die than non-Indigenous women, with a maternal mortality ratio of 16.4 deaths per 100,000 Indigenous women giving birth (2012–2020).

In Aotearoa New Zealand in 2016, 16.8 maternal deaths per 100,000 maternities were reported. The 3-year maternal mortality ratio for 2016 to 2018 was 11.6 per 100,000 maternities, occurring during either pregnancy or within 42 days of birth, with 16 being the highest number recorded, for 2018.[18]

Transgender and pregnancy

A transgender man is a person who identifies as male but whose sex may have been designated female at birth.[19] Not all people use the term transgender, preferring nonbinary terms such as genderqueer.[20] Transgender men have often been born with reproductive anatomy that aligns with the capacity to become pregnant.

Transgender people have unique and complex reproductive needs. Gender-affirming medical care may include hormone therapy, surgery or a combination of interventions. Gender-affirming medical care may affect future reproductive ability in the transgender population, but fertility-preserving options are available.[21] All transgender people should receive counselling on how hormone therapy and surgery may affect fertility to enable them to make an informed decision regarding preserving fertility. It is important to note that not all gender-affirming medical care makes future pregnancy impossible. Some transgender people can successfully conceive and carry a child. Transgender men who stop gender-affirming hormone therapy can become pregnant, and there are reports of successful chestfeeding (feeding from the breast) postpartum.

The experience of marginalisation of transgender people in the healthcare system has affected their health and wellbeing. There are significant gaps in the education of healthcare providers on the unique needs of transgender people, and this is even more apparent during pregnancy care. Transgender men's experiences of pregnancy have reported alienation, isolation and loneliness, with consequent significant risk to mental health.[19] Gender dysmorphia can be triggered by both the physical changes of pregnancy and the reactions of others to the changing body.[20] Equitable access to inclusive care, high-quality prenatal counselling and specialist health services are of utmost importance to support transgender men through pregnancy. Healthcare providers should create a welcoming environment for all people and seek education to better meet the needs of transgender people.

HEALTH EDUCATION

Leading a healthy lifestyle

Pregnancy is a time when women are generally receptive to positive health messages, due to their health and lifestyle affecting not only them but also their unborn child's short- and long-term health. Healthcare providers are well placed to influence the health of the woman and her family positively. Health promotion topics may include nutrition, exercise/physical activity and stopping or minimising alcohol consumption and smoking.

Nutrition

Nutrition is an essential part of every person's health. In pregnancy, the importance of a woman's diet for her and her developing baby is well recognised. Beginning pregnancy either underweight or obese and/or gaining excess weight during pregnancy can cause significant health risks for both the mother and her fetus/baby. Advice regarding a healthy diet during pregnancy can be based on national dietary guidelines (refer to Chapter 21), with specific advice regarding increased intake to be tailored to the woman depending on her weight, height and activity levels.[22] Advice about food avoidances include foods that may contain listeria bacteria such as soft cheeses, pre-prepared salads and raw, undercooked or pre-cooked meats. Raw eggs should not be consumed due to the risk of salmonella. Fish with high levels of mercury such as shark, marlin or swordfish should be avoided or consumed infrequently.[22]

Nutritional supplementation

There is robust evidence to support supplementing dietary folic acid as a risk reduction strategy for neural tube defects such as a 400-microgram oral supplement taken ideally from 1 month preconception through to 3 completed months of pregnancy. Although many women will take a multivitamin supplement, there is no supporting evidence of any benefit in the absence of identified deficiencies and it has the potential to cause harm (e.g. excess intake of vitamin A).[7]

Physical activity

Physical activity during pregnancy provides health benefits for the woman and her baby and has been shown to reduce several pregnancy-related complications. Pregnancy exercise guidelines recommend that pregnant women without contraindication should accumulate between 150 to 300 minutes of exercise across most days of the week. This exercise should be of moderate intensity and include aerobic, muscle-strengthening elements and pelvic floor exercises. Each woman should be evaluated individually by their healthcare provider in terms of suitability of their current or planned exercise regimen in the context of their pregnancy.[23]

Health professionals should support pregnant women to evaluate their physical activity and facilitate informed decision making about how they can modify their activity level during pregnancy. Some modification to exercise may be needed—for example, lifting heavy weights in a gym or running. Due to the physical changes over the duration of a pregnancy, women should be advised to consult with a health professional about modifying their exercise. Ideally positive changes made to physical activity levels will be maintained after the pregnancy is completed.[23]

Alcohol

National guidelines for both Australia and Aotearoa New Zealand advise that there is no safe level of alcohol consumption in pregnancy.[24,25] The risks to the unborn baby are well documented and include prematurity, low birthweight and a spectrum of developmental, behavioural and physical manifestations known as fetal alcohol syndrome, with lifelong effects for the child. Risk of fetal harm is highest with frequent large amounts of alcohol consumption. While there is some community awareness of the harmful effects of alcohol consumption, 30% of women continue to consume alcohol in pregnancy.[25] Women who are planning to become pregnant should be informed of the potential risk of alcohol consumption. Women who are concerned about early-pregnancy alcohol consumption should seek specialist medical advice. If a woman is unable to reduce alcohol consumption, they should be referred to drug and alcohol specialist care.

HEALTH EDUCATION cont'd

Tobacco smoking

Health promotional campaigns targeting smoking cessation have had a positive effect on smoking behaviours of women during pregnancy over time. However, smoking during pregnancy remains higher in Indigenous women, young women and those from disadvantaged areas.[8,9] Smoking cessation during pregnancy is the most common preventable risk factor for pregnancy complications. The risks of continuation of tobacco smoking in pregnancy are well documented and include birth defects, premature birth, low birthweight, stillbirth and sudden infant death. In addition, passive smoking also poses a risk during pregnancy, so when discussing smoking status, the health professional should include questions about partner and household members' smoking habits. Interventions to support smoking cessation in pregnancy are evidenced to be effective because women often have heightened motivation during this time.[26] Routine antenatal care visits provide further opportunity for consistent information and support. Even if the woman cannot stop smoking completely, reducing the number of cigarettes smoked can potentially lessen effects on the fetus.[26]

Nurse's role

- assess the woman's health literacy and readiness to adopt a healthy lifestyle—for example, not smoking, eating a healthy diet, not drinking alcohol, exercising daily
- help the person identify real or perceived barriers that may prevent adopting a healthy lifestyle
- arrange a referral for women who need help to stop smoking (Chapter 19)
- provide health information about smoking/vaping cessation as required
- refer to a GP/obstetrician/midwife for antenatal care.

More information

The following online resources have more information about healthy behaviours during pregnancy:

- Smoking cessation and pregnancy: http://www.tobaccoinaustralia.org.au/chapter-7-cessation/7-11-smoking-cessation-and-pregnancy
- Eat for health—Australian Dietary Guidelines: https://www.eatforhealth.gov.au/
- Evidence-based physical activity guidelines for pregnant women: https://www.health.gov.au/sites/default/files/documents/2021/05/evidence-based-physical-activity-guidelines-for-pregnant-women.pdf

Subjective data

The initial consultation may cause some anxiety because this may be the first time the woman has been pregnant. Conversely, the woman may not be certain she is pregnant, and her anxiety may be related to this uncertainty or to what to expect if she is pregnant. It is imperative that this consultation with the woman is conducted in a private room to provide an explanation of the initial history-taking process and the investigations available to her. It is essential that the woman is given information so she can make informed decisions related to her care.

Practice note

Before you start the assessment, introduce yourself to the person, confirm the person's identity, discuss the purpose and scope of the assessment, clarify any questions the person may have and get verbal consent from the person to perform the assessment.

ASSESSMENT GUIDELINES AND NORMAL FINDINGS	CLINICAL SIGNIFICANCE AND CLINICAL ALERTS
Menstrual history	
• *How old were you when you had your first period?* • *How often do you menstruate and how long for?* • *Do you experience regularity or irregularity of your menstrual cycle?* • *Do you experience a heavy loss or intermenstrual bleeding?* • *Do you experience chronic pelvic pain?* • *When was the first day of your last normal menstrual cycle?*	Issues related to the woman's menstrual cycle such as chronic pelvic pain may be due to hormonal conditions such as **endometriosis** or **adenomyosis**, conditions that are associated with potential pregnancy complications.[6] Using **Nägele's rule**, calculate the estimated date of birth from the first day of the last normal menstrual cycle by counting forwards 9 months and 7 days for a 28-day regular menstrual cycle.
Gynaecological history	
• *Have you ever had surgery of the genital tract, cervix or uterus?*	Cervical surgery may affect the integrity of the cervix during pregnancy, increasing risk of preterm birth. During labour it may impede cervical dilation. Uterine surgery increases the risk for uterine rupture during pregnancy and labour. There are four main types of female genital mutilation: • *type I:* partial or total removal of the clitoris and/or the prepuce (clitoridectomy) • *type II:* partial or total removal of the clitoris and the labia minora, with or without excision of the labia majora (excision) • *type III:* Narrowing of the vaginal orifice with creation of a covering seal by the cutting of and apposition of the labia minora and/or the labia majora, with or without excision of the clitoris (infibulation) • *type IV:* All other harmful procedures to the female genitalia for non-medical purposes such as pricking, piercing, incising, scraping and cauterisation. Women with genital mutilation are more likely to experience complications related to labour and birth such as caesarean section, postpartum haemorrhage, episiotomy, extended maternal hospital stay, resuscitation of the infant and inpatient perinatal death.[27]

ASSESSMENT GUIDELINES AND NORMAL FINDINGS	CLINICAL SIGNIFICANCE AND CLINICAL ALERTS
	Women with genital mutilation require discussion with appropriate healthcare providers about ongoing health after childbirth. Sometimes the woman goes through repeated opening and closing procedures, further increasing both immediate and long-term risks.[27]
• *When was your last cervical screening test?* • *Have you ever had an abnormal cervical screening test or a colposcopy?*	A **cervical screening test** is done every 5 years (if normal), and if the woman has not had one previously, suggest that it should be done. An abnormal cervical screening test in the past may have a negative effect on the pregnancy or birth depending on whether there was surgery of the cervix involved.
• *Do you have any history of fibroids or uterine abnormalities?*	**Fibroids** (non-cancerous growths found in the muscle wall) can increase risk for placental abruption, preterm labour and birth, and postpartum haemorrhage. Uterine abnormalities can include **double uterus, unicornuate or bicornuate uterus**, and **septate or subseptate uterus**. These can result in spontaneous abortion.
• *Have you ever had a sexually transmitted infection (STIs such as genital herpes, syphilis, chlamydia, gonorrhoea, pelvic inflammatory disease, trichomoniasis or genital warts)?* See Chapter 26 for more information about screening for STIs in women.	If untreated, STIs increase the risk of morbidity and mortality of the newborn. **Genital herpes** Newborn infants have an impaired immune response to herpes simplex virus types 1 and 2 and are at increased risk of morbidity (e.g. encephalitis, septicaemia) and mortality if the mother is infectious and experiences a vaginal birth. Management can include use of antiviral agents. **Maternal syphilis** left untreated can cause miscarriage, stillbirth or congenital syphilis infection. **Congenital syphilis** is a serious condition and can result in severe hepatic abnormality leading to stillbirth. Neonates with congenital syphilis may present with a variety of systemic disorders including skin lesions, jaundice, pneumonia, myocarditis and nephrosis.

ASSESSMENT GUIDELINES AND NORMAL FINDINGS	CLINICAL SIGNIFICANCE AND CLINICAL ALERTS
	Chlamydia is caused by the bacterium *Chlamydia trachomatis*. Genital chlamydial infection remains asymptomatic in most women, with a recent change of sexual partner placing the woman at risk. Complications that may arise for women include **pelvic inflammatory disease**, **infertility** and **ectopic pregnancy**.[7] **Gonorrhoea**—the causative organism is *Neisseria gonorrhoeae*—is transmitted through intimate contact; it may initially cause symptoms of mild vaginitis. If untreated it can lead to severe complications of pelvic inflammatory disease. Untreated in pregnancy, gonorrhoea can lead to ectopic pregnancy, septic miscarriage, chorioamnionitis and preterm labour. Transmission during birth to the neonate presents as severe eye infections. **Trichomoniasis** is a common STI. The woman can experience vulval itching, dysuria and vaginal discharge that is malodorous, though many are asymptomatic. **Genital warts**, caused by the human papillomavirus (HPV), have been a common STI. A vaccine is now administered to adolescent girls to prevent HPV infection. ***Clinical alert:*** Women with any of the above infections require referral to a medical practitioner for further treatment.[7]
• *Have you been tested for HIV? When? What was the result?* • *Have you ever had a blood transfusion?* • *Have you ever used intravenous drugs?* • *Have you ever had a sexual partner who had any HIV risk factors?*	Address HIV status to promote the health of the woman. Following a complete evaluation, a plan of HIV-related care should be provided, taking into account pregnancy-specific maternal or fetal safety issues. Early HIV diagnosis can reduce the risk of mother-to-child transmission and the rate of disease progression in the mother. Give the woman information about healthcare options so she can make an informed choice.
• *Are you in a sexual relationship with more than one person?* • *What is your sexual preference?*	The number of sexual partners and frequency of partner change increase the risk for STIs. People in a same-sex relationship may have used assisted reproduction or surrogacy.

ASSESSMENT GUIDELINES AND NORMAL FINDINGS	CLINICAL SIGNIFICANCE AND CLINICAL ALERTS
• *Have you had a mammogram, breast biopsy, breast implants, breast augmentation or breast reconstruction (reduction mammoplasty)?*	Previous breast surgery may have a significant effect on breastfeeding success. Surgery that involves the complete incision of the areola is the strongest predictor of inadequate milk supply; silicone implants have not resulted in significant adverse events.[11]
Obstetric history	
• *Do you have a history of infertility?* • *Have you used assisted reproductive technology (ART)—for example, sperm or egg donor and/or IVF?*	There is an increased rate of adverse pregnancy outcomes following ART, with both singleton and multiple gestations.[3]
• *Have you had a previous pregnancy?* • *How did you experience previous pregnancies?* • *What were your birthing outcomes?* • *What were the years of each birth?* • *Have you experienced any spontaneous miscarriages, elective abortions or ectopic pregnancies?* • *What were the postnatal outcomes?*	It is important to obtain from the woman her history of pregnancy because previous experiences can affect her emotions about the current pregnancy. The woman may require referral to other health professionals for care of her current pregnancy.
• *What were the birthweights of your babies?* • *What sex were they?* • *Were your babies born alive?* • *Were they born at term of pregnancy?*	A small infant may indicate prematurity or **intrauterine growth restriction**—complications that may be repeatable. A large infant may indicate **gestational diabetes mellitus**. Conversely, birthweights of other children may indicate a 'constitutional size'—for example, the tendency of a couple to conceive smaller but normal children.
• *Have you ever had a caesarean section?* If so: • *What was the indication?* • *What type of uterine incision was made?* • *Have you ever had a vaginal birth after a caesarean section (VBAC)?*	Although rare, women who have a vertical or 'classical' incision of uterus due to a previous caesarean section carry a higher risk of uterine rupture. This means that all subsequent births will be by caesarean section. The 'low transverse' or horizontal incision carries a low risk, and the woman can plan to have a VBAC. Note that the direction of the skin scar does not necessarily tell how the uterus was incised.

ASSESSMENT GUIDELINES AND NORMAL FINDINGS	CLINICAL SIGNIFICANCE AND CLINICAL ALERTS
• *Have you breastfed previously?* If so: • *How was that experience for you?* • *How long did you breastfeed for?* • *If you did not breastfeed previously, was this your choice or was it unsuccessful?* • *If unsuccessful in breastfeeding, what do you think were the factors?*	A woman's experience and knowledge of breastfeeding can influence the level of teaching and support required.
• *Do you have any history of breastfeeding problems such as mastitis?*	A problematic or painful previous breastfeeding experience increases the need for support after this pregnancy.
Current pregnancy	
The number of weeks of amenorrhoea (absence of menstrual bleeding) for the current pregnancy are elicited when taking the woman's health history at the first antenatal visit.	
• *What method of contraception did you use most recently, and when did you discontinue it?*	Recent use of oral contraception or other hormonal contraceptives may have delayed ovulation and irregular menses—consider when establishing the **estimated date of birth**. An intrauterine contraceptive device still in place after conception requires removal to reduce the risk of a mid-trimester abortion.
• *Was this pregnancy planned? How do you feel about it?*	Even a planned pregnancy represents loss for the woman—perhaps a loss of freedom, compromise of goals, loss of time with other children or her partner. This sense of loss can also be influenced by the impact of physiological and physical changes on how she feels about her pregnancy.
• *Do you have a partner?* • *How does your partner feel about the pregnancy?* • *How do other family members feel about the pregnancy?*	The woman may need assistance with her partner and support people so they can be more supportive of her. Support strategies include inviting the woman's partner or significant others to attend antenatal visits with her.
• *Have you experienced any recent vaginal bleeding?* • *When? How much? What colour was the loss (e.g. bright blood loss or dark in colour)?* • *Was it accompanied by any pain?*	***Clinical alert:*** Vaginal bleeding may indicate a threatened abortion in early pregnancy; later it could be related to a low-lying placenta. The woman requires referral for further investigation and care.

ASSESSMENT GUIDELINES AND NORMAL FINDINGS	CLINICAL SIGNIFICANCE AND CLINICAL ALERTS
• *Are you experiencing any nausea and/or vomiting?* Nausea and vomiting are symptoms of pregnancy that generally begin between 4 and 6 weeks, peak around weeks 8 to 12 and then usually resolve. Health education and promotion includes advice on small, frequent, low-fat meals to assist the woman in self-care.	 ***Clinical alert:*** **Hyperemesis gravidarum** is a serious and potentially life-threatening form of nausea and vomiting, occurring early in pregnancy, gradually resolving during the middle of the second trimester. Medical assistance is required for unremitting nausea and vomiting.
• *Have you experienced any abdominal pain?* • *When? Where in your abdomen?* • *Was the pain accompanied by vaginal bleeding?*	The most common causes of abdominal pain in early pregnancy are **spontaneous abortion**, **ectopic pregnancy**, UTI and round ligament discomfort. Causes of pain later in pregnancy include **preterm labour**, **placental abruption** and haemolysis, elevated liver enzymes and **low platelet syndrome (HELLP)** (Table 29.1). Also consider other medical and surgical causes for abdominal pain.
• *Have you had any recent unexplained itching, rash or skin infections?*	Itching is the most common dermatological symptom of pregnancy. Mild pruritus is common and frequently occurs over the abdomen. The woman requires support and information related to caring for her skin during pregnancy. If there are pre-existing skin disorders the woman is encouraged to consult a dermatologist.
• *Have you had any x-rays recently?* • *Are you taking any medication—prescribed, unprescribed or recreational drugs?*	Discuss the potential effect of any teratogenic exposure. Refer for expert counselling if necessary.
• *Have you experienced any visual changes such as the new onset of blurred vision or spots before your eyes?*	In the third trimester, this may be a sign of **pre-eclampsia**. Evaluate for other signs and symptoms of pre-eclampsia (Table 29.1).
• *Have you experienced any oedema? Where and under what circumstances?*	In the third trimester, differentiate the normal weight-dependent oedema of pregnancy from that of generalised oedema associated with pre-eclampsia.
• *Have you had any frequency or burning with urination? Any blood in your urine?* • *Do you pass small amounts of urine?* • *Do you have any history of UTIs, pyelonephritis or kidney stones?*	Differentiate the normal urinary frequency of the first and third trimesters from UTI, for which pregnant women are at increased risk. Confirm by urinalysis. UTIs increase the rate of preterm labour.
• *Do you have any vaginal burning or itching? Any foul-smelling or coloured discharge?*	If symptoms occur, refer to a midwife or medical practitioner.

ASSESSMENT GUIDELINES AND NORMAL FINDINGS	CLINICAL SIGNIFICANCE AND CLINICAL ALERTS
• *Are you feeling your baby move?*	Educate the woman to be aware of the normal pattern of her fetal movements each day. Changes in fetal activity may reflect hypoxaemia or placental insufficiency. If the woman has not felt normal fetal movements, advise her to contact her healthcare provider immediately.
• *Do you have cats in the home?*	Explain **toxoplasmosis** (a teratogenic disease transmitted through raw or undercooked meat, cat faeces and soil). To avoid exposure, ensure careful handwashing following contact with soil and when dealing with cat litter. Ensure thorough cooking of meat and wash hands after handling meat and fruit and vegetables because of soil contamination.
• *How do you plan to feed your baby?*	If planning to breastfeed, arrange breastfeeding resources including classes and other support for women who plan to breastfeed. Provide appropriate education for those planning to bottle feed. The support will differ for those who are first-time mothers.
Medical history	
• *Do you have allergies to medications or foods? If so, what type of reaction?*	Alerts for health professionals to avoid a prescribing error and to ensure foods causing allergies and for the woman to have specific dietary arrangements when admitted for care during labour, birth and the time following birth.
• *Do you have a history of asthma?* • *What is your immunisation status and/or immunity to rubella, chickenpox (varicella), whooping cough (pertussis), influenza and COVID-19?*	Women with asthma have been reported to have higher risks for complications of pregnancy such as pre-eclampsia, preterm labour and birth, low birthweight or intrauterine growth restriction of the fetus and perinatal mortality. If **rubella** is contracted during the first trimester, it can lead to congenital rubella syndrome. Preventing congenital infection relies on maintaining high levels of immunity to rubella in the general population. There is no treatment to prevent or reduce mother-to-child transmission of rubella once infection has been detected in pregnancy. Rubella vaccination is contraindicated in pregnancy.

ASSESSMENT GUIDELINES AND NORMAL FINDINGS	CLINICAL SIGNIFICANCE AND CLINICAL ALERTS
	Rarely, **varicella** causes congenital anomalies. A non-immune woman should avoid exposure. **Whooping cough** (pertussis) immunisation between 20 and 32 weeks of pregnancy is recommended to reduce the risk of pertussis in pregnant women and to provide passive immunity to the fetus, which is protective in the first months of life. **Influenza** can cause significant complications if contracted during pregnancy. The flu vaccine can be administered at any time during pregnancy and also provides passive immunity to the infant.[28,29] **COVID-19** in pregnancy increases the risk of severe disease. A booster immunisation is recommended in pregnancy if more than 6 months has elapsed since the last vaccine or COVID-19 infection. Antibodies may provide the infant with some protection in the first months of life.
• *Have you had any injury to your back or another weight-bearing part of your body?*	The localised and overall weight gain of pregnancy and the joint-softening property of progesterone may cause backache and other joint pain.
• *Do you smoke cigarettes? How many? For how many years? Have you ever tried to quit?* • *Do you drink alcohol? How many times per week?* • *Do you use any illicit substances such as methamphetamine, cocaine or heroin?*	Explain the health risks associated with these substances in pregnancy. Smoking increases the risk of ectopic pregnancy, spontaneous abortion, low birthweight, prematurity, preterm premature rupture of membranes, pregnancy-induced hypertension, placental abruption and sudden infant death syndrome. Alcohol increases the risk to the fetus of **fetal alcohol syndrome** (Table 21.13). Cocaine use during pregnancy is associated with congenital anomalies, fetal growth restriction and premature birth. Fetal exposure can result in long-term behavioural and cognitive impairment.[6] It is recommended that pregnant women are referred to drug and alcohol programs for consultation provided by a multidisciplinary team.

ASSESSMENT GUIDELINES AND NORMAL FINDINGS	CLINICAL SIGNIFICANCE AND CLINICAL ALERTS
• *Do you take any prescribed, non-prescribed (over-the-counter) or complementary or traditional medicines?*	Screen all medications (prescribed, non-prescribed, complementary and traditional) to establish safety during pregnancy.
• *Do you have a regular exercise program? What type of exercise program do you do?*	There are many positive physical and psychological benefits of regular exercise in pregnancy for both the woman and the fetus. Benefits include reduced risk of gestational diabetes, gestational hypertension and excessive pregnancy weight gain.
Family history	
• *What is your family medical history?*	The woman's family medical history is important in planning her care during pregnancy. Familial diseases such as hypertension and diabetes or congenital abnormalities may require a referral for genetic counselling and diagnostic procedures.
• *Do you have anxiety, depression or any other mental illness?*	Anxiety and depression can occur during pregnancy and after birth. Assessing the woman for psychosocial risk factors and symptoms of distress during pregnancy gives her the opportunity to link with appropriate services. Antenatal screening also seeks to identify whether a woman has experienced, or received treatment for, more severe mental health disorders. If this is affirmed, further understanding of current and future significance is indicated along with collaboration with relevant mental health professionals.
• *Is there a history of multiple births in your family?*	Approximately two-thirds of twins are **dizygotic** (fraternal), arising from multiple ovulation and one-third **monozygotic** (identical), derived from one fertilised oocyte. Older women are at risk of spontaneous dizygotic twinning.
• *Does anyone in your family have congenital anomalies? What is your ethnicity?* • *Does anyone in your partner's family have congenital anomalies? What is the ethnicity of your baby's father?*	Some anomalies, such as heart conditions, are familial. Offer a referral to genetic counselling to provide the woman and her family with options such as diagnostic procedures. Establishing ethnicity will indicate any increased risks for known problems such as sickle cell anaemia or thalassaemia.

ASSESSMENT GUIDELINES AND NORMAL FINDINGS	CLINICAL SIGNIFICANCE AND CLINICAL ALERTS
• *Do you have any specific thoughts about how you would like the pregnancy and birth to be managed?*	Establishing the woman's preferences will assist healthcare providers in meeting her particular needs.
General health history	
• *Do you have a pre-existing cardiovascular disease, such as vascular disease, a heart murmur or disease of a heart valve?*	Women with cardiac disease who become pregnant must be monitored carefully for signs of cardiac compromise. The profound alterations in the cardiorespiratory system and haemodynamics (e.g. blood volume increase of up to 50%) during pregnancy can result in morbidity and mortality for the woman and her fetus. It is recommended that the woman's care is provided with a multidisciplinary team approach.[3]
• *Have you ever had anaemia? What kind? When? How was it treated?*	Pregnancy worsens any pre-existing anaemia because iron is used extensively by the growing fetus. This can be managed with oral iron supplementation. **Sickle cell anaemia** (an inherited red blood cell disorder that affects haemoglobin) may worsen during pregnancy, thereby placing both the woman and her fetus at risk for complications as a result of the effects of haematological, cardiovascular, renal and respiratory changes. As the plasma volume increases during pregnancy, the woman can become more anaemic. Folic acid can be given during pregnancy and blood transfusions may be required for severe anaemia.
• *Have you had thrombophlebitis, pulmonary embolus (PE) or deep venous thrombosis (DVT)?*	Pregnancy is an acquired hypercoagulable state due to an increase of blood factors VII, VIII, IX, X and XII in preparation for birth. As a consequence of this increase, there is the risk of thrombosis in pregnancy. These include, for example, venous stasis in the lower extremities and the compression of the inferior vena cava by the enlarging uterus.[11]
• *Have you had hypertension or renal disease?*	Hypertensive disorders are one of the most common complications of pregnancy and include hypertension during pregnancy: • **chronic hypertension** • **pre-eclampsia** • **pre-eclampsia superimposed on chronic hypertension** • **gestational hypertension.**

ASSESSMENT GUIDELINES AND NORMAL FINDINGS	CLINICAL SIGNIFICANCE AND CLINICAL ALERTS
	Women with renal disease are at increased risk for pre-eclampsia (a dangerous complication of pregnancy characterised by high blood pressure), preterm birth and fetal growth restriction, but in mild disease their renal prognosis is not significantly altered. Women with moderate to severe renal disease are at risk of worsening renal function.[3]
• *Do you have pre-existing diabetes mellitus (type 1 or type 2)?* If so: • *When was the onset and how is it managed?* • *Did you experience gestational diabetes in your previous pregnancies?* • *Is there a family history of diabetes?*	A history of **diabetes** indicates that the woman will require increased monitoring and assessment throughout pregnancy. This approach also applies to women with a history of gestational diabetes and are at risk of developing type 2 diabetes later in life. Diabetes is carefully managed during pregnancy to avoid serious complications such as fetal macrosomia resulting in interventions during birth and/or operative birth. **Macrosomia** (a newborn who is much larger than average size) can contribute to maternal morbidity and fetal/infant morbidity and mortality (Table 29.2).
• *Do you have a history of a thyroid disorder?*	Thyroid disorders are the second most common endocrine disorders to gestational diabetes. Close monitoring of women with a history of thyroid dysfunction is required to ensure the woman remains in an euthyroid state, where her thyroid hormones are within normal levels.
• *Have you ever had a seizure?*	**Seizure disorders** are the most frequent neurological complication in pregnancy. Pre-pregnancy counselling is vital for women with epilepsy due to the potential teratogenic effect of some anti-convulsant medications. Close medical monitoring including dose adjustments are also required during pregnancy. With careful medical management most women with epilepsy will have a positive pregnancy outcome.[11]

ASSESSMENT GUIDELINES AND NORMAL FINDINGS	CLINICAL SIGNIFICANCE AND CLINICAL ALERTS
Do you have a history of UTIs?	**Urinary tract infection** may occur with increased frequency during pregnancy and is related to anatomical changes in the renal system. Asymptomatic bacteriuria can occur in some women and has the potential to develop into pyelonephritis if untreated. If this occurs, the woman can experience a preterm birth of a low-birthweight infant. Screening for asymptomatic bacteriuria has been shown to reduce pyelonephritis.[7]
• *Do you have hepatitis B virus (HBV) or hepatitis C (HCV)?*	Antenatal screening for HBV (transmitted sexually or parenterally) is recommended for all pregnant women. There is a risk of transmission of this disease to the fetus. All infants of HBV mothers are routinely prescribed both HBV immunoglobulin and vaccine at birth to prevent infection. HCV is a blood-borne disease that is one of the major causes of liver cirrhosis, hepatocellular carcinoma and liver failure. Perinatal transmission is the main source of hepatitis C in Australian children born to mothers who used intravenous drugs, had invasive procedures overseas or have tattoos. Knowledge of HCV status in pregnancy ensures interventions that increase the risk of transmission to the fetus and newborn can be avoided.[7]
• *Have you been exposed to tuberculosis (TB) or had a positive tuberculin skin test (TST)/ Mantoux test or chest x-ray?* • *Were your born outside of Australia?*	Pregnancy does not adversely affect the course of TB if appropriate therapy is instituted. In the setting of incomplete treatment and advanced or extrapulmonary TB, the chances of perinatal complications such as pre-eclampsia, intrauterine growth restriction, antepartum haemorrhage, low birthweight, preterm birth and perinatal mortality rates for neonates are increased.
• *What was your weight before pregnancy?* The woman's weight baseline is needed to evaluate changes over the course of pregnancy.	In the care of a woman who is obese, health professionals should address the issue of obesity but do so in a supportive and positive way to recognise individual needs and expectations. Excessive weight gain in pregnancy increases the risk of large-for-gestational-age babies, whereas low weight gain in pregnancy is associated with small-for-gestational-age babies.

ASSESSMENT GUIDELINES AND NORMAL FINDINGS	CLINICAL SIGNIFICANCE AND CLINICAL ALERTS
• *When did you last see the dentist? Tell me about your oral care routine.*	Gums may be puffy and bleed easily during pregnancy due to the impact of estrogen on the blood flow and consistency of connective tissue. There is an increase in gingivitis due to dental plaque, calculus and debris. Changes in saliva and the nausea and vomiting of pregnancy may increase the risk of caries. Periodontal disease has been associated with preterm birth and low-birthweight risk. The woman needs to take care with brushing her teeth and seek care from her dentist. She needs to advise her dentist of her pregnancy (Table 29.3).
• *Do you feel safe in your relationship or home environment?*	Domestic violence is relatively common during pregnancy. The frequency and severity of violence initiated by a male partner against a woman may be higher during pregnancy, resulting in a significant increase in risk for women. Intimate partner and sexual violence affects a large proportion of the population and has long-term and far-reaching outcomes.[7] Questioning the safety of the woman is part of care. Refer to Chapter 5 for a full discussion of screening for family violence.
Nutritional history	
• *Do you take vitamin D supplements? What is your exposure to natural sunlight?* Vitamin D is essential for bone development in children and skeletal health in adults. It regulates calcium and phosphate absorption and metabolism. Vitamin D is obtained through the direct action of sunlight on the skin (90%) or through dietary nutrients (10%), in particular dairy products, eggs and fish.	Reasons for vitamin D deficiency include people with darkly pigmented skin, successful skin protection including avoidance of sunlight and sunscreen use, less outdoor activity and diets lacking in vitamin D. Vitamin D deficiency in pregnancy is common and linked to several complications such as pre-eclampsia, gestational diabetes and fetal growth restriction. Vitamin D supplementation during pregnancy helps protect the skeletal health of both the mother and the baby and may improve clinical outcomes for conditions associated with vitamin D deficiency.[7]

ASSESSMENT GUIDELINES AND NORMAL FINDINGS	CLINICAL SIGNIFICANCE AND CLINICAL ALERTS
• *Do you follow a special diet? Are you a vegan?* During pregnancy, growth, development and optimal health rely on good nutrition and adequate quality and quantity of nutrients.	For a woman who follows a special diet (including vegan), encourage and support her to achieve adequate nutrition within the confines of her diet, including carbohydrates, proteins, fats, essential micronutrients, vitamins and minerals as well as water.
• *Do you have any food intolerances?*	A food intolerance may affect the woman and her fetus's nutrition, such as lactose intolerance limiting calcium intake. It is important the woman informs her healthcare provider of any food intolerances for referral to a dietitian for further support through health education and promotion.
• *Do you crave non-foods such as ice, paint chips, dirt or clay?* • *Do you experience food cravings or aversions?*	Craving for non-foods is called '**pica**' and is concerning if it prevents the woman from consuming nutrient-rich food. Women who experience this condition should be tested for possible iron-deficiency anaemia. Food cravings or aversions during pregnancy are common. For example, a woman may crave highly seasoned foods and develop an aversion to tea, coffee or alcohol. Alcohol consumption is contraindicated during pregnancy.
Environment/hazards	
• *What is your occupation? What are the physical demands of your work?* • *Are you exposed to any strong odours, chemicals, radiation or other harmful substances?*	If the woman's employment is strenuous, physical activity can contribute to fatigue and risk of a diet compromise. If there is heavy lifting or long periods of standing, then the woman may need to seek alternative work arrangements. Woman who do shift work where there are irregular hours can also experience a compromised diet due to changes in eating patterns. Establish any difficulties that the woman may have at work such as possible teratogenic exposures.
• *Do you consider your housing adequate?*	If appropriate, refer to state and federal programs to assist with housing or other needs.

ASSESSMENT GUIDELINES AND NORMAL FINDINGS	CLINICAL SIGNIFICANCE AND CLINICAL ALERTS
• *How do you wear your seatbelt when driving?*	For maternal and fetal safety, instruct pregnant women to place the lap belt below the uterus.
• *Do you have any other questions or concerns?*	Suggest women write down questions between visits or encourage them to have their partner or a support person accompany them to antenatal visits.
Additional history for transgender men	
Gender-affirming information • *Are you receiving gender-affirming hormone therapy? When was the last dose?* • *Have you had a gender-affirming surgical procedure?* If yes, ask: *Which one?* • *Do you have breast tenderness?* • *Was this a planned pregnancy?* • *Do you have partner support?* • *Do you have family support?* • *Do you plan to chestfeed or bottle feed?* Refer to questions about mental health in Chapter 11.	Testosterone can have a teratogenic effect on the fetus and must be stopped during pregnancy. Some gender-affirming surgeries may make it difficult to chestfeed.[30] Testosterone is not a form of birth control and unplanned pregnancy can occur.[30] Chest tissue growth can still occur after chest surgical procedures and the area may become tender. Transgender people are at high risk for depression and gender dysphoria as the body changes during the perinatal period.[19]

Objective data

The extent of the objective part of a health assessment during pregnancy depends on the stage of pregnancy. Physical examination involves checking the woman's blood pressure, performing an abdominal examination to estimate fundal height, determining fetal position and auscultating the fetal heart rate. The woman's lower limbs need to be checked for oedema, and a urine test is needed to rule out abnormalities. Other objective tests and examinations are performed according to the presenting symptoms and signs. When providing antenatal care services, it is also a good opportunity to discuss with the woman and her partner about pregnancy, labour, birth and the time following birth, as well as their expectations and beliefs (cultural and traditional).

Preparation

Outline the process for the physical examination and ask the woman for her consent to continue. Ask the woman to empty her bladder and obtain a urine specimen before the physical examination. Assist the woman into a supine position, but when the woman is in an advanced stage of pregnancy, she should be positioned in a slight left lateral position to prevent compression of the vena cava.

Equipment needed

Hand hygiene solution
Stethoscope, sphygmomanometer cuff
Centimetre measuring tape
Fetal Doppler
Urine collection containers

PROCEDURES AND NORMAL FINDINGS	ABNORMAL FINDINGS AND CLINICAL ALERTS
General inspection	
Observe the woman's state of nourishment and her grooming, posture, mood and affect, which reflect her mental state. Throughout the exam, observe her maturity and ability to attend and learn to plan your teaching of the information she needs to successfully complete a healthy pregnancy.	Undernourished or obese. Poor grooming can be a sign of a lack of resources. A slumped posture or flat affect can indicate that the woman is feeling unwell or experiencing depression and is at risk for postpartum depression. A lack of attention may indicate some preoccupation with a concern.
Measuring blood pressure	
Take the blood pressure when the woman is the most relaxed, in the upright position. Recheck an elevated pressure.	**Chronic hypertension** is defined when there is a documented history of high blood pressure before 20 weeks' gestation of pregnancy. Hypertension in pregnancy is defined as a systolic blood pressure greater than or equal to 140 mmHg and/or diastolic blood pressure greater than or equal to 90 mmHg (Korotkoff 5). These measurements should be confirmed by repeated readings over several hours. Elevations of both systolic and diastolic blood pressures are associated with adverse maternal and fetal outcomes.[31]
Inspecting and palpating the skin, mouth, neck and breasts	
Skin Observe the colour of the skin and any scars (particularly those from a previous caesarean delivery). Many women have skin changes during pregnancy that may spontaneously resolve after the pregnancy or skin lesions present on the upper body. Some women have **chloasma**, known as the 'mask of pregnancy', which is a butterfly-shaped pigmentation of the face. Note the presence of the **linea nigra**, a hyperpigmented line that begins at the sternal notch and extends down the abdomen through the umbilicus to the pubis (Figure 29.5). Also note **striae**, or stretch marks, in areas of weight gain, particularly on the abdomen, breasts and thighs. These marks are bright red when they first form, but they will shrink and lighten to a silvery colour (in the lightly pigmented woman) after the pregnancy (Figure 29.5).	Multiple bruises may suggest physical abuse and scars (tracks) along easily accessed veins can indicate intravenous drug use. Skin lesions include spider angiomas (also referred to as spider naevi) and palmar erythema usually seen in the first trimester. Skin changes tend to disappear or reduce in size following birth and are thought to be caused by estrogens.

PROCEDURES AND NORMAL FINDINGS	ABNORMAL FINDINGS AND CLINICAL ALERTS

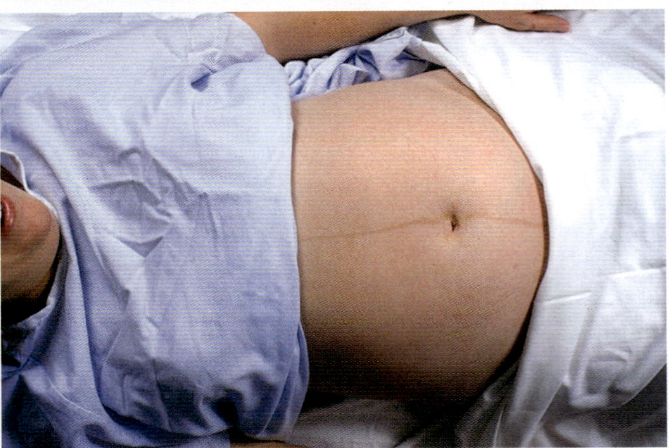

FIGURE 29.5 Linea nigra

Inspecting the mouth

Mucous membranes should be red and moist. Gingivitis occurs in most women occurring about the second month of pregnancy and peaking in the middle of the third trimester. Estrogen increases blood flow to the oral cavity and accelerates turnover of gum epithelial lining cells so they become highly vascularised, hyperplastic and oedematous. The woman can experience bleeding from her gums, particularly after brushing her teeth, discomfort with chewing food, increased periodontal disease and heartburn.

Pale mucous membranes are indicative of anaemia.

Inspecting the size and shape of the breasts

The breasts are enlarged during pregnancy (Figure 29.6), perhaps with resulting striae. The areolae and nipples enlarge and darken in pigmentation, the nipples become more erect and 'secondary areolae' (mottling around the areolae) may develop. The blood vessels of the breast enlarge and may shine blue through a seemingly more translucent than usual chest wall. Montgomery's tubercles, located around the areola and responsible for skin integrity of the areola, enlarge. Colostrum, a thick yellow fluid, may be expressed from the nipples.

PROCEDURES AND NORMAL FINDINGS	ABNORMAL FINDINGS AND CLINICAL ALERTS
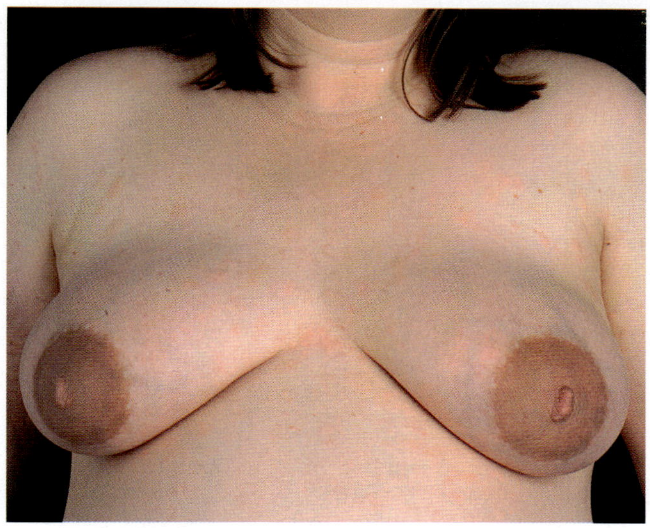 **FIGURE 29.6** Breasts are enlarged	
Palpating the breasts The breast tissue feels nodular as the mammary alveoli increase in size and may be very tender. Some women have an embryological remnant called a supernumerary nipple, which may or may not have breast tissue beneath it. It could possibly be mistaken previously for a mole. They occur under the arm or in a line directly underneath each nipple on the abdominal wall. This nipple and breast tissue may show the same changes of pregnancy.	Refer any unusual breast changes to a medical practitioner for further investigation.
Peripheral vascular assessment (hands, feet, legs)	
Inspect the hands, feet and legs for swelling The woman may have swelling of her fingers; her legs and feet may show diffuse, bilateral pitting oedema, particularly if the examination is occurring later in the day when she has been on her feet and especially during the third trimester. Varicose veins in the legs are common in the third trimester. (See also Chapter 14.)	Pregnant women with varicosities are at risk for thrombophlebitis. Carefully evaluate any red, hot, tender swelling to rule out phlebitis. It is recommended that the woman not wear restrictive clothing or sit without moving the legs for long periods. Varicosities will worsen with the weight and volume of pregnancy and support hosiery is recommended. **!** ***Clinical alert:*** Oedema, together with an increased blood pressure reading and proteinuria, are signs of pre-eclampsia. Refer to a medical practitioner.

PROCEDURES AND NORMAL FINDINGS	ABNORMAL FINDINGS AND CLINICAL ALERTS
Auscultating the heart and lungs	
Auscultating the heart Auscultation of the heart reveals an exaggerated split and loudness of both components of the first heart sounds (mitral and tricuspid valve closure), occurring during second trimester and resolving between 2 and 4 weeks after birth (Chapter 17). The woman's heart, due to displacement of the diaphragm and the effect of pregnancy on the shape of the rib cage, is displaced upwards and towards the left and rotates on its long axis moving the apex laterally. There is enlargement with the greatest change in the left atrium as the blood volume increases in the second and third trimesters.	The woman with pre-existing cardiac disease should be managed closely. Alternatively, the woman may be diagnosed with cardiac disease for the first time in pregnancy because of symptoms precipitated by increased demands on the system.
Auscultating the lungs The lungs are clear bilaterally on auscultation with no crackles or wheezing. Shortness of breath is common in the third trimester from pressure of the enlarged uterus on the diaphragm (Chapter 19). Changes in lung function during pregnancy related to ventilation, airflow and diffusing capacity. Increased minute volume and tidal volume along with a reduced functional residual capacity all contribute to meeting the increased oxygen requirements of pregnancy and consequently there is minimal effect on respiratory rate. The woman deepens her breathing rather than increasing the rate significantly. The hyperventilation of pregnancy and associated respiratory system alterations are also influenced by the interaction of the acid–base balance changes, increased breathing drive, increased central chemoreflex sensitivity, increased metabolism and decreased cerebral blood flow.	When a woman is in labour there is major impact related to muscular and metabolic activity and oxygen consumption.[3] Women need to be monitored carefully throughout pregnancy and in particular during labour.
Abdominal examination	
Abdominal examination of pregnant women includes inspection, palpation and auscultation of the fetus—after ensuring the woman's comfort by making sure she has an empty bladder and privacy. This examination is conducted to observe the signs of pregnancy, assess fetal size, growth, listen to the fetal heart and recognise any deviations from normal. The examiner should be considerate of the risk of possible **supine hypotension**, which can be precipitated by the woman lying flat. The weight of a pregnant uterus compresses the aorta and inferior vena cava, which lie slightly to the right of the maternal midline posteriorly. To avoid this, the examination should not be prolonged and the woman encouraged to report any symptoms such as feeling dizzy or lightheaded.	Should **supine hypotension** occur, the woman should be immediately moved into a left lateral position. Following completion, the examiner should give an explanation of findings, health education and promotion to facilitate self-care.

PROCEDURES AND NORMAL FINDINGS	ABNORMAL FINDINGS AND CLINICAL ALERTS
Inspecting the abdomen Inspect the size, shape and contours of the abdomen to discern the fetal position and to identify any incision scars from previous operations and striae. Ask the woman to lift her head. **Diastasis recti**, the separation of the rectus muscles, may be visible. This separation occurs during pregnancy, is most likely to occur in multiparous women or those with a multiple pregnancy or polyhydramnios. Diastasis recti can take up to 2 years to resolve.	
Palpating the abdomen The uterine fundus is usually palpable abdominally from 12 weeks' gestation. In using the ulnar border of your hand that is placed at the uppermost point of the fundus of the uterus, begin palpating centrally on the abdomen higher than where the uterus is expected to be and continue to palpate down until the fundus (the top of the uterus) is located. This is called fundal palpation and helps estimate gestation in terms of weeks in comparison with the size. Symphyseal fundal (S-F) height measurement is another method of estimating gestational age using a tape measure (described below). The next step for abdominal examination is to stand at the woman's right side facing her head (Figure 29.7). The palm of your right hand is placed on the curve of the uterus in the left lower quadrant, with your left palm on the curve of the uterus in the right lower quadrant. Follow the curve of the uterus and 'walk' your fingers of both hands until they meet centrally at the fundus. This is called lateral palpation and facilitates identification of the fetal back and head. Other palpation manoeuvres used later in pregnancy are presented below. 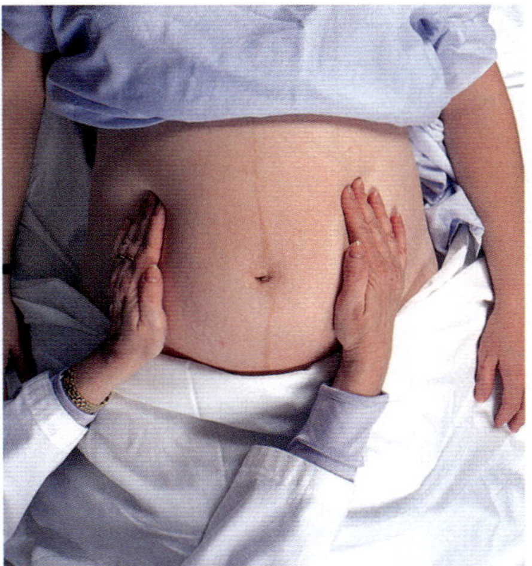 **FIGURE 29.7** Abdominal examination of the woman's right side facing her head	Palpation of the abdomen should be gently performed and after ensuring the woman's informed consent and physical comfort (i.e. empty bladder and privacy).

PROCEDURES AND NORMAL FINDINGS	ABNORMAL FINDINGS AND CLINICAL ALERTS

Note the fundal location by referring to landmarks and fingerbreadths, as described in Figure 29.2.

Note that individual variations of landmarks and examiner's variations using fingerbreadths make this measurement an inexact but helpful guide.

The fundal height measurement should be done with the woman lying flat with her head supported on a single pillow. It is recommended when using the S-F height assessment, that a consistent approach is adopted. The tape measure (non-elastic) is used with the scale placed downwards, starting from the fundus of the uterus to the fixed point of the symphysis pubis or vice versa (Figure 29.8). After 20 weeks, the number of centimetres should approximate the number of weeks of gestation. S-F measurement may provide a degree of reliability and consistency not given by palpation.[7]

Compare the finding with the previous assessments and measurements.

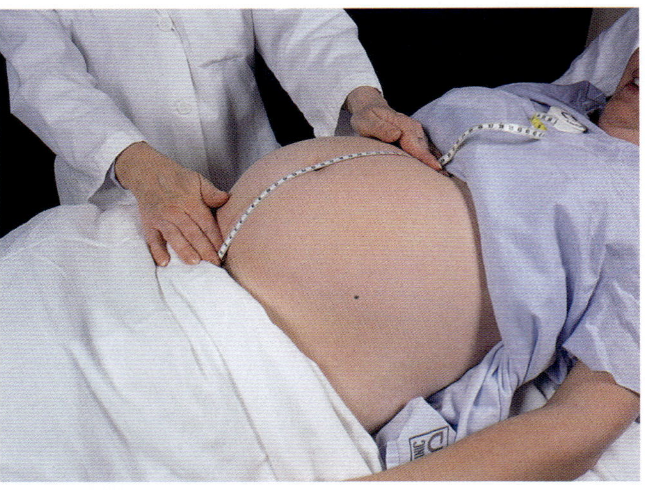

FIGURE 29.8 Assessing fundal height using a tape measure

At approximately 20 weeks' gestation, the examiner may feel fetal movements and from about 25 weeks affirm that fetal growth is consistent with the gestational age. As from 36 weeks' gestation, the presenting part, preferably the fetal head, can be ballotted (moved easily using an external manoeuvre).

PROCEDURES AND NORMAL FINDINGS	ABNORMAL FINDINGS AND CLINICAL ALERTS
The **palpation techniques** for identifying the fetal presenting part and other information in the late stages of pregnancy are presented below. In the **third trimester**, determine fetal size, presentation, lie, attitude, position and whether engagement of the presenting part has occurred at approximately 37 weeks in a primigravida woman. This information can be determined from fundal, lateral and pelvic palpations. When performing a fundal palpation, the examiner faces the woman's head and places both hands on the sides of the fundus of the uterus, with fingers held close together and gently curving round the upper border of the uterus (Figure 29.9). Gentle but deliberate pressure is applied to determine soft buttocks or a firm fetal head. The purpose of this palpation is to determine fetal size and presentation. A lateral palpation is used to locate the fetal back to assist in determining fetal position and fetal lie, the orientation of the fetal spine to the maternal spine (Figure 29.10). **Fetal lie** refers to the relationship between the longitudinal axis of the baby with respect to the longitudinal axis of the mother. The fetal lie is ideally a longitudinal one. **Presentation** describes the part of the fetus that is entering the pelvis first. **Attitude** refers to the position of fetal parts in relation to each other. Attitudes may include flexed, straight or extended. Ideally the presenting part should be the fetal head with the neck in a well-flexed position so the smallest diameter passes through the pelvis. **Position** designates the location of a fetal part in relation to the maternal pelvis. **Engagement** occurs when the widest diameter of the presenting part has passed through the maternal pelvic brim. 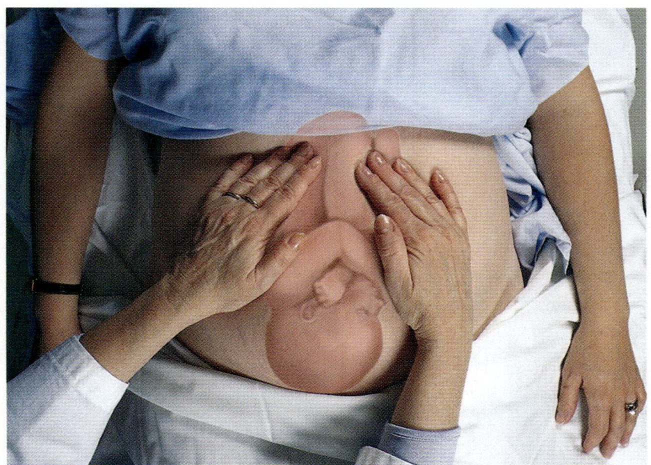 **FIGURE 29.9** Fundal palpation	 ***Clinical alert:*** Fetal size not equivalent to the number of weeks of gestation. If the woman is a **primigravida** and engagement of the presenting part has not occurred late in her pregnancy, this may require careful assessment and monitoring for possible cephalopelvic disproportion (Table 29.2).

PROCEDURES AND NORMAL FINDINGS	ABNORMAL FINDINGS AND CLINICAL ALERTS

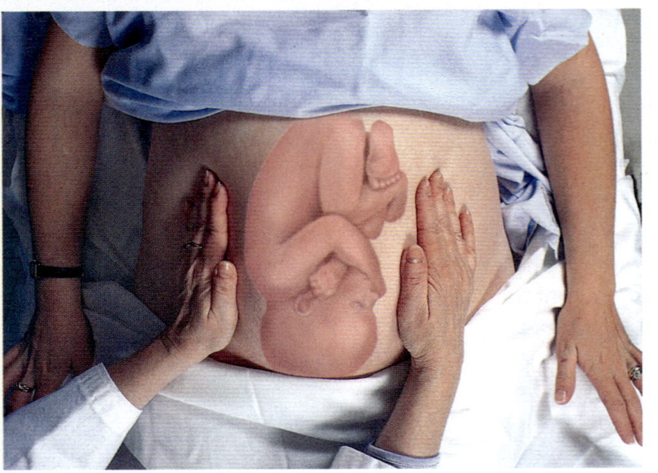

FIGURE 29.10 Lateral palpation

Lower abdominal palpation includes **Pawlik's manoeuvre** and deep pelvic palpation. These techniques assess what part of the fetus is presenting at the pelvis and the engagement of the presenting part in late pregnancy. For Pawlik's manoeuvre, the woman is requested to bend her knees up slightly (Figure 29.11) to relax her abdominal muscles and to breathe steadily and slowly to support relaxation. The examiner grasps the lower pole of the uterus between the fingers that are spread sufficiently wide to accommodate a fetal head, to assess mobility of the presenting part. If the presenting part is engaging, it will feel 'fixed'.

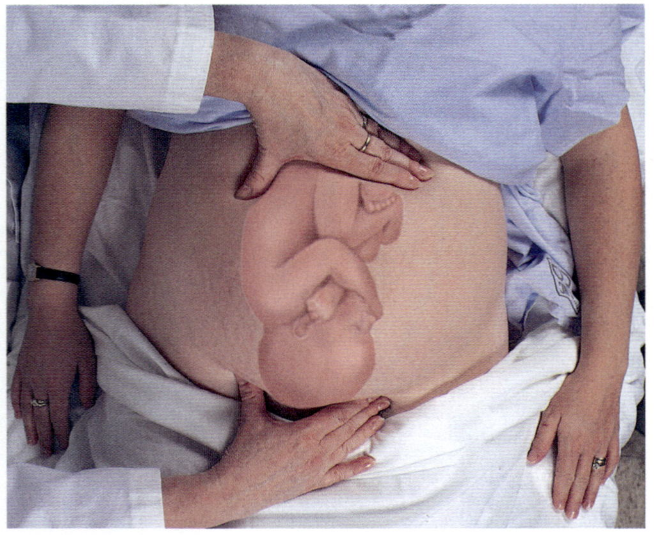

FIGURE 29.11 Pawlik's manoeuvre

PROCEDURES AND NORMAL FINDINGS	ABNORMAL FINDINGS AND CLINICAL ALERTS

Deep pelvic palpation assists in determining fetal presentation and the level of engagement by estimating the amount of the fetal head palpable above the maternal pelvic brim (Figure 29.12). This can be a most uncomfortable procedure for the woman and, once again, request her to bend her knees and breathe steadily and slowly to support relaxation.

To perform this procedure the examiner stands alongside the woman and faces towards her feet. The examiner places one hand on each side of the uterus just above the maternal pelvic brim to feel the fetal presentation. If the fetal head is immobile but broadens as you track back towards the fetal torso it is not yet engaged. To be engaged the broadest part has descended below the pelvic brim—this is felt as the fetal head narrowing as you track back towards the fetal torso.

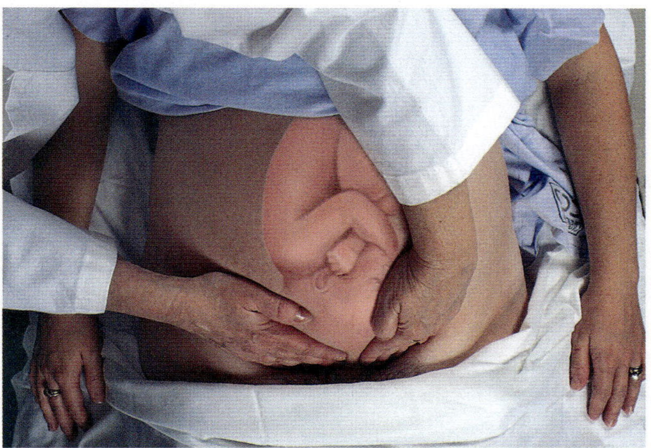

FIGURE 29.12 Pelvic palpation (fingers are directed inwards and downwards

See Figure 29.13 for various fetal positions and where to auscultate the fetal heart beats for each. At the end of pregnancy, 97% of fetal presentations are vertex, 2 to 3% are breech, and the remainder may present with the shoulder, brow or face.

The most common fetal presentations are:

- **vertex**—head-first
- **breech**—buttocks first.

See Table 29.4.

PROCEDURES AND NORMAL FINDINGS	ABNORMAL FINDINGS AND CLINICAL ALERTS

RSA LSA ROP LOP RMA ROA LMA LOA

RSA and LSA = right and left sacral anterior (breech)
RMA and LMA = right and left mentum anterior (face)
ROA and LOA = right and left occiput anterior (vertex)
ROP and LOP = right and left occiput posterior (vertex)

FIGURE 29.13 Fetal positions

Auscultating the fetal heart

Identifying the fetal heart rate is a positive sign of pregnancy and can be heard by fetal Doppler from 10 weeks' gestation. The fetal heart rate is best auscultated over the shoulder of the fetus. After identifying the position of the fetus (Figure 29.13), count the fetal heart beats for a complete minute (Figure 29.14). The normal rate is between 110 and 160 beats per minute.

The fetal heartbeat needs to be differentiated from the maternal heartbeat. This is easily done, in most cases, by noting the difference between the fetal heart rate and the maternal pulse rate.

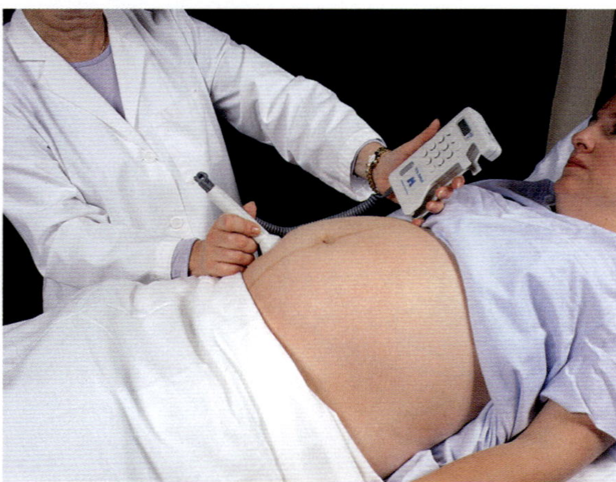

FIGURE 29.14 Auscultation of the fetal heart using a Doppler

! ***Clinical alert:*** If the presence of a fetal heartbeat is not confirmed or still in doubt, then an immediate ultrasound scan assessment of fetal cardiac activity must be undertaken.

Listening to the fetal heart does not provide any information about the health of the fetus. Any concern about fetal wellbeing requires further investigation.[7]

PROCEDURES AND NORMAL FINDINGS	ABNORMAL FINDINGS AND CLINICAL ALERTS
Screening for maternal and fetal health	
Before laboratory tests are carried out, it is essential to explain to the woman and her partner what screening tests are available and that results are confidential. This assists in an informed decision-making process. Further, give advice that there are processes for follow-up on positive test results and that any woman who declines testing is offered the opportunity to discuss concerns without being coerced to reconsider the test.[7]	
Maternal screening tests include blood group, haemoglobin, full blood examination, ferritin, glucose (between 24 and 28 weeks' gestation) and screening tests for HIV, syphilis, rubella, hepatitis B, hepatitis C and vitamin D.	For a woman with a **Rhesus-negative blood group**, it is recommended that the presence of Rhesus antibodies is identified. Rhesus antibodies form due to a feto-maternal haemorrhage when fetal Rhesus-positive cells are released into the maternal circulation. This can occur during procedures such as **amniocentesis or chorionic villi sampling, antepartum haemorrhage** or at the time of birth. When exchange of cells occurs, the administration of anti-D immunoglobin is administered. Anti-D immunoglobin is effective in preventing the production of antibodies and is recommended and administered according to guidelines.[32] Inform the woman that she needs to report any bleeding so anti-D is administered to protect the fetus from haemolysis. Blood needs to be tested for Rhesus antibody titres before administering anti-D. At 34 weeks, the titre level may be omitted if prophylactic anti-D was given at 28 weeks.[32] The National Notifiable Diseases Surveillance System must be advised of notifiable infections. These include HIV, hepatitis B, hepatitis C, rubella, syphilis and chlamydia.[7]
Clean catch specimen of urine Urinalysis for proteinuria and laboratory microbiology testing for asymptomatic bacteriuria.	Any abnormalities detected on dipstick urine testing should be referred to a medical practitioner for further investigation.

PROCEDURES AND NORMAL FINDINGS	ABNORMAL FINDINGS AND CLINICAL ALERTS
	The presence of proteinuria is potentially a sign of **pre-eclampsia,** a serious multisystem pregnancy disorder characterised by the new onset of hypertension and proteinuria or the new onset of hypertension plus significant end-organ dysfunction with or without proteinuria, typically presenting after 20 weeks' gestation or postpartum.
Vaginal swabs for chlamydia, bacterial vaginosis and group B streptococcal disease (GBS).	**Group B streptococcus infection:** up to 36% of women have GBS in their lower genital tract and rectum but are usually asymptomatic. The aim of this screening test is to prevent neonatal infection through administering antibiotic therapy to the woman. Early-onset GBS disease is defined as occurring in infants less than 1 week old and is acquired through vertical transmission from colonised mothers. Clinical presentations include sepsis, pneumonia and meningitis.
Weight and height measurement is performed at the first antenatal appointment and includes BMI calculation.[7]	
First trimester screening for chromosomal abnormality includes a maternal plasma test between 9 and 14 weeks combined with an ultrasound between the 11th and 14th weeks of pregnancy (when the fetus has a crown–rump length of 45 to 84 mm). In addition to this, an NIPT test is also an option, available from 10 weeks' gestation. This test analyses maternal blood for cell-free deoxyribonucleic acid, with a greater than expected number of relevant chromosome fragments present in genetic fetal abnormality such as Down syndrome. The NIPT test may be offered as a first-line test, combined with first trimester screening or in addition to first trimester screening where intermediate risk has been identified.[7] Women who present later in pregnancy (14 to 20 weeks) are offered second trimester maternal serum screening for fetal chromosomal anomaly. It needs to be explained to the woman what chromosomal abnormalities may be identified, the available tests, the gestation of pregnancy at which these should be undertaken, the process of the procedure and the risks involved.	A high-probability result requires genetic counselling regarding options for diagnostic testing, the process of the testing, risks, timeframe for results and options regarding continuing the pregnancy.[7]

PROCEDURES AND NORMAL FINDINGS	ABNORMAL FINDINGS AND CLINICAL ALERTS
None of these tests are diagnostic; the results offer a probability of fetal chromosomal abnormality.	
Ultrasound during the first trimester is usually conducted between 8 and 11 weeks' gestation and is used to: • confirm gestational age • check the pregnancy when there has been a complication such as bleeding • view the position of the placenta • confirm the presence of a multiple pregnancy • check fetal growth, physical development and viability. Ultrasound is available to women at 18 to 20 weeks' gestation to obtain information about anatomical structures including internal organs, head, limbs, spine and assessment of fetal growth.	Ultrasound can detect neural tube defects (e.g. anencephaly, an absence of a major portion of the brain; spina bifida, where spinal cord and meninges are exposed through a gap in the vertebrae), cardiac defects, gastrointestinal malformations (gastroschisis, a deficit in the abdominal wall resulting in herniation of gastric organs; exomphalos, herniation of abdominal organs due to a defect around the umbilical cord area), limb defects, central nervous system defects and urinary tract anomalies.
A **cervical screening test** is performed if the woman has not had screening within the recommended timeframe.	

Abnormal findings

TABLE 29.1 Pre-eclampsia

Pre-eclampsia is a multisystem disorder unique to human pregnancy characterised by hypertension and involvement of one or more other organ systems and/or the fetus when there is an impact on placental perfusion. It is a condition that is unique to human pregnancy with hypertension, but this is not always the first manifestation. Proteinuria is the most commonly recognised additional feature after hypertension but should not be considered mandatory to make the clinical diagnosis. Other features of this condition can include central nervous system irritability and possible coagulation or liver function abnormalities.

Women with pre-eclampsia may develop seizures (eclampsia) or a variant with abnormal liver function and thrombocytopenia referred to as **HELLP syndrome**.

The pathogenesis of pre-eclampsia is thought to be due to ischaemia or hypoxia of the placenta as a consequence of defective progression of spiral artery remodelling and placental angiogenesis.[3] Pre-eclampsia places the woman and her fetus at increased risk of morbidity and mortality.

Healthcare providers have an important role in providing the woman with information related to symptoms of pre-eclampsia such as severe headaches, visual disturbances, epigastric pain or sudden marked generalised oedema.[7,16]

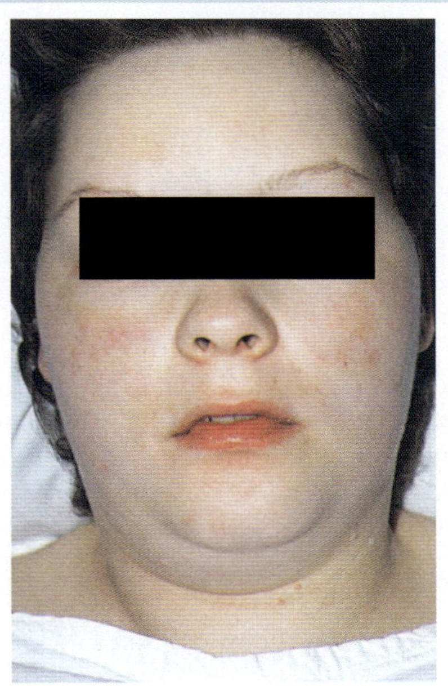

TABLE 29.2 Fetal size inconsistent with dates

Size small for dates	Fundal height measures smaller than expected for gestation or not increasing from previous measurements.
Inaccuracy of dates	Conception may have occurred later than originally thought. Reconsider the woman's menstrual history, sexual history, contraceptive use, early pregnancy testing, early sizing of the uterus, ultrasound results, timing of pregnancy symptoms (including the date of quickening) and the fundal height measurements. If, after this review, the estimated date of birth is correct, then further investigation is required.
Premature labour	Premature labour occurs before 37 completed weeks of gestation. Possible causes include previous preterm birth; preterm rupture of membranes, multiple pregnancy, antepartum haemorrhage, systemic infections, genital tract infections, cervical insufficiency and congenital uterine abnormalities.
Fetal growth restriction	Fetal growth restriction refers to the fetus not reaching the growth potential during pregnancy related to placental insufficiency. Fetal growth restriction is recognised by an estimated fetal weight or serial antenatal ultrasound evidence of growth restriction or growth arrest and is associated with fetal morbidity and mortality.[33]
Oligohydramnios	Oligohydramnios is a reduction in amniotic fluid volume and is seen in post-term gestations, a fetus diagnosed with fetal growth restriction and those with congenital anomalies. A low amniotic fluid index (0–5 cm) alone or in combination with other findings is a strong predictor of fetal intolerance of labour.[3]
Fetal position	Fetal position varies until about 34 weeks, when the vertex should settle into the pelvis and remain there. The fetus occupying a transverse lie, or shoulder presentation, results in the maternal abdomen widening from side to side and the fundal height diminishing. Fetal malposition may occur with lax maternal abdominal musculature (simply not holding the baby in close), an abnormality in the fetus (e.g. the enlarged head of the hydrocephalic infant), placenta praevia (the placenta being implanted over the cervix, blocking fetal descent) or a restricted maternal pelvis.
Size large for dates	Fundal height measures larger than expected for dates.
Inaccuracy of dates	Review the same findings as listed above.
Gestational trophoblastic disease	Gestational trophoblastic disease includes hydatidiform mole (complete mole) or molar pregnancy and choriocarcinoma. Hydatidiform mole occurs as a result of degeneration of the chorionic villi at an early age in pregnancy and where the embryo is absent. For this condition, the woman can experience an exacerbation of the minor disorders of pregnancy such as nausea and breast tenderness. Other findings include the uterus larger than for the gestational period and without location of fetal parts. The woman requires careful evacuation of the mole; intensive treatment of this condition may also include chemotherapy. Choriocarcinoma is a malignant, rapidly spreading disease of trophoblastic tissue that is fatal unless it is treated early.

TABLE 29.2 Fetal size inconsistent with dates cont'd

Multiple fetuses	The frequency of multiple fetuses increases with advanced maternal age and is enhanced by the increasing use of fertility drugs. The uterus enlarges where the fundal height may be beyond the calculated/expected gestational age. Ultrasound examination confirms the diagnosis.
Polyhydramnios	Polyhydramnios is determined by the amniotic fluid index based on the largest amniotic fluid pocket seen on ultrasound (≥ 25 cm at any gestational age or a maximum vertical pocket of ≥ 8 cm depth). The earlier polyhydramnios presents in pregnancy, the greater the amount of fluid. This condition can occur gradually during pregnancy or rapidly over a few days or weeks and is usually idiopathic but is associated with maternal disease, multiple gestation, immune and non-immune hydrops, trisomy 21 (Down syndrome) and fetal gastrointestinal, cardiac and neural tube anomalies.[3]
Fibroids (leiomyomas)	Fibroids are pre-existing benign smooth muscle tumours of the myometrium of which the woman may be unaware until they are identified during pregnancy. They may be located anywhere in the myometrium and the impact of fibroids on the woman's pregnancy is determined by the number, size and location. During pregnancy fibroid growth is estrogen- and probably progesterone-dependent and growth is unpredictable in pregnancy with the fibroids potentially becoming larger, smaller or remaining unchanged. During pregnancy issues caused by the presence of fibroids can include preterm labour, fetal malpresentation, obstructed labour and postpartum haemorrhage. Careful assessment supported by ultrasound can assist in a management plan for a childbearing woman. Fibroids stop growing and often calcify after menopause.[6]
Fetal macrosomia 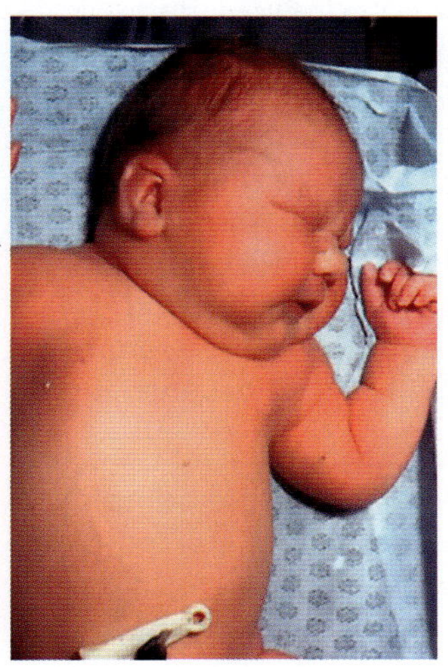	Macrosomia describes a newborn that is significantly larger than average—for example, birthweight greater than 4,000 gm in which the birthweight is above the 90th percentile. Fetal macrosomia is more typically associated with women with pre-existing diabetes or gestational diabetes where the maternal pancreas has increased insulin secretion to counter the pregnancy-induced insulin resistance. Maternal hyperglycaemia can lead to fetal hyperglycaemia and hyperinsulinaemia resulting in excessive fetal growth. It is therefore important that the woman maintains glycaemic control to reduce the risk of fetal macrosomia. Birth risks to the mother include an increased incidence for caesarean birth, bladder trauma and genital tract trauma. Fetal/neonatal risks include birth trauma such as fractured clavicle and brachial plexus nerve damage from shoulder dystocia, depressed Apgar scores, extended hospitalisations and possible mortality.

TABLE 29.3 Disorders of pregnancy

Disorder/Condition	Description
Vaginal bleeding	Some women will have bright red, pink or dark brown spotting at some time during the first trimester. This is not always a sign of pending pregnancy loss but may be from a blighted ovum, friable cervix, ectopic pregnancy, peri-gestational haemorrhage or cervical lesions. In the second and third trimester, vaginal bleeding may be indicative of placenta abruptio, placenta praevia, uterine rupture, cervical dilation or a friable cervix. Risk factors for placental abruption include increasing parity and maternal age, cigarette smoking, cocaine, trauma (e.g. motor vehicle crash) and preterm pre-labour rupture of membranes. This is defined as spontaneous rupture of the membranes before the onset of labour and prior to 37 weeks' gestation. Other possible causes of vaginal bleeding late in pregnancy include rapid uterine decompression associated with multiple gestation or polyhydramnios and maternal hypertensive conditions during pregnancy.
Cervical shortening and insufficiency	Cervical shortening (cervical length of 25 mm or less at 18–20 weeks' gestation) and cervical insufficiency (structural weakness of the cervix). Cervical insufficiency can occur as a consequence of disruption to the complex remodelling process of the cervix during pregnancy. It can result in pregnancy loss or preterm birth that is characterised by recurrent painless dilation of the cervix and is either a congenital or an acquired (e.g. by previous surgery) condition. Cervical length is most accurately measured by transvaginal ultrasound and only after the woman has emptied her bladder. The management can include conservative approaches such as vaginal progesterone or cervical surveillance (using transvaginal ultrasound serial scans).
Hyperemesis gravidarum	Hyperemesis gravidarum is a serious and potentially life-threatening form of nausea and vomiting, occurring early in pregnancy, gradually resolving during the middle of the second trimester. If not managed, this condition can interfere with electrolytes, acid–base balance and nutritional status. Dehydration and starvation may ensue and lead to fetal growth restriction. The exact cause of hyperemesis gravidarum is unknown but is believed to be related to the placenta and hCG; hyperthyroidism may be caused by high levels of hCG. Risk factors include a previous history of hyperemesis, multiple gestation and molar pregnancy. Women experiencing this condition require referrals to other health professionals to provide support for physical and emotional health and wellbeing.
Preterm labour	Preterm labour is labour occurring after 20 weeks and before completion of 37 weeks' gestation. Preterm labour is a major factor for fetal morbidity and mortality. Risk factors include previous preterm birth, preterm rupture of membranes, multiple pregnancy, obesity, diabetes, systemic infections, urogenital tract infections and cervical insufficiency.[7]

TABLE 29.3 Disorders of pregnancy cont'd

Disorder/Condition	Description
Decreased fetal movement	Maternal perception of fetal movement is an indicator of fetal wellbeing.[33] Pregnant women should be routinely given verbal and written information about normal fetal movements. This information should include a description of the changing patterns of movement as the fetus develops, normal wake–sleep cycles and factors that may modify the woman's perception of movements such as maternal weight and placental position. Women who are concerned by decreased or absent fetal movements are advised to make immediate contact with their healthcare provider. This assessment should be undertaken as soon as possible and preferably within 2 hours of the woman reporting her concern. Women who report decreased fetal movement should be assessed for the presence of other risk factors associated with an increased risk of stillbirth (e.g. fetal growth restriction, hypertension, diabetes, advanced maternal age).[33]

TABLE 29.4 Malpresentations of the fetus

Malpresentations may be detected by the hands of an experienced examiner, the fetal heart beat location and confirmed by ultrasound. Before 34 weeks' gestation, any position is normal. As assessed via abdominal examination a cephalic presentation is desirable thereafter because spontaneous turning becomes less likely as the fetus grows in proportion to the amount of space and fluid in the uterus and pelvis. Malpresentations of the fetus can include breech, shoulder, face and brow presentations.

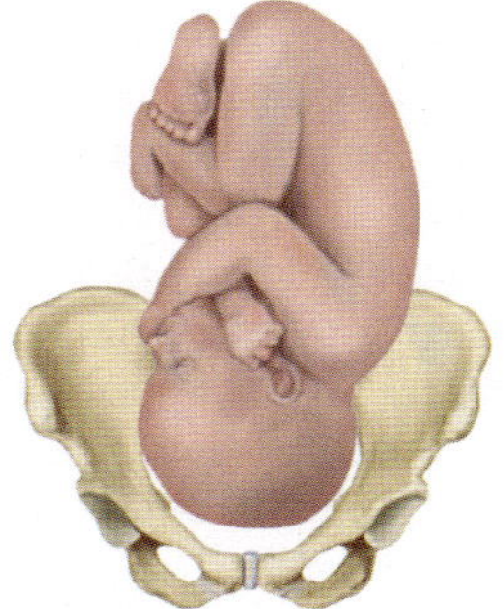

Vertex (for comparison)

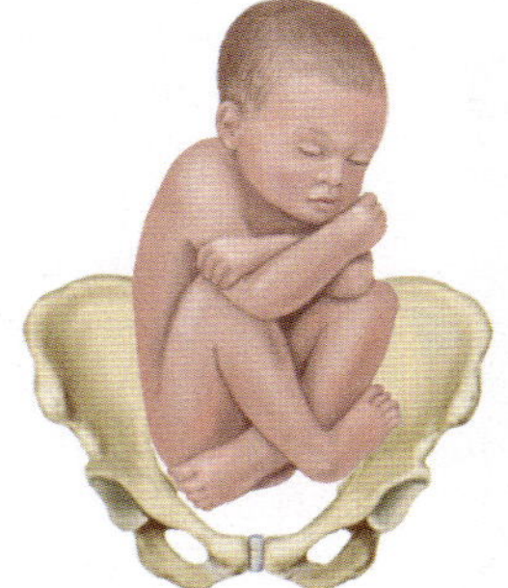

Complete breech

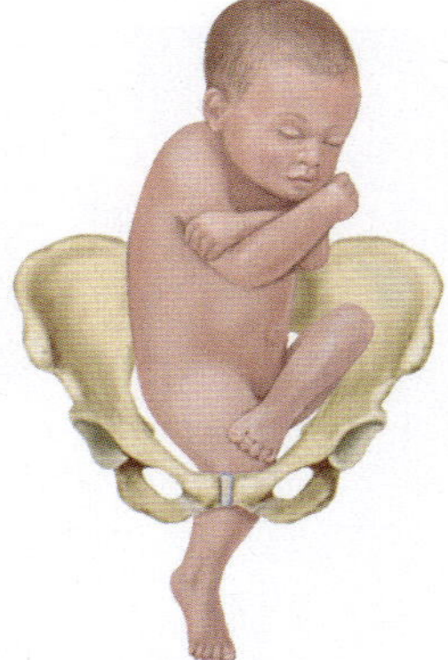

Footling breech

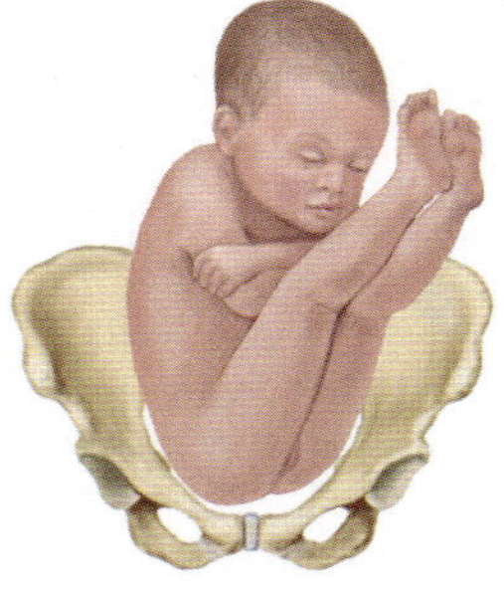

Frank breech

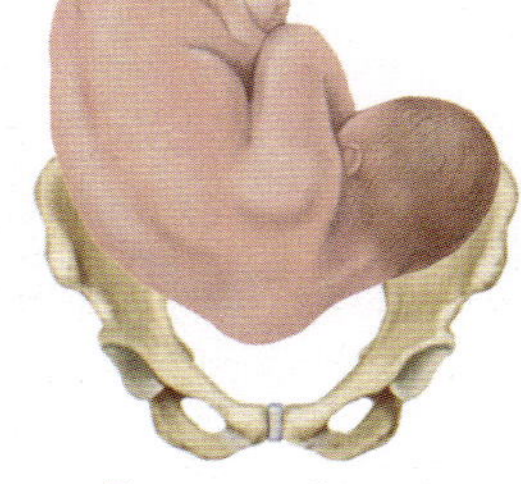

Transverse lie and shoulder presentation

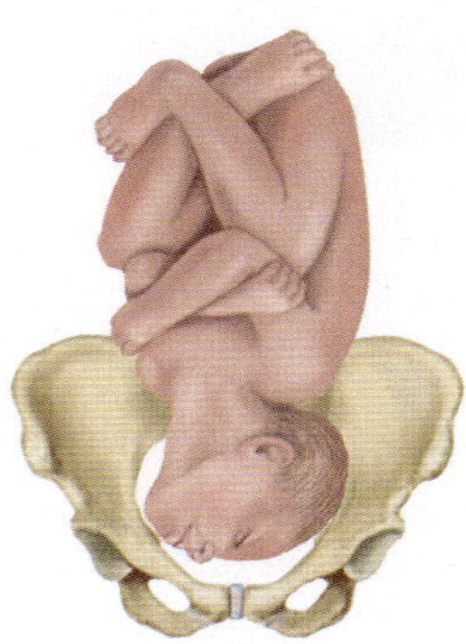

Face presentation

TABLE 29.4 Malpresentations of the fetus cont'd

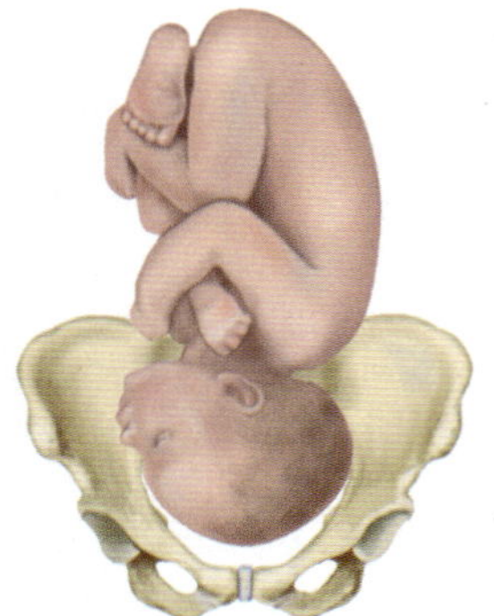

Brow presentation

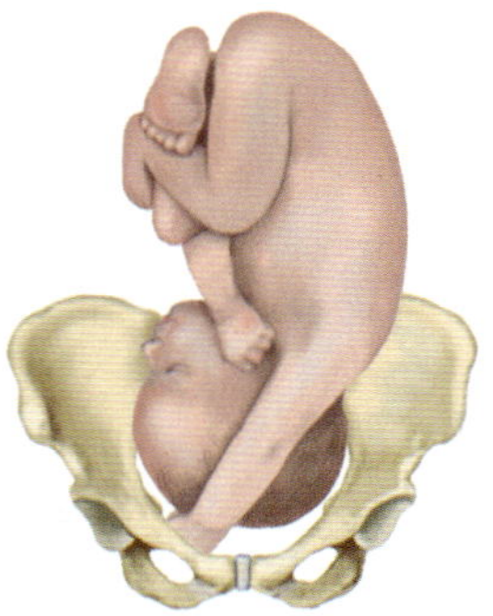

Compound presentation

Clinical reasoning and documentation

Case study 1 (continued)—Pregnancy

The following is a continuation of the case study provided at the beginning of this chapter and the clinical reasoning process including problem/issue identification. Consult a midwifery textbook for information about pregnancy care.

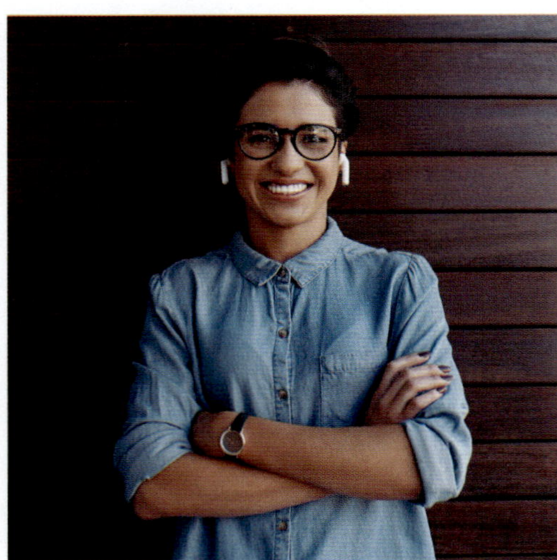

Context

You are a registered nurse working as a practice nurse in a general practice clinic.

Consider the patient's situation

Ms Imani Otieno, a 29-year-old woman, presents to the clinic reporting that she feels unwell and has missed her period.

Collect cues/information

Your further assessment reveals the following information.

Subjective data

Ms Otieno is gravida 1 para 1, married with a daughter (aged 3 years). Ms Otieno works part-time at a local supermarket. Her last normal menstrual period was 4 April of this year (certain of date), with an expected date of birth of 11 January of next year, thereby making her 10 weeks' gestation today. Her history includes a normal vaginal birth of a term female infant (Anna) 3 years ago, after a 12-hour-long labour. Ms Otieno sustained a small perineal tear that did not require suturing. She breastfed Anna for 1 year. The current pregnancy was planned. Ms Otieno feels well apart from nausea and some breast tenderness. The nausea resolves with dry biscuits and ginger tea. No past medical or surgical conditions are present. She has no known allergies. Ms Otieno has no significant family history relevant to pregnancy. Ms Otieno and her husband are happy with the pregnancy.

Objective data

General: Appears well nourished and is carefully groomed.
Skin: Dark skin tone, surface smooth with no lesions.
Mouth: Good dentition and oral hygiene. Oral mucosa pink, no gum hypertrophy.

Clinical reasoning and documentation cont'd

Chest: Expansion equal, respirations effortless. Lung sounds clear bilaterally.
Heart: Rate 76 bpm, regular rhythm, S_1 and S_2 are identified.
Breasts: Tender, without masses, with supple, everted nipples.
Abdomen: Bowel sounds present. No masses on palpation. Uterus nonpalpable.
Extremities: No varicosities, redness or oedema. BP 110/68 in semi-recumbent position.

Process information and identify health issues

Health issue

Suspected pregnancy for referral to GP for confirmation.

ADDITIONAL RESOURCES

You can further develop your knowledge and skills relevant to pregnancy assessment, related physiology, common health issues and nursing interventions by:

- reading chapters of a fundamentals of a midwifery textbook
- answering chapter multiple choice questions online. Log onto ClinicalKey Student and search for the text 'Health Assessment, 4th edition'. Choose the section titled 'Teaching material'. In this section you will find question and answer documents for each chapter. Please check instructions on the inside front cover of the book to access online resources.
- visiting websites

  Australian Breastfeeding Association: https://www.breastfeeding.asn.au

New Zealand Breastfeeding Alliance: https://www.babyfriendly.org.nz

Pregnancy Support Australia: https://pregnancyhelpaustralia.org.au/

Pregnancy, birth and baby hotline: https://www.health.gov.au/contacts/pregnancy-birth-and-baby-hotline

While you're pregnant: https://www.govt.nz/browse/family-and-whanau/having-a-baby/while-youre-pregnant/

Resources for pregnant women and new parents: https://www.healthpoint.co.nz/maternity/resources-for-pregnant-women-and-new-parents/.

REFERENCES

1. Nursing and Midwifery Board of Australia. Midwife Standards of Practice. 2018. Available at: https://www.nursingmidwiferyboard.gov.au/Codes-Guidelines-Statements/Professional-standards/Midwife-standards-for-practice.aspx
2. New Zealand College of Midwives. Standards of practice. 2019. Available at: https://www.midwife.org.nz/midwives/professional-practice/standards-of-practice/
3. Blackburn S. (2017). Maternal, Fetal, and Neonatal Physiology, 5th ed. Elsevier: Health Sciences Division.
4. Coad J, Pedley K, Dunstall M (2020). Anatomy and physiology for midwives (Fourth edition.). Elsevier.
5. Macdonald S, Magill-Cuerdan J, editors. Mayes' Midwifery. 15th ed. Edinburgh: Elsevier; 2017.

6. Cunningham FG, Leveno KJ, Dashe JS, Hoffman BL, Spong CY, Casey BM (2022). Williams Obstetrics (26th ed.). McGraw-Hill Education LLC.
7. Department of Health, Australian Government. Clinical practice guidelines: pregnancy care. Canberra: Australian Government; 2020. Available at: https://www.health.gov.au/resources/pregnancy-care-guidelines
8. Australian Institute of Health and Welfare (AIHW). Australia's mothers and babies. 2020. Available at: https://www.aihw.gov.au/reports/mothers-babies/australias-mothers-and-babies-2018-in-brief/summary
9. Ministry of Health, Report on Maternity 2017. New Zealand Government. Available at: https://www.health.govt.nz/publication/report-maternity-2017
10. Urale PW, O'Brien MA, Fouché CB. The relationship between ethnicity and fertility in New Zealand. Kōtuitui: New Zealand Journal of Social Science Online 2019;14(1):80–94. Available at: https://doi.org/10.1080/1177083X.2018.1534746
11. Landon MB, Galan HL, Jauniaux E, Driscoll DA, Berghella V, Grobman WA, et al. (2019). Gabbe's obstetrics essentials: normal and problem pregnancies. Elsevier.
12. Australian Institute of Health and Welfare (AIHW). Australia's mothers and babies: Maternal Deaths in Australia 2020. 2020. Available at: www.aihw.gov.au/reports/mothers-babies/maternal-deaths-australia
13. World Health Organization (WHO). Maternal mortality. Fact sheet updated Feb 2023. 2023. Available at: https://www.who.int/news-room/fact-sheets/detail/maternal-mortality
14. Australian Institute of Health and Welfare (AIHW). Australia's mothers and babies. Maternity models of care in Australia, 2022. Available at: https://www.aihw.gov.au/reports/mothers-babies/maternity-models-of-care/contents/what-do-maternity-models-of-care-look-like/maternity-carers
15. New Zealand College of Midwives. Midwifery in New Zealand. 2019. Available at: www.midwife.org.nz/in-new-zealand/midwifery-in-new-zealand
16. Pairman S, Tracy S, Dahlen G, et al. Midwifery: preparation for practice. 5th ed. Sydney: Elsevier; 2023.
17. COAG Health Council (Department of Health), Woman-centred care: Strategic directions for Australian maternity services, 2019. Available at: https://www.health.gov.au/sites/default/files/documents/2019/11/woman-centred-care-strategic-directions-for-australian-maternity-services.pdf
18. Health Quality and Safety Commission, New Zealand. Fourteenth Annual Report of the Perinatal and Maternal Mortality Review Committee, Te Pūrongo ā-Tau Tekau mā Whā o te Komiti Arotake Mate Pēpi, Mate Whaea Hoki, 2021. Available at: https://www.hqsc.govt.nz/resources/resource-library/fourteenth-annual-report-of-the-perinatal-and-maternal-mortality-review-committee-te-purongo-a-tau-tekau-ma-wha-o-te-komiti-arotake-mate-pepi-mate-whaea-hoki/
19. Charter R, Ussher JM, Perz J, Robinson K (2018). The transgender parent: experiences and constructions of pregnancy and parenthood for transgender men in Australia. International Journal of Transgenderism, 19(1), 64–77. https://doi.org/10.1080/15532739.2017.1399496
20. Gedzyk-Nieman SA, McMillian-Bohler J (2022). Inclusive care for birthing transgender men: a review of the literature. Journal of Midwifery & Women's Health, 67(5), 561–568. https://doi.org/10.1111/jmwh.13397
21. Rodriquez-Wallberg K, Obedin-Maliver J, Taylor B, Van Mello N, Tilleman K, Nahata L (2022). Reproductive health in transgender and gender diverse individuals: a narrative review to guide clinical care and international guidelines. International Journal of Transgender Health. https://doi.org/10.1080/26895269.2022.2035883
22. National Health and Medical Research Council (NHMRC) (2013). Eat for Health, Australian Dietary Guidelines. Australian Government, 2013. Available at: https://www.eatforhealth.gov.au
23. Brown WJ, Hayman M, Haakstad LAH, Mielke GI, Mena GP, Lamerton T, et al. Evidence-based

physical activity guidelines for pregnant women. Report for the Australian Government Department of Health, March 2020. Canberra: Australian Government Department of Health. Available at: https://www.health.gov.au/sites/default/files/documents/2021/05/evidence-based-physical-activity-guidelines-for-pregnant-women.pdf

24. Ministry of Health, Alcohol: Pregnancy and babies, 2018. New Zealand Government. Available at: https://www.health.govt.nz/your-health/healthy-living/addictions/alcohol-and-drug-abuse/alcohol/alcohol-pregnancy-and-babies
25. National Health and Medical Research Council (NHMRC) (2018) Australian guidelines to reduce health risks from drinking alcohol. Australian Government, 2018. Available at: https://www.nhmrc.gov.au/health-advice/alcohol
26. Jenkins S, Hanley-Jones S, Ford C, Greenhalgh EM. 7.11 Smoking cessation and pregnancy. In: Greenhalgh EM, Scollo MM, Winstanley MH [editors]. Tobacco in Australia: Facts and issues. Melbourne: Cancer Council Victoria; 2022. Available at: http://www.tobaccoinaustralia.org.au/chapter-7-cessation/7-11-smoking-cessation-and-pregnancy
27. World Health Organization (WHO). Female genital mutilation. 2023a. Available at: https://www.who.int/news-room/fact-sheets/detail/female-genital-mutilation
28. Department of Health & Aged Care, Australian Government. Australian Immunisation Handbook. Canberra: Australian Government, Department of Health & Aged Care; 2022. Available at: https://immunisationhandbook.health.gov.au/contents/vaccination-for-special-risk-groups/vaccination-for-women-who-are-planning-pregnancy-pregnant-or-breastfeeding
29. Ministry of Health, New Zealand, 2020. Immunisation of special groups. Available at: https://www.health.govt.nz/our-work/immunisation-handbook-2020/4-immunisation-special-groups#4-1
30. MacLean LR (2021). Preconception, pregnancy, birthing, and lactation needs of transgender men. Nursing for Women's Health, 25(2), 129–138.
31. Society of Obstetric Medicine of Australia and New Zealand (SOMANZ). The SOMANZ guideline for the management of hypertensive disorders of pregnancy. 2015. Available at: https://www.somanz.org/downloads/HTguidelineupdatedJune2015.pdf
32. Royal Australian and New Zealand College of Obstetricians and Gynaecologists. Guidelines for the use of Rh(D) immunoglobulin (anti-D) in obstetrics in Australia. 2019. Available at: https://ranzcog.edu.au/RANZCOG_SITE/media/RANZCOG-MEDIA/Women%27s%20Health/Statement%20and%20guidelines/Clinical-Obstetrics/Use-of-Rh(D)-Isoimmunisation-(C-Obs-6).pdf?ext=.pdf
33. Gardener G, Daly L, Bowring V, Burton G, Chadha Y, Ellwood D, et al. Clinical practice guideline for the care of women with decreased fetal movements. Brisbane: Centre of Research Excellence in Stillbirth; 2017.

CHAPTER 30

Using health assessment to promote safe and quality nursing care

Written by Elizabeth Watt and Helen Forbes

INTRODUCTION

In this final chapter we will further discuss the use of health assessment in nursing practice and its relationship to quality and safety in health care. By now you will have developed some knowledge, skill and confidence in health assessment and have had the opportunity to apply this in clinical practice. It takes time and practice to gain expertise and you will need to continually learn and challenge yourself. Take every opportunity to extend your knowledge and skills. However, skill in health assessment also requires you to continually work on developing your clinical reasoning skills so you can use the data to improve the quality and safety of nursing care.

In this chapter we will revisit the rationale for health assessment and its importance in nursing practice and how this contributes to safe and quality care. We will explore the use of ongoing and focused assessment to detect deterioration in a hospitalised patient. Finally, a clinical case study will be presented to illustrate the use of health assessment and clinical reasoning over time in an emergency department context.

Resources available

You will find additional resources and the reference list at the end of this chapter.

Case study

The following case study gives an example of a typical situation involving acute deterioration in a person's health status and the initial clinical reasoning process. It will help you identify your learning needs.

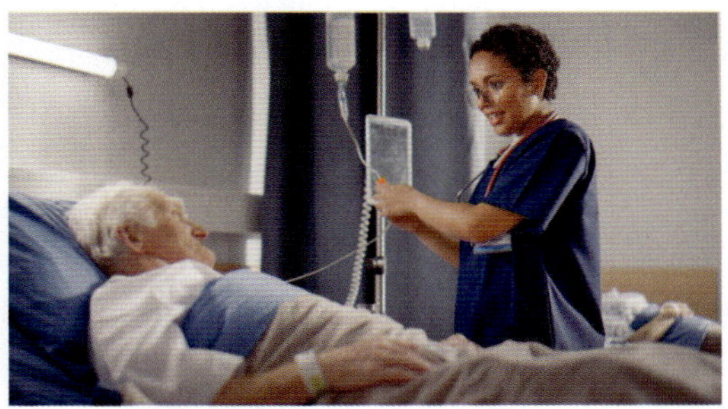

Context

You are a registered nurse working on an afternoon shift in an orthopaedic surgical ward.

Consider the patient's situation

Mr Antonio Giudice is an 89-year-old man who was admitted to the ward yesterday afternoon for insertion of a dynamic hip screw for his fractured left neck of femur that occurred after a fall in his garden at home.

He is scheduled to go the operating theatre later in the day and has been fasting since 8 am. During the shift handover, you are told that he is resting in bed, has been sleeping most of the morning and is receiving an intravenous narcotic infusion for pain relief (pain score 5/10). When you introduce yourself to him, he seems sleepy and distracted. He tells you he is ready to go to bed now, but he needs to make sure that he has fed his cat.

Questions to further your learning

- What are the possible things that might be going on with Mr Giudice?
- What knowledge do you need to be able to predict what might be going on?
- What approach to Mr Giudice's health assessment will you take?
- What questions (subjective data) will you ask Mr Giudice or a family member to extend the health history and why?
- What physical examination (objective data) will you conduct and why?
- What resources are available to assist in your assessment of Mr Giudice?

When to assess and why

Often pre-registration nursing students perceive that health assessment is an 'event' in the clinical day. They see experienced nurses working with patients in a fluid way and may not notice that the nurse is continually 'assessing' the health status of the person. Health assessment is a continuous process from the first time you see the person, patient or client. You are using a 'clinical gaze' with every interaction and using clinical reasoning to make sense of the information. Levett-Jones[1] refers to this as 'thinking like a nurse'.

You learned in Chapter 1 that the approach you take to health assessment will depend on the context of care and the reason for the assessment—a comprehensive health assessment, focused health assessment, ongoing assessment and primary survey. See Table 1.2 in Chapter 1 for a summary of assessment.

A **comprehensive health assessment** is performed at a patient's first entry in an outpatient setting or initial admission to the hospital or other health service. A comprehensive health assessment includes a complete health history (Chapter 8) and relevant physical examination (Chapters 9 and 10). It describes the person's current and past health and forms a baseline against which all future changes can be measured. A comprehensive health assessment also forms a basis by which a change in the person's health state can be measured.

A **focused health assessment** is a highly specific assessment of a symptom, sign or body system and is a frequently used assessment approach. Focused assessment aims to establish or add to existing health assessment data and is smaller in scope than the comprehensive health assessment. It helps identify priorities and areas for further investigation.

The purpose of **ongoing assessment** is to monitor for any change in the person's health status over time. This may be performed for potential short-term health risks—for example, in the acute care setting, assessing a person following a surgical procedure or frequent neurological observations (neuro obs) in a person who has an actual or potential change in conscious state. In a primary care setting the assessment may be related to, for example, ongoing monitoring of an asthma or diabetes plan. This type of assessment is used in all healthcare settings to follow up short-term or chronic health problems.

Finally, a **primary survey** involves a purposeful initial assessment of the person's health status, potential risks to the person and to the clinician. When you take over the care of a person at the beginning of a shift it is important to do a primary survey that includes airway, breathing, circulation, level of consciousness and environment.

You can see that health assessment is a vital and core role in nursing practice. It is a means by which nurses (and other health professionals) can ensure the person in their care is kept safe and is receiving quality person-centred care. Important functions of health assessment in any healthcare setting are to:

- gain an understanding of the person's health care or illness experience
- investigate any presenting signs and symptoms (cues)
- monitor the person's response to medical, nursing and allied health treatments
- identify any indicators of deterioration in the person's physiological, mental and cognitive health status.

Health assessment, clinical reasoning and patient safety

Throughout this textbook you have learnt that health assessment is critical to the quality and safety of health care and is a core standard of practice of the Nursing and Midwifery Board of Australia[2] Registered Nurse and Registered Midwife Standards of Practice,[3] the Nursing Council of New Zealand Competencies for Registered Nurses,[4] and the Midwifery Council of New Zealand[5] (Chapter 1). As stated previously, health assessment is an active process and not merely collecting and recording patient data. It is part of the clinical reasoning cycle,[1] which involves:

- considering the patient situation
- collecting patient cues and information
- processing the information (interpret, discriminate, relate, infer, matching, predicting)
- identifying actual or potential problem/issues
- establishing goals
- taking action
- evaluating the effectiveness of the intervention/therapies
- reflecting on the process and new learning (Chapter 2).

Monitoring of patient progress and identifying indicators of deterioration in health status is a core skill for all nurses regardless of the context in which they work. In Australia, the Australian Commission on Safety and Quality in Health Care developed the National Safety and Quality in Health Service Standards[6] to set a consistent standard of practice to protect patients from harm and to improve the quality of health service provision. There are eight standards including clinical governance, partnering with consumers, preventing and controlling infection, medication safety, comprehensive care, communicating for safety, blood management and recognising and responding to acute deterioration.

Recognising and responding to acute deterioration in health status

Standard 8, 'recognising and responding to acute deterioration', aims to ensure a person's acute deterioration is recognised promptly and appropriate action is taken. Acute deterioration includes physiological changes as well as changes in cognition and mental state that may indicate a worsening of the person's health status, which can occur over hours or days.[6] Assessing changes in vital signs and other observations over time plays a significant role in detecting acute deterioration.[6]

The monitoring of vital signs, including respiratory rate, heart rate, blood pressure, temperature, oxygen saturation, level of consciousness and new onset confusion or behaviour change, should be done at least once every 6 hours in Australian health services.[7] The frequency of observations should be consistent with the patient's clinical status and may be directed by a medical practitioner. But if a registered nurse is concerned about a patient's health status, they can make an independent decision to monitor the vital signs or to conduct other observations more frequently.

Sometimes family members may also note a significant change in a person's health state that is a trigger for further assessment. It is very important that health professionals take notice of and respond to a family member or carer's concern that a person's health status is getting worse, not doing as well as expected or not improving, or even if they just feel that 'something is not right'.[8–10]

While accurately taking and recording vital signs and documenting the findings on an appropriate chart is important, it is only the first part of the assessment process. The Australian Commission on Safety and Quality in Health Care[6] makes the point that recognising deterioration also requires:

- understanding and interpreting abnormal vital signs and other observations
- knowledge of the appropriate treatment for the cause of acute deterioration
- knowledge of when and how to escalate care—for example, initiate a medical emergency team (MET) call in the specific clinical setting (which may be different depending on the size and location of the healthcare setting)
- excellent clinical communication skills—to communicate their concern to other health practitioners and to advocate for the patient.

Recognising physiological deterioration

In the acute care hospital environment, patients have a variety of health problems, many of which can lead to unexpected clinical deterioration causing an acute critical illness, cardiac arrest or even death.[11] However, there is significant evidence that clinical deterioration is preceded by changes in the person's physiological status, which can be detected in changes to respiratory rate, heart rate, blood pressure and oxygen saturation (SpO_2).[8,12–14]

Tachypnoea (respiratory rate ≥ 20 breaths/min) has been found to be significantly associated with later deterioration in hospitalised patients, children and those in emergency departments.[12,13,15] An increased respiratory rate indicates a potential clinical instability, which is often anxiety, pain, stress, hypoxia, acidosis or infection-related, not necessarily resulting from complications within the respiratory system itself.[13]

Bradycardia (≤ 60 beats/min) or **tachycardia** (≥ 100 beats/min) is associated with clinical deterioration and increased mortality.[12,13] While there are many factors that can increase a person's heart rate—for example, pain, anxiety, a cardiac condition—tachycardia may also reflect a compensatory response to a reduction in circulating volume.

In a study by Bunkenborg and colleagues,[13] **older age** was also found to be significantly associated with clinical deterioration. Ageing is associated with a reduced ability to adapt to significant physiological challenges, and Bunkenborg and colleagues[13] advise that close attention to respiratory and heart rate changes in older people and prompt intervention might prevent some patients from severe deterioration.

The **adult deterioration detection system (ADDS) chart** is used throughout Australia[16] (Chapter 10) and the **adult early warning system chart** is used in Aotearoa New Zealand.[17] There is also an early warning system vital signs chart for use with infants, children and adolescents, for maternity care, subacute care and in-home care in Australia, although these are currently state/territory-based.[18–21] A paediatric early warning system chart is being implemented in Aotearoa New Zealand.[22]

These charts are designed to make it easier to identify trends in changing vital signs and give direction to the nurse (or other health professionals) about appropriate action to take when a significant trend or change has been identified. The chart has been designed to be personalised to the patient so specific modifications to acceptable vital sign changes can be made. For example, a change to a lower heart rate in people for whom this is a normal finding. For the chart to work effectively, vital signs and other observations need to be assessed and recorded accurately and consistently over time and care escalated if deterioration in the person's condition is noted.

People with COVID-19 can experience rapid clinical deterioration and respiratory failure. Health professionals need to be cautious in assessing these patients because they may have only minor abnormalities in other vital signs but have a worsening or low SpO_2 while receiving oxygen therapy. Therefore, these patients may not trigger the early warning score systems, as found as the ADDS chart, to quickly identify clinical deterioration and escalate a timely clinical review.[23]

Also, as with the need to respond to family members or carer's feelings that something is just 'not quite right', it is important for nurses to act on their concerns about a patient's condition, even if their vital signs are not indicating acute deterioration. A nurse's sense of concern or 'gut feeling' is described as a reaction to patient signs such as the person's colour, pain changes and behavioural observations, as well as a feeling based on the nurse's intuition gained through experience.[24] Apart from having experience and a sense of responsibility, important elements of being able to make the clinical judgement that there is something not quite right with the person is knowing them, interacting with them and performing assessments in a person-centred way. Through these activities, nurses will often notice changes even before vital signs or early warning scores indicate deterioration.[25] Most deterioration detection system charts also include a prompt to escalate care if a family member, carer or the health professional is concerned about the person's health state.

Recognising deterioration in mental state

The Australian Commission on Safety and Quality in Health Care[26] require that health professionals be alert for changes in mental and cognitive health in all patients, not just those with an identified risk. Mental state deterioration is a change in a person's perception, cognitive function or mood that negatively influences their capacity to function as they would typically choose.[26] In addition to validated mental health screening tools (as discussed in Chapter 11), Gaskin and Dagley[27] have identified five indicators of mental health deterioration:

- **reported change in mental state**—a person or someone close to the person reporting that there is a change for the worse in their mental state
- **distress**—a person shows signs of distress that is evident through observation and conversation
- **loss of touch with reality or consequences of behaviours**—a person is losing touch with reality or the consequences of their behaviour
- **loss of function**—a person is losing their ability to think clearly, communicate or engage in regular activities
- **evaluated risk to self, others or property**—a person's actions indicate an increased risk to self, others or property.

Two other important factors identified by Gaskin and Dagley[27] are the need for good-quality baseline information about the person's usual mental state and the need to ask for and listen closely to the person and their carers' perception of changes in the person's mental state.

An important contribution to potential deterioration in mental state is developing **delirium**. Delirium is an acute change in mental status that is often triggered by acute illness including infection, surgery, injury or adverse effects of medications.[28] Delirium is common in hospitalised patients, affecting one in four older hospitalised adults. It is a medical emergency and causes significant distress in patients and carers and greatly increases the risk of mortality and other complications[29] (Chapter 12). Therefore, nurses and other health professionals need to be alert to the risk of cognitive impairment in patients who either:[28]

- are aged 65 years or older (or aged 45 years or older for Aboriginal and Torres Strait Islander people)
- have known cognitive impairment or a formal diagnosis of dementia
- have a previous diagnosis of delirium
- have a severe illness or are at risk of dying
- have a current hip fracture.

Typical key signs of delirium to be alert for include your own observations of the person or reports from a family member, carer or support person about changes in a person's cognitive state.[28] The person may:

- be confused or have worsened concentration
- be agitated or restless
- appear sleepy or have an altered level of consciousness
- be less communicative or less responsive than usual
- have difficulty cooperating with reasonable requests or have other alterations in mood.

Delirium symptoms may vary throughout the day and develop over hours or days.[30] As with physical health deterioration, when a change in mental state is detected, nurses need to initiate a response. This may begin with using strategies to calm the person and de-escalate the situation and to mobilise the person's existing supports.[28] Escalating care by consulting and/or referring to more experienced or specialist geriatric or mental health practitioners may be required. In the case of delirium, the person's cognitive state can quickly deteriorate, so the person needs further assessment, identification of the causes of delirium and appropriate treatment.

Clinical reasoning and documentation

The following is a continuation of the case study provided at the beginning of this chapter and the clinical reasoning process including problem/issue identification. Consult a fundamentals of nursing or medical-surgical nursing text for information about goal setting, nursing interventions and evaluation.

Case study (continued)—Change in mental status

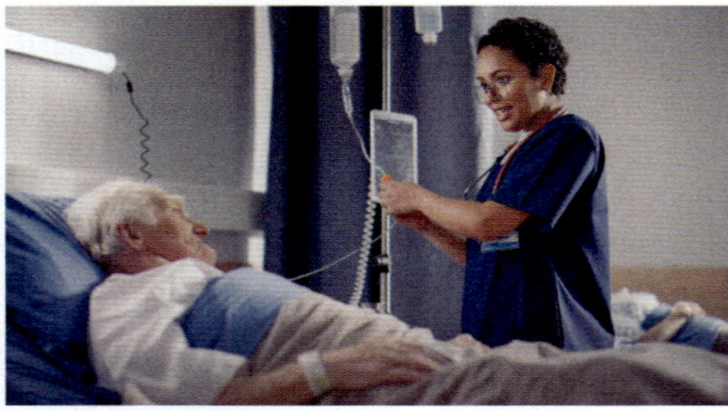

Context

You will recall from the case study described earlier in the chapter that you are a registered nurse working on an afternoon shift in an orthopaedic surgical ward.

Consider the patient's situation

Mr Antonio Giudice is an 89-year-old man who was admitted to the ward yesterday afternoon for insertion of a dynamic hip screw for a fractured left neck of femur after a fall in his garden.

Collect cues/information

Your further assessment reveals the following information.

Subjective data

His wife (85 years of age) reports that he lives at home with her. They manage with family assistance and some other help with shopping and general household tasks.

He has been generally healthy, with some osteoarthritis in his back, knees and hips. He maintains a large vegetable garden at home, loves catching up with his family and friends and has been an active member of the local Italian club.

Clinical reasoning and documentation cont'd

Objective data

Mr Giudice seems very sleepy and distracted. He responds to verbal commands—opening eyes on request. He can state his name but is confused about the time. He says he is ready to go to bed now, but he needs to make sure he has fed his cat (actual time 11 am). He is confused about where he is and why he is here. GCS 13/15

He has been resting in bed, sleeping most of the morning and is receiving an intravenous narcotic infusion for pain relief (pain score 5/10) 2 hours ago. Fasting for surgery this afternoon. Last void 3 hours ago—dark-yellow urine, approx. 250 mL. Urine dipstix: pH 6, SG 1030.

Process information and identify problems/issues

Collaborative problems

Change in cognitive state—potentially delirium related to advanced age, fractured neck of femur, pain, narcotic infusion and fasting state—need for urgent medical review

Probable fluid volume deficit—less than body requirements due to fasting for surgery

Problem statement/nursing diagnoses

Risk for injury related to change in conscious state

Inability to complete activities of daily living independently due to changed cognitive state

Complex case study—Recognising and responding to acute deterioration in physical health status

The following case study presents an example of Ms Emily Black, a 24-year-old woman who presented to an emergency department with abdominal pain (written by Bucknall, Hewitt and Guinane[31]). Take the time to read through the case study because it illustrates the use of focused assessment over time, clinical decision making, communication, documentation, patient deterioration and responding to patient deterioration (including initiating a MET call).

As you read through this case study consider the following at each step or time point:

- What are the possible things that might be going on with Ms Black?
- What knowledge do you need to be able to predict what might be going on?
- What questions (subjective data) will you ask to extend or clarify the health history and why?
- What physical assessment (objective data) will you conduct and why?
- Use an ADDS chart (see link in the 'Additional resources' section at the end of the chapter) to chart the vital signs and other observations as you progress through the case study.
- Identify the important changes in Ms Black's health status that indicate that her condition is deteriorating.
- Identify factors other than vital signs that may indicate that Ms Black's health state is deteriorating.
- When and what actions would you take to escalate further clinical review (by another clinician, a MET call or other intervention)? Give a rationale for your actions.

PRESENTING COMPLAINT
Abdominal pain

Time: 1000 (Emergency triage)

Patient states
Female, 24 yrs old
Generalised abdominal pain for 18/24
Lethargy
Mild nausea (nil vomiting)
Bowels normal
Reduced appetite
Feels 'off'
Mother with patient and states she 'looks unwell'

Triage nurse documents
Primary survey:
Airway: Patent
Breathing: Work of breathing effortless. Patient talking in sentences
Circulation: Slightly pale, skin warm and dry

Patient does not appear distressed. States generalised abdominal pain. Pain rated 3/10. Nil nausea or vomiting at triage. No difficulty passing urine
Past history: Endometriosis, tonsillectomy, asthma.
Triaged category 4 and sent to waiting room

Time: 1130 (Emergency waiting room)

Patient in waiting room for 1.5 h
Patient presents back to triage
States pain worse—now 6/10
Nausea increasing and states she had 1 vomit
Feels slightly dizzy

Assessment in waiting room by triage nurse
Time: 1135
Airway: Patient alert. Airway patent
Breathing: Effortless
Circulation: Skin pale, warm to touch, dry.
Nil diaphoresis
Pain more prominent right side of abdomen
BP = 110/70, HR = 80, RR = 15, SpO_2 = 100% Ra and Temp = 37.2°C
Taken to cubicle

Patient arrives in cubicle Time: 1145
Handover given to cubicle nurse from triage nurse
'Hi, Sally, this is Emily. Emily is 24 years old. She presents with generalised abdominal pain for the past 18 h. At triage her pain was 3/10 and she had no nausea or vomiting. When she was in the waiting room she stated the pain increased to 6/10, and became more prominent on her right side. She also had one vomit. She has a past history of endometriosis, tonsillectomy and asthma. She states the pain is different from the pain she gets with endometriosis. I brought her through now because she looks worse to me than when she arrived.'

Nursing assessment
Nurse documents:
Time: 1200
Airway: Airway patent. Nil obvious obstruction
Breathing: Slight increased work of breathing (talking in phrases associated with intermittent increases in pain)
Circulation: Skin, pale, warm, slightly sweaty on palpation
Patient appears slightly distressed from pain
Rates pain 6–7/10. More severe to right side of abdomen. Patient asks for analgesia
Mild nausea—no further vomiting since patient arrived in cubicle. Bowels open yesterday—diarrhoea. Bowels opened 0800 and described as normal by the patient. Patient's mother in attendance and states patient looks very pale to her and 'not right'

Medications: Oral contraceptive pill
Past history: Endometriosis, tonsillectomy, asthma
Allergies: None known

Vital signs
BP = 102/55
HR = 92
RR = 17
SpO_2 = 100% Ra
Temp = 37.6°C

IV cannula size 18 inserted. Blood taken and sent to the lab. Await medical review and results

Time: 1225
Nurse gets called away to help with another patient

↓

Time: 1245 Nurse returns to cubicle

Vitals signs re-taken
BP = 95/55
HR = 102
RR = 18
SpO_2 = 100% Ra
Temp = 37.8°C
Pain 8/10

Nurse documents: 'Pt groaning with pain. States pain increased to 8/10. Describes pain as "stabbing" pain to right side of abdomen. Reporting worsening nausea. Patient guarding stomach. Patient's mother expresses concern stating "she is used to pain with her endometriosis but this looks a lot worse". Doctor notified of pt condition and order for morphine 2.5 mg IV and Maxolon 10 mg given.'

Nurse goes to get analgesia and antiemetic—returns to cubicle

Nurse documents: 'Patient pale. Skin hot to touch. Patient is sweaty. Patient holding her abdomen. States pain remains 8/10. Patient had one further vomit. Nil blood or mucus in vomit. Patient given 2.5 mg IV morphine and 10 mg IV Maxolon. Doctor in charge notified of patient condition. Awaits review. Patient's mother becoming anxious and wanting to know how long until a doctor will review patient. Patient's mother notified patient is next to be seen.'

↓

Time: 1310 Nurse goes back to room to check on patient

Doctor is in the room assessing the patient. He states he will review the blood test results and has ordered an ultrasound. He leaves the room.

Nurse documents: 'Patient appears slightly more comfortable after analgesia. Vitals signs re-checked. Patient states pain reduced to 6/10 and requests more morphine for the pain. Nil vomiting. Nausea settled. Patient states pain localised to the right lower quadrant. Patient not voided since arrived to Emergency Department. Pt mother states she "looks so pale". Further morphine 2.5 mg given to patient.'

Vital signs
BP = 95/45
HR = 115
RR = 20
SpO_2 = 98% Ra
Temp = 38.1°C

Time: 1320 Nurse documents: 'Patient taken for ultrasound. Doctor notified that patient requests more analgesia and that further 2.5 mg IV morphine was given. Doctor stated he has notified the surgeon of her admission, and request for her to be admitted to the ward. Possible surgery tonight for ? appendicitis. The surgeon will review pt on the ward when he arrives at the hospital at 1500 h. If the ultrasound is normal she will remain in hospital for monitoring overnight.'

Nurse in charge states: Ward bed ready in 2South. Pt to be transferred to ward on her return from ultrasound.

Time: 1345 Patient returns to cubicle

Nurse documents: 'Patient returns to cubicle following ultrasound. Instructed by doctor and nurse in charge to transfer patient to the ward. Pt pale, skin hot to touch. Slightly sweating. Pt lying in the bed. Currently asleep. Seems comfortable. All belongings taken to ward.'

Time: 1400 Arrives to Ward 2, handover given to ward nurse at nurses' station

Nurse states: 'Hi, Kate, this is Emily. Emily is 24 years old. She has come into hospital today with abdominal pain. She has a past history of endometriosis, tonsillectomy and asthma. She states this pain is different from the pain she gets with endometriosis. The pain started about 18 h before she came into ED. She had one vomit in the waiting room but I gave her Maxolon when she came into the cubicle and has not vomited any more. Just before we transferred her to the ward she went to ultrasound. She was given 2.5 mg of IV morphine for her pain prior to the ultrasound. On return she looked a lot more settled. Before going for the ultrasound she was holding her stomach and groaning. She said the pain was generalised but more severe on her right side. Her mother has been here the whole time, and said to me she was concerned at how much pain she was in and how pale she was. Her last observations before ultrasound were: BP = 95/45, HR = 115, RR = 20, SpO_2 = 98% and Temp = 38.1°C. The plan is for a surgical review this afternoon and most likely theatre tonight for an appendicectomy. Blood tests were taken but I have not seen the results yet. The surgeon will review the ultrasound when he arrives. Her only regular medication is the oral contraceptive pill and she is not allergic to anything.'

Time: 1410 Ward nurse goes in to introduce herself to patient and do an assessment

On arrival to room patient appears to be asleep. RN Kate says hello and gently rubs on her shoulder. Pt groans and opens her eyes. RN Kate notices her skin is very hot to touch and she feels sweaty. RN Kate immediately takes patient's vital signs.

Vital signs
BP = 85/40
HR = 135
RR = 24
SpO_2 = 96% Ra
Temp = 38.9°C

Time: 1420 RN MAKES A MET CALL FOR HYPOTENSION, TACHYCARDIA AND FEVER

Time: 1425 MET arrive and conduct a patient assessment

Primary survey
Airway: Patent. Nil obvious obstruction to airway.
Breathing: Spontaneously breathing. Noted increased work of breathing. Use of accessory muscles. Respiratory rate is 22. Pt able to speak in phrases to sentences depending on pain levels.
Circulation: Skin pale, diaphoretic. Capillary refill is 3 s. Pulse strong, fast and regular.
Disability: GCS is fluctuating between 14 and 15. Pt drowsy but rouses to voice and touch. States pain 9/10 to right side of abdomen.
Exposure: Nil rash noted to limb or torso. Nil obvious abdominal mass. Nil lesions. Nil dilated veins.

Secondary survey (focused assessment)
Nurse conducts assessment of patient

When did it start?
'I have had this pain now for nearly 24 h.' Patient describes constant dull pain across entire abdomen. But now it is much more severe. It is sharp pain to right lower quadrant. She states 'It is so severe I feel like I can't breathe properly.'

Have you ever had this pain before?
'No. I have endometriosis but the pain is very different. That pain is lower down and is crampy—this feels so much worse.' Patient's mother adds: 'I have had to take my daughter to the GP before when she was in pain caused by her endometriosis, but it was nothing like this. I have never seen her in so much pain.'

What is the quality of the pain (sharp, dull, tender, cramping, burning)?
'It's sharp pain. My entire stomach is aching, it's very sharp and more prominent on the right side.'

Is it intermittent or continuous?
'The aching pain is continuous, and the sharp pain is intermittent.'

Does the pain travel anywhere (radiate) or is it localised?
'As I said my entire abdomen is sore. I can't tell anymore, it's just so painful. It hurts around into my back on the right side.' Patient indicates that pain is most severe in the lower right quadrant.

On a scale of 0 to 10 with 0 being no pain and 10 being the worst pain ever felt, what is your pain level right now?
'Right now, the pain is a 9. But when the severe pain comes it is 10/10.'

Does anything make the pain better or worse?
'No, it just hurts all the time. Well, the morphine took the edge off for a little while, but that only lasted about 45 min. I took Panadeine Forte at home. I usually take that when I get pain from my endometriosis and it works well. But this time, it did nothing. I have never felt this pain before. It didn't even touch the sides.'

Is the pain associated with eating? Has the pain affected your food intake and appetite?
'I'm not sure, I have not eaten since lunch time yesterday. I just have not wanted to eat, I've had no appetite.'

Have you had any recent weight loss? If so, was it planned weight loss or not planned?
'No, I have not lost any weight.'

Have you had any abdominal surgeries? If so, what was the procedure and what was the outcome of the procedure?
'I had a laparoscopy 2 years ago. That is when I found out I had endometriosis. As I said, I just take Panadeine Forte when the pain is bad, but it has been OK now for around 6 months.'

Have you had any menstrual irregularities recently? When was your last period?
'I have not had a period for 2 months. But that is normal for me. The last period was normal.'

Do you have any pain when having intercourse? Any vaginal discharge?
'No'.

Is there any chance you could be pregnant?
'No.'

Are there associated symptoms, such as nausea and vomiting and/or diarrhoea?
'I felt nauseated all night. I had one vomit in emergency. I felt better after I was given Maxolon, but now I feel really nauseated, like I will vomit anytime soon.'

Have you noticed any black stools or blood in your stool? Have your stools been white or chalky?
'No. Yesterday I had one episode of diarrhoea at 2 pm. I did not notice any blood in my stool. This morning I had a normal bowel action.'

Have you noticed blood in your urine? Do you have frequency?
'No, I haven't had any blood. But last time I went to the toilet was around 2 am. It was quite dark at that time. I have not been since then. I don't even feel like I need to go.'

Do you feel as though you have had a fever?
'I don't know. The nurse said I did. I know I have been sweating a lot. But I feel really cold. When I was having the ultrasound I was shaking. I couldn't stop it. I was so freezing.'

Physical examination
Nurse palpates patient's abdomen
Palpation: Involuntary rigidity noted suggestive of peritoneal inflammation. Abdomen is very firm and distended. Pain is reported to be greater with the withdrawal of the hands as compared to palpation itself, thus positive for rebound tenderness. Rebound tenderness could indicate peritoneal inflammation

Listens to patient's bowel sounds
Hypoactive bowel sounds

Listens to patient's chest
Chest clear. Equal air entry to bases. Nil wheeze. Nil crackles. Nil reported cough

↓

The following information is combined:
Subjective data from patient
Discussion with patient's mother
Physical assessment data including patient's visual appearance, assessment of circulation, skin, chest, abdomen and vital signs
Blood test results
Ultrasound report

Medical diagnosis: Peritonitis caused by perforated appendix

Problem statements
Pain related to perforated appendix
Risk for deficient fluid volume related to vomiting and inadequate fluid intake
Fever related to infection

Immediate plan
- Immediate surgery—to remove appendix and wash out blood and pus from the abdominal cavity
- IV antibiotics—tailored to the specific bacteria to kill the infection
- Intravenous fluids—to rehydrate the body and replace lost electrolytes
- Vital signs every 15 min until taken to the operating theatre
- Nil by mouth

Source: *Bucknall, Hewitt & Guinane 2012*[31]

ADDITIONAL RESOURCES

You can further develop your knowledge and skills relevant to health assessment, related pathophysiology, common health issues and nursing interventions by:

- reading chapters of a fundamentals of nursing or medical-surgical nursing textbook
- answering chapter multiple choice questions online. Log onto ClinicalKey Student and search for the text 'Health Assessment, 4th edition'. Choose the section titled 'Teaching material'. In this section you will find question and answer documents for each chapter. Please check instructions on the inside front cover of the book to access online resources.
- visiting websites:

Australian Commission on Safety and Quality in Health Care (ACSQHC)—Hip fracture clinical care standard: https://www.safetyandquality.gov.au/publications-and-resources/resource-library/hip-fracture-clinical-care-standard-2023

ACSQHC—Sepsis clinical care standard: https://www.safetyandquality.gov.au/standards/clinical-care-standards/sepsis-clinical-care-standard

ACSQHC—Adult deterioration detection system chart (ADDS): https://www.safetyandquality.gov.au/sites/default/files/migrated/ADDS-chart-with-blood-pressure-table-2012.pdf

Health Quality and Safety Commission NZ—Early warning score vital sign chart: https://www.hqsc.govt.nz/resources/resource-library/new-zealand-early-warning-score-vital-sign-chart-user-guide/

Clinical Excellence Commission—Between the flags: https://www.cec.health.nsw.gov.au/keep-patients-safe/between-the-flags

REFERENCES

1. Levett-Jones T. Clinical reasoning: Learning to think like a nurse. Richmond, Victoria: Pearson Australia; 2023.
2. Nursing and Midwifery Board of Australia. Registered Nurse Standards of Practice. 2016. Available from: https://www.nursingmidwiferyboard.gov.au/Codes-Guidelines-Statements/Professional-standards/registered-nurse-standards-for-practice.aspx
3. Nursing and Midwifery Board of Australia. Midwife Standards of Practice. 2018. Available from: https://www.nursingmidwiferyboard.gov.au/Codes-Guidelines-Statements/Professional-standards/Midwife-standards-for-practice.aspx
4. Nursing Council of New Zealand. Competencies for Registered Nurses. 2022 Available at: https://www.nursingcouncil.org.nz/Public/Nursing/Standards_and_guidelines/NCNZ/nursing-section/Standards_and_guidelines_for_nurses.aspx?hkey=9fc06ae7-a853-4d10-b5fe-992cd44ba3de
5. Midwifery Council of New Zealand. Standards of clinical & cultural competence and conduct. n.d. Available at: https://www.midwiferycouncil.health.nz/Public/Public/06.-I-am-a-registered-midwife/1.-Standards-of-Clinical-Cultural%20Competence-Conduct.aspx?hkey=b3251793-36c1-46b8-821f-afb858c8b04a

6. Australian Commission on Safety and Quality in Health Care. National Safety and Quality Health Service Standards. 2nd ed. Sydney: ACSQHC; 2021. Available at: https://www.safetyandquality.gov.au/publications-and-resources/resource-library/national-safety-and-quality-health-service-standards-second-edition
7. Australian Commission on Safety and Quality in Health Care. National Consensus Statement: Essential elements for recognising and responding to acute physiological deterioration (3rd ed.). Sydney: ACSQHC; 2021b. Available at: https://www.safetyandquality.gov.au/publications-and-resources/resource-library/national-consensus-statement-essential-elements-recognising-and-responding-acute-physiological-deterioration-third-edition
8. Australian Commission on Safety and Quality in Health Care. Recognising and responding to acute deterioration standard—detecting and recognising acute deterioration. National safety and quality health service standards. 2nd ed. Sydney: ACSQHC; 2021c. Available at:https://www.safetyandquality.gov.au/standards/nsqhs-standards/recognising-and-responding-acute-deterioration-standard/detecting-and-recognising-acute-deterioration-and-escalating-care/action-807
9. Thiele L, Flabouris A, Thompson C. Acute clinical deterioration and consumer escalation: the understanding and perceptions of hospital staff. Plos One. 2022 Jun 16;17(6):e0269921.
10. Flynn DE, Flynn H, Gifford S, Smith K. Can you hear me? Analysis of a Queensland patient-initiated escalation process and the importance of communication in surgical care. ANZ Journal of Surgery. 2022 Jun;92(6): 1371–1376.
11. Al-Moteri M, Plummer V, Cooper S, Symmons M. Clinical deterioration of ward patients in the presence of antecedents: a systematic review and narrative synthesis. Australian Critical Care. 2019 Sep 1;32(5):411–420.
12. Bartzak PJ. Inextricable Relationship Between Vital Signs and Clinical Deterioration. MEDSURG Nursing. 2022;31(1):65–66.
13. Bunkenborg G, Poulsen I, Samuelson K, Ladelund S, Akeson J. Bedside vital parameters that indicate early deterioration. International Journal of Health Care Quality Assurance 2019;32(1):262–272.
14. Kayser SA, Williamson R, Siefert G, Roberts D, Murray A. Respiratory rate monitoring and early detection of deterioration practices. British Journal of Nursing. 2023; 32(13): 620–627.
15. Daw W, Kaur R, Delaney M, Elphick H. Respiratory rate is an early predictor of clinical deterioration in children. Pediatric Pulmonology. 2020 Aug;55(8):2041–2049.
16. Australian Commission on Safety and Quality in Health Care. ADDS chart with blood pressure table. Sydney: ACSQHC; 2012. Available at: https://www.safetyandquality.gov.au/publications-and-resources/resource-library/adult-deterioration-detection-system-adds-chart-blood-pressure-table
17. Health Quality and Safety Commission NZ. Vital signs chart with early warning score. 2021. Available at: https://www.hqsc.govt.nz/resources/resource-library/vital-signs-chart-with-new-zealand-early-warning-score/
18. Government of SA, SA Health. Rapid Detection and Response (RDR) Observation Charts. 2022. Available at: https://www.sahealth.sa.gov.au/wps/wcm/connect/public+content/sa+health+internet/clinical+resources/clinical+programs+and+practice+guidelines/safety+and+wellbeing/clinical+deterioration/rapid+detection+and+response+rdr+observation+charts
19. The Royal Children's Hospital Melbourne. Observation and continuous monitoring. 2023. Available at: https://www.rch.org.au/rchcpg/hospital_clinical_guideline_index/Observation_and_Continuous_Monitoring/?epik=dj0yJnU9X3ZCZlZxaks2cEJGUzJ6d3BZbDlpX2ZTLXIzSnU1UU8mcD0wJm49NHhVc2daZFo2NFVQMWI1SmZzT1J5QSZ0PUFBQUFBR0FWR3hR
20. RCH The education hub—Victorian Children's Tool for Observation and Response (ViCTOR). 2023. Available at: https://education-hub.rch.org.au/education-programs-and-resources/victor/

21. Clinical Excellence Commission. NSW observation charts. NSW Government. 2023. Available at: https://www.cec.health.nsw.gov.au/keep-patients-safe/between-the-flags/observation-charts
22. Health Quality and Safety Commission NZ. Paediatric early warning system. 2023. Available at: https://www.hqsc.govt.nz/our-work/improved-service-delivery/patient-deterioration/workstreams/paediatric-early-warning-system/
23. Pimentel MA, Redfern OC, Hatch R, Young JD, Tarassenko L, Watkinson PJ. Trajectories of vital signs in patients with COVID-19. Resuscitation. 2020 Nov 1;156:99–106.
24. Jensen CS, Lisby M, Kirkegaard H, Loft MI. Signs and symptoms, apart from vital signs, that trigger nurses' concerns about deteriorating conditions in hospitalized paediatric patients: a scoping review. Nursing Open. 2022 Jan;9(1): 57–65.
25. Dresser S, Teel C, Peltzer J. Frontline Nurses' clinical judgment in recognizing, understanding, and responding to patient deterioration: a qualitative study. International Journal of Nursing Studies. 2023 Mar 1;139:104436.
26. Australian Commission on Safety and Quality in Health Care. National consensus statement: Essential elements for recognising and responding to deterioration in a person's mental state. Sydney: ACSQHC; 2017. Available at: https://www.safetyandquality.gov.au/sites/default/files/2019-06/national-consensus-statement-essential-elements-for-recognising-and-responding-to-deterioration-in-a-persons-mental-state-july-2017.pdf
27. Gaskin C, Dagley G. Recognising signs of deterioration in a person's mental state. Sydney: ACSQHC; 2018. Available at: https://www.safetyandquality.gov.au/sites/default/files/migrated/Recognising-Signs-of-Deterioration-in-a-Persons-Mental-State-Gaskin-Research-Final-Report.pdf.
28. Australian Commission on Safety and Quality in Health Care. Delirium clinical care standard. Sydney: ACSQHC; 2021. Available at: https://www.safetyandquality.gov.au/our-work/clinical-care-standards/delirium-clinical-care-standard
29. MacLullich AM, Hosie A, Tieges Z, Davis DH. Three key areas in progressing delirium practice and knowledge: recognition and relief of distress, new directions in delirium epidemiology and developing better research assessments. Age and Ageing. 2022 Nov;51(11):271.
30. Ormseth CH, LaHue SC, Oldham MA, Josephson SA, Whitaker E, Douglas VC. Predisposing and precipitating factors associated with delirium: a systematic review. JAMA Network Open. 2023 Jan 3;6(1):e2249950.
31. Bucknall T, Hewitt N, Guinane J. Focussed assessment. In: Forbes H, Watt, E (editors). Jarvis's physical examination and health assessment. 2nd ed. Chatswood, Elsevier. 2012. pp. 812–820.

Illustration credits

Original illustrations by Pat Thomas, CMI, FAMI
East Troy, Wisconsin
Assessment photographs by Kevin Strandberg
Professor of Art
Illinois Wesleyan University
Bloomington, Illinois

CHAPTER 2

Figure 2.1: Modified from Alfaro-LeFevre R: *Critical thinking and clinical judgement: a practical approach*, 4th edn. Philadelphia, 2008, Saunders.

CHAPTER 3

Art for Case Study: Stock photo ID:1270072400 https://www.istockphoto.com/photo/smiling-schoolboy-in-the-schoolyard-gm1270072400-373156139?searchscope=image%2Cfilm
Figure 3.3: Lissauer T, Clayden G, Craft A: *Illustrated textbook of paediatrics*, 4th edn. 2012, Elsevier.
Figure 3.4: Zitelli BJ, McIntire SC, Nowalk AJ: *Atlas of pediatric physical diagnosis*, 6th edn. Philadelphia, 2012, Elsevier Saunders.
Figure 3.7: CDC/Amanda Mills.
Figures 3.8, 3.9: © Photos.com, 2011.
Figures 3.10, 3.11: CDC/Amanda Mills.
Figure 3.12: CDC/Dawn Arlotta.
Figure 3.13: CDC/Amanda Mills.

CHAPTER 4

Figure 4.1: Shutterstock/JackQ; Shutterstock/sianc; Shutterstock/Tatiana Morozova; Shutterstock/Goodluz; Shutterstock/S L; Flickr/Mark Roy.
Figures 4.2 and 4.3: Cox L, Taua C, Drummond, A, Kidd, J. Enabling Cultural Safety. In Crisp J, Taylor C, Douglas C, et al, editors. Potter and Perry's fundamentals of nursing. 6e Chatswood, NSW: Elsevier; 2021, p. 59. ISBN 978-0-729-54341-5.
Box 4.9: Kleinman A. Patients and healers in the context of culture: an exploration of the borderland between anthropology, medicine, and psychiatry. Berkeley, CA, 1980, University of California Press.

CHAPTER 5

Art for Case Study: Stock photo ID:1499721340 https://www.istockphoto.com/photo/portrait-of-a-sad-woman-gm1499721340-521348832?searchscope=image%2Cfilm
Table 5.1: Full Stop Australia (2024).Types of domestic and family violence. Available at: https://fullstop.org.au
Figure 5.1: National Ageing Research Institute (NARI) Australian Elder Abuse Screening Instrument (AUSI) DRAFT. (2023). Available at: https://www.nari.net.au/Handlers/Download.ashx?IDMF=b793ff77-d3ff-4440-91df-bd883a1ba86d
Box 5.1: World Health Organization. Child Maltreatment: World Health Organization; 2022 [Available from: https://www.who.int/news-room/fact-sheets/detail/child-maltreatment
Table 5.2: Australian Government Institute of Family studies. 2023. What is child abuse and neglect? Available at: https://aifs.gov.au/resources/policy-and-practice-papers/what-child-abuse-and-neglect
Table 5.3: World Health Organization. Child Maltreatment: World Health Organization;

2022 [Available from: https://www.who.int/news-room/fact-sheets/detail/child-maltreatment

Table 5.4: Reprinted with permission from Elsevier (Yon Y, Mikton CR, Gassoumis ZD, Wilber KH. Elder abuse prevalence in community settings: a systematic review and meta-analysis. The Lancet Global Health. 2017;5(2):e147–e156.)

Table 5.5: World Health Organization. Violence against women. Geneva: World Health Organization; 2021. Available at: https://www.who.int/news-room/fact-sheets/detail/violence-against-women

Table 5.6: Victorian Government 2023. Maram Practice Guides. Responsibility 2: identification of family violence risk. Available at: https://www.vic.gov.au/maram-practice-guides-and-resources

Table 5.7: Family Safety Victoria. (2018). Family violence multi-agency risk assessment and management framework: a shared responsibility for assessing and managing family violence risk. Melbourne, Australia: Victorian Government. Available at: https://www.vic.gov.au/family-violence-multi-agency-risk-assessment-and-management

Table 5.8: Sheridan DJ, Nash KR. Acute injury patterns of intimate partner violence victims. Trauma, Violence, & Abuse. 2007 Jul;8(3):281–9. Miller-Keane, M. Miller-Keane Encyclopedia & Dictionary of Medicine, Nursing & Allied Health 7th Edition 2003. Retrieved June August 29, 2023 from https://www.elsevier.com/books/miller-keane-encyclopediaand-dictionary-of-medicine-+nursing-and-allied-health/millerkeane/978-0-7216-9791-8

CHAPTER 6

Figure 6.1: National Health and Medical Research Council (representing the Commonwealth of Australia).

Table 6.2: Adapted from Diagnostic and statistical manual of mental disorders: DSM-5 5th ed. American Psychiatric Association 2013. doi-org.db29.linccweb.org/10.1176/appi

Art for Case Study: ID:1409200993 https://www.istockphoto.com/photo/woman-sitting-on-couch-at-home-feeling-sad-life-difficulties-gm1409200993-459831917

Table 6.1: Australian Institute of Health and Welfare. National Drug Strategy Household Survey 2019. Canberra, Australia: 2020. Available at: https://www.aihw.gov.au/reports/illicit-use-of-drugs/national-drug-strategy-household-survey-2019/contents/summary

Figure 6.2: Australian Institute of Health and Welfare. Alcohol, tobacco & other drugs in Australia: Harm minimization. 2023. Australian Government. Available at: https://www.aihw.gov.au/reports/alcohol/alcohol-tobacco-other-drugs-australia/contents/harm-minimisation

Table 6.3: Diagnostic and statistical manual of mental disorders: DSM-5 5th ed. American Psychiatric Association 2013. doi-org.db29.linccweb.org/10.1176/appi

Table 6.4: Gould GS, Oncken C, Medelsohn CP. Management of smoking in pregnant women. Australian Family Physician. 2014; 43(1). Available at: https://www.racgp.org.au/afp/2014/january-february/smoking-in-pregnant-women

Table 6.5: Babor TF, Higgins-Biddle JC, Saunders JB, Monteiro G. AUDIT: The Alcohol Use Disorders Identification Test Guidelines for Use in Primary Care, Second Edition, 2001. World Health Organization. Geneva.

Table 6.6: Van Gils Y, Franck E, Dierckx E, Van Alphen SP, Saunders JB, Dom G. Validation of the AUDIT and AUDIT-C for hazardous drinking in community-dwelling older adults. International Journal of Environmental Research and Public Health. 2021 Sep 2;18(17):9266.

Table 6.7: Shenoi RP, Linakis JG, Bromberg JR, Casper TC, Richards R, Mello MJ, et al. Predictive Validity of the CRAFFT for Substance Use Disorder. Pediatrics. 2019; 144(2). DOI: 10.1542/peds.2018-3415

Table 6.8: Corniello A, Skowronsky C. Clinical institute withdrawal assessment alcohol scale-revised (CIWA-Ar). Clinical Nurse Specialist. 2012;26(2).

Table 6.9: The Regents of the University of Michigan. Short Michigan Alcoholism Screening Test-Geriatric Version (SMAST-G). 1991. Available at: https://consultgeri.org/try-this/general-assessment/issue-17.pdf

Table 6.10: Skinner HA (1982). The Drug Abuse Screening Test. Addictive Behaviour 7(4):363–371. DOI: 10.1016/0306-4603(82)90005-3

Table 6.11: National Institute on Drug Abuse, 2021. Words matter: Preferred language for talking about addiction. Available at: https://nida.nih.gov/nidamed-medical-health-professionals/health-professions-education/words-matter-terms-to-use-avoid-when-talking-about-addiction

CHAPTER 7

Art for Case Study: Stock photo ID:1133502771 https://www.istockphoto.com/photo/woman-selling-tea-at-a-street-of-khartoum-gm1133502771-300856159?phrase=sudanese+woman&searchscope=image%2Cfilm

Figure 7.1: iStockphoto.com/Ergin Yalcin

Figure 7.2: Shutterstock/NotarYES.

Figure 7.3: Science Photo Library/Jim Varney.

Figure 7.4: Shutterstock/Photographee.eu.

Figure 7.5: © Newspix/News Ltd/Chloe Erlich.

CHAPTER 8

Art for Case Study 8.1: Katiekk2/iStockPhoto.com

Art for Case Study 8.2: Stock photo ID:1133502771 https://www.istockphoto.com/photo/woman-selling-tea-at-a-street-of-khartoum-gm1133502771-300856159?phrase=sudanese+woman&searchscope=image%2Cfilm

Figure 8.1: Adapted with permission from the NCCN Clinical Practice Guidelines in Oncology (NCCN Guidelines®) for Distress Management V.2.2024. © 2024 National Comprehensive Cancer Network, Inc. All rights reserved. The NCCN Guidelines® and illustrations herein may not be reproduced in any form for any purpose without the express written permission of NCCN. To view the most recent and complete version of the NCCN Guidelines, go online to NCCN.org. The NCCN Guidelines are a work in progress that may be refined as often as new significant data becomes available. NCCN makes no warranties of any kind whatsoever regarding their content, use or application and disclaims any responsibility for their application or use in any way.

Figure 8.2: Adapted from The American Society of Human Genetics. www.ashg.org, 2004.

Figure 8.3: Adapted from Katz S, Down TD, Cash HR et al, The Gerontological Society of America: Progress in the development of the index of ADL, *Gerontologist*, 10:20–30, 1970.

Figure 8.4: Goldenring JM, Rosen DS: Getting into adolescent heads: an essential update, *Contemporary Pediatrics*, 21(1): 64–68, 70, 73–74, 2004.

CHAPTER 9

Figure 9.1: Reproduced from: https://healthywa.wa.gov.au/Articles/F_I/Facts-about-hand-hygiene

Art for Case Study 9.1: Stock photo ID:1133502771 https://www.istockphoto.com/photo/woman-selling-tea-at-a-street-of-khartoum-gm1133502771-300856159?phrase=sudanese+woman&searchscope=image%2Cfilm
Art for Case Study 9.2: Stock photo ID:1133502771 https://www.istockphoto.com/photo/woman-selling-tea-at-a-street-of-khartoum-gm1133502771-300856159?phrase=sudanese+woman&searchscope=image%2Cfilm
Figure 9.9: Stock photo ID:1727918713 https://www.istockphoto.com/photo/mature-male-patient-sits-alone-in-the-hospital-room-gm1727918713-541475569
Figure 9.7: iStockphoto/NormaF.

CHAPTER 10

Figure 10.1: iStockphoto.com/fatcamera.
Figure 10.2: © Commonwealth of Australia 2012.
Figure 10.3: iStockphoto.com/monkeybusinessimages.
Figure 10.5: iStockphoto.com/aldomurillo.
Figure 10.6: iStockphoto.com/tbradford.
Figure 10.7: iStockphoto.com/Image Source.
Figure 10.11: Stock photo ID:154959351 https://www.istockphoto.com/photo/digital-medical-thermometer-isolated-gm154959351-16290250
Figure 10.12: Stock photo ID:1148643391 https://www.istockphoto.com/photo/doctor-checking-patients-temperature-in-the-ear-with-tympanic-thermometer-inside-the-gm1148643391-310264176
Figure 10.13: Kathy Bonewit-West. Clinical Procedures for Medical Assistants, 11th edition. Saunders; 2024.
Figure 10.14: Stock photo ID:1414763881 https://www.istockphoto.com/photo/the-child-has-a-fever-gm1414763881-463375399
Figure 10.17: Science Photo Library/BSIP/Astier.
Figure 10.23: Arlene M. Adler, Richard R. Carlton. Introduction to Radiologic and Imaging Sciences and Patient Care, 7th edition. Saunders; 2020.

CHAPTER 11

Figure 11.1: Colucci E. et al., (2018). Suicide first aid guidelines for assisting persons from immigrant or refugee background: a Delphi study. Advances in Mental Health, 16(2), 105–116 https://doi.org/10.1080/18387357.2018.1469383
Art for Clinical Case Study: Shutterstock/Irina Borsuchenko.
Table 11.13: http://www.stanford.edu/~yesavage/GDS.html
Table 11.14: https://dementiaresearch.org.au/wp-content/uploads/2016/06/PAS.pdf
Table 11.15: Cox JL, Holden JM Sagovsky R (1987) Detection of postnatal depression: development of the 10-item Edinburgh postnatal depression scale. Brit J Psychiatry 150:782–786. Reproduced with permission.

CHAPTER 12

Art for Case Study: Stock photo ID:1479592011 https://www.istockphoto.com/photo/portrait-of-aboriginal-australian-mother-gm1479592011-507529303
Table 12.1: Adapted from Institute of Neurological Sciences. (2015). Glasgow Coma Scale: Do it this way. NHS Greater Glasgow and Clyde. https://www.glasgowcomascale.org/downloads/GCS-Assessment-Aid-English.pdf?v53; Mehta, R., & Chinthapalli, K. (2019). Glasgow coma scale explained. BMJ, 365, l1296.
Figure 12.9: © Pat Thomas, 2014.
Figure 12.13: Adapted from Institute of Neurological Sciences, 2015.
Figures 12.51, 12.52: Murray SS, McKinney ES: *Foundations of maternal-newborn and*

women's health nursing, 5th edn. St Louis, 2010, Saunders.
Figure 12.63B: Fenichel GM: *Clinical pediatric neurology*, Philadelphia, 1988, Saunders.
Art for Table 12.12: © Pat Thomas, 2010.
Art for Table 12.14: (Decorticate rigidity) © Pat Thomas, 2006; (Decerebrate rigidity) © Pat Thomas, 2006; (Flaccid quadriplegia) © Pat Thomas, 2006; (Opisthotonos) © Pat Thomas, 2006.
Art for Table 12.16: (Snout) © Pat Thomas, 2006; (Sucking) © Pat Thomas, 2006; (Grasp) © Pat Thomas, 2006.
Art for Table 12.17: (Parkinson's syndrome) Glynn M, Drake WM: *Hutchison's clinical methods: an integrated approach to clinical practice,* 23rd edn. Philadelphia, 2012, Elsevier Saunders; (Bell's palsy [right side]) Swartz MH: *Textbook of physical diagnosis: history and examination,* 5th edn. Philadelphia, 2006, Saunders; (Stroke) Nolte J, Sundsten J: *The Human brain: an introduction to its functional anatomy,* 6th edn. Philadelphia, 2009, Elsevier Mosby.
Art for Clinical Case Study: iStockphoto.com/RAUL RODRIGUEZ.

CHAPTER 13

Figure 13.4: (Reflexive sympathetic dystrophy) © Pat Thomas, 2010.
Figure 13.5: © Pat Thomas, 2018.
Figures 13.6, 13.7: McAffery M, Pasero C: *Pain: clinical manual,* 2nd edn. St Louis, 1999, Mosby.
Figure 13.8: Acute Pain Management Guideline Panel, 1992.
Figure 13.9: Abbey J, De Bellis A, Piller N et al: Funded by the JH & JD Gunn Medical Research Foundation 1998–2002.
Figure 13.10: Warden, V., Hurley, A. C., & Voticer, L. (2003). Development and psychometric evaluation of the Pain Assessment in Advanced Dementia (PAINAD) Scale. *J Am Med Dir Assoc. 4*(1), 9–15.
Figure 13.11: Hicks CL, von Baeyer CL, Spafford P et al: Faces Pain Scale—Revised: toward a common metric in pediatric pain measurement, *Pain,* 93:173–183, 2001. Copyright 2001 the International Association for the Study of Pain (IASP).
From Hockenberry MJ, Wilson D, Winkelstein ML: Wong's essentials of pediatric nursing, 7th edn. St. Louis, 2005, p. 470. Used with permission. Copyright, Mosby.
Figure 13.12: Krechel SW, Bildner J: CRIES: a neonatal postoperative pain measurement score: initial testing of validity and reliability, *Pediatric Anesthesia*, 5:53–61, 1995.
Figure 13.13: Voepel-Lewis, T., Zanotti, J., Dammeyer, J. A., et al. (2010). Reliability and validity of the face, legs, activity, cry, consolability behavioral tool in assessing acute pain in critically ill patients. *Am J Crit Care*, 19(1), 55–61.
Art for Clinical Case Study 1: Shutterstock.com/De Visu.
Art for Clinical Case Study 2: Shutterstock.com/AJP.

CHAPTER 14

Figure 14.1: © Pat Thomas, 2006.
Figure 14.3: © Pat Thomas, 2006.
Figure 14.4: © Pat Thomas, 2006.
Figure 14.10: Lemmi and Lemmi, 2011.
Figure 14.11: Kidd DP, Newman NJ, Biousse V: *Neuro-ophthalmology*. Copyright © 2008 by Butterworth–Heinemann, an imprint of Elsevier Inc.
Figure 14.14: Zitelli BJ, Davis HW: *Atlas of pediatric physical diagnosis,* 5th edn. St Louis, 2007, Mosby.
Figure 14.15: Albert DM, Jakobiec FA: *Principles and practice of ophthalmology,* Philadelphia, 1994, Saunders.
Figure 14.16: Swartz MH: *Textbook of physical diagnosis: history and examination,* 5th edn. Philadelphia, 2005, Saunders.

Figure 14.29: Heather Boyd-Monk and Wills Eye Hospital, Philadelphia.
Figures 14.30, 14.31: Lemmi and Lemmi, 2011.
Figure 14.32: Douglas G, Nicol F, Robertson C: *Macleod's clinical examination*, 13th edn. Elsevier Churchill Livingstone, 2013.
Figure 14.33: Friedman N, Kaiser PK, Pineda R: *The Massachusetts Eye and Ear Infirmary illustrated manual of ophthalmology*, 4th edn. Philadelphia, 2014, Saunders.
Art for Table 14.1: (Left esotropia) Zitelli BJ, Davis HW: *Atlas of pediatric physical diagnosis*, 5th edn. St Louis, 2007, Mosby; (Exotropia) Zitelli BJ, Davis HW: *Atlas of pediatric physical diagnosis*, 5th edn. St Louis, 2007, Mosby.
Art for Table 14.2: (Periorbital oedema) Ibsen OAC, Phelan JA: *Oral pathology for the dental hygienist,* 2nd edn. Philadelphia, 1992, Saunders; (Orbital cellulitis) Uddin JM, Scawn RL: *Pediatric ophthalmology and strabismus*, 4th edn. Elsevier, 2013; (Exophthalmos [protruding eyes]) Lemmi and Lemmi, 2011; (Ptosis [drooping upper lid]) Lemmi and Lemmi, 2011; (Upward palpebral slant) Hockenberry MJ, Wilson D: *Wong's essentials of pediatric nursing*, 9th edn. St Louis, 2013, Mosby; (Ectropion) Albert DM, Jakobiec FA: *Principles and practice of ophthalmology*, Philadelphia, 1994, Saunders; (Entropion) Albert DM, Jakobiec FA: *Principles and practice of ophthalmology*, Philadelphia, 1994, Saunders.
Art for Table 14.3: (Blepharitis [inflammation of the eyelids]) Friedman N, Kaiser PK, Pineda R: *The Massachusetts Eye and Ear Infirmary illustrated manual of ophthalmology*, 4th edn. Philadelphia, 2014, Saunders; (Chalazion) Heather Boyd-Monk and Wills Eye Hospital, Philadelphia; (Hordeolum [stye]) Lemmi and Lemmi, 2011; (Basal cell carcinoma) Friedman NJ, Kaiser PK, Pineda R: *The Massachusetts Eye and Ear Infirmary illustrated manual of ophthalmology,* 4th edn. Philadelphia, 2014, Saunders Elsevier; (Squamous cell carcinoma) Krachmer JH: *Cornea atlas*, 3rd edn. Elsevier, 2014.
Art for Table 14.6: (Conjunctivitis) Lemmi and Lemmi, 2011; (Subconjunctival haemorrhage) Lemmi and Lemmi, 2011; (Iritis [circumcorneal redness]) Scheie HG, Albert DM: *Textbook of ophthalmology*, 9th edn. Philadelphia, 1977, Saunders; (Primary angle-closure glaucoma) Atkinson P, Kendall R, Rensburg LV: *Emergency medicine: an illustrated color text.* Philadelphia, 2011, Churchill Livingstone; (Herpes simplex virus) Friedman NJ, Kaiser PK, Pineda R: *The Massachusetts Eye and Ear Infirmary Illustrated Manual of Ophthalmology*, 4th edn. Philadelphia, 2014, Saunders Elsevier.
Art for Table 14.7: (Pterygium) Lemmi and Lemmi, 2011; (Corneal abrasion) Heather Boyd-Monk and Wills Eye Hospital, Philadelphia; (Hyphaema) Lemmi and Lemmi, 2011; (Hypopyon) Scheie HG, Albert DM: *Textbook of ophthalmology*, 9th edn. Philadelphia, 1977, Saunders.
Art for Table 14.8: (Central grey opacity—nuclear cataract) Friedman N, Pineda R: *The Massachusetts Eye and Ear Infirmary illustrated manual of ophthalmology*. Philadelphia, 1998, Saunders; (Star-shaped opacity—cortical cataract) Friedman N, Pineda R: *The Massachusetts Eye and Ear Infirmary illustrated manual of ophthalmology*. Philadelphia, 1998, Saunders.
Art for Table 14.9: (Optic atrophy [disc pallor]) Friedman NJ, Kaiser PK, Pineda R: *The Massachusetts Eye and Ear Infirmary illustrated manual of ophthalmology*, 4th edn. Philadelphia, 2014, Saunders Elsevier; (Papillo-oedema) Friedman NJ, Kaiser PK, Pineda R: *The Massachusetts Eye and Ear Infirmary illustrated manual of ophthalmology*,

4th edn. Philadelphia, 2014, Saunders Elsevier; (Excessive cup–disc ratio) Friedman NJ, Kaiser PK, Pineda R: *The Massachusetts Eye and Ear Infirmary illustrated manual of ophthalmology*, 4th edn. Philadelphia, 2014, Saunders Elsevier.

Art for Table 14.10: (Arteriovenous crossing [nicking]) Friedman N, Kaiser PK, Pineda R: *The Massachusetts eye and ear infirmary illustrated manual of ophthalmology*, 4th edn. Philadelphia, 2014, Saunders; (Narrow [attenuated] arteries) Lemmi and Lemmi, 2011; (Diabetic retinopathy) Friedman N, Kaiser PK, Pineda R: *The Massachusetts eye and ear infirmary illustrated manual of ophthalmology*, 4th edn. Philadelphia, 2014, Saunders.

Art for Clinical Case Study: iStockphoto.com/seb_ra.

CHAPTER 15

Art for Table 15.2a: © Custom Medical Stock Photo/SCIENCE PHOTO LIBRARY

Art for Table 15.4g: © Pat Thomas, 2010

Figure 15.4: Hreib KK, Choi E, Catalano PJ: 'Cranial Nerve VIII: Auditory and Vestibular' in Jones HR et al: *Netter's Neurology*, 2nd edn. Philadelphia, 2012, Saunders.

Figure 15.8: Lemmi and Lemmi, 2011.

Figure 15.13: Casey JR, Bluestone CD: 'Otitis Media' in Cherry J, Demmler-Harrison GJ, Kaplan SL et al: *Feigin and Cherry's Textbook of Pediatric Infectious Diseases*. Philadelphia, 2019, Elsevier.

Art for Table 15.1: (Frostbite) Science Photo Library/Custom Medical Stock; (Otitis externa [swimmer's ear]) Lemmi and Lemmi, 2011; (Branchial remnant and ear deformity) Liebert PS: *Color atlas of pediatric surgery,* 2nd edn. Philadelphia, 1996, Saunders.

Art for Table 15.2: (Sebaceous cyst) Liebert PS: *Color atlas of pediatric surgery,* 2nd edn. Philadelphia, 1996, Saunders; (Tophi) Science Photo Library; (Chondrodermatitis nodularis helicus) Habif TP, Campbell JL, Dinulos JGH et al: *Skin disease: diagnosis and treatment,* 2nd edn. St Louis, 2005, Mosby; (Keloid) Lemmi and Lemmi, 2011; (Carcinoma) Ameerally PJ, Colver GB: Cutaneous cryotherapy in maxillofacial surgery, *Journal of Oral and Maxillofacial Surgery*, 65(9): 1785–1792, 2007.

Art for Table 15.3: (Excessive cerumen) © Pat Thomas, 2010; (Otitis externa) Lim EKS, Thompson AM, Loke YK: *Medicine & surgery: an integrated textbook.* New York, 2007, Churchill Livingstone; (Osteoma) © Pat Thomas, 2010; (Foreign body) Swartz MH: *Textbook of physical diagnosis*, 2nd edn. Philadelphia, 2014, Elsevier; (Exostosis) © Pat Thomas, 2010; (Furuncle) © Pat Thomas, 2010; (Polyp) © Pat Thomas, 2010.

Art for Table 15.4: (Retracted drum) Adams GL, Boies LR Jr, Hilger PA: *Boies fundamentals of otolaryngology: a textbook of ear, nose and throat diseases*, 6th edn. Philadelphia, 1989, Saunders; (Otitis media with effusion [OME]) Swartz MH: *Textbook of physical diagnosis: history and examination*, 5th edn. Philadelphia, 2005, Saunders; (Acute [purulent] otitis media) Adams GL, Boies LR Jr, Hilger PA: *Boies fundamentals of otolaryngology: a textbook of ear, nose and throat disease,* 6th edn. Philadelphia, 1989, Saunders; (Perforation) Dhillon RS, East CA: *Ear, nose and throat and head and neck surgery*, 4th edn. Philadelphia, 2013, Churchill Livingstone; (Insertion of tubes [grommets]) Fireman P: *Atlas of allergies*, 2nd edn. London, 1996, Mosby; (Cholesteatoma) Swartz MH: *Textbook of physical diagnosis: history and examination,* 5th edn. Philadelphia, 2005, Saunders; (Scarred drum) Lim EKS, Thompson AM, Loke YK: *Medicine & surgery: an integrated textbook.* New York, 2007, Churchill Livingstone; (Blue drum [haemotympanum]) Dhillon RS, East CA: *Ear, nose and throat and head and neck surgery*, 4th edn. Philadelphia, 2013, Churchill Livingstone; (Bullous myringitis) Swartz MH: *Textbook of*

physical diagnosis: history and examination, 5th edn. Philadelphia, 2005, Saunders; (Fungal infection [otomycosis]) © Pat Thomas, 2010.
Art for Clinical Case Study 1: iStockphoto.com/Techin24
Art for Clinical Case Study 2: iStockphoto.com/RichLegg

CHAPTER 16

Art for Case Study: Stock photo ID:1401214649 https://www.istockphoto.com/photo/senior-woman-sitting-on-chair-and-looking-through-the-window-gm1401214649-454536202
Art for Table 16.2e: Anna R Dover, J. Alastair Innes, Karen Fairhurst. Macleod's Clinical Examination, 15th edition. Elsevier; 2024.
Figures 16.1–16.4, 16.6: © Pat Thomas, 2010.
Figure 16.5: © Pat Thomas, 2014.
Figure 16.18B: Bloom A, Watkins, PH, Ireland J: *Color atlas of diabetes*, 2nd edn. St Louis, 1992, Mosby.
Figure 16.20B: Lemmi and Lemmi, 2011.
Art for Table 16.2: (Arteriosclerosis—ischaemic ulcer) Dockery GL: *Cutaneous disorders of the lower extremity*. Philadelphia, 1997, Saunders; (Venous [stasis] ulcer) Lookingbill DP, Marks JG: *Principles of dermatology*, 2nd edn. Philadelphia, 1993, Saunders; (Diabetic [neuropathic] related foot ulcer) Lemmi and Lemmi, 2011; (Superficial varicose veins) Lemmi and Lemmi, 2011; (Deep vein thrombophlebitis) Cronenwett JL, Johnston KW: *Rutherford's vascular surgery*, 8th edn, 2014, Saunders.
Art for Table 16.4: (Raynaud's phenomenon) Lemmi and Lemmi, 2011; (Lymphoedema) Walsh TD, Caraceni AT, Fainsinger R et al: *Palliative medicine*. Philadelphia, 2009, Saunders.
Art for Table 16.5: © Pat Thomas, 2010.
Art for Clinical Case Study: iStockphoto.com/Grigorev_Vladimir.

CHAPTER 17

Figures 17.3–17.5, 17.8–17.10, 17.13: © Pat Thomas, 2006.
Figure 17.15: Lakatta EG: Cardiovascular function in later life, *Cardiovascular Medicine*, 10:37–40, 1985.
Art for Table 17.2: Adapted from Zitkus BS: Take chest pain to heart, *Nurse Practitioner*, 35(9):41–47, 2010.
Art for Tables 17.9–17.11: © Pat Thomas, 2006.
Art for Clinical Case Study: Shutterstock.com/Pablo Rogat.

CHAPTER 18

Figures 18.2, 18.3: © Pat Thomas.
Figure 18.6B: Fireman P: *Atlas of allergies*, 2nd edn. London, 1996, Mosby.
Figure 18.11: Zitelli BJ, Davis HW: *Atlas of pediatric physical diagnosis,* 5th edn. St Louis, 2007, Mosby.
Figure 18.17: © Burghart Messtechnik GmbH.
Figure 18.18: © Amy Johnston.
Art for Table 18.1: (Foreign body) Fireman P: *Atlas of allergies*, 2nd edn. London, 1996, Mosby; (Perforated septum) Science Photo Library/Dr P Marazzi; (Acute rhinitis) Fireman P: *Atlas of allergies*, 2nd edn. London, 1996, Mosby; (Allergic rhinitis) Fireman P: *Atlas of allergies*, 2nd edn. London, 1996, Mosby; (Nasal polyps) Fireman P: *Atlas of allergies*, 2nd edn. London, 1996, Mosby; (Carcinoma) Rosai J: *Rosai & Ackerman's surgical pathology*, 10th edn. 2011, Elsevier.
Art for Table 18.2: (Cleft palate) Zitelli BJ, Davis HW: *Atlas of pediatric physical diagnosis*, 4th edn. St Louis, 2002, Mosby, Courtesy of Dr Michael Sherlock; (Bifid uvula) Neville BW, Damm DD, Allen CM et al: *Oral and maxillofacial pathology*, 2009, Elsevier Saunders; (Oral Kaposi's sarcoma) Flint PW, Haughey BH, Lund VJ et al: *Otolaryngology head & neck surgery*, 5th edn. Philadelphia, 2010, Saunders; (Acute

tonsillitis and pharyngitis) Science Photo Library/Dr P Marazzi.
Art for Clinical Case Study: iStockphoto.com/romrodinka.

CHAPTER 19

Figures 19.1, 19.2, 19.10: © Pat Thomas, 2010.
Figure 19.11: © Pat Thomas, 2006.
Figure 19.12: From Hall JE. Guyton and Hall Textbook of Medical Physiology. 13th ed. Philadelphia, PA: Saunders; 2016. https://cdn.clinicalkey.com/ck-thumbnails/C20130099677/B9780323287531000118/f011-023-9780323287531-t.gif
Figure 19.13: © Copyright 2013 GSK. All rights reserved.
Art for Table 19.7: Wahls SA: Causes and evaluation of chronic dyspnea, *American family physician*, 86(2): 173–180, 2012.
Art for Clinical Case Study: Shutterstock.com/Lopolo.

CHAPTER 20

Art for Case Study: Stock photo ID:1204788026 https://www.istockphoto.com/photo/close-up-shot-of-hand-with-arthritis-outside-gm1204788026-346801092
Art for Table 20-07c: Stock illustration ID:1266684098 https://www.istockphoto.com/vector/spine-x-ray-gm1266684098-371397537
Figures 20.2–20.4, 20.7–20.14: © Pat Thomas, 2006.
Figure 20.15: Douglas G, Nicol F, Robertson C: *Macleod's clinical examination*, 13th edn. Elsevier Churchill Livingstone, 2013.
Figures 20.34C, 20.35B: Dieppe PA, Cooper C, McGill N: *Arthritis and rheumatism in practice*, London, 1991, Gower Medical Publishing.
Figure 20.44: © Pat Thomas, 2006.
Figure 20.50: Zitelli BJ, Davis HW*: Atlas of pediatric physical diagnosis*, 4th edn. St Louis, 2002, Mosby.
Art for Table 20.2: (Atrophy) Science Photo Library/Dr P Mazarri; (Dislocated shoulder) Roberts JR: *Roberts and Hedges' Clinical Procedures in Emergency Medicine*, 6th edn. 2014, Elsevier Saunders; (Joint effusion) Science Photo Library/Dr P Mazarri; (Tear of rotator cuff) Waldman SD: *Physical diagnosis of pain: an atlas of signs and symptoms,* 2nd edn. Philadelphia, 2010, Saunders; (Frozen shoulder—adhesive capsulitis) Peñas CF, Cleland JA, Huijbregts PAL: *Neck and arm pain syndromes: evidence-informed screening, diagnosis and management.* Philadelphia, 2011, Churchill Livingstone.
Art for Table 20.3: (Olecranon bursitis) Stanley D, Trail IA: *Operative elbow surgery.* 2012, Elsevier Churchill Livingstone; (Gouty arthritis) Polley HF, Hunder GG: *Physical examination of the joints,* 2nd edn. Philadelphia, 1978, Saunders; (Subcutaneous nodules) Callen JP et al. *Color atlas of dermatology.* Philadelphia, 1993, Saunders; (Epicondylitis—tennis elbow) Skirven TM, Osterman AL, Fedorczyk JM et al: *Rehabilitation of the hand and upper extremity,* 6th edn. St Louis, 2011, Mosby.
Art for Table 20.4: (Ganglion cyst) Callen JP et al. *Color atlas of dermatology.* Philadelphia, 1993, Saunders; (Carpal tunnel syndrome with atrophy of thenar eminence) Science Photo Library/Mike Devlin; (Ankylosis) Slutsky DJ: *Principles and practice of wrist surgery.* Philadelphia, 2010, Saunders; (Dupuytren's contracture) Canale ST, Beaty JH: *Campbell's operative orthopaedics,* 12th edn. St Louis, 2013, Mosby; (Swan-neck and boutonnière deformity) Reprinted from the Clinical Slide Collection on the Rheumatic Diseases. Copyright © 1991, 1995, 1997. Used by permission of the American College of Rheumatology; (Ulnar deviation or drift) Walker JM, Helewa A: *Physical therapy in arthritis.* Philadelphia, 1996, Saunders; (Degenerative joint disease or osteoarthritis)

Walker JM, Helewa A: *Physical therapy in arthritis.* Philadelphia, 1996, Saunders; (Syndactyly) Liebert PS: *Color atlas of pediatric surgery,* 2nd edn. Philadelphia, 1996, Saunders; (Polydactyly) Liebert PS: *Color atlas of pediatric surgery,* 2nd edn. Philadelphia, 1996, Saunders.

Art for Table 20.5: (Mild synovitis) Dieppe PA, Cooper C, McGill N: *Arthritis and rheumatism in practice.* London, 1991, Gower Medical Publishing; (Prepatellar bursitis) Science Photo Library/Dr P Marazzi; (Swelling of menisci) Jones A, Owen R: *Color atlas of clinical orthopaedics,* 2nd edn. London, 1995, Mosby; (Osgood-Schlatter disease) Zitelli BJ, Davis HW: *Atlas of pediatric physical diagnosis,* 4th edn. St Louis, 2002, Mosby.

Art for Table 20.6: (Achilles tenosynovitis) Science Photo Library/CMSP/Dr P Marazzi; (Tophi with chronic gout) Dockery GL: *Cutaneous disorders of the lower extremity.* Philadelphia, 1997, Saunders; (Acute gout) Science Photo Library/Dr P Marazzi; (Hallux valgus with bunion and hammertoes) Walker JM, Helewa A: *Physical therapy in arthritis.* Philadelphia, 1996, Saunders.

Art for Table 20.7: (Scoliosis) Zitelli BJ, Davis HW: *Atlas of pediatric physical diagnosis,* 4th edn. St Louis, 2002, Mosby; (Herniated nucleus pulposus) Polley HF, Hunder GG: *Physical examination of the joints,* 2nd edn. Philadelphia, 1978, Saunders.

Art for Table 20.8: (Developmental hip dysplasia) Zitelli BJ, Davis HW: *Atlas of pediatric physical diagnosis,* 4th edn. St Louis, 2002, Mosby; (Talipes equinovarus [clubfoot]) Dr AE Chudley, MD; (Spina bifida) Thompson DNP: Spinal dysraphic anomalies; classification, presentation and management, *Paediatrics and Child Health,* 20(9): 397–403, 2010.

Art for Clinical Case Study: Shutterstock.com/Phovoir.

CHAPTER 21

Figure 21.1: © Pat Thomas, 2010.
Figure 21.3: © Pat Thomas, 2006.
Figure 21.5: © Commonwealth of Australia 2014, Creative Commons Attribution 3.0 Australia License.
Figure 21.6: *Food and Nutritional Health for Adults, Risk Screening and Monitoring Outline,* Department of Health & Human Services, State Government of Victoria, 2012.
Figure 21.10: Ibsen OAC, Phelan JA: *Oral pathology for the dental hygienist,* 2nd edn. Philadelphia, 1996, Saunders.
Figures 21.11, 21.16B: Lemmi and Lemmi, 2011.
Figure 21.12: © Pat Thomas, 2006.

Art for Table 21.4: (Starved appearance) Hall R, Evered DC: *Color atlas of endocrinology,* 2nd edn. London, 1990, Mosby.

Art for Table 21.5: (Pellagra) Latham MC et al: *Scope manual on nutrition.* Kalamazoo, 1980, The Upjohn Company, copyright Thomas Spies, MD; (Follicular hyperkeratosis) Taylor KB, Anthony LE: *Clinical nutrition.* New York, 1983, McGraw-Hill, copyright by Harold H Sandstead; (Scorbutic gums) Taylor KB, Anthony LE: *Clinical nutrition.* New York, 1983, McGraw-Hill, copyright by The Upjohn Company; (Bitot's spots) Taylor KB, Anthony LE: *Clinical nutrition.* New York, 1983, McGraw-Hill, copyright by Helen Keller International, Inc; (Rickets) Nunn T, Rollinson P, Scott B: Blount's disease, *Orthopaedics and Trauma,* 25(6):454–461, 2011; (Magenta tongue) McLaren DS: *Color atlas of nutritional disorders.* London, 1981, Wolfe Medical, copyright by CE Butterworth, Jr.

Art for Table 21.6: (Cleft lip) Ibsen OAC, Phelan JA: *Oral pathology for the dental hygienist,* 2nd edn. Philadelphia, 1996, Saunders; (Herpes simplex 1) Callen JP et al: *Color atlas of dermatology.* Philadelphia, 1993, Saunders; (Angular cheilitis [stomatitis, perlèche]) Callen JP et al: *Color atlas of* *dermatology*. Philadelphia, 1993, Saunders; (Carcinoma) Science Photo Library/Dr P Marazzi; (Retention 'cyst' [mucocoele]) Zitelli BJ, McIntire SC, Nowalk AJ: *Atlas of pediatric physical diagnosis*, 6th edn. Philadelphia, 2012, Elsevier Saunders.

Art for Table 21.7: (Baby bottle tooth decay) Courtesy of F Ferguson, Department of Children's Dentistry, School of Dental Medicine, SUNY at Stony Brook, Stony Brook, NY 11733; (Dental caries) Courtesy of A McWhorter, Pediatric Dentistry, Baylor College of Dentistry, The Texas A & M University System, Dallas, TX; (Epulis) Ibsen OAC, Phelan JA: *Oral pathology for the dental hygienist*, 2nd edn. Philadelphia, 1996, Saunders; (Gingival hyperplasia) Ibsen OAC, Phelan JA: *Oral pathology for the dental hygienist*, 2nd edn. Philadelphia, 1996, Saunders; (Gingivitis) Callen JP et al: *Color atlas of dermatology*. Philadelphia, 1993, Saunders; (Meth mouth) Neville BW et al: *Oral and maxillofacial pathology*, 3rd edn. St Louis, 2009, Saunders.

Art for Table 21.8: (Ankyloglossia) Ibsen OAC, Phelan JA: *Oral pathology for the dental hygienist*, 2nd edn. Philadelphia, 1996, Saunders; (Fissured or scrotal tongue) Lemmi and Lemmi, 2011; (Geographic tongue [migratory glossitis]) Lemmi and Lemmi, 2011; (Smooth, glossy tongue [atrophic glossitis]) Adams GL, Bois LR, Hilger PA: *Boies fundamentals of otolaryngology: a textbook of ear, nose, and throat diseases*, 6th edn. Philadelphia, 1989, Saunders; (Black hairy tongue) Callen JP et al: *Color atlas of dermatology*. Philadelphia, 1993, Saunders; (Enlarged tongue [macroglossia]) Zitelli BJ, Davis HW: *Atlas of pediatric physical diagnosis*, 4th edn. St Louis, 2002, Mosby, courtesy of Dr Christine Williams; (Carcinoma) Wenig BM, Heffess CS, Adair CF: *Atlas of endocrine pathology*. Philadelphia, 1997, Saunders.

Art for Table 21.9: (Aphthous ulcers) Lemmi and Lemmi, 2011; (Koplik's spots) Feigin RD, Cherry JD: *Textbook of pediatric infectious diseases*, 4th edn. Philadelphia, 1998, Saunders; (Leucoplakia) Sleisinger MH, Fordtran JS: *Gastrointestinal diseases: pathophysiology, diagnosis, and management*, vol 1, 5th edn. Philadelphia, 1993, Saunders; (Candidiasis or monilial infection) Callen JP et al: *Color atlas of dermatology*. Philadelphia, 1993, Saunders.

Art for Table 21.10: (Metabolic syndrome [MetS]) Ford ES, Li C, Zhao G et al: Prevalence of the metabolic syndrome among U.S. adolescents using the definition from the International Diabetes Federation, *Diabetes Care*, 31(3):587–589, 2008 and Mozumdar A, Liguori G: Persistent increase in prevalence of metabolic syndrome among U.S. adults: NHANES III to NHANES 1999–2006, *Diabetes Care*, 34(1):216–219, 2011.

Art for Table 21.12: (Thyroid—multiple nodules) Swartz MH: *Textbook of physical diagnosis: history and examination*, 5th edn. Philadelphia, 2006, Saunders; (Parotid gland enlargement) Swartz MH: *Textbook of physical diagnosis: history and examination*, 5th edn. Philadelphia, 2006, Saunders; (Fetal alcohol syndrome) © Pat Thomas, 2006; (Congenital hypothyroidism) Zitelli BJ, Davis HW: *Atlas of pediatric physical diagnosis*, 4th edn. St Louis, 2002, Mosby, courtesy of Dr Thomas P Foley Jr; (Hyperthyroidism) Swartz MH: *Textbook of physical diagnosis: history and examination*, 5th edn. Philadelphia, 2006, Saunders; Myxoedema [hypothyroidism]) Hall R, Evered DC: *Color atlas of endocrinology*, 2nd edn. London, 1990, Mosby.

Art for Clinical Case Study: Shutterstock.com/Zurijeta.

CHAPTER 22

Art for Table 22.2 A & B: Carolyn Jarvis & Ann L. Eckhardt. Physical Examination and Health Assessment, 9th Edition. Elsevier; 2024.

Figure 22.3AB: Lookingbill DP, Marks JG: *Principles of dermatology*, 2nd edn. Philadelphia, 1993, Saunders.
Figures 22.4A, 22.4B: Hurwitz S: *Clinical pediatric dermatology: a textbook of skin disorders of childhood and adolescence*, 2nd edn. Philadelphia, 1993, Saunders.
Figure 22.4C: Lookingbill DP, Marks JG: *Principles of dermatology*, 2nd edn. Philadelphia, 1993, Saunders.
Figure 22.5: Patton KT, Thibodeau GA, Douglas MM: *Essentials of anatomy & physiology*. St Louis, 2012, Mosby.
Figures 22.7–22.12: Lemmi and Lemmi, 2011.
Figure 22.13: Bowden VR, Dickey SB, Greenburg CS: *Children and their families: the continuum of care*, Philadelphia, 1998, Saunders.
Figures 22.14, 22.15: Hurwitz S: *Clinical pediatric dermatology: a textbook of skin disorders of childhood and adolescence*, 2nd edn. Philadelphia, 1993, Saunders.
Figure 22.16: Lemmi and Lemmi, 2011.
Figure 22.17: Hurwitz S: *Clinical pediatric dermatology: a textbook of skin disorders of childhood and adolescence*, 2nd edn. Philadelphia, 1993, Saunders.
Figure 22.18: Murray SS, McKinney ES: *Foundations of maternal-newborn and women's health nursing*, 5th edn. Philadelphia, 2010, Saunders.
Figures 22.19A, B: Habif TP, Campbell JL, Dinulos JGH et al: *Skin disease: diagnosis and treatment,* 2nd edn. St Louis, 2005, Mosby.
Figure 22.20: Lookingbill DP, Marks JG: *Principles of dermatology*, 2nd edn. Philadelphia, 1993, Saunders.
Figure 22.21: Lemmi and Lemmi, 2011.
Figure 22.22: Habif TP, Campbell JL, Dinulos JGH et al: *Skin disease: diagnosis and treatment,* 2nd edn. St Louis, 2005, Mosby.
Figure 22.23: Lookingbill DP, Marks JG: *Principles of dermatology*, 2nd edn. Philadelphia, 1993, Saunders.
Figure 22.24: Callen JP et al: *Color atlas of dermatology*. Philadelphia, 1993, Saunders.
Art for Table 22.4: (Macule and patch) © Pat Thomas, 2010. Photos courtesy Lemmi and Lemmi, 2011; (Papule and plaque) Pat Thomas, 2010. Photos courtesy Lemmi and Lemmi, 2011; (Nodule tumour and Wheal) © Pat Thomas, 2010. Photos courtesy Lemmi and Lemmi, 2011; (Urticaria [hives]) © Pat Thomas, 2010. Fireman P: *Atlas of allergies*, 2nd edn. St Louis, 1996, Mosby; (Vesicle and bulla) © Pat Thomas, 2010. Photos courtesy Lemmi and Lemmi, 2011; (Cyst) © Pat Thomas, 2010. Photos courtesy Lemmi and Lemmi, 2011; (Pustule) © Pat Thomas, 2010. Photos courtesy Lemmi and Lemmi, 2011.
Art for Table 22.5: (Crust) © Pat Thomas, 2010. Photo courtesy Lemmi and Lemmi, 2011; (Scale) © Pat Thomas, 2010. Photo courtesy Lemmi and Lemmi, 2011; (Fissure) © Pat Thomas, 2010. Photo courtesy Lemmi and Lemmi, 2011; (Erosion) © Pat Thomas, 2010. Photo courtesy Lemmi and Lemmi, 2011; (Ulcer) © Pat Thomas, 2010. Photo courtesy Lemmi and Lemmi, 2011; (Excoriation) © Pat Thomas, 2010. Photo courtesy Lemmi and Lemmi, 2011; (Scar) © Pat Thomas, 2010. Photo courtesy Lemmi and Lemmi, 2011; (Atrophic scar) © Pat Thomas, 2010. Photo courtesy Lemmi and Lemmi, 2011; (Lichenification) © Pat Thomas, 2010. Photo courtesy Lemmi and Lemmi, 2011; (Keloid) © Pat Thomas, 2010. Photo courtesy Lemmi and Lemmi, 2011.
Art for Table 22.6: (Pressure injury [decubitus ulcer] Stage I) Potter PA, Perry AG: *Fundamentals of nursing*, 7th edn. St Louis, 2009, Mosby; (Pressure injury [decubitus ulcer] Stage II) Potter PA, Perry AG: *Fundamentals of nursing*, 7th edn. St Louis, 2009, Mosby; (Pressure injury

[decubitus ulcer] Stage III) Potter PA, Perry AG: *Fundamentals of nursing*, 7th edn. St Louis, 2009, Mosby; (Pressure injury [decubitus ulcer] Stage IV) Potter PA, Perry AG: *Fundamentals of nursing*, 7th edn. St Louis, 2009, Mosby.

Art for Table 22.8: (Port-wine stain [naevus flammeus]) Paller AS, Mancini AJ: *Hurwitz clinical pediatric dermatology: a textbook of skin disorders of childhood and adolescence*, 4th edn. Philadelphia, 2011, Saunders; (Strawberry mark [immature haemangioma]) Lookingbill DP, Marks JG: *Principles of dermatology*, 2nd edn. Philadelphia, 1993, Saunders; (Cavernous haemangioma [mature]) Habif TP, Campbell JL, Dinulos JGH et al: *Skin disease: diagnosis and treatment,* 2nd edn. St Louis, 2005, Mosby; (Telangiectasia) Lemmi and Lemmi, 2011; (Spider or star angioma) Lemmi and Lemmi, 2011; (Venous lake) Habif TP, Campbell JL, Dinulos JGH et al: *Skin disease: diagnosis and treatment,* 2nd edn. St Louis, 2005, Mosby; (Petechiae) Dockery GL: *Cutaneous disorders of the lower extremity*, Philadelphia, 1997, Saunders; (Ecchymosis) Lemmi and Lemmi, 2011; (Purpura) Paller AS, Mancini AJ: *Hurwitz clinical pediatric dermatology: a textbook of skin disorders of childhood and adolescence*, 4th edn. Philadelphia, 2011, Saunders.

Art for Table 22.9: (Nappy dermatitis) Paller AS, Mancini AJ: *Hurwitz clinical pediatric dermatology: a textbook of skin disorders of childhood and adolescence*, 4th edn. Philadelphia, 2011, Saunders; (Intertrigo [candidiasis]) Lemmi and Lemmi, 2011; (Impetigo) Lemmi and Lemmi, 2011; (Atopic dermatitis [eczema]) Paller AS, Mancini AJ: *Hurwitz clinical pediatric dermatology: a textbook of skin disorders of childhood and adolescence*, 4th edn. Philadelphia, 2011, Saunders; (Measles [rubeola] in dark skin) Feigin RD, Cherry JD: *Textbook of pediatric infectious diseases*, 4th edn. Philadelphia, 1998, Saunders; (Measles [rubeola] in light skin) Lemmi and Lemmi, 2011; (German measles [rubella]) Paller AS, Mancini AJ: *Hurwitz clinical pediatric dermatology: a textbook of skin disorders of childhood and adolescence*, 4th edn. Philadelphia, 2011, Saunders; (Chickenpox [varicella]) Callen JP et al: *Color atlas of dermatology*. Philadelphia, 1993, Saunders.

Art for Table 22.10: (Primary contact dermatitis) Lookingbill DP, Marks JG: *Principles of dermatology*, 2nd edn. Philadelphia, 1993, Saunders; (Allergic drug reaction) Lookingbill DP, Marks JG: *Principles of dermatology*, 2nd edn. Philadelphia, 1993, Saunders; (Tinea corporis [ringworm of the body]) Paller AS, Mancini AJ: *Hurwitz clinical pediatric dermatology: a textbook of skin disorders of childhood and adolescence*, 4th edn. Philadelphia, 2011, Saunders; (Tinea pedis [ringworm of the foot]) Lemmi and Lemmi, 2011; (Psoriasis) Lookingbill DP, Marks JG: *Principles of dermatology*, 2nd edn. Philadelphia, 1993, Saunders; (Tinea versicolor) Lemmi and Lemmi, 2011; (Labial herpes simplex [cold sores]) Lemmi and Lemmi, 2011; (Herpes zoster [shingles]) Lemmi and Lemmi, 2011; (Lyme disease) Swartz MH: *Textbook of physical diagnosis: history and examination,* 5th edn. Philadelphia, 2005, Saunders.

Art for Table 22.11: (Basal cell carcinoma) Lookingbill DP, Marks JG: *Principles of dermatology*, 2nd edn. Philadelphia, 1993, Saunders; (Squamous cell carcinoma) Habif TP, Campbell JL, Dinulos JGH et al: *Skin disease: diagnosis and treatment,* 2nd edn. St Louis, 2005, Mosby; (Malignant melanoma) Lookingbill DP, Marks JG: *Principles of dermatology*, 2nd edn. Philadelphia, 1993, Saunders.

Art for Table 22.12: (AIDS-related Kaposi's sarcoma: patch stage) Friedman-Kien AE: *Color atlas of AIDS*. Philadelphia, 1989, Saunders.

Art for Table 22.13: (Seborrhoeic dermatitis [cradle cap]) Hurwitz S: *Clinical pediatric dermatology: a textbook of skin disorders of childhood and adolescence*, 2nd edn. Philadelphia, 1993, Saunders; (Tinea capitis [scalp ringworm]) Lookingbill DP, Marks JG: *Principles of dermatology*, 2nd edn. Philadelphia, 1993, Saunders; (Toxic alopecia) Hurwitz S: *Clinical pediatric dermatology: a textbook of skin disorders of childhood and adolescence*, 2nd edn. Philadelphia, 1993, Saunders; (Alopecia areata) Hurwitz S: *Clinical pediatric dermatology: a textbook of skin disorders of childhood and adolescence*, 2nd edn. Philadelphia, 1993, Saunders; (Traumatic alopecia: traction alopecia) Hurwitz S: *Clinical pediatric dermatology: a textbook of skin disorders of childhood and adolescence*, 2nd edn. Philadelphia, 1993, Saunders; (Trichotillomania) Callen JP et al: *Color atlas of dermatology*. Philadelphia, 1993, Saunders; (Pediculosis capitis [head lice]) Callen JP et al: *Color atlas of dermatology*, Philadelphia, 1993, Saunders; (Furuncle and abscess) Lookingbill DP, Marks JG: *Principles of dermatology*, 2nd edn. Philadelphia, 1993, Saunders.
Art for Table 22.14: (Scabies) Lemmi and Lemmi, 2011; (Paronychia) Lemmi and Lemmi, 2011; (Beau's line) Callen JP et al: *Color atlas of dermatology*. Philadelphia, 1993, Saunders; (Splinter haemorrhages) Callen JP et al: *Color atlas of dermatology*. Philadelphia, 1993, Saunders; (Late clubbing) Reprinted from the Clinical Slide Collection on the Rheumatic Diseases. Copyright © 1991, 1995, 1997. Used by permission of the American College of Rheumatology; (Onycholysis) Lemmi and Lemmi, 2011; (Pitting) Lemmi and Lemmi, 2011; (Habit–tic dystrophy) Lemmi and Lemmi, 2011.
Art for Clinical Case Study 1: Shutterstock.com/Steve Buckley
Art for Clinical Case Study 2: iStock Image ID 77021236

CHAPTER 23

Art for Case Study: Stock photo ID:1373258287 https://www.istockphoto.com/photo/pulse-oximeter-on-senior-patients-hand-at-hospital-gm1373258287-442152162
Art for Table 23.4d: Emily Slone McKinney, Susan Rowen James, Sharon Smith Murray, et al. Maternal-Child Nursing, 6th edition. Elsevier; 2022.
Figures 23.1–23.6: © Pat Thomas, 2006.
Art for Table 23.2: © Pat Thomas, 2014.
Art for Table 23.4: (Umbilical hernia) Zitelli BJ, Davis HW: *Atlas of pediatric physical diagnosis*, 4th edn. St Louis, 2002, Mosby, courtesy of Dr Thomas P Foley, Jr; (Epigastric hernia) Conroy K, Malata CM: Epigastric hernia following DIEP flap breast reconstruction: Complication or coincidence? *Journal of Plastic, Reconstructive & Aesthetic Surgery*, 65(3):387–391, 2012; (Incisional hernia) Lemmi and Lemmi, 2011; (Diastasis recti) Clark DA: *Atlas of neonatology*, 7th edn. Philadelphia, 2000, Saunders.
Art for Tables 23.5–23.7: © Pat Thomas.
Art for Clinical Case Study: iStockphoto.com/Juanmonino.

CHAPTER 24

Figures 24.1, 24.2: © Pat Thomas, 2006.
Figure 24.3: Brown D, Edwards H: *Lewis's medical–surgical nursing*, 3rd edn. Chatswood NSW, 2011, Elsevier.
Figure 24.4: © Pat Thomas.
Figure 24.5: © Pat Thomas, 2010.
Table 24.1: Courtesy Connie Cooper.
Art for Table 24.2: © Pat Thomas.
Art for Clinical Case Study: iStockphoto.com/torwai.
Figure 24.6: Health direct https://www.healthdirect.gov.au/urine-colour-chart

CHAPTER 25

Art for Case Study 25.1: Stock photo ID:912333918 https://www.istockphoto.com/photo/lonely-senior-man-at-a-nursing-home-lying-in-bed-with-a-sad-expression-gm912333918-251167021
Art for Case Study 25.2: Stock photo ID:938640778 https://www.istockphoto.com/photo/relaxing-gm938640778-256674535
Figures 25.1, 25.2: © Pat Thomas.
Figure 25.3: Bristol Stool Scale, CC BY SA 3.0, Wikipedia/Kyle Thompson. Based on the Bristol Stool Scale developed by Dr Ken Heaton at the University of Bristol.
Art for Table 25.2: © Pat Thomas.
Art for Clinical Case Study: iStockphoto.com/SilviaJansen.

CHAPTER 26

Figures 26.1, 26.2: © Pat Thomas.
Figure 26.3: Adapted from Figure 47-8 in Brown D, Edwards H, Buckley T: *Lewis's medical surgical nursing*, 4th edn. Sydney, 2014, Mosby Elsevier.
Figures 26.11, 26.12, 26.17, 26.22: © Pat Thomas.
Figure 26.14: © 2017 Victorian Cytology Service Limited (ACN 609 597 408). These materials are subject to copyright and are protected by the Copyright Laws of Australia. All rights are reserved. Any copying or distribution of these materials without the written permission of the copyright owner is not authorized.
Art for Table 26.1: Adapted from Tanner JM: *Growth at adolescence*. Oxford, England, 1962, Blackwell Scientific.
Art for Table 26.2: (Pediculosis pubis [crab lice]) from Callen JP et al: *Color atlas of dermatology*. Philadelphia, 1993, Saunders; (Herpes simplex virus—type 2 [herpes genitalis]) Lemmi and Lemmi, 2011; (Syphilitic chancre) Reprinted from Emond R, Rowland HAK, Welsby P: *Colour atlas of infectious diseases,* 3rd edn. London, 1995, Mosby; (Red rash—contact dermatitis) Courtesy of Pfizer Laboratories Division, Pfizer Inc, New York. From *A close look at VD*: a slide presentation produced as a public service; (Human papillomavirus [HPV] genital warts) Habif TP, Campbell JL, Chapman JS et al: *Skin disease: diagnosis and treatment*. St Louis, 2001, Mosby; (Abscess of Bartholin's gland) Reprinted from Emond R, Rowland HAK, Welsby P: *Colour atlas of infectious diseases*, 3rd edn. London, 1995, Mosby; (Urethral caruncle) Rimsza ME: An illustrated guide to adolescent gynecology, *Pediatric Clinics of North America*, 36(3):641, 1989.
Art for Table 26.3: (Cystocele) Lemmi and Lemmi, 2011; (Uterine prolapse) Symonds EM, McPherson MBA: *Diagnosis in color: obstetrics and gynecology*. London, 1997, Mosby-Wolfe.
Art for Table 26.4: (Human papillomavirus [HPV, condylomata]) Symonds EM, McPherson MBA: *Diagnosis in color: obstetrics and gynecology*. London, 1997, Mosby-Wolfe; (Polyp) Lemmi and Lemmi, 2011; (Cervical cancer) Symonds EM, McPherson MBA: *Diagnosis in color: obstetrics and gynecology*. London, 1997, Mosby-Wolfe.
Art for Table 26.5: (Candidiasis (moniliasis)] Lemmi and Lemmi, 2011; (Gonorrhoea) Courtesy of Pfizer Laboratories Division, Pfizer Inc, New York. From *A close look at VD*: a slide presentation produced as a public service.
Art for Table 26.8: (Ambiguous genitalia) Moore KL, Persaud TN: *Before we are born: essentials of embryology and birth defects*, 5th edn. Philadelphia, 1998, Saunders; (Vulvovaginitis in child) Muram D, Simmons KJ: Pattern recognition in pediatric and adolescent gynecology—a case for

formal education, *Journal of Pediatric and Adolescent Gynecology*, (21)2:103–108, 2008.
Art for Clinical Case Study: iStockphoto.com/FatCamera.

CHAPTER 27

Art for Table 27.2e: Stock photo ID 1445382269. https://www.istockphoto.com/photo/monkeypox-lesions-in-the-thigh-of-asian-child-gm1445382269-483806845?phrase=monkey%2Bpox
Figures 27.1–27.3, 27.15: © Pat Thomas.
Figure 27.6: Science Photo Library/Dr P. Marazzi.
Figure 27.9B: Lemmi and Lemmi, 2011.
Art for Table 27.1: Adapted from Tanner JM: *Growth at adolescence*, Oxford, 1962, Blackwell Scientific Publications.
Art for Table 27.2: (Genital herpes—HSV-2 infection) Lemmi and Lemmi, 2011; (Syphilitic chancre) Reprinted from Emond R, Rowland HAK, Welsby P: *Colour atlas of infectious diseases*, 3rd edn. London, 1995, Mosby; (Genital warts) Habif TP, Campbell JL, Dinulos JGH et al: *Skin disease: diagnosis and treatment,* 2nd edn. St Louis, 2005, Mosby; (Carcinoma) Callen JP et al: *Color atlas of dermatology*. Philadelphia, 1993, Saunders; (Urethritis [urethral discharge and dysuria]) Reprinted from Emond R, Rowland, HAK, Welsby P: *Colour atlas of infectious diseases*, 3rd edn. London, 1995, Mosby.
Art for Table 27.3: (Phimosis) Liebert PS: *Color atlas of pediatric surgery*, 2nd edn. Philadelphia, 1996, Saunders; (Paraphimosis) Keys C, Lam JPH: Foreskin and penile problems in childhood, *Surgery* (Oxford) 31(3):130–134, 2013; (Hypospadias) Liebert PS: *Color atlas of pediatric surgery*, 2nd edn. Philadelphia, 1996, Saunders; (Epispadias) Zitelli BJ, Davis HW: *Atlas of pediatric physical diagnosis*, 4th edn. St Louis, 2002, Mosby; (Peyronie's disease) Courtesy of Dr Hans Stricker, Department of Urology, Henry Ford Hospital, Detroit, MI.
Art for Tables 27.4–27.5: © Pat Thomas, 2006.
Art for Clinical Case Study: iStockphoto.com/stray_cat.

CHAPTER 28

Figures 28.1, 28.2: © Pat Thomas, 2010.
Figure 28.4: © Pat Thomas, 2014.
Figure 28.6: From Callen JP et al: *Color atlas of dermatology*. Philadelphia, 1993, Saunders.
Figure 28.17: Moore KL, Persaud TVN: *Before we are born: essentials of embryology and birth defects*, 7th edn. Philadelphia, 2008, Saunders.
Art for Table 28.1: © Pat Thomas.
Art for Table 28.3: (Dimpling) Evans AJ et al: *Atlas of breast disease management: 50 illustrative cases*. Philadelphia, 1998, Saunders; (Oedema [peau d'orange]) Mansel R: *Color atlas of breast diseases*. London, 1995, Mosby; (Deviation in nipple pointing) Mansel R: *Color atlas of breast diseases*. London, 1995, Mosby; (Fixation) Mansel R: *Color atlas of breast diseases*. London, 1995, Mosby.
Art for Table 28.4: © Pat Thomas.
Art for Table 28.6: (Mammary duct ectasia) Mansel R: *Color atlas of breast diseases*. London, 1995, Mosby; (Intraductal papilloma) Mansel R: *Color atlas of breast diseases*. London, 1995, Mosby; (Carcinoma) Evans AJ et al: *Atlas of breast disease management: 50 illustrative cases*. Philadelphia, 1998, Saunders; (Paget's disease [intraductal carcinoma]) Mansel R: *Color atlas of breast diseases*. London, 1995, Mosby.
Art for Table 28.7: (Breast abscess) Mansel R: *Color atlas of breast diseases*. London, 1995, Mosby; (Mastitis) Mansel R: *Color atlas of breast diseases*. London, 1995, Mosby.

Art for Table 28.8: (Gynaecomastia) Lorenzo GD, Autorino R, Perdonà S et al: Management of gynaecomastia in patients with prostate cancer: a systematic review, *Lancet* 6(12): 972–979, 2005; (Carcinoma) Elshafieya ME, Zeeneldinb AA, Elsebaia HI et al: Epidemiology and management of breast carcinoma in Egyptian males: experience of a single Cancer Institute, *Journal of the Egyptian National Cancer Institute*, 23(3):115–122, 2011.
Art for Clinical Case Study: iStockphoto.com/JohnnyGreig.

CHAPTER 29

Art for Case Study: ID:1357577027 https://www.istockphoto.com/photo/shot-of-an-attractive-young-businesswoman-standing-alone-on-the-balcony-with-her-gm1357577027-431440009
Figures 29.1, 29.2: © Pat Thomas, 2018.
Figure 29.4: Black M, Ambros-Rudolph CM, Edwards L et al: *Obstetric and gynecologic dermatology*, 3rd edn. St Louis, 2008, Mosby.
Figures 29.9–29.12: © Pat Thomas, 2018.
Art for Table 29.1: Symonds EM, McPherson MBA: *Diagnosis in color: obstetrics and gynecology*. London, 1997, Mosby-Wolfe.
Art for Table 29.2: Meur S, Mann NP: Infant outcomes following diabetic pregnancies, *Paediatrics and Child Health*, (17)6:217–222, 2007.
Art for Table 29.4: © Pat Thomas.
Art for Clinical Case Study: iStockphoto.com/michaeljung.

CHAPTER 30

Art for Case Study: Stock photo ID:1353357764 https://www.istockphoto.com/photo/friendly-female-head-nurse-making-rounds-does-checkup-on-elderly-patient-resting-in-gm1353357764-428478699
Art for scenarios: (1. Mr Micha Krawiec) Shutterstock/Budimir Jevtic; (2. Ms Josephine Magliore) Shutterstock/jeep5d; (3. Mrs Jennifer Guyatt) Shutterstock/Fotoluminate LLC; (4. Mr Max Smith) Shutterstock/A Master Image; (5. Mr Bill Craven) Shutterstock/Laurin Rinder; (6. Mrs Christine Thomas) Shutterstock/Kamira.

Index

Page numbers followed by *b* indicate boxes, *f* indicate figures, and *t* indicate tables.

B

D

E

G

H

N

Q

R

T

U

V

W

X

Z